YOUR GUIDE TO

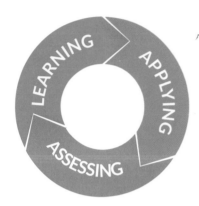

Psychiatric Mental Health Nursing

Everything you need to succeed...
in class, in clinical, on exams and on the NCLEX®

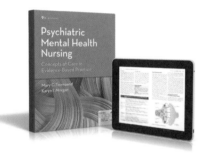

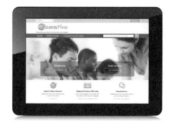

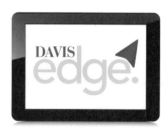

LEARNING

Your text provides the foundational knowledge you need to know.

APPLYING

Davis*Plus* features interactive clinical scenarios that show you how theory applies to practice.

ASSESSING

Davis Edge is the online Q&A review platform that evaluates your mastery of the material and builds your test-taking skills.

Your journey to success
BEGINS HERE!

Your text works together with Davis*Plus* and Davis Edge to make this often intimidating, but must-know content easier to master.

Don't miss everything that's waiting online to make learning less stressful...and save you time. Follow the instructions on the inside front cover to use the access code to unlock your resources today.

LEARNING

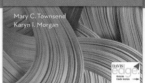

9th EDITION

Psychiatric
Mental Health
Nursing

Concepts of Care in
Evidence-Based Practice

Mary C. Townsend
Karyn I. Morgan

DAVIS edge
Access Code Inside

STEP #1
Build a solid foundation.

Communication Exercises let you practice your communication skills with vignettes and questions that prepare you for clinical and practice.

 Communication Exercises

1. Hal, a patient on the psychiatric unit, has a diagnosis of schizophrenia. He lives in a halfway house, where last evening he began yelling that "aliens were on the way to take over our bodies! The message is coming through loud and clear!" The residence supervisor became frightened and called 911. Hal tells the nurse, "I'm special! I get messages from a higher being! We are in for big trouble!"

One of the Quality and Safety in Nursing Education (QSEN) criteria identified by the Institute of Medicine (IOM) (2003) stresses that the patient must be at the center of decisions about treatment (patient-centered care), and this type of assessment tool provides an opportunity to actively engage the patient in describing what medications have been effective or ineffective and identifying side effects that may impact willingness to adhere to a medication regimen.

Quality and Safety Education for Nurses (QSEN) activities and content, highlighted with a special icon, help you attain the knowledge, skills, and attitudes required to fulfill the initiative's quality and safety competencies.

NEW! "Real People. Real Stories" features interviews with patients to bring their experiences to life.

 MOVIE CONNECTIONS

I Never Promised You a Rose Garden (schizophrenia) • *A Beautiful Mind* (schizophrenia) • *The Fisher King* (schizophrenia) • *Bennie & Joon* (schizophrenia) • *Out of Darkness* (schizophrenia) • *Conspiracy Theory* (delusional disorder) • *The Fan* (delusional disorder)

Movie Connections list films that demonstrate the conditions and behaviors you may not encounter in clinical.

Therapeutic Communication Icon identifies helpful interventions and guidance on how to speak with your patients. Look for this icon in Care Plan sections.

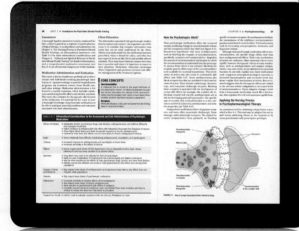

Table 24-4 | CARE PLAN FOR THE CLIENT WITH SCHIZOPHRENIA

NURSING DIAGNOSIS: DISTURBED SENSORY PERCEPTION: AUDITORY/VISUAL
RELATED TO: Panic anxiety, extreme loneliness, and withdrawal into the self
EVIDENCED BY: Inappropriate responses, disordered thought sequencing, rapid mood swings, poor concentration, disorientation

OUTCOME CRITERIA	NURSING INTERVENTIONS	RATIONALE
Short-Term Goal • Client will discuss content of hallucinations with nurse or therapist within 1 week. **Long-Term Goal** • Client will be able to define and test reality, reducing or eliminating the occurrence of hallucinations. This goal may not be realistic for the individual with severe and persistent illness who has experienced auditory hallucinations for many years. A more realistic goal may be: • Client will verbalize understanding that the voices are a result of his or her illness and demonstrate ways to	1. Observe client for signs of hallucinations (listening pose, laughing or talking to self, stopping in midsentence). Ask, "Are you hearing the voices again?" 2. Avoid touching the client without warning him or her that you are about to do so. 3. An attitude of acceptance will encourage the client to share the content of the hallucination with you. Ask, "What do you hear the voices saying to you?" 4. Do not reinforce the hallucination. Use "the voices" instead of words like "they" that imply validation. Let client know	1. Early intervention may prevent aggressive response to command hallucinations. 2. Client may perceive touch as threatening and may respond in an aggressive manner. 3. This is important to prevent possible injury to the client or others from command hallucinations. 4. It is important for the nurse to be honest, and the client must accept the perception as unreal before hallucinations can be eliminated.

A FREE ebook version of your text is available with each new printed book to make studying and reviewing easier. Use the access code on the inside front cover.

APPLYING

APPLYING · LEARNING · ASSESSING

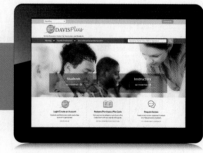

STEP #2
Practice in a safe environment.

Clinical Scenarios on www.DavisPlus.com walk you through the nursing process with client summaries, multiple-choice questions with rationales, drag- and drop activities, and so much more.

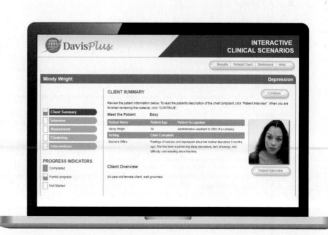

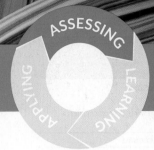
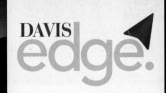
STEP #3

Study smarter, not harder.

Davis Edge is the interactive, online Q&A review platform that provides the practice you need to master course content and to improve your scores on classroom exams. Access it from a laptop, tablet, or mobile device for review and study on the go.

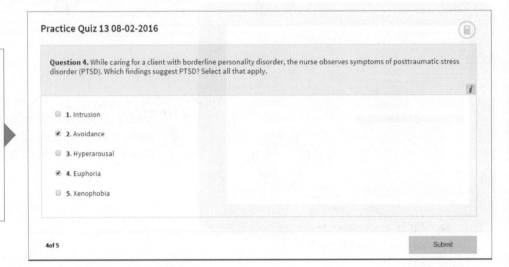

Practice Quiz 13 08-02-2016

Question 4. While caring for a client with borderline personality disorder, the nurse observes symptoms of posttraumatic stress disorder (PTSD). Which findings suggest PTSD? Select all that apply.

- ☐ 1. Intrusion
- ☑ 2. Avoidance
- ☐ 3. Hyperarousal
- ☑ 4. Euphoria
- ☐ 5. Xenophobia

4of 5   Submit

Question 4. While caring for a client with borderline personality disorder, the nurse observes symptoms of posttraumatic stress disorder (PTSD). Which findings suggest PTSD? Select all that apply.

Course Topic: Personality Disorders | **Concept(s):** Mood; Self | **Cognitive Level:** Application [Applying]

- ✗ ☐ 1. Intrusion
- ✓ ☑ 2. Avoidance
- ✗ ☐ 3. Hyperarousal
- ✗ ☑ 4. Euphoria
- ☐ 5. Xenophobia

Rationale

Option 1:	Intrusion is a posttraumatic symptom in which the client occasionally reexperiences the trauma. This finding supports the nurse's assumption.
Option 2:	The client avoids places, activities, and people in order to avoid reexperiencing the traumatic event. This finding supports the nurse's assumption.
Option 3:	Hyperarousal is the state in which the client has difficulty in sleeping and has difficulty in concentrating due to a traumatic experience. This finding supports the nurse's assumption.
Option 4:	Euphoria is the state in which the client appears cheerful with an expansive mood. It is not a symptom of posttraumatic event; instead, it is a symptom of mania.
Option 5:	Xenophobia is the condition in which the client has a fear of strangers. It is not a symptom of a posttraumatic event; instead, it is a symptom of anxiety.

Assignments are made by your instructor. Or, create your own practice quizzes to review before an exam.

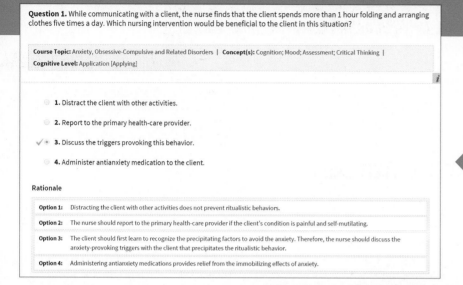

Question 1. While communicating with a client, the nurse finds that the client spends more than 1 hour folding and arranging clothes five times a day. Which nursing intervention would be beneficial to the client in this situation?

Course Topic: Anxiety, Obsessive-Compulsive and Related Disorders | **Concept(s):** Cognition; Mood; Assessment; Critical Thinking | **Cognitive Level:** Application [Applying]

- ○ **1.** Distract the client with other activities.
- ○ **2.** Report to the primary health-care provider.
- ✓ ● **3.** Discuss the triggers provoking this behavior.
- ○ **4.** Administer antianxiety medication to the client.

Rationale

Option 1:	Distracting the client with other activities does not prevent ritualistic behaviors.
Option 2:	The nurse should report to the primary health-care provider if the client's condition is painful and self-mutilating.
Option 3:	The client should first learn to recognize the precipitating factors to avoid the anxiety. Therefore, the nurse should discuss the anxiety-provoking triggers with the client that precipitates the ritualistic behavior.
Option 4:	Administering antianxiety medications provides relief from the immobilizing effects of anxiety.

Comprehensive rationales explain why your responses are correct or incorrect. Page-specific references direct you to the relevant content in *Psychiatric Mental Health Nursing.*

The Success Center offers a snapshot of your progress and identifies your strengths and weaknesses.

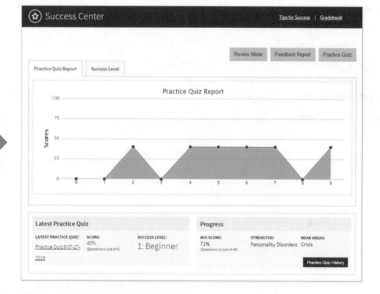

The Feedback Report drills down to show your performance in individual content areas. It's easy to create new practice quizzes that focus on your areas of weakness or to select the topics or concepts you want to study.

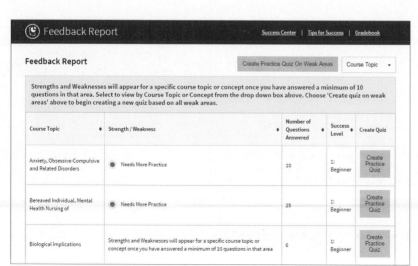

Psychiatric Mental Health Nursing:

Concepts of Care in Evidence-Based Practice

NINTH EDITION

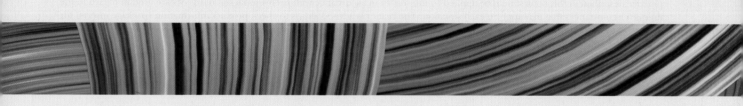

Mary C. Townsend, DSN, PMHCNS-BC

Clinical Specialist/Nurse Consultant
Adult Psychiatric Mental Health Nursing

Former Assistant Professor and
Coordinator, Mental Health Nursing
Kramer School of Nursing
Oklahoma City University
Oklahoma City, Oklahoma

Karyn I. Morgan, RN, MSN, CNS

Psychiatric Clinical Nurse Specialist
Professor of Instruction, Mental Health Nursing
The University of Akron
Akron, OH

F.A. Davis Company • Philadelphia

F. A. Davis Company
1915 Arch Street
Philadelphia, PA 19103
www.fadavis.com

Copyright © 2018 by F. A. Davis Company

Printed in the United States of America

Last digit indicates print number: 10 9 8 7 6 5 4 3 2 1

Senior Acquisitions Editor: Susan R. Rhyner
Content Project Manager II: Amy M. Romano
Electronic Project Editor: Samantha Olin
Cover Design: Carolyn O'Brien

As new scientific information becomes available through basic and clinical research, recommended treatments and drug therapies undergo changes. The author(s) and publisher have done everything possible to make this book accurate, up to date, and in accord with accepted standards at the time of publication. The author(s), editors, and publisher are not responsible for errors or omissions or for consequences from application of the book, and make no warranty, expressed or implied, in regard to the contents of the book. Any practice described in this book should be applied by the reader in accordance with professional standards of care used in regard to the unique circumstances that may apply in each situation. The reader is advised always to check product information (package inserts) for changes and new information regarding dose and contraindications before administering any drug. Caution is especially urged when using new or infrequently ordered drugs.

Library of Congress Control Number: 2014944300
ISBN: 978-0-8036-6054-0

Library of Congress Cataloging-in-Publication Data

Names: Townsend, Mary C., 1941- author. | Morgan, Karyn I., author.
Title: Psychiatric mental health nursing : concepts of care in evidence-based
  practice / Mary C. Townsend, Karyn I. Morgan.
Description: Ninth edition. | Philadelphia, PA : F. A. Davis Company, [2018]

  | Includes bibliographical references (p.) and index.
Identifiers: LCCN 2017009564| ISBN 9780803660540 | ISBN 0803660545
Subjects: | MESH: Psychiatric Nursing—methods | Mental Disorders—nursing |

  Evidence-Based Nursing
Classification: LCC RC440 | NLM WY 160 | DDC 616.89/0231—dc23 LC record available at https://lccn.loc.gov/2017009564

THIS BOOK IS DEDICATED TO:

FRANCIE

God made sisters for sharing laughter

and wiping tears

–Mary Townsend

To my friend and mentor, Chaplain (Colonel) Thomas W. Elsey

He was dearly loved and will be deeply missed

October 26, 1942–November 10, 2015

–Karyn Morgan

Reviewers

Theresa Aldelman
Bradley University
Peoria, Illinois

Fredrick Astle
University of South Carolina
Columbia, South Carolina

Carol Backstedt
Baton Rouge Community College
Baton Rouge, Louisiana

Elizabeth Bailey
Clinton Community College
Pittsburgh, New York

Sheryl Banak
Baptist Health Schools – Little Rock
Little Rock, Arkansas

Joy A. Barham
Northwestern State University
Shreveport, Louisiana

Barbara Barry
Cape Fear Community College
Wilmington, North Carolina

Carole Bomba
Harper College
Palatine, Illinois

Judy Bourrand
Samford University
Birmingham, Alabama

Susan Bowles
Barton Community College
Great Bend, Kansas

Wayne Boyer
College of the Desert
Palm Desert, California

Joyce Briggs
Ivy Tech Community College
Columbus, Indiana

Toni Bromley
Rogue Community College
Grants Pass, Oregon

Terrall Bryan
North Carolina A & T State University
Greensboro, North Carolina

Ruth Burkhart
New Mexico State University/Dona Ana Community
College
Las Cruces, New Mexico

Annette Cannon
Platt College
Aurora, Colorado

Deena Collins
Huron School of Nursing
Cleveland, Ohio

Martha Colvin
Georgia College & State University
Milledgeville, Georgia

Mary Jean Croft
St. Joseph School of Nursing
Providence, Rhode Island

Connie Cupples
Union University
Germantown, Tennessee

Karen Curlis
State University of New York Adirondack
Queensbury, New York

Nancy Cyr
North Georgia College and State University
Dahlonega, Georgia

Carol Danner
Baptist Health Schools Little Rock – School of Nursing
Little Rock, Arkansas

Carolyn DeCicco
Our Lady of Lourdes School of Nursing
Camden, New Jersey

Leona Dempsey, PhD, APNP (ret.), PMHCS-BC
University of Wisconsin Oshkosh
Oshkosh, Wisconsin

Debra J. DeVoe
Our Lady of Lourdes School of Nursing
Camden, New Jersey

Victoria T. Durkee, PhD, APRN
University of Louisiana at Monroe
Monroe, Louisiana

J. Carol Elliott
St. Anselm College
Fairfield, California

Sandra Farmer
Capital University
Columbus, Ohio

Patricia Freed
Saint Louis University
St. Louis, Missouri

Diane Gardner
University of West Florida
Pensacola, Florida

Maureen Gaynor
Saint Anselm College
Manchester, New Hampshire

Denise Glenore
West Coast University
Riverside, California

Sheilia R. Goodwin
Winston Salem State University
Salem, North Carolina

Janine Graf-Kirk
Trinitas School of Nursing
Elizabeth, New Jersey

Susan B. Grubbs
Francis Marion University
Florence, South Carolina

Elizabeth Gulledge
Jacksonville State University
Jacksonville, Alabama

Kim Gurcan
Columbus Practical School of Nursing
Columbus, Ohio

Patricia Jean Hedrick Young
Washington Hospital School of Nursing
Washington, Pennsylvania

Melinda Hermanns
University of Texas at Tyler
Tyler, Texas

Alison Hewig
Victoria College
Victoria, Texas

Cheryl Hilgenberg
Millikin University
Decatur, Illinois

Lori Hill
Gadsden State Community College
Gadsden, Alabama

Ruby Houldson
Illinois Eastern Community College
Olney, Illinois

Eleanor J. Jefferson
Community College of Denver
Platt College
Metropolitan St. College
Denver, Colorado

Dana Johnson
Mesa State College/Grand Junction Regional Center
Grand Junction, Colorado

Janet Johnson
Fort Berthold Community College
New Town, North Dakota

Nancy Kostin
Madonna University
Livonia, Michigan

Linda Lamberson
University of Southern Maine
Portland, Maine

Irene Lang
Bristol Community College
Fall River, Massachusetts

Rhonda Lansdell
Northeast MS Community College
Baldwyn, Mississippi

Jacqueline Leonard
Franciscan University of Steubenville
Steubenville, Ohio

Judith Lynch-Sauer
University of Michigan
Ann Arbor, Michigan

Glenna Mahoney
University of Saint Mary
Leavenworth, Kansas

Jacqueline Mangnall
Jamestown College
Jamestown, North Dakota

Lori A. Manilla
Hagerstown Community College
Hagerstown, Maryland

Patricia Martin
West Kentucky Community and Technical College
Paducah, Kentucky

Christine Massey
Barton College
Wilson, North Carolina

Joanne Matthews
University of Kentucky
Lexington, Kentucky

Joanne McClave
: Wayne Community College
Goldsboro, North Carolina

Mary McClay
: Walla Walla University
Portland, Oregon

Susan McCormick
: Brazosport College
Lake Jackson, Texas

Shawn McGill
: Clovis Community College
Clovis, New Mexico

Margaret McIlwain
: Gordon College
Barnesville, Georgia

Nancy Miller
: Minneapolis Community and Technical College
Minneapolis, Minnesota

Vanessa Miller
: California State University Fullerton
Fullerton, California

Mary Mitsui
: Emporia State University
Emporia, Kansas

Cheryl Moreland, MS, RN
: Western Nevada College
Carson City, Nevada

Daniel Nanguang
: El Paso Community College
El Paso, Texas

Susan Newfield
: West Virginia University
Morgantown, West Virginia

Dorothy Oakley
: Jamestown Community College
Olean, New York

Christie Obritsch
: University of Mary
Bismarck, North Dakota

Sharon Opsahl
: Western Technical College
La Crosse, Wisconsin

Vicki Paris
: Jackson State Community College
Jackson, Tennessee

Lillian Parker
: Clayton State University
Morrow, Georgia

JoAnne M. Pearce, MS, RN
: Idaho State University
Pocatello, Idaho

Karen Peterson
: DeSales University
Center Valley, Pennsylvania

Carol Pool
: South Texas College
McAllen, Texas

William S. Pope
: Barton College
Wilson, North Carolina

Karen Pounds
: Northeastern University
Boston, Massachusetts

Konnie Prince
: Victoria College
Victoria, Texas

Cheryl Puntil
: Hawaii Community College
Hilo, Hawaii

Larry Purnell
: University of Delaware
Newark, Delaware

Susan Reeves
: Tennessee Technological University
Cookeville, Tennessee

Debra Riendeau
: Saint Joseph's College of Maine
Lewiston, Maine

Sharon Romer
: South Texas College
McAllen, Texas

Lisa Romero
: Solano Community College
Fairfield, California

Donna S. Sachse
: Union University
Germantown, Tennessee

Betty Salas
: Otero Junior College
La Junta, Colorado

Sheryl Samuelson, PhD, RN
: Millikin University
Decatur, Illinois

John D. Schaeffer
: San Joaquin Delta College
Stockton, California

Mindy Schaffner
Pacific Lutheran University
Tacoma, Washington

Becky Scott
Mercy College of Northwest Ohio
Toledo, Ohio

Janie Shaw
Clayton State University
Morrow, Georgia

Lori Shaw
Nebraska Methodist College
Omaha, Nebraska

Joyce Shea
Fairfield University
Fairfield, Connecticut

Judith Shindul-Rothschild
Boston College
Chestnut Hill, Massachusetts

Audrey Silveri
UMass Worcester Graduate School of Nursing
Worcester, Massachusetts

Brenda Smith, MSN, RN
North Georgia College and State University
Dahlonega, Georgia

Janet Somlyay
University of Wyoming
Laramie, Wyoming

Charlotte Strahm, DNSc, RN, CNS-PMH
Purdue North Central
Westville, Indiana

Jo Sullivan
Centralia College
Centralia, Washington

Kathleen Sullivan
Boise State University
Boise, Idaho

Judy Traynor
Jefferson Community College
Watertown, New York

Claudia Turner
Temple College
Temple, Texas

Suzanne C. Urban
Mansfield University
Mansfield, Pennsylvania

Dorothy Varchol
Cincinnati State
Cincinnati, Ohio

Connie M. Wallace
Nebraska Methodist College
Omaha, Nebraska

Sandra Wardell
Orange County Community College
Middletown, New York

Susan Warmuskerken
West Shore Community College
Scottville, Michigan

Roberta Weseman
East Central College
Union, Missouri

Margaret A. Wheatley
Case Western Reserve University, FPB School
of Nursing
Cleveland, Ohio

Jeana Wilcox
Graceland University
Independence, Missouri

Jackie E. Williams
Georgia Perimeter College
Clarkston, Georgia

Rita L. Williams, MSN, RN, CCM
Langston University School of Nursing & Health
Professions
Langston, Oklahoma

Rodney A. White
Lewis and Clark Community College
Godfrey, Illinois

Vita Wolinsky
Dominican College
Orangeburg, New York

Marguerite Wordell
Kentucky State University
Frankfort, Kentucky

Jan Zlotnick
City College of San Francisco
San Francisco, California

Acknowledgments

Amy M. Romano, Content Project Manager, Nursing, F.A. Davis Company, for all your help and support in preparing the manuscript for publication.

Sharon Y. Lee, Production Editor, for your support and competence in the final editing and production of the manuscript.

The nursing educators, students, and clinicians, who provide critical information about the usability of the textbook and offer suggestions for improvements. Many changes have been made on the basis of your input.

To those individuals who critiqued the manuscript for this edition and shared your ideas, opinions, and suggestions for enhancement. I sincerely appreciate your contributions to the final product.

My husband, Jim, and children and grandchildren, Kerry and Ryan, Tina and Jonathan, Meghan, Matthew, and Catherine for showing me what life is truly all about.

Mary C. Townsend

First of all, sincere thanks to Mary Townsend for having the confidence in me to be included in authoring this exceptional text. I have the utmost respect for what you have created and for your foresight in recognizing the most relevant issues in the changing face of psychiatric mental health nursing care.

My thanks also to Susan Rhyner for the encouragement, humor, and passion that have made this work enjoyable. Thanks to Amy Romano, Andrea Miller, and Christine Becker for your expertise and accessibility in preparing the manuscript. I, too, appreciate all the reviewers who have offered feedback and their unique expertise. Thanks to Jennifer Feldman, MLIS, AHIP, for sharing your skills and research assistance. I have learned just how true it is that it "takes a village" and I am grateful for each of you.

Special thanks to Erin Barnard, Alan Brunner, Fred Frese, Emmy Strong, and the others who courageously allowed their stories to be told. Your contributions to student learning and to breaking down the barriers of stigmatization are immeasurable.

I appreciate each of you more than I can say.

Karyn I. Morgan

Contents

UNIT 5
Psychiatric Mental Health Nursing of Special Populations   731

Ebook Bonus Chapters

To the Instructor

Currently in progress, implementation of the recommendations set forth by the New Freedom Commission on Mental Health has given enhanced priority to mental health care in the United States. Moreover, at the 65th meeting of the World Health Assembly (WHA) in May 2012, India, Switzerland, and the United States cosponsored a resolution requesting that the World Health Organization, in collaboration with member countries, develop a global mental health action plan. This resolution was passed at the 66th WHA in May 2013. By their support of this resolution, member countries have expressed their commitment for "promotion of mental health, prevention of mental disorders, and early identification, care, support, treatment, and recovery of persons with mental disorders." With the passage of this resolution, mental health services may now be available for millions who have been without this type of care. More recently, national initiatives have sought to address the growing crises of deaths related to suicide and opiate overdoses. Mental health and mental illness continue to gain attention globally in the wake of these and other critical issues but much still needs to be done to reduce stigmatization and premature loss of life in this population.

Many nurse leaders see this period of mental health-care reform as an opportunity for nurses to expand their roles and assume key positions in education, prevention, assessment, and referral. Nurses are, and will continue to be, in key positions to assist individuals to attain, maintain, or regain optimal emotional wellness.

As it has been with each new edition of *Psychiatric Mental Health Nursing: Concepts of Care in Evidence-Based Nursing*, the goal of this ninth edition is to bring to practicing nurses and nursing students the most up-to-date information related to neurobiology, psychopharmacology, and evidence-based nursing interventions. This edition includes changes associated with the latest(fifth) edition of the American Psychiatric Association's *Diagnostic and Statistical Manual of Mental Disorders (DSM-5)*.

Content and Features New to the Ninth Edition

All content has been updated to reflect the current state of the discipline of nursing.

All nursing diagnoses are current with the NANDA-I *2015–2017 Nursing Diagnoses Definitions and Classifications*.

Communication Exercises are included in Chapters 13, Crisis Intervention; 17, Suicide Prevention; 21, The Recovery Model; 22, Neurocognitive Disorders; 23, Substance Use and Addictive Disorders; 24, Schizophrenia Spectrum and Other Psychotic Disorders; 25, Depressive Disorders; 26, Bipolar and Related Disorders; 27, Anxiety, Obsessive-Compulsive, and Related Disorders; 30, Issues Related to Human Sexuality; 31, Eating Disorders; 32, Personality Disorders; 35, Survivors of Abuse or Neglect; and 37, The Bereaved Individual. These exercises portray clinical scenarios that allow the student to practice communication skills with clients. Examples of answers appear in an appendix at the back of the book.

A new feature, "Real People, Real Stories," includes interviews conducted by one of the authors, Karyn Morgan, in which individuals discuss their experience of living with a mental illness and their thoughts on important information for nurses to know. These discussions can be used with students to explore communication issues and interventions to combat stigmatization and to build empathy through understanding individuals' unique experiences. "Real People, Real Stories" interviews are in Chapters 8, Therapeutic Communication; 17, Suicide Prevention; 23, Substance Use and Addictive Disorders; 24, Schizophrenia Spectrum and Other Psychotic Disorders; 25, Depressive Disorders; 30, Issues Related to Human Sexuality and Gender Dysphoria; and 38, Military Families.

New QSEN icons (in addition to the existing QSEN Teaching Strategy boxes) have been added selectively throughout chapters to highlight content that reflects application of one or more of the six QSEN competencies (patient-centered care, evidence-based practice, teamwork and collaboration, maintaining safety, quality improvement, and informatics).

Chapter 4, Psychopharmacology, has been moved from DavisPlus to the textbook. While each class of psychoactive substances is discussed in this chapter, lists of commonly used agents have been retained in the chapters that discuss specific disorders. For example, a list of commonly used antipsychotic agents (along with dosage ranges, half-life, and pregnancy categories) appears in Chapter 24, Schizophrenia Spectrum and Other Psychotic Disorders. These lists also appear online at DavisPlus.

New content on motivational interviewing appears in Chapters 8 and 23.

New content describing the concept of emotional intelligence is included in Chapter 14, Assertiveness Training.

New content on RAISE (Recovery After an Initial Schizophrenia Episode), based on the NIMH initiative is included in Chapter 24.

New content on gender dysphoria and transgender issues appears in Chapter 21.

Updated and new psychotropic drugs approved since the publication of the eighth edition are included in the specific diagnostic chapters to which they apply.

Features That Have Been Retained in the Ninth Edition

The concept of **holistic nursing** is retained in the ninth edition. An attempt has been made to ensure that the physical aspects of psychiatric-mental health nursing are not overlooked. In all relevant situations, the mind/body connection is addressed.

Nursing process is retained in the ninth edition as the tool for delivery of care to the individual with a psychiatric disorder or to assist in the primary prevention or exacerbation of mental illness symptoms. The six steps of the nursing process, as described in the American Nurses Association *Standards of Clinical Nursing Practice,* are used to provide guidelines for the nurse. These standards of care are included for the *DSM-5* diagnoses, as well as those on the aging individual, the bereaved individual, survivors of abuse and neglect, and military families, and as examples in several of the therapeutic approaches. The six steps include:

Assessment: Background assessment data, including a description of symptomatology, provides an extensive knowledge base from which the nurse may draw when performing an assessment. Several assessment tools are also included.

Diagnosis: Nursing diagnoses common to specific psychiatric disorders are derived from analysis of assessment data.

Outcome Identification: Outcomes are derived from the nursing diagnoses and stated as measurable goals.

Planning: A plan of care is presented with selected nursing diagnoses for the *DSM-5* diagnoses, as well as for the elderly client, the bereaved individual, victims of abuse and neglect, military veterans and their families, the elderly homebound client, and the primary caregiver of the client with a chronic mental illness. The planning standard also includes tables that list topics for educating clients and families about mental illness. Concept map care plans are included for all major psychiatric diagnoses.

Implementation: The interventions that have been identified in the plan of care are included along with rationales for each. Case studies at the end of each *DSM-5* chapter assist the student in the practical application of theoretical material. Also included as a part of this particular standard is Unit 3, Therapeutic Approaches in Psychiatric Nursing Care. This section of the textbook addresses psychiatric nursing intervention in depth and frequently speaks to the differentiation in scope of practice between the basic-level psychiatric nurse and the advanced practice–level psychiatric nurse.

Evaluation: The evaluation standard includes a set of questions that the nurse may use to assess whether the nursing actions have been successful in achieving the objectives of care.

Following are additional features of this ninth edition:

- **Internet references** for each *DSM-5* diagnosis, with website listings for information related to the disorder.
- **Tables that list topics for client/family education** (in the clinical chapters).
- **Boxes that include current research studies** with implications for evidence-based nursing practice (in the clinical chapters).
- **Assigning nursing diagnoses to client behaviors** (diagnostic chapters).
- **Taxonomy and diagnostic criteria from the *DSM-5* (2013).** Used throughout the text.
- **All references have been updated throughout the text.** Classical references are distinguished from general references.
- **Boxes with definitions of core concepts** appear throughout the text.
- **Comprehensive glossary.**
- **Answers to end-of-chapter review questions** (Appendix A).
- **Answers to communication exercises** (Appendix B).
- **Sample client teaching guides** (online at www .davisplus.com).
- **Website.** An F.A. Davis/Townsend website that contains additional nursing care plans that do not appear in the text, links to psychotropic medications, concept map care plans, and neurobiological content and illustrations, as well as student resources including practice test questions, learning activities, concept map care plans, and client teaching guides.

Additional Educational Resources

Faculty may also find the teaching aids that accompany this textbook helpful. These Instructor Resources are located at www.davisplus.com:

- **Multiple choice questions** (including new format questions reflecting the latest NCLEX blueprint).
- **Lecture outlines** for all chapters

- **Learning activities** for all chapters (including answer key)
- **Answers to the Critical Thinking Exercises** from the textbook
- **PowerPoint Presentation** to accompany all chapters in the textbook
- **Answers to the Homework Assignment Questions** from the textbook
- **Case studies for use with student teaching**

Additional chapters on Theories of Personality Development, Relaxation Therapy, Complementary and Psychosocial Therapies, and Forensic Nursing are presented online at www.davisplus.com.

It is hoped that the revisions and additions to this ninth edition continue to satisfy a need within psychiatric-mental health nursing practice. The mission of this textbook has been, and continues to be, to provide both students and clinicians with up-to-date information about psychiatric-mental health nursing. The user-friendly format and easy-to-understand language, for which we have received many positive comments, have been retained in this edition. We hope that this ninth edition continues to promote and advance the commitment to psychiatric/mental health nursing.

Mary C. Townsend

Karyn I. Morgan

Basic Concepts in Psychiatric-Mental Health Nursing

1 The Concept of Stress Adaptation

CHAPTER OUTLINE

KEY TERMS

OBJECTIVES

After reading this chapter, the student will be able to:

1. Define *adaptation* and *maladaptation*.
2. Identify physiological responses to stress.
3. Explain the relationship between stress and "diseases of adaptation."
4. Describe the concept of stress as an environmental event.
5. Explain the concept of stress as a transaction between the individual and the environment.
6. Discuss adaptive coping strategies in the management of stress.

HOMEWORK ASSIGNMENT

Please read the chapter and answer the following questions:

1. How are the body's physiological defenses affected when under sustained stress? Why?
2. In the view of stress as an environmental event, what aspects are missing when considering an individual's response to a stressful situation?
3. In their study, what event did Miller and Rahe (1997) find produced the highest level of stress reaction in their participants?
4. What is the initial step in stress management?

Psychologists and others have struggled for many years to establish an effective definition of the term *stress*. This term is used loosely today and still lacks a definitive explanation. Stress may be viewed as an individual's reaction to any change that requires an adjustment or response, which can be physical, mental, or emotional. Responses directed at stabilizing internal biological processes and preserving self-esteem can be viewed as healthy adaptations to stress.

Roy (1976), a nursing theorist, defined an **adaptive response** as behavior that maintains the integrity of the individual. Adaptation is viewed as positive and is correlated with a healthy response. When behavior disrupts the integrity of the individual, it is perceived as maladaptive. **Maladaptive responses** by the individual are considered to be negative or unhealthy.

Various 20th-century researchers contributed to several different concepts of stress. Three of these concepts include stress as a biological response, stress as an environmental event, and stress as a transaction between the individual and the environment. This chapter includes an explanation of each of these concepts.

CORE CONCEPT

Stressor

A biological, psychological, social, or chemical factor that causes physical or emotional tension and may contribute to the development of certain illnesses.

Stress as a Biological Response

In 1956, Hans Selye published the results of his research on the physiological response of a biological system to an imposed change on the system. Since his initial publication, his definition of stress has evolved to "the state manifested by a specific syndrome which consists of all the nonspecifically induced changes within a biologic system" (Selye, 1976). This combination of symptoms has come to be known as the **fight-or-flight syndrome.** Schematics of these biological responses, both initially and with sustained stress, are presented in Figures 1–1 and 1–2. Selye called this phenomenon the **general adaptation syndrome.** He described three distinct stages of the reaction:

1. **Alarm reaction stage:** During this stage, the physiological responses of the fight-or-flight syndrome are initiated.

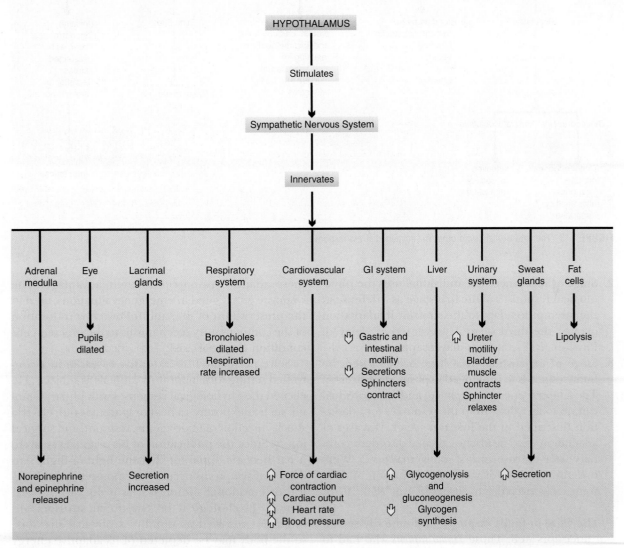

FIGURE 1–1   The fight-or-flight syndrome: The initial stress response.

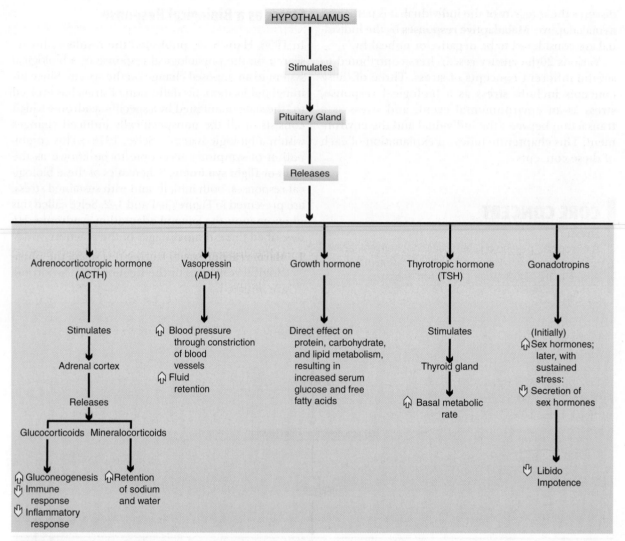

FIGURE 1–2 The fight-or-flight syndrome: The sustained stress response.

2. **Stage of resistance:** The individual uses the physiological responses of the first stage as a defense in the attempt to adapt to the stressor. If adaptation occurs, the third stage is prevented or delayed. Physiological symptoms may disappear.

3. **Stage of exhaustion:** This stage occurs when the body responds to prolonged exposure to a stressor. The adaptive energy is depleted, and the individual can no longer draw from the resources for adaptation described in the first two stages. Diseases of adaptation (e.g., headaches, mental disorders, coronary artery disease, ulcers, colitis) may occur. Without intervention for reversal, exhaustion and, in some cases, even death, ensues (Selye, 1956, 1974).

The fight-or-flight response undoubtedly served our ancestors well. Those *Homo sapiens* who had to face the giant grizzly bear or the saber-toothed tiger as part of their struggle for survival must have used

these adaptive resources to their advantage. The response was elicited in emergency situations, used in the preservation of life, and followed by restoration of the compensatory mechanisms to the preemergent condition (homeostasis).

Selye performed his extensive research in a controlled setting with laboratory animals as subjects. He elicited the physiological responses with physical stimuli, such as exposure to heat or extreme cold, electric shock, injection of toxic agents, restraint, and surgical injury. Since the publication of his original research, it has become apparent that the fight-or-flight syndrome of symptoms occurs in response to psychological or emotional stimuli just as it does to physical stimuli. Psychological or emotional stressors are often not resolved as rapidly as physical stressors, so the body may be depleted of its adaptive energy more readily than it is from physical stressors. The fight-or-flight response may be inappropriate or even dangerous in our modern lifestyle in which stress has been described as a pervasive, chronic, and relentless psychosocial state. When the stress response becomes chronic, the body's existence in the aroused condition for extended time periods promotes susceptibility to disease.

■ CORE CONCEPT

Adaptation

Adaptation is said to occur when an individual's physical or behavioral response to any change in his or her internal or external environment results in preservation of individual integrity or timely return to equilibrium.

Stress as an Environmental Event

A second concept defines stress as an "event" that triggers an individual's adaptive physiological and psychological responses. The event creates change in the life pattern of the individual, requires significant adjustment in lifestyle, and taxes available personal resources. The change can be either positive, such as outstanding personal achievement, or negative, such as being fired from a job. The emphasis here is on *change* from the existing steady state of the individual's life pattern.

Miller and Rahe (1997) have updated the original Social Readjustment Rating Scale devised by Holmes and Rahe in 1967 to reflect an increased number of modern stressors. Just as in the earlier version, numerical values are assigned to various common life events based on the stress these events create. In their research, Miller and Rahe found that women react to life stress events at higher levels than do men, and unmarried people gave higher scores than married people for most of the events. Younger participants rated more events at a higher stress level than did older participants. A high score on the Recent Life Changes Questionnaire (RLCQ) places the individual at greater susceptibility to physical or psychological illness. The questionnaire may be completed considering life stressors within a 6-month or 1-year period. Six-month totals equal to or greater than 300 life change units (LCUs) or 1-year totals equal to or greater than 500 LCUs are considered indicative of a high level of recent life stress, thereby increasing the individual's risk of illness. The RLCQ is presented in Table 1–1.

It is unknown whether stress overload merely predisposes a person to illness or actually precipitates it, but there does appear to be a link (Amirkhan, 2012). Individuals differ in their reactions to life events, and these variations are related to the degree to which the change is perceived as stressful. Life changes

TABLE 1–1 The Recent Life Changes Questionnaire

LIFE CHANGE EVENT	LCU	LIFE CHANGE EVENT	LCU
HEALTH		Troubles at work:	
An injury or illness which:	74	With your boss	29
Kept you in bed a week or more, or sent you to the hospital		With coworkers	35
Was less serious than above	44	With persons under your supervision	35
		Other work troubles	28
Major dental work	26	Major business adjustment	60
Major change in eating habits	27	Retirement	52
Major change in sleeping habits	26	Loss of job:	
Major change in your usual type/amount of recreation	28	Laid off from work	68
		Fired from work	79
WORK		Correspondence course to help you in your work	18
Change to a new type of work	51	**PERSONAL AND SOCIAL**	
Change in your work hours or conditions	35	Change in personal habits	26
Change in your responsibilities at work:		Beginning or ending school or college	38
More responsibilities	29	Change of school or college	35
Fewer responsibilities	21	Change in political beliefs	24
Promotion	31	Change in religious beliefs	29
Demotion	42		
Transfer	32		

Continued

TABLE 1–1 The Recent Life Changes Questionnaire—cont'd

LIFE CHANGE EVENT	LCU	LIFE CHANGE EVENT	LCU
Change in social activities	27	Spouse beginning or ending work	46
Vacation	24	Child leaving home:	
New, close, personal relationship	37	To attend college	41
Engagement to marry	45	Due to marriage	41
Girlfriend or boyfriend problems	39	For other reasons	45
Sexual difficulties	44	Change in arguments with spouse	50
"Falling out" of a close personal relationship	47	In-law problems	38
An accident	48	Change in the marital status of your parents:	
Minor violation of the law	20	Divorce	59
Being held in jail	75	Remarriage	50
Death of a close friend	70	Separation from spouse:	
Major decision regarding your immediate future	51	Due to work	53
Major personal achievement	36	Due to marital problems	76
HOME AND FAMILY		Divorce	96
Major change in living conditions	42	Birth of grandchild	43
Change in residence:		Death of spouse	119
Move within the same town or city	25	Death of other family member:	
Move to a different town, city, or state	47	Child	123
Change in family get-togethers	25	Brother or sister	102
Major change in health or behavior of family member	55	Parent	100
Marriage	50	**FINANCIAL**	
Pregnancy	67	Major change in finances:	
Miscarriage or abortion	65	Increased income	38
Gain of a new family member:		Decreased income	60
Birth of a child	66	Investment and/or credit difficulties	56
Adoption of a child	65	Loss or damage of personal property	43
A relative moving in with you	59	Moderate purchase	20
		Major purchase	37
		Foreclosure on a mortgage or loan	58

LCU, life change unit.

SOURCE: Miller, M.A., & Rahe, R.H. (1997). Life changes scaling for the 1990s. *Journal of Psychosomatic Research, 43*(3), 279-292, with permission.

questionnaires have been criticized because they do not consider the individual's perception of the event. These types of instruments also fail to consider cultural variations, the individual's coping strategies, and available support systems at the time when the life change occurs. Amirkhan (2012) developed a tool to assess stress overload that attempts to correct for these limitations by asking a series of 30 questions that all begin with "In the past week have you felt . . ." followed by choices such as calm, inadequate, depressed, and others. The emphasis in this tool is on the individual's perception of events rather than on the events themselves. Although the approaches to assessing for stress and vulnerability vary, it is clear that positive coping mechanisms and strong social or familial support can reduce the intensity of stressful life changes and promote a more adaptive response.

Stress as a Transaction Between the Individual and the Environment

The concept of stress as a transaction between the individual and the environment emphasizes the *relationship* between internal variables (within an individual) and external variables (within the environment). This concept parallels the modern concept of disease etiology. No longer is causation viewed solely as an external entity; whether or not illness occurs depends also on the receiving organism's susceptibility. Similarly, to predict psychological stress as a reaction, the internal characteristics of the person in relation to the environment must be considered.

Precipitating Event

Lazarus and Folkman's seminal theory (1984) defines stress (and potentially illness) as a psychological phenomenon in which the relationship between the person and the environment is appraised by the person as taxing or exceeding his or her resources and endangering his or her well-being. A **precipitating event** is a stimulus arising from the internal or external environment and perceived by the individual in a specific manner. Determination of an event as stressful depends on the individual's cognitive appraisal of the situation. *Cognitive appraisal* is an individual's evaluation of the personal significance of the event or occurrence. The event "precipitates" a response on the part of the individual, and the response is influenced by the individual's perception of the event. The *cognitive response* consists of a primary appraisal and a secondary appraisal.

Individual's Perception of the Event

Primary Appraisal

Lazarus and Folkman (1984) identify three types of primary appraisal: irrelevant, benign-positive, and stressful. An event is judged *irrelevant* when the outcome holds no significance for the individual. A *benign-positive* outcome is one that is perceived as producing pleasure for the individual. *Stress appraisals* include harm or loss, threat, and challenge. *Harm* or *loss* appraisals refer to damage or loss already experienced by the individual. Appraisals of a *threatening* nature are perceived as anticipated harms or losses. When an event is appraised as *challenging*, the individual focuses on potential for gain or growth rather than on risks associated with the event. Challenge produces stress even though the emotions associated with it (eagerness and excitement) are viewed as positive, and coping mechanisms must be

called upon to face the new encounter. Challenge and threat may occur together when an individual experiences these positive emotions along with fear or anxiety over possible risks associated with the challenging event.

When stress is produced in response to harm or loss, threat, or challenge, a secondary appraisal is made by the individual.

Secondary Appraisal

The secondary appraisal is an assessment of skills, resources, and knowledge that the person possesses to deal with the situation. The individual evaluates by considering the following:

■ Which coping strategies are available to me?
■ Will the option I choose be effective in this situation?
■ Do I have the ability to use that strategy in an effective manner?

The interaction between the primary appraisal of the event that has occurred and the secondary appraisal of available coping strategies determines the quality of the individual's adaptation response to stress.

Predisposing Factors

A variety of elements influence how an individual perceives and responds to a stressful event. These **predisposing factors** strongly influence whether the response is adaptive or maladaptive. Types of predisposing factors include genetic influences, past experiences, and existing conditions.

Genetic influences are those circumstances of an individual's life that are acquired through heredity. Examples include family history of physical and psychological conditions (strengths and weaknesses) and temperament (behavioral characteristics present at birth that evolve with development).

Past experiences are occurrences that result in learned patterns that can influence an individual's adaptation response. They include previous exposure to the stressor or other stressors, learned coping responses, and degree of adaptation to previous stressors.

Existing conditions incorporate vulnerabilities that influence the adequacy of the individual's physical, psychological, and social resources for dealing with adaptive demands. Examples include current health status, motivation, developmental maturity, severity and duration of the stressor, financial and educational resources, age, existing coping strategies, and a caring support system. Hobfoll's conservation of resources theory (Hobfoll 1989; Hobfoll, Schwarzer, & Chon, 1998) adds that as existing conditions (loss or lack of resources) exceed the person's perception of adaptive capabilities, the person not only experience stress in the present but also becomes more

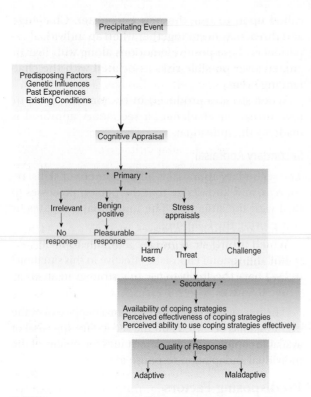

FIGURE 1–3 Transactional model of stress and adaptation.

vulnerable to the effects of stress in the future due to a "weaker resource reservoir to call on to meet future demand" (Hobfoll et al., 1998, p. 191). All of the preceding concepts and theories are foundational to the transactional model of stress and adaptation that serves as the framework for the process of nursing in this text. A graphic display of the model is presented in Figure 1–3.

CORE CONCEPT

Maladaptation

Maladaptation occurs when an individual's physical or behavioral response to any change in his or her internal or external environment results in disruption of individual integrity or in persistent disequilibrium.

Stress Management*

The growth of stress management into a multimillion-dollar-a-year industry unto itself attests to its importance in our society. Stress management involves the use of coping strategies in response to stressful situations. Coping strategies are adaptive when they

---

*Some stress management techniques are discussed at greater length in Unit 3 of this text and in the Complementary and Psychosocial Therapies chapter available online at www.DavisPlus.com.

---

protect the individual from harm (or additional harm) or strengthen the individual's ability to meet challenging situations. Adaptive responses help restore homeostasis to the body and impede the development of diseases of adaptation. Positive adaptation, particularly in response to adversity, has also been referred to as *resilience.*

Responses are considered maladaptive when the conflict goes unresolved or intensifies. Energy resources become depleted as the body struggles to compensate for the chronic physiological and psychological arousal experienced in response to the stressful event. The effect is a significant vulnerability to physical or psychological illness. One key to stress management is to identify factors and practices that contribute to adaptive coping and resilience.

Adaptive Coping Strategies

Awareness

The initial step in managing stress is awareness—to become aware of the factors that create stress and the feelings associated with a stressful response. Stress can be controlled only when one recognizes the signs that it is occurring. As an individual becomes aware of stressors, he or she can choose to omit, avoid, or accept them.

Relaxation

Individuals experience relaxation in different ways. Some people relax by engaging in large motor activities, such as sports, jogging, and physical exercise. Others use techniques such as breathing exercises and progressive relaxation. A discussion of relaxation therapy may be found online at Davis*Plus.*

Meditation

Meditation has been shown to produce a lasting reduction in blood pressure and other stress-related symptoms when practiced for 20 minutes once or twice a day (Scott, 2016). The practice of mindfulness meditation is foundational to many psychosocial interventions aimed at reducing anxiety and improving engagement in problem-solving. Meditation involves assuming a comfortable position, closing the eyes, casting off all other thoughts, and concentrating on a single word, sound, or phrase that has positive meaning to the individual. It may also involve concentrating on one's breathing or other mindfulness practices. The technique of meditation is described in detail online at Davis*Plus.*

Interpersonal Communication

As previously mentioned, the strength of an individual's available support system is an existing condition that significantly influences his or her adaptation when coping with stress. Sometimes just "talking the problem out" with an empathetic individual can interrupt escalation of the stress response. Writing about one's feelings in a journal or diary can also be therapeutic.

Problem-Solving

Problem-solving is an adaptive coping strategy in which the individual is able to view the situation objectively (or to seek assistance from another individual to accomplish this if the anxiety level is too high to concentrate) and then apply a problem-solving and decision-making model such as the following:

■ Assess the facts of the situation.
■ Formulate goals for resolution of the stressful situation.
■ Study the alternatives for dealing with the situation.
■ Determine the risks and benefits of each alternative.
■ Select an alternative.
■ Implement the alternative selected.
■ Evaluate the outcome of the alternative implemented.
■ If the first choice is ineffective, select and implement a second option.

Pets

Studies show that those who care for pets, especially dogs and cats, are better able to cope with the stressors of life (Mayo Clinic, 2015). The physical act of stroking a dog's or cat's fur can be therapeutic, giving the animal an intuitive sense of being cared for and providing the individual the calming feeling of warmth, affection, and interdependence with a reliable, trusting being. Studies have also shown that individuals with companion pets demonstrate improvements in heart health, allergies, anxiety, and mental illnesses such as depression (Casciotti & Zuckerman, 2016, Donehy, 2015).

Music

It is true that music can "soothe the savage beast." Studies have shown multiple benefits of listening to music, including relieving pain, improving motivation and performance, improving sleep, enhancing blood vessel function, reducing stress, relieving symptoms of depression, improving cognition, and easing recovery in stroke patients (Christ, 2013).

Summary and Key Points

■ Stress has become a chronic and pervasive condition in the United States.
■ Adaptive behavior is a stress response that maintains the integrity of the individual with a timely return to equilibrium. It is viewed as positive and is correlated with a healthy response.
■ When behavior disrupts the integrity of the individual or results in persistent disequilibrium, it is perceived as maladaptive. Maladaptive responses by the individual are unhealthy.

■ A stressor is defined as a biological, psychological, social, or chemical factor that causes physical or emotional tension and may be a factor in the etiology of certain illnesses.
■ Hans Selye identified the biological changes associated with a stressful situation as the fight-or-flight syndrome.
■ Selye called the general reaction of the body to stress the "general adaptation syndrome," which occurs in three stages: the alarm reaction stage, the stage of resistance, and the stage of exhaustion.
■ When individuals remain in the aroused response to stress for an extended period of time, they become susceptible to diseases, including headaches, mental disorders, coronary artery disease, ulcers, and colitis.
■ Stress may also be viewed as an environmental event, which results when a change from the existing steady state of the individual's life pattern occurs.
■ When an individual experiences a high level of life change events, he or she becomes susceptible to physical or psychological illness.
■ Limitations of the environmental concept of stress include failure to consider the individual's perception of the event, coping strategies, and available support systems at the time when the life change occurs.
■ Stress is more appropriately expressed as a transaction between the individual and the environment that is appraised by the individual as taxing or exceeding his or her resources and endangering his or her well-being.
■ The individual makes a cognitive appraisal of the precipitating event to determine the personal significance of the event or occurrence.
■ Primary cognitive appraisals may be irrelevant, benign-positive, or stressful.
■ Secondary cognitive appraisals include assessment and evaluation by the individual of skills, resources, and knowledge to deal with the stressful situation.
■ Predisposing factors influence how an individual perceives and responds to a stressful event. They include genetic influences, past experiences, and existing conditions.
■ Stress management involves the use of adaptive coping strategies in response to stressful situations in an effort to impede the development of diseases of adaptation.
■ Examples of adaptive coping strategies include developing awareness, relaxation, meditation, interpersonal communication with caring other, problem-solving, pets, and music.

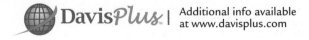

DavisPlus | Additional info available at www.davisplus.com

Review Questions
Self-Examination/Learning Exercise

Select the answer that is most appropriate for each of the following questions.

1. Sondra, who lives in Maine, hears on the evening news that 25 people were killed in a tornado in south Texas. Sondra experiences no anxiety upon hearing of this stressful situation. What is the most likely reason that Sondra experiences no anxiety?
   a. She is selfish and does not care what happens to other people.
   b. She appraises the event as irrelevant to her own situation.
   c. She assesses that she has the skills to cope with the stressful situation.
   d. She uses suppression as her primary defense mechanism.

2. Cindy regularly develops nausea and vomiting when she is faced with a stressful situation. Which of the following is most likely a predisposing factor to this maladaptive response by Cindy?
   a. Cindy inherited her mother's "nervous" stomach.
   b. Cindy is fixed in a lower level of development.
   c. Cindy has never been motivated to achieve success.
   d. When Cindy was a child, her mother pampered her and kept her home from school when she was ill.

3. When an individual's stress response is sustained over a long period, the endocrine system involvement results in which of the following?
   a. Decreased resistance to disease
   b. Increased libido
   c. Decreased blood pressure
   d. Increased inflammatory response

4. Why is stress management extremely important in today's society?
   a. Evolution has diminished the human capability for fight-or-flight responses.
   b. The stressors of today tend to be ongoing, resulting in a sustained response.
   c. We have stress disorders that did not exist in the days of our ancestors.
   d. One never knows when one will have to face a grizzly bear or saber-toothed tiger in today's society.

5. Elena has just received a promotion on her job. She is very happy and excited about moving up in her company, but she has been experiencing anxiety since receiving the news. Her primary appraisal is that she most likely views the situation as which of the following?
   a. Benign-positive
   b. Irrelevant
   c. Challenging
   d. Threatening

6. John comes to the mental health clinic with reports of anxiety and depression. According to the transactional model of stress and adaptation, which of the following are important to consider when assessing John's complaints? (Select all that apply.)
   a. John's perception of precipitating events
   b. Past stressors and degree of positive coping abilities
   c. Existing social supports
   d. Physical strength
   e. Pupillary adaptation to light

References

Amirkhan, J.H. (2012). Stress overload: A new approach to the assessment of stress. *American Journal of Community Psychology, 49*(1-2), 55-71. doi:10.1007/s10464-011-9438-x

Casciotti, D., & Zuckerman, D. (2016). The benefits of pets for human health. Retrieved from http://center4research.org/healthy-living-prevention/pets-and-health-the-impact-of-companion-animals

Christ, S. (2013). 20 surprising science-backed health benefits of music. Retrieved from www.usatoday.com/story/news/health/2013/12/17/health-benefits-music/4053401

Donehy, K. (2015). Pets for depression and health. Retrieved from www.webmd.com/depression/features/pets-depression

Mayo Clinic. (2015). Pet therapy: Man's best friend as healer. Retrieved from www.mayoclinic.org/healthy-lifestyle/consumer-health/in-depth/pet-therapy/art-20046342

Scott, E. (2016). Meditation research and benefits. Retrieved from www.verywell.com/meditation-research-and-benefits-3144996

Classical References

Hobfoll, S. (1989). Conservation of resources: A new attempt at conceptualizing stress. *American Psychologist 44*(3), 513-524. doi:http://dx.doi.org/10.1037/0003-066X.44.3.513

Hobfoll, S., Schwarzer, R., & Chon, K. (1998). Disentangling the stress labyrinth: Interpreting the meaning of stress as it is studied in the health context. *Anxiety, Stress, and Coping, 11*(3), 181-212. doi:http://dx.doi.org/10.1080/10615809808248311

Holmes, T., & Rahe, R. (1967). The social readjustment rating scale. *Journal of Psychosomatic Research, 11*(2), 213-218. doi:http://dx.doi.org/10.1016/0022-3999(67)90010-4

Lazarus, R.S., & Folkman, S. (1984). *Stress, appraisal and coping.* New York: Springer Publishing.

Miller, M.A., & Rahe, R.H. (1997). Life changes scaling for the 1990s. *Journal of Psychosomatic Research, 43*(3), 279-292. doi:10.1016/S0022-3999(97)00118-9

Roy, C. (1976). *Introduction to nursing: An adaptation model.* Englewood Cliffs, NJ: Prentice-Hall.

Selye, H. (1956). *The stress of life.* New York: McGraw-Hill.

Selye, H. (1974). *Stress without distress.* New York: Signet Books.

Selye, H. (1976). *The stress of life* (rev. ed.). New York: McGraw Hill.

2 Mental Health and Mental Illness: Historical and Theoretical Concepts

CHAPTER OUTLINE

KEY TERMS

anticipatory grieving

bereavement overload

defense mechanisms

   compensation

   denial

   displacement

   identification

   intellectualization

introjection

isolation

projection

rationalization

reaction formation

regression

repression

sublimation

suppression

undoing

humors

mental health

mental illness

neurosis

psychosis

OBJECTIVES

After reading this chapter, the student will be able to:

1. Discuss the history of psychiatric care.
2. Define *mental health* and *mental illness*.
3. Discuss cultural elements that influence attitudes toward mental health and mental illness.
4. Describe psychological adaptation responses to stress.
5. Correlate adaptive and maladaptive responses to the mental health/mental illness continuum.

HOMEWORK ASSIGNMENT

Please read the chapter and answer the following questions:

1. Explain the concepts of *incomprehensibility* and *cultural relativity*.
2. Describe some symptoms of panic anxiety.
3. Jane was involved in an automobile accident in which both her parents were killed. When you ask her about it, she says she has no memory of the accident. What ego defense mechanism is she using?
4. In what stage of the grieving process is the individual with delayed or inhibited grief fixed?

The consideration of mental health and mental illness has its basis in the cultural beliefs of the society in which the behavior takes place. Some cultures are quite liberal in the range of behaviors that are considered acceptable, whereas others have very little tolerance for behaviors that deviate from the cultural norms.

A study of the history of psychiatric care reveals some shocking truths about past treatment of individuals with mental illness. Many were kept in control by means that today could be considered less than humane.

This chapter deals with the evolution of psychiatric care from ancient times to the present. **Mental health** and **mental illness** are defined, and the psychological adaptation to stress is explained in terms of the two major responses: anxiety and grief. Behavioral responses are conceptualized along the mental health/mental illness continuum.

Historical Overview of Psychiatric Care

Primitive beliefs regarding mental disturbances took several views. Some cultures thought that an individual with mental illness had been dispossessed of his or her soul and wellness could be achieved only if the soul was returned. Others believed that evil spirits or supernatural or magical powers had entered the body. The "cure" for these individuals involved a ritualistic exorcism to purge the body of these unwanted forces. This purging often consisted of brutal beatings, starvation, or other torturous means. Still other cultures considered that the individual with mental illness may have broken a taboo or sinned against another individual or God, for which ritualistic purification was required or various types of retribution were demanded. The correlation of mental illness to demonology led to some individuals with mental illness being burned at the stake.

These ancient beliefs evolved with increasing knowledge about mental illness and changes in cultural, religious, and sociopolitical attitudes. Around 400 BC, the work of Hippocrates was the first to place mental illness in a physical rather than supernatural context. Hippocrates theorized that mental illness was caused by irregularity in the interaction of the four body fluids: blood, black bile, yellow bile, and phlegm. He called these body fluids **humors** and associated each with a particular disposition. Disequilibrium among these four humors was often treated by inducing vomiting and diarrhea with potent cathartic drugs.

During the Middle Ages (AD 500 to 1500), the association of mental illness with witchcraft and the supernatural continued to prevail in Europe. During this period, many people with mental illness were set to sea alone in sailing boats with little guidance to search for their lost rationality, a practice from which the expression "ship of fools" was derived. But in Middle Eastern countries, a change in attitude began to occur that led to the perception of mental illness as a medical problem rather than a result of supernatural forces. This notion gave rise to the establishment of special units for clients with mental illness within general hospitals as well as residential institutions specifically designed for this purpose. They can likely be considered the first asylums for individuals with mental illness.

Colonial Americans tended to reflect the attitudes of the European communities from which they had emigrated. Particularly in the New England area, individuals were punished for behavior attributed to witchcraft. In the 16th and 17th centuries, institutions for people with mental illness did not exist in the United States, and care of these individuals became a family responsibility. Those without family or other resources became the responsibility of the communities in which they lived and were incarcerated in places where they could do no harm to themselves or others.

The first hospital in America to admit clients with mental illness was established in Philadelphia in the middle of the 18th century. Benjamin Rush, often called the father of American psychiatry, was a physician at the hospital. He initiated the provision of humanistic treatment and care for clients with mental illness. But although he included kindness, exercise, and socialization in his care, he also employed harsh methods such as bloodletting, purging, various types of physical restraints, and extremes of temperatures, reflecting the medical therapies of that era.

The 19th century brought the establishment of a system of state asylums, largely the result of the work of Dorothea Dix, a former New England schoolteacher who lobbied tirelessly on behalf of the mentally ill population. She was unfaltering in her belief that mental illness was curable and that state hospitals should provide humanistic therapeutic care. This system of hospital care for individuals with mental illness grew, but the mentally ill population grew faster. The institutions became overcrowded and understaffed, and conditions deteriorated. Therapeutic care reverted to custodial care in state hospitals, which provided the largest resource for individuals with mental illness until the initiation of the community health movement of the 1960s (see Chapter 36, Community Mental Health Nursing).

The emergence of psychiatric nursing began in 1873 with the graduation of Linda Richards from the nursing program at the New England Hospital for Women and Children in Boston. She has come to be known as the first American psychiatric nurse. During her career, Richards was instrumental in the establishment of a number of psychiatric hospitals and the first school of psychiatric nursing at the McLean Asylum in Waverly, Massachusetts, in 1882. This school and others like it provided training in custodial care for clients in psychiatric asylums—training that did not include the study of psychological concepts. Significant change in psychiatric nursing education did not occur until 1955, when incorporation of psychiatric nursing into the curricula became a requirement for all undergraduate schools of nursing. This new curricula emphasized the importance of the nurse–patient relationship and therapeutic communication techniques. Nursing intervention in the somatic therapies (e.g., insulin and electroconvulsive therapy) provided impetus for the incorporation of these concepts into the profession's body of knowledge.

With the increasing need for psychiatric care in the aftermath of World War II, the government passed the National Mental Health Act of 1946. This legislation provided funds for the education of psychiatrists, psychologists, social workers, and psychiatric nurses. Graduate-level education in psychiatric nursing was established during this period. Around the same time, the introduction of antipsychotic medications made it possible for clients with psychoses to more readily participate in their treatment, including nursing therapies.

Knowledge of the history of psychiatric-mental health care contributes to the understanding of the concepts presented in this chapter and those in the online chapter (available at www.DavisPlus.com), which describe the theoretical models of personality development according to various 19th- and 20th-century leaders in the mental health movement. Modern American psychiatric care has its roots in ancient times. A great deal of opportunity exists for continued advancement of this specialty within the practice of nursing.

Mental Health

A number of theorists have attempted to define the concept of mental health. Many of these concepts deal with various aspects of individual functioning. Maslow (1970) emphasized an individual's motivation in the continuous quest for self-actualization. He identified a "hierarchy of needs," with the most basic needs requiring fulfillment before those at higher levels can be achieved and with self-actualization defined as fulfillment of one's highest potential. An individual's position within the hierarchy may revert from a higher level to a lower level based on life circumstances. For example, an individual facing major surgery who has been working to achieve self-actualization may become preoccupied, if only temporarily, with the need for physiological safety. A representation of this needs hierarchy is presented in Figure 2–1.

Maslow described self-actualization as being "psychologically healthy, fully human, highly evolved, and fully mature." He believed that self-actualized individuals possess the following characteristics:

- An appropriate perception of reality
- The ability to accept oneself, others, and human nature
- The ability to manifest spontaneity
- The capacity for focusing concentration on problem-solving
- A need for detachment and desire for privacy
- Independence, autonomy, and a resistance to enculturation
- An intensity of emotional reaction
- A frequency of "peak" experiences that validate the worthwhileness, richness, and beauty of life
- An identification with humankind
- The ability to achieve satisfactory interpersonal relationships
- A democratic character structure and strong sense of ethics
- Creativeness
- A degree of nonconformance

Jahoda (1958) identified a list of six indicators that are a reflection of mental health:

1. **A positive attitude toward self:** This indicator refers to an objective view of self, including knowledge and acceptance of strengths and limitations. The individual feels a strong sense of personal identity and security within his or her environment.
2. **Growth, development, and the ability to achieve self-actualization:** This indicator correlates with whether the individual successfully achieves the tasks associated with each level of development (see Erikson, in the online chapter Theoretical Models of Personality Development). With successful achievement in each level, the individual gains motivation for advancement to his or her highest potential.
3. **Integration:** The focus of this indicator is on maintaining equilibrium or balance among various life processes. Integration includes the ability to adaptively respond to the environment and the development of a philosophy of life, both of which help the individual maintain a manageable anxiety level in response to stressful situations.
4. **Autonomy:** This indicator refers to the individual's ability to perform in an independent, self-directed manner. He or she makes choices and accepts responsibility for the outcomes.
5. **Perception of reality:** Accurate reality perception is a positive indicator of mental health. It includes

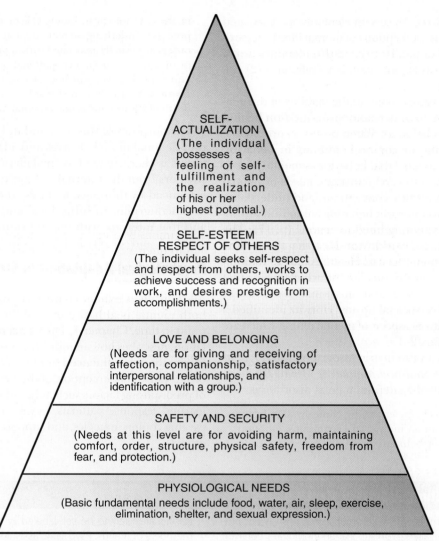

FIGURE 2-1 Maslow's hierarchy of needs.

perception of the environment without distortion as well as the capacity for empathy and social sensitivity—a respect and concern for the wants and needs of others.

6. **Environmental mastery:** This indicator suggests that the individual has achieved a satisfactory role within the group, society, or environment and is able to love and accept the love of others. When faced with life situations, the individual is able to strategize, make decisions, change, adjust, and adapt. Life offers satisfaction to the individual who has achieved environmental mastery.

Black and Andreasen (2014) describe mental health as a state of being that is relative rather than absolute but marked by the successful performance of mental functions such as adapting to change, coping with stressors, fulfilling relationships with others, and the accomplishing productive activities.

Robinson (1983) offers the following definition of mental health:

> A dynamic state in which thought, feeling, and behavior that is age-appropriate and congruent with the local and cultural norms is demonstrated. (p. 74)

For purposes of this text, and in keeping with the framework of stress and adaptation, a modification of Robinson's definition of mental health is considered. Thus, *mental health* is viewed as "the successful adaptation to stressors from the internal or external environment, evidenced by thoughts, feelings, and behaviors that are age-appropriate and congruent with local and cultural norms."

Mental Illness

Arriving at a universal concept of mental illness is difficult because of the cultural factors that influence such a definition. However, certain elements are associated with individuals' perceptions of mental illness, regardless of cultural origin. Horwitz (2010) identifies two of these elements as (1) incomprehensibility and (2) cultural relativity.

Incomprehensibility relates to the inability of the general population to understand the motivation behind an individual's behavior. When observers are unable to find meaning or comprehensibility in behavior, they are likely to label that behavior as mental illness. Horwitz states, "Observers attribute labels of mental illness when the rules, conventions, and understandings they use to interpret behavior fail to find any intelligible motivation behind an action" (p. 17). The element of *cultural relativity* considers that these rules, conventions, and understandings are conceived within an individual's own particular culture. Behavior that is considered "normal" and "abnormal" is defined by one's cultural or societal norms. Horwitz identified a number of cultural aspects of mental illness, which are presented in Box 2–1.

The American Psychiatric Association (2013), in its *Diagnostic and Statistical Manual of Mental Disorders, Fifth Edition (DSM-5)*, defines mental disorder as

> a syndrome characterized by clinically significant disturbance in an individual's cognitions, emotion regulation, or behavior that reflects a dysfunction in the psychological, biological, or developmental processes underlying mental functioning. Mental disorders are usually associated with significant distress or disability in social, occupational, or other important activities. An expected or culturally approved response to a common stressor or loss such as the death of a loved one is not a mental disorder. (p. 20)

For purposes of this text, and in keeping with the transactional model of stress and adaptation, mental illness is characterized as "maladaptive responses to stressors from the internal or external environment, evidenced by thoughts, feelings, and behaviors that are incongruent with the local and cultural norms and that interfere with the individual's social, occupational, and/or physical functioning."

Psychological Adaptation to Stress

All individuals exhibit characteristics associated with both mental health and mental illness at any given point in time. Chapter 1, The Concept of Stress Adaptation, describes how an individual's response to stressful situations is influenced by physiological factors, his or her personal perception of the event, and a variety of predisposing factors such as heredity, temperament, learned response patterns, developmental maturity, existing coping strategies, and support systems of caring others.

BOX 2–1 Cultural Aspects of Mental Illness

1. Usually, members of the community, not a psychiatric professional, initially recognizes that an individual's behavior deviates from societal norms.
2. People who are related to an individual or who are of the same cultural or social group are less likely to label an individual's behavior as mentally ill than are people who are relationally or culturally distant. Relatives and those who share a culture try to normalize the behavior by looking for an explanation.
3. Often, psychiatrists see a person with mental illness only when the family members can no longer deny the illness. Recognition or acknowledgment of possible mental illness typically occurs when behavior is at its worst as defined by local or cultural norms.
4. Individuals in lower socio-economic classes usually display more mental illness symptoms than do people in higher socio-economic classes. However, they tend to tolerate a wider range of behaviors that deviate from societal norms and are less likely to consider these behaviors as indicative of mental illness. Mental illness labels are most often applied by psychiatric professionals.
5. The higher the social class, the greater the recognition of mental illness behaviors. Members of the higher social classes are likely to be self-labeled or labeled by family members or friends. Psychiatric assistance is sought near the first signs of emotional disturbance.
6. The more highly educated the person, the greater the recognition of mental illness behaviors. However, even more relevant than the *amount* of education is the *type* of education. Individuals in the more humanistic professions (lawyers, social workers, artists, teachers, nurses) are more likely to seek psychiatric assistance than are professionals such as business executives, computer specialists, accountants, and engineers.
7. Women are more likely than men to recognize the symptoms of mental illness and seek assistance.
8. The greater the cultural distance from the *mainstream* of society (i.e., the fewer the ties with *conventional* society), the greater the likelihood of negative societal response to mental illness. For example, immigrants have a greater distance from the mainstream than the native born, ethnic minorities greater than the dominant culture, and "bohemians" greater than the bourgeoisie. These groups are more likely to be subjected to coercive treatment, and involuntary psychiatric commitments are more common.

Adapted from Horwitz, A.V. (2010). The social control of mental illness. Clinton Corners, NY: Percheron Press.

Anxiety and grief have been described as two primary psychological response patterns to stress. A variety of thoughts, feelings, and behaviors are associated with each of these response patterns. Adaptation is determined by the degree to which the thoughts, feelings, and behaviors interfere with an individual's functioning.

CORE CONCEPT
Anxiety
A diffuse, vague apprehension that is associated with feelings of uncertainty and helplessness.

Anxiety

Feelings of anxiety are so common in our society that they are almost considered universal. Anxiety arises from the chaos and confusion that exists in the world. Fear of the unknown and conditions of ambiguity offer a perfect breeding ground for anxiety to take root and grow. Low levels of anxiety are adaptive and can provide the motivation required for survival. Anxiety becomes problematic when the individual is unable to prevent his or her response from escalating to a level that interferes with the ability to meet basic needs.

Peplau (1963) described four levels of anxiety: mild, moderate, severe, and panic. It is important for nurses to be able to recognize the symptoms associated with each level to plan for appropriate intervention with anxious individuals.

■ **Mild anxiety:** This level of anxiety is seldom a problem for the individual. It is associated with the tension experienced in response to the events of day-to-day living. Mild anxiety prepares people for action. It sharpens the senses, increases motivation for productivity, increases the perceptual field, and results in a heightened awareness of the environment. Learning is enhanced, and the individual is able to function at his or her optimal level.

■ **Moderate anxiety:** As the level of anxiety increases, the extent of the perceptual field diminishes. The moderately anxious individual is less alert to events occurring in the environment. The individual's attention span and ability to concentrate decrease, although he or she may still attend to needs with direction. Assistance with problem-solving may be required. Increased muscular tension and restlessness are evident.

■ **Severe anxiety:** The perceptual field of the severely anxious individual is so greatly diminished that concentration centers on one particular detail only or on many extraneous details. Attention span is extremely limited, and the individual has difficulty completing even the simplest task. Physical symptoms (e.g., headaches, palpitations, insomnia) and emotional symptoms (e.g., confusion, dread, horror) may be evident. Discomfort is experienced to the degree that virtually all overt behavior is aimed at relieving the anxiety.

■ **Panic anxiety:** In this most intense state of anxiety, the individual is unable to focus on even one detail in the environment. Misperceptions are common, and a loss of contact with reality may occur. The individual may experience hallucinations or delusions. Behavior may be characterized by wild and desperate actions or extreme withdrawal. Human functioning and communication with others is ineffective. Panic anxiety is associated with a feeling of terror, and individuals may be convinced that they have a life-threatening illness or fear that they are "going crazy," are losing control, or are emotionally weak. Prolonged panic anxiety can lead to physical and emotional exhaustion and can be a life-threatening situation.

A synopsis of the characteristics associated with each of the four levels of anxiety is presented in Table 2–1.

Behavioral Adaptation Responses to Anxiety

A variety of behavioral adaptation responses occur at each level of anxiety. Figure 2–2 depicts these behavioral responses on a continuum of anxiety ranging from mild to panic.

Mild Anxiety

At the mild level, individuals employ any of a number of coping behaviors that satisfy their needs for comfort. Menninger (1963) described the following types of coping mechanisms that individuals use to relieve anxiety in stressful situations:

■ Sleeping
■ Yawning
■ Eating
■ Drinking
■ Physical exercise
■ Daydreaming
■ Smoking
■ Laughing
■ Crying
■ Cursing
■ Pacing
■ Nail biting
■ Foot swinging
■ Finger tapping
■ Fidgeting
■ Talking to someone with whom one feels comfortable

Undoubtedly, there are many more responses too numerous to mention here, considering that each individual develops his or her own unique ways to relieve mild anxiety. Some of these behaviors are more adaptive than others.

Mild-to-Moderate Anxiety

Sigmund Freud (1961) identified the ego as the reality component of the personality, governing

TABLE 2–1	**Levels of Anxiety**			
LEVEL	PERCEPTUAL FIELD	ABILITY TO LEARN	PHYSICAL CHARACTERISTICS	EMOTIONAL AND BEHAVIORAL CHARACTERISTICS
Mild	Heightened perception (e.g., noises may seem louder; details within the environment are clearer) Increased awareness Increased alertness	Learning is enhanced	Restlessness Irritability	May remain superficial with others Rarely experienced as distressful Motivation is increased
Moderate	Reduction in perceptual field Reduced alertness to environmental events (e.g., someone talking may not be heard; part of the room may not be noticed)	Learning still occurs but not at optimal ability Decreased attention span Decreased ability to concentrate	Increased restlessness Increased heart and respiration rates Increased perspiration Gastric discomfort Increased muscular tension Increase in speech rate, volume, and pitch	A feeling of discontent May lead to a degree of impairment in interpersonal relationships as individual begins to focus on self and the need to relieve personal discomfort
Severe	Greatly diminished; only extraneous details are perceived, or fixation on a single detail may occur May not take notice of an event even when attention is directed by another	Extremely limited attention span Unable to concentrate or problem-solve Effective learning cannot occur	Headaches Dizziness Nausea Trembling Insomnia Palpitations Tachycardia Hyperventilation Urinary frequency Diarrhea	Feelings of dread, loathing, horror Total focus on self and intense desire to relieve the anxiety
Panic	Unable to focus on even one detail within the environment Misperceptions of the environment common (e.g., a perceived detail may be elaborated and out of proportion)	Learning cannot occur Unable to concentrate Unable to comprehend even simple directions	Dilated pupils Labored breathing Severe trembling Sleeplessness Palpitations Diaphoresis and pallor Muscular incoordination Immobility or purposeless hyperactivity Incoherence or inability to verbalize	Sense of impending doom Terror Bizarre behavior, including shouting, screaming, running about wildly, clinging to anyone or anything from which a sense of safety and security is derived Hallucinations, delusions Extreme withdrawal into self

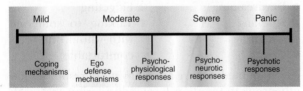

FIGURE 2–2 Adaptation responses on a continuum of anxiety.

problem-solving and rational thinking. As the level of anxiety increases, the strength of the ego is tested, and energy is mobilized to confront the threat. Anna Freud (1953) identified a number of **defense mechanisms** employed by the ego in the face of

threat to biological or psychological integrity. Some of these ego defense mechanisms are more adaptive than others, but all are used either consciously or unconsciously as protective devices for the ego in an effort to relieve mild-to-moderate anxiety. The mechanisms become maladaptive when used by an individual to such a degree that there is interference with the ability to deal with reality, effective interpersonal relations, or occupational performance. Maladaptive use of defense mechanisms promotes disintegration of the ego. The major ego defense mechanisms identified by Anna Freud are summarized in Table 2–2.

TABLE 2–2 Ego Defense Mechanisms

DEFENSE MECHANISM	EXAMPLE	DEFENSE MECHANISM	EXAMPLE
COMPENSATION Covering up a real or perceived weakness by emphasizing a trait one considers more desirable	A physically handicapped boy is unable to participate in football, so he compensates by becoming a great scholar.	**RATIONALIZATION** Attempting to make excuses or formulate logical reasons to justify unacceptable feelings or behaviors	John tells the rehab nurse, "I drink because it's the only way I can deal with my bad marriage and my worse job."
DENIAL Refusing to acknowledge the existence of a real situation or the feelings associated with it	A woman drinks alcohol every day and cannot stop, failing to acknowledge that she has a problem.	**REACTION FORMATION** Preventing unacceptable or undesirable thoughts or behaviors from being expressed by exaggerating opposite thoughts or types of behaviors	Jane hates nursing. She attended nursing school to please her parents. During career day, she speaks to prospective students about the excellence of nursing as a career.
DISPLACEMENT The transfer of feelings from one target to another that is considered less threatening or that is neutral	A client is angry with his physician, does not express it, but becomes verbally abusive with the nurse.	**REGRESSION** Retreating in response to stress to an earlier level of development and the comfort measures associated with that level of functioning	When 2-year-old Jay is hospitalized for tonsillitis he will drink only from a bottle, even though his mother states he has been drinking from a cup for 6 months.
IDENTIFICATION An attempt to increase self-worth by acquiring certain attributes and characteristics of an individual one admires	A teenager who required lengthy rehabilitation after an accident decides to become a physical therapist as a result of his experiences.	**REPRESSION** Involuntarily blocking unpleasant feelings and experiences from one's awareness	An accident victim can remember nothing about his accident.
INTELLECTUALIZATION An attempt to avoid expressing actual emotions associated with a stressful situation by using the intellectual processes of logic, reasoning, and analysis	Sarah's husband is being transferred with his job to a city far away from her parents. She hides anxiety by explaining to her parents the advantages associated with the move.	**SUBLIMATION** Rechanneling of drives or impulses that are personally or socially unacceptable into activities that are constructive	A mother whose son was killed by a drunk driver channels her anger and energy into being the president of the local chapter of Mothers Against Drunk Driving.
INTROJECTION Integrating the beliefs and values of another individual into one's own ego structure	Children integrate their parents' value system into the process of conscience formation. A child says to a friend, "Don't cheat. It's wrong."	**SUPPRESSION** The voluntary blocking of unpleasant feelings and experiences from one's awareness	Scarlett says, "I don't want to think about that now. I'll think about that tomorrow."
ISOLATION Separating a thought or memory from the feeling, tone, or emotion associated with it	A young woman describes being attacked and raped without showing any emotion.	**UNDOING** Symbolically negating or canceling out an experience that one finds intolerable	Joe is nervous about his new job and yells at his wife. On his way home he stops and buys her some flowers.
PROJECTION Attributing feelings or impulses unacceptable to one's self to another person	Sue feels a strong sexual attraction to her track coach and tells her friend, "He's coming on to me!"		

Moderate-to-Severe Anxiety

Anxiety at the moderate-to-severe level that remains unresolved over an extended period of time can contribute to a number of physiological disorders. The *DSM-5* (APA, 2013) describes these disorders under the category "Psychological Factors Affecting Other Medical Conditions." The psychological factors may exacerbate symptoms of, delay recovery from, or interfere with treatment of the medical condition. The condition may be initiated or exacerbated by an environmental situation that the individual perceives as stressful. Measurable pathophysiology can be demonstrated. It is thought that psychological and behavioral factors may affect the course of almost every major category of disease, including but not limited to cardiovascular, gastrointestinal, neoplastic, neurological, and pulmonary conditions.

Severe Anxiety

Extended periods of repressed severe anxiety can result in psychoneurotic behavior patterns. **Neurosis** is no longer considered a separate category of mental disorder. However, the term is still used in the literature to further describe the symptomatology of certain disorders and to differentiate from behaviors that occur at the more serious level of *psychosis*. Neuroses are psychiatric disturbances characterized by excessive anxiety that is expressed directly or altered through defense mechanisms. It appears as a symptom such as an obsession, a compulsion, a phobia, or a sexual dysfunction (Sadock, Sadock, & Ruiz, 2015). The following are common characteristics of people with neuroses:

■ They are aware that they are experiencing distress.
■ They are aware that their behaviors are maladaptive.
■ They are unaware of any possible psychological causes of the distress.
■ They feel helpless to change their situation.
■ They experience no loss of contact with reality.

The following disorders are examples of psychoneurotic responses to anxiety as they appear in the *DSM-5:*

■ **Anxiety disorders:** Disorders in which the characteristic features are symptoms of anxiety and avoidance behavior (e.g., phobias, panic disorder, generalized anxiety disorder, and separation anxiety disorder).
■ **Somatic symptom disorders:** Disorders in which the characteristic features are physical symptoms for which there is no demonstrable organic pathology. Psychological factors are judged to play a significant role in the onset, severity, exacerbation, or maintenance of the symptoms (e.g., somatic symptom disorder, illness anxiety disorder, conversion disorder, and factitious disorder).
■ **Dissociative disorders:** Disorders in which the characteristic feature is a disruption in the usually integrated functions of consciousness, memory, identity, or perception of the environment (e.g., dissociative amnesia, dissociative identity disorder, and depersonalization-derealization disorder).

Panic Anxiety

At this extreme level of anxiety, an individual is not capable of processing what is happening in the environment and may lose contact with reality. **Psychosis** is defined as a significant thought disturbance in which reality testing is impaired, resulting in delusions, hallucinations, disorganized speech, or catatonic behavior (Black & Andreasen, 2014). The following are common characteristics of people with psychoses:

■ They exhibit minimal distress (emotional tone is flat, bland, or inappropriate).
■ They are unaware that their behavior is maladaptive.
■ They are unaware of any psychological problems (anosognosia).
■ They are exhibiting a flight from reality into a less stressful world or one in which they are attempting to adapt.

Examples of psychotic responses to anxiety include schizophrenic, schizoaffective, and delusional disorders.

CORE CONCEPT
Grief
Grief is a subjective state of emotional, physical, and social responses to the loss of a valued entity.

Grief

Most individuals experience intense emotional anguish in response to a significant personal loss. A loss is anything that is perceived as such by the individual. Losses may be real, in which case they can be substantiated by others (e.g., death of a loved one, loss of personal possessions), or they may be perceived by the individual alone, unable to be shared or identified by others (e.g., loss of the feeling of femininity following mastectomy). Any situation that creates change for an individual can be identified as a loss. Failure (either real or perceived) also can be viewed as a loss.

The loss or anticipated loss of anything of value to an individual can trigger the grief response. This period of characteristic emotions and behaviors is called *mourning*. The "normal" mourning process is adaptive and is characterized by feelings of sadness, guilt, anger, helplessness, hopelessness, and despair. An absence of mourning after a loss may be considered maladaptive.

Stages of Grief

Kübler-Ross (1969), in extensive research with terminally ill patients, identified five stages of feelings and behaviors that individuals experience in response to a real, perceived, or anticipated loss:

Stage 1—Denial: This is a stage of shock and disbelief. The response may be one of "No, it can't be true!" The reality of the loss is not acknowledged. Denial is a protective mechanism that allows the individual to cope in an immediate time frame while organizing more effective defense strategies.

Stage 2—Anger: "Why me?" and "It's not fair!" are comments often expressed during the anger stage. Envy and resentment toward individuals not affected by the loss are common. Anger may be directed at the self or displaced on loved ones, caregivers, and even God. There may be a preoccupation with an idealized image of the lost entity.

Stage 3—Bargaining: During this stage, which is usually not visible or evident to others, a "bargain" is made with God in an attempt to reverse or postpone the loss: "If God will help me through this, I promise I will go to church every Sunday and volunteer my time to help others." Sometimes the promise is associated with feelings of guilt for not having performed satisfactorily, appropriately, or sufficiently.

Stage 4—Depression: During this stage, the full impact of the loss is experienced. The sense of loss is intense, and feelings of sadness and depression prevail. This is a time of quiet desperation and disengagement from all association with the lost entity. It differs from *pathological* depression, which occurs when an individual becomes fixed in an earlier stage of the grief process. Rather, stage 4 of the grief response represents advancement toward resolution.

Stage 5—Acceptance: The final stage brings a feeling of peace regarding the loss that has occurred. It is a time of quiet expectation and resignation. The focus is on the reality of the loss and its meaning for the individuals affected by it.

Not all individuals experience each of these stages in response to a loss, nor do they necessarily experience them in this order. Some individuals' grieving behaviors may fluctuate and even overlap between stages.

Anticipatory Grief

When a loss is anticipated, individuals often begin the work of grieving before the actual loss occurs. Most people reexperience the grieving behaviors once the loss occurs, but preparing for the loss in advance can facilitate the process of mourning, actually decreasing the length and intensity of the response. Problems arise, particularly in anticipating the death of a loved one, when family members experience **anticipatory grieving** and complete the mourning process prematurely. They disengage emotionally from the dying person, who may then experience feelings of rejection by loved ones at a time when this psychological support is so necessary.

Resolution

The grief response can last from weeks to years. It cannot be hurried, and individuals must be allowed to progress at their own pace. In the loss of a loved one, grief work usually lasts for at least a year, during which the grieving person experiences each significant anniversary or holiday for the first time without the loved one present.

Length of the grief process may be prolonged by a number of factors. If the relationship with the lost entity was marked by ambivalence or if there had been an enduring love–hate association, reaction to the loss may be burdened with guilt. Guilt lengthens the grief reaction by promoting feelings of anger toward oneself for having committed a wrongdoing or behaved in an unacceptable manner toward a lost loved one. He or she may even feel that the negative behavior contributed to the loss.

Anticipatory grieving may shorten the grief response in individuals who are able to work through some of the feelings before the loss occurs. If the loss is sudden and unexpected, mourning may take longer than it would if individuals were able to grieve in anticipation of the loss.

Length of the grieving process is also affected by the number of recent losses experienced by an individual and whether he or she is able to complete one grieving process before another loss occurs. This is particularly true for elderly individuals who may experience numerous losses in a span of a few years, including spouse, friends, other relatives, independent functioning, home, personal possessions, and pets. Grief accumulates into a **bereavement overload,** which for some individuals is perceived as difficult or even impossible to overcome.

The process of mourning may be considered resolved when an individual is able to regain a sense of organization, redefine his or her life in the absence of the lost person or object, and pursue new interests and relationships. Disorganization and emotional pain have been experienced and tolerated. Preoccupation with the lost entity has been replaced with a renewed energy and new resolve about ways to keep the memory of the lost one alive. Most grief, however, does not permanently disappear but will reemerge from time to time in response to triggers such as anniversary dates (Sadock et al., 2015).

Maladaptive Grief Responses

Maladaptive responses to loss occur when an individual is not able to satisfactorily progress through the stages of grieving to achieve resolution. These responses usually occur when an individual becomes fixed in the denial or anger stage of the grief process. Several types of grief responses have been identified as pathological, including those that are prolonged, delayed, inhibited, or distorted. The *prolonged* response is characterized by an intense preoccupation with memories of the lost entity for *many years after the loss has occurred.* Behaviors associated with the stages of denial or anger are manifested, and disorganization of functioning and intense emotional pain related to the lost entity are evidenced.

In the *delayed* or *inhibited* response, the individual becomes fixed in the denial stage of the grieving process. The emotional pain associated with the loss is not experienced, but anxiety disorders (e.g., phobias, somatic symptom disorders) or sleeping and eating disorders (e.g., insomnia, anorexia) may be evident. The individual may remain in denial for many years until the grief response is triggered by a reminder of the loss or even by an unrelated loss.

The individual who experiences a *distorted* response is fixed in the anger stage of grieving. In the distorted response, all the normal behaviors associated with grieving, such as helplessness, hopelessness, sadness, anger, and guilt, are exaggerated out of proportion to the situation. The individual turns the anger inward on the self, is consumed with overwhelming despair, and is unable to function in normal activities of daily living. Pathological depression is a distorted grief response.

Mental Health/Mental Illness Continuum

Anxiety and grief have been described as two primary responses to stress. In Figure 2–3, both of these responses are presented on a continuum according to degree of symptom severity. Disorders as they appear in the *DSM-5* are identified at their appropriate placement along the continuum.

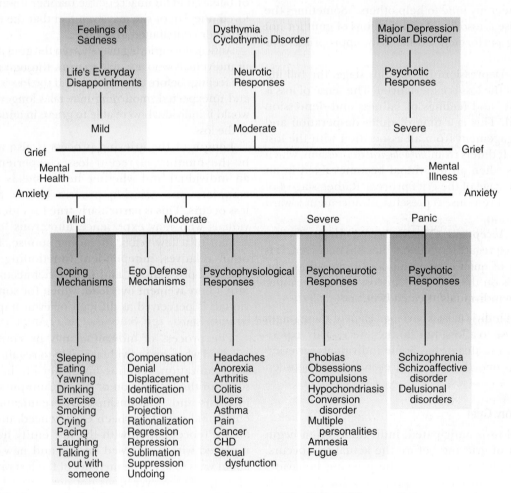

FIGURE 2–3 Conceptualization of anxiety and grief responses along the mental health/mental illness continuum.

Summary and Key Points

■ Psychiatric care has its roots in ancient times, when etiology was based in superstition and ideas related to the supernatural.

■ Treatments were often inhumane and included brutal beatings, starvation, or torture.

■ Hippocrates associated insanity and mental illness with an irregularity in the interaction of the four body fluids (humors): blood, black bile, yellow bile, and phlegm.

■ Conditions for care of the mentally ill have improved, largely because of the influence of leaders such as Benjamin Rush, Dorothea Dix, and Linda Richards, whose endeavors provided a model for more humanistic treatment.

■ Maslow identified a hierarchy of needs that individuals seek to fulfill in their quest to self-actualization (one's highest potential).

■ For purposes of this text, the definition of *mental health* is "the successful adaptation to stressors from the internal or external environment, evidenced by thoughts, feelings, and behaviors that are age-appropriate and congruent with local and cultural norms."

■ Most cultures label behavior as mental illness on the basis of incomprehensibility and cultural relativity.

■ When observers are unable to find meaning or comprehensibility in behavior, they are likely to label that behavior as mental illness. The meaning of behaviors is determined within individual cultures. For purposes of this text, the definition of *mental illness* is viewed as "maladaptive responses to stressors from the internal or external environment, evidenced by thoughts, feelings, and behaviors that are incongruent with the local and cultural norms, and that interfere with the individual's social, occupational, and/or physical functioning."

■ Anxiety and grief have been described as two primary psychological response patterns to stress.

■ Peplau defined anxiety by levels of symptom severity: mild, moderate, severe, and panic.

■ Behaviors associated with levels of anxiety include coping mechanisms, ego defense mechanisms, psychophysiological responses, psychoneurotic responses, and psychotic responses.

■ Grief is described as a response to loss of a valued entity. Loss is anything that is perceived as such by the individual.

■ Kübler-Ross, in extensive research with terminally ill patients, identified five stages of feelings and behaviors that individuals experience in response to a real, perceived, or anticipated loss: denial, anger, bargaining, depression, and acceptance.

■ Anticipatory grief is grief work that begins and sometimes ends before the loss occurs.

■ Resolution is thought to occur when an individual is able to remember and accept both the positive and negative aspects associated with the lost entity.

■ Grieving is thought to be maladaptive when the mourning process is prolonged, delayed or inhibited, or becomes distorted and exaggerated out of proportion to the situation. Pathological depression is considered to be a distorted reaction.

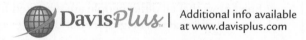 Additional info available at www.davisplus.com

Review Questions
Self-Examination/Learning Exercise

Select the answer that is most appropriate for each of the following questions.

1. Anna's dog, Lucky, her pet for 16 years, was killed by a car 3 years ago. Since that time, Anna has lost weight, rarely leaves her home, and talks excessively about Lucky. Why would Anna's behavior be considered maladaptive?
   a. It has been more than 3 years since Lucky died.
   b. Her grief is too intense over the loss of a dog.
   c. Her grief is interfering with her functioning.
   d. Cultural norms typically do not comprehend grief over the loss of a pet.

Continued

Review Questions—cont'd
Self-Examination/Learning Exercise

2. Anna states that Lucky was her closest friend, and since his death, there is no one who could ever replace the relationship they had. According to Maslow's hierarchy of needs, which level of need is not being met?
   a. Physiological needs
   b. Self-esteem needs
   c. Safety and security needs
   d. Love and belonging needs

3. Anna's daughter notices that Anna appears to be listening to another voice when just the two of them are in a room together. When questioned, Anna admits that she hears someone telling her that she was a horrible caretaker for Lucky and did not deserve to ever have a pet. Which of the following best describes what Anna is experiencing?
   a. Neurosis
   b. Psychosis
   c. Depression
   d. Bereavement

4. Anna, who is 72 years old, is of the age when she may have experienced several losses in a short time. What is this called?
   a. Bereavement overload
   b. Normal mourning
   c. Isolation
   d. Cultural relativity

5. Anna has been grieving the death of Lucky for 3 years. She is unable to take care of her normal activities because she insists on visiting Lucky's grave daily. What is the most likely reason that Anna's daughter has put off seeking help for Anna?
   a. Women are less likely than men to seek help for emotional problems.
   b. Relatives often try to normalize behavior rather than label it mental illness.
   c. She knows that all older people are expected to be a little depressed.
   d. She is afraid that the neighbors will think her mother is "crazy."

6. Lucky's accident occurred when he got away from Anna while they were taking a walk. He ran into the street and was hit by a car. Anna cannot remember the circumstances of his death. This is an example of what defense mechanism?
   a. Rationalization
   b. Suppression
   c. Denial
   d. Repression

7. Lucky sometimes refused to obey Anna's commands to come back to her, including when he ran into the street on the day of the accident. But Anna continues to insist, "He was the very best dog. He always minded me. He always did everything I told him to do." Which defense mechanism is Anna exhibiting?
   a. Sublimation
   b. Compensation
   c. Reaction formation
   d. Undoing

8. Anna has been a widow for 20 years. Her maladaptive grief response to the loss of her dog may be attributed to which of the following? (Select all that apply.)
   a. Unresolved grief over loss of her husband
   b. Loss of several relatives and friends over the last few years
   c. Repressed feelings of guilt over the way Lucky died
   d. Inability to prepare in advance for the loss

Review Questions—cont'd
Self-Examination/Learning Exercise

9. For what reason would Anna's illness be considered a neurosis rather than a psychosis?
   a. She is unaware that her behavior is maladaptive.
   b. She exhibits inappropriate affect (emotional tone).
   c. She experiences no loss of contact with reality.
   d. She tells the nurse, "There is nothing wrong with me!"

10. Which of the following statements by Anna might suggest that she is achieving resolution of her grief over Lucky's death?
    a. "I don't cry anymore when I think about Lucky."
    b. "It's true. Lucky didn't always mind me. Sometimes he ignored my commands."
    c. "I remember how it happened now. I should have held tighter to his leash!"
    d. "I won't ever have another dog. It's just too painful to lose them."

References

American Psychiatric Association. (2013). *Diagnostic and statistical manual of mental disorders* (5th ed.). Washington, DC: American Psychiatric Publishing.

Black, D.W., & Andreasen, N.C. (2014). *Introductory textbook of psychiatry* (6th ed.). Washington, DC: American Psychiatric Publishing.

Horwitz, A.V. (2010). *The social control of mental illness.* Clinton Corners, NY: Percheron Press.

Sadock, B.J., Sadock, V.A., & Ruiz, P. (2015). *Synopsis of psychiatry: Behavioral sciences/clinical psychiatry* (11th ed.). Philadelphia: Lippincott Williams & Wilkins.

Classical References

Freud, A. (1953). *The ego and mechanisms of defense.* New York: International Universities Press.

Freud, S. (1961). The ego and the id. In *Standard edition of the complete psychological works of Freud* (Vol. XIX). London: Hogarth Press.

Jahoda, M. (1958). *Current concepts of positive mental health.* New York: Basic Books.

Kübler-Ross, E. (1969). *On death and dying.* New York: Macmillan.

Maslow, A. (1970). *Motivation and personality* (2nd ed.). New York: Harper & Row.

Menninger, K. (1963). *The vital balance.* New York: Viking Press.

Peplau, H. (1963). A working definition of anxiety. In S. Burd & M. Marshall (Eds.), *Some clinical approaches to psychiatric nursing.* New York: Macmillan.

Robinson, L. (1983). *Psychiatric nursing as a human experience* (3rd ed.). Philadelphia: WB Saunders.

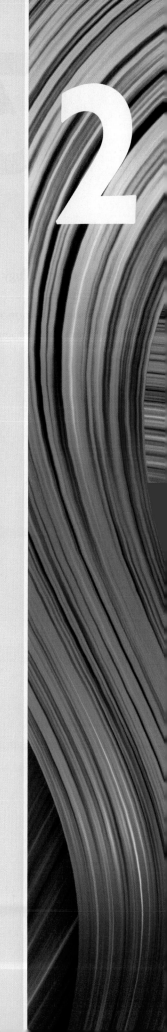

UNIT

2

Foundations for Psychiatric-Mental Health Nursing

3 Concepts of Psychobiology

CHAPTER OUTLINE

KEY TERMS

axon
cell body
circadian rhythms
dendrites

genotype
limbic system
neuron
neurotransmitter

phenotype
receptor sites
synapse

OBJECTIVES

After reading this chapter, the student will be able to:

1. Identify gross anatomical structures of the brain and describe their functions.
2. Discuss the physiology of neurotransmission in the central nervous system.
3. Describe the role of neurotransmitters in human behavior.
4. Discuss the association of endocrine functioning to the development of psychiatric disorders.
5. Describe the role of genetics in the development of psychiatric disorders.
6. Discuss the correlation of altered brain function to various psychiatric disorders.
7. Identify diagnostic procedures used to detect alteration in biological functioning that may contribute to psychiatric disorders.
8. Discuss the influence of psychological factors on the immune system.
9. Describe the biological mechanisms of psychoactive drugs at neural synapses.
10. Recognize theorized influences in the development of psychiatric disorders, including brain physiology, genetics, endocrine function, immune system, and psychosocial and environmental factors.
11. Discuss the implications of psychobiological concepts for the practice of psychiatric-mental health nursing.

HOMEWORK ASSIGNMENT

Please read the chapter and answer the following questions:

1. A dramatic reduction in which neurotransmitter is most closely associated with Alzheimer's disease?
2. Anorexia nervosa has been associated with a primary dysfunction of which structure of the brain?
3. Many psychotropic medications work by blocking the reuptake of neurotransmitters. Describe the process of *reuptake*.
4. What psychiatric disorder may be linked to chronic hypothyroidism?

In recent years, increased emphasis has been placed on the organic basis for psychiatric illness. This "neuroscientific revolution" studies the biological basis of behavior, and several mental illnesses are now considered physical disorders resulting from malfunctions and/or malformations of the brain. That some psychiatric illnesses and associated behaviors can be traced to biological factors does not imply that psychosocial and sociocultural influences are totally discounted. For example, there is evidence that *psychological* interventions have an influence on brain activity that is similar to that of psychopharmacological intervention (Flor, 2014; Furmark et al., 2002). Other evidence indicates that lifestyle choices such as marijuana use can precipitate mental illness (psychosis) in individuals with genetic vulnerability (National Institutes of Health, 2017). Ongoing research will build a better understanding of the complex interplay of neural activities within the brain and interaction with one's environment.

The systems of biology, psychology, and sociology are not mutually exclusive—they are interacting systems. This interaction is clearly indicated by the fact that individuals experience biological changes in response to environmental events. One or several of these systems may at various times explain behavioral phenomena.

This chapter focuses on the role of neurophysiological, neurochemical, genetic, and endocrine influences on psychiatric illness. An introduction to psychopharmacology is included (discussed in more detail in Chapter 4, Psychopharmacology), and various diagnostic procedures used to detect alteration in biological function that may contribute to psychiatric illness are identified. The implications for psychiatric-mental health nursing are discussed.

CORE CONCEPT

Psychobiology

The study of the biological foundations of cognitive, emotional, and behavioral processes.

The Nervous System: An Anatomical Review

The Brain

The brain has three major divisions, subdivided into six major parts:

1. Forebrain
   a. Cerebrum
   b. Diencephalon
2. Midbrain
   a. Mesencephalon
3. Hindbrain
   a. Pons
   b. Medulla
   c. Cerebellum

Each of these structures is discussed individually. A summary is presented in Table 3–1.

Cerebrum

The cerebrum consists of a right and left hemisphere and constitutes the largest part of the human brain. The two hemispheres are separated by a deep groove and connected to each other by a band of 200 million axons (nerve fibers) called the *corpus callosum*. Because

TABLE 3–1 **Structure and Function of the Brain**	
STRUCTURE	**PRIMARY FUNCTION**
I. FOREBRAIN A. Cerebrum	Composed of two hemispheres connected by a band of nerve tissue that houses a band of 200 million axons called the *corpus callosum*. The outer layer is called the *cerebral cortex*. It is extensively folded and consists of billions of neurons. The left hemisphere appears to deal with logic and solving problems. The right hemisphere may be called the "creative" brain and is associated with affect, behavior, and spatial-perceptual functions. Each hemisphere is divided into four lobes
1. Frontal lobes	Voluntary body movement, including movements that permit speaking, thinking and judgment formation, and expression of feelings
2. Parietal lobes	Perception and interpretation of most sensory information (including touch, pain, taste, and body position)
3. Temporal lobes	Hearing, short-term memory, and sense of smell; expression of emotions through connection with limbic system
4. Occipital lobes	Visual reception and interpretation

Continued

TABLE 3–1	**Structure and Function of the Brain—cont'd**
STRUCTURE	PRIMARY FUNCTION
B. Diencephalon	Connects cerebrum with lower brain structures
1. Thalamus	Integrates all sensory input (except smell) on way to cortex; some involvement with emotions and mood
2. Hypothalamus	Regulates anterior and posterior lobes of pituitary gland; exerts control over actions of the autonomic nervous system; regulates appetite and temperature
3. Limbic system	Consists of medially placed cortical and subcortical structures and the fiber tracts connecting them with one another and with the hypothalamus. It is sometimes called the "emotional brain"—associated with feelings of fear and anxiety; anger and aggression; love, joy, and hope; and with sexuality and social behavior
II. MIDBRAIN	
A. Mesencephalon	Responsible for visual, auditory, and balance ("righting") reflexes
III. HINDBRAIN	
A. Pons	Regulation of respiration and skeletal muscle tone; ascending and descending tracts connect brainstem with cerebellum and cortex
B. Medulla	Pathway for all ascending and descending fiber tracts; contains vital centers that regulate heart rate, blood pressure, and respiration; reflex centers for swallowing, sneezing, coughing, and vomiting
C. Cerebellum	Regulates muscle tone and coordination and maintains posture and equilibrium

each hemisphere controls different functions, information is processed through the corpus callosum so that each hemisphere is aware of the activity of the other.

The surface of the cerebrum consists of gray matter and is called the *cerebral cortex*. The gray matter is composed of neuron cell bodies that appear gray to the eye. These cell bodies are thought to be the actual "thinking" structures of the brain. The *basal ganglia*, four subcortical nuclei of gray matter (the striatum, the pallidum, the substantia nigra, and the subthalamic nucleus), are found deep within the cerebral hemispheres. They are responsible for certain subconscious aspects of voluntary movement, such as swinging the arms when walking, gesturing while speaking, and regulating muscle tone (Scanlon & Sanders, 2015).

The cerebral cortex is identified by numerous folds called *gyri* and deep grooves between the folds called *sulci*. This extensive folding extends the surface area of the cerebral cortex to permit the presence of millions more neurons than could not be accommodated without the folds (as is the case in the brains of some animals, such as dogs and cats). Each hemisphere of the cerebral cortex is divided into the frontal lobe, parietal lobe, temporal lobe, and occipital lobe. These lobes, which are named for the overlying bones in the cranium, are identified in Figure 3–1.

The Frontal Lobes

Voluntary body movement is controlled by impulses through the frontal lobes. The right frontal lobe controls motor activity on the left side of the body, and the left frontal lobe controls motor activity on the right side of the body. The frontal lobe may also play a role in the emotional experience, as evidenced by changes in mood and character after damage to this area. The prefrontal cortex (the front part of the frontal lobe) plays an essential role in the regulation and adaptation of our emotions to new situations and may have implications for moral and spiritual responses (Sadock, Sadock, & Ruiz, 2015). Neuroimaging tests suggest there may be decreased activity in the frontal lobes of people with schizophrenia (Butler et al., 2012).

The Parietal Lobes

The parietal lobes manage somatosensory input, including touch, pain, pressure, taste, temperature, perception of joint and body position, and visceral sensations. The parietal lobes also contain association fibers linked to the primary sensory areas through which interpretation of sensory-perceptual information is made. Language interpretation is associated with the left hemisphere of the parietal lobe.

The Temporal Lobes

The upper anterior temporal lobe is concerned with auditory functions, and the lower part is dedicated to short-term memory. The sense of smell has a connection to the temporal lobes, as the impulses carried by the olfactory nerves end in this area of the brain. The temporal lobes also play a role in the expression of

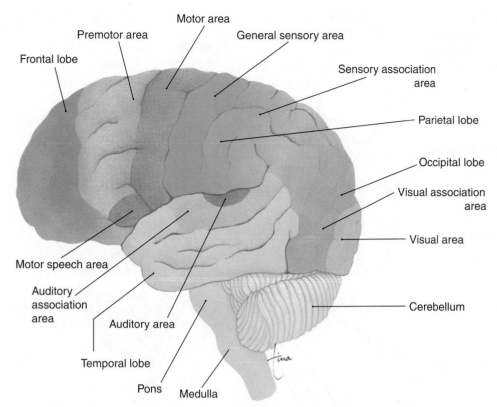

FIGURE 3–1 Left cerebral hemisphere showing some of the functional areas that have been mapped. (Adapted from Scanlon, V.C., & Sanders, T. [2015]. *Essentials of anatomy and physiology* [7th ed.]. Philadelphia: F.A. Davis Company, with permission.)

emotions through an interconnection with the limbic system. The left temporal lobe and the left parietal lobe are involved in language interpretation.

The Occipital Lobes

The occipital lobes are the primary area of visual reception and interpretation. Visual perception, the ability to judge spatial relationships such as distance and to see in three dimensions, is also processed in this area. Language interpretation is affected by the visual processing that occurs in the occipital lobes.

Diencephalon

The second part of the forebrain is the diencephalon, which connects the cerebrum with lower structures of the brain. The major components of the diencephalon include the thalamus and the hypothalamus, which are part of a neuroanatomical loop of structures known as the **limbic system.** These structures are identified in Figures 3–1 and 3–2.

Thalamus

The thalamus integrates all sensory input (except smell) on its way to the cortex. This integration allows for rapid interpretation of the whole rather than individual perception of each sensation. The thalamus is also involved in temporarily blocking minor sensations so that an individual can concentrate on one important event when necessary. For example, an individual who is studying for an examination may be unaware of the clock ticking in the room or another person entering because the thalamus has temporarily blocked these incoming sensations from the cortex. The impact of dopamine in the thalamus is associated with several neuropsychiatric disorders.

Hypothalamus

The hypothalamus is located just below the thalamus and just above the pituitary gland. It has a number of diverse functions.

1. **Regulation of the pituitary gland:** The pituitary gland consists of two lobes—the posterior lobe and the anterior lobe.
   a. The *posterior lobe* of the pituitary gland is actually extended tissue from the hypothalamus. The posterior lobe stores antidiuretic hormone (which helps to maintain blood pressure through regulation of water retention) and oxytocin (the hormone responsible for stimulation of the uterus during labor and the release of milk from the mammary glands). Both of these hormones are produced in the hypothalamus. When the hypothalamus detects the body's need for these hormones, it sends nerve impulses to the posterior pituitary for their release.

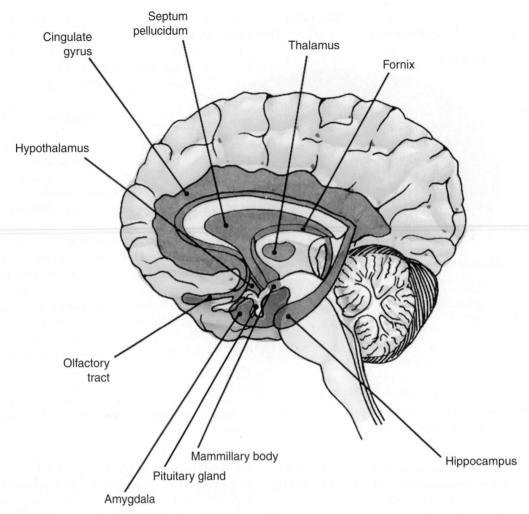

FIGURE 3–2 Structures of the limbic system. (From Scanlon, V.C., & Sanders, T. [2011]. *Essentials of anatomy and physiology* [6th ed.]. Philadelphia: F.A. Davis Company, with permission.)

b. The *anterior lobe* of the pituitary gland consists of glandular tissue that produces a number of hormones used by the body. These hormones are regulated by *releasing factors* from the hypothalamus. When the hormones are required by the body, the releasing factors stimulate the release of the hormone from the anterior pituitary, and the hormone in turn stimulates its target organ to carry out its specific functions.

2. **Direct neural control over the actions of the autonomic nervous system:** The hypothalamus regulates the appropriate visceral responses during various emotional states. The actions of the autonomic nervous system are described later in this chapter.

3. **Regulation of appetite, temperature, blood pressure, thirst, and circadian rhythms:** Appetite is regulated through response to blood nutrient levels.

4. **Regulation of temperature:** The hypothalamus senses internal temperature changes in the blood that flows through the brain. It receives information through sensory input from the skin about external temperature changes and uses this information to promote certain types of responses (e.g., sweating or shivering) that help maintain body temperature within the normal range.

Limbic System

The part of the brain known as the limbic system consists of portions of the cerebrum and the diencephalon. Its major components include the medially placed cortical and subcortical structures and the fiber tracts connecting them with one another and with the hypothalamus. The limbic system is a group of structures including the amygdala, mammillary body, olfactory tract, hypothalamus, cingulate gyrus, septum pellucidum, thalamus, hippocampus, and fornix. This system has been called the "emotional brain" and is associated with feelings of fear and anxiety; anger, rage, and aggression; love, joy, and hope; and sexuality and social behavior. The amygdala seems to be a primary gateway for processing emotional stimuli, particularly responses to fear, anxiety, and panic.

Mesencephalon

Structures of major importance in the mesencephalon, or midbrain, include nuclei and fiber tracts. The mesencephalon extends from the pons to the hypothalamus and is responsible for integration of various reflexes, including visual reflexes (e.g., automatically turning away from a dangerous object when it comes into view), auditory reflexes (e.g., automatically turning toward a sound that is heard), and righting reflexes (e.g., automatically keeping the head upright and maintaining balance).

Pons

The pons is a bulbous structure that lies between the midbrain and the medulla as part of the brainstem (Fig. 3–1). It is composed of large bundles of fibers and forms a major connection between the cerebellum and the brainstem. The pons is a relay station that transmits messages between various parts of the nervous system, including the cerebrum and cerebellum. It contains the central connections of cranial nerves V through VIII and centers for respiration and skeletal muscle tone. The pons is also associated with sleep and dreaming.

Medulla

The medulla is the connecting structure between the spinal cord and the pons, and all of the ascending and descending fiber tracts pass through it. The vital centers are contained in the medulla, and it is responsible for regulation of heart rate, blood pressure, and respiration. The medulla contains reflex centers for swallowing, sneezing, coughing, and vomiting, as well as nuclei for cranial nerves IX through XII. The medulla, pons, and midbrain form the structure known as the *brainstem.*

Cerebellum

The cerebellum is separated from the brainstem by the fourth ventricle but is connected to it through bundles of fiber tracts (Fig. 3–1). The cerebellum is associated with involuntary aspects of movement such as coordination, muscle tone, and the maintenance of posture and equilibrium.

Nerve Tissue

The tissue of the central nervous system (CNS) consists of nerve cells called *neurons* that generate and transmit electrochemical impulses. The structure of a neuron is composed of a cell body, an axon, and dendrites. The **cell body** contains the nucleus and is essential for the continued life of the neuron. The **dendrites** are processes that transmit impulses toward the cell body, and the **axon** transmits impulses away from the cell body. The axons and dendrites are covered by layers of cells called *neuroglia* that form a coating, or "sheath," of myelin. *Myelin* is a phospholipid that provides insulation against short-circuiting of the neurons during their electrical activity and increases the velocity of the impulse. The white matter of the brain and spinal cord is so called because of the whitish appearance of the myelin sheath over the axons and dendrites. The gray matter is composed of cell bodies that contain no myelin.

The three classes of neurons include afferent (sensory), efferent (motor), and interneurons. The *afferent neurons* carry impulses from receptors in the internal and external periphery to the CNS, where they are then interpreted into various sensations. The *efferent neurons* carry impulses from the CNS to *effectors* in the periphery, such as muscles (that respond by contracting) and glands (that respond by secreting).

Interneurons exist entirely within the CNS, and 99 percent of all nerve cells belong to this group. They may carry only sensory or motor impulses, or they may serve as integrators in the pathways between afferent and efferent neurons. They account in large part for thinking, feelings, learning, language, and memory.

Synapses

Information is transmitted through the body from one neuron to another. Some messages may be processed through only a few neurons, whereas others may require thousands of neuronal connections. The neurons that transmit the impulses do not actually touch each other. The junction between two neurons is called a **synapse.** The small space between the axon terminals of one neuron and the cell body or dendrites of another is called the *synaptic cleft.* Neurons conducting impulses toward the synapse are called *presynaptic neurons,* and those conducting impulses away are called *postsynaptic neurons.*

Chemicals that act as **neurotransmitters** are stored in the axon terminals of the presynaptic neuron. An electrical impulse through the neuron causes the release of this neurotransmitter into the synaptic cleft. The neurotransmitter then diffuses across the synaptic cleft and combines with **receptor sites** that are situated on the cell membrane of the postsynaptic neuron. The type of combination determines whether or not another electrical impulse is generated. If an electrical impulse is generated, the result is called an *excitatory response* and the electrical impulse moves on to the next synapse, where the same process recurs. If an electrical impulse is not generated by the neurotransmitter-receptor site combination, the result is called an *inhibitory response,* and synaptic transmission is terminated. Activity at the neural synapse is relevant in the study of psychiatric disorders because excessive or deficient activity of neurotransmitters influences a variety of cognitive and emotional symptoms. The synapse is also believed to be the primary site of activity for psychotropic drugs.

The cell body of the postsynaptic neuron also contains a chemical *inactivator* that is specific to the neurotransmitter released by the presynaptic neuron. When the synaptic transmission has been completed, the chemical inactivator quickly inactivates the neurotransmitter to prevent unwanted, continuous impulses until a new impulse from the presynaptic neuron releases more of the neurotransmitter. Continuous impulses can result in excessive activity of neurotransmitters such as dopamine, which is believed to be responsible for symptoms such as hallucinations and delusions seen in people with schizophrenia. A schematic representation of a synapse is presented in Figure 3–3.

Autonomic Nervous System

The autonomic nervous system (ANS) is considered part of the peripheral nervous system. Its regulation is modulated by the hypothalamus, and emotions exert a great deal of influence over its functioning. For this reason, the ANS has been implicated in the etiology of a number of psychophysiological disorders.

The ANS has two divisions: the sympathetic and the parasympathetic. The sympathetic division is dominant in stressful situations and prepares the body for the fight-or-flight response (discussed in Chapter 1, The Concept of Stress Adaptation). The neuronal cell bodies of the sympathetic division originate in the thoracolumbar region of the spinal cord. Their axons extend to the chains of sympathetic ganglia where they synapse with other neurons that subsequently innervate the visceral effectors. This results in an increase in heart rate and respiration and a decrease in digestive secretions and peristalsis. Blood is shunted to the vital organs and skeletal muscles to ensure adequate oxygenation.

The neuronal cell bodies of the parasympathetic division originate in the brainstem and the sacral segments of the spinal cord and extend to the parasympathetic ganglia where the synapse takes place either very close to or actually in the visceral organ being innervated. In this way, a very localized response is possible. The parasympathetic division dominates when an individual is in a relaxed, nonstressful condition. The heart and respirations are

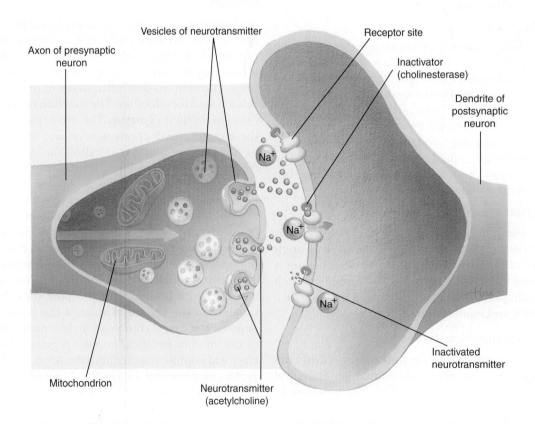

FIGURE 3–3 Impulse transmission at a synapse. The arrow indicates the direction of electrical impulses. (From Scanlon, V.C., & Sanders, T. [2015]. *Essentials of anatomy and physiology* [7th ed.]. Philadelphia: F.A. Davis Company, with permission.)

maintained at a normal rate, and secretions and peristalsis increase for normal digestion. Elimination functions are promoted. A schematic representation of the ANS is presented in Figure 3–4.

Neurotransmitters

Although neurotransmitters were described during the explanation of synaptic activity, they are discussed here separately and in detail because of the essential function they perform in the role of human emotion

and behavior. Neurotransmitters are also central to the therapeutic action of many psychotropic medications.

Neurotransmitters are chemicals that convey information across synaptic clefts to neighboring target cells. They are stored in small vesicles in the axon terminals of neurons. When the action potential, or electrical impulse, reaches this point, the neurotransmitters are released from the vesicles. They cross the synaptic cleft and bind with receptor sites on the cell body or dendrites of the adjacent neuron to allow the impulse

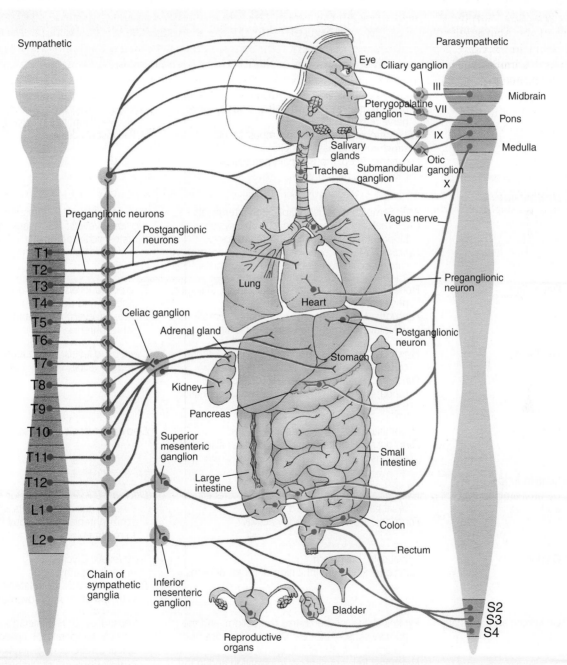

FIGURE 3–4   The autonomic nervous system. The sympathetic division is shown on the left, and the parasympathetic division is shown on the right (both divisions are bilateral). (From Scanlon, V.C., & Sanders, T. [2015]. *Essentials of anatomy and physiology* [7th ed.]. Philadelphia: F.A. Davis Company, with permission.)

to continue its course or to prevent the impulse from continuing. After the neurotransmitter has performed its function in the synapse, it either returns to the vesicles to be stored and used again or is inactivated and dissolved by enzymes. The process of being stored for reuse is called *reuptake*, a function that holds significance for understanding the mechanism of action of certain psychotropic medications.

Many neurotransmitters exist in the central and peripheral nervous systems, but only a limited number have implications for psychiatry. Major categories include cholinergics, monoamines, amino acids, and neuropeptides. Each of these is discussed separately and summarized in Table 3–2.

Cholinergics

Acetylcholine

Acetylcholine was the first chemical to be identified as and proven to be a neurotransmitter. It is a major effector chemical in the ANS, producing activity

TABLE 3–2 Neurotransmitters in the Central Nervous System

NEUROTRANSMITTER	LOCATION AND FUNCTION	POSSIBLE IMPLICATIONS FOR MENTAL ILLNESS
I. CHOLINERGICS A. Acetylcholine	*ANS:* Sympathetic and parasympathetic presynaptic nerve terminals; parasympathetic postsynaptic nerve terminals *CNS:* Cerebral cortex, hippocampus, limbic structures, and basal ganglia *Functions:* Sleep, arousal, pain perception, movement, memory	*Increased levels:* Depression *Decreased levels:* Alzheimer's disease, Huntington's disease, Parkinson's disease
II. MONOAMINES A. Norepinephrine	*ANS:* Sympathetic postsynaptic nerve terminals *CNS:* Thalamus, hypothalamus, limbic system, hippocampus, cerebellum, cerebral cortex *Functions:* Mood, cognition, perception, locomotion, cardiovascular functioning, and sleep and arousal	*Decreased levels:* Depression *Increased levels:* Mania, anxiety states, schizophrenia
B. Dopamine	Frontal cortex, limbic system, basal ganglia, thalamus, posterior pituitary, spinal cord *Functions:* Movement and coordination, emotions, voluntary judgment, release of prolactin	*Decreased levels:* Parkinson's disease and depression *Increased levels:* Mania and schizophrenia
C. Serotonin	Hypothalamus, thalamus, limbic system, cerebral cortex, cerebellum, spinal cord *Functions:* Sleep and arousal, libido, appetite, mood, aggression, pain perception, coordination, judgment	*Decreased levels:* Depression *Increased levels:* Anxiety states
D. Histamine	Hypothalamus *Functions:* Wakefulness; pain sensation, inflammatory response	*Decreased levels:* Depression
III. AMINO ACIDS A. Gamma-aminobutyric acid	Hypothalamus, hippocampus, cortex, cerebellum, basal ganglia, spinal cord, retina *Functions:* Slowdown of body activity	*Decreased levels:* Huntington's disease, anxiety disorders, schizophrenia, and various forms of epilepsy
B. Glycine	Spinal cord, brainstem *Functions:* Recurrent inhibition of motor neurons	*Toxic levels:* Glycine encephalopathy *Decreased levels:* Correlated with spastic motor movements
C. Glutamate and aspartate	Pyramidal cells of the cortex, cerebellum, and the primary sensory afferent systems; hippocampus, thalamus, hypothalamus, spinal cord *Functions:* Relay of sensory information and in the regulation of various motor and spinal reflexes Glutamate also has a role in memory and learning.	*Increased levels:* Huntington's disease, temporal lobe epilepsy, spinal cerebellar degeneration, anxiety disorders, depressive disorders *Decreased levels:* Schizophrenia

TABLE 3-2	**Neurotransmitters in the Central Nervous System—cont'd**	
NEUROTRANSMITTER	**LOCATION AND FUNCTION**	**POSSIBLE IMPLICATIONS FOR MENTAL ILLNESS**
D. D-Serine	Cerebral cortex, forebrain, hippocampus, cerebellum striatum, thalamus *Functions:* Binds at NMDA receptors and, with glutamate, is a coagonist whose functions include mediating NMDA receptor transmission, synaptic plasticity, neurotoxicity	*Decreased levels:* Schizophrenia
IV. NEUROPEPTIDES A. Endorphins and enkephalins	Hypothalamus, thalamus, limbic structures, midbrain, brainstem; enkephalins are also found in the gastrointestinal tract *Functions:* Modulation of pain and reduced peristalsis (enkephalins)	Modulation of dopamine activity by opioid peptides may indicate some link to the symptoms of schizophrenia
B. Substance P	Hypothalamus, limbic structures, midbrain, brainstem, thalamus, basal ganglia, spinal cord; also found in gastrointestinal tract and salivary glands *Function:* Regulation of pain	*Decreased levels:* Huntington's disease, Alzheimer's disease *Increased levels:* Depression
C. Somatostatin	Cerebral cortex, hippocampus, thalamus, basal ganglia, brainstem, spinal cord *Function:* Depending on part of the brain affected, stimulates release of dopamine, serotonin, norepinephrine, and acetylcholine, and inhibits release of norepinephrine, histamine, and glutamate; also acts as a neuromodulator for serotonin in the hypothalamus	*Decreased levels:* Alzheimer's disease *Increased levels:* Huntington's disease

ANS, autonomic nervous system, CNS, central nervous system, NMDA, *N*-methyl D-aspartate.

at all sympathetic and parasympathetic presynaptic nerve terminals and all parasympathetic postsynaptic nerve terminals. It is highly significant in the neurotransmission that occurs at the junctions of nerves and muscles. Acetylcholinesterase is the enzyme that destroys acetylcholine or inhibits its activity.

In the CNS, acetylcholine neurons innervate the cerebral cortex, hippocampus, and limbic structures. The pathways are especially dense through the area of the basal ganglia in the brain.

Functions of acetylcholine are manifold and include sleep, arousal, pain perception, the modulation and coordination of movement, and memory acquisition and retention. Cholinergic mechanisms may have some role in certain disorders of motor behavior and memory, such as Parkinson's disease, Huntington's disease, and Alzheimer's disease.

Monoamines

Norepinephrine

Norepinephrine is the neurotransmitter that produces activity at the sympathetic postsynaptic nerve terminals in the ANS, resulting in fight-or-flight responses in the effector organs. In the CNS, norepinephrine pathways originate in the pons and medulla and innervate the thalamus, dorsal hypothalamus, limbic system, hippocampus, cerebellum, and cerebral cortex. When norepinephrine is not returned for storage in the vesicles of the axon terminals, it is metabolized and inactivated by the enzymes monoamine oxidase (MAO) and catechol-*O*-methyl-transferase (COMT).

The functions of norepinephrine include the regulation of mood, cognition, perception, locomotion, cardiovascular functioning, and sleep and arousal. The activity of norepinephrine also has been implicated in certain mood disorders such as depression and mania, in anxiety states, and in schizophrenia (Sadock et al., 2015).

Dopamine

Dopamine pathways arise from the midbrain and hypothalamus and terminate in the frontal cortex, limbic system, basal ganglia, and thalamus. As with norepinephrine, the inactivating enzymes for dopamine are MAO and COMT.

Dopamine functions include regulation of movements and coordination, emotions, and voluntary decision-making ability. Because of its influence on the pituitary gland, it inhibits the release of prolactin (Sadock et al., 2015). Increased levels of dopamine are associated with mania and schizophrenia.

Serotonin

Serotonin pathways originate from cell bodies located in the pons and medulla and project to areas including the hypothalamus, thalamus, limbic system, cerebral cortex, cerebellum, and spinal cord. Serotonin that is not returned to be stored in the axon terminal vesicles is catabolized by the enzyme MAO.

Serotonin may play a role in sleep and arousal, libido, appetite, mood, aggression, and pain perception. The serotoninergic system has been implicated in the etiology of certain psychopathological conditions including anxiety states, mood disorders, and schizophrenia (Sadock et al., 2015).

Histamine

The role of histamine in mediating allergic and inflammatory reactions has been well documented. Its role in the CNS as a neurotransmitter has only recently been confirmed, and the availability of information on this function is limited. The highest concentrations of histamine are found within various regions of the hypothalamus. Histaminic neurons in the posterior hypothalamus are associated with sustaining wakefulness. The enzyme that catabolizes histamine is MAO. Although the exact processes mediated by histamine in the CNS are uncertain, some data suggest that histamine may play a role in depressive illness.

Amino Acids

Inhibitory Amino Acids

Gamma-Aminobutyric Acid Gamma-aminobutyric acid (GABA) has a widespread distribution in the CNS, with high concentrations in the hypothalamus, hippocampus, cortex, cerebellum, and basal ganglia of the brain; in the gray matter of the dorsal horn of the spinal cord; and in the retina. GABA is catabolized by the enzyme GABA transaminase.

Inhibitory neurotransmitters such as GABA prevent postsynaptic excitation, interrupting the progression of the electrical impulse at the synaptic junction. This function is significant when slowdown of body activity is advantageous. Enhancement of the GABA system is the mechanism of action by which the benzodiazepines produce their calming effect.

Alterations in the GABA system have been implicated in the etiology of anxiety disorders, movement disorders (e.g., Huntington's disease), and various forms of epilepsy.

Glycine The highest concentrations of glycine in the CNS are found in the spinal cord and brainstem. Little is known about the possible enzymatic metabolism of glycine.

Glycine appears to be the neurotransmitter of recurrent inhibition of motor neurons within the spinal cord and is possibly involved in the regulation of spinal and brainstem reflexes. It has been implicated in the pathogenesis of certain types of spastic disorders and in *glycine encephalopathy,* which is known to occur with toxic accumulation of the neurotransmitter in the brain and cerebrospinal fluid (Van Hove, Coughlin, & Sharer, 2013).

Excitatory Amino Acids

Glutamate and Aspartate Glutamate and aspartate appear to be primary excitatory neurotransmitters in the pyramidal cells of the cortex, the cerebellum, and the primary sensory afferent systems. They are also found in the hippocampus, thalamus, hypothalamus, and spinal cord. Glutamate and aspartate are inactivated by uptake into the tissues and through assimilation in various metabolic pathways.

Glutamate and aspartate function in the relay of sensory information and in the regulation of various motor and spinal reflexes. Alteration in these systems has been implicated in the etiology of certain neurodegenerative disorders, such as Huntington's disease, temporal lobe epilepsy, and spinal cerebellar degeneration. Recent studies have implicated increased levels of glutamate in anxiety and depressive disorders and decreased levels in schizophrenia (Ouellet-Plamondon & George, 2012). Glutamate also plays a role in memory and learning. Another amino acid, D-serine, has been identified as a neurotransmitter that, with glutamate, may act as a coagonist at NMDA (*N*-methyl D-aspartate) receptors. Hypofunction of these neurotransmitters may be associated with schizophrenia (Balu et al., 2013; Wolosker et al., 2008).

Neuropeptides

Neuropeptides act as signaling molecules in the CNS. Their activities include regulating processes related to sex, sleep, stress and pain, emotion, and social cognition. They may contribute to symptoms and behaviors associated with psychosis, mood disorders, dementia, and autism spectrum disorders (Sadock et al., 2015). Hormonal neuropeptides are discussed in the section of this chapter on neuroendocrinology.

Opioid Peptides

Opioid peptides, which include the endorphins and enkephalins, have been widely studied. They are found in various concentrations in the hypothalamus, thalamus, limbic structures, midbrain, and brainstem. Enkephalins are also found in the gastrointestinal tract. Opioid peptides have natural morphine-like properties and are thought to have a role in pain modulation. Released in response to painful stimuli, they may be responsible for producing the analgesic effect that results from acupuncture. Opioid peptides alter the release of dopamine and affect the spontaneous activity of the dopaminergic neurons. These findings may have some implication for opioid peptide-dopamine interaction in the etiology of schizophrenia.

Substance P

Substance P, the first neuropeptide to be discovered, is present in high concentrations in the hypothalamus, limbic structures, midbrain, and brainstem. It is also found in the thalamus, basal ganglia, and spinal cord. Substance P plays a role in sensory transmission, particularly in the regulation of pain. Recent studies demonstrated that people with depression and posttraumatic stress disorder (PTSD) had elevated levels of substance P in cerebral spinal fluid (Sadock et al., 2015).

Somatostatin

Somatostatin (also called *growth hormone–inhibiting hormone [GHIH]*) is found in the cerebral cortex, hippocampus, thalamus, basal ganglia, brainstem, and spinal cord, and has multiple effects on the CNS. In its function as a neurotransmitter, somatostatin exerts both stimulatory and inhibitory effects. Depending on the part of the brain affected, it has been shown to stimulate dopamine, serotonin, norepinephrine, and acetylcholine and to inhibit norepinephrine, histamine, and glutamate. It also acts as a neuromodulator for serotonin in the hypothalamus, thereby regulating its release. Somatostatin may serve this function for other neurotransmitters as well. High concentrations of somatostatin have been reported in brain specimens of clients with Huntington's disease, and low concentrations have been found in those with Alzheimer's disease.

CORE CONCEPTS

Neuroendocrinology

The study of the interaction between the nervous system and the endocrine system and the effects of various hormones on cognitive, emotional, and behavioral functioning.

Neuroendocrinology

Human endocrine functioning has a strong foundation in the CNS under the direction of the hypothalamus, which has direct control over the pituitary gland. The pituitary gland has two major lobes—the interior lobe (also called the *adenohypophysis*) and the posterior lobe (also called the *neurohypophysis*). The pituitary gland is only about the size of a pea, but despite its size and because of the powerful control it exerts over endocrine functioning in humans, it is sometimes called the "master gland." Figure 3–5 shows the hormones of the pituitary gland and their target organs. Many of the hormones subject to hypothalamus-pituitary regulation may have implications for behavioral functioning. Discussion of these hormones is summarized in Table 3–3.

Pituitary Gland

The Posterior Pituitary (Neurohypophysis)

The hypothalamus has direct control over the posterior pituitary through efferent neural pathways. Two hormones are found in the posterior pituitary: vasopressin (antidiuretic hormone) and oxytocin. They are actually produced by the hypothalamus and stored in the posterior pituitary. Their release is mediated by neural impulses from the hypothalamus (Fig. 3–6).

Antidiuretic Hormone

The main function of antidiuretic hormone (ADH) is to conserve body water and maintain normal blood pressure. The release of ADH is stimulated by pain, emotional stress, dehydration, increased plasma concentration, and decreases in blood volume. An alteration in the secretion of this hormone is related to the polydipsia seen in patients with diabetes. This may be one of many factors contributing to the polydipsia and water intoxication (a state of hyperhydration related to excessive consumption of water) observed in about 10 to 20 percent of patients with severe mental illness, particularly those with schizophrenia. Other factors correlated with this behavior include adverse effects of psychotropic medications and features of the behavioral disorder itself. Many factors may influence excessive intake of water in patients with severe psychiatric illness. Severe water intoxication can result in electrolyte imbalance and death (Kohli, Shishir, & Sharma, 2011). ADH also may play a role in learning and memory, alteration of the pain response, and modification of sleep patterns.

Oxytocin

Oxytocin causes contraction of the uterus at the end of pregnancy and stimulates release of milk from the mammary glands (Scanlon & Sanders, 2015). It is also released in response to stress and during sexual arousal. Oxytocin may promote bonding between sexes and has been used experimentally with autistic children to increase socialization (Sadock et al., 2015). Its role in behavioral functioning is unclear, although it is possible that oxytocin may stimulate the release of adrenocorticotropic hormone (ACTH) in certain situations, thereby playing a key role in the overall hormonal response to stress.

The Anterior Pituitary (Adenohypophysis)

The hypothalamus produces releasing hormones that pass through capillaries and veins of the hypophyseal portal system to capillaries in the anterior

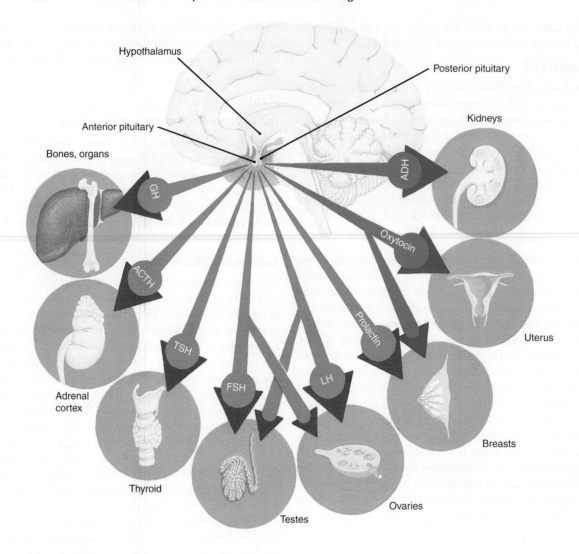

FIGURE 3–5   Hormones of the pituitary gland and their target organs. (From Scanlon, V.C., & Sanders, T. [2015]. *Essentials of anatomy and physiology* [7th ed.]. Philadelphia: F.A. Davis Company, with permission.)

TABLE 3–3 **Hormones of the Neuroendocrine System**				
HORMONE	**LOCATION AND STIMULATION OF RELEASE**	**TARGET ORGAN**	**FUNCTION**	**POSSIBLE BEHAVIORAL CORRELATION TO ALTERED SECRETION**
Antidiuretic hormone (ADH)	Posterior pituitary; release stimulated by dehydration, pain, stress	Kidney (causes increased reabsorption)	Conservation of body water; maintenance of blood pressure	Polydipsia; altered pain response; modified sleep pattern
Oxytocin	Posterior pituitary; release stimulated by end of pregnancy; stress; during sexual arousal	Uterus; breasts	Contraction of the uterus for labor; release of breast milk	May perform role in stress response by stimulation of ACTH

TABLE 3–3	Hormones of the Neuroendocrine System—cont'd			
HORMONE	LOCATION AND STIMULATION OF RELEASE	TARGET ORGAN	FUNCTION	POSSIBLE BEHAVIORAL CORRELATION TO ALTERED SECRETION
Growth hormone (GH)	Anterior pituitary; release stimulated by growth hormone–releasing hormone from hypothalamus	Bones and tissues	Growth in children; protein synthesis in adults	Anorexia nervosa
Thyroid-stimulating hormone (TSH)	Anterior pituitary; release stimulated by thyrotropin-releasing hormone from hypothalamus	Thyroid gland	Stimulation of secretion of needed thyroid hormones for metabolism of food and regulation of temperature	*Increased levels of thyroid hormones (decreased secretion of TSH):* Insomnia, anxiety, emotional lability *Decreased levels of thyroid hormones (increased secretion of TSH):* Fatigue, depression
Adrenocorticotropic hormone (ACTH)	Anterior pituitary; release stimulated by corticotropin-releasing hormone from hypothalamus	Adrenal cortex	Stimulation of secretion of cortisol, which performs a role in response to stress	*Increased levels*: Mood disorders, psychosis *Decreased levels*: Depression, apathy, fatigue
Prolactin	Anterior pituitary; release stimulated by prolactin-releasing hormone from hypothalamus	Breasts	Stimulation of milk production	*Increased levels*: Depression, anxiety, decreased libido, irritability
Gonadotropic hormones	Anterior pituitary; release stimulated by gonadotropin-releasing hormone from hypothalamus	Ovaries and testes	Stimulation of secretion of estrogen, progesterone, and testosterone; role in ovulation and sperm production	*Decreased levels*: Depression, anorexia nervosa *Increased testosterone*: Increased sexual behavior and aggressiveness
Melanocyte-stimulating hormone (MSH)	Anterior pituitary; release stimulated by onset of darkness	Pineal gland	Stimulation of secretion of melatonin	*Increased levels*: Depression

pituitary, where they stimulate secretion of specialized hormones. The hormones of the anterior pituitary gland regulate multiple body functions and include growth hormone, thyroid-stimulating hormone, ACTH, prolactin, gonadotropin-stimulating hormone, and melanocyte-stimulating hormone. Most of these hormones are regulated by a *negative feedback mechanism.* Once the hormone has exerted its effects, the information is "fed back" to the anterior pituitary, which inhibits the release and ultimately decreases the effects of the stimulating hormones.

Growth Hormone

The release of growth hormone (GH), also called *somatotropin,* is stimulated by growth hormone–releasing hormone (GHRH) from the hypothalamus. Its release is inhibited by GHIH, or somatostatin, also from the hypothalamus. It is responsible for growth in children and continued protein synthesis throughout life. During periods of fasting, it stimulates the release of fat from the adipose tissue to increase energy. The release of GHIH is stimulated in response to periods of hyperglycemia. GHRH is stimulated in response to hypoglycemia and to stressful situations. During prolonged stress, GH has a direct effect on protein, carbohydrate, and lipid metabolism, resulting in increased serum glucose and free fatty acids to be used for increased energy. GH deficiency has been noted in many patients with major depressive disorder, and several GH abnormalities have been noted in patients with anorexia nervosa.

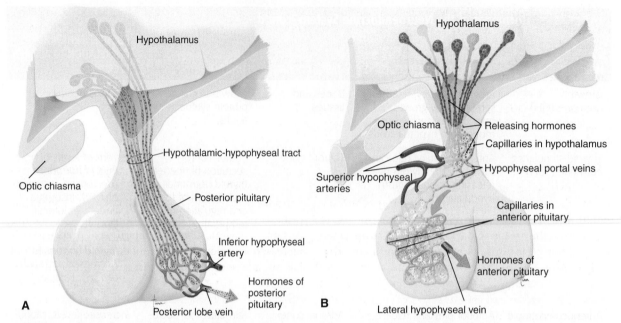

FIGURE 3-6 Structural relationships of hypothalamus and pituitary gland. (A) Posterior pituitary stores hormones produced in the hypothalamus. (B) Releasing hormones of the hypothalamus circulate directly to the anterior pituitary and influence its secretions. Notice the two networks of capillaries. (From Scanlon, V.C., & Sanders, T. [2015]. *Essentials of anatomy and physiology* [7th ed.]. Philadelphia: F.A. Davis Company, with permission.)

Thyroid-Stimulating Hormone

Thyrotropin-releasing hormone (TRH) from the hypothalamus stimulates the release of thyroid-stimulating hormone (TSH), or thyrotropin, from the anterior pituitary. TSH stimulates the thyroid gland to secrete triiodothyronine (T_3) and thyroxine (T_4). Thyroid hormones are integral to the metabolism of food and the regulation of temperature.

A correlation between thyroid dysfunction and altered behavioral functioning has been well documented. Common symptoms of hyperthyroidism include irritability, insomnia, anxiety, restlessness, weight loss, and emotional lability, in some instances progressing to delirium or psychosis. Symptoms of fatigue, decreased libido, memory impairment, depression, and suicidal ideation have been associated with chronic hypothyroidism. Studies have correlated various forms of thyroid dysfunction with mood disorders, anxiety, eating disorders, schizophrenia, and dementia.

Adrenocorticotropic Hormone

Corticotropin-releasing hormone (CRH) from the hypothalamus stimulates the release of ACTH from the anterior pituitary. ACTH stimulates the adrenal cortex to secrete cortisol. CRH, ACTH, and cortisol levels all rise in response to stress. Disorders of the adrenal cortex have been associated with mood disorders, PTSD, Alzheimer's dementia, and substance use disorders.

Addison's disease is the result of hyposecretion of the hormones of the adrenal cortex. Behavioral symptoms of hyposecretion include mood changes with apathy, social withdrawal, impaired sleep, decreased concentration, and fatigue. Hypersecretion of cortisol results in Cushing's disease and is associated with behaviors that include depression, mania, psychosis, and suicidal ideation. Cognitive impairments also have been observed.

Prolactin

Prolactin is mainly involved in reproductive functions and milk production in the mammary glands during pregnancy. First-generation antipsychotic medications increase prolactin levels and may be responsible for the undesired side effect of lactation. High prolactin levels are also associated with depression, decreased libido, anxiety, irritability, and the negative symptoms of schizophrenia. Prolactin levels in psychotic patients have been positively correlated with severity of tardive dyskinesia (Sadock et al., 2015).

Gonadotropic Hormones

The gonadotropic hormones are so called because they produce an effect on the gonads—the ovaries and the testes. The gonadotropins include follicle-stimulating hormone (FSH) and luteinizing hormone (LH). In women, FSH initiates maturation of ovarian follicles into ova and stimulates their secretion of estrogen. LH is responsible for ovulation and the secretion of progesterone from the corpus luteum. In men, FSH initiates sperm production in the testes, and LH increases secretion of testosterone by the interstitial cells of the testes (Scanlon & Sanders, 2015).

Limited evidence exists to correlate gonadotropins to behavioral functioning, although some observations have been made that warrant hypothetical consideration. Studies have indicated decreased levels of testosterone, LH, and FSH in men who have depression. Increased sexual behavior and aggressiveness have been linked to elevated testosterone levels in both men and women. Decreased plasma levels of LH and FSH commonly occur in patients with anorexia nervosa. Supplemental estrogen therapy has resulted in improved mentation and mood in some depressed women.

Melanocyte-Stimulating Hormone

Melanocyte-stimulating hormone (MSH) from the hypothalamus stimulates the pineal gland to secrete melatonin. The release of melatonin appears to depend on the onset of darkness and is suppressed by light. Studies of this hormone have indicated that environmental light can affect neuronal activity and influence circadian rhythms. Correlation between abnormal secretion of melatonin and symptoms of depression has led to the implication of melatonin in the etiology of seasonal affective disorder, in which individuals become depressed only during the fall and winter months when the amount of daylight decreases.

Circadian Rhythms

Human biological rhythms are largely determined by genetic coding, with input from the external environment influencing the cyclic effects. **Circadian rhythms** in humans follow a near-24-hour cycle and may influence a variety of regulatory functions, including the sleep–wakefulness cycle, body temperature regulation, patterns of activity such as eating and drinking, and hormone secretion. The 24-hour rhythms in humans are affected to a large degree by the cycles of lightness and darkness. This occurs because of a "pacemaker" in the brain that sends messages to other systems in the body and maintains the 24-hour rhythm. This endogenous pacemaker appears to be the suprachiasmatic nuclei of the hypothalamus. These nuclei receive projections of light through the retina and in turn stimulate electrical impulses to various other systems in the body, mediating the release of neurotransmitters or hormones that regulate bodily functioning.

Most of the biological rhythms of the body operate over a period of about 24 hours, but cycles of longer lengths have been studied. For example, women of menstruating age show monthly cycles of progesterone levels in the saliva, of skin temperature over the breasts, and of prolactin levels in the plasma of the blood (Hughes, 1993).

Some rhythms may even last as long as a year. These circannual rhythms are particularly relevant to certain medications, such as cyclosporine, which appears to be more effective at some times than others during a period of about 12 months (Hughes, 1993). Clinical studies have shown that administration of chemotherapy during the appropriate circadian phase and at the appropriate time of day can significantly increase the efficacy and decrease the toxic effects of certain cytotoxic agents (Garlapow, 2016; Lis et al., 2003).

The Role of Circadian Rhythms in Psychopathology

Circadian rhythms may play a role in psychopathology. Abnormal circadian rhythms have been associated with a variety of mental illnesses including depression, bipolar disorder, and seasonal affective disorder. Because many hormones have been implicated in behavioral functioning, it is reasonable to believe that peak secretion times could be influential in predicting certain behaviors. The association of depression with increased secretion of melatonin during darkness hours has already been discussed. External manipulation of the light–dark cycle and removal of external time cues often have beneficial effects on mood disorders.

Symptoms that occur in the premenstrual cycle have been linked to disruptions in biological rhythms. A number of the symptoms associated with premenstrual dysphoric disorder (PMDD) strongly resemble those attributed to depression, and hormonal changes have been implicated in the etiology. Some of these changes include progesterone–estrogen imbalance, increase in prolactin and mineralocorticoids, high level of prostaglandins, decrease in endogenous opiates, changes in metabolism of biogenic amines (serotonin, dopamine, norepinephrine, acetylcholine), and variations in secretion of glucocorticoids or melatonin.

Because the sleep–wakefulness cycle is probably the most fundamental of biological rhythms, and sleep disturbances are common in both depression and PMDD, it will be discussed in greater detail. A representation of bodily functions affected by 24-hour biological rhythms is presented in Figure 3–7.

Sleep

The sleep–wakefulness cycle is genetically determined rather than learned and is established some time after birth. Even when environmental cues such as the ability to detect light and darkness are removed, the human sleep–wakefulness cycle generally develops about a 25-hour periodicity, which is close to the 24-hour normal circadian rhythm.

Sleep can be measured by the types of brain waves that occur during various stages of sleep activity. Dreaming episodes are characterized by rapid eye movement (REM) and are called REM sleep. The sleep–wakefulness cycle is represented by six distinct stages.

Stage 0—Alpha rhythm: This stage of the sleep–wakefulness cycle is characterized by a relaxed, waking state with eyes closed. The alpha brain wave rhythm has a frequency of 8 to 12 cycles per second.

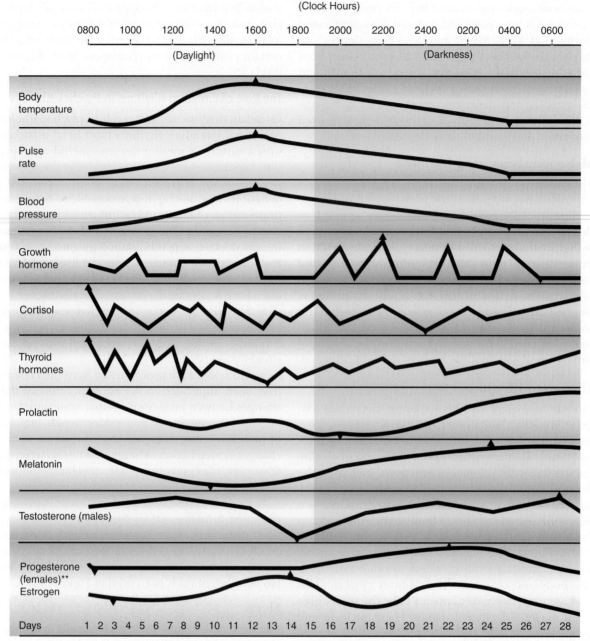

FIGURE 3–7 Circadian biological rhythms.

* ▼ indicates low point and ▲ indicates peak time of these biological factors within a 24-hour circadian rhythm.
** The female hormones are presented on a monthly rhythm because of their influence on the reproductive cycle. Daily rhythms of female gonadotropins are difficult to assay and are probably less significant than monthly.

Stage 1—Beta rhythm: Stage 1 characterizes the transition into sleep, a period of dozing in which thoughts wander and the person drifts in and out of sleep. Beta brain wave rhythm has a frequency of 18 to 25 cycles per second.

Stage 2—Theta rhythm: This stage comprises about half of time spent sleeping. Eye movement and muscular activity are minimal. Theta brain wave rhythm has a frequency of 4 to 7 cycles per second.

Stage 3—Delta rhythm: This is a period of deep and restful sleep. Muscles are relaxed, heart rate and

blood pressure fall, and breathing slows. No eye movement occurs. Delta brain wave rhythm has a frequency of 1.5 to 3 cycles per second.

Stage 4—Delta rhythm: This is the stage of deepest sleep. Individuals who suffer from insomnia or other sleep disorders often do not experience this stage of sleep. Eye movement and muscular activity are minimal. Delta waves predominate.

REM sleep—Beta rhythm: The dream cycle occurs during REM sleep. Eyes dart about beneath closed eyelids, moving more rapidly than when awake.

The brain wave pattern is similar to that of stage 1 sleep. Heart and respiration rates increase, and blood pressure may increase or decrease. Muscles are hypotonic during REM sleep.

Stages 2 through REM repeat themselves throughout the cycle of sleep. One is more likely to experience longer periods of stages 3 and 4 sleep early in the cycle and longer periods of REM sleep later in the sleep cycle. Most people experience REM sleep about four to five times during the night. The amount of REM sleep and deep sleep decreases with age, and the time spent in drowsy wakefulness and dozing increases.

Neurochemical Influences

A number of neurochemicals have been shown to influence the sleep–wakefulness cycle. Several studies have revealed information about the sleep-inducing characteristics of serotonin. L-Tryptophan, the amino acid precursor to serotonin, has been used for many years as an effective sedative-hypnotic to induce sleep in individuals with sleep-onset disorder. Serotonin and norepinephrine both appear to be most active during non-REM sleep, whereas the neurotransmitter acetylcholine is activated during REM sleep (Skudaev, 2009). The exact role of GABA in sleep facilitation is unclear, although the sedative effects of drugs that enhance GABA transmission, such as benzodiazepines, suggest that this neurotransmitter plays an important role in regulation of sleep and arousal. Some studies have suggested that acetylcholine induces and prolongs REM sleep, whereas histamine appears to have an inhibitory effect. Neuroendocrine mechanisms seem to be more closely tied to circadian rhythms than to the sleep–wakefulness cycle. One exception is growth hormone secretion, which increases during the stage 3 sleep period and may be associated with slow-wave sleep (Van Cauter & Plat, 1996).

CORE CONCEPT
Genetics
The study of the biological transmission of certain physical and/or behavioral characteristics from parent to offspring.

Genetics

Human behavioral genetics seeks to understand both the genetic and environmental contributions to individual variations in human behavior. This type of study is complicated by the fact that behaviors, like all complex traits, involve *multiple genes*.

The term **genotype** refers to the total set of genes present in an individual and coded in the DNA at the time of conception. The physical manifestations of a particular genotype are designated by characteristics that specify a **phenotype.** Examples of phenotypes include eye color, height, blood type, sound of voice, and hair type. As evident by the examples presented, phenotypes are not *only* genetic but may also be acquired (i.e., influenced by the environment) or a combination of both. It is likely that many psychiatric disorders are the result of a combination of genetics and environmental influences.

Investigators who study the etiological implications for psychiatric illness may explore several risk factors. Studies to determine if an illness is *familial* compare the percentage of family members with the illness to those in the general population or within a control group of unrelated individuals. These studies estimate the prevalence of psychopathology among relatives and make predictions about the predisposition to an illness based on familial risk factors. Schizophrenia, bipolar disorder, major depressive disorder, anorexia nervosa, panic disorder, somatic symptom disorder, antisocial personality disorder, and alcoholism are examples of psychiatric illness in which familial tendencies have been indicated.

Studies that are purely genetic search for a specific gene that causes a particular illness. A number of disorders exist in which the mutation of a specific gene or change in the number or structure of chromosomes has been associated with the etiology. Examples include Huntington's disease, cystic fibrosis, phenylketonuria, Duchenne's muscular dystrophy, and Down syndrome.

The search for pure genetic links to certain psychiatric disorders continues. Risk factors for early-onset Alzheimer's disease have been linked to mutations on chromosomes 21, 14, and 1 (National Institute on Aging, 2015). Other studies have linked a gene in the region of chromosome 19 that produces apolipoprotein E (ApoE) with late-onset Alzheimer's disease. One large study (National Institute of Mental Health, 2013) found similar genetic variations in patients with five mental disorders that were previously considered completely distinct. Autism, attention-deficit/hyperactivity disorder (ADHD), bipolar disorder, major depression, and schizophrenia all showed some common gene variations, including differences in two genes that regulate the flow of calcium into cells. Although these findings are intriguing, they do not clearly explain all the genetic risks for mental illness, the nongenetic risks, or the interaction between the two. Future research will continue to search for answers with the ultimate goal of improving diagnosis and treatment and perhaps uncovering keys to prevention of mental illness. In addition to familial and purely genetic investigations, other types of studies have been conducted to estimate the existence and degree of genetic and environmental contributions to the etiology of certain psychiatric disorders. Twin studies and adoption studies have been successfully employed for this purpose.

Twin studies examine the frequency of a disorder in monozygotic (genetically identical) and dizygotic (not genetically identical) twins. Twins are called *concordant* when both members suffer from the disorder in question. Concordance in monozygotic twins is considered stronger evidence of genetic involvement than it is in dizygotic (fraternal) twins. Twin studies have supported genetic vulnerability in the etiology of several mental illnesses, including adjustment disorders, PTSD, substance abuse, schizophrenia, bipolar disorder, major depression, obsessive compulsive disorder, risk for suicide, and others (Sadock et al., 2015).

Adoption studies allow researchers to compare the influence of genetics versus environment on the development of a psychiatric disorder. Knowles (2003) describes the four types of adoption studies that have been conducted:

1. The study of adopted children whose biological parent(s) had a psychiatric disorder but whose adoptive parent(s) did not.
2. The study of adopted children whose adoptive parent(s) had a psychiatric disorder but whose biological parent(s) did not.
3. The study of adoptive and biological relatives of adopted children who developed a psychiatric disorder.
4. The study of monozygotic twins reared apart by different adoptive parents.

Disorders in which adoption studies have suggested a possible genetic link include alcoholism, schizophrenia, major depression, bipolar disorder, suicide risk, ADHD, and antisocial personality disorder (Sadock et al., 2015).

A summary of various psychiatric disorders and the possible biological influences discussed in this chapter is presented in Table 3–4. Various diagnostic procedures used to detect alteration in biological functioning that may contribute to psychiatric disorders are presented in Table 3–5.

CORE CONCEPT

Psychoneuroimmunology

The study of the relationship between the immune system, the nervous system, and psychological processes such as thinking and behavior.

TABLE 3–4 Biological Implications of Psychiatric Disorders

ANATOMICAL BRAIN STRUCTURES INVOLVED	NEUROTRANSMITTER HYPOTHESIS	POSSIBLE ENDOCRINE CORRELATION	IMPLICATIONS OF CIRCADIAN RHYTHMS	POSSIBLE GENETIC LINK
SCHIZOPHRENIA Frontal cortex, temporal lobes, limbic system	Dopamine hyperactivity; decreased glutamate	Decreased prolactin levels	May correlate antipsychotic medication administration to times of lowest level	Twin, familial, and adoption studies suggest genetic link
DEPRESSIVE DISORDERS Frontal lobes, limbic system, temporal lobes	Decreased levels of norepinephrine, dopamine, and serotonin; increased glutamate	Increased cortisol levels; thyroid hormone hyposecretion; increased melatonin	DST* used to predict effectiveness of antidepressants; melatonin linked to depression during periods of darkness	Twin, familial, and adoption studies suggest a genetic link
BIPOLAR DISORDER Frontal lobes, limbic system, temporal lobes	Increased levels of norepinephrine and dopamine in acute mania	Some indication of elevated thyroid hormones in acute mania	Abnormal circadian rhythms have been associated with bipolar disorder	Twin, familial, and adoption studies suggest a genetic link
PANIC DISORDER Limbic system, midbrain	Increased levels of norepinephrine; decreased GABA activity	Elevated levels of thyroid hormones	May have some application for times of medication administration	Twin and familial studies suggest a genetic link

TABLE 3–4 Biological Implications of Psychiatric Disorders—cont'd

ANATOMICAL BRAIN STRUCTURES INVOLVED	NEUROTRANSMITTER HYPOTHESIS	POSSIBLE ENDOCRINE CORRELATION	IMPLICATIONS OF CIRCADIAN RHYTHMS	POSSIBLE GENETIC LINK
ANOREXIA NERVOSA Limbic system, particularly the hypothalamus	Decreased levels of norepinephrine, serotonin, and dopamine	Decreased levels of gonadotropins and growth hormone; increased cortisol levels	DST often shows same results as in depression	Twin and familial studies suggest a genetic link
OBSESSIVE-COMPULSIVE DISORDER Limbic system, basal ganglia (specifically caudate nucleus)	Decreased levels of serotonin	Increased cortisol levels	DST often shows same results as in depression	Twin studies suggest a possible genetic link
ALZHEIMER'S DISEASE Temporal, parietal, and occipital regions of cerebral cortex; hippocampus	Decreased levels of acetylcholine, norepinephrine, serotonin, and somatostatin	Decreased corticotropin-releasing hormone	Decreased levels of acetylcholine and serotonin may inhibit hypothalamic-pituitary axis and interfere with hormonal releasing factors	Familial studies suggest a genetic predisposition; late-onset disorder linked to marker on chromosome 19; early-onset to chromosomes 21, 14, and 1

*DST, dexamethasone suppression test. Dexamethasone is a synthetic glucocorticoid that suppresses cortisol secretion via the feedback mechanism. In this test, 1 mg of dexamethasone is administered at 11:30 p.m., and blood samples are drawn at 8:00 a.m., 4:00 p.m., and 11:00 p.m. on the following day. A plasma value greater than 5 mcg/dL suggests that the individual is not suppressing cortisol in response to the dose of dexamethasone. This is a positive result for depression and may have implications for other disorders as well.
GABA, gamma-aminobutyric acid.

TABLE 3–5 Diagnostic Procedures Used to Detect Altered Brain Functioning

EXAMINATION	TECHNIQUE USED	PURPOSE AND POSSIBLE FINDINGS
Electroencephalography (EEG)	Electrodes are placed on the scalp in a standardized position. Amplitude and frequency of beta, alpha, theta, and delta brain waves are graphically recorded on paper by ink markers for multiple areas of the brain surface.	Measures brain electrical activity; identifies dysrhythmias, asymmetries, or suppression of brain rhythms; used in the diagnosis of epilepsy, neoplasm, stroke, metabolic, or degenerative disease.
Computerized EEG mapping	EEG tracings are summarized by computer-assisted systems in which various regions of the brain are identified and functioning is interpreted by color coding or gray shading.	Measures brain electrical activity; used largely in research to represent statistical relationships between individuals and groups or between two populations of subjects (e.g., patients with schizophrenia vs. control subjects).
Computed tomographic (CT) scan	CT scan may be used with or without contrast medium. X-rays are taken of various transverse planes of the brain while a computerized analysis produces a precise reconstructed image of each segment.	Measures accuracy of brain structure to detect possible lesions, abscesses, areas of infarction, or aneurysm. CT has also identified various anatomical differences in patients with schizophrenia, organic mental disorders, and bipolar disorder.

Continued

TABLE 3–5 Diagnostic Procedures Used to Detect Altered Brain Functioning—cont'd

EXAMINATION	TECHNIQUE USED	PURPOSE AND POSSIBLE FINDINGS
Magnetic resonance imaging (MRI)	Within a strong magnetic field, the nuclei of hydrogen atoms absorb and reemit electromagnetic energy that is computerized and transformed into image information. No radiation or contrast medium is used.	Measures anatomical and biochemical status of various segments of the brain; detects brain edema, ischemia, infection, neoplasm, trauma, and other changes such as demyelination. Morphological differences have been noted in brains of patients with schizophrenia as compared with control subjects.
Positron emission tomography (PET)	The patient receives an intravenous (IV) injection of a radioactive substance (type depends on brain activity to be visualized). The head is surrounded by detectors that relay data to a computer that interprets the signals and produces the image.	Measures specific brain functioning, such as glucose metabolism, oxygen utilization, blood flow, and, of particular interest in psychiatry, neurotransmitter-receptor interaction.
Single photon emission computed tomography (SPECT)	The technique is similar to PET, but longer-acting radioactive substance must be used to allow time for a gamma-camera to rotate about the head and gather the data, which are then computer assembled into a brain image.	Measures various aspects of brain functioning, as with PET; has also been used to image activity of cerebrospinal fluid circulation.

Psychoneuroimmunology

Normal Immune Response

Cells responsible for *nonspecific* immune reactions include neutrophils, monocytes, and macrophages. They work to destroy the invasive organism and initiate and facilitate the healing of damaged tissue. If these cells do not accomplish a satisfactory healing response, *specific* immune mechanisms take over.

Cytokines are one such mechanism. These molecules, which regulate immune and inflammatory responses, become active when an individual is fighting an infection and the resultant inflammatory processes. Recent research has also demonstrated that cytokines are active in mood disorders such as depression and bipolar disorder. Current research focuses on the impact of cytokines as part of an essential and complex system of responses that are crucial for reducing inflammation and bolstering the immune response. Studies are also attempting to identify what happens when inflammation is not resolved and cytokines remain active or cross the blood-brain barrier. There is evidence that these maladaptations may be implicated in a multitude of illnesses (Ratnayake et al., 2013).

Implications of the Immune System in Psychiatric Illness

Studies of the biological response to stress have hypothesized that individuals become more susceptible to physical illness following exposure to a stressful stimulus or life event (see Chapter 1). This response is thought to be caused by increased glucocorticoid release from the adrenal cortex following stimulation from the hypothalamic-pituitary-adrenal axis during stressful situations. The result is a suppression in lymphocyte proliferation and function.

Studies have shown that nerve endings exist in tissues of the immune system. The CNS has connections in both bone marrow and the thymus, where immune system cells are produced, and in the spleen and lymph nodes, where those cells are stored.

GH, which may be released in response to certain stressors, may enhance immune functioning, whereas testosterone is thought to inhibit immune functioning. Increased production of epinephrine and norepinephrine occurs in response to stress and may decrease immunity. Serotonin has been described as an immunomodulator because it has demonstrated both enhancing and inhibitory effects on inflammation and immunity (Arreola et al., 2015).

Studies have correlated a decrease in lymphocyte function with periods of grief, bereavement, and depression, associating the degree of altered immunity with severity of the depression. A number of research studies have attempted to correlate the onset of schizophrenia to abnormalities of the immune system. These studies have considered autoimmune responses, viral infections, and immunogenetics (Sadock et al., 2015). The role of these factors in the onset and course of schizophrenia remains unclear. Attempts to identify a neurotoxic virus that triggers the manifestations of schizophrenia have not been successful; however, there is clear evidence of higher incidence of schizophrenia following viral epidemics.

Immunological abnormalities have also been investigated in a number of other psychiatric illnesses, including alcoholism, autism spectrum disorder, and neurocognitive disorder.

Evidence exists to support a correlation between psychosocial stress and the onset of illness. Research is still required to determine the specific processes involved in stress-induced modulation of the immune system.

Psychopharmacology and the Brain

Understanding the brain and the biological processes involved in thoughts, feelings, and behavior has positive ramifications beyond better understanding of psychopharmacological treatment options. As mentioned earlier, future research may continue to demonstrate the impact of psychological interventions on brain activity and neurotransmitters, which would open opportunities to hone psychological treatments and avoid the troubling side effects that accompany many medications. Furthermore, continued research in areas such as psychoneuroimmunology may reveal causes of mental illness, which would provide the opportunity for primary prevention.

In spite of these opportunities, psychopharmacology remains a primary treatment modality for mental disorders. Understanding, as best we can with current evidence, the biological mechanisms at work in psychoactive drugs is essential to nursing practice. Figure 3–8 shows the biological mechanism of psychoactive drugs at the neural synapse. Psychopharmacology, the classes of psychoactive drugs, and relevant nursing implications are discussed in detail in Chapter 4.

Implications for Nursing

The discipline of psychiatric-mental health nursing has always championed its role in holistic health care, but historical review reveals that emphasis has been placed on treatment approaches that focus on psychological and social factors. Psychiatric nurses must integrate knowledge of the biological sciences into their practices if they are to ensure safe and effective care to people with mental illness. In the hallmark Surgeon General's Report on Mental Health (U.S. Department of Health and Human Services, 1999), Dr. David Satcher wrote:

> The mental health field is far from a complete understanding of the biological, psychological, and sociocultural bases of development, but development clearly involves interplay among these influences. Understanding the process of development requires knowledge, ranging from the most fundamental level—that of gene expression and interactions between molecules and cells—all the way up to the highest levels of cognition, memory, emotion, and language. The challenge requires integration of concepts from many different disciplines. A fuller understanding of development is not only important in its own right, but it is expected to pave the way for our ultimate understanding of mental health and mental illness and how different factors shape their expression at different stages of the life span. (pp. 61–62)

To ensure a smooth transition from a strictly psychosocial focus to one of *bio*psychosocial emphasis, nurses must have a clear understanding of the following:

- **Neuroanatomy and neurophysiology:** The structure and functioning of the various parts of the brain and their correlation to human behavior and psychopathology
- **Neuronal processes:** The various functions of the nerve cells, including the role of neurotransmitters, receptors, synaptic activity, and information pathways
- **Neuroendocrinology:** The interaction of the endocrine and nervous systems and the role that the endocrine glands and their respective hormones play in behavioral functioning
- **Circadian rhythms:** The regulation of biochemical functioning over periods of rhythmic cycles and its influence in predicting certain behaviors
- **Genetic influences:** The hereditary factors that predispose individuals to certain psychiatric disorders
- **Psychoneuroimmunology:** The influence of stress on the immune system and its role in the susceptibility to illness
- **Psychopharmacology:** The increasing use of psychotropic drugs in the treatment of mental illness, demanding greater knowledge of psychopharmacological principles and nursing interventions necessary for safe and effective management
- **Diagnostic technology:** The importance of keeping informed about the latest in technological procedures for diagnosing alterations in brain structure and function

Why are these concepts important to the practice of psychiatric-mental health nursing? The interrelationship between psychosocial adaptation and physical functioning has been established. Integrating biological and behavioral concepts into psychiatric nursing practice is essential for nurses to meet the complex needs of clients with mental illness. Psychobiological perspectives must be incorporated into nursing practice, education, and research to attain the evidence-based outcomes necessary for the delivery of competent care.

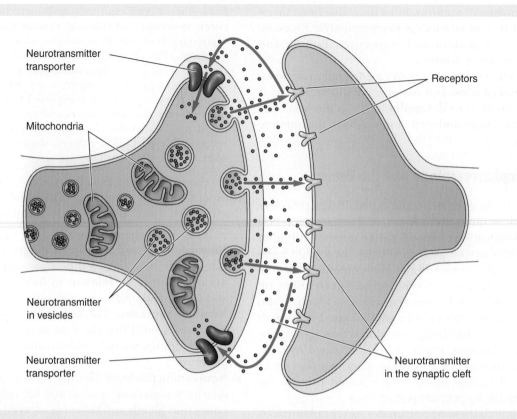

FIGURE 3–8 Area of synaptic transmission that is altered by drugs.

The transmission of electrical impulses from the axon terminal of one neuron to the dendrite of another is achieved by the controlled release of neurotransmitters into the synaptic cleft. Neurotransmitters include serotonin, norepinephrine, acetylcholine, dopamine, glutamate, gamma-aminobutyric acid (GABA), and histamine, among others. Prior to its release, the neurotransmitter is concentrated into specialized synaptic vesicles. Once fired, the neurotransmitter is released into the synaptic cleft where it encounters receptors on the postsynaptic membrane. Each neurotransmitter has receptors specific to it alone. Some neurotransmitters are considered to be *excitatory,* whereas others are *inhibitory,* a feature that determines whether another action potential will occur. In the synaptic cleft, the neurotransmitter rapidly diffuses, is catabolized by enzymatic action, or is taken up by the neurotransmitter transporters and returned to vesicles inside the axon terminal to await another action potential.

Psychotropic medications exert their effects in various ways in this area of synaptic transmission. Reuptake inhibitors block *reuptake* of the neurotransmitters by the transporter proteins, resulting in elevated levels of extracellular neurotransmitter. Drugs that inhibit catabolic enzymes promote excess buildup of the neurotransmitter at the synaptic site.

Some drugs cause *receptor blockade,* resulting in a reduction in transmission and decreased neurotransmitter activity. These drugs are called *antagonists.* Drugs that increase neurotransmitter activity by *direct stimulation* of the specific receptors are called *agonists.*

Summary and Key Points

- It is important for nurses to understand the interaction between biological and behavioral factors in the development and management of mental illness.
- Psychobiology is the study of the biological foundations of cognitive, emotional, and behavioral processes.
- The limbic system has been called the "emotional brain." It is associated with feelings of fear and anxiety; anger, rage, and aggression; love, joy, and hope; and with sexuality and social behavior.

- The three classes of neurons include afferent (sensory), efferent (motor), and interneurons. The junction between two neurons is called a *synapse.*
- Neurotransmitters are chemicals that convey information across synaptic clefts to neighboring target cells. Many neurotransmitters have implications in the etiology of emotional disorders and in the pharmacological treatment of those disorders.
- Major categories of neurotransmitters include cholinergics, monoamines, amino acids, and neuropeptides.

■ The endocrine system plays an important role in human behavior through the hypothalamic-pituitary axis.

■ Hormones and their circadian rhythms of regulation significantly influence a number of physiological and psychological life cycle phenomena, such as moods, sleep and arousal, stress response, appetite, libido, and fertility.

■ Research continues to validate the role of genetics in psychiatric illness.

■ Familial, twin, and adoption studies suggest that genetics may be implicated in the etiology of schizophrenia, bipolar disorder, depressive disorder, panic disorder, anorexia nervosa, alcoholism, and obsessive-compulsive disorder. Genetic studies, however, fail to entirely explain the complex factors involved in the development of these illnesses.

■ Psychoneuroimmunology examines the relationship between psychological factors, the immune system, and the nervous system.

■ Evidence exists to support a link between psychosocial stressors and suppression of the immune response.

■ Technologies such as magnetic resonance imagery, computed tomographic scan, positron emission tomography, and electroencephalography are used as diagnostic tools for detecting alterations in psychobiological functioning.

■ Psychotropic medications act at the neural synapse to affect neurotransmitter activity and have been associated with improvement in symptoms of many mental disorders.

■ Integrating knowledge of the expanding biological focus into psychiatric nursing is essential if nurses are to meet the changing needs of today's psychiatric clients.

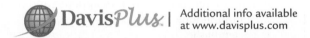

DavisPlus | Additional info available at www.davisplus.com

Review Questions
Self-Examination/Learning Exercise

Select the answer that is most appropriate for each of the following questions:

1. Which of the following parts of the brain is associated with multiple feelings and behaviors and is sometimes referred to as the "emotional brain"?
   a. Frontal lobe
   b. Thalamus
   c. Hypothalamus
   d. Limbic system

2. Which of the following parts of the brain is concerned with visual reception and interpretation?
   a. Frontal lobe
   b. Parietal lobe
   c. Temporal lobe
   d. Occipital lobe

3. Which of the following parts of the brain is associated with voluntary body movement, thinking and judgment, and expression of feeling?
   a. Frontal lobe
   b. Parietal lobe
   c. Temporal lobe
   d. Occipital lobe

4. Which of the following parts of the brain integrates all sensory input (except smell) on the way to the cortex?
   a. Temporal lobe
   b. Thalamus
   c. Limbic system
   d. Hypothalamus

Continued

Review Questions—cont'd
Self-Examination/Learning Exercise

5. Which of the following parts of the brain deals with sensory perception and interpretation?
   a. Hypothalamus
   b. Cerebellum
   c. Parietal lobe
   d. Hippocampus

6. Which of the following parts of the brain is concerned with hearing, short-term memory, and sense of smell?
   a. Temporal lobe
   b. Parietal lobe
   c. Cerebellum
   d. Hypothalamus

7. Which of the following parts of the brain has control over the pituitary gland and autonomic nervous system, as well as regulation of appetite and temperature?
   a. Temporal lobe
   b. Parietal lobe
   c. Cerebellum
   d. Hypothalamus

8. At a synapse, the determination of further impulse transmission is accomplished by means of which of the following?
   a. Potassium ions
   b. Interneurons
   c. Neurotransmitters
   d. The myelin sheath

9. A decrease in which of the following neurotransmitters has been implicated in depression?
   a. Gamma-aminobutyric acid, acetylcholine, and aspartate
   b. Norepinephrine, serotonin, and dopamine
   c. Somatostatin, substance P, and glycine
   d. Glutamate, histamine, and opioid peptides

10. Which of the following hormones has been implicated in the etiology of mood disorder with seasonal pattern?
    a. Increased levels of melatonin
    b. Decreased levels of oxytocin
    c. Decreased levels of prolactin
    d. Increased levels of thyrotropin

11. Psychotropic medications may act at the neural synapse to accomplish which of the following? (Select all that apply)
    a. Inhibit the reuptake of certain neurotransmitters, creating more availability
    b. Inhibit catabolic enzymes, promoting more availability of a neurotransmitter
    c. Block receptors, resulting in less neurotransmitter activity
    d. Add synthetic neurotransmitters found in the drug

12. Psychoneuroimmunology is a branch of science that involves which of the following? (Select all that apply.)
    a. The impact of psychoactive medications at the neural synapse
    b. The relationships between the immune system, the nervous system, and psychological processes including mental illness
    c. The correlation between psychosocial stress and the onset of illness
    d. The potential role of viruses in the onset of schizophrenia
    e. The genetic factors that influence prevention of mental illness

References

Arreola, R., Becerril-Villanueva, E., Cruz-Fuentes, C., Velasco-Velázquez, M.A., Garcés-Alvarez, M.E., Hurtado-Alvarado, G., . . . Pavón, L. (2015). Immunomodulatory effects mediated by serotonin. *Journal of Immunology Research*. doi:http://dx.doi.org/10.1155/2015/354957

Balu, D.T., Li, Y., Puhl, M.D., Benneyworth, M.A., Basu, A.C, Takagi, S., . . . Coyle, J.T. (2013). Multiple risk pathways for schizophrenia converge in serine racemase knockout mice, a mouse model of NMDA receptor hypofunction. *Proceedings of the National Academy of Sciences of the United States of America, 110*(26), E2400-2409. doi:10.1073/pnas.1304308110

Butler, T., Weisholtz, D., Isenberg, N., Harding, E., Epstein, J., Stern, E., & Silbersweig, D. (2012). Neuroimaging of frontal-limbic dysfunction in schizophrenia and epilepsy-related psychosis: Toward a convergent neurobiology. *Epilepsy Behavior, 23*(2), 113-122. doi:10.1016/j.yebeh.2011.11.004

Flor, H. (2014). Psychological pain interventions and neurophysiology: Implications for a mechanism-based approach. *American Psychologist, 69*(2), 188-196. doi:http://dx.doi.org/10.1037/a0035254

Furmark, T., Tilfors, M., Martiensdottir, I., Fischer, H., Pissiota, A., Långström, B., & Fredrikson, M. (2002). Common changes in cerebral blood flow in patients with social phobia treated with citalopram or cognitive behavior therapy. *Archives of General Psychiatry, 59*(5), 425-430. doi:10.1001/archpsyc.59.5.425

Garlapow, M. (2016). Timing chemotherapy administration to circadian rhythm improves drug effectiveness. *Oncology Nurse Advisor.* Retrieved from www.oncologynurseadvisor.com/side-effect-management/chemotherapy-more-effective-when-synced-with-circadian-rhythm/article/504455

Hughes, M. (1993). *Body clock: The effects of time on human health.* New York: Facts on File.

Knowles, J.A. (2003). Genetics. In R.E. Hales & S.C. Yudofsky (Eds.), *Textbook of psychiatry* (2th ed.). Washington, DC: American Psychiatric Publishing.

Kohli, A., Shishir, V., & Sharma, A. (2011). Psychogenic polydipsia. *Indian Journal of Psychiatry, 53*(2),166-167. doi:10.4103/0019-5545.82554

Lis, C.G., Grutsch, J.F., Wood, P., You, M., Rich, I., & Hrushesky, W.J. (2003). Circadian timing in cancer treatment: The biological foundation for an integrative approach. *Integrative Cancer Therapies, 2*(2), 105-111. doi:10.1177/1534735403253766

National Institutes of Health (NIH). (2017). Is there a link between marijuana use and mental illness? Retrieved from www.drugabuse.gov/publications/research-reports/marijuana/there-link-between-marijuana-use-mental-illness

National Institute of Mental Health (NIMH). (2013). Five major mental disorders share genetic roots. Retrieved from www.nimh.nih.gov/news/science-news/2013/five-major-mental-disorders-share-genetic-roots.shtml

National Institute on Aging. (2015). Alzheimer's disease genetics. The Alzheimer's Disease Education and Referral Center. Retrieved from www.nia.nih.gov/alzheimers/publication/alzheimers-disease-genetics-fact-sheet

Ouellet-Plamondon, C., & George, T.P. (2012). Glutamate and psychiatry in 2012—Up, up and away! *Psychiatric Times, 29*(12), 1-5. doi:10.3389/fphar.2012.00195

Ratnayake, U., Quinn, T., Walker, D.W., & Dickinson, H. (2013). Cytokines and the neurodevelopmental basis of mental illness. *Frontiers of Neuroscience, 7.* doi:10.3389/fnins.2013.00180

Sadock, B.J., Sadock, V.A., & Ruiz, P.(2015). *Synopsis of psychiatry: Behavioral sciences/clinical psychiatry* (11th ed.). Philadelphia: Lippincott Williams & Wilkens.

Scanlon, V.C., & Sanders, T. (2015). *Essentials of anatomy and physiology* (7th ed.). Philadelphia: F.A. Davis.

Skudaev, S. (2009). The neurophysiology and neurochemistry of sleep. Retrieved from www.healthstairs.com/sleep3.php

Van Cauter, E., & Plat, L. (1996). Physiology of growth hormone secretion during sleep. *Journal of Pediatrics,128*(5), 32-37. doi:10.1016/S0022-3476(96)70008-2

Van Hove, J., Coughlin, C., & Sharer, G. (2013). Glycine encephalopathy. *GeneReviews.* National Library of Medicine. Retrieved from www.ncbi.nlm.nih.gov/books/NBK1357

Wolosker, H., Dumin, E., Balan, L., & Foltyn, V.N. (2008). D-Amino acids in the brain: D-serine in neurotransmission and neurodegeneration. *The FEBS Journal, 275*(14), 3514-3526. doi:10.1111/j.1742-4658.2008.06515.x

Classical References

Sage, D.L. (Producer) (1984). *The Brain: Madness.* [Television Broadcast] Washington, DC: Public Broadcasting Company.

U.S. Department of Health and Human Services. (1999). *Mental health: A report of the Surgeon General—Executive summary.* Rockville, MD: U.S. Department of Health and Human Services.

4

Psychopharmacology

KEY TERMS

agranulocytosis	extrapyramidal symptoms	oculogyric crisis
akathisia	gynecomastia	priapism
akinesia	hypertensive crisis	retrograde ejaculation
amenorrhea	neuroleptic malignant	serotonin syndrome
dystonia	syndrome	tardive dyskinesia

OBJECTIVES
After reading this chapter, the student will be able to:

1. Discuss historical perspectives related to psychopharmacology.
2. Describe indications, actions, contraindications, precautions, side effects, and nursing implications for the following classifications of drugs:
   a. Antianxiety agents
   b. Antidepressants
   c. Mood-stabilizing agents
   d. Antipsychotics
   e. Antiparkinsonian agents
   f. Sedative-hypnotics
   g. Agents for attention-deficit/hyperactivity disorder
3. Apply the steps of the nursing process to the administration of psychotropic medications.

HOMEWORK ASSIGNMENT
Please read the chapter and answer the following questions:

1. Identify three priority safety concerns for each class of psychotropic medications.
2. Differentiate primary actions and side effects for traditional versus atypical antipsychotics.
3. Differentiate primary actions and side effects for tricyclic versus SSRI antidepressants.

The middle of the 20th century identifies a pivotal period in the treatment of individuals with mental illness with the introduction of the phenothiazine class of antipsychotics in the United States. They were previously used in France as preoperative medications.

As Dr. Henri Laborit (1914–1995) of the Hospital Boucicaut in Paris stated,

> It was our aim to decrease the anxiety of the patients to prepare them in advance for their postoperative recovery. With these new drugs, the phenothiazines,

we were seeing a profound psychic and physical relaxation . . . a real indifference to the environment and to the upcoming operation. It seemed to me these drugs must have an application in psychiatry. (Sage, 1984)

As Laborit foresaw, phenothiazines have had a significant application in psychiatry. Not only have they helped many individuals to function effectively, but they have also provided researchers and clinicians with information to study the origins and etiologies of mental illness. Knowledge gained from learning how these drugs work has promoted advancement in understanding how behavioral disorders develop. Dr. Arnold Scheibel, director of the UCLA Brain Research Institute, stated,

[When these drugs came out] there was a sense of disbelief that we could actually do something substantive for the patients . . . see them for the first time as sick individuals and not as something bizarre that we could literally not talk to. (Sage, 1984)

This chapter explores historical perspectives in the use of psychotropic medications in the treatment of mental illness. Seven classifications of medications are discussed, and their implications for psychiatric nursing are presented in the context of the steps of the nursing process.

CORE CONCEPT

Psychotropic Medication
Medication that affects psychic function, behavior, or experience.

Historical Perspectives

Historically, reaction to and treatment of individuals with mental illness ranged from benign involvement to interventions that some would consider inhumane. Individuals with mental illness were feared because of common beliefs associating them with demons or the supernatural. They were looked upon as loathsome and often were mistreated.

Beginning in the late 18th century, a type of moral reform in the treatment of persons with mental illness began to occur. Community and state hospitals concerned with the needs of persons with mental illness were established. Considered a breakthrough in the humanization of care, these institutions, however well intentioned, fostered the concept of custodial care. Clients were ensured food and shelter but received little or no hope of change for the future. As they became increasingly dependent on the institution to fulfill their needs, the likelihood of their return to the family or community diminished.

The early part of the 20th century saw the advent of the somatic therapies in psychiatry. Individuals with mental illness were treated with insulin shock therapy, wet sheet packs, ice baths, electroconvulsive therapy, and psychosurgery. Before 1950, sedatives and amphetamines were the only significant psychotropic medications available. Even these drugs had limited use because of their toxicity and addictive effects. Since the 1950s, the development of psychopharmacology has expanded to include widespread use of antipsychotic, antidepressant, antianxiety, and mood-stabilizer medications. Research into how these drugs work has provided an understanding of the biochemical influences in many psychiatric disorders.

Psychotropic medications are not a cure for mental illness. Most mental health practitioners who prescribe these medications for their clients use them as an adjunct to individual or group psychotherapy. Although their contribution to psychiatric care cannot be minimized, it must be emphasized that psychotropic medications relieve some physical and behavioral symptoms. They do not eliminate mental disorders.

The Role of the Nurse in Psychopharmacology

Ethical and Legal Implications

Nurses must understand the ethical and legal implications associated with the administration of psychotropic medications. Laws differ from state to state, but most adhere to the client's right to refuse treatment. Exceptions exist in emergency situations when it has been determined that clients are likely to harm themselves or others. Many states have adopted laws that allow courts to order outpatient treatment, which may include medication, in circumstances where an individual is not seeking treatment and has a history of violent, aggressive behavior. The original law, called Kendra's law, was enacted after a young woman named Kendra Webdale was pushed in front of a New York City subway train by a man who lived in the community but was not seeking treatment for his mental illness (New York State Office of Mental Health, 2006). This law is perhaps more developed than those in other states but also includes a medication grant clause that provides uninterrupted medication for those transitioning from hospitals or correctional facilities. Some states do not have similar laws, so nurses must be informed about local, state, and federal laws when working in any health-care setting or correctional facility and providing care to a client with a psychiatric disorder.

Assessment

A thorough baseline assessment must be conducted before a client is placed on a regimen of psychopharmacological therapy. A nursing history and assessment (see Chapter 9, The Nursing Process in Psychiatric-Mental Health Nursing), an ethnocultural assessment (see Table 4–1 for some ethnocultural considerations and Chapter 6, Cultural and Spiritual Concepts Relevant to Psychiatric-Mental Health Nursing for detailed information), and a comprehensive medication assessment (see Box 4–1) are all essential components of this database.

Medication Administration and Evaluation

The nurse is the key health-care professional in direct contact with individuals receiving psychotropic medication in inpatient settings, in partial hospitalization programs, day treatment centers, home health care, and other settings. Medication administration is followed by a careful evaluation, which includes continuous monitoring for side effects and adverse reactions. The nurse also evaluates the therapeutic effectiveness of the medication. It is essential for the nurse to have a thorough knowledge of psychotropic medications to be able to anticipate potential problems and outcomes associated with their administration.

Client Education

The information associated with psychotropic medications is copious and complex. An important role of the nurse is to translate that complex information into terms that can be easily understood by the client. Clients must understand why the medication has been prescribed, when it should be taken, and what they may expect in terms of side effects and possible adverse reactions. They must know whom to contact when they have a question and when it is important to report to their physician. Medication education encourages client cooperation and promotes accurate and effective management of the treatment regimen.

CORE CONCEPTS

Neurotransmitter

A chemical that is stored in the axon terminals of the presynaptic neuron. An electrical impulse through the neuron stimulates the release of the neurotransmitter into the synaptic cleft, which in turn determines whether another electrical impulse is generated.

Receptors

Molecules situated on the cell membrane that are binding sites for neurotransmitters.

TABLE 4–1	**Ethnocultural Considerations in the Assessment and Safe Administration of Psychotropic Medications**
African Americans	■ Metabolize alcohol, psychotropic drugs, beta blockers, antihypertensives, and caffeine differently than European Americans ■ Higher incidence of extrapyramidal side effects with haloperidol decanoate than European Americans ■ Show higher blood levels and faster therapeutic response to tricyclic antidepressants ■ Experience more toxic side effects and are more prone to tricyclic antidepressant delirium
Arabs	■ Some individuals have difficulty metabolizing antidepressants, neuroleptics, and opioid agents
Chinese	■ Increased response to antidepressants and neuroleptics at lower doses ■ Increased sensitivity to the effects of alcohol
Japanese	■ Many are poor metabolizers of mephenytoin (an anticonvulsant) and related medications ■ May be more sensitive to the effects of many psychotropic drugs, alcohol, and some beta blockers ■ Opiates may be less effective and produce more gastrointestinal side effects than among white populations
Hispanic (Cuban and Mexican)	■ May require lower doses of antidepressants and experience more intense side effects than non-Hispanic white populations
Koreans	■ May require lower doses of psychotropic medications
Vietnamese	■ Increased sensitivity to sedative effects of benzodiazepines ■ May require lower doses of tricyclic antidepressants ■ More sensitive to gastrointestinal side effects of analgesics ■ Generally consider American medicine more concentrated than Asian medicine and may be inclined to reduce the dose from that which is prescribed

SOURCE: Adapted from Purnell, L.D. (2014). *Guide to culturally competent health care* (3rd ed.). Philadelphia: F.A. Davis.

How Do Psychotropics Work?

Most psychotropic medications affect the neuronal synapse, producing changes in neurotransmitter release and the receptors to which they bind (see Figure 4–1). Researchers hypothesize that most antidepressants work by blocking the reuptake of neurotransmitters, specifically, serotonin and norepinephrine. *Reuptake* is the process of neurotransmitter inactivation by which the neurotransmitter is reabsorbed into the presynaptic neuron from which it was released. Blocking the reuptake process allows more of the neurotransmitter to be available for neuronal transmission. This mechanism of action may also result in undesirable side effects (see Table 4–2). Some antidepressants also block receptor sites that are unrelated to their mechanisms of action. These include α-adrenergic, histaminergic, and muscarinic cholinergic receptors. Blocking these receptors is associated with the development of certain side effects; for example, this explains why individuals treated with tricyclic antidepressants are at risk for developing postural hypotension. The specific type of receptor that medications bind to is also relevant to its level of antianxiety, antidepressant, and sedative properties (see Table 4–2).

Antipsychotic medications block dopamine receptors, and some affect muscarinic cholinergic, histaminergic, and α-adrenergic receptors. The *atypical* (or novel) antipsychotics focus primarily on blocking specific serotonin receptors. Benzodiazepines facilitate the transmission of the inhibitory neurotransmitter gamma-aminobutyric acid (GABA). Psychostimulants work by increasing norepinephrine, serotonin, and dopamine release.

Although each psychotropic medication affects neurotransmission, the specific drugs within each class have varying neuronal effects. Their exact mechanisms of action are unknown. Many neuronal effects occur rapidly; however, therapeutic effects of some medications, such as antidepressants and atypical antipsychotics, may take weeks. Acute alterations in neuronal function do not fully explain how these medications work. Long-term neuropharmacological reactions to increased norepinephrine and serotonin levels may better explain their mechanisms of action. Recent research suggests that the therapeutic effects are related to the nervous system's adaptation to increased levels of neurotransmitters. These adaptive changes result from a homeostatic mechanism, much like a thermostat, that regulates the cell and maintains equilibrium.

Applying the Nursing Process in Psychopharmacological Therapy

An assessment tool for obtaining a drug history is provided in Box 4–1. This tool may be adapted for use by staff nurses admitting clients to the hospital or by nurse practitioners with prescriptive privileges.

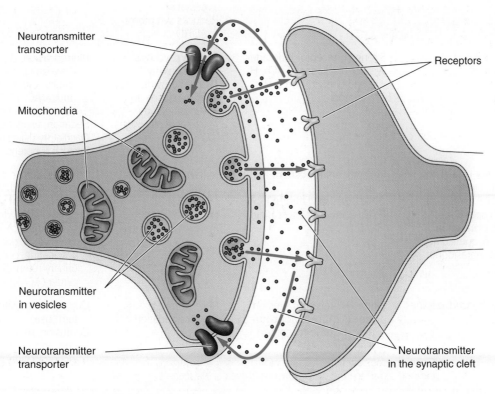

FIGURE 4–1   Area of synaptic transmission that is altered by drugs.

TABLE 4–2 Effects of Psychotropic Medications on Neurotransmitters

EXAMPLE OF MEDICATION	ACTION ON NEUROTRANSMITTER AND/OR RECEPTOR	DESIRED EFFECTS	SIDE EFFECTS
SSRIs	Inhibit reuptake of serotonin (5-HT)	Reduce depression Control anxiety Control obsessions	Nausea, agitation, headache, sexual dysfunction
Tricyclic antidepressants	Inhibit reuptake of serotonin (5-HT) Inhibit reuptake of NE Block NE (α_1) receptor Block ACh receptor Block histamine (H_1) receptor	Reduce depression Relieve severe pain Prevent panic attacks	Sexual dysfunction (NE & 5-HT) Sedation, weight gain (H_1) Dry mouth, constipation, blurred vision, urinary retention (ACh) Postural hypotension and tachycardia (α_1)
MAOIs	Increase NE and 5-HT by inhibiting the enzyme that degrades them (MAO-A)	Reduce depression Control anxiety	Sedation, dizziness Sexual dysfunction Hypertensive crisis (interaction with tyramine)
Trazodone and nefazodone	5-HT reuptake block 5-HT$_2$ receptor antagonism Adrenergic receptor blockade	Reduce depression Reduce anxiety	Nausea (5-HT) Sedation (5-HT$_2$) Orthostasis (α_1) Priapism (α_2)
SNRIs: venlafaxine, desvenlafaxine, duloxetine, and levomilnacipran	Potent inhibitors of serotonin and norepinephrine reuptake Weak inhibitors of dopamine reuptake	Reduce depression Relieve pain of neuropathy (duloxetine) Relieve anxiety (venlafaxine)	Nausea (5-HT) ↑ Sweating (NE) Insomnia (NE) Tremors (NE) Sexual dysfunction (5-HT)
Bupropion	Inhibits reuptake of NE and D	Reduces depression Aids in smoking cessation Reduces symptoms of ADHD	Insomnia, dry mouth, tremor, seizures
Antipsychotics: phenothiazines and haloperidol	Strong D$_2$ receptor blockades Weaker blockades of ACh, H$_1$, α_1-adrenergic, and 5-HT$_2$ receptors	Relieve psychosis Relieve anxiety (Some) provide relief from nausea and vomiting and intractable hiccoughs	Blurred vision, dry mouth, ↓ sweating, constipation, urinary retention, tachycardia (ACh) EPS (D$_2$) ↑ Plasma prolactin (D$_2$) Sedation; weight gain (H$_1$) Ejaculatory difficulty (5-HT$_2$) Postural hypotension (α; H$_1$)
Antipsychotics (novel): aripiprazole, asenapine, brexpiprazole, cariprazine, clozapine, iloperidone, lurasidone, olanzapine, paliperidone, quetiapine, risperidone, ziprasidone	Receptor antagonism of 5-HT$_1$ and 5-HT$_2$ D$_1$–D$_5$ (varies with drug) H$_1$,α_1-adrenergic muscarinic (ACh)	Relieve psychosis (with minimal or no EPS) Relieve anxiety Relieve acute mania	Potential with some of the drugs for mild EPS (D$_2$) Sedation, weight gain (H$_1$) Orthostasis and dizziness (α-adrenergic) Blurred vision, dry mouth, ↓ sweating, constipation, urinary retention, tachycardia (ACh)
Antianxiety: benzodiazepines	Bind to BZ receptor sites on the GABA$_A$ receptor complex; increase receptor affinity for GABA	Relieve anxiety Produce sedation	Dependence (with long-term use) Confusion, memory impairment, motor incoordination

TABLE 4–2 Effects of Psychotropic Medications on Neurotransmitters–cont'd

EXAMPLE OF MEDICATION	ACTION ON NEUROTRANSMITTER AND/OR RECEPTOR	DESIRED EFFECTS	SIDE EFFECTS
Antianxiety: buspirone	5-HT_{1A} agonist D_2 agonist D_2 antagonist	Relieves anxiety	Nausea, headache, dizziness Restlessness

5-HT, 5-hydroxytryptamine (serotonin); ACh, acetylcholine; ADHD, attention deficit-hyperactivity disorder; BZ, benzodiazepine; D, dopamine; EPS, extrapyramidal symptoms; GABA, gamma-aminobutyric acid; H, histamine; MAO, monoamine oxidase; MAO-A, monoamine oxidase A; MAOI, monoamine oxidase inhibitor; NE, norepinephrine; SNRI, serotonin-norepinephrine reuptake inhibitor; SSRI, selective serotonin reuptake inhibitor.

One of the Quality and Safety Education for Nurses (QSEN) criteria culminating from the Institute of Medicine (IOM) (2003) report on essential competencies for health care professionals stresses that the patient must be at the center of decisions about treatment (patient-centered care), and this type of assessment tool provides an opportunity to actively engage the patient in describing what medications have been effective or ineffective and identifying side effects that may impact willingness to adhere to a medication regimen.

Antianxiety Agents

Background Assessment Data

Indications

Antianxiety drugs are also called *anxiolytics* and historically were referred to as *minor tranquilizers*. They are used in the treatment of anxiety disorders, anxiety symptoms, acute alcohol withdrawal, skeletal muscle spasms, convulsive disorders, status epilepticus, and preoperative sedation. They are most appropriate for

BOX 4–1 Medication Assessment Tool

Date _____ Client's Name _____ Age _____

Marital Status _____ Children _____ Occupation _____

Presenting Symptoms (subjective & objective) _____

_____

Diagnosis (DSM-5) _____

Current Vital Signs: Blood Pressure: Sitting _____/_____ ; Standing _____/_____ ; Pulse_____ ;

Respirations _____ Height _____ Weight _____

CURRENT/PAST USE OF PRESCRIPTION DRUGS (Indicate with "c" or "p" beside name of drug whether current or past use):

Name	Dosage	How Long Used	Why Prescribed	By Whom	Side Effects/Results
_____	_____	_____	_____	_____	_____
_____	_____	_____	_____	_____	_____
_____	_____	_____	_____	_____	_____

CURRENT/PAST USE OF OVER-THE-COUNTER DRUGS (Indicate with "c" or "p" beside name of drug whether current or past use):

Name	Dosage	How Long Used	Why Prescribed	By Whom	Side Effects/Results
_____	_____	_____	_____	_____	_____
_____	_____	_____	_____	_____	_____
_____	_____	_____	_____	_____	_____

CURRENT/PAST USE OF STREET DRUGS, ALCOHOL, NICOTINE, AND/OR CAFFEINE (Indicate with "c" or "p" beside name of drug):

Name	Amount Used	How Often Used	When Last Used	Effects Produced
_____	_____	_____	_____	_____
_____	_____	_____	_____	_____
_____	_____	_____	_____	_____

Any allergies to food or drugs?_____

Any special diet considerations?_____

Continued

BOX 4–1 **Medication Assessment Tool–cont'd**

Do you have (or have you ever had) any of the following? If yes, provide explanation on the back of this sheet.

	Yes No		Yes No		Yes No
Difficulty swallowing	__ __	Chest pain	__ __	Sexual dysfunction	__ __
Delayed wound healing	__ __	Blood clots/pain in legs	__ __	Lumps in your breasts	__ __
Constipation problems	__ __	Fainting spells	__ __	Blurred or double vision	__ __
Urination problems	__ __	Swollen ankles/legs/hands	__ __	Ringing in the ears	__ __
Recent change in		Asthma		Insomnia	__ __
elimination patterns	__ __	Varicose veins	__ __	Skin rashes	__ __
Weakness or tremors	__ __	Numbness/tingling		Diabetes	__ __
Seizures	__ __	(location?)	__ __	Hepatitis (or other liver	
Headaches	__ __	Ulcers	__ __	disease)	__ __
Dizziness	__ __	Nausea/vomiting	__ __	Kidney disease	__ __
High blood pressure	__ __	Problems with diarrhea	__ __	Glaucoma	__ __
Palpitations	__ __	Shortness of breath	__ __		

Are you pregnant or breast feeding?_____ Date of last menses_____ Type of contraception used_____

Describe any restrictions/limitations that might interfere with your use of medication for your current problem. _____
_____

Prescription orders: Patient teaching related to medications prescribed:

Lab work or referrals prescribed:

Nurse's signature _____ **Client's signature** _____

---

the treatment of acute anxiety states rather than long-term treatment, as their use and efficacy for longer than 4 months has not been evaluated. For long-term management of anxiety disorders, antidepressants are often used as the first line of treatment because they are not addictive. (A table of current FDA-approved antianxiety agents, pregnancy categories, half-life, and daily dosage ranges can be found online at Davis*Plus* and in Chapter 27, Anxiety, Obsessive-Compulsive, and Related Disorders.)

Action

Antianxiety drugs depress subcortical levels of the central nervous system (CNS), particularly the limbic system and reticular formation. They may potentiate the effects of the powerful inhibitory neurotransmitter GABA in the brain, thereby producing a calming effect. All levels of CNS depression can be affected, from mild sedation to hypnosis to coma. The most commonly prescribed antianxiety agents are benzodiazepines, including clonazepam (Klonopin), diazepam (Valium), and alprazolam (Xanax). Benzodiazepines are much like alcohol in their effects on GABA receptors, which explains why benzodiazepines may be used for the management of alcohol withdrawal. Buspirone (BuSpar) is an antianxiety agent but not a benzodiazepine and does not depress the CNS. Although its action is unknown, the drug is believed to produce

the desired effects through interactions with serotonin, dopamine, and other neurotransmitter receptors. Clients should be instructed that buspirone has a lag period of 7 to 10 days before full therapeutic benefits are achieved. It does not have the addiction potential of the other antianxiety agents and therefore may be a better option for clients with anxiety disorders who have also struggled with substance use disorders.

Interactions

■ Increased effects of antianxiety agents can occur when they are taken concomitantly with alcohol, barbiturates, narcotics, antipsychotics, antidepressants, antihistamines, neuromuscular blocking agents, cimetidine, or disulfiram.
■ Increased effects can also occur with herbal depressants (e.g., kava, valerian, lemon verbena, L-tryptophan, melatonin, and chamomile).
■ Decreased effects can be noted with cigarette smoking and caffeine consumption.

Diagnosis

The following nursing diagnoses may be considered for clients receiving therapy with antianxiety agents:

■ Risk for injury related to seizures, panic anxiety, acute agitation from alcohol withdrawal (indications), abrupt withdrawal from the medication after long-term use, or effects of medication intoxication or overdose

■ Anxiety (specify) related to threat to physical integrity or self-concept

■ Risk for activity intolerance related to side effects of sedation, confusion, and/or lethargy

■ Disturbed sleep pattern related to situational crises, physical condition, or severe level of anxiety

Safety Issues in Planning and Implementing Care

 The IOM (2003) identifies *ensuring safety* as a core competency for nursing. Table 4–3 notes some of the significant safety issues to be considered for clients taking antianxiety agents. Nursing interventions related to each side effect are noted in the right-hand column.

Outcome Criteria and Evaluation

The following criteria may be used for evaluating the effectiveness of therapy with antianxiety agents.

The client:

■ Demonstrates a reduction in anxiety, tension, and restless activity

■ Experiences no seizure activity

■ Experiences no physical injury

■ Is able to tolerate usual activities without excessive sedation

■ Exhibits no evidence of confusion

■ Tolerates the medication without gastrointestinal distress

■ Verbalizes understanding of the need for, side effects of, and regimen for self-administration

■ Verbalizes possible consequences of abrupt withdrawal from the medication

Antidepressants

Sorting out information on antidepressant medications can be particularly confusing because there are several types of antidepressant medications, some of which are also prescribed to treat anxiety disorders. The first "antidepressant" drug was a monoamine oxidase inhibitor (MAOI), isoniazid, which was used to treat tuberculosis. When patients began describing their increased feelings of well-being on these drugs, MAOIs were developed specifically for the treatment of depression. Unfortunately, they were also potentially deadly for anyone who ate foods

TABLE 4–3 Safety Issues and Nursing Interventions for Patients Taking Antianxiety Agents	
SAFETY ISSUES	**NURSING INTERVENTIONS**
Tolerance and physical dependence may develop. **Abrupt withdrawal can be life threatening** (except with buspirone); signs include sweating, agitation, tremors, nausea and vomiting, delirium, seizures.	Instruct client not to stop taking the drug abruptly. Assess the client for signs of developing tolerance (requiring higher doses of medication to achieve effects). Educate the client about symptoms of withdrawal. Contact the doctor immediately if symptoms of withdrawal are assessed.
Drowsiness, confusion, and lethargy are the most common side effects.	Instruct client not to drive or operate dangerous machinery while taking this medication.
Effects of other CNS depressants are increased.	Instruct the client not to drink alcohol or take other CNS depressants, antihistamines, cimetidine, antidepressants, neuromuscular blocking agents, or disulfiram while taking these drugs.
Antianxiety agents may **aggravate symptoms of depression.**	Assess the client's mood and assess for suicide risk.
Orthostatic hypotension may occur.	Instruct the client to rise slowly from a sitting to standing position to minimize risk for falls. Monitor lying and standing blood pressures to assess for orthostatic hypotension.
Paradoxical excitement (opposite from the desired effect) may occur. Especially the elderly may be at higher risk for agitation and increased anxiety.	Hold the medication and notify the doctor.
Blood dyscrasias, although rare, can be serious or life threatening.	Assess for sore throat, fever, bruising, or unusual bleeding. Hold medication and report these symptoms immediately to the doctor.
Congenital malformations have been associated with use of these drugs during the first trimester of pregnancy.	Instruct the female client who is pregnant or anticipating pregnancy while on these drugs to explore alternative treatment options with her physician.

high in tyramine while taking these drugs, and several serious interactions occurred with other drugs. Because MAOIs increase the availability of norepinephrine, researchers focused on developing drugs that impacted norepinephrine without the need for food restrictions, leading to introduction of the *tricyclic antidepressants.*

Tricyclics were the first line of treatment for depression for many years but were effective for only about 70 percent of those treated. In addition, because all neurotransmitters bind to various receptor sites, increasing the availability of norepinephrine with tricyclics also has anticholinergic effects and increases the potential for postural hypotension. This created limitations for the elderly and those with cardiovascular problems.

In the late 1980s and early 1990s, *serotonin reuptake inhibitors* (SSRIs) and *serotonin-norepinephrine reuptake inhibitors* (SNRIs) were developed in response to research indicating that serotonin, an antianxiety hormone and neurotransmitter, could promote improvement in depression and anxiety without significant anticholinergic side effects. SSRIs and SNRIs became the preferred first line of treatment for depression.

The most recent additions to the pharmacological treatments for depression and anxiety are actually atypical antipsychotics that increase the availability of serotonin and dopamine. These medications are promoted as adjunctive to antidepressant therapy. The most popular example is aripiprazole (Abilify). In a recent large study sponsored by the National Institute of Mental Health, the combination of Abilify with venlafaxine demonstrated a 44 percent improvement in elderly adults who were not responding to antidepressants alone. This finding is important for treatment of elderly clients because more than half of older adults with clinical depression do not respond to antidepressants alone (Lenze et al., 2015).

Despite these developments and client-subjective reports of improvement with antidepressant medications, our understanding of the exact mechanisms of action remains theoretical because, currently, the levels of neurotransmitters in the brain cannot be measured. Further, a large study funded by the National Institute of Mental Health (STAR*D) found that two-thirds of patients with at least moderate depression on antidepressant medication did not experience full recovery after initial treatment with an SSRI (NIMH, 2006).

Research continues with the goal of identifying more broadly effective antidepressant therapies. Several of the newest drugs on the market for treatment of depression are not significantly different from existing products. For example, a "new" antidepressant approved by the FDA in 2016, Oleptro, is a reformulation of trazodone. But new mechanisms are being explored, and some are in clinical trials. Drugs that impact specific types of glutamate receptors (*N*-methyl-D-aspartate (NMDA) receptors) are being studied for potential antidepressant effects, ketamine and midazolam (Versed, a benzodiazepine with transient effects similar to those of ketamine) are being explored as potentially faster-acting treatments, drugs that act on melatonin receptors are currently in clinical trials for use in depression (one is already approved for use in Europe), and a new group of antidepressants called *triple reuptake inhibitors* that simultaneously block reuptake of serotonin, norepinephrine, and dopamine is in preliminary phases of research (Tartakovsky, 2016).

Current research also continues to explore genetic testing to identify factors that may influence whether an individual is more likely to respond to one type of antidepressant than another. If reliability is established, the research will provide a valuable resource for making decisions about which antidepressant to prescribe first.

Background Assessment Data

Indications

In addition to the obvious indications for antidepressant medications in the treatment of major depressive and dysthymic disorders, some atypical drugs, such as the SSRIs, have received FDA approval for the treatment of most anxiety disorders, bulimia nervosa, premenstrual dysphoric disorder, borderline personality disorder, obesity, smoking cessation, and alcoholism A hallmark review of the research on antidepressants (Fournier et al., 2010) found that the benefits of antidepressant therapy for patients with mild to moderate symptoms of depression may be minimal or nonexistent but that, for clients with severe depression, the benefits when compared with placebo effects are substantial. Therefore, these medications are particularly indicated when an individual is identified as having severe depression. (A table of current FDA-approved antidepressants, pregnancy categories, half-life, and daily dosage ranges can be found online at Davis*Plus* and in Chapter 25, Depressive Disorders.)

Action

Antidepressant drugs ultimately work to increase the concentration of norepinephrine, serotonin, and/or dopamine in the body. This is accomplished in the brain by blocking the reuptake of these neurotransmitters by the neurons (tricyclics [TCAs], tetracyclics, SSRIs, and SNRIs). It also occurs when an enzyme, monoamine oxidase (MAO), known to inactivate norepinephrine, serotonin, and dopamine, is *inhibited* at various sites in the nervous system (MAOIs).

> **CLINICAL PEARL** All antidepressants carry an FDA black-box warning for increased risk of suicidality in children and adolescents.

Interactions

Tables 4–4, 4–5, 4–6, and 4–7 identify some of the significant, dangerous interactions between antidepressant and other drugs or foods. It is important to recognize that new information about drug interactions is discovered and published frequently. To fully understand safety issues related to medication administration, nurses need to access the most current, evidence-based informatics on drug interaction information.

Other Atypical Antidepressants

Other atypical antidepressants include bupropion (Wellbutrin), mirtazapine (Remeron), and trazodone (Desyrel). Common SNRIs include desvenlafaxine (Pristiq), duloxetine (Cymbalta), levomilnacipran (Fetzima), and venlafaxine (Effexor). Drug interactions vary widely within these groups; following are several examples.

- Concomitant use with MAOIs results in serious, sometimes fatal, effects resembling **neuroleptic malignant syndrome.** Coadministration is contraindicated.
- **Serotonin syndrome** may occur when any of the following are used together: St. John's wort, sumatriptan, sibutramine, trazodone, nefazodone, venlafaxine, duloxetine, levomilnacipran, SSRIs, 5-HT-receptor agonists (triptans).

TABLE 4–4 Drug Interactions With SSRIs

INTERACTING DRUGS	ADVERSE EFFECTS
Buspirone (BuSpar), tricyclic antidepressants (especially clomipramine), selegiline (Eldepryl), St. John's wort	Serotonin syndrome*
Monoamine oxidase inhibitors	Hypertensive crisis
Warfarin, NSAIDs	Increased risk of bleeding
Alcohol, benzodiazepines	Increased sedation
Antiepileptics	Lowered seizure threshold

*Serotonin syndrome is a potentially fatal syndrome of serotonin overstimulation with rapid onset that progresses from diarrhea, restlessness, agitation, hyperreflexia, fluctuations in vital signs to later symptoms of myoclonus, seizures, hyperthermia, uncontrolled shivering, muscle rigidity, and ultimately can lead to delirium, coma, status epilepticus, cardiovascular collapse, and death. Immediate cessation of offending drugs and comprehensive supportive intervention is essential (Sadock, Sadock, & Ruiz, 2015).

TABLE 4–5 Drug Interactions With Tricyclic Antidepressants (TCAs)

INTERACTING DRUGS	ADVERSE EFFECTS
Monoamine oxidase inhibitors	High fever, convulsions, death
St. John's wort, tramadol (Ultram)	Seizures, serotonin syndrome
Clonidine (Catapres), epinephrine	Severe hypertension
Acetylcholine blockers	Paralytic ileus
Alcohol and carbamazepine (Tegretol)	Blocks antidepressant action, increases sedation
Cimetidine (Tagamet), bupropion (BuSpar)	Increased TCA blood levels and increased side effects

TABLE 4–6 Drug Interactions With Monoamine Oxidase Inhibitors (MAOIs)

INTERACTING DRUGS	ADVERSE EFFECTS
Selective serotonin reuptake inhibitor, tricyclic antidepressants, atomoxetine (Strattera), duloxetine (Cymbalta), dextromethorphan (an ingredient in many cough syrups), venlafaxine (Effexor), St. John's wort, ginkgo biloba	Serotonin syndrome
Morphine and other narcotic pain relievers, antihypertensives	Hypotension
All other antidepressants, pseudoephedrine, amphetamines, cocaine cyclobenzaprine (Flexeril), dopamine, methyldopa, levodopa, epinephrine, buspirone (BuSpar)	Hypertensive crisis (these side effects can occur even if taken within 2 weeks of stopping MAOIs)
Buspirone	Psychosis, agitation, seizures
Antidiabetics	Hypoglycemia
Tegretol	Fever, hypertension, seizures

- Increased effects of haloperidol, clozapine, and desipramine may occur with concomitant use of venlafaxine.
- Increased effects of levomilnacipran may occur with concomitant use of CYP3A4 inhibitors.
- Increased effects of venlafaxine may occur with concomitant use of cimetidine.

TABLE 4–7	**Diet Restrictions for Clients on MAOI Therapy**	
FOODS CONTAINING TYRAMINE		
HIGH TYRAMINE CONTENT (AVOID WHILE ON MAOI THERAPY)	**MODERATE TYRAMINE CONTENT (MAY EAT OCCASIONALLY WHILE ON MAOI THERAPY)**	**LOW TYRAMINE CONTENT (LIMITED QUANTITIES PERMISSIBLE WHILE ON MAOI THERAPY)**
Aged cheeses (cheddar, Swiss, Camembert, blue cheese, parmesan, provolone, Romano, brie)	Gouda cheese, processed American cheese, mozzarella	Pasteurized cheeses (cream cheese, cottage cheese, ricotta)
Raisins, fava beans, flat Italian beans, Chinese pea pods	Yogurt, sour cream	Figs
Red wines (chianti, burgundy, cabernet sauvignon)	Avocados, bananas	Distilled spirits (in moderation)
Liqueurs	Beer, white wine, coffee, colas, tea, hot chocolate	
Smoked and processed meats (salami, bologna, pepperoni, summer sausage)	Meat extracts, such as bouillon	
Caviar, pickled herring, corned beef, chicken or beef liver	Chocolate	
Soy sauce, brewer's yeast, meat tenderizer (MSG)		
Sauerkraut		

SOURCE: Sadock, B.J., Sadock, V.A., & Ruiz, P. (2015). *Synopsis of psychiatry: Behavioral sciences/clinical psychiatry* (11th ed.). Philadelphia: Lippincott Williams & Wilkins; Vallerand, A.H., Sanoski, C.A., & Deglin, J.H. (2016). *Davis drug guide for nurses* (15th ed.). Philadelphia: F.A. Davis.

■ Increased effects of duloxetine may occur with concomitant use of CYP1A2 inhibitors (e.g., fluvoxamine, quinolone antibiotics) or CYP2D6 inhibitors (e.g., fluoxetine, quinidine, paroxetine).

■ Risk of liver injury is increased with concomitant use of alcohol and duloxetine.

■ Risk of toxicity or adverse effects from drugs extensively metabolized by CYP2D6 (e.g., flecainide, phenothiazines, propafenone, tricyclic antidepressants, thioridazine) is increased when these drugs are used concomitantly with duloxetine or bupropion.

■ Decreased effects of bupropion and trazodone may occur with concomitant use of carbamazepine.

■ The anticoagulant effect of warfarin may be altered with concomitant use of bupropion, venlafaxine, desvenlafaxine, duloxetine, levomilnacipran, or trazodone.

■ Risk of seizures is increased when bupropion is coadministered with drugs that lower the seizure threshold (e.g., antidepressants, antipsychotics, systemic steroids, theophylline, tramadol).

■ Effects of midazolam are decreased with concomitant use of desvenlafaxine.

■ Effects of desvenlafaxine and levomilnacipran are increased with concomitant use of potent CYP3A4 inhibitors (e.g., ketoconazole).

Diagnosis

The following nursing diagnoses may be considered for clients receiving therapy with antidepressant medications:

■ Risk for suicide related to depressed mood
■ Risk for injury related to side effects of sedation, lowered seizure threshold, orthostatic hypotension, **priapism,** photosensitivity, arrhythmias, **hypertensive crisis,** or serotonin syndrome
■ Social isolation related to depressed mood
■ Risk for constipation related to side effects of the medication
■ Insomnia related to depressed mood and elevated level of anxiety

Safety Issues in Planning and Implementing Care

Some of the common but manageable side effects of antidepressant medications include dry mouth, sedation, and nausea. General nursing interventions such as offering hard candies, ice, and frequent sips of water are helpful in alleviating dry mouth. Clients may find that sedation is less bothersome if they take the daily dose of antidepressant at bedtime; they should be encouraged to discuss the time of day that their medication should be taken with the prescribing physician or nurse practitioner. Taking antidepressant medication with food may help minimize nausea.

Some patients taking SSRIs or SNRIs complain of sexual dysfunction. Men may report abnormal ejaculation or impotence, and women may report loss of orgasm. This side effect sometimes results in clients stopping the medication abruptly, which may put them at risk for discontinuation syndrome and worsen symptoms of depression. Nurses must develop an open attitude regarding discussion and assessment of client sexual concerns, and clients who are particularly troubled by this side effect can be encouraged to explore alternative medication with their physician or nurse practitioner.

Other side effects or adverse reactions may be dangerous or even fatal. Many of these are related to drug–drug or drug–food interactions, as discussed previously. Because there is so much information and new drug development is ongoing, practicing nurses should assure that they are accessing evidence-based informatics to keep up to date on side effects as well. Many health-care organizations provide online medication resources to employees, and mobile device applications provide a readily available resource for updated drug information. Some important safety issues and nursing interventions are listed in Table 4–8.

TABLE 4–8 Safety Issues and Nursing Interventions for Patients Taking Antidepressants	
SAFETY ISSUES	NURSING INTERVENTIONS
Drug interactions (multiple, as discussed in the text)	Instruct clients to inform their physician or nurse practitioner of *all* medications they are taking, including herbal preparations, over-the-counter drugs, and any medications they have stopped taking within the previous 2 weeks. Notify the physician immediately when any symptoms of serotonin syndrome are assessed. Do not administer the offending agent. ■ Monitor vital signs. ■ Protect from injury secondary to muscle rigidity or change in mental status. ■ Provide cooling blankets for temperature regulation. ■ Monitor intake and output. The condition usually resolves when the offending agent is promptly discontinued but can be fatal without intervention (Cooper & Sejnowski, 2013).
Increased risk for suicide	Assess frequently for presence or worsening of suicide ideation. Initiate suicide precautions as needed. Monitor clients' use of medication as prescribed, since these medications can be lethal in overdose.
Sedation	Instruct clients not to drive or operate dangerous machinery when experiencing sedation.
Discontinuation syndrome: SSRIs—dizziness, lethargy, headache, nausea TCAs—hypomania, akathisia, cardiac arrhythmias, gastrointestinal upset, panic attacks MAOIs—flu-like symptoms, confusion, hypomania	Instruct clients that all antidepressants have some potential for discontinuation syndrome and should not be stopped abruptly but rather tapered off (Schatzberg, Cole, & DeBattista, 2010).
Photosensitivity	Instruct clients of their vulnerability to severe sunburn and recommend sunscreen.
Orthostatic hypotension (TCAs)	Instruct clients to rise slowly from sitting to standing. Monitor blood pressure to assess for symptoms.
Tachycardia, arrhythmias (TCAs)	Monitor vital signs, especially in elderly with preexisting cardiovascular disorders.
Hyponatremia (SSRIs) especially among the elderly (potentially life threatening)	Instruct clients to report any symptoms of nausea, malaise, lethargy, muscle cramps. Assess for disorientation or restlessness. Monitor sodium levels: ■ <120 mEq/L risk for seizure, coma, respiratory arrest ■ Withhold medication, contact physician, restrict water intake (Jacob & Spinier, 2006)
Blurred vision (TCAs and atypicals)	Instruct clients to avoid driving, and reassure them that this side effect usually resolves within 3 weeks. Monitor blood pressure to rule out symptoms of hypertension.
Constipation	Recommend a high-fiber diet and regular exercise, and instruct clients to report any symptoms of ongoing difficulty with bowel movements.

MAOI, monoamine oxidase inhibitor; SSRI, selective serotonin reuptake inhibitor; TCA, tricyclic antidepressant.

CLINICAL PEARL As antidepressant drugs take effect and mood begins to lift, the individual may have increased energy with which to implement a suicide plan. Suicide potential may increase as level of depression decreases. The nurse should be particularly alert to sudden lifts in mood.

Outcome Criteria and Evaluation

The following criteria may be used for evaluating the effectiveness of therapy with antidepressant medications.

The client:

■ Has not harmed self
■ Has not experienced injury caused by side effects
■ Exhibits vital signs within normal limits
■ Manifests symptoms of improvement in mood (presents brighter affect, interacts with others, demonstrates improved hygiene, expresses clear thought, conveys hopefulness, shows improved ability to make decisions)
■ Willingly participates in activities and interacts appropriately with others

Mood-Stabilizing Agents

Background Assessment Data

For many years, the drug of choice for treatment and management of bipolar mania was lithium carbonate. In recent years, several other medications have demonstrated effectiveness either alone or in combination with lithium. Most notably are drugs in the class of anticonvulsant medications, which are now FDA approved for mood stabilization. Some second-generation atypical antipsychotics have also demonstrated benefits for management of this disorder.

Bipolar disorder is characterized by cycles of depression and manic episodes, which may manifest as grandiose thinking and behavior, rapid thoughts, hyperactivity, and/or impulsive agitation. The effective medication treatment for this disorder is one that reduces the rollercoaster of "ups and downs" often described by clients; thus, the name "mood stabilizer" is an apt description of their purpose. Lithium was first identified as an antimanic but was also recognized as successful for stabilizing the mood swings of bipolar disorder.

Lithium is a salt present in mineral springs and added to spa baths. Although it was also used for other medicinal purposes, in 1949, Australian physician John Cade reported using lithium to treat manic excitement. He found it so successful that some of his patients became symptom free and were able to be discharged after years of institutionalization (Shorter, 2009). It remains true that people who respond to lithium and remain on the medication may show no evidence of bipolar mood swings. While it is not a cure, it is often described as "like insulin to a diabetic" in that proper use and response can reduce or eliminate symptoms. Unfortunately, not everyone responds with the same degree of success, and too much lithium can be fatal. Today, however, we are able to measure the blood levels of lithium and be confident of its safety when maintained within the specified therapeutic range (0.6–1.2 mEq/L). The exact mechanism of action remains unknown, but it is believed to have an impact on the same neurotransmitters (serotonin, norepinephrine, glutamate, GABA, and dopamine) as previously discussed.

In 1995, the FDA approved valproate (Depakote) as a mood stabilizer; since then, a great shift toward this group of anticonvulsant mood stabilizers (including carbamazepine, clonazepam, topiramate, and lamotrigine) and away from lithium has occurred (Shorter, 2009). The mechanism of action for these drugs as well as for lithium is unclear. Impact on cellular sodium transport, GABA modulation, and raising of the seizure threshold have all been advanced as possible explanations for their effectiveness. Both first-generation and second-generation antipsychotics have been used alone or as adjuncts to other medication treatment for bipolar mania. Since lithium has a lag period of 7 to 10 days, first-generation antipsychotics such as haloperidol may be helpful in that their sedative effects are more immediate and may bring relief from manic symptoms before lithium reaches therapeutic levels. They also increase the effects of lithium, so monitoring blood serum levels is especially important in the initial phase of treatment when these two drugs are used in combination. (A table of current FDA-approved mood-stabilizer medications, pregnancy categories, half-life, and daily dosage ranges can be found online at Davis*Plus* and in Chapter 26, Bipolar and Related Disorders.)

Interactions

One of the interesting things about drug interactions with mood stabilizers is that many drugs either increase or decrease their effectiveness, as shown in Table 4–9. Understanding that lithium is a salt is relevant in explaining some of these interactions. Because lithium is an imperfect substitute for sodium, anything that depletes sodium will make more receptor sites available to lithium and increase the risk for lithium toxicity. This is also the rationale behind maintenance of regular dietary sodium and fluid intake, because major fluctuations impact lithium levels. For example, significant increases in dietary sodium intake may reduce the effectiveness of lithium because sodium will bind at more receptor sites and lithium will be excreted. Other drugs that increase serum sodium levels also have an impact on lithium levels.

TABLE 4–9 Drug Interactions With Mood-Stabilizing Agents

THE EFFECTS OF:	ARE INCREASED BY:	ARE DECREASED BY:	CONCURRENT USE MAY RESULT IN:
ANTIMANIC: Lithium	Carbamazepine, fluoxetine, haloperidol, loop diuretics, methyldopa, NSAIDs, and thiazide diuretics	Acetazolamide, osmotic diuretics, theophylline, and urinary alkalinizers	Increased effects of neuromuscular blocking agents and tricyclic antidepressants; decreased pressor sensitivity of sympathomimetics; neurotoxicity may occur with phenothiazines or calcium channel blockers
ANTICONVULSANTS: Clonazepam	CNS depressants, cimetidine, hormonal contraceptives, disulfiram, fluoxetine, isoniazid, ketoconazole, metoprolol, propranolol, valproic acid, probenecid	Rifampin, theophylline (↓ sedative effects), phenytoin	Increased phenytoin levels; decreased efficacy of levodopa
Carbamazepine	Verapamil, diltiazem, propoxyphene, erythromycin, clarithromycin, SSRIs, tricyclic antidepressants, cimetidine, isoniazid, danazol, lamotrigine, niacin, acetazolamide, dalfopristin, valproate, nefazodone	Cisplatin, doxorubicin, felbamate, rifampin, barbiturates, hydantoins, primidone, theophylline	Decreased levels of corticosteroids, doxycycline, quinidine, warfarin, estrogen-containing contraceptives, cyclosporine, benzodiazepines, theophylline, lamotrigine, valproic acid, bupropion, haloperidol, olanzapine, tiagabine, topiramate, voriconazole, ziprasidone, felbamate, levothyroxine, or antidepressants; increased levels of lithium; life-threatening hypertensive reaction with MAOIs
Valproic acid	Chlorpromazine, cimetidine, erythromycin, felbamate, salicylates	Rifampin, carbamazepine, cholestyramine, lamotrigine, phenobarbital, ethosuximide, hydantoins	Increased effects of tricyclic antidepressants, carbamazepine, CNS depressants, ethosuximide, lamotrigine, phenobarbital, warfarin, zidovudine, hydantoins
Lamotrigine	Valproic acid	Primidone, phenobarbital, phenytoin, rifamycin, succinimides, oral contraceptives, oxcarbazepine, carbamazepine, acetaminophen	Decreased levels of valproic acid; increased levels of carbamazepine and topiramate
Topiramate	Metformin, hydrochlorothiazide	Phenytoin, carbamazepine, valproic acid, lamotrigine	Increased risk of CNS depression with alcohol or other CNS depressants; increased risk of kidney stones with carbonic anhydrase inhibitors; increased effects of phenytoin, metformin, amitriptyline; decreased effects of oral contraceptives, digoxin, lithium, risperidone, and valproic acid
Oxcarbazepine		Carbamazepine, phenobarbital, phenytoin, valproic acid, verapamil	Increased concentrations of phenobarbital and phenytoin; decreased effects of oral contraceptives, felodipine, and lamotrigine

Continued

TABLE 4–9 **Drug Interactions With Mood-Stabilizing Agents—cont'd**

THE EFFECTS OF:	ARE INCREASED BY:	ARE DECREASED BY:	CONCURRENT USE MAY RESULT IN:
CALCIUM CHANNEL BLOCKER: Verapamil	Amiodarone, beta blockers, cimetidine, ranitidine, and grapefruit juice	Barbiturates, calcium salts, hydantoins, rifampin, and antineoplastics	Increased effects of beta blockers, disopyramide, flecainide, doxorubicin, benzodiazepines, buspirone, carbamazepine, digoxin, dofetilide, ethanol, imipramine, nondepolarizing muscle relaxants, prazosin, quinidine, sirolimus, tacrolimus, and theophylline; altered serum lithium levels
ANTIPSYCHOTICS: Olanzapine	Fluvoxamine and other CYP1A2 inhibitors, fluoxetine	Carbamazepine and other CYP1A2 inducers, omeprazole, rifampin	Decreased effects of levodopa and dopamine agonists; increased hypotension with antihypertensives; increased CNS depression with alcohol or other CNS depressants
Aripiprazole	Ketoconazole and other CYP3A4 inhibitors; quinidine, fluoxetine, paroxetine, or other potential CYP2D6 inhibitors	Carbamazepine, famotidine, valproate	Increased CNS depression with alcohol or other CNS depressants; increased hypotension with antihypertensives
Chlorpromazine	Beta blockers, paroxetine	Centrally acting anticholinergics	Increased effects of beta blockers; excessive sedation and hypotension with meperidine; decreased hypotensive effect of guanethidine; decreased effect of oral anticoagulants; decreased or increased phenytoin levels; increased orthostatic hypotension with thiazide diuretics; increased CNS depression with alcohol or other CNS depressants; increased hypotension with antihypertensives; increased anticholinergic effects with anticholinergic agents
Quetiapine	Cimetidine; ketoconazole, itraconazole, fluconazole, erythromycin, or other CYP3A4 inhibitors	Phenytoin, thioridazine	Decreased effects of levodopa and dopamine agonists; increased CNS depression with alcohol or other CNS depressants; increased hypotension with antihypertensives
Risperidone	Clozapine, fluoxetine, paroxetine, or ritonavir	Carbamazepine	Decreased effects of levodopa and dopamine agonists; increased effects of clozapine and valproate; increased CNS depression with alcohol or other CNS depressants; increased hypotension with antihypertensives
Ziprasidone	Ketoconazole and other CYP3A4 inhibitors	Carbamazepine	Life-threatening prolongation of QT interval with quinidine, dofetilide, other class Ia and III antiarrhythmics, pimozide, sotalol, thioridazine, chlorpromazine, pentamidine, arsenic trioxide, mefloquine, dolasetron, tacrolimus, droperidol, gatifloxacin, or moxifloxacin; decreased effects of levodopa and dopamine agonists; increased CNS depression with alcohol or other CNS depressants; increased hypotension with antihypertensives

TABLE 4–9 Drug Interactions With Mood-Stabilizing Agents–cont'd

THE EFFECTS OF:	ARE INCREASED BY:	ARE DECREASED BY:	CONCURRENT USE MAY RESULT IN:
Asenapine	Fluvoxamine, imipramine, valproate	Carbamazepine, cimetidine, paroxetine	Increased effects of paroxetine and dextromethorphan; increased CNS depression with alcohol or other CNS depressants; increased hypotension with antihypertensives; additive effects of QT interval prolongation with quinidine, dofetilide, other class Ia and III antiarrhythmics, pimozide, sotalol, thioridazine, chlorpromazine, pentamidine, arsenic trioxide, mefloquine, dolasetron, tacrolimus, droperidol, gatifloxacin, or moxifloxacin

CNS, central nervous system; MAOI, monoamine oxidase inhibitor; SSRI, selective serotonin reuptake inhibitor.

Diagnosis

The following nursing diagnoses may be considered for clients receiving therapy with mood-stabilizing agents:

■ Risk for injury related to manic hyperactivity
■ Risk for self-directed or other-directed violence related to unresolved anger turned inward on the self or outward on the environment
■ Risk for injury related to lithium toxicity
■ Risk for injury related to adverse effects of mood-stabilizing drugs
■ Risk for activity intolerance related to side effects of drowsiness and dizziness

Planning and Implementing Care

One of the primary safety issues with lithium is its narrow therapeutic range. A description of lithium toxicity, other safety concerns with mood-stabilizing agents, and relevant nursing interventions are discussed in Table 4–10.

Lithium Maintenance

Clients who respond to lithium typically remain on the medication indefinitely. To assure safe maintenance and prevent lithium toxicity, client education and regular monitoring are essential. Monitoring includes but

TABLE 4–10 Safety Issues and Nursing Interventions for Clients Taking Mood Stabilizers

SAFETY ISSUES	NURSING INTERVENTIONS

Lithium toxicity (blood levels >1.2 mEq/L) or <1.2 in elderly or debilitated but most common at 1.5 mEq/L
■ Early signs: vomiting, diarrhea
■ Over 2 mEq/L: tremors, sedation, confusion
■ Levels over 3.5 mEq/L: delirium, seizures, coma, cardiovascular collapse, death
    Chlorpromazine (Thorazine) may mask early signs of lithium toxicity
    (Vallerand, Sanoski, & Deglin, 2016)
	Instruct clients to report all medications, herbals, and caffeine use to physician or nurse practitioner to evaluate for drug interactions.
	Encourage clients to maintain fluid intake at 2,000–3,000 ml/day and avoid activities in which excessive sweating and fluid loss are a risk, since inadequate fluid intake can impact lithium levels.
	Instruct clients about the importance of regular monitoring of serum lithium levels.
	Blood levels should be drawn 12 hours after the last dose.

Increased risk of suicide for all antiepileptics (FDA, 2008)	Assess for suicide risk regularly and inform clients of risks associated with anticonvulsants.
Hyponatremia (lithium, carbamazepine)	Instruct clients to maintain usual dietary intake of sodium. Assess for and educate clients to report any episodes of nausea, vomiting, headache, muscle weakness, confusion, seizures, since these may be signs of hyponatremia.
Stevens-Johnson syndrome (especially with lamotrigine and carbamazepine) This toxic skin necrolysis can be life threatening	Assess for and educate clients to report any signs of rash or unusual skin breakdown.

Continued

TABLE 4–10 Safety Issues and Nursing Interventions for Clients Taking Mood Stabilizers–cont'd	
SAFETY ISSUES	NURSING INTERVENTIONS
Hypotension, arrhythmias (lithium)	Monitor vital signs and instruct clients to report any symptoms of dizziness or palpitations.
Blood dyscrasias (valproic acid, carbamazepine)	Educate clients to report infections or other illness while on these medications. Ensure that platelet counts and bleeding time are determined before initiation of therapy. Monitor for spontaneous bleeding or bruising.
Increased risk of birth defects (anticonvulsant mood stabilizers)	Inform female clients of the risks of birth defects and provide education about contraception as desired.
Drowsiness (lithium and all anticonvulsants)	Instruct clients to avoid driving or operating dangerous machinery when experiencing this side effect. Assess clients' mental status for level of alertness.

is not limited to evaluating serum lithium levels to assure that they remain within the therapeutic range. The usual ranges of therapeutic serum concentrations differ for initiation of treatment in an acute manic state and maintenance (Facts and Comparisons [Firm], 2014; Schatzberg, Cole, & DeBattista, 2010):

■ For acute mania: 1.0 to 1.5 mEq/L
■ For maintenance: 0.6 to 1.2 mEq/L

Serum lithium levels should be monitored once or twice a week after initial treatment until dosage and serum levels are stable and then monthly during maintenance therapy. Blood samples should be drawn 12 hours after the last dose is taken.

At times, clients complain that they miss the "high" feeling of being in a manic or hypomanic state once they begin mood-stabilizer medications. They may be at risk for self-adjusting medication or discontinuing it all together. Open discussion and exploring the benefits versus disadvantages of medication treatment promotes patient-centered care and enables the nurse to troubleshoot with the client ways to minimize risks.

Another generally undesirable side effect of lithium is weight gain. Clients should be educated about this potential, and weight should be monitored at regular intervals. It may be helpful to discuss low-calorie diets while stressing the importance of not making large changes in sodium intake because of its impact on serum blood levels of lithium.

CLINICAL PEARL The U.S. Food and Drug Administration requires that all antiepileptic (anticonvulsant) drugs carry a warning label indicating that use of the drugs increases risk for suicidal thoughts and behaviors. Patients treated with these medications should be monitored for the emergence or worsening of depression, suicidal thoughts or behavior, or any unusual changes in mood or behavior.

Outcome Criteria and Evaluation

The following criteria may be used for evaluating the effectiveness of therapy with mood stabilizing agents.

The client:

■ Is maintaining stability of mood
■ Has not harmed self or others
■ Has experienced no injury from hyperactivity
■ Is able to participate in activities without excessive sedation or dizziness
■ Is maintaining appropriate weight
■ Exhibits no signs of lithium toxicity
■ Verbalizes importance of taking medication regularly and reporting for regular laboratory blood tests

Antipsychotic Agents
Background Assessment Data

Antipsychotic medications are also called *neuroleptics*. Historically, they have been referred to as major tranquilizers and clearly have sedative effects. The term *antipsychotics* is most descriptive because the primary benefit over time is the alleviation of psychotic symptoms such as hallucinations and delusions. Antipsychotic agents were introduced into the United States in the 1950s with the phenothiazines. Other drugs in this classification soon followed. Unfortunately, this group of medications was found to have the potential for side effects that interfere with normal movements, including acute **dystonias** (muscle spasms) that can be life threatening, Parkinson-like symptoms, and **tardive dyskinesia** (later-onset involuntary movement disorders primarily in the tongue, lips, and jaw that may also involve other movement disturbances). Some of these side effects can be permanent, continuing even after the drug is discontinued. Since that discovery, a second generation of medications has been developed with less potential for extrapyramidal side effects (EPS) such as those mentioned above. These drugs have become the first line of treatment for clients with psychotic disorders such as schizophrenia. This group of drugs may also be effective for treating negative symptoms of schizophrenia and alleviating positive symptoms like hallucinations, delusions, and agitation. More recently, aripiprazole (Abilify), an atypical antipsychotic, has been described as a third-generation antipsychotic because of its unique functional profile with dopamine receptors and minimal risk for EPS (Brust et al., 2015). The typical antipsychotics include the phenothiazines, haloperidol, loxapine, pimozide, and thiothixene. The atypical antipsychotics include aripiprazole, asenapine, clozapine, olanzapine, quetiapine, risperidone, paliperidone, iloperidone, lurasidone, ziprasidone, brexpiprazole (Rexulti), cariprazine (Vraylar), and pimavanserin (Nuplazid) indicated for hallucinatins and delusions associated with Parkinson's disease psychosis.

Indications

Antipsychotics are used in the treatment of schizophrenia and other psychotic disorders. Selected agents are used in the treatment of bipolar mania (see previous section, "Mood-Stabilizing Agents"). Others are used as antiemetics (chlorpromazine, perphenazine, prochlorperazine), in the treatment of intractable hiccoughs (chlorpromazine), and for the control of tics and vocal utterances in Tourette's disorder (haloperidol, pimozide). Selected atypical antipsychotics, including aripiprazole (Abilify), are being identified as adjuncts to the treatment of major depressive disorders. (A table of current FDA-approved antipsychotics, pregnancy categories, half-life, and daily dosage ranges, as well as antiparkinsonian agents used to treat extrapyramidal side effects of antipsychotic medication, can be found online at Davis*Plus* and in Chapter 24, Schizophrenia Spectrum and Other Psychotic Disorders.)

Action

Typical antipsychotics work by blocking postsynaptic dopamine receptors in the basal ganglia, hypothalamus, limbic system, brainstem, and medulla. They also demonstrate varying affinity for cholinergic, alpha$_1$-adrenergic, and histaminic receptors. Antipsychotic effects may be related to inhibition of dopamine-mediated transmission of neural impulses at the synapses.

Atypical antipsychotics are weaker dopamine receptor antagonists than conventional antipsychotics but are more potent antagonists of the serotonin type 2A ($5HT_{2A}$) receptors. They also exhibit antagonism for cholinergic, histaminic, and adrenergic receptors. As mentioned previously, aripiprazole (Abilify) is a dopamine receptor antagonist but seems to have a unique way of accomplishing its action and thus has a minimal risk of extrapyramidal side effects.

Contraindications and Precautions

Certain individuals may be at greater risk for experiencing side effects associated with antipsychotic agents. The elderly have been identified as an at-risk population because of accounts of stroke and sudden death while taking antipsychotic medication. Studies have indicated that elderly patients with psychosis related to neurocognitive disorder (NCD) who are treated with antipsychotic drugs are at increased risk of death compared with those taking a placebo (Steinberg & Lyketsos, 2012). Causes of death are most commonly related to infections or cardiovascular problems. All antipsychotic drugs now carry blackbox warnings to this effect. They are not approved for treatment of elderly patients with NCD-related psychosis.

Typical antipsychotics are contraindicated in clients with known hypersensitivity (cross-sensitivity may exist among phenothiazines). They should not be used in comatose states or when CNS depression is evident; when blood dyscrasias exist; in clients with Parkinson's disease or narrow-angle glaucoma; for those with liver, renal, or cardiac insufficiency; in individuals with poorly controlled seizure disorders; or in elderly clients with dementia-related psychosis. Caution should be taken in administering these drugs to clients who are elderly, severely ill, or debilitated and to clients with diabetes or with respiratory insufficiency, prostatic hypertrophy, or intestinal obstruction.

Atypical antipsychotics are contraindicated in hypersensitivity, comatose or severely depressed patients, elderly patients with dementia-related psychosis, and lactation. Ziprasidone, risperidone, paliperidone, asenapine, and iloperidone are contraindicated in patients with a history of QT prolongation or cardiac arrhythmias, recent myocardial infarction (MI), uncompensated heart failure, and concurrent use with other drugs that prolong the QT interval. Clozapine is contraindicated in patients with myeloproliferative disorders, with a history of clozapine-induced **agranulocytosis** or severe granulocytopenia, and in uncontrolled epilepsy. Lurasidone is contraindicated in concomitant use with strong inhibitors of cytochrome P450 isozyme 3A4 (CYP3A4) (e.g., ketoconazole, an antifungal) and strong CYP3A4 inducers (e.g., rifampin, an antitubercular).

Caution should be taken in administering these drugs to elderly or debilitated patients; patients with cardiac, hepatic, or renal insufficiency; those with a history of seizures; patients with diabetes or risk factors for diabetes; clients exposed to temperature extremes; pregnant clients and children (safety not established); and under conditions that cause hypotension (dehydration, hypovolemia, treatment with antihypertensive medication). The risk for metabolic disturbances such as weight gain can be particularly dangerous in the elderly.

Interactions

Table 4–11 highlights some drug interactions that warrant monitoring and assessment by nurses.

Diagnosis

The following nursing diagnoses may be considered for clients receiving antipsychotic therapy:

- Risk for other-directed violence related to panic anxiety and mistrust of others
- Risk for injury related to medication side effects of sedation, photosensitivity, reduction of seizure threshold, agranulocytosis, **extrapyramidal symptoms,** tardive dyskinesia, neuroleptic malignant syndrome, and/or QT prolongation
- Risk for activity intolerance related to medication side effects of sedation, blurred vision, and/or weakness
- Noncompliance with medication regimen related to suspiciousness and mistrust of others

Safety Issues in Planning and Implementing Care

Table 4–12 discusses some significant safety issues to consider and relevant nursing interventions for clients taking antipsychotic medication.

TABLE 4–11 Drug Interactions With Antipsychotic Medications	
DRUG INTERACTION	ADVERSE EFFECT
Antihypertensives, CNS depressants Epinephrine or dopamine in combination with haloperidol or phenothiazines	Additive and potentially severe hypotension
Oral anticoagulants with phenothiazines	Less effective anticoagulant effects
Drugs that prolong QT intervals	Additive effects
Drugs that trigger orthostatic hypotension	Additive hypotension
Drugs with anticholinergic effects, prescription and OTC drugs	Additive anticholinergic effects, including anticholinergic toxicity, signs of which are ■ Flushing ■ Dry mouth ■ Mydriasis ■ Altered mental status ■ Tachycardia ■ Urinary retention ■ Tremulousness ■ Hypertension (Ramnarine & Ahmed, 2015)

TABLE 4–12 Safety Issues and Nursing Interventions for Clients Taking Antipsychotic Medication	
SAFETY ISSUES	NURSING INTERVENTIONS
Extrapyramidal side effects[a] (see Table 4–13 for relative risk among specific medications)	Instruct client to report any signs of muscle stiffness or spasms. Hold the medication if this occurs. Administer antiparkinsonian agents as ordered and immediately when signs of acute dystonia are present. Assess the patient for abnormal involuntary movements (see Box 4–2). (See "Additional Issues for Client Education" for further discussion.)
Hyperglycemia, weight gain, and diabetes (more common with atypical antipsychotic agents)	Assess for history of diabetes. Evaluate blood sugars. Instruct the client in these risks and the importance of diet and exercise. Assess for signs of hyperglycemia including polydipsia, polyphagia, polyuria, and weakness.
Hypotension	Educate the client about risk for hypotension. Monitor blood pressure.
Orthostatic hypotension (see Table 4–13 for level of risk by specific medications)	Instruct client to rise slowly from sitting to standing. Monitor blood pressure lying and then standing to assess for postural changes.
Lower seizure threshold (especially with clozapine)	Assess client for history of seizure disorder. Monitor client for evidence of seizure activity and report to prescribing physician or nurse practitioner.

TABLE 4–12 Safety Issues and Nursing Interventions for Clients Taking Antipsychotic Medication–cont'd

SAFETY ISSUES	NURSING INTERVENTIONS
Prolonged QT interval[b] especially ziprasidone, thioridazine, pimozide, haloperidol, paliperidone, iloperidone, asenapine, and clozapine.	Assess for history of arrhythmias, recent MI, heart failure, and report to prescribing physician or nurse practitioner because these events are contraindications. Assess for other medications the client is taking that prolong QT interval (there are many; online resources such as www.crediblemeds.org provide a composite list for comparison), but note that erythromycin and clarithromycin are two that are commonly prescribed. Instruct client to reported any rapid heartbeat, dizziness, or fainting. Check baseline EKG before beginning treatment.
Anticholinergic effects (see Table 4–13 for relative risk among medications)	Instruct client about additive effects of other anticholinergic drugs in combination with antipsychotics, and to report any other medications taken including over-the-counter and herbal remedies. For minor symptoms such as dry mouth, recommend hard candies, sips of water. Instruct client regarding the importance of good oral hygiene. Instruct client to report and assess for any evidence of urinary retention, tachycardia, tremulousness, or hypertension, which may be signs of anticholinergic toxicity.
Sedation	Educate client about this side effect and instruct client not to drive or operate dangerous machinery if experiencing sedation.
Photosensitivity	Instruct client to use sunblock and sunglasses and to wear protective clothing when in the sun because of the increased risk for severe sunburn while on these medications.
Agranulocytosis (more common with typical antipsychotics but especially with the atypical antipsychotic agent clozapine)	Instruct the client receiving clozapine that regular monitoring of white blood cell and absolute neutrophil counts is essential. Instruct the client to report any signs of sore throat, fever, or malaise. (See additional guidelines in the section on Issues in Antipsychotic Maintenance Therapy.)
Neuroleptic malignant syndrome (NMS)[c]	Instruct client to report immediately any fever, muscle rigidity, diaphoresis, tachycardia. Assess vital signs regularly, including temperature. Assess for deteriorating mental status or any other sign of NMS. Presence of any of these signs requires holding the medication and contacting the prescribing physician or nurse practitioner immediately, as well as monitoring vital signs and intake and output.

[a]Acute dystonias can be life threatening (more common with typical antipsychotic agents).
[b]Potentially life-threatening.
[c]Rare but potentially life-threatening side effect characterized by muscle rigidity, severe hyperthermia, and cardiac effects that can progress rapidly over 24–72 hours.

Additional Issues for Client Education

A comparison of side effects among antipsychotic agents is presented in Table 4–13. Clients should be apprised of health risks, including the following:

■ Smoking increases the metabolism of antipsychotics, requiring an adjustment in dosage to achieve a therapeutic effect. Encourage clients to discuss this issue with the prescribing physician or nurse practitioner.

■ Body temperature is harder to maintain with this medication, so clients should be encouraged to dress warmly in cold weather and avoid extended exposure to very high or low temperatures.

■ Alcohol and antipsychotic drugs potentiate each other's effects, so clients should be advised to avoid drinking alcohol while on antipsychotic therapy.

■ Many medications contain substances that interact with antipsychotics in a way that may be harmful. Clients should avoid taking other medications, including over-the-counter products, without the physician's approval.

■ A significant number of clients on clozapine report excessive salivation. Sugar-free gum and medications (anticholinergic or alpha$_2$-adrenoceptor agonists) may alleviate symptoms. Encourage clients to discuss these options with the prescribing physician or nurse practitioner.

■ Safe use of antipsychotics during pregnancy has not been established. Antipsychotics are thought to readily cross the placental barrier; if so, a fetus could experience adverse effects of the drug. Clients should

TABLE 4–13 Comparison of Side Effects Among Antipsychotic Agents

CLASS	GENERIC (TRADE) NAME	EPS	SEDATION	ANTICHOLINERGIC	ORTHOSTATIC HYPOTENSION	WEIGHT GAIN
TYPICAL ANTIPSYCHOTIC AGENTS	Chlorpromazine	3	4	3	4	*
	Fluphenazine	5	2	2	2	
	Haloperidol (Haldol)	5	2	2	2	
	Loxapine	3	2	2	2	*
	Perphenazine	4	2	2	2	*
	Pimozide (Orap)	4	2	2	2	*
	Prochlorperazine	3	2	2	2	*
	Thioridazine	2	4	4	4	*
	Thiothixene (Navane)	4	2	2	2	*
	Trifluoperazine	4	2	2	2	*
ATYPICAL ANTIPSYCHOTIC AGENTS	Aripiprazole (Abilify)	1	2	1	3	2
	Asenapine (Saphris)	1	3	1	3	4
	Clozapine (Clozaril)	1	5	5	4	5
	Iloperidone (Fanapt)	1	3	2	3	3
	Lurasidone (Latuda)	1	3	1	3	3
	Olanzapine (Zyprexa)	1	3	2	2	5
	Paliperidone (Invega)	1	2	1	3	2
	Quetiapine (Seroquel)	1	3	1	3	4
	Risperidone (Risperdal)	1	2	1	3	4
	Ziprasidone (Geodon)	1	3	1	2	2

Key: 1 = Very low; 2 = Low; 3 = Moderate; 4 = High; 5 = Very high.
*Weight gain occurs, but incidence is unknown.
EPN = extrapyramidal symptoms.
SOURCE: Adapted from Black, D.W., & Andreasen, N.C. (2014). *Introductory textbook of psychiatry* (6th ed.). Washington, DC: American Psychiatric Publishing; Facts and Comparisons (Firm) & Wolters Kluwer Health. (2014). *Drug facts and comparisons.* St. Louis, MO: Wolters Kluwer; Schatzberg, A.F., Cole, J.O., & DeBattista, C. (2010). *Manual of clinical psychopharmacology* (7th ed.). Washington, DC: American Psychiatric Publishing.

be aware of the possible risks and should inform the physician immediately if pregnancy occurs, is suspected, or is planned.

Issues in Antipsychotic Maintenance Therapy

The nurse must understand the management of side effects associated with antipsychotic medication in order to conduct a thorough assessment and minimize risks. In addition, some of these side effects can be difficult for clients to manage or understand, particularly when they are struggling with impaired mental status including psychosis and cognitive deficits. Three of these are discussed below.

Clozaril and the Risk for Agranulocytosis Agranulocytosis is a potentially fatal blood disorder in which the client's white blood cell (WBC) count can drop to extremely low levels. A baseline WBC count and absolute neutrophil count (ANC) must be taken before initiation of treatment with clozapine and weekly for the first 6 months of treatment. Only a 1-week supply of medication is dispensed at one time. If the counts remain within the acceptable levels (i.e., WBC count at least 3,500/mm³ and ANC at least 2,000/mm³) during the 6-month period, blood counts may be monitored biweekly and a 2-week supply of medication may be dispensed. If the counts remain within the acceptable level for the biweekly period (6 months),

counts may then be monitored every 4 weeks. When the medication is discontinued, weekly WBC counts are continued for an additional 4 weeks.

While the benefits of clozapine can be profound, this medication is typically used when clients fail to respond to other antipsychotics because of the strict protocols for adherence. If the client agrees to this option, the nurse can be a vital link in assuring that support services, both professional and personal (such as family members or peers), are engaged to assist the client with follow-through as needed.

Extrapyramidal Side Effects (See Table 4–13 for differences between typical and atypical antipsychotics.) To conduct a thorough assessment, the nurse must be familiar with the several distinct types of extrapyramidal side effects:

■ **Pseudoparkinsonism:** Symptoms of pseudoparkinsonism—tremor, shuffling gait, drooling, rigidity—may appear 1 to 5 days following initiation of antipsychotic medication. This side effect occurs most often in women, the elderly, and dehydrated clients.

■ **Akinesia:** Absence or impairment in voluntary movement.

■ **Akathisia:** Continuous restlessness and fidgeting, or **akathisia,** occurs most often in women and may manifest 50 to 60 days after therapy begins. Combining second generation antipsychotics has demonstrated a three-fold risk for developing akathisia as compared to monotherapy with a single second generation antipsychotic (Berna et al., 2015)

■ **Dystonia:** This side effect—involuntary muscle spasms in the face, arms, legs, and neck—occurs most often in men and those younger than age 25. **Dystonia** should be treated as an emergency situation because laryngospasm follows these symptoms and can be fatal. The physician should be contacted, and intravenous or intramuscular benztropine mesylate (Cogentin) is commonly administered (see Table 4–13 for a list of antiparkinsonian agents used to treat extrapyramidal symptoms). Stay with the client and offer reassurance and support during this frightening time.

■ **Oculogyric crisis:** Uncontrolled rolling back of the eyes, or **oculogyric crisis,** is a symptom of acute dystonia and can be mistaken for seizure activity. As with other symptoms of acute dystonia, this side effect should be treated as a medical emergency.

■ **Tardive dyskinesia:** This extrapyramidal side effect involves bizarre face and tongue movements, stiff neck, and difficulty swallowing. It may occur with all classifications but most commonly takes place with typical antipsychotics. All clients receiving antipsychotic therapy for months or years are at risk. Symptoms are potentially irreversible. Nurses should immediately report to the prescribing physician or nurse practitioner earliest signs of **tardive dyskinesia** (usually vermiform movements of the tongue) as the drug is often discontinued, changed to a different antipsychotic, or the dosage is altered. In 2017 the FDA approved the first drug for treating tardive dyskinesia; valbenazine (Ingrezza). It is hoped that this novel drug will effectively reduce this troubling condition and its sometimes stigmatizing effects (FDA, 2017). The involuntary movements associated with tardive dyskinesia can be measured by the Abnormal Involuntary Movement Scale (AIMS), developed in the 1970s by the National Institute of Mental Health. AIMS aids in early detection of movement disorders and provides means for ongoing surveillance. AIMS is featured in Box 4–2.

BOX 4–2 Abnormal Involuntary Movement Scale (AIMS)

NAME _____ **RATER NAME** _____ **DATE** _____

INSTRUCTIONS: Complete the examination procedure before making ratings. For movement ratings, circle the highest severity observed. Rate movements that occur upon activation one less than those observed spontaneously. Circle movement as well as code number that applies.

Code: 0 = None
1 = Minimal, may be normal
2 = Mild
3 = Moderate
4 = Severe

Facial and Oral Movements	1. Muscles of Facial Expression (e.g., movements of forehead, eyebrows, periorbital area, cheeks, including frowning, blinking, smiling, grimacing)	0 1 2 3 4
	2. Lips and Perioral Area (e.g., puckering, pouting, smacking)	0 1 2 3 4
	3. Jaw (e.g., biting, clenching, chewing, mouth opening, lateral movement)	0 1 2 3 4
	4. Tongue (Rate only increases in movement both in and out of mouth. NOT inability to sustain movement. Darting in and out of mouth.)	0 1 2 3 4
Extremity Movements	5. Upper (arms, wrists, hands, fingers) Include choreic movements (i.e., rapid, objectively purposeless, irregular, spontaneous) and athetoid movements (i.e., slow, irregular, complex serpentine). *Do not include tremor* (i.e., repetitive, regular, rhythmic)	0 1 2 3 4
	6. Lower (legs, knees, ankles, toes) (e.g., lateral knee movement, foot tapping, heel dropping, foot squirming, inversion and eversion of foot)	0 1 2 3 4
Trunk Movements	7. Neck, shoulders, hips (e.g., rocking, twisting, squirming, pelvic gyrations)	0 1 2 3 4
Global Judgments	8. Severity of abnormal movements overall	0 1 2 3 4
	9. Incapacitation due to abnormal movements	0 1 2 3 4

Continued

BOX 4–2 Abnormal Involuntary Movement Scale (AIMS)—cont'd

	10. Patient's awareness of abnormal movements		
	(Rate only the client's report)		
	No awareness		0
	Aware, no distress		1
	Aware, mild distress		2
	Aware, moderate distress		3
	Aware, severe distress		4
Dental Status	11. Current problems with teeth and/or dentures?	No	Yes
	12. Are dentures usually worn?	No	Yes
	13. Edentia?	No	Yes
	14. Do movements disappear in sleep?	No	Yes

AIMS EXAMINATION PROCEDURE

Either before or after completing the Examination Procedure, observe the client unobtrusively, at rest (e.g., in waiting room). The chair to be used in this examination should be a hard, firm one without arms.

1. Ask client to remove shoes and socks.
2. Ask client whether there is anything in his/her mouth (i.e., gum, candy, etc.), and if there is, to remove it.
3. Ask client about the current condition of his/her teeth. Ask client if he/she wears dentures. Do teeth or dentures bother client now?
4. Ask client whether he/she notices any movements in mouth, face, hands, or feet. If yes, ask to describe and to what extent they currently bother client or interfere with his/her activities.
5. Have client sit in chair with both hands on knees, legs slightly apart, and feet flat on floor. (Look at entire body for movements while in this position.)
6. Ask client to sit with hands hanging unsupported. If male, between legs, if female and wearing a dress, hanging over knees. (Observe hands and other body areas.)
7. Ask client to open mouth. (Observe tongue at rest within mouth.) Do this twice.
8. Ask client to protrude tongue. (Observe abnormalities of tongue movement.) Do this twice.
9. Ask client to tap thumb with each finger as rapidly as possible for 10 to 15 seconds; separately with right hand, then with left hand. (Observe facial and leg movements.)
10. Flex and extend client's left and right arms (one at a time). (Note any rigidity.)
11. Ask client to stand up. (Observe in profile. Observe all body areas again, hips included.)
12. Ask client to extend both arms outstretched in front with palms down. (Observe trunk, legs, and mouth.)
13. Have client walk a few paces, turn, and walk back to chair. (Observe hands and gait.) Do this twice.

INTERPRETATION OF AIMS SCORE

Add client scores and note areas of difficulty.
Score of:

- 0 to 1 = Low risk
- 2 in only ONE of the areas assessed = borderline/observe closely
- 2 in TWO or more of the areas assessed **or** 3 to 4 in ONLY ONE area = indicative of TD

From U.S. Department of Health and Human Services. Available for use in the public domain.

Some extrapyramidal side effects can be life-threatening, and those that are not can sometimes be permanent. The abnormal movements in the tongue and lips are sometimes very visible and severe enough to interfere with a person's ability to speak or swallow.

 The nurse's empathic approach in listening to the client's wishes with regard to medication and advocating for exploring other options for management of symptoms is one way to promote patient-centered care, an essential nursing competency, (!OM, 2003) and to promote a recovery model that empowers the client to make decisions about management of the illness. There is evidence that remaining on antipsychotic medication can reduce the frequency of hospitalization, so educating the client about this fact is important in assisting him or her to make an informed decision about medication treatment.

Hormonal Side Effects These may occur with all classifications but are more common with typical antipsychotics. Sexual side effects that may accompany these medications include decreased libido, **retrograde ejaculation,** and **gynecomastia** in men and

amenorrhea in women. These side effects can be troubling for anyone, but for a client struggling with thought disturbances, they can become the foundation for delusions. A male client with gynecomastia, for example, might begin to believe that external forces are taking over his body and turning him into a woman. An amenorrheic woman may begin to believe that she has been divinely impregnated. It is important for the nurse to be clear that these are side effects of the medication and offer reassurance that they are reversible. Women with amenorrhea should be instructed that this side effect does not indicate cessation of ovulation, so contraception use should continue as usual. Clients should be encouraged to explore alternative treatment if these side effects are deemed intolerable.

Current Developments in Psychopharmacological Treatment of Schizophrenia

One of the identified limitations of medication treatments available for schizophrenia is the cognitive deficits that are core symptoms of this illness, including deficits in working memory and long-term memory, reduced processing speed, limited verbal fluency, and impaired executive functions. Some atypical antipsychotics have demonstrated efficacy in lessening cognitive deficits but do not eliminate residual effects.

A drug recently approved by the FDA, *cariprazine* (Vraylor), has demonstrated efficacy in treating the negative symptoms of schizophrenia, including flat affect, social withdrawal, and apathy (Harrison, 2015). Although the atypical antipsychotics have been identified as better than typical antipsychotics in treating these symptoms, no drugs have yet been shown to eliminate them. Ongoing evaluation is needed to determine the effectiveness of cariprazine in this regard.

Outcome Criteria and Evaluation

The following criteria may be used for evaluating the effectiveness of therapy with antipsychotic medications.

The client:

- Has not harmed self or others
- Has not experienced injury caused by side effects of lowered seizure threshold or photosensitivity
- Maintains a WBC count within normal limits
- Exhibits no symptoms of extrapyramidal side effects, tardive dyskinesia, neuroleptic malignant syndrome, or hyperglycemia
- Maintains weight within normal limits
- Tolerates activity unaltered by the effects of sedation or weakness
- Takes medication willingly
- Verbalizes understanding of medication regimen and the importance of regular administration

Sedative-Hypnotics
Background Assessment Data
Indications

Sedative-hypnotics are used in the short-term management of various anxiety states and to treat insomnia. Selected agents are used as anticonvulsants (pentobarbital, phenobarbital) and preoperative sedatives (pentobarbital, secobarbital) and to reduce anxiety associated with alcohol withdrawal (chloral hydrate). (A table of current FDA-approved sedative-hypnotics, pregnancy categories, half-life, and daily dosage ranges can be found online at Davis*Plus*.) Examples of commonly used sedative-hypnotics are presented in Table 4–14.

Action

Sedative-hypnotics cause generalized CNS depression. They may produce tolerance with chronic use and have the potential for psychological or physical dependence.

> **EXCEPTION:** Ramelteon (Rozerem) is not a controlled substance. It does not produce tolerance or physical dependence. Sleep-promoting properties are the result of ramelteon's agonist activity on selective melatonin receptors.

Contraindications and Precautions

Sedative-hypnotics are contraindicated in individuals with hypersensitivity to the drug or to any drug within the chemical class; in pregnancy (exceptions may be made in certain cases based on benefit-to-risk ratio); during lactation; in severe hepatic, cardiac, respiratory, or renal disease; and in children younger than age 15 for flurazepam and those younger than age 18 for estazolam, quazepam, temazepam, triazolam. Triazolam is contraindicated in concurrent use with ketoconazole, itraconazole, or nefazodone, medications that impair the metabolism of triazolam by cytochrome P4503A (CYP3A). Ramelteon is contraindicated in concurrent use with fluvoxamine. Zolpidem, zaleplon, eszopiclone, and ramelteon are contraindicated in children. Chloral hydrate is contraindicated in persons with esophagitis, gastritis, or peptic ulcer disease and in those with hepatic, renal, or cardiac impairment.

Caution should be used in administering these drugs to clients with cardiac, hepatic, renal, or respiratory insufficiency. They should be used with caution in clients who may be suicidal or who previously may have been addicted to drugs. Hypnotic use should be short term. Elderly clients may be more sensitive to CNS depressant effects, and dosage reduction may be required. Chloral hydrate should be used with caution in clients susceptible to acute intermittent porphyria.

TABLE 4–14 Sedative-Hypnotic Agents

CHEMICAL CLASS	GENERIC (TRADE) NAME	CONTROLLED CATEGORIES	PREGNANCY CATEGORIES/ HALF-LIFE (hr)	DAILY DOSAGE RANGE (mg)
Barbiturates	Amobarbital	CII	D/16–40	60–200
	Butabarbital (Butisol)	CIII	D/66–140	45–120
	Pentobarbital (Nembutal)	CII	D/15–50	150–200
	Phenobarbital (Luminal; Solfoton)	CIV	D/53–118	30–200
	Secobarbital (Seconal)	CII	D/15–40	100 (hypnotic) 200–300 (preoperative sedation)
Benzodiazepines	Estazolam	CIV	X/8–28	1–2
	Flurazepam	CIV	X/2–3 (active metabolite: 47–100)	15–30
	Quazepam (Doral)	CIV	X/39 (active metabolite: 73)	7.5–15 mg
	Temazepam (Restoril)	CIV	X/9–15	15–30 mg
	Triazolam (Halcion)	CIV	X/1.5–5.5	0.125–0.5
Miscellaneous	Chloral hydrate	CIV	C/7–10	500–1,000
	Eszopiclone (Lunesta)	CIV	C/6	1–3
	Ramelteon (Rozerem)		C/1–2.6	8
	Zaleplon (Sonata)	CIV	C/1	5–20
	Zolpidem (Ambien)	CIV	C/2–3	5–10 (immediate release), 12.5 (extended release)

Interactions

Barbiturates The effects of barbiturates are increased with concomitant use of alcohol, other CNS depressants, MAOIs, or valproic acid. The effects of barbiturates may be decreased with rifampin. Possible decreased effects of the following drugs may occur when used concomitantly with barbiturates: anticoagulants, beta blockers, carbamazepine, clonazepam, oral contraceptives, corticosteroids, digitoxin, doxorubicin, doxycycline, felodipine, fenoprofen, griseofulvin, metronidazole, phenylbutazone, quinidine, theophylline, or verapamil. Concomitant use with methoxyflurane may enhance renal toxicity.

Benzodiazepines The effects of the benzodiazepine hypnotics are increased with concomitant use of alcohol or other CNS depressants, cimetidine, oral contraceptives, disulfiram, isoniazid, or probenecid. The effects of the benzodiazepine hypnotics are decreased with concomitant use of rifampin, theophylline, carbamazepine, or St. John's wort and with cigarette smoking. The effects of digoxin or phenytoin are increased when used concomitantly with benzodiazepines. Bioavailability of triazolam is increased with concurrent use of macrolides.

Eszopiclone Additive effects of eszopiclone occur with alcohol or other CNS depressants. Decreased effects of eszopiclone occur with CYP3A4 inducers (e.g., rifampin, phenytoin, carbamazepine, phenobarbital), with lorazepam, or following a high-fat or heavy meal. Increased effects of eszopiclone occur with CYP3A4 inhibitors (e.g., ketoconazole, clarithromycin, nefazodone, ritonavir). There are decreased effects of lorazepam with concomitant use.

Zaleplon Additive effects of zaleplon occur with alcohol or other CNS depressants. Decreased effects of zaleplon occur with CYP3A4 inducers (e.g., rifampin, phenytoin, carbamazepine, phenobarbital) or following a high-fat or heavy meal. There are increased effects of zaleplon with cimetidine.

Zolpidem Increased effects of zolpidem occur with alcohol or other CNS depressants, azole antifungals, ritonavir, or SSRIs. Decreased effects of zolpidem occur with flumazenil, rifampin, and with food. There is a risk of life-threatening cardiac arrhythmias with concomitant use of amiodarone.

Ramelteon Increased effects of ramelteon occur with alcohol, ketoconazole (and other CYP3A4 inhibitors), or fluvoxamine (and other CYP1A2 inhibitors). Decreased effects of ramelteon occur with rifampin (and other CYP3A4 inducers) and following a heavy or high-fat meal.

Diagnosis

The following nursing diagnoses may be considered for clients receiving therapy with sedative hypnotics:

■ Risk for injury related to abrupt withdrawal from long-term use or decreased mental alertness caused by residual sedation

■ Disturbed sleep pattern and/or insomnia related to situational crises, physical condition, or severe level of anxiety
■ Risk for activity intolerance related to side effects of lethargy, drowsiness, and dizziness
■ Risk for acute confusion related to action of the medication on the CNS

Safety Issues in Planning and Implementing Care

Refer to the earlier discussion of safety issues in the section "Antianxiety Agents." In addition to the side effects listed in that section, abnormal thinking and behavioral changes, including aggressiveness, hallucinations, and suicidal ideation, have also been noted in some individuals taking sedative-hypnotics. Certain complex behaviors, such as sleep-driving, preparing and eating food, and making phone calls, with amnesia for the behavior, have occurred. Although a direct correlation to the behavior with the use of sedative-hypnotics cannot be made, the emergence of any new behavioral sign or symptom of concern requires careful and immediate evaluation.

Outcome Criteria and Evaluation

The following criteria may be used for evaluating the effectiveness of therapy with sedative-hypnotic medications.

The client:

■ Demonstrates a reduction in anxiety, tension, and restless activity
■ Falls asleep within 30 minutes of taking the medication and remains asleep for 6 to 8 hours without interruption
■ Is able to participate in usual activities without residual sedation
■ Experiences no physical injury
■ Exhibits no evidence of confusion
■ Verbalizes understanding of taking the medication on a short-term basis
■ Verbalizes understanding of potential for development of tolerance and dependence with long-term use

Agents for Attention-Deficit/Hyperactivity Disorder (ADHD)
Background Assessment Data
Indications

The medications in this section are used for ADHD in children and adults. Amphetamines are also used in the treatment of narcolepsy and exogenous obesity. Bupropion is used in the treatment of major depression and for smoking cessation (Zyban only). Clonidine and guanfacine are used to treat hypertension. (A table of current FDA-approved agents for ADHD, pregnancy categories, half-life, and daily dosage ranges can be found online at Davis*Plus* and in Chapter 33, Children and Adolescents.)

Action

CNS stimulants increase levels of neurotransmitters (probably norepinephrine, dopamine, and serotonin) in the CNS. They produce CNS and respiratory stimulation, dilated pupils, increased motor activity and mental alertness, diminished sense of fatigue, and brighter spirits. The CNS stimulants discussed in this section include dextroamphetamine sulfate, methamphetamine, lisdexamfetamine, amphetamine mixtures, methylphenidate, and dexmethylphenidate. Action in the treatment of ADHD is unclear. However, recent research indicates that their effectiveness in the treatment of hyperactivity disorders is based on the activation of dopamine D_4 receptors in the basal ganglia and thalamus, which depress rather than enhance motor activity (Erlij et al., 2012).

Atomoxetine inhibits the reuptake of norepinephrine, and bupropion blocks the neuronal uptake of serotonin, norepinephrine, and dopamine. Clonidine and guanfacine stimulate central alpha-adrenergic receptors in the brain, resulting in reduced sympathetic outflow from the CNS. The exact mechanism by which these nonstimulant drugs produce the therapeutic effect in ADHD is unclear.

Contraindications and Precautions

CNS stimulants are contraindicated in individuals with hypersensitivity to sympathomimetic amines. They should not be used in patients with advanced arteriosclerosis, cardiovascular disease, hypertension, hyperthyroidism, glaucoma, or agitated or hyperexcitability states; in clients with a history of drug abuse; during or within 14 days of receiving therapy with MAOIs; in children younger than age 3; or in pregnancy and lactation. Atomoxetine and bupropion are contraindicated in clients with hypersensitivity to the drugs or their components, in lactation, and in concomitant use with or within 2 weeks of using MAOIs. Atomoxetine is contraindicated in clients with narrow-angle glaucoma. Bupropion is contraindicated in individuals with known or suspected seizure disorder, in the acute phase of MI, and in clients with bulimia or anorexia nervosa. Alpha agonists are contraindicated in clients with known hypersensitivity to the drugs.

Caution is advised in using CNS stimulants in children with psychosis; in Tourette's disorder; in clients with anorexia or insomnia; in elderly, debilitated, or asthenic clients; and in clients with a history of suicidal or homicidal tendencies. Prolonged use may result in tolerance and physical or psychological dependence. Use atomoxetine and bupropion cautiously in clients with urinary retention, hypertension, or hepatic, renal, or cardiovascular disease; in suicidal clients; during pregnancy; and in elderly and debilitated clients. Alpha agonists should be used with caution in clients with coronary insufficiency, recent MI, or cerebrovascular disease; in chronic renal or hepatic failure; in the elderly; and in pregnancy and lactation.

Interactions

CNS Stimulants (Amphetamines) Effects of amphetamines are increased with furazolidone or urinary alkalinizers. Hypertensive crisis may occur with concomitant use of (and up to several weeks after discontinuing) MAOIs. Increased risk of serotonin syndrome occurs with coadministration of SSRIs. Decreased effects of amphetamines occur with urinary acidifiers, and decreased hypotensive effects of guanethidine occur with amphetamines.

Dexmethylphenidate and Methylphenidate Effects of antihypertensive agents and pressor agents (e.g., dopamine, epinephrine, phenylephrine) are decreased with concomitant use of the methylphenidates. Effects of coumarin anticoagulants, anticonvulsants (e.g., phenobarbital, phenytoin, primidone), tricyclic antidepressants, and SSRIs are increased with the methylphenidates. Hypertensive crisis may occur with coadministration of MAOIs.

Atomoxetine Effects of atomoxetine are increased with concomitant use of CYP2D6 inhibitors (e.g., paroxetine, fluoxetine, quinidine). Potentially fatal reactions may occur with concurrent use of (or within 2 weeks of discontinuation of) MAOIs. Risk of cardiovascular effects is increased with concomitant use of albuterol or vasopressors.

Bupropion Effects of bupropion are increased with amantadine, levodopa, or ritonavir. Effects of bupropion are decreased with carbamazepine. There is increased risk of acute toxicity with MAOIs. Increased risk of hypertension may occur with nicotine replacement agents, and adverse neuropsychiatric events may occur with alcohol. Increased anticoagulant effects of warfarin and increased effects of drugs metabolized by CYP2D6 (e.g., nortriptyline, imipramine, desipramine, paroxetine, fluoxetine, sertraline, haloperidol, risperidone, thioridazine, metoprolol, propafenone, and flecainide) occur with concomitant use.

Alpha Agonists Synergistic pharmacologic and toxic effects, possibly causing atrioventricular block, bradycardia, and severe hypotension, may occur with concomitant use of calcium channel blockers or beta-blockers. Additive sedation occurs with CNS depressants, including alcohol, antihistamines, opioid analgesics, and sedative-hypnotics. Effects of clonidine may be decreased with concomitant use

of tricyclic antidepressants and prazosin. Decreased effects of levodopa may occur with clonidine, and effects of guanfacine are decreased with barbiturates or phenytoin.

Diagnosis

The following nursing diagnoses may be considered for clients receiving therapy with agents for ADHD:

■ Risk for injury related to overstimulation and hyperactivity (CNS stimulants) or seizures (possible side effect of bupropion)
■ Risk for suicide secondary to major depression related to abrupt withdrawal after extended use (CNS stimulants)
■ Risk for suicide (children and adolescents) as a side effect of atomoxetine and bupropion (black-box warning)
■ Imbalanced nutrition, less than body requirements, related to side effects of anorexia and weight loss (CNS stimulants)
■ Insomnia related to side effects of overstimulation
■ Nausea related to side effects of atomoxetine or bupropion
■ Pain related to side effect of abdominal pain (atomoxetine, bupropion) or headache (all agents)
■ Risk for activity intolerance related to side effects of sedation and dizziness with atomoxetine or bupropion

Planning and Implementation

The plan of care should include monitoring for the following side effects from agents for ADHD. Nursing implications related to each side effect are designated by an asterisk (*).

■ Overstimulation, restlessness, insomnia (CNS stimulants)
  *Assess mental status for changes in mood, level of activity, degree of stimulation, and aggressiveness.
  *Ensure that the client is protected from injury.
  *Keep stimuli low and environment as quiet as possible to discourage overstimulation.
  *To prevent insomnia, administer the last dose at least 6 hours before bedtime. Administer sustained-release forms in the morning.
■ Palpitations, tachycardia (CNS stimulants, atomoxetine, bupropion, clonidine), or bradycardia (clonidine, guanfacine)
  *Monitor and record vital signs at regular intervals (two or three times a day) throughout therapy. Report significant changes to the physician immediately.

  NOTE: The FDA has issued warnings associated with CNS stimulants and atomoxetine of the risk for sudden death in patients who have cardiovascular disease. A careful personal and family history of heart disease, heart defects, or hypertension should be obtained before these medications are prescribed. Careful monitoring of cardiovascular function during administration must be ongoing.

■ Anorexia, weight loss (CNS stimulants, atomoxetine, bupropion)

*To reduce anorexia, the medication may be administered immediately after meals.

*The client should be weighed regularly (at least weekly) when receiving therapy with CNS stimulants, atomoxetine, or bupropion because of the potential for anorexia and weight loss and temporary interruption of growth and development.

■ Tolerance, physical and psychological dependence (CNS stimulants)

*In children with ADHD, a drug "holiday" should be attempted periodically under direction of the physician to determine the effectiveness of the medication and the need for continuation.

*The drug should not be withdrawn abruptly. To do so could initiate a syndrome of symptoms with nausea, vomiting, abdominal cramping, headache, fatigue, weakness, mental depression, suicidal ideation, increased dreaming, and psychotic behavior.

■ Nausea and vomiting (atomoxetine and bupropion)

*Recommend taking medication with food to minimize gastrointestinal upset.

■ Constipation (atomoxetine, bupropion, clonidine, guanfacine)

*Recommend increasing fiber and fluid in diet if not contraindicated.

■ Dry mouth (clonidine and guanfacine)

*Offer the client sugarless candy, ice, frequent sips of water.

*Strict oral hygiene is very important.

■ Sedation (clonidine and guanfacine)

*Warn the client that this effect is increased by concomitant use of alcohol and other CNS drugs.

*Warn the client to refrain from driving or performing hazardous tasks until response has been established.

■ Potential for seizures (bupropion)

*Protect the client from injury if seizure should occur.

*Instruct family and significant others of clients on bupropion therapy how to protect the client during a seizure if one should occur.

*Ensure that doses of the immediate-release medication are administered at least 4 to 6 hours apart and doses of the sustained-release medication at least 8 hours apart.

■ Severe liver damage (with atomoxetine)

*Monitor for the following side effects and report to physician immediately: itching, dark urine, right upper quadrant pain, yellow skin or eyes, sore throat, fever, malaise.

■ New or worsened psychiatric symptoms (with CNS stimulants and atomoxetine)

*Monitor for psychotic symptoms (e.g., hearing voices, paranoid behaviors, delusions).

*Monitor for manic symptoms, including aggressive and hostile behaviors.

■ Rebound syndrome (with clonidine and guanfacine)

*The client should be instructed not to discontinue therapy abruptly. To do so may result in symptoms of nervousness, agitation, headache, tremor, and a rapid rise in blood pressure. In addition, sudden withdrawal from stimulants may increase the risk for depression and suicide.

Dosage should be tapered gradually under the supervision of the physician.

Client and Family Education

Instruct the client and/or family that the client should:

■ Use caution when driving or operating dangerous machinery. Drowsiness, dizziness, and blurred vision can occur.

■ Not stop taking CNS stimulants abruptly. To do so could produce serious withdrawal symptoms.

■ Avoid taking CNS stimulants late in the day to prevent insomnia. Take medication no later than 6 hours before bedtime.

■ Not take other medications (including over-the-counter drugs) without physician's approval. Many medications contain substances that, in combination with agents for ADHD, can be harmful.

■ Monitor blood sugar two or three times a day or as instructed by the physician if the client is diabetic. Be aware of the need for possible alteration in insulin requirements because of changes in food intake, weight, and activity.

■ Avoid consumption of large amounts of caffeinated products (coffee, tea, colas, chocolate), as they may enhance the CNS stimulant effect.

■ Notify physician if restlessness, insomnia, anorexia, or dry mouth becomes severe or if rapid, pounding heartbeat becomes evident.

■ Report any of the following side effects to the physician immediately: shortness of breath, chest pain, jaw/left arm pain, fainting, seizures, sudden vision changes, weakness on one side of the body, slurred speech, confusion, itching, dark urine, right-upper quadrant pain, yellow skin or eyes, sore throat, fever, malaise, increased hyperactivity, believing things that are not true, or hearing voices.

■ Be aware of possible risks of taking agents for ADHD during pregnancy. Safe use during pregnancy and lactation has not been established. Inform the physician immediately if pregnancy is suspected or planned.

■ Be aware of potential side effects of agents for ADHD. Refer to written materials furnished by health-care providers for safe self-administration.

■ Carry a card or other identification at all times describing medications being taken.

Outcome Criteria and Evaluation

The following criteria may be used for evaluating the effectiveness of therapy with agents for ADHD.

The client:

■ Does not exhibit excessive hyperactivity
■ Has not experienced injury
■ Is maintaining expected parameters of growth and development
■ Verbalizes understanding of safe self-administration and the importance of not withdrawing medication abruptly

Summary and Key Points

■ Psychotropic medications are intended to be used as adjunctive therapy to individual or group psychotherapy.

■ *Antianxiety agents* are used in the treatment of anxiety disorders and to alleviate acute anxiety symptoms. Benzodiazepines are the most commonly used group. They are CNS depressants and have a potential for physical and psychological dependence. They should not be discontinued abruptly following long-term use because they can produce a life-threatening withdrawal syndrome. The most common side effects are drowsiness, confusion, and lethargy.

■ *Antidepressants* elevate mood and alleviate other symptoms associated with moderate-to-severe depression. These drugs work to increase the concentration of norepinephrine and serotonin in the body.

■ The tricyclics and related drugs accomplish their effect by blocking the reuptake of norepinephrine by the neurons.

■ Another group of antidepressants inhibits MAO, an enzyme that is known to inactivate norepinephrine and serotonin. They are called MAOIs.

■ A third category of drugs blocks neuronal reuptake of serotonin and has minimal or no effect on reuptake of norepinephrine or dopamine. SSRIs.

■ Antidepressant medications may take up to 2 weeks before desired effects are noticed and may take up to 4 weeks to produce full therapeutic benefits.

The most common side effects are anticholinergic effects, sedation, and orthostatic hypotension. They can also reduce the seizure threshold. MAOIs can cause hypertensive crisis if products containing tyramine are consumed while taking these medications.

■ Lithium carbonate is widely used as a *mood-stabilizing agent*. Its mechanism of action is not fully understood, but it is thought to enhance the reuptake of norepinephrine and serotonin in the brain, thereby lowering the levels in the body, resulting in decreased hyperactivity. The most common side effects are dry mouth, gastrointestinal upset, polyuria, and weight gain.

■ There is a very narrow margin between the therapeutic and toxic levels of lithium. Serum levels must be drawn regularly to monitor for toxicity. Symptoms of lithium toxicity begin to appear at serum levels of approximately 1.5 mEq/L. If left untreated, lithium toxicity can be life threatening.

■ Several other medications are used as mood-stabilizing agents. Two groups, anticonvulsants (carbamazepine, clonazepam, valproic acid, lamotrigine, oxcarbazepine, and topiramate) and the calcium channel blocker verapamil, have been used with some effectiveness. Their action in the treatment of bipolar mania is not well understood.

■ Most recently, several atypical antipsychotic medications have been used with success in the treatment of bipolar mania. These include olanzapine, aripiprazole, quetiapine, risperidone, asenapine, and ziprasidone. The phenothiazine chlorpromazine has also been used effectively. The action of antipsychotics in the treatment of bipolar mania is not understood.

■ *Antipsychotic drugs* are used in the treatment of acute and chronic psychoses. The action of phenothiazines is caused by blocking postsynaptic dopamine receptors in the basal ganglia. Their most common side effects include anticholinergic effects, sedation, weight gain, reduction in seizure threshold, photosensitivity, and extrapyramidal symptoms. A newer generation of antipsychotic medications, which includes clozapine, risperidone, paliperidone, olanzapine, quetiapine, aripiprazole, asenapine, iloperidone, lurasidone, and ziprasidone, may have an effect on dopamine, serotonin, and other neurotransmitters. They show promise of greater efficacy with fewer side effects.

■ *Antiparkinsonian agents* are used to counteract the extrapyramidal symptoms associated with antipsychotic medications. Antiparkinsonian drugs work to restore the natural balance of acetylcholine and dopamine in the brain. The most common side effects of these drugs are the anticholinergic effects. They may also cause sedation and orthostatic hypotension.

■ *Sedative-hypnotics* are used in the management of anxiety states and to treat insomnia. These CNS depressants (except ramelteon) have the potential for physical and psychological dependence. They are indicated for short-term use only. Side effects and nursing implications are similar to those described for antianxiety medications.

■ Several medications have been designated as *agents for treatment of ADHD*. These include CNS stimulants, which have the potential for physical and psychological dependence. Tolerance develops quickly with CNS stimulants, and they should not be withdrawn abruptly because they can produce serious withdrawal symptoms. The most common side effects are restlessness, anorexia, and insomnia. Other medications that have shown to be effective with ADHD include atomoxetine, bupropion, and the α-adrenergic agonists clonidine and guanfacine. Their mechanism of action in the treatment of ADHD is not clear.

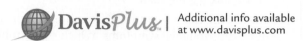

DavisPlus | Additional info available at www.davisplus.com

Review Questions
Self-Examination/Learning Exercise

Select the answer that is most appropriate for each of the following questions.

1. How do antianxiety medications, such as benzodiazepines, produce a calming effect?
   a. Depressing the CNS
   b. Decreasing levels of norepinephrine and serotonin in the brain
   c. Decreasing levels of dopamine in the brain
   d. Inhibiting production of the enzyme MAO

2. Tam has a new diagnosis of panic disorder. Dr. S has written a prn order for alprazolam (Xanax) for when Tam is feeling anxious. She says to the nurse, "Dr. S prescribed buspirone for my friend's anxiety. Why did he order something different for me?" The nurse's answer is based on which of the following?
   a. Buspirone is not an antianxiety medication.
   b. Alprazolam and buspirone are essentially the same medication, so either one is appropriate.
   c. Buspirone has delayed onset of action and cannot be used on a prn basis.
   d. Alprazolam is the only medication that really works for panic disorder.

3. Education for the client who is taking MAOIs should include which of the following?
   a. Fluid and sodium replacement when appropriate, frequent drug blood levels, signs and symptoms of toxicity
   b. Lifetime of continuous use, possible tardive dyskinesia, advantages of an injection every 2 to 4 weeks
   c. Short-term use, possible tolerance to beneficial effects, careful tapering of the drug at end of treatment
   d. Tyramine-restricted diet, prohibitive concurrent use of over-the-counter medications without physician notification

4. There is a very narrow margin between the therapeutic and toxic levels of lithium carbonate. Symptoms of toxicity are most likely to appear if the serum levels exceed:
   a. 0.15 mEq/L
   b. 1.5 mEq/L
   c. 15.0 mEq/L
   d. 150 mEq/L

5. Initial symptoms of lithium toxicity include:
   a. Constipation, dry mouth
   b. Dizziness, thirst
   c. Vomiting, diarrhea
   d. Anuria, arrhythmias

Continued

Review Questions—cont'd
Self-Examination/Learning Exercise

6. Antipsychotic medications are thought to decrease psychotic symptoms by:
   a. Blocking reuptake of norepinephrine and serotonin
   b. Blocking the action of dopamine in the brain
   c. Inhibiting production of the enzyme MAO
   d. Depressing the CNS

7. Part of the nurse's continual assessment of the client taking antipsychotic medications is to observe for extrapyramidal symptoms. Which of the following are examples of extrapyramidal symptoms?
   a. Muscular weakness, rigidity, tremors, facial spasms
   b. Dry mouth, blurred vision, urinary retention, orthostatic hypotension
   c. Amenorrhea, gynecomastia, retrograde ejaculation
   d. Elevated blood pressure, severe occipital headache, stiff neck

8. If the foregoing extrapyramidal symptoms should occur, which of the following would be a priority nursing intervention?
   a. Notify the physician immediately.
   b. Administer prn trihexyphenidyl (Artane).
   c. Withhold the next dose of antipsychotic medication.
   d. Explain to the client that these symptoms are only temporary and will disappear shortly.

9. A concern with children on long-term therapy with CNS stimulants for ADHD is:
   a. Addiction
   b. Weight gain
   c. Substance abuse
   d. Growth suppression

10. Doses of bupropion should be administered at least 4 to 6 hours apart and never doubled when a dose is missed in order to prevent:
    a. Orthostatic hypotension
    b. Seizures
    c. Hypertensive crisis
    d. Extrapyramidal symptoms

References

Berna, F., Misdrahi, D., Boyer, L., Aouizerate, B., Brunel, L., Capdevielle, D., Liorca, P.M. (2015). Prevalence and risk factors in a community dwelling sample of patients with Schizophrenia. Results from the FACE-SZ dataset. *Schizophrenia Research, 169*(1-3), 255-261.

Black, D.W., & Andreasen, N.C. (2014). *Introductory textbook of psychiatry* (6th ed.). Washington, DC: American Psychiatric Publishing.

Brust, T.F., Hayes, M.P., Roman, D.L., & Watts, V.J. (2015). New functional activity of aripiprazole revealed: Robust antagonism of D2 dopamine receptor-stimulated Gβγ signaling. *Biochemical Pharmacology, 93*(1), 85-91. doi:10.1016/j.bcp.2014.10.014

Cooper, B.E., & Sejnowski, C.A. (2013). Serotonin syndrome: Recognition and treatment. *AACN Advanced Critical Care, 24*(1), 15-20. doi:10.1097/NCI.0b013e31827eecc6

Erlij, D., Acosta-Garcia, J., Rojas-Marquez, M., Gonzalez-Hernandez, B., Escartin-Perez, E., Aceves, J., & Floran, B. (2012). Dopamine D4 receptor stimulation in GABAergic projections of the globus pallidus to the reticular thalamic nucleus and the substantia nigra reticulata of the rat decreases locomotor activity. *Neuropharmacology, 62*(2), 1111-1118. doi:10.1016/j.neuropharm.2011.11.001

Facts and Comparisons (Firm) & Wolters Kluwer Health. (2014). *Drug facts and comparisons.* St. Louis, MO: Wolters Kluwer.

FDA (Food and Drug Administration). (2017). *FDA approves first drug to treat tardive dyskinesia.* Retrieved from https://www.fda.gov/NewsEvents/Newsroom/PressAnnouncements/ucm552418.htm

FDA (U.S. Food and Drug Administration). (2008). FDA requires warnings about risk of suicidal thoughts and behavior for antiepileptic medications. Retrieved from https://www.fda.gov/Drugs/DrugSafety/PostmarketDrugSafetyInformationforPatientsandProviders/ucm100197.htm

Fournier, J.C., DeRubeis, R.J., Hollon, S.D., Dimidjian, S., Amsterdam, J.D., Shelton, R.C., & Fawcett, J. (2010). Antidepressant drug effects and depression severity: A patient-level meta-analysis. *Journal of the American Medical Association, 303*(1), 47-53. doi:10.1001/jama.2009.1943

Harrison, P. (2015). Novel drug first to treat negative symptoms in schizophrenia. Retrieved from www.medscape.com/viewarticle/850701

Institute of Medicine. (2003). *Health professions education: A bridge to quality*. Washington, DC: Author.

Jacob, S., & Spinier, S.A. (2006). Hyponatremia associated with selective serotonin-inhibitors in older adults. *Annals of Pharmacotherapy, 40*(9), 1618-1622. doi:10.1345/aph.1G293

Lenze, E.J., Mulsant, B.H., Blumberger, D.M., Karp, J.F., Newcomer, J.W., Anderson, S.J., . . . Reynolds, C.F. (2015). Efficacy, safety, and tolerability of augmentation pharmacotherapy with aripiprazole for treatment resistant depression in late life: A randomized placebo-controlled study. *Lancet, 386*(10011), 2404-2412. doi:http://dx.doi.org/10.1016/So140-6736(15)00308-6

National Institute of Mental Health (NIMH). (2006). *Questions and answers about the NIMH sequenced treatment alternatives to relieve depression (STAR*D) study—all medication levels*. Retrieved from https://www.nimh.nih.gov/funding/clinical-research/practical/stard/allmedicationlevels.shtml

New York State Office of Mental Health. (2006). An explanation of Kendra's law. Retrieved from https://www.omh.ny.gov/omhweb/Kendra_web/Ksummary.htm

Purnell, L.D. (2014). *Guide to culturally competent health care* (3rd ed.). Philadelphia: F.A. Davis.

Ramnarine, M., & Ahmed, D. (2015). Anticholinergic toxicity. Retrieved from http://emedicine.medscape.com/article/812644-overview

Sadock, B.J., Sadock, V.A., & Ruiz, P. (2015). *Synopsis of psychiatry: Behavioral sciences/clinical psychiatry* (11th ed.). Philadelphia: Lippincott Williams & Wilkins.

Sage, D.L. (Producer). (1984). *The brain: Madness* [television broadcast]. Washington, DC: Public Broadcasting Company.

Schatzberg, A.F., Cole, J.O., & DeBattista, C. (2010). *Manual of clinical psychopharmacology* (7th ed.). Washington, DC: American Psychiatric Publishing.

Shorter, E. (2009). The history of lithium therapy. *Bipolar Disorders, 11*(Suppl. 2), 4-9. doi:10.1111/j.1399-5618.2009.00706.x

Steinberg, M., & Lyketsos, C.G. (2012). Atypical antipsychotic use in patients with dementia: Managing safety concerns. *American Journal of Psychiatry, 169*(9), 900-906. doi:10.1176/appi.aip.2012.12030342

Tartakovsky, M. (2016). *Depression: New medications on the horizon*. Retrieved from https://psychcentral.com/lib/depression-new-medications-on-the-horizon/

Vallerand, A.H., Sanoski, C.A., & Deglin, J.H. (2016). *Davis drug guide for nurses* (15th ed.). Philadelphia: F.A. Davis.

5

Ethical and Legal Issues

CORE CONCEPTS

Bioethics

Ethics

Moral Behavior

Right

Values

Values Clarification

CHAPTER OUTLINE

Objectives   Legal Considerations

Homework Assignment   Summary and Key Points

Ethical Considerations   Review Questions

KEY TERMS

advocacy	ethical dilemma	negligence
assault	ethical egoism	nonmaleficence
autonomy	ethics	privileged communication
battery	false imprisonment	right
beneficence	informed consent	slander
bioethics	justice	statutory law
Christian ethics	Kantianism	tort
civil law	libel	utilitarianism
common law	malpractice	values
criminal law	moral behavior	values clarification
defamation of character	natural law theory	veracity

OBJECTIVES
After reading this chapter, the student will be able to:

1. Differentiate among *ethics, morals, values,* and *rights.*
2. Discuss ethical theories, including *utilitarianism, Kantianism, Christian ethics, natural law theories,* and *ethical egoism.*
3. Define *ethical dilemma.*
4. Discuss the ethical principles of *autonomy, beneficence, nonmaleficence, justice,* and *veracity.*
5. Use an ethical decision-making model to make an ethical decision.
6. Describe ethical issues relevant to psychiatric-mental health nursing.
7. Define *statutory law* and *common law.*
8. Differentiate between *civil law* and *criminal law.*
9. Discuss legal issues relevant to psychiatric-mental health nursing.
10. Differentiate between *malpractice* and *negligence.*
11. Identify behaviors relevant to the psychiatric-mental health setting for which specific malpractice action could be taken.

HOMEWORK ASSIGNMENT
Please read the chapter and answer the following questions:

1. Malpractice and negligence are examples of what kind of law?
2. What charges may be brought against a nurse for confining a client against his or her wishes (outside of an emergency situation)?
3. Which ethical theory espouses that what is right and good is what is best for the individual making the decision?
4. Name the three major elements of informed consent.

Nurses are constantly faced with the challenge of making difficult decisions regarding good and evil or life and death. Complex situations frequently arise in caring for individuals with mental illness, and nurses are held to the highest level of legal and ethical accountability in their professional practice. This chapter presents basic ethical and legal concepts and their relationship to psychiatric-mental health nursing. A discussion of ethical theory is presented as a foundation upon which ethical decisions may be made. The American Nurses Association (ANA) (2015) has established a code of ethics for nurses to use as a framework within which to make ethical choices and decisions (Box 5–1). These recently revised provisions and interpretive guidelines have been expanded to address some of the complexities of the current health-care environment and include ethical principles regarding the nurse's duty not only to the patient but also to himself or herself and all people with whom he or she interacts. All relationships should be conducted within a culture of respect and civility.

◆ The ANA Code of Ethics interpretive guidelines include a discussion of the importance of teamwork and collaboration, which is consistent with one of the recommendations of the Institute of Medicine (IOM) (2003) for improving the future of health care and has become one of the Quality and Safety in Education for Nurses (QSEN) standards.

The ANA, in cooperation with the American Psychiatric Nurses Association and the International Society of Psychiatric-Mental Health Nurses (2014), has published a scope and standards of practice manual specifically for psychiatric-mental health nursing. It maintains consistency with the ANA code of ethics and applies those provisions to psychiatric-mental health nursing issues. Knowledge about the *Code of Ethics for Nurses* (ANA, 2015) and *Psychiatric-Mental Health Nursing: Scope and Standards of Practice* (ANA et al., 2014) are essential for guiding practice because they clarify the accepted expectations of the nurse in this field.

Because legislation determines what is *right* or *good* within a society, legal issues pertaining to psychiatric-mental health nursing are also discussed in this chapter. Definitions are presented along with rights of psychiatric clients of which nurses must be aware. Nursing competency and client care accountability are compromised when the nurse has inadequate knowledge about the laws that regulate the practice of nursing.

Knowledge of the legal and ethical concepts presented in this chapter will enhance the quality of care the nurse provides in his or her psychiatric-mental

BOX 5–1 American Nurses Association Code of Ethics for Nurses

1. The nurse practices with compassion and respect for the inherent dignity, worth, and unique attributes of every person.
2. The nurse's primary commitment is to the patient whether an individual, family, group, community, or population.
3. The nurse promotes, advocates for, and strives to protect the health, safety, and rights of the patient.
4. The nurse has authority, accountability, and responsibility for nursing practice; makes decisions; and takes action consistent with the obligation to promote health and to provide optimal care.
5. The nurse owes the same duties to self as to others, including the responsibility to promote health and safety, preserve wholeness of character and integrity, maintain competence, and continue personal and professional growth.
6. The nurse, through individual and collective effort, establishes, maintains, and improves the ethical environment of the work setting and conditions of employment that are conducive to safe, quality health care.
7. The nurse, in all roles and settings, advances the profession through research and scholarly inquiry, professional standards development, and the generation of both nursing and health policy.
8. The nurse collaborates with other health professionals and the public to protect human rights, promote health diplomacy, and reduce health disparities.
9. The profession of nursing, collectively through its professional organizations, must articulate nursing values, maintain the integrity of the profession and integrate principles of social justice into nursing and health policy.

Reprinted with permission from American Nurses Association (ANA). (2015). Code of Ethics for Nurses with Interpretive Statements. Silver Spring, MD: ANA. © 2015.

health nursing practice and will also protect the nurse within the parameters of legal accountability. The right to practice nursing carries with it the responsibility to maintain a specific level of competency and to practice in accordance with certain ethical and legal standards of care.

CORE CONCEPTS

Ethics is a branch of philosophy that deals with systematic approaches to distinguishing right from wrong behavior (Butts & Rich, 2016). **Bioethics** is the term applied to these principles when they refer to concepts within the scope of medicine, nursing, and allied health.

Moral behavior is conduct that results from serious critical thinking about how individuals ought to treat others. Moral behavior reflects the way a person interprets basic respect for other persons, such as the respect for autonomy, freedom, justice, honesty, and confidentiality.

Values are personal beliefs about what is important and desirable (Butts & Rich, 2016). Values clarification is a process of self-exploration through which individuals identify and rank their own personal values. This process increases awareness about why individuals behave in certain ways. Values clarification is important in nursing to increase understanding about why certain choices and decisions are made over others and how values affect nursing outcomes.

A right is "a valid, legally recognized claim or entitlement, encompassing both freedom from government interference or discriminatory treatment and an entitlement to a benefit or service" (Levy & Rubenstein, 1996). A right is *absolute* when there is no restriction whatsoever on the individual's entitlement. A *legal right* is one on which the society has agreed and formalized into law. Both the National League for Nursing (NLN) and the American Hospital Association (AHA) have established guidelines of patients' rights. Although these are not considered legal documents, nurses and hospitals are responsible for upholding these patients' rights.

Ethical Considerations

Theoretical Perspectives

An *ethical theory* is a moral principle or a set of moral principles that can be used in assessing what is morally right or morally wrong (Ellis & Hartley, 2012). These principles provide frameworks for ethical decision-making.

Utilitarianism

The basis of **utilitarianism** is the "greatest-happiness principle." This principle holds that actions are right to the degree that they tend to promote happiness and are wrong as they tend to produce the reverse of happiness. Thus, the good is happiness and the right is that which promotes the good. Conversely, the wrongness of an action is determined by its tendency to bring about unhappiness. An ethical decision based on the utilitarian view looks at the end results of the decision. Action is taken on the basis of the end results that will produce the most good (happiness) for the most people.

Kantianism

Named for philosopher Immanuel Kant, **Kantianism** is directly opposed to utilitarianism. Kant argued that it is not the consequences or end results that make an action right or wrong; rather it is the principle or motivation on which the action is based that is the morally decisive factor. Kantianism suggests that our actions are bound by a sense of duty. This theory is often called *deontology* (from the Greek word *deon,* which means "that which is binding; duty"). Kantian-directed ethical decisions are made out of respect for moral law. For example, "I make this choice because it is morally right and my duty to do so" (not because of consideration for a possible outcome).

Christian Ethics

This approach to ethical decision-making is focused on the way of life and teachings of Jesus Christ. It advances the importance of virtues such as love, forgiveness, and honesty. One basic principle often associated with Christian ethics is known as the golden rule: "Do unto others as you would have them do unto you." The imperative demand of **Christian ethics** is that all decisions about right and wrong should be centered in love for God and in treating others with the same respect and dignity with which we would expect to be treated.

Natural Law Theory

Natural law theory is based on the writings of St. Thomas Aquinas. It advances the idea that decisions about right versus wrong are self-evident and determined by human nature. The theory espouses that, as rational human beings, we inherently know the difference between good and evil (believed to be knowledge that is given to man from God), and this knowledge directs our decision-making.

Ethical Egoism

Ethical egoism espouses that what is right and good is what is best for the individual making the decision. An individual's actions are determined by what is to his or her own advantage. The action may not be best for anyone else involved, but consideration is only for the individual making the decision.

Ethical Dilemmas

An **ethical dilemma** in nursing is a situation that requires the nurse to make a choice between two equally unfavorable alternatives (Catalano, 2015). Evidence exists to support both moral "rightness" and moral "wrongness" related to a certain action. The individual who must make the choice experiences conscious conflict regarding the decision.

Not all ethical issues are dilemmas. An ethical dilemma arises when there is no clear reason to choose one action over another. Ethical dilemmas generally create a great deal of emotion. Often, the reasons supporting each side of the argument for action are logical and appropriate. The actions associated with both sides are desirable in some respects and undesirable in others. In most situations, taking no action is considered an action taken. For example, consider a patient who refuses to take a prescribed cardiac medication, claiming that he does not believe it is necessary. Although each patient has the right to refuse medication under ordinary circumstances, if the same patient is known to be depressed and suicidal, might he be intending self-harm by his refusal to take such a medication? And, if so, what is the best course of action? Many health-care settings have established guidelines for how to proceed should an ethical question or dilemma arise. Hospitals typically have a formal committee to explore and analyze ethical issues from several vantage points. Nurses can improve their critical-thinking and clinical judgment skills by identifying such issues and seeking clarification through collaborative exploration with others and through ethics committee involvement.

Ethical Principles

Ethical principles are fundamental guidelines that influence decision-making. The ethical principles of autonomy, beneficence, nonmaleficence, veracity, and justice are helpful and are used frequently by health-care workers to assist with ethical decision-making.

Autonomy

The principle of **autonomy** arises from the Kantian view of persons as autonomous moral agents whose right to determine their destinies should always be respected. This presumes that individuals are always capable of making their own independent choices. Health-care workers know this is not always the case. Children, comatose individuals, and people with serious mental illness are incapable of making informed choices. In these instances, a representative of the individual is usually asked to intervene and give consent. However, health-care workers must ensure that respect for an individual's autonomy is not disregarded in favor of what another person may view as best for the client.

Beneficence

Beneficence refers to one's duty to benefit or promote the good of others. Health-care workers who act in their clients' interests are beneficent, provided their actions really do serve the client's best interest. In fact, some duties do take preference over other duties. For example, the duty to respect the autonomy of an individual may be overridden when that individual has been deemed harmful to self or others. "Doing good" for the patient should not be confused with "doing whatever the patient wants" (What do I

do now?, 2013). Good care must include a holistic focus that considers the patient's beliefs, feelings, and wishes; the wishes of the family and significant others; and considerations about competent nursing care (Catalano, 2015). Despite the above-mentioned guidelines, it is not always clear which action *is* in the best interest of the client. When such dilemmas occur, nurses should reach out to available resources, such as an ethics committee or a supervisor, to build confidence that their decisions have explored the necessary vantage points.

Peplau (1991) recognized client **advocacy** as an essential role for the psychiatric nurse. The term *advocacy* means acting in another's behalf as a supporter or defender. Being a client advocate in psychiatric nursing means helping clients fulfill needs that, without assistance and because of their illness, may go unfulfilled. Individuals with mental illness are not always able to speak for themselves. Nurses serve in this manner to protect clients' rights and interests. Strategies include educating clients and their families about their legal rights, ensuring that clients have sufficient information to make informed decisions or to give informed consent, assisting clients to consider alternatives, and supporting them in the decisions they make. Additionally, nurses may act as advocates by speaking on behalf of individuals with mental illness to secure essential mental health services.

Nonmaleficence

Nonmaleficence is the requirement that health-care providers do no harm to their clients, either intentionally or unintentionally. Some philosophers suggest that this principle is more important than beneficence; that is, they support the notion that it is more important to avoid doing harm than it is to do good. In any event, ethical dilemmas arise when a conflict exists between an individual's rights and what is thought to best represent the welfare of the individual. An example of this conflict might occur when a psychiatric client refuses antipsychotic medication (consistent with his or her rights), and the nurse must then decide how to maintain client safety while psychotic symptoms continue.

Justice

The principle of **justice** has been referred to as the "justice as fairness" principle. It is sometimes called *distributive justice,* and its basic premise lies with the right of individuals to be treated equally and fairly regardless of race, gender, marital status, medical diagnosis, social standing, economic level, or religious belief (Catalano, 2015). When applied to health care, the principle of justice suggests that all resources (including health-care services) ought to be distributed equally to all people. Thus, according to this principle, the vast disparity in the quality of care dispensed to the various socioeconomic classes within our society would be considered unjust. *Retribution* or *restorative justice* refers to the rules for responding when expectations for fairness are violated. *Social justice* can be summarized as the principle that rules for both distribution and rules for retribution should be fair and people should play by the rules (Maiese, 2013). It is important for nurses to recognize that in the latest revision of the *Code of Ethics for Nurses* (ANA, 2015), a new focus in one of the provisions states that nursing should integrate principles of social justice both in practice and in developing health policy.

Veracity

The principle of **veracity** refers to one's duty to always be truthful. Catalano (2015) states that veracity "requires the health-care provider to tell the truth and not intentionally deceive or mislead clients" (p. 126). There are times when limitations must be placed on this principle, such as when the truth would knowingly produce harm or interfere with the recovery process. Being honest is not always easy, but rarely is lying justified. Clients have the right to know about their diagnosis, treatment, and prognosis.

A Model for Making Ethical Decisions

The following steps may be used in making an ethical decision. These steps closely resemble the steps of the nursing process.

1. **Assessment:** Gather the subjective and objective data about a situation. Consider personal values as well as values of others involved in the ethical dilemma.
2. **Problem identification:** Identify the conflict between two or more alternative actions.
3. **Planning:**
   a. Explore the benefits and consequences of each alternative.
   b. Consider principles of ethical theories.
   c. Select an alternative.
4. **Implementation:** Act on the decision made, and communicate the decision to others.
5. **Evaluation:** Evaluate outcomes.

A schematic of this model is presented in Figure 5–1. A case study using this decision-making model is presented in Box 5–2. If the outcome is acceptable, action continues in the manner selected. If the outcome is unacceptable, benefits and consequences of the remaining alternatives are reexamined, and steps 3 through 7 in Box 5–2 are repeated.

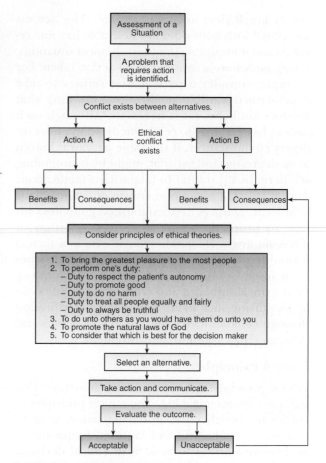

FIGURE 5–1 Ethical decision-making model.

Ethical and Legal Issues in Psychiatric-Mental Health Nursing

The Right to Treatment

Anyone who is admitted to the hospital has the right to treatment. Consequently, a psychiatric patient cannot legally be hospitalized and then denied appropriate treatment. The American Hospital Association (AHA) has also identified the rights of hospitalized patients. The AHA patient bill of rights was originally written with an emphasis on protecting the patient from a breach of reasonable standards while hospitalized. These guidelines were revised in 2003 to create an emphasis on the importance of the collaborative relationship between the client and the hospital health-care team. Titled "The Patient Care Partnership," this document informs patients of their rights to high-quality care while hospitalized, to a clean and safe environment, to be involved in their own care, to have their privacy protected, to get help when leaving the hospital, and to get help with their billing claims (AHA, 2003). Nurses practicing in hospital settings need to be aware of and adhere to legal statutes,

BOX 5-2 Ethical Decision-Making—A Case Study

STEP 1. ASSESSMENT

Tonja is a 17-year-old girl who is currently on the psychiatric unit with a diagnosis of conduct disorder. Tonja reports that she has been sexually active since she was 14. She had an abortion when she was 15 and a second one just 6 weeks ago. She states that her mother told her she has "had her last abortion" and that she has to start taking birth control pills. She asks her nurse, Kimberly, to give her some information about the pills and to tell her how to go about getting some. Kimberly believes Tonja desperately needs information about birth control pills and other types of contraceptives, but the psychiatric unit is part of a Catholic hospital, and hospital policy prohibits distributing this type of information.

STEP 2. PROBLEM IDENTIFICATION

A conflict exists between the client's need for information, the nurse's desire to provide that information, and the institution's policy prohibiting the provision of that information.

STEP 3. ALTERNATIVES—BENEFITS AND CONSEQUENCES

Alternative 1: Give the client information and risk losing job.

Alternative 2: Do not give client information and compromise own values of holistic nursing.

Alternative 3: Refer client to another source outside the hospital and risk reprimand from supervisor.

STEP 4. CONSIDER PRINCIPLES OF ETHICAL THEORIES

Alternative 1: Giving the client information would certainly respect the client's autonomy and would benefit the client by decreasing her chances of becoming pregnant again. It would not be to the best advantage of Kimberly in that she would likely lose her job. According to the beliefs of the Catholic hospital, the natural laws of God would be violated.

Alternative 2: Withholding information restricts the client's autonomy. It has the potential for doing harm in that without the use of contraceptives, the client may become pregnant again (and she implies that this is not what she wants). Kimberly's Christian ethic is violated in that this action is not what she would want "done unto her."

Alternative 3: A referral would respect the client's autonomy, would promote good, would do no harm (except perhaps to Kimberly's ego from the possible reprimand), and would comply with Kimberly's Christian ethic.

STEP 5. SELECT AN ALTERNATIVE

Alternative 3 is selected on the basis of the ethical theories of utilitarianism (does the most good for the greatest number of people), Christian ethics (Kimberly's belief of "Do unto others as you would have others do unto you"), and Kantianism (to perform one's duty) and on the basis of the ethical principles of autonomy, beneficence, and nonmaleficence. The success of this decision depends on the client's follow-through with the referral and compliance with use of the contraceptives.

STEP 6. TAKE ACTION AND COMMUNICATE

Taking action involves providing information in writing for Tonja or perhaps making a phone call to set up an appointment for her with Planned Parenthood. Communicating suggests sharing the information with Tonja's mother. The referral should be documented in the client's chart.

STEP 7. EVALUATE THE OUTCOME

An acceptable outcome might indicate that Tonja kept her appointment at Planned Parenthood and is complying with the prescribed contraceptive regimen. It might also include Kimberly's input into the change process in her institution to implement these types of referrals to other clients who request them.

An unacceptable outcome might be indicated by Tonja's lack of follow-through with the appointment at Planned Parenthood or lack of compliance in using the contraceptives, resulting in another pregnancy. Kimberly may also view a reprimand from her supervisor as an unacceptable outcome, particularly if she is told that she must select other alternatives should this situation arise in the future. Kimberly's disagreement with the institution's policy may motivate her to make another decision—that of seeking employment in an institution that supports a philosophy more consistent with her own.

---

accepted standards of practice, and organizational policies with regard to a client's rights during hospital treatment.

The Right to Refuse Treatment (Including Medication)

Legally, patients have the right to refuse treatment unless immediate intervention is required to prevent death or serious harm to the patient or another person (Sadock, Sadock, & Ruiz, 2015). The U.S. Constitution and several of its amendments affirm this right (e.g., the First Amendment, which addresses the rights of speech, thought, and expression; the Eighth Amendment, which grants the right to freedom from cruel and unusual punishment; and the Fifth and Fourteenth Amendments, which grant due process of law and equal protection for all). In psychiatry, however, both ethical and legal issues must be considered. Sometimes patients are involuntarily hospitalized because they are at risk of harm to themselves or others and do not recognize the severity of their symptoms. In emergency cases, sedative medication may be administered without the patients' consent in order to protect them from harming themselves or others. Because laws vary from state to state, nurses must know the laws that pertain in their local jurisdictions. Organizational policies in the nurse's practice setting should also guide decision-making.

Although many courts support a client's right to refuse medications in the psychiatric area, exceptions do exist. Regarding decision-making about forced medication, Weiss-Kaffie and Purtell (2001) stated:

> The treatment team must determine that three criteria be met to force medication without client consent. The client must exhibit behavior that is dangerous to self or others; the medication ordered by the physician must have a reasonable chance of providing help to the client; and clients who refuse medication must be judged incompetent to evaluate the benefits of the treatment in question. (p. 361)

More recently, some states have adopted laws that allow a court to mandate outpatient treatment for people with mental illness who have a history of violent behavior. In New York City, this law, known as *Kendra's law*, also includes a provision for ordering an individual to take medication as part of the treatment plan.

The Right to the Least-Restrictive Treatment Alternative

The right to the least-restrictive treatment alternative means that clients who can be adequately treated in an outpatient setting should not be hospitalized, and if they are hospitalized, they should not be sedated, restrained, or secluded unless less restrictive measures were unsuccessful. In other words, the client has a right to whatever level of treatment is effective and least restricts his or her freedom. The restrictiveness of psychiatric therapy can be described in the context of a continuum based on severity of illness. Clients may be treated on an outpatient basis, in day hospitals, or through voluntary or involuntary hospitalization. Symptoms may be treated with verbal rehabilitative techniques and move successively to behavioral techniques, chemical interventions, mechanical restraints, or electroconvulsive therapy. However, ethical issues arise in selecting the least-restrictive means among involuntary chemical intervention, seclusion, and mechanical restraints. Sadock and associates (2015) state:

> Distinguishing among these interventions on the basis of restrictiveness proves to be a purely subjective exercise fraught with personal bias. Moreover, each of these three interventions is both more and

less restrictive than each of the other two. Nevertheless, the effort should be made to think in terms of restrictiveness when deciding how to treat patients. (p. 1386)

While the right to the least restrictive treatment may seem reasonable and expected, it is important to recognize that clients with mental illness have historically been hospitalized against their will simply because they had a mental illness. In the case of *O'Connor v. Donaldson* (1976), the Supreme Court ruled that harmless mentally ill individuals cannot be confined against their will if they are able to remain safe outside of a hospital setting. They must be considered dangerous to themselves or others or be so unable to care for themselves that their safety and survival are at risk. In 1981, the case of *Roger v. Oken* culminated in the ruling that all patients, even those involuntarily hospitalized, are competent to refuse treatment, but a legal guardian may authorize treatment (Sadock et al., 2015). These laws and policies have better attempted to protect the rights of clients with mental illness while still recognizing that, at times, an individual with acute mental illness may be unable to make decisions in the interest of his or her safety and survival.

Ideally, a person recognizes his or her need for treatment and agrees voluntarily to be hospitalized if this measure is recommended by the health-care provider. The client who is voluntarily hospitalized typically signs a consent to treatment upon admission, but it remains the client's right as a voluntary patient to revoke that consent and to be discharged from the hospital if he or she so choose.

Legal Considerations

The Patient Self-Determination Act, as part of the Omnibus Budget Reconciliation Act of 1990, went into effect on December 1, 1991. Cady (2010) states:

> The Patient Self-determination Act requires health-care facilities to provide clear written information for every patient concerning his/her legal rights to make healthcare decisions, including the right to accept or refuse treatment. (p. 118)

Box 5–3 lists the rights of patients affirmed by this law.

Nurse Practice Acts

The legal parameters of professional and practical nursing are defined within each state by the state's nurse practice act. These documents are passed by the state legislature and in general are concerned with provisions such as

■ The definition of important terms, including nursing itself and the various types of nurses.

BOX 5–3 Patient Self-Determination Act–Patient Rights

1. The right to appropriate treatment and related services in a setting and under conditions that are the most supportive of such person's personal liability and that restrict such liberty only to the extent necessary consistent with such person's treatment needs, applicable requirements of law, and applicable judicial orders.
2. The right to an individualized, written treatment or service plan (such plan to be developed promptly after admission of such person), the right to treatment based on such plan, the right to periodic review and reassessment of treatment and related service needs, and the right to appropriate revision of such plan, including any revision necessary to provide a description of mental health services that may be needed after such person is discharged from such program or facility.
3. The right to ongoing participation, in a manner appropriate to a person's capabilities, in the planning of mental health services to be provided (including the right to participate in the development and periodic revision of the plan).
4. The right to be provided, in terms and language appropriate to a person's condition and ability to understand, a reasonable explanation of the person's general mental and physical (if appropriate) condition, the objectives of treatment, the nature and significant possible adverse effects of recommended treatment, the reasons a particular treatment is considered appropriate, the reasons access to certain visitors may not be appropriate, and any appropriate and available alternative treatments, services, and types of providers of mental health services.
5. The right not to receive a mode or course of treatment in the absence of informed, voluntary, written consent to treatment except during an emergency situation or as permitted by law when the person is being treated as a result of a court order.
6. The right not to participate in experimentation in the absence of informed, voluntary, written consent (includes human subject protection).
7. The right to freedom from restraint or seclusion, other than as a mode or course of treatment or restraint or seclusion during an emergency situation with a written order by a responsible mental health professional.
8. The right to a humane treatment environment that affords reasonable protection from harm and appropriate privacy with regard to personal needs.
9. The right to access, on request, to such person's mental health-care records.
10. The right, in the case of a person admitted on a residential or inpatient care basis, to converse with others privately, to have convenient and reasonable access to the telephone and mail, and to see visitors during regularly scheduled hours. (For treatment purposes, specific individuals may be excluded.)
11. The right to be informed promptly and in writing at the time of admission of these rights.
12. The right to assert grievances with respect to infringement of these rights.
13. The right to exercise these rights without reprisal.
14. The right of referral to other providers upon discharge.

Adapted from the U.S. Code, Title 42, Section 10841, The Public Health and Welfare, 1991.

■ A statement of the education and other training or requirements for licensure and reciprocity.
■ Broad statements that describe the scope of practice for various levels of nursing (APN, RN, LPN).
■ Conditions under which a nurse's license may be suspended or revoked and instructions for appeal.
■ The general authority and powers of the state board of nursing.

Most nurse practice acts are general in their terminology and do not provide specific guidelines for practice. Nurses must understand the scope of practice protected by their license and should seek assistance from legal counsel if they are unsure about the proper interpretation of a nurse practice act.

Types of Law

The two general categories of law that are of most concern to nurses are statutory law and common law. These laws are identified by their source or origin.

Statutory Law

A **statutory law** is a law that has been enacted by a legislative body, such as a county or city council, state legislature, or the U.S. Congress. An example of statutory law is the nurse practice acts.

Common Law

Common laws are derived from decisions made in previous cases. These laws apply to a body of principles that evolve from court decisions resolving various controversies. Because common law in the United States has been developed on a state basis, the law on specific subjects may differ from state to state. An example of a common law might be how different states deal with a nurse's refusal to provide care for a specific client.

Classifications Within Statutory and Common Law

Broadly speaking, there are two kinds of unlawful acts: civil and criminal. Both statutory law and common law have civil and criminal components.

Civil Law

Civil law protects the private and property rights of individuals and businesses. Private individuals or groups may bring a legal action to court for breach of civil law. These legal actions are of two basic types: torts and contracts.

Torts

A **tort** is a violation of a civil law in which an individual has been wronged. In a tort action, one party asserts that wrongful conduct on the part of the other has caused harm and seeks compensation. A tort may be *intentional* or *unintentional*. Examples of unintentional torts are malpractice and negligence actions. An example of an intentional tort is the touching of another person without that person's consent. Intentional touching (e.g., a medical treatment) without the client's consent can result in a charge of battery, an intentional tort.

Contracts

In a contract action, one party asserts that the other party, in failing to fulfill an obligation, has breached the contract, and either compensation or performance of the obligation is sought as remedy. An example is an action by a mental health professional whose clinical privileges have been reduced or terminated in violation of an implied contract between the professional and a hospital.

Criminal Law

Criminal law provides protection from conduct deemed injurious to the public welfare. It provides for punishment of those found to have engaged in such conduct, which commonly includes imprisonment, parole conditions, a loss of privilege (such as a license), a fine, or any combination of these (Ellis & Hartley, 2012). An example of a violation of criminal law is the theft by a hospital employee of supplies or drugs.

Legal Issues in Psychiatric-Mental Health Nursing

Confidentiality and Right to Privacy

The Fourth, Fifth, and Fourteenth Amendments to the U.S. Constitution protect an individual's privacy. Most states have statutes protecting the confidentiality of client records and communications. Nurses must recognize that the only individuals who have a right to observe a client or have access to medical information are those involved in the client's medical care. The client must provide written consent for health-care information to be shared with anyone outside the current treatment team.

HIPAA

Until 1996, client confidentiality in medical records was not protected by federal law. In August 1996, President Clinton signed the Health Insurance Portability and Accountability Act (HIPAA) into law. This federal privacy rule pertains to data that is called *protected health information* (PHI) and applies to most individuals and institutions involved in health care. PHI is individually identifiable health information indicators that "relate to past, present, or future physical or mental health or condition of the individual, or the past, present, or future payment for the provision of health care to an individual; and (1) that identifies the individual; or (2) with respect to which there is a reasonable basis to believe the information can be used to identify the individual" (U.S. Department of Health and Human Services, 2003). These specific identifiers are listed in Box 5–4.

Under HIPAA, individuals have the rights to access their medical records, to have corrections made to their medical records, and to decide with whom their medical information may be shared. The actual document belongs to the facility or the therapist, but the information contained therein belongs to the client. The passage of HIPAA increased the level of control clients have over the information maintained in their

---

BOX 5–4 Protected Health Information (PHI): Individually Identifiable Indicators

1. Names
2. Postal address information (except state), including street address, city, county, precinct, and zip code
3. All elements of dates (except year) for dates directly related to an individual, including birth date, admission date, discharge date, date of death; and all ages over 89 and all elements of dates (including year) indicative of such age, except that such ages and elements may be aggregated into a single category of age 90 or older
4. Telephone numbers
5. Fax numbers
6. Electronic mail addresses
7. Social Security numbers
8. Medical record numbers
9. Health plan beneficiary numbers
10. Account numbers
11. Certificate/license numbers
12. Vehicle identifiers and serial numbers, including license plate numbers
13. Device identifiers and serial numbers
14. Web Universal Resource Locators (URLs)
15. Internet protocol (IP) address numbers
16. Biometric identifiers, including finger and voice prints
17. Full face photographic images and any comparable images
18. Any other unique identifying number, characteristic, or code

From U.S. Department of Health and Human Services (HHS). (2003). Standards for privacy of individually identifiable health information. Washington, DC: HHS.

medical records. Notice of privacy policies must be provided to clients upon entry into the health-care system.

In 2013, HIPAA privacy and security rules were again expanded to afford more rights to patients with regard to their medical information and to assure greater security of a person's health information. In some cases, such as when paying out of pocket for care, patients can tell a provider that they do not want treatment information shared with their health insurance plan (U.S. Department of Health &Human Services, 2013). Nurses in any practice setting need to be aware of these HIPAA laws and any new provisions in law that will impact the conduct of their practice.

Pertinent medical information may be released without consent in a life-threatening situation. If information is released in an emergency, the following information must be recorded in the client's record: date of disclosure, person to whom information was disclosed, reason for disclosure, reason written consent could not be obtained, and the specific information disclosed.

Most states have statutes that pertain to the doctrine of **privileged communication.** Although the codes differ markedly from state to state, most grant certain professionals privileges under which they may refuse to reveal information about and communications with clients. In most states, the doctrine of privileged communication applies to psychiatrists and attorneys; in some instances, psychologists, clergy, and nurses are also included.

In certain instances, nurses may be called on to testify in cases in which the medical record is used as evidence. In most states, the right to privacy of these records is exempted in civil or criminal proceedings. Therefore, it is important that nurses document with these possibilities in mind. Strict recordkeeping using objective and nonjudgmental statements, care plans that are specific in their prescriptive interventions, and documentation that describes those interventions and their subsequent evaluation, all serve the best interests of the client, the nurse, and the institution should questions regarding care arise. Documentation very often weighs heavily in malpractice case decisions.

The right to confidentiality is a basic one, especially in psychiatry. Although societal attitudes are improving, individuals have experienced discrimination in the past for no other reason than a history of mental illness. Nurses working in psychiatric-mental health nursing must guard the privacy of their clients with great diligence.

Exception: A Duty to Warn (Protection of a Third Party)

There are exceptions to the laws of privacy and confidentiality. One of these exceptions stems from the 1974 case of *Tarasoff v. Regents of the University of California.* The incident from which this case evolved came about in the late 1960s. A young man from Bengal, India (Mr. P.), who was a graduate student at the University of California (UC), Berkeley, fell in love with another university student (Ms. Tarasoff). Because she was not interested in an exclusive relationship with Mr. P., he became resentful and angry. He began to stalk her and record some of their conversations in an effort to determine why she did not love him. He soon became very depressed and neglected his health, appearance, and studies.

Ms. Tarasoff spent the summer of 1969 in South America. During this time, Mr. P. entered therapy with a psychologist at UC. He confided in the psychologist that he intended to kill his former girlfriend (identifying Ms. Tarasoff by name) when she returned from vacation. The psychologist recommended civil commitment for Mr. P., claiming he was suffering from acute and severe paranoid schizophrenia. Mr. P. was picked up by the campus police but released a short time later because he appeared rational and promised to stay away from Ms. Tarasoff. Neither Ms. Tarasoff nor her parents received any warning of Mr. P.'s stated intention to kill her.

When Ms. Tarasoff returned to campus in October 1969, Mr. P. resumed his stalking behavior and eventually stabbed her to death. Ms. Tarasoff's parents sued the psychologist, several psychiatrists, and the university for failure to warn the family of the danger. The case was referred to the California Supreme Court, which ruled that a mental health professional has a duty not only to a client but also to individuals who are being threatened by that client. The Court stated:

> Once a therapist does in fact determine, or under applicable professional standards should have determined, that a patient poses a serious danger of violence to others, he bears a duty to exercise reasonable care to protect the foreseeable victim of that danger. While the discharge of this duty of due care will necessarily vary with the facts of each case, in each instance the adequacy of the therapist's conduct must be measured against the traditional negligence standard of reasonable care under the circumstances. (*Tarasoff v. Regents of University of California*, 1974a)

The defendants argued that warning the woman or her family would have breached professional ethics and violated the client's right to privacy. But the court ruled that "the confidential character of patient-psychotherapist communications must yield to the extent that disclosure is essential to avert danger to others. The protective privilege ends where the public peril begins" (*Tarasoff v. Regents of University of California*, 1974b).

In 1976, the California Supreme Court expanded the original case ruling (now referred to as *Tarasoff I*). The second ruling (known as *Tarasoff II*) broadened the ruling of "duty to warn" to include "duty to protect." It stated that under certain circumstances, a therapist might be required to warn an individual, notify police, or take whatever steps are necessary to protect the intended victim from harm. This duty to protect can also occur in instances when patients must be protected by health-care providers because they are vulnerable due to their inability to identify harmful situations (Guido, 2014).

The *Tarasoff* rulings created a great deal of controversy in the psychiatric community regarding breach of confidentiality and the subsequent negative impact on the client-therapist relationship. However, most states now recognize that therapists have ethical and legal obligations to prevent their clients from harming themselves or others. Many states have passed their own variations on the original "protect and warn" legislation, but in most cases, courts have outlined the following guidelines for therapists to follow in determining their obligation to take protective measures:

1. Assessment of a threat of violence by a client toward another individual
2. Identification of the intended victim
3. Ability to intervene in a feasible, meaningful way to protect the intended victim

When these guidelines apply to a specific situation, it is reasonable for the therapist to notify the victim, law enforcement authorities, and/or relatives of the intended victim. They may also consider initiating voluntary or involuntary commitment of the client in an effort to prevent potential violence.

Implications for Nursing While the original decision in the *Tarasoff* ruling was directed toward psychotherapists, it has since been more broadly applied. Not all states identify registered nurses as having a duty to warn, but other statutes include a duty to warn for nurses at all levels, from licensed practical nurses to advanced practice nurses. As of 2015, three states (Maine, Nevada, and North Dakota) have not yet addressed the issue of duty to warn. One state (North Carolina) does not recognize the duty to warn (National Conference of State Legislatures, 2016). But even in states that do not recognize a duty to warn, practitioners still need to make a decision about warning a potential victim. Every nurse, not just those practicing in psychiatric nursing, should be informed about the laws in his or her state regarding duty to warn. As Henderson (2015) notes, emergency nurses are often the front-line health-care workers and thus are in a position to identify persons at risk for violence and to protect

the safety of the patient and others. In psychiatric-mental health nursing practice, if a client confides in the nurse about the potential for harm to an intended victim, it is the nurse's duty to report this information to the psychiatrist and to other team members. This is not a breach of confidentiality, and the nurse may be considered negligent for failure to report. All members of the treatment team must be made aware of the potential danger that the client poses to self or others. Detailed written documentation of the situation is also required.

Exception: Suspected Child or Elder Abuse

Every state requires that health-care professionals—and in many jurisdictions, every citizen—report suspicion of child abuse to legal authorities (Hartsell & Bernstein, 2013). Many jurisdictions also have statutes requiring that suspected elder abuse or neglect be reported. At times, health-care professionals may be reluctant to report, fearing that they may be liable for false allegations, but reporting statutes generally grant immunity to anyone making a good faith report about a reasonable suspicion. In addition, in some jurisdictions, it is a criminal act *not* to report, "so declining to report should not be considered an option" (Hartsell & Bernstein, 2013, p. 170).

Implications for Nursing There is often an element of clinical judgment about whether a patient's communication raises a reasonable suspicion of abuse. For example, when a person is experiencing hallucinations or delusions, his or her perception about events may be distorted. The nurse has a responsibility to explore all patient perceptions of abuse or mistreatment and discuss these with other health-care team members to identify the most appropriate decision with consideration of all legal, ethical, and clinical factors.

Informed Consent

According to law, all individuals have the right to decide whether to accept or reject medical treatment. A health-care provider can be charged with assault and battery for providing life-sustaining treatment to a client when the client has not agreed to the treatment. The rationale for the doctrine of **informed consent** is the preservation and protection of individual autonomy in determining what will and will not happen to a person's body (Guido, 2014).

Informed consent is permission granted by a client for a physician to perform a therapeutic procedure. Before the procedure, the client is presented written information about the treatment and given adequate time to consider the pros and cons. The client should receive information such as what treatment alternatives are available; why the physician believes this treatment is most appropriate; the possible outcomes, risks, and adverse effects; the possible outcome should the client select another treatment alternative; and the possible outcome should the client choose to decline all treatment. An example of a psychiatric treatment that requires informed consent is electroconvulsive therapy.

Under some conditions, treatment may be performed without obtaining informed consent. A client's refusal to accept treatment may be challenged under the following circumstances (Guido, 2014; Levy & Rubenstein, 1996):

1. When a client is mentally incompetent to make a decision and treatment is necessary to preserve life or avoid serious harm
2. When refusing treatment endangers the life or health of another
3. During an emergency in which a client is in no condition to exercise judgment
4. When the client is a child (consent is obtained from parent or surrogate)
5. In the case of therapeutic privilege, information about a treatment may be withheld if the physician can show that full disclosure would
   a. hinder or complicate necessary treatment,
   b. cause severe psychological harm, or
   c. be so upsetting as to render a rational decision by the client impossible

Although most clients in psychiatric-mental health facilities are competent and capable of giving informed consent, those with severe psychiatric illness do not possess the cognitive ability to do so. If an individual has been legally determined mentally incompetent, consent is obtained from the legal guardian. Difficulty arises when no legal determination has been made, but the individual's current mental state prohibits informed decision-making (e.g., a person who is psychotic, unconscious, or inebriated). In these instances, informed consent is usually obtained from the individual's nearest relative, or if none exist and time permits, the physician may ask the court to appoint a conservator or guardian. When time does not permit court intervention, permission may be sought from the hospital administrator.

A client or guardian always has the right to withdraw consent after it has been given. When this occurs, the physician should inform (or reinform) the client about the consequences of refusing treatment. If treatment has already been initiated, the physician should terminate treatment in a way least likely to cause injury to the client and inform the client or guardian of the risks associated with interrupted treatment (Guido, 2014).

The nurse's role in obtaining informed consent is usually defined by agency policy. A nurse may sign the consent form as witness for the client's signature. However, legal liability for informed consent lies with the physician. The nurse acts as client advocate, ensuring that the following three major elements of informed consent have been addressed:

1. **Knowledge:** The client has received adequate information on which to base his or her decision.
2. **Competency:** The individual's cognition is not impaired to an extent that would interfere with decision-making, or he or she has a legal representative.
3. **Free will:** The individual has given consent voluntarily without pressure or coercion from others.

Restraints and Seclusion

An individual's privacy and personal security are protected by the Patient Self-Determination Act of 1991. This legislation includes a set of patient rights, including an individual's right to freedom from restraint or seclusion except in an emergency. The use of seclusion and restraint as a therapeutic intervention for psychiatric patients has long been controversial. Many efforts have been made through federal and state regulations and through standards set forth by accrediting bodies to minimize or eliminate the use of this type of intervention.

In addition, there is an element of moral decision-making when any kind of treatment is coerced, as is often the case with seclusion and restraint. Landeweer, Abma, and Widdershoven (2011) point out that although coercion may sometimes be necessary, it can be detrimental to the patient, as it may produce trauma and mistrust. One advantage of using a forum such as a hospital-based ethics committee to guide moral decision-making is that by exploring issues such as the use of seclusion and restraint with a diverse group of people who have different vantage points, alternative treatments can be identified and explored.

Because injuries and deaths have been associated with restraint and seclusion, this treatment requires careful attention whenever it is deemed necessary. Further, the laws, regulations, accreditation standards, and hospital policies are frequently revised, so anyone practicing in inpatient psychiatric settings must be well informed in each of these areas.

In psychiatry, the term *restraints* generally refers to a set of leather straps used to restrain the extremities of an individual whose behavior is out of control and who poses an immediate risk to the physical safety and psychological well-being of himself or herself and others. It is important to note that the currently accepted definition of restraint refers not only to leather restraints but also to any manual method or medication used to restrict a person's freedom of movement. Restraints are never to be used as punishment or for the convenience of staff. Other measures to decrease agitation, such as "talking down" (verbal intervention) and chemical restraints (tranquilizing medication), are usually tried first. If these interventions are ineffective, mechanical restraints may be instituted (although some controversy exists as to whether chemical restraints are indeed less restrictive than mechanical restraints). *Seclusion* is another type of physical restraint in which the client is confined alone in a room from which he or she is unable to leave. The room is usually minimally furnished with items to promote the client's comfort and safety.

The Joint Commission, an association that accredits health-care organizations, has established standards regarding the use of seclusion and restraint. Some examples of current standards include the following (The Joint Commission, 2015):

1. Seclusion or restraint is discontinued as soon as possible regardless of when the order is scheduled to expire.
2. Unless state law is more restrictive, orders for restraint or seclusion must be renewed every 4 hours for adults ages 18 and older, every 2 hours for children and adolescents ages 9 to 17, and every hour for children younger than 9 years. Orders may be renewed according to these time limits for a maximum of 24 consecutive hours.
3. An in-person evaluation (by a physician, clinical psychologist, or other licensed independent practitioner responsible for the care of the patient) must be conducted within 1 hour of initiating restraint or seclusion. Appropriately trained registered nurses and physician assistants may also conduct this assessment, but they must consult with the physician.
4. Patients who are simultaneously restrained and secluded must be continuously monitored by trained staff, either in person or through audio or video equipment positioned near the patient.
5. Staff who are involved in restraining and secluding patients are trained to monitor the physical and psychological well-being of the patient including but not limited to respiratory and circulatory status, skin integrity, and vital signs.

The laws, regulations, accreditation standards, and hospital policies pertaining to restraint and seclusion share a common priority of maintaining patient safety for a procedure that has the potential to incur injury or death. The importance of close and careful monitoring cannot be overstated.

False imprisonment is the deliberate and unauthorized confinement of a person within fixed limits by the use of verbal or physical means (Ellis & Hartley, 2012). Health-care workers may be charged with false imprisonment for restraining or secluding—against the wishes of the client—anyone admitted to the hospital voluntarily. Should a voluntarily admitted client decompensate to a point that restraint or seclusion for protection of self or others is necessary, court intervention to determine competency and involuntary commitment is required to preserve the client's rights to privacy and freedom.

Hospitalization
Voluntary Admissions

Each year, more than 1 million people are admitted to health-care facilities for psychiatric treatment; of these admissions, approximately two-thirds are considered voluntary. To be admitted voluntarily, an individual makes direct application to the institution for services and may stay as long as treatment is deemed necessary. He or she may sign out of the hospital at any time unless the health-care professional determines that the client may be harmful to self or others following a mental status examination and recommends that admission status be changed from voluntary to involuntary. Even when an admission is considered voluntary, it is important to ensure that the individual comprehends the meaning of his or her actions, has not been coerced in any manner, and is willing to proceed with admission.

Involuntary Commitment

Although the term *involuntary hospitalization* is preferred by some over the term *involuntary commitment*, this process needs to be conducted with respect to state and federal law. Because involuntary hospitalization results in substantial restrictions of the rights of an individual, the admission process is subject to the guarantee of the Fourteenth Amendment to the U.S. Constitution that provides citizens protection against loss of liberty and ensures due process rights (Weiss-Kaffie & Purtell, 2001). Involuntary hospitalizations may be made for various reasons. Most states commonly cite the following criteria:

■ The person is imminently dangerous to himself or herself (i.e., suicidal intent).
■ The person is a danger to others (i.e., physically aggressive, violent, or homicidal).
■ The person is unable to take care of basic personal needs (the "gravely disabled").

Under the Fourth Amendment, individuals are protected from unlawful searches and seizures without probable cause. Therefore, the individual recommending involuntary hospitalization must show probable cause why the client should be hospitalized against his or her wishes; that is, the person must show that there is cause to believe that the client would be dangerous to self or others, is mentally ill and in need of treatment, or is gravely disabled.

Emergency Commitments

Emergency commitments are sought when an individual manifests behavior that is clearly and imminently dangerous to self or others. These admissions are usually instigated by relatives or friends of the individual or by police officers, the court, or health-care professionals. Emergency commitments are time-limited, and a court hearing for the individual is scheduled, usually within 72 hours. At that time, the court may decide that the client may be discharged or, if deemed necessary and voluntary admission is refused by the client, an additional period of involuntary hospitalization may be ordered. In most instances, another hearing is scheduled for a specified time (usually in 7 to 21 days).

The Mentally Ill Person in Need of Treatment

A second type of involuntary commitment is for the observation and treatment of mentally ill persons in need of treatment. These commitments typically last longer than emergency commitments. Most states have established definitions of what constitutes "mentally ill" for purposes of state involuntary admission statutes. Some examples include individuals who, because of severe mental illness, are

■ Unable to make informed decisions concerning treatment.
■ Likely to cause harm to self or others.
■ Unable to fulfill basic personal needs necessary for health and safety.

In determining whether commitment is required, the court looks for substantial evidence of abnormal conduct—evidence that cannot be explained by a physical cause. There must be "clear and convincing evidence" as well as probable cause to substantiate the need for involuntary hospitalization to ensure that an individual's constitutional rights are protected. As mentioned earlier, the U.S. Supreme Court, in *O'Connor v. Donaldson,* held that the existence of mental illness alone does not justify involuntary hospitalization. State standards require a specific impact or consequence caused by mental illness that involves danger or an inability to care for one's own needs. These clients are entitled to court hearings with representation, at which time determination of commitment and length of stay are considered. Legislative statutes governing involuntary commitments vary among states.

Involuntary Outpatient Commitment

Involuntary outpatient commitment (IOC) is a court-ordered mechanism used to compel a person with mental illness to submit to treatment on an outpatient basis. A number of eligibility criteria for commitment to outpatient treatment have been cited (Appelbaum, 2001; Csere, 2013; Maloy, 1996; Torrey & Zdanowicz, 2001). Some of these include

■ A history of repeated decompensation requiring involuntary hospitalization.
■ Likelihood that without treatment the individual will deteriorate to the point of requiring inpatient commitment.
■ Presence of severe and persistent mental illness (e.g., schizophrenia or bipolar disorder) and limited awareness of the illness or need for treatment.
■ The presence of severe and persistent mental illness contributing to a risk of becoming homeless, incarcerated, or violent, or of committing suicide.
■ The existence of an individualized treatment plan likely to be effective and a service provider who has agreed to provide the treatment.
■ A danger to self or others. Although this is also a criterion for inpatient commitment, the American Psychiatric Association recommends outpatient commitment as an option when there is an acceptable treatment plan and access to a community provider (Harvard Health, 2008).
■ The risk for relapse and hospitalization related to noncompliance with treatment.

Most states have already enacted IOC legislation or currently have agenda resolutions that speak to this topic. Most commonly, clients who are committed into the IOC programs are those with severe and persistent mental illness such as schizophrenia. The rationale behind the legislation is to improve preventive care and reduce the number of readmissions and lengths of hospital stays for these clients. The need for this kind of legislation arose after it was recognized that patients with schizophrenia who did not meet criteria for involuntary hospital treatment were in some cases ultimately dangerous to themselves or others. In New York, public attention to this need arose after a man with schizophrenia who had stopped taking his medication pushed a young woman into the path of a subway train. He would not have met criteria for involuntary hospitalization until he was deemed dangerous to others, but advocates for this legislation argued that there should be provisions to prevent violence rather than waiting until it happens. The subsequent law governing IOC in New York became known as Kendra's law in reference to the woman who was pushed to her death. Opponents of this legislation fear that it may violate the individual rights of psychiatric clients without significant improvement in outcomes.

Some research studies have attempted to evaluate whether IOC (sometimes abbreviated as OPC, which refers simply to outpatient commitment) improves care, reduces lengths of stay in the hospital, and/or reduces episodes of violence. Most studies have shown positive outcomes, including a decrease in hospital readmissions, with IOC (Swartz & Swanson, 2008). Continuing research is required to determine whether IOC will ultimately improve treatment compliance and enhance quality of life in the community for individuals with severe and persistent mental illness.

The Gravely Disabled Client

A number of states have statutes that specifically define the "gravely disabled" client. For those that do not use this label, the description of the individual who is unable to take care of basic personal needs because of mental illness is very similar.

Gravely disabled is generally defined as a condition in which an individual, as a result of mental illness, is in danger of serious physical harm resulting from inability to provide for basic needs such as food, clothing, shelter, medical care, and personal safety. Inability to care for oneself cannot be established by showing that an individual lacks the resources to provide the necessities of life. Rather, it is the inability to make use of available resources.

Should it be determined that an individual is gravely disabled, a guardian, conservator, or committee will be appointed by the court to ensure the management of the person and his or her estate. To legally restore competency requires another court hearing to reverse the previous ruling. The individual whose competency is being determined has the right to be represented by an attorney.

Nursing Liability

Mental health practitioners—psychiatrists, psychologists, psychiatric nurses, and social workers—have a duty to provide appropriate care based on the standards of their professions and the standards set by law. The standards of care for psychiatric-mental health nursing are presented in Chapter 9, The Nursing Process in Psychiatric-Mental Health Nursing.

Malpractice and Negligence

The terms **malpractice** and **negligence** are often used interchangeably. Negligence has been defined as

> the failure to exercise the standard of care that a reasonably prudent person would have exercised in a similar situation; any conduct that falls below the legal standard established to protect others against unreasonable risk of harm, except for conduct that is intentionally, wantonly, or willfully disregardful of others' rights. (Garner, 2014)

Any person may be negligent. In contrast, malpractice is a specialized form of negligence caused only by professionals. *Black's Law Dictionary* defines malpractice as

> an instance of negligence or incompetence on the part of a professional. To succeed in a malpractice

claim, a plaintiff must also prove proximate cause and damages. (Garner, 2014)

In the absence of state statutes, common law is the basis of liability for injuries to clients caused by acts of malpractice and negligence by individual practitioners. In other words, most decisions of negligence in the professional setting are based on legal precedent (decisions that have been made previously about similar cases) rather than on any specific action taken by the legislature.

To summarize, when a breach of duty is characterized as malpractice, the action is weighed against the professional standard. When it is brought forth as negligence, the action is contrasted with what a reasonably prudent professional would have done in the same or similar circumstances.

Austin (2011) cites the following basic elements of a nursing malpractice lawsuit:

1. A duty to the patient existed, based on the recognized standard of care.
2. A breach of duty occurred, meaning that the care rendered was not consistent with the recognized standard of care.
3. The client was injured.
4. The injury was directly caused by the breach of a standard of care.

For the client to prevail in a malpractice claim, each of these elements must be proven. Jury decisions are generally based on the testimony of expert witnesses because members of the jury are laypeople who cannot be expected to know what nursing interventions should have taken place. Without the testimony of expert witnesses, a favorable verdict usually goes to the defendant nurse.

Types of Lawsuits That Occur in Psychiatric Nursing

Most malpractice suits against nurses are civil actions, which means they are considered breach of conduct actions on the part of the professional for which compensation is sought. The nurse in a psychiatric setting should be aware of the types of behavior that may result in malpractice charges.

The hospitalized psychiatric client has a basic right to confidentiality and privacy. A nurse may be charged with *breach of confidentiality* for revealing aspects about a client's case or even for revealing that an individual has been hospitalized if the client can show that making this information known resulted in harm.

When shared information is detrimental to the client's reputation, the person sharing the information may be liable for **defamation of character.** When the information is in writing, the action is called **libel.** Oral defamation is called **slander.** Defamation of character involves communication that is malicious and false (Ellis & Hartley, 2012). Occasionally, libel arises out of critical, judgmental statements written in the client's medical record. Nurses need to be very objective in their charting, backing up all statements with factual evidence.

Invasion of privacy is a charge that may result when a client is searched without probable cause. Many institutions conduct body searches on clients with mental illness as a routine intervention. In these cases, there should be a physician's order and written rationale showing probable cause for the intervention. Many institutions are reexamining their policies regarding this procedure.

Assault is an act that results in a person's genuine fear and apprehension that he or she will be touched without consent. **Battery** is the unconsented touching of another person. These charges can result when a treatment is administered to a client against his or her wishes and outside of an emergency situation. Harm or injury need not have occurred for these charges to be legitimate.

For confining a client against his or her wishes outside of an emergency situation, the nurse may be charged with false imprisonment. Examples of actions that may invoke these charges include locking an individual in a room, taking a client's clothes for purposes of detainment against his or her will, and restraining a competent voluntary client who demands to be released.

Avoiding Liability

Catalano (2015) suggests the following proactive nursing actions in an effort to avoid nursing malpractice and the risk of lawsuits:

1. *Effective communication* with patients and other caregivers. The SBAR model of reporting information, which stands for situation, background, assessment, and recommendations, has been identified as a useful tool for effective communication with caregivers. Establishing rapport with clients encourages open and honest communication.
2. *Accurate and complete documentation in the medical record.*

   The electronic health record (EHR) has been identified as the best way to document and share this information. The use of best informatics sources is identified as an essential nursing competency (Institute of Medicine, 2003) and an important standard for quality and safety in nursing education (QSEN Institute, 2013).

3. *Complying with standards of care,* including those established within the profession (such as ANA standards) and those identified by specific hospital policies.
4. *Knowing the client,* which includes helping the client become involved in his or her care as well as

understanding and responding to aspects of care in which the client is dissatisfied.
5. *Practicing within the nurse's level of competence and scope of practice,* which includes not only adhering to professional standards (those of the ANA and state boards of nursing) but also keeping knowledge and nursing skills current through evidence-based literature, in-services, and continuing education.

Some clients appear to be more "suit prone" than others. Suit-prone clients are often very critical, complaining, uncooperative, and even hostile. A natural staff response to these clients is to become defensive or withdrawn. Either of these behaviors increases the likelihood of a lawsuit should an unfavorable event occur (Ellis & Hartley, 2012). No matter how high the nurse's technical competence and skill, his or her insensitivity to a client's complaints and failure to meet the client's emotional needs often influence whether or not a lawsuit is generated. A great deal depends on the psychosocial skills of the health-care professional.

CLINICAL PEARLS
- Always put the client's rights and welfare first.
- Develop and maintain a good interpersonal relationship with each client and his or her family.

Summary and Key Points

- *Ethics* is a branch of philosophy that addresses methods for determining the rightness or wrongness of one's actions.
- *Bioethics* is the term applied to these principles when they refer to concepts within the scopes of medicine, nursing, and allied health.
- *Moral behavior* is conduct that results from serious critical thinking about how individuals ought to treat others.
- *Values* are personal beliefs about what is important or desirable
- A *right* is "a valid, legally recognized claim or entitlement, encompassing both freedom from government interference or discriminatory treatment and an entitlement to a benefit or service" (Levy & Rubenstein, 1996).
- The ethical theory of utilitarianism is based on the premise that what is right and good is that which produces the most happiness for the most people.
- The ethical theory of Kantianism suggests that actions are bound by a sense of duty and that ethical decisions are made out of respect for moral law.
- The code of Christian ethics is that all decisions about right and wrong should be centered in love for God and in treating others with the same respect and dignity with which we would expect to be treated.

■ The moral precept of the natural law theory is "do good and avoid evil." Good is viewed as that which is inscribed by God into the nature of things. Evil acts are never condoned, even if they are intended to advance the noblest of ends.

■ Ethical egoism espouses that what is right and good is what is best for the individual making the decision.

■ Ethical principles include autonomy, beneficence, nonmaleficence, veracity, and justice.

■ An ethical dilemma is a situation that requires an individual to make a choice between two equally unfavorable alternatives.

■ Ethical issues may arise in psychiatric-mental health nursing around the client's right to refuse medication and right to the least-restrictive treatment alternative.

■ Statutory laws are those that have been enacted by legislative bodies, and common laws are derived from decisions made in previous cases. Both types of laws have civil and criminal components.

■ Civil law protects the private and property rights of individuals and businesses, and criminal law provides protection from conduct deemed injurious to the public welfare.

■ Legal issues in psychiatric-mental health nursing center around confidentiality and the right to privacy, informed consent, restraints and seclusion, and commitment issues.

■ Nurses are accountable for their own actions in relation to legal issues, and violation can result in malpractice lawsuits against the physician, the hospital, and the nurse.

■ Developing and maintaining a good interpersonal relationship with the client and his or her family appears to be a positive factor when the question of malpractice is being considered.

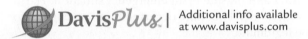 **DavisPlus** | Additional info available at www.davisplus.com

Review Questions
Self-Examination/Learning Exercise

Select the answer that is most appropriate for each of the following questions.

1. The nurse decides to go against family wishes and tell the client of his terminal status because that is what she would want if she were the client. Which of the following ethical theories is considered in this decision?
   a. Kantianism
   b. Christian ethics
   c. Natural law theories
   d. Ethical egoism

2. The nurse decides to respect family wishes and not tell the client of his terminal status because that would bring the most happiness to the most people. Which of the following ethical theories is considered in this decision?
   a. Utilitarianism
   b. Kantianism
   c. Christian ethics
   d. Ethical egoism

3. The nurse decides to tell the client of his terminal status because she believes it is her duty to do so. Which of the following ethical theories is considered in this decision?
   a. Natural law theories
   b. Ethical egoism
   c. Kantianism
   d. Utilitarianism

4. The nurse assists the physician with electroconvulsive therapy on a client who has refused to give consent. With which of the following legal actions might the nurse be charged because of this nursing action?
   a. Assault
   b. Battery
   c. False imprisonment
   d. Breach of confidentiality

Review Questions—cont'd
Self-Examination/Learning Exercise

5. A competent, voluntary client has stated he wants to leave the hospital. The nurse hides his clothes in an effort to keep him from leaving. With which of the following legal actions might the nurse be charged because of this nursing action?
   a. Assault
   b. Battery
   c. False imprisonment
   d. Breach of confidentiality

6. Joe is very restless and is pacing the room. The nurse says to Joe, "If you don't sit down in the chair and be still, I'm going to put you in restraints!" With which of the following legal actions might the nurse be charged because of this nursing action?
   a. Defamation of character
   b. Battery
   c. Breach of confidentiality
   d. Assault

7. An individual may be considered *gravely disabled* for which of the following reasons? (Select all that apply.)
   a. A person, because of mental illness, cannot fulfill basic needs.
   b. A mentally ill person is in danger of physical harm based on inability to care for himself or herself.
   c. A mentally ill person lacks the resources to provide the necessities of life.
   d. A mentally ill person is unable to make use of available resources to meet daily living requirements.

8. Which of the following statements is correct regarding the use of restraints? (Select all that apply.)
   a. Restraints may never be initiated without a physician's order.
   b. Orders for restraints must be reissued by a physician every 2 hours for children and adolescents.
   c. Clients in restraints must be observed and assessed every hour for issues regarding circulation, nutrition, respiration, hydration, and elimination.
   d. An in-person evaluation must be conducted within 1 hour of initiating restraints.

9. Guidelines relating to "duty to warn" state that a therapist should consider taking action to warn a third party when his or her client does which of the following? (Select all that apply.)
   a. Threatens violence toward another individual
   b. Identifies a specific intended victim
   c. Is having command hallucinations
   d. Reveals paranoid delusions about another individual

10. Attempting to calm an angry client by using "talk therapy" is an example of which of the following clients' rights?
   a. The right to privacy
   b. The right to refuse medication
   c. The right to the least-restrictive treatment alternative
   d. The right to confidentiality

11. The Quality and Safety Education for Nurses guidelines identify that student nurses need to be well schooled on informatics. This most directly refers to which of the following?
   a. Learning how to effectively communicate information using electronic health records
   b. Learning the SBAR method of reporting information
   c. Learning guidelines for preventing lawsuits
   d. Learning information about new treatments to keep nursing skills current

References

American Hospital Association (AHA). (2003). The patient care partnership: Understanding expectations, rights, and responsibilities. Retrieved from www.aha.org/advocacy-issues/communicatingpts/pt-care-partnership.shtml

American Nurses Association (ANA). (2015). *Code of ethics for nurses with interpretive statements.* Silver Spring, MD: ANA.

American Nurses Association (ANA), American Psychiatric Nurses Association, & International Society of Psychiatric-Mental Health Nurses. (2014). *Psychiatric–mental health nursing: Scope and standards of practice* (2nd ed.). Silver Spring, MD: ANA.

Appelbaum, P.S. (2001). Thinking carefully about outpatient commitment. *Psychiatric Services, 52*(3), 347-350. doi:10.1176/appi.ps.52.3.347

Austin, S. (2011). Stay out of court with proper documentation. *Nursing2011, 41*(4), 25-29. doi:10.1097/01.NURSE.0000395202.86451.d4

Butts, J., & Rich, K. (2016). *Nursing ethics: Across the curriculum and into practice* (4th ed.). Burlington, MA: Jones & Bartlett.

Cady, R.F. (2010). A review of basic patient rights in psychiatric care. *JONA's Healthcare Law, Ethics, and Regulation, 12*(4), 117-125. doi:10.1097/NHL.0b013e3181f4d357

Catalano, J.T. (2015). *Nursing now! Today's issues, tomorrow's trends* (7th ed.). Philadelphia: F.A. Davis.

Csere, M. (2013). Updated report: involuntary outpatient mental health treatment laws. *OLR Research Report.* Retrieved from https://www.cga.ct.gov/2013/rpt/2013-R-0105.htm

Ellis, J.R., & Hartley, C.L. (2012). *Nursing in today's world: Challenges, issues, and trends* (10th ed.). Philadelphia: Wolters Kluwer Health/Lippincott Williams & Wilkins.

Garner, B.A. (Ed.). (2014). *Black's law dictionary* (10th ed.). St. Paul, MN: Thompson West.

Guido, G.W. (2014). *Legal and ethical issues in nursing* (6th ed.). Upper Saddle River, NJ: Pearson.

Hartsell, T.L., & Bernstein, B.E. (2013). *The portable lawyer for mental health professionals: An A-Z guide to protecting your clients, your practice, and yourself* (3rd ed.). Hoboken, NJ: Wiley & Sons.

Henderson, E. (2015). Potentially dangerous patients: A review of the duty to warn. *Journal of Emergency Nursing, 41*(3), 193-200. doi:http://dx.doi.org/10.1016/j.jen.2014.08.012

Institute of Medicine. (2003). *Health professions education: A bridge to quality.* Washington, DC: Institute of Medicine.

Landeweer, E., Abma, T.A., & Widdershoven, G. (2011). Moral margins concerning the use of coercion in psychiatry. *Nursing Ethics, 18*(3), 304-316. doi:10.1177/0969733011400301

Maiese, M. (2013 [originally posted July 2003]). Principles of justice and fairness. *Beyond intractability.* Eds. C. Burgess & H. Burgess. Conflict Information Consortium, University of Colorado, Boulder. Retrieved from www.beyondintractability.org/essay/principles-of-justice

Maloy, K.A. (1996). Does involuntary outpatient commitment work? In B.D. Sales & S.A. Shah (Eds.), *Mental health and law: Research, policy and services* (pp. 41-74). Durham, NC: Carolina Academic Press.

National Conference of State Legislatures. (2016). Mental health professionals' duty to warn. Retrieved from www.ncsl.org/research/health/mental-health-professionals-duty-to-warn.aspx

QSEN Institute. (2013). *Competencies.* Retrieved from http://qsen.org/competencies/

Sadock, B.J., Sadock, V.A., & Ruiz, P. (2015). *Synopsis of psychiatry: Behavioral sciences/clinical psychiatry* (11th ed.). Philadelphia, PA: Lippincott Williams & Wilkins.

Swartz, M.S., & Swanson, J.W. (2008). Outpatient commitment: When it improves patient outcomes. *Current Psychiatry, 7*(4), 25-35. doi:http://dx.doi.org/10.1176/appi.ps.52.3.325

Tarasoff v. Regents of University of California et al. (1974a), 551 P.d 345.

Tarasoff v. Regents of University of California et al. (1974b), 554 P.d 347.

The Joint Commission. (2015). *The comprehensive accreditation manual for hospitals (CAMH).* Oakbrook Terrace, IL: Joint Commission Resources.

Torrey, E.F., & Zdanowicz, M. (2001). Outpatient commitment: What, why, and for whom. *Psychiatric Services, 52*(3), 337-341. doi:http://dx.doi.org/10.1176/appi.ps.52.3.337

U.S. Code, Title 42, Section 10841, The Public Health and Welfare, 1991.

U.S. Department of Health & Human Services (HHS). (2003). *Standards for privacy of individually identifiable health information.* Washington, DC: HHS.

U.S. Department of Health & Human Services (HHS). (2013, Jan. 17). New rule protects patient privacy, secures health information [press release]. Retrieved from www.hhs.gov/news/press/2013pres/01/20130117b.html

Weiss-Kaffie, C.J., & Purtell, N.E. (2001). Psychiatric nursing. In M.E. O'Keefe (Ed.), *Nursing practice and the law: Avoiding malpractice and other legal risks* (pp. 352-371). Philadelphia: F.A. Davis.

What do I do now? Ethical dilemmas in nursing and health care. (2013). *ISNA Bulletin, 13*(2), 5-12.

Classical References

Levy, R.M., & Rubenstein, L.S. (1996). *The rights of people with mental disabilities.* Carbondale: Southern Illinois University Press.

Patient Self-Determination Act—Patient Rights. (1991). U.S. Code, Title 42, Section 10841, The Public Health and Welfare.

Peplau, H.E. (1991). *Interpersonal relations in nursing: A conceptual frame of reference for psychodynamic nursing.* New York: Springer.

Cultural and Spiritual Concepts Relevant to Psychiatric-Mental Health Nursing

6

CORE CONCEPTS

Culture
Ethnicity
Religion
Spirituality

KEY TERMS

acculturate	density	shaman
assimilate	distance	spirituality
collectivist culture	enculturation	stereotyping
culture	ethnicity	territoriality
cultural syndromes	folk medicine	yin and yang
curandera	individualist culture	
curandero	religion	

OBJECTIVES
After reading this chapter, the student will be able to:

1. Define and differentiate between *culture, race,* and *ethnicity.*
2. Identify cultural differences based on six characteristic phenomena.
3. Describe cultural variances, based on the six phenomena, for the following:
   a. Northern European Americans
   b. African Americans
   c. American Indian and Alaska Natives
   d. Asian and Pacific Islander Americans
   e. Latino Americans
   f. Western European Americans
   g. Arab Americans
   h. Jewish Americans
4. Apply the nursing process in the care of individuals from various cultural groups.
5. Define and differentiate between *spirituality* and *religion.*
6. Identify clients' spiritual and religious needs.
7. Apply the six steps of the nursing process to individuals with spiritual and religious needs.

HOMEWORK ASSIGNMENT
Please read the chapter and answer the following questions.

1. Which cultural group may use a medicine man (or woman) called a *shaman*?
2. Restoring a balance between opposite forces is a fundamental concept of Asian health practices. What is this called?
3. Name five types of human spiritual needs.
4. What is the largest ethnic minority group in the United States?
5. What is the perception of mental illness in the Arab culture?

Cultural Concepts

What is culture? What is race? How does it differ from ethnicity? Why are these questions important? The answers lie in the changing face of America. Immigration is not new in the United States. Most U.S. citizens are either immigrants or descendants of immigrants, and the number of foreign-born residents in this country continues to grow each year. This pattern persists because of the many individuals who want to take advantage of the technological growth and upward mobility that exists in this country.

CORE CONCEPTS

Culture describes a particular society's entire way of living, encompassing shared patterns of belief, feeling, and knowledge that guide people's conduct and are passed down from generation to generation. **Ethnicity** relates to groups of people who identify with each other because of a shared social and cultural heritage passed on to each successive generation (Giger, 2017). **Race** may be understood as a more biological term, describing a group of people who share similar inherited characteristics such as skin color, facial features, and blood groups.

Knowledge related to culture and ethnicity is important because these influences affect human behavior, its interpretation, and the response to it. Therefore, it is essential for nurses to understand the effects of cultural influences if they are to work effectively with the diverse population. Generalizations about a cultural group in this context can be beneficial. As Sue and Sue (2016) state, "Generalizations are necessary for us; without them we would become inefficient creatures. However, they are guidelines for our behaviors, to be tentatively applied in new situations, and they should be open to change and challenge" (p. 245). Caution must be taken, however, not to assume that all individuals who share a culture or ethnic group are identical or exhibit behaviors perceived as characteristic of the group. Such assumptions constitute **stereotyping** and must be avoided.

Many variations and subcultures occur within a culture. These differences may be related to status, ethnic background, residence, religion, education, or other factors. People of many different cultures reside in the United States. Some maintain traditional cultural practices, whereas others **acculturate** to dominant cultural practices (give up cultural practices or values as a result of contact with another group) and **assimilate** by incorporating practices and values of the dominant culture. Every individual must be appreciated for his or her uniqueness and assessed carefully to identify his

or her preferences with regard to cultural and spiritual practices.

Race is a controversial term because of its association with racism or prejudicial views about a group of people based on their appearance. Some scientists argue that no group of individuals is genetically pure enough to define race as a set of biological distinctions. Other scientists argue the benefit of understanding racial differences in determining response to treatments such as medications (see Chapter 4, Psychopharmacology, for a discussion of this topic). The U.S. Census Bureau collects data on racial demographics, and they clarify that the data is based on self-reported, self-identified affiliations (U.S. Census Bureau, 2013). In 2000, the Census Bureau also began including a category that allows for individuals to identify with two or more races. A breakdown of these demographics is presented in Figure 6–1.

This chapter explores the ways in which various cultures differ. The nursing process is applied to the delivery of psychiatric-mental health nursing care for individuals from the following cultural groups: Northern European Americans, African Americans, American Indian and Alaska Natives, Asian and Pacific Islander Americans, Latino Americans, Arab Americans, and Jewish Americans.

How Do Cultures Differ?

It is difficult to generalize about any specific group in a country that is known for its heterogeneity. Within

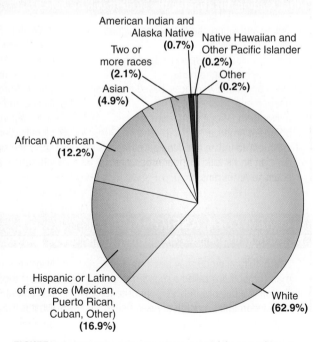

FIGURE 6–1 U.S. Census Bureau report on racial demographics. (From U.S. Census Bureau, 2010–2014 American Community Survey 5-Year estimates [2016].)

our American "melting pot," any or all characteristics could apply to individuals within any or all of the cultural groups represented. As these differences continue to be integrated, one American culture will eventually emerge. This integration is already evident in some regions of the country today, particularly in the urban coastal areas. However, some differences still exist, and it is important for nurses to be aware of cultural influences that may affect individuals' behaviors and beliefs, particularly as they apply to health care.

Giger (2017) describes six cultural phenomena that vary with application and use yet are evidenced among all cultural groups: (1) communication, (2) space, (3) social organization, (4) time, (5) environmental control, and (6) biological variations.

Communication

All verbal and nonverbal behavior in connection with another individual is communication. Therapeutic communication has always been considered an essential part of the nursing process and represents a critical element in most nursing school curricula. Communication has its roots in culture. Cultural mores, norms, ideas, and customs provide the basis for our way of thinking. Cultural values are learned and differ from society to society. Communication is expressed through language (the spoken and written word), paralanguage (the voice quality, intonation, rhythm, and speed of the spoken word), and gestures (touch, facial expression, eye movements, body posture, and physical appearance). The nurse who is planning care must have an understanding of the client's needs and expectations as they are being communicated. As a third party, an interpreter often complicates matters but may be necessary when the client does not speak the same language as the nurse. Interpreting is a very complex process, however, that requires a keen sensitivity to cultural nuances and not just translating words into another language. Technology has facilitated access to interpreters through such devices as telephone services, video remote interpretation, and Internet document translation, but these technologies do not negate the importance of culturally sensitive, respectful nursing care. Tips for facilitating the communication process when using an interpreter are presented in Box 6–1.

Space

Spatial determinants relate to the place where the communication occurs and encompass the concepts of *territoriality, density,* and *distance.* **Territoriality** is the innate tendency to own space. The need for territoriality is met only if the individual has control of a

---

BOX 6–1 **Using an Interpreter**

When using an interpreter, keep the following points in mind:

• Whenever possible, use a certified interpreter with a background in health care. Avoid using relatives or children as interpreters because they may not be objective or may have difficulty relaying information about sensitive topics.
• Address the client directly and maintain eye contact with the client (rather than the interpreter) to engage the client in interaction with the health-care provider.
• Do not interrupt or rush the client and the interpreter. Allow time for interpretation and response before asking another question.
• Ask the interpreter to give you verbatim translations so that you can assess and document exactly what the client has stated in response to questions.
• Avoid using medical jargon or colloquialisms that the interpreter or client may not understand.
• Avoid talking separately with the interpreter at length; the client may feel left out and distrustful.
• Always ask permission to discuss emotional or sensitive topics first, and prepare the interpreter for the content of the interview.
• When possible, allow the client and the interpreter to meet each other before the interview, and if possible, try to use the same interpreter for all subsequent interviews with the client.
• If possible, request an interpreter of the same gender as the client and of similar age or older.
• Discuss the interview questions with the interpreter ahead of time to facilitate flow of the interview.

SOURCES: Gorman, L.M., & Sultan, D. (2008). Psychosocial nursing for general patient care. *Philadelphia: F.A. Davis; Purnell, L.D. (2013).* Transcultural health care: A culturally competent approach *(4th ed.). Philadelphia: F.A. Davis.*

---

space, can establish rules for that space, and is able to defend the space against invasion or misuse by others. **Density,** which refers to the number of people within a given environmental space, can influence interpersonal interaction. **Distance** is the means by which various cultures use space to communicate. Hall (1966) identified three primary dimensions of space in interpersonal interactions in the Western culture: the intimate zone (0 to 18 inches), the personal zone (18 inches to 3 feet), and the social zone (3 to 6 feet).

Social Organization

Cultural behavior is socially acquired through a process called **enculturation,** also called *socialization,* which involves acquiring knowledge and internalizing values of the group (Giger, 2017). Children are enculturated by observing adults within their social organizations. Social organizations include, among others, families, religious groups, and ethnic groups.

Time

An awareness of the concept of time is a gradual learning process. Some cultures place great importance on values measured by clock time. Punctuality and efficiency are highly valued in the United States, whereas some cultures are actually scornful of clock time. For example, some rural people in Algeria label the clock as the "devil's mill" and therefore have no notion of scheduled appointment times or meal times (Giger, 2017). They are indifferent to the passage of clock time and despise haste in all human endeavors. Other cultural implications regarding time have to do with perception of time orientation. Whether individuals are present oriented or future oriented in their perception of time influences many aspects of their lives.

Environmental Control

The variable of environmental control has to do with the degree to which individuals perceive that they have control over their environments. Cultural beliefs and practices influence how an individual responds to his or her environment during periods of wellness and illness. To provide culturally appropriate care, the nurse should not only respect the individual's unique beliefs, but also have an understanding of how these beliefs can be used to promote optimal health in the client's environment.

Biological Variations

Biological differences exist among people in various racial groups. These differences include body structure (both size and shape), skin color, physiological responses to medication, electrocardiographic patterns, susceptibility to disease, and nutritional preferences and deficiencies. Giger (2017) suggests that nurses who provide care for diverse cultural groups need to be aware of basic biological differences to give nonharmful, competent, and culturally appropriate care.

Application of the Nursing Process

Background Assessment Data

A cultural assessment tool for gathering information related to culture and ethnicity that is important in the planning of client care is provided in Box 6–2.

Northern European Americans

Northern European Americans include people who originate from England, Ireland, Iceland, Wales, Finland, Sweden, Norway, Denmark, and the Baltic states of Estonia, Latvia, and Lithuania. English is the primary language for those living in the United States. Their language may also include words and phrases that reflect the influence of the languages spoken in the countries of their heritages. The descendants of these immigrants comprise the dominant cultural

---

BOX 6–2 Cultural Assessment Tool

Client's name _____ Ethnic origin _____
Address _____ Birthdate _____
Name of significant other _____ Relationship _____
Primary language spoken _____ Second language spoken _____
How does client usually communicate with people who speak a different language? _____
Is an interpreter required? _____ Available? _____
Highest level of education achieved: _____ Occupation: _____
Presenting problem: _____
Has this problem ever occurred before? _____
If so, in what manner was it handled previously? _____
What is the client's usual manner of coping with stress? _____
Who is (are) the client's main support system(s)? _____
Describe the family living arrangements: _____
Who is the major decision maker in the family? _____
Describe client's/family members' roles within the family. _____

Describe religious beliefs and practices: _____
   Are there any religious requirements or restrictions that place limitations on the client's care? _____
   If so, describe: _____
Who in the family takes responsibility for health concerns? _____
Describe any special health beliefs and practices: _____

From whom does family usually seek help in addressing health care concerns when needed? _____

BOX 6–2 Cultural Assessment Tool—cont'd

Describe client's usual emotional/behavioral response to:
 Anxiety: _____
 Anger: _____
 Loss/change/failure: _____
 Pain: _____
 Fear: _____
Describe any topics that are particularly sensitive or that the client is unwilling to discuss (because of cultural taboos):
_____
Describe any activities in which the client is unwilling to participate (because of cultural customs or taboos):
_____
What are the client's personal feelings regarding touch? _____
What are the client's personal feelings regarding eye contact? _____
What is the client's personal orientation to time? (past, present, future) _____
What are the client's practices regarding punctuality and scheduled appointment times? _____
_____
Describe any particular illnesses to which the client may be biologically susceptible (e.g., hypertension and sickle cell anemia in African Americans):
_____
Describe any nutritional deficiencies to which the client may be biologically susceptible (e.g., lactose intolerance in Native and Asian Americans) _____
Describe client's favorite foods: _____
Are there any foods the client requests or refuses because of cultural beliefs related to this illness (e.g., "hot" and "cold" foods for Latino Americans and Asian Americans)? If so, please describe: _____
_____
What does the client typically do to balance his or her diet? _____
Describe client's perception of the problem and expectations of health care: _____
_____
_____

---

group in the United States today. Specific dialects and rate of speech are common to various regions of the country. All cultures can be described on a continuum from individualistic to collectivistic, which describes, in part, the degree of focus on self versus group. **Individualistic cultures** stress independence, self-reliance, and freedom, and traditional European American culture in the United States is a highly individualistic culture (Purnell, 2013). Northern European Americans value territory. Personal space preference is about 18 inches to 3 feet.

Data collected on the U.S. population can be revealing about cultural values and trends, which influence perceptions about American culture both within and outside the country. Data on marriage and divorce in the United States show that about half of first marriages end in divorce (Centers for Disease Control and Prevention [CDC], 2015a). The CDC also identifies that the marriage rate has steadily declined over the past 14 years, from 8.2 per 1000 population in 2000 to 6.9 per 1000 in 2014.

The value that was once placed on religion and the organized church also seems to be diminishing in the American culture. According to Gallup polls, over the last four decades there has been a steady decline in Americans' confidence in religion. The organized church reached an all-time low confidence rating of 42 percent in 2015 (Gallup, 2015). A 2012 Pew Research poll noted that church attendance has also shown a similar decline but that some individuals still report a religious affiliation even though they do not attend church. Among the variables cited for lack of church attendance were disagreements with the church and being too busy (Lipka, 2013). Although the majority of Americans still identify as affiliated with some branch of Christianity, the percentage declined from 78.4 percent in 2014 to 70.6 percent in 2014. The number of Americans identifying as agnostic, atheist, or "nothing in particular" increased from 16.1 percent to 22.8 percent over the same time period (Pew Research Center, 2015). These findings suggest that while a majority of Americans may still value faith and worship, their mechanisms for expressing those values are undergoing cultural change.

Northern European Americans, particularly those who achieve middle-class socioeconomic status, value preventive medicine and primary health care. This value follows with the socioeconomic group's educational level, successful achievement, and financial capability to maintain a healthy lifestyle. Most recognize the importance of regular physical exercise. Punctuality and efficiency are valued aspects of mainstream American work ethic, and in general, individual needs are considered subservient to the needs of the organization (Purnell, 2013). However, as Purnell points out, in the current postmodern movement with its lack of adherence to truths as "absolute" and an emphasis on worldviews based on perception and social context, the face of mainstream American culture is changing.

A typical diet for many Northern European Americans is high in fats and cholesterol and low in fiber. Americans, in general, are learning about the health benefits of reducing fats and increasing nutrients in their diet. However, they still enjoy fast food, which conforms to their fast-paced lifestyles.

Changing Trends in Dominant American Culture and Nurse Self-Awareness

Nurses who identify with the dominant culture will benefit from reflecting on the values and practices considered important within this context. Much attention is placed on understanding values and practices of people of different cultures, but self-awareness is vitally important as well. Asking clients to describe their expectations for health-care provision and the role of the nurse can begin to lay the groundwork for discussing differences in cultural values and interacting as individuals within a culturally sensitive context. For example, a nurse who identifies with the dominant, individualistic culture may have the belief that people should take responsibility for themselves and do what they want to do independent of the opinions of family and community. If the nurse communicates this expectation to someone from a collectivist cultural framework, the nurse and client may encounter difficulty establishing a working relationship because their basic values are at odds with one another.

The United States, viewed as a melting pot of multiple worldwide ethnic groups, has its own unique blended culture that impacts the health and care of individuals. It is important that the nurse is aware—and self-aware of these conscious and unconscious attitudes and values within the U.S. culture when caring for clients and understands how these characteristics can impact mental health and mental illness. Characteristics common to the U.S. culture are presented in Box 6–3.

African Americans

The African American or black population in the United States numbers 46.3 million according to the most recent US Census data. Of those, 2.2 million are

---

BOX 6–3 **American Culture**

General: The United States is the third-largest country and one of the most culturally diverse. The vast majority of Americans speak and understand at least some English. The majority (83%) identify as being of the Christian faith, and the second-largest group (13%) identifies as having no religious affiliation. Judaism is the second-largest religion (1.7%), and Islam is the third (0.6%). Football and baseball are identified as favorite pastimes. Marketing products to people in their homes and other countries now constitutes one of the biggest industries.

Work and economy: Equality and economic mobility are valued, and several laws protect equality rights, but there is still evidence of stratification and segregation (e.g., urban versus suburban neighborhoods). Most Americans are not opposed to social security benefits, but welfare for the poor is controversial. Work and competition are valued; being "on the go" is more valued than idle time.

Time and orientation: Making the best use of time is important and may be connected to work ethics (e.g., "time is money"). Being on time for meetings is expected. Most Americans are future oriented; from a young age, children are taught to focus on what they "want to be" when they grow up.

Individuality: Developing one's own goals and not relying too heavily on others is valued. Independent achievements are rewarded.

Privacy: Privacy and having some "alone time" are valued. Personal thoughts and feelings are considered by most to be private. It is often considered rude to ask about someone's finances or their age.

Informality: Casual lifestyle is common. Greetings and farewells are usually short and friendly but superficial; friendships are often casual (e.g., easily developed and easily ended).

Social: Personal restraint of one's body is common; physical distance is common in interaction, especially among men. Breastfeeding, yawning, and expelling gas in public are considered rude.

Death: Most Americans are uncomfortable with their own mortality. Death is considered difficult to talk about, and funerals are typically sad and solemn occasions.

SOURCES: Beane, M. (no date). An adventure in American culture and values. International Student Guide to the United States of America. Retrieved from www.internationalstudentguidetotheusa.com/articles/culture.htm; Countries & Their Cultures Forum. (2017). United States of America. Retrieved from www.everyculture.com/To-Z/United-States-of-America.html; Zimmerman, K.A. (2015). American culture: Traditions and customs of the United States. Live Science. Retrieved from www.livescience.com/28945-american-culture.html.

---

military veterans, and 84.7% over the age of 25 hold a high school diploma or higher level of education. Despite these favorable statistics, the US Census also reports that 25.4% of the US black population remains below the poverty level.

Despite decades of civil rights advances, patterns of discrimination against African Americans continue, and evidence of segregation still exists, usually in the form of predominantly black neighborhoods, churches, and schools, which are still visible in most U.S. cities. Some African Americans find it difficult to assimilate into the mainstream culture and choose to remain within their own social organization.

The most recent survey by the U.S. Census Bureau revealed that 40.4 percent of African American family households were headed by a woman (U.S. Census Bureau, 2015). Social support systems may be large and include sisters, brothers, aunts, uncles, cousins, boyfriends, girlfriends, neighbors, and friends. Many African Americans have a strong religious orientation, with the vast majority practicing some form of Protestantism. However, the declining rate of those who identify themselves as Christians and the concurrent rise in numbers who identify themselves as having no affiliation with organized religion is similar among many demographic groups, including African Americans (Pew Research Center, 2015).

African Americans who have assimilated into the dominant culture are likely to be well educated, professional, and future oriented. Some who have not become assimilated may believe that planning for the future is hopeless, a belief based on their previous experiences and encounters with racism and discrimination (Cherry & Giger, 2013). Among this group, some may be unemployed or have low-paying jobs with little expectation for improvement.

Some African Americans, particularly those from lower socio-economic groups, may have limited access to primary care services, and may be more receptive to folk medicine practices as an alternative. Incorporated into the system of **folk medicine** is the belief that health is a gift from God, whereas illness is a punishment from God or a retribution for sin and evil. Historically, African Americans have sometimes pursued folk medicine remedies because the cost of mainstream medical treatment was prohibitive, or because of the insensitive treatment by caregivers in the health-care delivery system.

Hypertension occurs more frequently and sickle cell disease occurs predominantly in African Americans. Hypertension carries a strong hereditary risk factor, and sickle cell disease is genetically derived. Alcoholism is a serious problem among members of the black community, leading to a high incidence of alcohol-related illness and death (Cherry & Giger, 2013).

American Indian and Alaska Natives

The federal government currently recognizes 566 American Indian (AI) tribes and Alaska Native (AN) groups. Approximately 200 tribal languages are still spoken, some by only a few individuals and others by many (Bureau of Indian Affairs, 2016). Fewer than half of these individuals still live on reservations, but many return regularly to participate in family and tribal life and sometimes to retire. American Indians and Alaska Natives are often grouped together in statistical reporting about Native Americans, but they are a diverse group, and some Alaska Natives prefer not to be referred to as Native Americans (Purnell, 2014). The AI/AN group is described as a *collectivist culture,* which stresses their close dependence on and interconnectedness with family and tribe.

Touch is an aspect of communication that is not the same among AI/AN groups as in the dominant American culture. Some AI/AN groups view the traditional handshake as somewhat aggressive. Instead, if a hand is offered to another, it may be accepted with a light touch or just a passing of hands. Some AI/AN groups will not touch a dead person (Hanley, 2017).

American Indians and Alaska Natives may appear silent and reserved. They may be uncomfortable expressing emotions because the culture encourages keeping private thoughts to oneself. In conversation, most prefer a distance of greater than 2 feet, and for some it may be up to 6 feet, so it is important to pay attention to cues from the client (Purnell, 2014).

The concept of space is very concrete to AI/AN culture. Living space is often crowded with members of both nuclear and extended families. A large network of kin is very important to American Indians and Alaska Natives. However, a need for extended space exists, as demonstrated by a distance of many miles between individual homes or camps.

The primary social organizations of AI/AN groups are the family and the tribe. From infancy, AI/AN children are taught the importance of these units. Traditions are passed down by the elders, and children are taught to respect tradition and to honor wisdom.

Most AI/AN individuals are present-time oriented. The concept of time is very casual, and tasks are accomplished not with the notion of a particular time in mind but in a present-oriented time frame. AI/AN individuals typically are not ruled by the clock, and some do not even own clocks.

Religion and health practices are intertwined in the AI/AN culture. The medicine man (or woman), generally called the shaman (although some tribes prefer different terms) may use a variety of methods in his or her practice. Some use crystals to diagnose illness, some sing and perform healing ceremonies, and some use herbs and other plants or roots to create remedies with healing properties. The American Indian healers and U.S. Indian Health Service have worked together with mutual respect for many years. Hanley (2017) relates that an AI/AN healer may confer with a physician regarding the care of a client in the hospital. Research studies have continued to show the importance of each of these health-care approaches and collaborative practice in the overall wellness of AI/AN client (Hanley, 2017).

The risks of illness and premature death from alcoholism, diabetes, tuberculosis, heart disease, accidents, homicide, suicide, pneumonia, and influenza are dramatically higher for American Indians and Alaska Natives than for the U.S. population as a whole. The Indian Health Service (2015) reports that American Indians and Alaska Natives are "more likely to report past-year alcohol and substance use disorders than any other race, and suicide rates are 1.7 times higher than the U.S. all-races rate." Domestic violence, too, is a significant behavioral health concern in this group, with 39 percent of women experiencing intimate partner violence. Nutritional deficiencies are not uncommon among tribal AI/AN populations. Fruits and green vegetables are often scarce in many of the federally defined Indian geographical regions. Meat and corn products are identified as preferred foods. Fiber intake is relatively low, while fat intake is often of the saturated variety. Approximately 276 of the tribes recognized by the federal or state government receive commodity foods supplied by the U.S. Department of Agriculture's food distribution program (U.S. Department of Agriculture, 2015).

Asian Pacific Islander Americans

Asian Americans comprise 4.9 percent of the U.S. population. The Asian American culture includes peoples (and their descendants) from Japan, China, Vietnam, the Philippines, Thailand, Cambodia, Korea, Laos, India, and the Pacific Islands. Although this discussion relates to this population as a single culture, it is important to keep in mind that a multiplicity of differences regarding attitudes, beliefs, values, religious practices, and language exist among these subcultures.

Many Asian Americans, particularly Japanese, are third- and even fourth-generation Americans. These individuals are likely to be acculturated to the U.S. culture. Kuo and Roysircar-Sodowsky (2000) describe three patterns common to Asian Americans in their attempt to adjust to the American culture. Some older-generation Asians tend to hold on to the traditional values and practices of their native culture. They have strong, internalized Asian values. Primary allegiance is to their biological family. Frequently,

members of the younger generation may reject the traditional values of their ancestral culture, and totally embrace Western culture. Finally, some Asian Americans strike a balance, incorporating traditional values and beliefs with Western values and beliefs. They are—or become—integrated into the American culture while maintaining a connection with their ancestral culture.

The languages and dialects of Asian Americans are very diverse. In general, they share a similar belief in harmonious interaction. To raise one's voice is likely to be interpreted as a sign of loss of control. The English language is very difficult to master, and even bilingual Asian Americans who are recent immigrants may encounter communication problems because of the differences in meaning assigned to nonverbal cues such as facial gestures, verbal intonation and speed, and body movements. In Asian cultures, touching during communication has historically been considered unacceptable. However, with the advent of Western acculturation, younger generations of Asian Americans accept touching as more appropriate than did their ancestors. Acceptable personal and social spaces are larger than in the dominant American culture. Some Asian Americans have a great deal of difficulty expressing emotions. Because of their reserved public demeanor, Asian Americans may be misperceived as shy, cold, or uninterested.

The family is the ultimate social organization in traditional Asian American culture, and loyalty to family is emphasized above all else. Children are expected to obey and honor their parents. Misbehavior is perceived as bringing dishonor to the entire family. Filial piety (one's social obligation or duty to one's parents) is held in high regard. Failure to fulfill these obligations can create a great deal of guilt and shame in an individual. A chronological hierarchy exists with the elderly maintaining positions of authority. Several generations or even extended families may share a single household.

Although education is highly valued among traditional Asian Americans, many remain undereducated. Religious beliefs and practices are diverse and exhibit influences of Taoism, Buddhism, Confucianism, Islam, Hinduism, and Christianity.

Many Asian Americans value both a past and a present orientation. Emphasis is placed on the wishes of one's ancestors while adjusting to demands of the present. Prompt adherence to schedules or rigid standards of activities may or may not be valued.

Restoring the balance of **yin and yang** is the fundamental concept of Asian health practices. Yin and yang represent opposite forces of energy, such as negative/positive, dark/light, cold/hot, hard/soft, and feminine/masculine. The belief is that illness occurs when there is a disruption in the balance of these energy forces. In medicine, the opposites are expressed as "hot" and "cold," and health is the result of a balance between hot and cold elements (Chang, 2017). Food, medicines, and herbs are classified according to their hot and cold properties and are used to restore balance between yin and yang (cold and hot), thereby restoring health.

Rice, vegetables, and fish were the traditional main staple foods of many Asian diets. Milk is seldom consumed because a large majority of Asian Americans experience lactose intolerance. With Western acculturation, their diet is changing, and unfortunately, the percentage of fat in the diet is increasing as more meat is consumed.

Some Asian cultures believe that psychiatric illness is merely behavior that is out of control. They view this as a great shame to the individual and the family. They often attempt to manage the ill person on their own until they can no longer handle the situation. It is not uncommon for Asian Americans to somaticize. Expressing mental distress through various physical ailments may be viewed as more acceptable than expressing true emotions.

The incidence of alcohol dependence is low among Asians. This may be a result of a possible genetic intolerance of the substance. Some Asians develop unpleasant symptoms, such as flushing, headaches, and palpitations, from drinking alcohol. Research indicates that this is due to an isoenzyme variant that quickly converts alcohol to acetaldehyde and the absence of an isoenzyme that is needed to oxidize acetaldehyde. This results in a rapid accumulation of acetaldehyde that produces the unpleasant symptoms (Wall et al., 1997).

Latino Americans

Latino Americans are the fastest-growing group of people in the United States, comprising 16.9 percent of the population (U.S. Census Bureau, 2016). They represent the largest ethnic minority group. Recent presidential debates highlighted public confusion about the correct terminology to describe different groups (Garcia-Navarro, 2015). The U.S. Census Bureau clarifies that Latino or Hispanic peoples comprise many different races. It would not be correct, for example, to refer to someone as a member of the Latin race, since there are a variety of races among Latin American countries. Latin Americans are those who currently reside in Latin American countries. Latino Americans are those who come from Latin American countries but currently reside in the United States. *Latino American* is often shortened to *Latino*, but individual preferences about this term vary. The term *Hispanic* is used to refer to people who share the common language of Spanish. Brazilian people, for example, would be offended by being referred to as Hispanic, since their primary language is Portuguese (Garcia-Navarro, 2015). Preferences as to what constitutes appropriate descriptive terms can vary depending on geographic location. Asking clients how *they* would describe their cultural identity is in the interest of averting an unintentional insult and demonstrates cultural sensitivity.

Latino Americans trace their ancestry to countries such as Mexico, Spain, Puerto Rico, Cuba, and other countries of Central and South America. Touch is a common form of communication among Latinos; however, they can also be very modest and are likely to withdraw from any infringement on their modesty.

Traditional Latino Americans, as a collectivist culture, are very group oriented and often interact with large groups of relatives. Touching and embracing are common modes of communication. The family is the primary social organization and includes nuclear family members as well as numerous extended family members. The traditional nuclear family is male dominated, and the father possesses ultimate authority.

Latino Americans tend to be focused on the present time. The concept of being punctual and giving attention to activities that concern the future are perceived as less important than activities in the present.

Roman Catholicism is the predominant religion among Latino Americans. Most Latinos identify with the Roman Catholic Church, even if they do not attend services. Religious beliefs and practices are likely to be strong influences in their lives. Especially in times of crisis, such as in cases of illness and hospitalization, Latino Americans rely on priests and the family to carry out important religious rituals, such as promise making, offering candles, visiting shrines, and offering prayers (Spector, 2013).

Folk beliefs regarding health are a combination of elements incorporating views of Roman Catholicism and Indian and Spanish beliefs. The folk healer is called a **curandero** (male) or **curandera** (female). Among traditional Latino Americans, the *curandero* is believed to have a gift from God for healing the sick and is often the first contact made when illness is encountered. Treatments used include massage, diet, rest, suggestions, practical advice, indigenous herbs, prayers, magic, and supernatural rituals (McMurry et al., 2017). Many Latino Americans still subscribe to the "hot and cold theory" of disease. This concept is similar to the Asian perception of yin and yang discussed earlier in this chapter. Diseases and the foods and medicines used to treat them are classified as "hot" or "cold," and the intention is to restore the body to a balanced state.

National studies have revealed that the lifetime prevalence for selected psychiatric disorders is higher for U.S.-born Latinos (52.5%) than for Latino immigrants (30.9%), suggesting that there may be a protective context associated with living in their country of origin before immigrating (Alegria et al., 2008; Alegria et al., 2007). This has been referred to as the "immigration paradox" (Alegria et al., 2008), since the stresses of immigration might seem to confer more risk of mental disorders, while the reverse is actually true. The contributing factors are not well understood, and there is variation among some Latino subgroups. Among Mexicans, the immigration paradox holds true for mood, anxiety, and substance disorders, but among Cubans and other Latino subgroups, it holds true only for substance disorders. This paradox does not hold true for migrant versus U.S.-born Puerto Ricans (Alegria et al., 2008). In general, Latino Americans have demonstrated a lower lifetime prevalence of mental disorders than their non-Hispanic white counterparts, but it should be noted that the CDC (2015b) reports that the risk for suicide attempts among teenage girls is higher among Latino girls (15.1%) than non-Hispanic white teenage girls (9.8%). As this cultural group, and particularly U.S.-born Latino Americans, continues to grow in number, mental health professionals will need to develop awareness of risks for illness and sensitivity to the cultural values that may impact seeking treatment.

Arab Americans*

Arab Americans trace their ancestry and traditions to the nomadic desert tribes of the Arabian Peninsula. The Arab countries include Algeria, Bahrain, Comoros, Djibouti, Egypt, Iraq, Jordan, Kuwait, Lebanon, Libya, Mauritania, Morocco, Oman, Palestine, Qatar, Saudi Arabia, Somalia, Sudan, Syria, Tunisia, United Arab Emirates, and Yemen.

First-wave immigrants, primarily Christians, came to the United States between 1887 and 1913 seeking economic opportunity. These immigrants and their descendants typically resided in urban centers of the

Northeast. Second-wave immigrants entered the United States after World War II. Most are refugees from nations beset by war and political instability. This group includes a large number of professionals and individuals seeking educational degrees who have subsequently remained in the United States. Most are Muslims and favor professional occupations.

Arabic is the official language of the Arab world. Although English is a common second language, language and communication can pose formidable problems in health-care settings. Communication is highly contextual, where unspoken expectations are more important than the actual spoken words. While conversing, individuals stand close together, maintain steady eye contact, and touch (only between members of the same gender) the other's hand or shoulder.

Speech may be loud and expressive and characterized by repetition and gesturing, particularly when in serious discussion. Observers witnessing impassioned communication may incorrectly assume that members of this culture are argumentative, confrontational, or aggressive. Privacy is valued, and many resist disclosure of personal information to strangers, especially when it relates to familial disease conditions. Among friends and relatives, Arabs express feelings freely. Devout Muslim men may not shake hands with women. When an Arab man is introduced to an Arab woman, the man may wait for the woman to extend her hand.

Gender roles are often clearly defined. The man is traditionally the head of the household, and women are subordinate to men. Men are traditionally breadwinners, protectors, and decision makers, and women traditionally are responsible for the care and education of children and for the maintenance of a successful marriage by tending to their husbands' needs.

The family is the primary social organization, and children are loved and indulged. The father is the disciplinarian, and the mother is an ally and mediator. Loyalty to one's family takes precedence over personal needs. Sons are responsible for supporting elderly parents.

Women value modesty, especially devout Muslims, for whom modesty is expressed with attire. Many Muslim women view the practice of *hijab*, covering the body except for one's face and hands, offering them protection in situations in which the genders mix.

Sickle cell disease and the thalassemias (a type of inherited blood disorder) are common in the eastern Mediterranean. Sedentary lifestyle and high fat intake among Arab Americans place them at higher risk for cardiovascular diseases. The rates of cholesterol testing, colorectal cancer screening, and uterine cancer

---

*This section on Arab Americans is adapted from Kulwicki, A.D., & Ballout, S. (2013). People of Arab heritage. In L.D. Purnell (Ed.), *Transcultural health care: A culturally competent approach* (4th ed.). © F.A. Davis. Used with permission.

screening are low; however, in recent years, the rate of mammography screening has increased.

Arab cooking shares many general characteristics. Spices and herbs include cinnamon, allspice, cloves, ginger, cumin, mint, parsley, bay leaves, garlic, and onions. Bread accompanies every meal and is viewed as a gift from God. Lamb and chicken are the most popular meats. Muslims are prohibited from eating pork and pork products. Food is eaten with the right hand because it is regarded as clean. Eating and drinking at the same time is viewed as unhealthy. Eating properly, consuming nutritious foods, and fasting are believed to cure disease. Gastrointestinal complaints are the most frequent reason for seeking health care. Lactose intolerance is common.

Most Arabs are Muslims. Islam is the religion of most Arab countries, and in Islam there is no separation of church and state; a certain amount of religious participation is obligatory. Many Muslims believe in combining spiritual medicine, performing daily prayers, and reading or listening to the Qur'an with conventional medical treatment. The devout client may request that his or her chair or bed be turned to face Mecca and that a basin of water be provided for ritual washing or ablution before praying. Sometimes illness is considered punishment for one's sins.

Mental illness is a major social stigma. Psychiatric symptoms may be denied or attributed to "bad nerves" or evil spirits. When individuals suffering from mental distress seek medical care, they are likely to present with a variety of vague complaints such as abdominal pain, lassitude, anorexia, and shortness of breath. Clients often expect and may insist on somatic treatment, often vitamins and tonics. When mental illness is accepted as a diagnosis, treatment with medications rather than counseling is preferred.

Jewish Americans

To be Jewish is to belong to a specific group of people and a specific religion. The term *Jewish* does not refer to a race. The Jewish people came to the United States mostly from Spain, Portugal, Germany, and Eastern Europe (Bralock & Padgham, 2017). More than 5 million Jewish Americans live in the United States, primarily in the larger urban areas.

Four main Jewish religious groups exist today: Orthodox, Reform, Conservative, and Reconstructionist. Orthodox Jews adhere to strict interpretation and application of Jewish laws and ethics. They believe that the laws outlined in the Torah (the five books of Moses) are divine, eternal, and unalterable.

Reform Judaism is the largest Jewish religious group in the United States. The Reform group believes in the autonomy of the individual in interpreting the Jewish code of law, and a more liberal interpretation is followed. Conservative Jews also accept a less strict interpretation. They believe that the code of laws come from God, but they accept flexibility and adaptation of those laws to absorb aspects of the culture while remaining true to Judaism's values. The Reconstructionists have modern views that generally override traditional Jewish laws. They do not believe that Jews are God's chosen people and reject the notion of divine intervention. Reconstructionists are generally accepting of interfaith marriage.

The primary language of Jewish Americans is English. Hebrew, the official language of Israel and the Torah, is used for prayers and taught in Jewish religious education. Early Jewish immigrants spoke a Judeo-German dialect called Yiddish, and some of those words have become part of American English (e.g., *klutz, kosher, tush, chutzpah, mazel tov*).

Although traditional Jewish law is clearly male oriented, with acculturation, little difference is seen today with regard to gender roles. Formal education is a highly respected value among the Jewish people. Over one-third of Jewish Americans hold advanced degrees and are employed as professionals (e.g., science, medicine, law, education), more than any other group within the U.S. white population.

Although most Jewish people live for today and plan for and worry about tomorrow, they are raised with stories of their past, especially of the Holocaust. They are warned to "never forget" lest history be repeated. Therefore, their time orientation is simultaneously to the past, the present, and the future (Selekman, 2013).

Children are considered blessings and valued treasures, treated with respect, and deeply loved. They play an active role in most holiday celebrations and services. Respecting and honoring one's parents is one of the Ten Commandments. Children are expected to be forever grateful to their parents for giving them the gift of life (Selekman, 2013). The rite of passage into adulthood occurs during a religious ceremony called a *bar* or *bat mitzvah* (son or daughter of the commandment) and is usually commemorated by a family celebration.

Because of the respect afforded physicians and the emphasis on keeping the body and mind healthy, Jewish Americans tend to be health conscious. In general, they practice preventive health care, with routine physical, dental, and vision screening. Circumcision for male infants is both a medical procedure and a religious rite and is performed on the eighth day of life. The procedure is usually performed at home and is considered a family festivity.

A number of genetic diseases are more common in the Jewish than among other populations, including Tay-Sachs disease, Gaucher's disease, and familial dysautonomia. Other conditions that occur with increased incidence in the Jewish population include inflammatory bowel disease (ulcerative colitis and Crohn's disease), colorectal cancer, and breast and ovarian cancer. Jewish people have a higher rate of side effects from the antipsychotic clozapine. About 20 percent develop agranulocytosis, the cause of which has been attributed to a specific genetic haplotype (Selekman, 2013).

Alcohol, especially wine, is an essential part of religious holidays and festive occasions. It is viewed as appropriate and acceptable as long as it is used in moderation. For Jewish people who follow the dietary laws, a tremendous amount of attention is given to the slaughter of livestock and the preparation and consumption of food. Religious laws dictate which foods are permissible. The term *kosher* means "fit to eat," and following these guidelines is considered a commandment of God. Meat may be eaten only if the permitted animal has been slaughtered, cooked, and served following kosher guidelines. Pigs are considered unclean, and pork and pork products are forbidden. Dairy products and meat may not be mixed together in cooking, serving, or eating.

Judaism opposes discrimination against people with physical, mental, and developmental conditions. The maintenance of one's mental health is considered just as important as the maintenance of one's physical health. Mental incapacity has always been recognized as grounds for exemption from all obligations under Jewish law (Selekman, 2013).

A summary of information related to the six cultural phenomena as they apply to the cultural groups discussed here is presented in Table 6–1.

Cultural Syndromes

Cultural syndromes are those that are specific to a cultural group and do not share an exact correlation to any diagnostic categories listed in the *Diagnostic and Statistical Manual of Mental Disorders, Fifth Edition (DSM-5)* (Sue & Sue, 2016). These syndromes have historically been described as culture-bound syndromes, but as Sadock, Sadock, and Ruiz (2015) point out, "The clear implication was that Western psychiatric categories were not culture bound . . . [when in fact] culture suffuses all forms of psychological distress,

the familiar as well as the unfamiliar" (p. 145). It is important for nurses to understand the physical and behavioral manifestations of these cultural syndromes. Ataques de nervios (attack of nerves), a Latin American cultural syndrome, may sound similar to the *DSM-5* category of panic attacks, but it is a distinct syndrome with distinct treatment implications (Sue & Sue, 2016). Examples of cultural syndromes are presented in Table 6–2.

Diagnosis and Outcome Identification

Nursing diagnoses are selected on the basis of information gathered during the assessment process. With background knowledge of cultural variables and information uniquely related to the individual, the following nursing diagnoses may be appropriate:

■ Impaired verbal communication related to cultural differences, evidenced by inability to speak the dominant language
■ Anxiety (moderate to severe) related to entry into an unfamiliar health-care system and separation from support systems, evidenced by apprehension and suspicion, restlessness, and trembling
■ Imbalanced nutrition, less than body requirements, related to refusal to eat unfamiliar foods provided in the health-care setting, evidenced by loss of weight
■ Spiritual distress related to inability to participate in usual religious practices because of hospitalization, evidenced by alterations in mood (e.g., anger, crying, withdrawal, preoccupation, anxiety, hostility, apathy)

Outcome criteria related to these nursing diagnoses may include the following:

The client:

1. Has all basic needs fulfilled
2. Communicates with staff through an interpreter
3. Maintains anxiety at a manageable level by having family members stay with him or her during hospitalization
4. Maintains weight by eating foods that he or she likes brought to the hospital by family members
5. Has restored spiritual strength through use of cultural rituals and beliefs and visits from a spiritual leader

Planning and Implementation

The following interventions have special cultural implications for nursing:

■ Use an interpreter, if necessary, to ensure that there are no barriers to communication. Be careful with nonverbal communication because it may be

TABLE 6-1 Summary of Six Cultural Phenomena in Comparison of Various Cultural Groups

CULTURAL GROUP AND COUNTRIES OF ORIGIN	COMMUNICATION	SPACE	SOCIAL ORGANIZATION	TIME	ENVIRONMENTAL CONTROL	BIOLOGICAL VARIATIONS
Northern European Americans (England, Ireland, and others)	National languages (although many learn English very quickly) Dialects (often regional) English More verbal than nonverbal	Territory valued Personal space: 18 inches to 3 feet Uncomfortable with personal contact and touch	Families: Nuclear and extended Religions: Jewish and Christian Organizations: Social community	Future oriented	Most value preventive medicine and primary health care through traditional health-care delivery system Alternative methods on the increase	Health concerns: Cardiovascular disease Cancer Diabetes mellitus
African Americans (Largely descendants of Africans brought forcibly to America as slaves). There are cultural differences between long-standing African Americans and those recently immigrating form Africa.	National languages Primary language is English Highly verbal and nonverbal	Close personal space Comfortable with touch	Large, extended families Many female-headed households Traditionally strong religious orientation, mostly Protestant Community social organizations	Present-time oriented	Traditional health-care delivery system Some individuals prefer to use folk practitioner Home remedies	Health concerns: Cardiovascular disease Hypertension Sickle cell disease Diabetes mellitus Lactose intolerance
American Indians and Alaska Natives (North America, Alaska, Aleutian Islands)	200 tribal languages recognized Comfortable with silence	Large, extended space important Uncomfortable with touch	Families: Nuclear and extended Children taught importance of tradition Social organizations: Tribe and family most important	Present-time oriented	Religion and health practices intertwined Nontraditional healer (shaman) uses folk practices to heal Shaman may work with modern medical practitioner	Health concerns: Alcoholism Tuberculosis Accidents Diabetes mellitus Heart disease
Asian/Pacific Islander Americans (Japan, China, Korea, Vietnam, Philippines, Thailand, Cambodia, Laos, Pacific Islands, others)	More than 30 different languages spoken Comfortable with silence Nonverbal connotations may be misunderstood	Large personal space Uncomfortable with touch	Families: Nuclear and extended Children taught importance of family loyalty and tradition Many religions: Taoism, Buddhism, Islam, Hinduism, Christianity Community social organizations	Present-time oriented Past is important and valued	Traditional health-care delivery system Some prefer to use folk practices (e.g, yin and yang, herbal medicine, and moxibustion)	Health concerns: Hypertension Cancer Diabetes mellitus Thalassemia Lactose intolerance

Continued

TABLE 6–1 Summary of Six Cultural Phenomena in Comparison of Various Cultural Groups—cont'd

CULTURAL GROUP AND COUNTRIES OF ORIGIN	COMMUNICATION	SPACE	SOCIAL ORGANIZATION	TIME	ENVIRONMENTAL CONTROL	BIOLOGICAL VARIATIONS
Latino Americans (Mexico, Spain, Cuba, Puerto Rico, other countries of Central and South America)	Spanish, with many dialects	Close personal space Lots of touching and embracing Very group oriented	Families: Nuclear and large extended families Strong ties to Roman Catholicism Community social organizations	Present-time oriented	Traditional health-care delivery system Some prefer to use folk practitioner, called *curandero* or *curandera* Folk practices include hot and cold herbal remedies	Health concerns: Heart disease Cancer Diabetes mellitus Accidents Lactose intolerance
Arab Americans (Algeria, Bahrain, Comoros, Djibouti, Egypt, Iraq, Jordan, Kuwait, Lebanon, Libya, Mauritania, Morocco, Oman, Palestine, Qatar, Saudi Arabia, Somalia, Sudan, Syria, Tunisia, United Arab Emirates, Yemen)	Arabic English	Large personal space between members of the opposite gender outside of the family Touching common between members of same gender	Families: Nuclear and extended Religion: Muslim and Christianity	Past and present-time oriented	Traditional health-care delivery system Authority of physician is seldom challenged or questioned Adverse outcomes are attributed to God's will Mental illness may be viewed as a social stigma	Health concerns: Sickle cell disease Thalassemia Cardiovascular disease Cancer
Jewish Americans (Spain, Portugal, Germany, Eastern Europe)	English, Hebrew, Yiddish	Touch forbidden between opposite genders in the Orthodox tradition Closer personal space common among non-Orthodox Jews	Families: Nuclear and extended Community social organizations	Past, present-time, and future oriented	Great respect for physicians Emphasis on keeping body and mind healthy Practice preventive health care	Health concerns: Tay-Sachs disease Gaucher's disease Familial dysautonomia Ulcerative colitis Crohn's disease Colorectal cancer Breast cancer Ovarian cancer

SOURCES: Giger, J.N. (2017). *Transcultural nursing: Assessment and intervention* (7th ed.). St. Louis, MO: Mosby; Murray, R.B., Zentner, J.P., & Yakimo, R. (2009). *Health promotion strategies through the life span* (8th ed.). Upper Saddle River, NJ: Prentice Hall; Purnell, L.D. (2013). *Transcultural health care: A culturally competent approach* (4th ed.). Philadelphia: F.A. Davis; Purnell, L.D. (2014). *Guide to culturally competent health care* (3rd ed.). Philadelphia: F.A. Davis; Spector, R.E. (2013). *Cultural diversity in health and illness* (8th ed.). Upper Saddle River: Prentice Hall.

TABLE 6–2 Examples of Cultural Syndromes

SYNDROME	CULTURE	SYMPTOMS
Amok	Malaysia, Laos, Philippines, Polynesia, Papua New Guinea, Puerto Rico, and among the Navajo (may be precipitated by the perception that they have been insulted in some way)	A state of depression followed by violent or homicidal behavior and ending with a period of exhaustion, somnolence, and amnesia; persecutory ideas are also common
Ataque de nervios	Latin America, Latin Caribbean, and Mediterranean (often occurs in response to a stressful family event such as death or divorce)	Uncontrollable shouting, crying, trembling, verbal or physical aggression, sometimes accompanied by dissociative experiences, seizure-like or fainting episodes, and suicidal gestures
Brain fag	West Africa (usually occurring in high school or university students during periods of academic stress)	Difficulty concentrating, poor memory retention, pain and pressure around head and neck, blurred vision; students often complain of "brain fatigue"
Ghost sickness	American Indian tribes	Preoccupation with death and the deceased; symptoms include anxiety, confusion, weakness, feelings of danger, anorexia, and bad dreams; sometimes associated with witchcraft
Hwa-byung	Korea (often attributed to suppression of anger)	Symptoms closely related to those of depression, including insomnia, fatigue, indigestion, dysphoria, anorexia, bodily aches, and loss of interest
Koro	Southern and Eastern Asia	Intense anxiety associated with fear that the penis (in males) or the vulva and nipples (in females) will retract into the body and cause the person to die
Pibloktoq	Eskimo cultures	Sometimes called *arctic hysteria,* an abrupt episode of extreme excitement, preceded by withdrawal or mild irritability, and followed by seizure activity and coma. During the attack the individual engages in aberrant and bizarre verbal and motor behavior; afterward, usually reports complete amnesia for the attack
Shenjing Shuairuo (neurasthenia)	China	Weakness, emotional excitement, nervous symptoms, and sleep disturbances; this condition is featured in the *Chinese Classification of Mental Disorders* under a section called "other neuroses"
Shen-k'uei or Shenkui	Taiwan, China	Panic anxiety and somatic symptoms; sexual dysfunctions are common but without identified physical cause. Attributed to fear of excessive semen loss related to frequent sexual activity; semen is considered part of one's vital essence
Susto	Latin America	Appetite and sleep disturbances, sadness, pains, headache, stomachache, and diarrhea. The soul is thought to leave the body (during dreams or following a traumatic event), resulting in unhappiness and illness
Taijin kyofusho	Japan	Intense anxiety and fear about possibly offending others, particularly with their body functions, appearance, or odor

SOURCES: Giger, J.N. (2017). *Transcultural nursing: Assessment and intervention* (7th ed.). St. Louis, MO: Mosby; Purnell, L.D. (2013). *Transcultural health care: A culturally competent approach* (4th ed.). Philadelphia: F.A. Davis; Sadock, B.J., Sadock, V.A., & Ruiz, P. (2015). *Synopsis of psychiatry: Behavioral sciences/clinical psychiatry* (11th ed.). Philadelphia: Lippincott Williams & Wilkins; Spector, R.E. (2013). *Cultural diversity in health and illness* (8th ed.). Upper Saddle River: Prentice Hall; Sue, D.W., & Sue, D. (2016). *Counseling the culturally diverse* (7th ed.). Hoboken, NJ: Wiley.

interpreted differently by different cultures (e.g., Asians and American Indians may be uncomfortable with touch, whereas Latinos and Western Europeans perceive touch as a sign of caring).

■ Make allowances for individuals from other cultures to have family members around them and even to participate in their care. Large numbers of extended family members are very important to African Americans, American Indians, Asian Americans, Latino Americans, and Western European Americans. To deny access to these family support systems could interfere with the healing process.

■ Ensure that the individual's spiritual needs are being met. Religion is an important source of support for many individuals, and the nurse must be tolerant of various rituals that may be connected with different cultural beliefs about health and illness.

■ Be aware of the differences in concept of time among the various cultures. Most members of the dominant American culture are future oriented and place a high value on punctuality and efficiency. Other cultures may be more present-time oriented. Nurses must be aware that such individuals may not share the value of punctuality. They may be late to appointments and appear to be indifferent to some aspects of their therapy. Nurses must be accepting of these differences and refrain from allowing existing attitudes to interfere with delivery of care.

■ Be aware of different beliefs about health care among the various cultures, and recognize the importance of these beliefs to the healing process. If an individual from another culture has been receiving health care from a spiritualist, curandero, or other nontraditional healer, it is important for the nurse to listen to what has been done in the past and even to consult with these cultural healers about the care being given to the client.

■ Follow the health-care practices the client views as essential, provided they do no harm and do not interfere with the healing process. For example, the concepts of yin and yang and the hot and cold theory of disease are very important to the well-being of some Asians and Latinos, respectively. Try to ensure that a balance of these foods are included in the diet as an important reinforcement for traditional medical care.

■ Be aware of favorite foods of individuals from different cultures. The health-care setting may seem strange and somewhat isolated, and for some individuals, it feels good to have anything around them that is familiar. They may even refuse to eat unfamiliar foods. If it does not interfere with his or her care, allow family members to provide favorite foods for the client.

■ The nurse working in psychiatry must realize that psychiatric illness is stigmatized in some cultures. Individuals who believe that expressing emotions is unacceptable will present unique problems as clients in a psychiatric setting. Nurses must have patience and work slowly to establish trust in order to provide these individuals with the assistance they require.

Evaluation

Evaluation of nursing actions is directed at achievement of the established outcomes. Part of the evaluation process is continuous reassessment to ensure that the selected actions are appropriate and the goals and outcomes are realistic. Including the family and extended support systems in the evaluation process is essential if cultural implications of nursing care are to be measured. Modifications to the plan of care are made as the need is determined.

Spiritual Concepts

CORE CONCEPT

Spirituality

The human quality that gives meaning and sense of purpose to an individual's existence. Spirituality exists within each individual regardless of belief system and serves as a force for interconnectedness between the self and others, the environment, and a higher power.

Spirituality is difficult to describe. Historically, it has had distinctly religious connections, with a spiritual person being described as "someone with whom the Spirit of God dwelt." Koenig (2012) describes spirituality as distinguished by its connection to that which is considered sacred and transcendent. He identifies spirituality as connected to the supernatural, the mystical, and to organized religion but extending beyond and beginning before organized religion. In other words, spirituality may be considered a quest for the transcendent that might lead to staunch belief or nonbelief.

In the treatment of mental illness, some of the earliest practices focused on spiritual treatment because insanity was considered a disruption of mind and spirit (Reeves & Reynolds, 2009). However, Freud (often described as a forefather of psychiatric treatment) believed that religion had a negative effect on mental health and that it was linked to a host of psychiatric symptoms. Thus, religion and spiritually have been avoided rather than embraced as a valuable aspect of treatment. More recently, the focus is changing once again. Reeves and Reynolds (2009) note that the large volume of contemporary research (more than 60 studies) demonstrating the value of spirituality for both medical and psychiatric patients is influencing this change. Nursing has embraced this new focus by the inclusion of nursing responsibility for spiritual care in the International Council of Nurses *Code of Ethics* and in the American Holistic Nurses Association *Standards for Holistic Nursing Practice*. The inclusion of spiritual care is also evidenced by two current NANDA International nursing diagnoses: Spiritual distress and Readiness for enhanced spiritual well-being (Herdman & Kamitsuru, 2014).

Smucker (2001) stated:

> Spirituality is the recognition or experience of a dimension of life that is invisible, and both within us and yet beyond our material world, providing a sense of connectedness and interrelatedness with the universe. (p. 5)

Smucker (2001) identified the following five factors as types of spiritual needs associated with human beings:

1. Meaning and purpose in life
2. Faith or trust in someone or something beyond ourselves
3. Hope
4. Love
5. Forgiveness

Spiritual Needs

Meaning and Purpose in Life

Humans by nature appreciate order and structure in their lives. Having a purpose in life gives one a sense of control and the feeling that life is worth living. Each nurse's exploration of his or her own spirituality and efforts to grow spiritually are foundational to being responsive to those needs in others. Walsh (1999) describes seven perennial practices that he believes promote enlightenment, aid in transformation, and encourage spiritual growth:

1. **Transform your motivation:** Reduce craving and find your soul's desire.
2. **Cultivate emotional wisdom:** Heal your heart and learn to love.
3. **Live ethically:** Feel good by doing good.
4. **Concentrate and calm your mind:** Accept the challenge of mastering attention and mindfulness.
5. **Awaken your spiritual vision:** See clearly and recognize the sacred in all things.
6. **Cultivate spiritual intelligence:** Develop wisdom and understand life.
7. **Express spirit in action:** Embrace generosity and the joy of service. (p. 14)

In the final analysis, each individual must determine his or her own perception of what is important and what gives meaning to life. Throughout one's existence, the meaning of life will undoubtedly be challenged many times. A solid spiritual foundation may help an individual confront the challenges that result from life's experiences.

Faith

Faith is often thought of as the acceptance of a belief in the absence of physical or empirical evidence. Smucker (2001) stated:

> For all people, faith is an important concept. From childhood on, our psychological health depends on having faith or trust in something or someone to help meet our needs. (p. 7)

Having faith requires that individuals rise above that which they can experience only through the five senses. Faith transcends the appearance of the physical world. An increasing amount of medical and scientific research is showing that what individuals believe exists can have as powerful an impact as what actually exists. Karren and associates (2010) stated:

> [There is a] growing appreciation of the healing power of faith among members of the medical community. Belief strongly impacts health outcomes, and belief of a large majority of Americans is connected to their religious commitments. Seventy-five percent of Americans say that their religious faith forms the foundation for their approach to life. Seventy-three percent of Americans say that prayer is an important part of their daily life. Religious belief provides power for an individual. With such beliefs so prevalent, it is no surprise that religious faith plays a significant role in healing. (p. 360)

Evidence suggests that faith, combined with conventional treatment and an optimistic attitude, can be a very powerful element in the healing process.

Hope

Hope has been defined as a special kind of positive expectation (Karren, Smith, & Gordon, 2013). With hope, individuals look at a situation, and no matter how negative, find something positive on which to focus. Hope functions as an energizing force. In addition, research indicates that hope may promote healing, facilitate coping, and enhance quality of life (Enayati, 2013; Nekolaichuk, Jevne, & Maguire, 1999).

Kübler-Ross (1969), in her classic study of dying patients, stressed the importance of hope. She suggested that even though these patients could not hope for a cure, they could hope for additional time to live, to be with loved ones, for freedom from pain, or for a peaceful death with dignity. She found hope to be a satisfaction unto itself, whether or not it was fulfilled. She stated, "If a patient stops expressing hope, it is usually a sign of imminent death" (p. 140).

Researchers in the field of psychoneuroimmunology have found that the attitudes we have and the emotions we experience have a definite effect on the body. An optimistic feeling of hope is not just a mental state. Hope and optimism produce positive physical changes in the body that can influence the immune system and the functioning of specific body organs. The medical literature abounds with countless examples of individuals with terminal conditions who suddenly improve when they find something to live for. Conversely, there are many accounts of patients whose conditions deteriorate when they lose hope.

Love

Love may be identified as a projection of one's own good feelings onto others. To love others, one must first experience love of self and then be able and willing to project that warmth and affectionate concern for others (Karren et al., 2013).

Smucker (2001) stated:

> Love, in its purest unconditional form, is probably life's most powerful force and our greatest spiritual need. Not only is it important to receive love, but equally important to give love to others. Thinking about and caring for the needs of others keeps us from being too absorbed with ourselves and our needs to the exclusion of others. We all have experienced the good feelings that come from caring for and loving others. (p. 10)

Love may be a very important key in the healing process. Thaik, a cardiologist, states that love, as one of many strong human emotions, releases a cascade of hundreds or thousands of neuropeptides and hormones that can affect physical and mental health (2013). Among the beneficial effects, Thaik reports:

1. Love counteracts the fight-or-flight syndrome and decreases production of the stress hormone cortisol.
2. Love encourages the production of oxytocin, the "feel good" hormone, which can reduce cardiovascular stress and improve the immune system.
3. Love increases the production of norepinephrine and dopamine and may stave off depression.
4. Love decreases inflammation, which affects immune function and pain relief.

Some researchers suggest that love has a positive effect on the immune system. This has been shown to be true in adults and children and also in animals (Fox & Fox, 1988; Ornish, 1998; Pace et al., 2009). The giving and receiving of love may also result in higher levels of endorphins, thereby contributing to a sense of euphoria and helping to reduce pain.

In a classic long-term study, researchers Werner and Smith (1992) studied children who were reared in impoverished environments. Their homes were troubled by discord, desertion, or divorce or were marred by parental alcoholism or mental illness. The participants were studied at birth, childhood, adolescence, and adulthood. Two out of three of these high-risk children had developed serious learning and/or behavioral problems by age 10 or had a record of delinquencies, mental health problems, or pregnancies by age 18. A quarter of them had developed "very serious" physical and psychosocial problems. By the time they reached adulthood, more than three-fourths of them suffered from profound psychological and behavioral problems, and even more were in poor physical health. But of particular interest to the researchers were the 15 to 20 percent who remained resilient and well despite their impoverished and difficult existence. These children had experienced a warm and loving relationship with another person during their first year of life, whereas the children who developed serious psychological and physical problems did not. This research indicates that the earlier people have the benefit of a strong, loving relationship, the better they seem able to resist the effects of a deleterious lifestyle.

Forgiveness

Forgiveness has been defined as the letting go of resentments and thoughts of revenge (Mayo Clinic, 2014). Feelings of bitterness and resentment take a physical toll on an individual by generating stress hormones, which, when maintained for long periods, can have a detrimental effect on health. Forgiveness enables a person to cast off resentment and begin the pathway to healing. Owen, as cited by Harrison (2011), conducted research with patients who were HIV positive to study the effects of forgiveness on the immune system and found that forgiveness was correlated with improvements in immune function.

Forgiveness is not easy. Individuals often have great difficulty when called upon to forgive others and even greater difficulty in attempting to forgive themselves. Many people carry throughout their lives a sense of guilt for having committed a mistake for which they do not believe they have been forgiven or for which they have not forgiven themselves.

To forgive is not necessarily to condone or excuse one's own or someone else's inappropriate behavior. Karren and associates (2013) suggest that forgiveness is an attitude of owning responsibility for one's own perceptions in order to move beyond the perception of being a helpless victim to the perception of being empowered in choosing one's own responses to hurts and offenses.

Holding on to grievances causes pain, suffering, and conflict. Forgiveness (of self and others) is a gift to oneself. It offers freedom and peace of mind.

Current research supports that spiritual issues such as love and forgiveness are important to address not only because of their impact on psychological and spiritual healing but also because they are deeply connected to neuroendocrine and immune system healing.

It is important for nurses to be able to assess the spiritual needs of their clients. Nurses need not serve the role of professional counselor or spiritual guide, but because of the closeness of their relationship with clients, nurses may be the part of the health-care team to whom clients may reveal the most intimate details of their lives. Smucker (2001) stated:

> Just as answering a patient's question honestly and with accurate information and responding to his needs in a timely and sensitive manner communicates caring, so also does high-quality professional nursing care reach beyond the physical body or the illness to that part of the person where identity, self-worth, and spirit lie. In this sense, good nursing care is also good spiritual care. (pp. 11–12)

Religion

Religion is one way an individual's spirituality may be expressed. There are more than 6500 religions in the world (Bronson, 2005). Some individuals seek out various religions in an attempt to find answers to fundamental questions that they have about life and, indeed, about their very existence. Others, although they may regard themselves as spiritual, choose not to affiliate with an organized religious group. In either situation, however, it is inevitable that questions related to life and the human condition arise during the progression of spiritual maturation.

Brodd (2015) suggested that all religious traditions manifest seven dimensions: experiential, mythic, doctrinal, ethical, ritual, social, and material. He explains that these seven dimensions are intertwined and complementary. Depending on the particular religion, certain dimensions are emphasized more than others. For example, Zen Buddhism has a strong experiential dimension but says little about doctrines. Roman Catholicism is strong in both ritual and doctrine. The social dimension is a significant aspect of religion, as it provides a sense of community from belonging to a group such as a parish or a congregation, which is empowering for some individuals.

CORE CONCEPT

Religion

A set of beliefs, values, rites, and rituals adopted by a group of people. The practices are usually grounded in the teachings of a spiritual leader.

Evidence supports that affiliation with a religious group is a health-enhancing endeavor (Karren et al., 2013). A number of studies indicate a correlation between religious faith/church attendance and increased chance of survival following serious illness, fewer instances of depression and mental illness, longer life, and overall better physical and mental health. In an extensive review of the literature, Levin (2010) concludes that the weight of the evidence across studies suggests that religious involvement is a generally protective factor for mental illness and psychological distress.

It is unknown how religious participation protects health and promotes well-being. Some churches actively promote healthy lifestyles and discourage behavior that would be harmful to health or would interfere with treatment of disease. Graham and Crown (2014) conducted a study to identify what aspects of religion most contributed to happiness and a sense of well-being. They found that those who sought religion for social purpose (as opposed to social interaction) were happiest regardless of religious affiliation or service attendance. Certainly, participation in religious activities also provides opportunities for social interaction. Despite these findings, confidence in organized religion and church attendance, as previously discussed, has been showing a steady decline in American society.

Addressing Spiritual and Religious Needs Through the Nursing Process

Assessment

It is important for nurses to consider spiritual and religious needs when planning care for their clients. The Joint Commission requires that nurses address the psychosocial, spiritual, and cultural variables that influence the perception of illness. Dossey (1998) has developed a spiritual assessment tool (Box 6–4) about which she stated,

> The Spiritual Assessment Tool provides reflective questions for assessing, evaluating, and increasing awareness of spirituality in patients and their significant others. The tool's reflective questions can facilitate healing because they stimulate spontaneous, independent, meaningful initiatives to improve the patient's capacity for recovery and healing. (p. 45)

Assessing the spiritual needs of a client with a psychotic disorder can pose some additional challenges. Approximately 25 percent of people with schizophrenia and 15 to 22 percent of people with bipolar disorder have religious delusions (Koenig, 2012). Sometimes these delusions can be difficult to differentiate from general religious or cultural beliefs, but nonpsychotic religious activity may actually

BOX 6–4 **Spiritual Assessment Tool**

The following reflective questions may assist you in assessing, evaluating, and increasing awareness of spirituality in yourself and others.

MEANING AND PURPOSE

These questions assess a person's ability to seek meaning and fulfillment in life, manifest hope, and accept ambiguity and uncertainty.

- What gives your life meaning?
- Describe your sense of purpose in life.
- How does your illness affect your life goals?
- How hopeful are you about obtaining a better degree of health?
- How would you describe your role in maintaining your health?
- What kind of changes will you be able to make in your life to maintain your health?
- Describe your level of motivation to get well.
- What is the most important or powerful thing in your life?

INNER STRENGTHS

These questions assess a person's ability to manifest joy and recognize strengths, choices, goals, and faith.

- What brings you joy and peace in your life?
- What can you do to feel alive and full of spirit?
- What traits do you like about yourself?
- What are your personal strengths?
- What choices are available to you to enhance your healing?
- What life goals have you set for yourself?
- What do you think is the role of stress, if any, in your illness?
- How aware were you of your body before you became sick?
- What do you believe in?
- How has your illness influenced your faith?
- How important is faith in your overall health and sense of well-being?

INTERCONNECTIONS

These questions assess a person's positive self-concept, self-esteem, and sense of self; sense of belonging in the world with others; capacity to pursue personal interests; and ability to demonstrate love of self and self-forgiveness.

- How do you feel about yourself right now?
- How do you feel when you have a true sense of yourself?
- Describe any activities of personal interest that you pursue.
- What do you do to show love for yourself?
- Can you forgive yourself?
- What do you do to heal your spirit?

RELATIONSHIPS

These questions assess a person's ability to connect in life-giving ways with family, friends, and social groups and to engage in the forgiveness of others.

- Who are the significant people in your life?
- Who are your readily available, nearby, support people?
- Who are the people to whom you are closest?
- Describe any groups in which you are an active participant.
- How comfortable are you with asking people for help when you need it?
- How comfortable are you with sharing your feelings with others?
- What are some of the most loving things that others have done for you?
- What are the loving things that you do for other people?
- What are your thoughts about forgiving others?

BEHAVIOR AND ACTIVITIES

These questions assess a person's capacity for finding meaning in worship or religious activities and a connectedness with a divinity.

- How important is worship to you?
- What do you consider the most significant act of worship in your life?
- Describe any religious activities in which you are an active participant.
- Describe any spiritual activities, if any, that you find meaningful.
- Do you find prayer meaningful?
- To whom do you turn for support?
- Describe any activities in which you engage for coping and support.
- Describe any activities in which you have previously engaged and have not found helpful.

ENVIRONMENT

These questions assess a person's ability to experience a sense of connection with life and nature, an awareness of the effects of the environment on life and well-being, and a capacity or concern for the health of the environment.

- How does your environment have an impact on your state of well-being?
- What are your environmental stressors at work and at home?
- What strategies reduce your environmental stressors?
- Do you have any concerns for the state of your immediate environment?
- Are you involved with environmental issues such as recycling environmental resources at home, work, or in your community?
- Are you concerned about the survival of the planet?

SOURCES: Burkhardt, M.A. (1989). Spirituality: An analysis of the concept. Holistic Nursing Practice, 3(3), 69-77; Dossey, B.M., & American Holistic Nurses' Association. (1995). Holistic nursing: A handbook for practice (2nd ed.). Gaithersburg, MD: Aspen. From Dossey, B.M. (1998). Holistic modalities and healing moments, American Journal of Nursing, 98(6), 44-47, with permission.

improve long-term prognosis in patients with psychotic disorders (Koenig, 2012). Engaging family members and significant others in the assessment process can be a great help in determining which religious beliefs and activities have been beneficial to the patient and which have been detrimental to their progress.

Diagnoses and Outcome Identification

Nursing diagnoses that may be used when addressing spiritual and religious needs of clients include the following:

■ Risk for spiritual distress
■ Spiritual distress
■ Readiness for enhanced spiritual well-being
■ Risk for impaired religiosity
■ Impaired religiosity
■ Readiness for enhanced religiosity

The following outcomes may be used as guidelines for care and to evaluate effectiveness of the nursing interventions.

The client:

■ Identifies meaning and purpose in life that reinforce hope, peace, and contentment
■ Verbalizes acceptance of self as a worthwhile human being
■ Accepts and incorporates change into life in a healthy manner
■ Expresses understanding of relationship between difficulties in current life situation and interruption in previous religious beliefs and activities
■ Discusses beliefs and values about spiritual and religious issues
■ Expresses desire and ability to participate in beliefs and activities of desired religion

Planning and Implementation

NANDA International information related to the diagnoses Risk for spiritual distress and Risk for impaired religiosity is provided in the subsections that follow.

Risk for Spiritual Distress

Definition "Vulnerable to an impaired ability to experience and integrate meaning and purpose in life through connectedness within self, literature, nature, and/or a power greater than oneself which may compromise health" (Herdman & Kamitsuru, 2014, p. 374).

Risk factors

Physical: Physical/chronic illness; substance abuse
Psychosocial: Low self-esteem; depression; anxiety; stress; poor relationships; separate from support systems; blocks to experiencing love; inability to forgive; loss; racial or cultural conflict; change in religious rituals; change in spiritual practices
Developmental: Life changes
Environmental: Environmental changes; natural disasters

Risk for Impaired Religiosity

Definition "Vulnerable to impaired ability to exercise reliance on religious beliefs and/or participate in rituals of a particular faith tradition which may compromise health" (Herdman & Kamitsuru, 2014, p. 371).

Risk factors

Physical: Illness/hospitalization; pain
Psychological: Ineffective support, coping, caregiving; depression; lack of security
Sociocultural: Lack of social interaction; cultural barrier to practicing religion; social isolation
Spiritual: Suffering
Environmental: Lack of transportation; environmental barriers to practicing religion
Developmental: Life transitions

A plan of care addressing client's spiritual and/or religious needs is presented in Table 6–3. Selected nursing diagnoses are presented along with appropriate nursing interventions and rationales for each.

Evaluation

Evaluation of nursing actions is directed at achievement of the established outcomes. Part of the evaluation process is continuous reassessment to ensure that the selected actions are appropriate and the goals and outcomes are realistic. Including the family and extended support systems in the evaluation process is essential if spiritual and religious implications of nursing care are to be measured. Modifications to the plan of care are made as the need is determined.

Table 6–3 | CARE PLAN FOR THE CLIENT WITH SPIRITUAL AND RELIGIOUS NEEDS*

NURSING DIAGNOSIS: RISK FOR SPIRITUAL DISTRESS

RELATED TO: Life changes; environmental changes; stress; anxiety; depression

OUTCOME CRITERIA	NURSING INTERVENTIONS	RATIONALE
Client identifies meaning and purpose in life that reinforce hope, peace, contentment, and self-satisfaction.	1. Assess current situation.	1–8. Thorough assessment is necessary to develop an accurate care plan for the client.
	2. Listen to client's expressions of anger, concern, self-blame.	
	3. Note reason for living and whether it is directly related to situation.	
	4. Determine client's religious and/or spiritual orientation, current involvement, and presence of conflicts, especially in current circumstances.	
	5. Assess sense of self-concept, worth, ability to enter into loving relationships.	
	6. Observe behavior indicative of poor relationships with others.	
	7. Determine support systems available to and used by client and significant others.	
	8. Assess substance use/abuse.	
	9. Establish an environment that promotes free expression of feelings and concerns.	9. Trust is the basis of a therapeutic nurse-client relationship.
	10. Have client identify and prioritize current/immediate needs.	10. Helps client focus on what needs to be done and identify manageable steps to take.
	11. Discuss philosophical issues related to impact of current situation on spiritual beliefs and values.	11. Helps client to understand that certain life experiences can cause individuals to question personal values and that this response is not uncommon.
	12. Use therapeutic communication skills of reflection and active listening.	12. Helps client find own solutions to concerns.
	13. Review coping skills used and their effectiveness in current situation.	13. Identifies strengths to incorporate into plan and techniques that need revision.
	14. Provide a role model (e.g., nurse, individual experiencing similar situation).	14. Sharing of experiences and hope assists client to deal with reality.

Table 6–3 | CARE PLAN FOR THE CLIENT WITH SPIRITUAL AND RELIGIOUS NEEDS*—cont'd

OUTCOME CRITERIA	NURSING INTERVENTIONS	RATIONALE
	15. Suggest use of journaling.	15. Journaling can assist in clarifying beliefs and values and in recognizing and resolving feelings about current life situation.
	16. Discuss client's interest in the arts, music, literature.	16. Provides insight into meaning of these issues and how they are integrated into an individual's life.
	17. Role-play new coping techniques. Discuss possibilities of taking classes, becoming involved in discussion groups, cultural activities of client's choice.	17. These activities will help to enhance integration of new skills and necessary changes in client's lifestyle.
	18. Refer client to appropriate resources for help.	18. Client may require additional assistance with an individual who specializes in these types of concerns.

NURSING DIAGNOSIS: RISK FOR IMPAIRED RELIGIOSITY
RELATED TO: Suffering; depression; illness; life transitions

OUTCOME CRITERIA	NURSING INTERVENTIONS	RATIONALE
Client expresses achievement of support and personal satisfaction from spiritual and/or religious practices.	1. Assess current situation (e.g., illness, hospitalization, prognosis of death, presence of support systems, financial concerns).	1. This information identifies problems client is dealing with in the moment that is affecting desire to be involved with religious activities.
	2. Listen nonjudgmentally to client's expressions of anger and possible belief that illness or condition may be a result of lack of faith.	2. Individuals often blame themselves for what has happened and reject previous religious beliefs and/or God.
	3. Determine client's usual religious and/or spiritual beliefs, current involvement in specific church activities.	3. This information is important background for establishing a database.
	4. Note quality of relationships with significant others and friends.	4. Individual may withdraw from others in relation to the stress of illness, pain, and suffering.
	5. Assess substance use/abuse.	5. When in distress, individuals often turn to use of various substances, which can affect the ability to deal with problems in a positive manner.
	6. Develop nurse-client relationship in which individual can express feelings and concerns freely.	6. Trust is the basis for a therapeutic nurse-client relationship.
	7. Use therapeutic communication skills of active listening, reflection, and "I" messages.	7. Helps client to find own solutions to problems and concerns and promotes sense of control.

Continued

Table 6–3 | CARE PLAN FOR THE CLIENT WITH SPIRITUAL AND RELIGIOUS NEEDS*–cont'd

OUTCOME CRITERIA	NURSING INTERVENTIONS	RATIONALE
	8. Be accepting and nonjudgmental when client expresses anger and bitterness toward God. Stay with the client.	8. The nurse's presence and non-judgmental attitude increase the client's feelings of self-worth and promote trust in the relationship.
	9. Encourage client to discuss previous religious practices and how these practices provided support in the past.	9. A nonjudgmental discussion of previous sources of support may help the client work through current rejection of them as potential sources of support.
	10. Allow the client to take the lead in initiating participation in religious activities, such as prayer.	10. Client may be vulnerable in current situation and needs to be allowed to decide own resumption of these actions.
	11. Contact spiritual leader of client's choice, if he or she requests.	11. These individuals serve to provide relief from spiritual distress and often can do so when other support persons cannot.

*The interventions for this care plan were adapted from Doenges, M.E., Moorhouse, M.F., & Murr, A.C. (2013). *Nursing diagnosis manual: Planning, individualizing, and documenting client care* (4th ed.). Philadelphia: F.A. Davis.

Summary and Key Points

- Culture encompasses shared patterns of belief, feeling, and knowledge that guide people's conduct and are passed down from generation to generation.
- Some cultures, such as the dominant culture in the United States, are described as **individualistic cultures** and value independence, personal responsibility, and freedom.
- Cultures such as Latin American, Asian, and AI/AN groups can be described as **collectivistic** cultures in that they place a high value on interconnectedness and interreliance on family, community, and/or tribal affiliation.
- Ethnic groups are tied together by a shared heritage.
- Cultural groups differ in terms of communication, space, social organization, time, environmental control, and biological variations.
- America is often described as the melting pot of cultural diversity. People of many different cultures reside in the United States; some maintain traditional cultural practices, whereas others acculturate to dominant cultural practices (give up cultural practices or values as a result of contact with another group) and assimilate by incorporating practices and values of the dominant culture.

- Northern European Americans are the descendants of the first immigrants to the United States and make up the current dominant cultural group. They value punctuality, work responsibility, and a healthy lifestyle.
- Some African Americans trace their roots in the United States to the days of slavery. Most have large support systems and a strong religious orientation. Many have assimilated into and have many of the same characteristics as the dominant culture.
- Many American Indians and Alaska Natives still live on reservations. They speak many different languages and dialects. They often appear silent and reserved, and many are uncomfortable with touch and expressing emotions. Health care may be delivered by a healer called a *shaman.*
- Asian American languages are very diverse. Touching during communication has historically been considered unacceptable. Asian Americans may have difficulty expressing emotions and appear cold and aloof. Family loyalty is emphasized. Psychiatric illness is viewed as behavior that is out of control and brings shame on the family.
- Latino Americans are those who have origins in Latin American countries but now reside in the United States. Many can be referred to as Hispanic,

which implies their primary language is Spanish. Large family groups are important, and touch is a common form of communication. The predominant religion is Roman Catholicism, and the church is often a source of strength in times of crisis. Health care may be delivered by a folk healer called a *curandero* or a *curandera,* who uses various forms of treatment to restore the body to a balanced state.

■ Arab Americans trace their ancestry and traditions to the nomadic desert tribes of the Arabian Peninsula. Arabic is the official language of the Arab world, and the dominant religion is Islam. Mental illness is considered a social stigma, and symptoms are often somaticized.

■ The Jewish people came to the United States predominantly from Spain, Portugal, Germany, and Eastern Europe. Four main Jewish religious groups exist today: Orthodox, Reform, Conservative, and Reconstructionist. The primary language is English. A high value is placed on education. Jewish Americans are very health conscious and practice preventive health care. The maintenance of one's mental health is considered just as important as the maintenance of one's physical health.

■ Cultural syndromes are clusters of physical and behavioral symptoms considered as illnesses or "afflictions" by specific cultures that do not readily fit into the Western conventional diagnostic categories.

■ Spirituality is the human quality that gives meaning and sense of purpose to an individual's existence.

■ Individuals possess a number of spiritual needs that include meaning and purpose in life, faith or trust in someone or something beyond themselves, hope, love, and forgiveness.

■ Religion is a set of beliefs, values, rites, and rituals adopted by a group of people.

■ Religion is one way in which an individual's spirituality may be expressed.

■ Affiliation with a religious group has been shown to be a health-enhancing endeavor.

■ Nurses must consider cultural, spiritual, and religious needs when planning care for their clients.

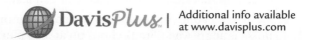 **Davis*Plus*** | Additional info available at www.davisplus.com

Review Questions
Self-Examination/Learning Exercise

Select the answer that is most appropriate for each of the following questions.

1. Miss Lee is an Asian American on the psychiatric unit. She tells the nurse, "I must have the hot ginger root for my headache. It is the only thing that will help." What cultural belief is likely associated with Miss Lee's request?
   a. She is being obstinate and wants control over her care.
   b. She believes that ginger root has magical qualities.
   c. She subscribes to the restoration of health through the balance of yin and yang.
   d. Asian Americans refuse to take traditional medicine for pain.

2. Miss Lee, an Asian American on the psychiatric unit, says she is afraid that no one from her family will visit her. On what belief does Miss Lee base her statement?
   a. Many Asian Americans do not believe in hospitals.
   b. Many Asian Americans do not have close family support systems.
   c. Many Asian Americans believe the body will heal itself if left alone.
   d. Many Asian Americans view psychiatric problems as bringing shame to the family.

3. Joe, an American Indian, appears at the community health clinic with an oozing stasis ulcer on his lower right leg. It is obviously infected, and he tells the nurse that the shaman has been treating it with herbs. The nurse determines that Joe needs emergency care, but Joe states he will not go to the emergency department (ED) unless the shaman is allowed to help treat him. How should the nurse handle this situation?
   a. Contact the shaman and have him meet them at the ED to consult with the attending physician.
   b. Tell Joe that the shaman is not allowed in the ED.
   c. Explain to Joe that the shaman is at fault for his leg being in the condition it is in now.
   d. Have the shaman try to talk Joe into going to the ED without him.

Continued

Review Questions—cont'd
Self-Examination/Learning Exercise

4. Joe, an American Indian, goes to the emergency department (ED) because he has an oozing stasis ulcer on his leg. He is accompanied by the tribal shaman, who has been treating Joe on the reservation. As a greeting, the physician extends his hand to the shaman, who lightly touches the physician's hand, then quickly moves away. What cultural norm among American Indians most likely explains the shaman's behavior?
   a. The shaman is snubbing the physician.
   b. The shaman is angry at Joe for wanting to go to the ED.
   c. The shaman does not believe in traditional medicine.
   d. The shaman does not feel comfortable with touch.

5. Sarah is an African American woman who receives a visit from the psychiatric home health nurse. A referral for a mental health assessment was made by the public health nurse, who noticed that Sarah was becoming exceedingly withdrawn. When the psychiatric nurse arrives, Sarah says to her, "No one can help me. I was an evil person in my youth, and now I must pay." How might the nurse assess this statement?
   a. Sarah is having delusions of persecution.
   b. Some African Americans believe illness is God's punishment for their sins.
   c. Sarah is depressed and just wants to be left alone.
   d. African Americans do not believe in psychiatric help.

6. Frank is a Latino American who has an appointment at the community health center for 1 p.m. The nurse is angry when Frank shows up at 3:30 p.m. stating, "I was visiting with my brother." How must the nurse interpret this behavior?
   a. Frank is being passive-aggressive by showing up late.
   b. This is Frank's way of defying authority.
   c. Frank is a member of a cultural group that is present-time oriented.
   d. Frank is a member of a cultural group that rejects traditional medicine.

7. The nurse must give Frank, a Latino American, a physical examination. She asks him to remove his clothing and put on an examination gown. Frank refuses. What cultural norm among Latino Americans most likely explains Frank's response?
   a. Frank does not believe in taking orders from a woman.
   b. Frank is modest and embarrassed to remove his clothes.
   c. Frank does not understand why he must remove his clothes.
   d. Frank does not think he needs a physical examination.

8. Maria is an Italian American who is in the hospital after having suffered a miscarriage at 5 months' gestation. Her room is filled with relatives who have brought a variety of foods and gifts for Maria. They are all talking, seemingly at the same time, and some, including Maria, are crying. They repeatedly touch and hug Maria and each other. How should the nurse handle this situation?
   a. Explain to the family that Maria needs her rest and they must all leave.
   b. Allow the family to remain and continue their activity as described, as long as they do not disturb other clients.
   c. Explain that Maria will not get over her loss if they keep bringing it up and causing her to cry so much.
   d. Call the family priest to come and take charge of this family situation.

9. Mark, who has come to the mental health clinic with symptoms of depression, says to the nurse, "My father is dying. I have always hated my father. He physically abused me when I was a child. We haven't spoken for many years. He wants to see me now, but I don't know if I want to see him." With which spiritual need is Joe struggling?
   a. Forgiveness
   b. Faith
   c. Hope
   d. Meaning and purpose in life

Review Questions—cont'd
Self-Examination/Learning Exercise

10. As a child, Joe was physically abused by his father. The father is now dying and has expressed a desire to see his son before he dies. Joe is depressed and says to the mental health nurse, "I'm so angry! Why did God have to give me a father like this? I feel cheated of a father! I've always been a good person. I deserved better. I hate God!" From this subjective data, which nursing diagnosis might the nurse apply to Joe?
    a. Readiness for enhanced religiosity
    b. Risk for impaired religiosity
    c. Readiness for enhanced spiritual well-being
    d. Spiritual distress

References

Alegria, M., Canino, G,. Shrout, P.E., Woo, M. Duan, N., Vila, D., & Meng, X.L. (2008). Prevalence of mental illness in immigrant and non-immigrant U.S. Latino groups. *American Journal of Psychiatry, 165*(3), 359-369. doi:10.1176/appi.ajp.2007.07040704

Alegria, M., Mulvaney-Day, N., Torres, M., Polo, A., Cao, Z., & Canino, G. (2007). Prevalence of psychiatric disorders across Latino subgroups in the United States. *American Journal of Public Health, 97*(1), 68-75. doi:10.2105/AJPH.2006.087205

Beane, M. (no date). An adventure in American culture and values. *International Student Guide to the United States of America.* Retrieved from www.internationalstudentguidetotheusa.com/articles/culture.htm

Bralock, A.R., & Padgham, C.S. (2017). Jewish Americans. In J.N. Giger (Ed.), *Transcultural nursing: Assessment & intervention* (7th ed., pp. 511-533). St. Louis, MO: Mosby.

Brodd, J. (2015). *World religions: A voyage of discovery* (4th ed.). Winona, MN: Saint Mary's Press.

Bronson, M. (2005). Why are there so many religions? Retrieved from www.biblehelp.org/relig.htm

Bureau of Indian Affairs (BIA). (2016). Who we are. Retrieved from www.indianaffairs.gov/WhoWeAre/index.htm

Burkhardt, M.A. (1989). Spirituality: An analysis of the concept. *Holistic Nursing Practice, 3*(3), 69-77.

Centers for Disease Control (CDC). (2015a). National marriage and divorce rates and trends. Retrieved from www.cdc.gov/nchs/nvss/marriage_divorce_tables.htm

Centers for Disease Control and Prevention (CDC). (2015b). High school youth risk behavior survey data (1991–2015). Retrieved from http://nccd.cdc.gov/youthonline

Chang, K. (2017). Chinese Americans. In J.N. Giger (Ed.), *Transcultural nursing: Assessment and intervention* (7th ed., pp. 388-407). St. Louis, MO: Mosby.

Cherry, B., & Giger, J.N. (2013). African-Americans. In J.N. Giger (Ed.), *Transcultural nursing: Assessment and intervention* (6th ed., pp. 162-206). St. Louis, MO: Mosby.

Countries & Their Cultures Forum. (2017). United States of America. Retrieved from www.everyculture.com/To-Z/United-States-of-America.html

Doenges, M.E., Moorhouse, M.F., & Murr, A.C. (2013). *Nursing diagnosis manual: Planning, individualizing, and documenting client care* (4th ed.). Philadelphia: F.A. Davis.

Dossey, B.M. (1998). Holistic modalities and healing moments. *American Journal of Nursing, 98*(6), 44-47.

Dossey, B.M., & American Holistic Nurses' Association. (1995). *Holistic nursing: A handbook for practice* (2nd ed.). Gaithersburg, MD: Aspen.

Enayati, A. (2013). How hope can help you heal. Retrieved from www.cnn.com/2013/04/11/health/hope-healing-enayati

Gallup. (2015). Religion. Retrieved from www.gallup.com/poll/1690/religion.aspx

Garcia-Navarro, L. (2015). Hispanic or Latino? A guide for the U.S. presidential campaign. Retrieved from www.npr.org/sections/parallels/2015/08/27/434584260/hispanic-or-latino-a-guide-for-the-u-s-presidential-campaign

Giger, J.N. (2017). *Transcultural nursing: Assessment and intervention* (7th ed.). St. Louis, MO: Mosby.

Gorman, L. M., & Sultan, D. (2008). *Psychosocial nursing for general patient care,* Philadelphia: F.A. Davis.

Graham, C., & Crown, S. (2014). Religion and well-being around the world: Social purpose, social time, or social insurance? *International Journal of Well-Being, 4*(1), 1-27. doi:10.5502/ijw.v4i1.1

Hanley, C.E. (2017). Navajos. In J.N. Giger (Ed.), *Transcultural nursing: Assessment and intervention* (7th ed., pp. 242-261). St. Louis, MO: Mosby.

Harrison, P. (2011). Forgiveness can improve immune function. Retrieved from www.medscape.com/viewarticle/742198

Herdman, T.H., & Kamitsuru, S. (Eds.). (2014). *NANDA-I nursing diagnoses: Definitions and classification, 2015–2017.* Oxford: Wiley Blackwell.

Indian Health Service (IHS). (2015). Behavioral health. Retrieved from https://www.ihs.gov/newsroom/factsheets/behavioralhealth

Karren, K.J., Hafen, B.Q., Smith, N.L., & Jenkins, K.J. (2010). *Mind/body health: The effects of attitudes, emotions, and relationships* (4th ed.). San Francisco, CA: Benjamin Cummings.

Karren, K.J., Smith, N.L., & Gordon, K. (2013). *Mind/body health: The effects of attitudes, emotions, and relationships* (5th ed.). San Francisco: Pearson.

Koenig, H.G. (2012). Religion, spirituality, and health: The research and clinical implications. *International Scholarly Research Notices, 2012.* doi:http://dx.doi.org/10.5402/2012/278730

Kulwicki, A.D., & Ballout, S. (2013). People of Arab heritage. In L.D. Purnell (Ed.), *Transcultural health care: A culturally competent approach* (4th ed., pp. 159-177). Philadelphia: F.A. Davis.

Kuo, P.Y., & Roysircar-Sodowsky, G. (2000). Political ethnic identity versus cultural ethnic identity: An understanding of research on Asian Americans. In D.S. Sandhu (Ed.), *Asian and Pacific Islander Americans: Issues and concerns for counseling and psychotherapy.* Hauppauge, NY: Nova Science Publishers.

Levin, J. (2010). Religion and mental health: Theory and research. *International Journal of Applied Psychoanalytic Studies.* doi:10.1002/aps.240

Lipka, M. (2013). What surveys say about worship attendance— And why some stay home. Retrieved from www.pewresearch. org/fact-tank/2013/09/13/what-surveys-say-about-worship-attendance-and-why-some-stay-home

Mayo Clinic. (2014). Forgiveness: Letting go of grudges and bitterness. Retrieved from www.mayoclinic.org/healthy-lifestyle/adult-health/in-depth/forgiveness/art-20047692

McMurry, L., Song, H., Owen, D.C., Gonzalez, E.W., & Esperat, C.R. (2017). Mexican Americans. In J.N. Giger (Ed.). *Transcultural nursing: Assessment and intervention* (6th ed., pp. 208-241). St. Louis, MO: Mosby.

Murray, R.B., Zentner, J.P., & Yakimo, R. (2009). *Health promotion strategies through the life span* (8th ed.). Upper Saddle River, NJ: Prentice Hall.

Pace, T.W., Negi, T.L., Adame, D.D., Cole, S.P., Sivilli, T.I., Brown, T.D., . . . Raison, C.L. (2009). Effect of compassion meditation on neuroendocrine, innate immune and behavioral responses to psychosocial stress. *Psychoneuroendocrinology, 34*(1), 87-98. doi:10.1016/j.psyneuen.2008.08.011

Pew Research Center. (2015). America's changing religious landscape. Retrieved from www.pewforum.org/2015/05/12/americas-changing-religious-landscape

Purnell, L.D. (2013). *Transcultural health care: A culturally competent approach* (4th ed.). Philadelphia: F.A. Davis.

Purnell, L.D. (2014). *Guide to culturally competent health care* (3rd ed.). Philadelphia: F.A. Davis.

Reeves, R., & Reynolds, M. (2009). What is the role of spirituality in mental health treatment? *Journal of Psychosocial Nursing, 54*(5), 8-9. doi:10.3928/02793695-20090301-05

Sadock, B.J., Sadock, V.A., & Ruiz, P. (2015). *Synopsis of psychiatry: Behavioral sciences/clinical psychiatry* (11th ed.). Philadelphia: Lippincott Williams & Wilkins.

Selekman, J. (2013). People of Jewish heritage. In L.D. Purnell (Ed.), *Transcultural health care: A culturally competent approach* (4th ed., pp. 339-356). Philadelphia: F.A. Davis.

Smucker, C.J. (2001). Overview of nursing the spirit. In D.L. Wilt & C.J. Smucker (Eds.), *Nursing the spirit: The art and science of applying spiritual care* (pp. 1-18). Washington, DC: American Nurses Publishing.

Spector, R.E. (2013). *Cultural diversity in health and illness* (8th ed.). Upper Saddle River: Prentice Hall.

Sue, D.W., & Sue, D. (2016). *Counseling the culturally diverse* (7th ed.). Hoboken, NJ: Wiley.

Thaik, C. (2013). *Love heals!* Retrieved from www.huffingtonpost. om/dr-cynthia-thaik/love-health-benefits_b_3131370.html

U.S. Census Bureau. (2013). Race. Retrieved from www. census.gov/topics/population/race/about.html

U.S. Census Bureau. (2015). American families and living arrangements: 2015: Households. Retrieved from www. census.gov/hhes/families/data/cps2015H.html

U.S. Census Bureau. (2016). 2010–2014 American Community Survey 5-year estimates. Retrieved from http://factfinder. census.gov/faces/tableservices/jsf/pages/productview. xhtml?pid=ACS_14_5YR_DP05&src=pt

U.S. Department of Agriculture. (2015). Food distribution program on Indian reservations. Retrieved from www.fns. usda.gov/fdd/programs/fdpir/about_fdpir.htm

Zimmerman, K.A. (2015). American culture: Traditions and customs of the United States. *Live Science.* Retrieved from www.livescience.com/28945-american-culture.html

Classical References

Fox, A. & Fox, B. (1988). *Wake up! You're alive.* Deerfield Beach, FL: Health Communications.

Hall, E.T. (1966). *The hidden dimension.* Garden City, NY: Doubleday.

Kübler-Ross, E. (1969). *On death and dying.* New York: Macmillan.

Nekolaichuk, C.L., Jevne, R.F., & Maguire, T.O. (1999). Structuring the meaning of hope in health and illness. *Social Science and Medicine, 48*(5), 591-605. doi:http://dx.doi.org/10.1016/S0277-9536(98)00348-7

Ornish, D. (1998). *Love and survival: Eight pathways to intimacy and health.* New York: Harper Perennial.

Wall, T.L., Peterson, C.M., Peterson, K.P., Johnson, M.L., Thomasson, H.R., Cole, M., & Ehlers, C.L. (1997). Alcohol metabolism in Asian-American men with genetic polymorphisms of aldehyde dehydrogenase. *Annals of Internal Medicine,* 127:376-379.

Walsh, R. (1999). *Essential spirituality.* New York: Wiley.

Werner, E.E., & Smith, R.S. (1992). *Overcoming the odds: High risk children from birth to adulthood.* Ithaca, NY: Cornell University Press.

Therapeutic Approaches in Psychiatric Nursing Care

7

Relationship Development

KEY TERMS

attitude	countertransference	sympathy
belief	empathy	transference
concrete thinking	genuineness	unconditional positive regard
confidentiality	rapport	values

OBJECTIVES

After reading this chapter, the student will be able to:

1. Describe the relevance of a therapeutic nurse-client relationship.
2. Discuss the dynamics of a therapeutic nurse-client relationship.
3. Discuss the importance of self-awareness in the nurse-client relationship.
4. Identify goals of the nurse-client relationship.
5. Identify and discuss essential conditions for a therapeutic relationship to occur.
6. Describe the phases of relationship development and the tasks associated with each phase.

HOMEWORK ASSIGNMENT

Please read the chapter and answer the following questions:

1. When the nurse's verbal and nonverbal interactions are congruent, he or she is thought to be expressing which characteristic of a therapeutic relationship?
2. During which phase of the nurse-client relationship do each of the following occur:
   a. The nurse may become angry and anxious in the presence of the client.
   b. A plan of action for dealing with stress is established.
   c. The nurse examines personal feelings about working with the client.
   d. Nurse and client establish goals of care.
3. What is the goal of using the Johari Window?
4. How do sympathy and empathy differ?
5. Write a one-page journal entry reflecting on patterns you notice in your relationships with others. How might you use this awareness in developing therapeutic relationship skills?

The nurse-client relationship is the foundation on which psychiatric nursing is established. It is a relationship in which both participants must recognize each other as unique and important human beings. It is also a relationship in which mutual learning occurs. In today's health-care environment, patient-centered care is promoted as central to quality and safety, and the therapeutic relationship remains at the foundation of this tenet. Concepts that were advanced over 60 years ago (by Hildegard Peplau in 1952) and have been the core of nursing practice to the present day are now recognized by the larger medical community as not only still relevant but critical to improving quality and safety in the future of health care. Peplau (1991) stated:

> Shall a nurse do things *for* a patient or can participant relationships be emphasized so that a nurse comes to do things *with* a patient as her share of an agenda of work to be accomplished in reaching a goal—health. *It is likely that the nursing process is educative and therapeutic when nurse and patient can come to know and to respect each other, as persons who are alike, and yet, different, as persons who share in the solution of problems.* (p. 9, emphasis in original)

This chapter examines the role of the psychiatric nurse and the use of self as the therapeutic tool in the nursing care of clients with mental illness. Phases of the therapeutic relationship are explored, and conditions essential to the development of a therapeutic relationship are discussed. The importance of values clarification in the development of self-awareness is emphasized.

CORE CONCEPT

Therapeutic Relationship
An interaction between two people (usually a caregiver and a care receiver) in which input from both participants contributes to a climate of healing, growth promotion, and/or illness prevention.

Role of the Psychiatric Nurse

What is a nurse? Undoubtedly, this question would elicit as many different answers as the number of people to whom it was presented. Nursing as a *concept* has probably existed since the beginning of the civilized world, with the provision of "care" for the ill or infirm by anyone in the environment who took the time to administer to those in need. However, the emergence of nursing as a *profession* only began in the late 1800s with the graduation of Linda Richards from the New England Hospital for Women and Children in Boston upon achievement of the diploma in nursing. Since that time, the nurse's role has evolved from that of

custodial caregiver and physician's handmaiden to recognition as a unique, independent member of the professional health-care team.

Peplau (1991) identified several subroles within the nursing role:

1. **The stranger:** A nurse is at first a stranger to the client. The client is also a stranger to the nurse. Peplau (1991) stated:

> Respect and positive interest accorded a stranger is at first nonpersonal and includes the same ordinary courtesies that are accorded to a new guest who has been brought into any situation. This principle implies: (1) accepting the patient as he is; (2) treating the patient as an emotionally able stranger and relating to him on this basis until evidence shows him to be otherwise. (p. 44)

2. **The resource person:** According to Peplau, "A resource person provides specific answers to questions usually formulated with relation to a larger problem" (p. 47). In the role of resource person, the nurse explains, in language that the client can understand, information related to the client's health care.

3. **The teacher:** In this subrole, the nurse identifies learning needs and provides information required by the client or family to improve the health situation.

4. **The leader:** According to Peplau, "Democratic leadership in nursing situations implies that the patient will be permitted to be an active participant in designing nursing plans for him" (p. 49). Autocratic leadership promotes overvaluation of the nurse and clients' substitution of the nurse's goals for their own. Laissez-faire leaders convey a lack of personal interest in the client.

5. **The surrogate:** Outside of their awareness, clients often perceive nurses as symbols of other individuals. They may view the nurse as a mother figure, a sibling, a former teacher, or another nurse who has provided care in the past. This perception occurs when a client is placed in a situation that generates feelings similar to ones he or she has experienced previously. Peplau (1991) explained that the nurse-client relationship progresses along a continuum. When a client is acutely ill, he or she may incur the role of infant or child, while the nurse is perceived as the mother surrogate. Peplau (1991) stated, "Each nurse has the responsibility for exercising her professional skill in aiding the relationship to move forward on the continuum, so that person to person relations compatible with chronological age levels can develop" (p. 55).

6. **The technical expert:** The nurse understands various professional devices and possesses the clinical skills necessary to perform interventions that are in the best interest of the client.

7. **The counselor:** The nurse uses "interpersonal techniques" to assist clients in adapting to difficulties or changes in life experiences. Peplau (1991) stated, "Counseling in nursing has to do with helping the patient to remember and to understand fully what is happening to him in the present situation, so that the experience can be integrated with, rather than dissociated from, other experiences in life" (p. 64).

Peplau (1962) believed that the emphasis in psychiatric nursing is on the counseling subrole. How then does this emphasis influence the role of the nurse in the psychiatric setting? Many sources define the *nurse therapist* as a person with graduate preparation in psychiatric-mental health nursing. He or she has developed skills through intensive, supervised educational experiences to provide helpful individual, group, or family therapy.

Peplau suggested that it is essential for the *staff nurse working in psychiatry* to have a general knowledge of basic counseling techniques. A therapeutic or "helping" relationship is established through use of these interpersonal techniques and is based on a sound knowledge of theories of personality development and human behavior.

Sullivan (1953) believed that emotional problems stem from difficulties with interpersonal relationships. Interpersonal theorists, such as Peplau and Sullivan, emphasize the importance of relationship development in the provision of emotional care. Through establishment of a satisfactory nurse-client relationship, individuals learn to generalize the ability to achieve satisfactory interpersonal relationships to other aspects of their lives.

Dynamics of a Therapeutic Nurse-Client Relationship

Travelbee (1971), who expanded on Peplau's theory of interpersonal relations in nursing, stated that only when each individual in the interaction perceives the other as a unique human being is a relationship possible. She refers not to a nurse-client relationship but rather to a human-to-human relationship, which she describes as a "mutually significant experience." That is, both the nurse and the recipient of care have needs met when each views the other as a unique human being, not as "an illness," as "a room number," or as "all nurses" in general.

Therapeutic relationships are goal oriented. Ideally, the nurse and client decide together what the goal of the relationship will be. Most often, the goal is promotion of learning and growth in an effort to bring about change in the client's life. In general, the goal of a therapeutic relationship may be based on a problem-solving model.

EXAMPLE

Goal

The client will demonstrate more adaptive coping strategies for dealing with (specific life situation).

Interventions

- Identify what is troubling the client at the present time.
- Encourage the client to discuss changes he or she would like to make.
- Discuss with the client which changes are possible and which are not possible.
- Have the client explore feelings about aspects of his or her life that cannot be changed and alternative ways of coping more adaptively.
- Discuss alternative strategies for creating changes the client desires to make.
- Weigh the benefits and consequences of each alternative.
- Assist the client to select an alternative.
- Encourage the client to implement the change.
- Provide positive feedback for the client's attempts to create change.
- Assist the client to evaluate outcomes of the change and make modifications as required.

Therapeutic Use of Self

Travelbee (1971) described the instrument for delivery of interpersonal nursing as the *therapeutic use of self*, which she defined as "the ability to use one's personality consciously and in full awareness in an attempt to establish relatedness and to structure nursing intervention" (p. 19).

Use of the self in a therapeutic manner requires that the nurse have a great deal of self-awareness and self-understanding, having arrived at a philosophical belief about life, death, and the overall human condition. The nurse must understand that the ability to and the extent to which one can effectively help others in time of need is strongly influenced by this internal value system—a combination of intellect and emotions.

Gaining Self-Awareness
Values Clarification

Knowing and understanding oneself enhances the ability to form satisfactory interpersonal relationships. Self-awareness requires that an individual recognize and accept what he or she values and learn to accept the uniqueness of and differences in others. This concept is important in everyday life and in the nursing profession in general, but it is *essential* in psychiatric nursing.

An individual's value system is established very early in life and has its foundations in the value system held by the primary caregivers. It is culturally oriented; consists of beliefs, attitudes, and values; and may change many times over the course of a lifetime. Values clarification is one process by which an individual may gain self-awareness.

Beliefs

A **belief** is an idea that one holds true, and it can take any of several forms:

■ *Rational beliefs* are ideas for which objective evidence exists to substantiate their truth.

EXAMPLE

Alcoholism is a disease.

■ *Irrational beliefs* are ideas that an individual holds as true despite the existence of objective contradictory evidence. Delusions can be a form of irrational beliefs.

EXAMPLE

Once an alcoholic has been through detoxification and rehabilitation, he or she can drink socially if desired.

■ *Faith* (sometimes called *blind beliefs*) is a belief in something or someone that does not require proof.

EXAMPLE

Belief in a higher power can help an alcoholic stop drinking.

■ *Stereotype* is a socially shared belief that describes a concept in an oversimplified or undifferentiated matter.

EXAMPLE

All alcoholics are skid-row bums.

Attitudes

An **attitude** is a frame of reference around which an individual organizes knowledge about his or her world. An attitude also has an emotional component. It can be a prejudgment and may be selective and biased. Attitudes fulfill the need to find meaning in life and to provide clarity and consistency for the individual. The prevailing stigma attached to mental illness is an example of a negative attitude. An associated belief might be that "all people with mental illness are dangerous."

Values

Values are abstract standards, positive or negative, that represent an individual's ideal mode of conduct and ideal goals. Examples of ideal modes of conduct include seeking truth and beauty; being clean and orderly; and behaving with sincerity, justice, reason, compassion, humility, respect, honor, and loyalty. Examples of ideal goals are security, happiness, freedom, equality, ecstasy, fame, and power.

Values differ from attitudes and beliefs in that they are action oriented or action producing. One may hold many attitudes and beliefs without behaving in a way that shows they hold those attitudes and beliefs. For example, a nurse may believe that all clients have the right to be told the truth about their diagnosis; however, he or she may not always act on the belief by telling all clients the complete truth about their conditions. Only when the belief is acted on does it become a value.

Attitudes and beliefs flow out of one's set of values. An individual may have thousands of beliefs and hundreds of attitudes, but his or her values probably number only in the dozens. Values may be viewed as a kind of core concept or basic standard that determines one's attitudes, beliefs, and ultimately, behavior. Raths, Harmin, and Simon (1978) identified a seven-step process of valuing that can be used to help clarify personal values. This process is presented in Table 7–1. The process can be used by applying these seven steps to an attitude or belief that one holds. When an attitude or belief has met each of the seven criteria, it can be considered a value.

TABLE 7–1 **The Process of Values Clarification**			
LEVEL OF OPERATIONS	**CATEGORY**	**CRITERIA**	**EXPLANATION**
Cognitive	Choosing	1. Freely 2. From alternatives 3. After careful consideration of the consequences	"This value is mine. No one forced me to choose it. I understand and accept the consequences of holding this value."
Emotional	Prizing	4. Satisfied; pleased with the choice 5. Making public affirmation of the choice, if necessary	"I am proud that I hold this value, and I am willing to tell others about it."
Behavioral	Acting	6. Taking action to demonstrate the value behaviorally 7. Demonstrating this pattern of behavior consistently and repeatedly	The value is reflected in the individual's behavior for as long as he or she holds it.

The Johari Window

The self arises out of self-appraisal and the appraisal of others. It represents each individual's unique pattern of values, attitudes, beliefs, behaviors, emotions, and needs. Self-awareness is the recognition of these aspects and understanding about their impact on the self and others. The Johari Window, presented in Figure 7–1, is a representation of the self and a tool that can be used to increase self-awareness (Luft, 1970). The Johari Window is divided into four quadrants (four aspects of the self): the open self, the unknowing self, the private self, and the unknown self.

The Open or Public Self

The upper-left quadrant of the window represents the part of the self that is public; that is, aspects of the self about which both the individual and others are aware.

EXAMPLE

Susan, a nurse who is the adult child of an alcoholic, has strong feelings about helping alcoholics to achieve sobriety. She volunteers her time as a support person on call to help recovering alcoholics. She is aware of her feelings and her desire to help others. Members of the Alcoholics Anonymous group in which she volunteers her time are also aware of Susan's feelings, and they feel comfortable calling her when they need help with refraining from drinking.

The Unknowing Self

The upper-right quadrant of the window represents the part of the self that is known to others but remains hidden from the awareness of the individual.

EXAMPLE

When Susan takes care of patients in detoxification, she does so without emotion, tending to the technical aspects of the task in a way that the patients perceive as cold and judgmental. She is unaware that she comes across to patients in this way.

The Private Self

The lower-left quadrant of the window represents the part of the self that is known to the individual but which the individual deliberately and consciously conceals from others.

EXAMPLE

Susan would prefer not to take care of the clients in detoxification because doing so provokes painful memories from her childhood. However, because she does not want the other staff members to know about these feelings, she volunteers to take care of the detoxification clients whenever they are assigned to her unit.

The Unknown Self

The lower-right quadrant of the window represents the part of the self that is unknown to both the individual and to others.

EXAMPLE

Susan felt very powerless as a child growing up with an alcoholic father. She seldom knew in what condition she would find her father or what his behavior would be. She learned over the years to find small ways to maintain control over her life situation, and she left home as soon as she graduated from high school. The need to stay in control has always been very important to Susan, and she is unaware that working with recovering alcoholics helps to fulfill this need. The people she is helping are also unaware that Susan is satisfying an unfulfilled personal need as she provides them with assistance.

The goal of increasing self-awareness by using the Johari Window is to increase the size of the quadrant that represents

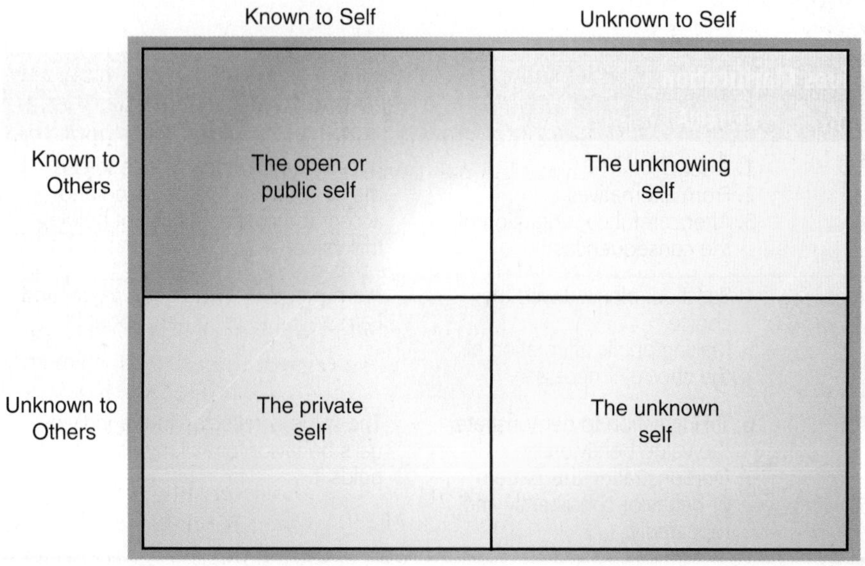

	Known to Self	Unknown to Self
Known to Others	The open or public self	The unknowing self
Unknown to Others	The private self	The unknown self

FIGURE 7–1 The Johari window. (From Luft, J. [1970]. *Group processes: An introduction to group dynamics* [3rd ed.]. Palo Alto, CA: Mayfield Publishing, 1984, with permission.)

the open or public self. The individual who is open to self and others has the ability to be spontaneous and to share emotions and experiences with others. This individual also has a greater understanding of personal behavior and of others' responses to him or her. Increased self-awareness allows an individual to interact comfortably with others, to accept the differences in others, and to observe each person's right to respect and dignity.

Conditions Essential to Development of a Therapeutic Relationship

Several characteristics that enhance the achievement of a therapeutic relationship have been identified. These concepts are highly significant to the use of self as the therapeutic tool in interpersonal relationship development.

Rapport

Getting acquainted and establishing **rapport** is the primary task in relationship development. Rapport implies special feelings on the part of both the client and the nurse based on acceptance, warmth, friendliness, common interest, a sense of trust, and a nonjudgmental attitude. Establishing rapport may be accomplished by discussing non-health-related topics. Travelbee (1971) states:

> [To establish rapport] is to create a sense of harmony based on knowledge and appreciation of each individual's uniqueness. It is the ability to be still and experience the other as a human being—to appreciate the unfolding of each personality one to the other. The ability to truly care for and about others is the core of rapport. (pp. 152; 155)

Trust

To trust another, one must feel confidence in that person's presence, reliability, integrity, veracity, and sincere desire to provide assistance when requested. As discussed in the chapter Theoretical Models of Personality Development (available online at www.davisplus.com), trust is the initial developmental task described by Erikson. If the task has not been achieved, this component of relationship development becomes more difficult. That is not to say that trust cannot be established, but only that additional time and patience may be required on the part of the nurse.

CLINICAL PEARL The nurse must convey an aura of trustworthiness, which requires that he or she possess a sense of self-confidence. Confidence in the self is derived from knowledge gained through achievement of personal and professional goals as well as the ability to integrate these roles and to function as a unified whole.

Trust cannot be presumed; it must be earned. Trustworthiness is demonstrated through nursing interventions that convey a sense of warmth and caring to the client. These interventions are initiated simply and concretely and directed toward activities that address the client's basic needs for physiological and psychological safety and security. Many psychiatric clients experience **concrete thinking,** which focuses their thought processes on specifics rather than generalities and on immediate issues rather than eventual outcomes. Examples of nursing interventions that promote trust in an individual who is thinking concretely include the following:

- Providing a blanket when the client is cold
- Providing food when the client is hungry
- Keeping promises
- Being honest (e.g., saying "I don't know the answer to your question, but I'll try to find out") and then following through
- Simply and clearly providing reasons for certain policies, procedures, and rules
- Providing a written, structured schedule of activities
- Attending activities with the client if he or she is reluctant to go alone
- Being consistent in adhering to unit guidelines
- Listening to the client's preferences, requests, and opinions and making collaborative decisions concerning his or her care whenever possible
- Ensuring **confidentiality;** providing reassurance that what is discussed will not be repeated outside the boundaries of the health-care team

Trust is the basis of a therapeutic relationship. The nurse working in psychiatry must perfect the skills that foster the development of trust. Trust must be established in order for the nurse-client relationship to progress beyond the superficial level of tending to the client's immediate needs.

Respect

To show respect is to believe in the dignity and worth of an individual regardless of his or her unacceptable behavior. The psychologist Carl Rogers called this **unconditional positive regard** (Raskin, Rogers, & Witty, 2014). The attitude is nonjudgmental, and the respect is unconditional in that it does not depend on the behavior of the client to meet certain standards. The nurse, in fact, may not approve of the client's lifestyle or behavior patterns. However, with unconditional positive regard, the client is accepted and respected for no other reason than that he or she is considered to be a worthwhile and unique human being.

Many psychiatric clients have very little self-respect. Sometimes lack of self-respect is related to the low self-esteem that accompanies illnesses such as clinical depression, and sometimes it is related to rejection and stigmatization by others. Recognition that they are unconditionally accepted and respected as unique, valuable individuals can elevate feelings of self-worth and self-respect. The nurse can convey an attitude of respect by

- Calling the client by name (and title, if he or she prefers).
- Spending time with the client.
- Allowing sufficient time to answer the client's questions and concerns.
- Promoting an atmosphere of privacy during therapeutic interactions with the client and during physical examination or therapy.
- Always being open and honest with the client, even when the truth may be difficult to discuss.
- Listening to the client's ideas, preferences, and opinions and making collaborative decisions concerning his or her care whenever possible.
- Striving to understand the motivation behind the client's behavior regardless of how unacceptable it may seem.

Genuineness

The concept of **genuineness** refers to the nurse's ability to be open, honest, and "real" in interactions with the client. To be real is to be aware of what one is experiencing internally and to allow the quality of this inner experience to be apparent in the therapeutic relationship. When one is genuine, there is *congruence* between what is felt and what is expressed (Raskin et al., 2014). The nurse who is genuine responds to the client with truth and honesty rather than with responses he or she may consider more "professional" or ones that merely reflect the "nursing role."

Genuineness may call for a degree of *self-disclosure* on the part of the nurse. This is not to say that the nurse must disclose to the client *everything* he or she is feeling or *all* personal experiences that relate to what the client is going through. Indeed, care must be taken when using self-disclosure to avoid reversing the roles of nurse and client. For example, when a client tells the nurse, "I just get so upset when someone disrespects me; sometimes you have to smack someone to teach them a lesson," the nurse might respond, "I get upset by that, too. Let's talk about some different ways to respond to your anger rather than hitting someone." In this example, the nurse discloses a common feeling while maintaining a focus on the client's need for problem-solving. When the nurse uses self-disclosure, a quality of "humanness" is revealed to the client, creating a role for the client to model in similar situations. The client may then feel more comfortable revealing personal information to the nurse.

Most individuals have an uncanny ability to detect when others are artificial. When the nurse does not bring genuineness and respect to the relationship, a reality basis for trust cannot be established. These qualities are essential to helping the client actualize his or her potential within the nurse-client relationship and for change and growth to occur (Raskin et al., 2014).

Empathy

Empathy is the ability to see beyond outward behavior and understand the situation from the client's point of view. With empathy, the nurse can accurately perceive and comprehend the meaning and relevance of the client's thoughts and feelings. The nurse must also be able to communicate this perception to the client by attempting to translate words and behaviors into feelings.

It is not uncommon for the concept of empathy to be confused with that of **sympathy.** The major difference is that with *empathy* the nurse "accurately perceives or understands" what the client is feeling and encourages the client to explore these feelings. With *sympathy* the nurse actually "shares" what the client is feeling and experiences a need to alleviate distress. Schuster (2000) stated:

> Empathy means that you remain emotionally separate from the other person, even though you can see the patient's viewpoint clearly. This is different from sympathy. Sympathy implies taking on the other's needs and problems as if they were your own and becoming emotionally involved to the point of losing your objectivity. To empathize rather than sympathize, you must show feelings but not get caught up in feelings or overly identify with the patient's and family's concerns. (p. 102)

Empathy is considered to be one of the most important characteristics of a therapeutic relationship. Accurate empathetic perceptions on the part of the nurse assist the client to identify feelings that may have been suppressed or denied. Positive emotions are generated as the client realizes that he or she is truly understood by another. As the feelings surface and are explored, the client learns aspects about self of which he or she may have been unaware. This contributes to the process of personal identification and the promotion of positive self-concept.

With empathy, while understanding the client's thoughts and feelings, the nurse is able to maintain sufficient objectivity to allow the client to achieve problem resolution with minimal assistance. With sympathy, the nurse actually feels what the client is feeling, objectivity is lost, and the nurse may become focused on relief of personal distress rather than on helping the client resolve the problem at hand. The following is an example of an empathetic and sympathetic response to the same situation.

EXAMPLE

Situation: BJ is a client on the psychiatric unit with a diagnosis of persistent depressive disorder (dysthymia). She is 5′5½″ tall and weighs 295 pounds. BJ has been overweight all her life. She is single, has no close friends, and has never had an intimate relationship with another person. It is her first day on the unit, and she is refusing to come out of her room. When she appeared for lunch in the dining room following admission, she was embarrassed when several of the other clients laughed out loud and called her "fatso."

Sympathetic response: Nurse: "I can certainly identify with what you are feeling. I've been overweight most of my life, too. I just get so angry when people act like that. They are so insensitive! It's just so typical of skinny people to act that way. You have a right to want to stay away from them. We'll just see how loud they laugh when *you* get to choose what movie is shown on the unit after dinner tonight."

Empathetic response: Nurse: "You feel angry and embarrassed by what happened at lunch today." As tears fill BJ's eyes, the nurse encourages her to cry if she feels like it and to express her anger at the situation. She stays with BJ but does not dwell on her *own* feelings about what happened. Instead, she focuses on BJ and what the client perceives are her most immediate needs at this time.

Rapport, trust, respect, genuineness, and empathy all are essential to forming therapeutic relationships, and they can be assets in social relationships, too. The primary differences between social and therapeutic relationships are that therapeutic relationships always remain focused on the health-care needs of the client, are never for the purpose of addressing the nurse's personal needs, and progress through identified phases of development for the purpose of helping the client solve health-related problems.

Phases of a Therapeutic Nurse-Client Relationship

Psychiatric nurses use interpersonal relationship development as the primary intervention with clients in psychiatric-mental health settings. This is congruent with Peplau's (1962) identification of *counseling* as the major subrole of nursing in psychiatry. Sullivan (1953), from whom Peplau patterned her own interpersonal theory of nursing, strongly believed that many emotional problems were closely related to difficulties with interpersonal relationships. With this concept in mind, this role of the nurse in psychiatry becomes especially meaningful and purposeful—an integral part of the total therapeutic regimen.

The therapeutic interpersonal relationship is the means by which the nursing process is implemented. Through the relationship, problems are identified and resolution is sought. Tasks of the relationship have been categorized into four phases: (1) the preinteraction phase, (2) the orientation (introductory) phase, (3) the working phase, and (4) the termination phase. Although each phase is presented as specific and distinct from the others, there may be some overlap of tasks, particularly when the interaction is limited. The major nursing goals during each phase of the nurse-client relationship are listed in Table 7–2.

The Preinteraction Phase

The preinteraction phase involves preparation for the first encounter with the client. Tasks include

■ Obtaining available information about the client from his or her chart, significant others, or other health-care team members. From this information, the initial assessment begins. The nurse may also become aware of personal responses to knowledge about the client.

■ Examining one's feelings, fears, and anxieties about working with a particular client. For example, the nurse may have been reared in an alcoholic family and have ambivalent feelings about caring for a client who is dependent on alcohol. All individuals bring attitudes and feelings from prior experiences to the clinical setting. The nurse needs to be aware of how these preconceptions may affect his or her ability to care for individual clients.

The Orientation (Introductory) Phase

During the orientation phase, the nurse and client become acquainted. Tasks include

■ Creating an environment for the establishment of trust and rapport.

■ Establishing a contract for intervention that details the expectations and responsibilities of both nurse and client.

TABLE 7–2	**Phases of Relationship Development and Major Nursing Goals**
PHASE	**GOALS**
1. Preinteraction	Explore self-perceptions
2. Orientation (introductory)	Establish trust Formulate contract for intervention
3. Working	Promote client change
4. Termination	Evaluate goal attainment Ensure therapeutic closure

■ Gathering assessment information to build a strong client database.
■ Identifying the client's strengths and limitations.
■ Formulating nursing diagnoses.
■ Setting goals that are mutually agreeable to the nurse and client.
■ Developing a plan of action that is realistic for meeting the established goals.
■ Exploring feelings of both the client and nurse in terms of the introductory phase.

Introductions are often uncomfortable, and the participants may experience some anxiety until a degree of rapport has been established. Interactions may remain on a superficial level until anxiety subsides. Several interactions may be required to fulfill the tasks associated with this phase.

The Working Phase

The therapeutic work of the relationship is accomplished during this phase. Tasks include

■ Maintaining the trust and rapport established during the orientation phase.
■ Promoting the client's insight and perception of reality.
■ Problem-solving using the model presented earlier in this chapter.
■ Overcoming resistance behaviors on the part of the client as the level of anxiety rises in response to discussion of painful issues.
■ Continuously evaluating progress toward goal attainment.

Transference and Countertransference

Transference and countertransference are common phenomena that often arise during the course of a therapeutic relationship.

Transference

Transference occurs when the client unconsciously displaces (or "transfers") to the nurse feelings formed toward a person from his or her past (Sadock, Sadock, & Ruiz, 2015). These feelings may be triggered by something about the nurse's appearance or personality characteristics that reminds the client of another person. Transference can interfere with the therapeutic interaction when the feelings expressed include anger and hostility. Anger toward the nurse can be manifested by uncooperativeness and resistance to therapy.

Transference can also take the form of overwhelming affection for or excessive dependency on the nurse. The nurse is overvalued, and the client forms unrealistic expectations of the nurse. When the nurse is unable to fulfill those expectations or meet the excessive dependency needs, the client becomes angry and hostile.

Interventions for Transference

Hilz (2013) states:

> In cases of transference, the relationship does not usually need to be terminated, except when the transference poses a serious barrier to therapy or safety. The nurse should work with the patient in sorting out the past from the present, assist the patient into identifying the transference, and reassign a new and more appropriate meaning to the current nurse-patient relationship. The goal is to guide patients toward independence by teaching them to assume responsibility for their own behaviors, feelings, and thoughts, and to assign the correct meanings to their relationships based on present circumstances instead of the past.

Countertransference

Countertransference refers to the nurse's behavioral and emotional responses to the client in which the nurse transfers feelings (often unconscious) about past experiences or people onto the patient. These responses may be related to unresolved feelings toward significant others from the nurse's past, or they may be generated in response to transference feelings on the part of the client. It is not easy to refrain from becoming angry when the client is consistently antagonistic, to feel flattered when showered with affection and attention by the client, or even to feel quite powerful when the client exhibits excessive dependency on the nurse. These feelings can interfere with the therapeutic relationship when they initiate the following types of behaviors:

■ The nurse overidentifies with the client's feelings, as they remind him or her of problems from the nurse's past or present.
■ The nurse and client develop a social or personal relationship.
■ The nurse begins to give advice or attempts to "rescue" the client.
■ The nurse encourages and promotes the client's dependence.
■ The nurse's anger engenders feelings of disgust toward the client.
■ The nurse feels anxious and uneasy in the presence of the client.
■ The nurse is bored and apathetic in sessions with the client.
■ The nurse has difficulty setting limits on the client's behavior.
■ The nurse defends the client's behavior to other staff members.

The nurse may be completely unaware or only minimally aware of the countertransference as it is occurring (Hilz, 2013).

Interventions for Countertransference

Hilz (2013) states:

The relationship usually should not be terminated in the presence of countertransference. Rather, the nurse or staff member experiencing the countertransference should be supportively assisted by other staff members to identify his or her feelings and behaviors and recognize the occurrence of the phenomenon. It may be helpful to have evaluative sessions with the nurse after his or her encounter with the patient, in which both the nurse and other staff members (who are observing the interactions) discuss and compare the exhibited behaviors in the relationship.

The Termination Phase

Termination of the relationship may occur for a variety of reasons: the mutually agreed-on goals may have been reached, the client may be discharged from the hospital, or, in the case of a student nurse, the clinical rotation ends. Termination can be difficult for both the client and nurse. The main task involves bringing a therapeutic conclusion to the relationship. This occurs when

■ Progress has been made toward attainment of mutually set goals.

■ A plan for continuing care or for assistance during stressful life experiences is mutually established by the nurse and client.

■ Feelings about termination of the relationship are recognized and explored. Both the nurse and client may experience feelings of sadness and loss. The nurse should share his or her feelings with the client. Through these interactions, the client learns that it is acceptable to have these kinds of feelings at a time of separation. With this knowledge, the client experiences growth during the process of termination. This is also a time when both nurse and client may evaluate and summarize the learning that occurred as an outgrowth of their relationship.

> **CLINICAL PEARL** When the client feels sadness and loss, behaviors to delay termination may become evident. If the nurse experiences the same feelings, he or she may allow the client's behaviors to delay termination. For therapeutic closure, the nurse must establish the reality of the separation and resist being manipulated into repeated delays by the client.

Boundaries in the Nurse-Client Relationship

A boundary indicates a border that determines the extent of acceptable limits. Many types of boundaries exist, such as the following:

■ **Material boundaries:** These are physical property that can be seen, such as fences that border land.

■ **Social boundaries:** These are established within a culture and define how individuals are expected to behave in social situations.

■ **Personal boundaries:** These are boundaries that individuals define for themselves. They include *physical distance boundaries,* or just how close individuals will allow others to invade their physical space; and *emotional boundaries,* or how much individuals choose to disclose of their most private and intimate selves to others.

■ **Professional boundaries:** These boundaries limit and outline expectations for appropriate professional relationships with clients. "Professional boundaries are the spaces between a nurse's power and the patient's vulnerability" (National Council of State Boards of Nursing [NCSBN], 2014). Nurses must recognize that they have an imbalance of power with their patients by virtue of their role and the patient information to which they have access. They must be consistently conscientious in avoiding any circumstance in which they might achieve personal gain within that relationship. Concerns regarding professional boundaries are commonly related to the following issues:

■ **Self-disclosure:** Self-disclosure on the part of the nurse may be appropriate when the information may therapeutically benefit the client. It should never be undertaken to meet the nurse's needs.

■ **Gift-giving:** Individuals who are receiving care often feel indebted toward health-care providers. Indeed, gift-giving may be part of the therapeutic process for people who receive care (College and Association of Registered Nurses of Alberta, 2011). Cultural beliefs and values may also enter into the decision of whether to accept a gift from a client. In some cultures, failure to do so would be interpreted as an insult (Pies, 2012). Accepting financial gifts is never appropriate, but in some instances nurses may be permitted to suggest instead a donation to a charity of the client's choice. If acceptance of a small gift of gratitude is deemed appropriate, the nurse may choose to share it with other staff members who have been involved in the client's care. In all instances, nurses should exercise professional judgment when deciding whether to accept a gift from a client. Attention should be given to what the gift-giving means to the client, as well as to institutional policy, the American Nurses Association (ANA) *Code of Ethics for Nurses,* and the ANA *Scope and Standards of Practice.*

■ **Touch:** Nursing by its very nature involves touching clients. Touching is required to perform the therapeutic procedures involved in the physical care of clients. Caring touch is the touching of clients when there is no physical need to do so. Touching or hugging can be beneficial when it is implemented with therapeutic intent and client consent. When using caring touch, make sure it is appropriate, supportive, and welcomed (College of Registered Nurses of British Columbia, 2015). Caring touch may provide comfort or encouragement, but some vulnerable clients may misinterpret its meaning. In certain cultures, such as within Navajo Indian, Chinese, and Japanese heritages, touch is not considered acceptable unless the parties know each other very well (Purnell, 2014). The nurse must be sensitive to these cultural nuances and aware when touch is crossing a personal boundary. Additionally, clients who are experiencing high levels of anxiety or suspicious or psychotic behavior may interpret touch as aggressiveness. These are times when touch should be avoided or considered with extreme caution.

■ **Friendship or romantic association:** When a nurse is acquainted with a client, the relationship must move from a personal nature to professional. If the nurse is unable to accomplish this separation, he or she should withdraw from the nurse-client relationship. Likewise, nurses must guard against personal relationships developing as a result of the nurse-client relationship. Romantic, sexual, or otherwise intimate personal relationships are never appropriate between nurse and client.

Certain warning signs indicate that professional boundaries of the nurse-client relationship may be in jeopardy. These may include (Coltrane & Pugh, 1978)

■ Favoring one client's care over that of another.
■ Keeping secrets with a client.
■ Changing dress style for working with a particular client.
■ Swapping assignments to care for a particular client.
■ Giving special attention or treatment to one client over others.
■ Spending free time with a client.
■ Frequently thinking about the client when away from work.
■ Sharing personal information or work concerns with the client.
■ Receipt of gifts or continued contact or communication with the client after discharge.

Boundary crossing can threaten the integrity of the nurse-client relationship. Nurses must gain self-awareness and insight to recognize when professional integrity is compromised. Although some variables, such as the care setting, community influences, patient needs, and the nature of therapy, affect how boundaries are delineated, "any actions that overstep the established boundaries to meet the needs of the nurse are boundary violations" (NCSBN, 2014).

Summary and Key Points

■ Nurses who work in the psychiatric-mental health field use special skills, or "interpersonal techniques," to assist clients in adapting to difficulties or changes in life experiences. Therapeutic nurse-client relationships are goal oriented, and the problem-solving model is used to try to bring about some type of change in the client's life.

■ The instrument for delivery of the process of interpersonal nursing is the therapeutic use of self, which requires that the nurse possess a strong sense of self-awareness and self-understanding.

■ Hildegard Peplau identified seven subroles within the role of nurse: stranger, resource person, teacher, leader, surrogate, technical expert, and counselor.

■ Characteristics that enhance the achievement of a therapeutic relationship include rapport, trust, respect, genuineness, and empathy.

■ Phases of a therapeutic nurse-client relationship include the preinteraction phase, the orientation (introductory) phase, the working phase, and the termination phase.

■ Transference occurs when the client unconsciously displaces (or "transfers") to the nurse feelings formed toward a person from the past.

■ Countertransference refers to the nurse's behavioral and emotional response to the client in which the nurse transfers feelings (often unconscious) about past experiences or people onto the patient. These responses may be related to unresolved feelings toward significant others from the nurse's past, or they may be generated in response to transference feelings on the part of the client.

■ Types of boundaries include material, social, personal, and professional.

■ Concerns associated with professional boundaries include self-disclosure, gift-giving, touch, and developing a friendship or romantic association.

■ Boundary crossings can threaten the integrity of the nurse-client relationship.

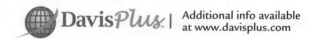 **DavisPlus** | Additional info available at www.davisplus.com

Review Questions
Self-Examination/Learning Exercise

Select the answer that is most appropriate for each of the following questions.

1. Nurse Mary has been providing care for Tom during his hospital stay. On Tom's day of discharge, his wife brings a bouquet of flowers and box of chocolates to his room. He presents these gifts to Nurse Mary, saying, "Thank you for taking care of me." What is a correct response by the nurse?
   a. "I don't accept gifts from patients."
   b. "Thank you so much! It is so nice to be appreciated."
   c. "Thank you. I will share these with the rest of the staff."
   d. "Hospital policy forbids me to accept gifts from patients."

2. Elisa says to the nurse, "I worked as a secretary to put my husband through college, and as soon as he graduated, he left me. I hate him! I hate all men!" Which of the following is an empathetic response by the nurse?
   a. "You are very angry now. This is a normal response to your loss."
   b. "I know what you mean. Men can be very insensitive."
   c. "I understand completely. My husband divorced me, too."
   d. "You are depressed now, but you will feel better in time."

3. Which of the following behaviors suggest a possible breach of professional boundaries? (Select all that apply.)
   a. The nurse repeatedly requests to be assigned to a specific client.
   b. The nurse shares the details of her divorce with the client.
   c. The nurse makes arrangements to meet the client outside of the therapeutic environment.
   d. The nurse shares how she dealt with a similar difficult situation.

4. Which of the following tasks are associated with the orientation phase of relationship development? (Select all that apply.)
   a. Promoting the client's insight and perception of reality
   b. Creating an environment for the establishment of trust and rapport
   c. Using the problem-solving model toward goal fulfillment
   d. Obtaining available information about the client from various sources
   e. Formulating nursing diagnoses and setting goals

5. Nurse Rosetta, who is the adult child of an alcoholic, is working with John, a client who abuses alcohol. John has experienced a successful detoxification process and is beginning a rehabilitation program. He says to Rosetta, "I'm not going to go to those stupid AA meetings. They don't help anything." Rosetta, whose father died of complications from alcoholism, responds with anger: "Don't you even care what happens to your children?" Rosetta's response is an example of which of the following?
   a. Transference
   b. Countertransference
   c. Self-disclosure
   d. A breach of professional boundaries

6. Nurse Jones is working with Kim, a client in the anger-management program. Which of the following identifies actions associated with the working phase of the therapeutic relationship?
   a. Kim tells Nurse Jones she wants to learn more adaptive ways to handle her anger. Together, they set some goals.
   b. The goals of therapy have been met, but Kim cries and says she has to keep coming to therapy in order to be able to handle her anger appropriately.
   c. Nurse Jones reads Kim's previous medical records. She explores her feelings about working with a woman who has abused her child.
   d. Nurse Jones helps Kim practice various techniques to control her angry outbursts. She gives Kim positive feedback for attempting to improve maladaptive behaviors.

Continued

Review Questions—cont'd
Self-Examination/Learning Exercise

7. When there is congruence between what is felt and what is expressed, the nurse is exhibiting which of the following characteristics?
   a. Trust
   b. Respect
   c. Genuineness
   d. Empathy

8. When the nurse shows unconditional acceptance of an individual as a worthwhile and unique human being, he or she is exhibiting which of the following characteristics?
   a. Trust
   b. Respect
   c. Genuineness
   d. Empathy

9. Hildegard Peplau identified seven subroles within the role of the nurse. She believed the emphasis in psychiatric nursing was on which of the subroles?
   a. The resource person
   b. The teacher
   c. The surrogate
   d. The counselor

10. Which of the following behaviors are associated with the phenomenon of *transference*? (Select all that apply.)
   a. The client attributes toward the nurse feelings associated with a person from the client's past.
   b. The nurse attributes toward the client feelings associated with a person from the nurse's past.
   c. The client forms an overwhelming affection for the nurse.
   d. The client becomes excessively dependent on the nurse and forms unrealistic expectations of him or her.

References

College and Association of Registered Nurses of Alberta (CARNA). (2011). *Professional boundaries for registered nurses: Guidelines for the nurse-client relationship.* Edmonton, AB: CARNA.

College of Registered Nurses of British Columbia (CRNBC). (2015). Boundaries in the nurse-client relationship. Retrieved from https://www.crnbc.ca/Standards/PracticeStandards/Pages/boundaries.aspx

Hilz, L.M. (2013). Transference and countertransference. *Kathi's Mental Health Review.* Retrieved from www.toddlertime.com/mh/terms/countertransference-transference-3.htm

National Council of State Boards of Nursing (NCSBN). (2014). A nurse's guide to professional boundaries. Retrieved from https://www.ncsbn.org/ProfessionalBoundaries_Complete.pdf

Pies, R.W. (2012). The patient gift conundrum. *Medscape Psychiatry & Mental Health.* Retrieved from www.medscape.com/viewarticle/775575

Purnell, L.D. (2014). *Guide to culturally competent health care* (3rd ed.). Philadelphia: F.A. Davis.

Raskin, N.J., Rogers, C.R., & Witty, M.C. (2014). Client-centered therapy. In D. Wedding & R.J. Corsini (Eds.), *Current psychotherapies* (10th ed., pp. 95-145). Belmont, CA: Brooks/Cole.

Sadock, B.J., Sadock, V.A., & Ruiz, P. (2015). *Synopsis of psychiatry: Behavioral sciences/clinical psychiatry* (11th ed.). Philadelphia: Lippincott Williams & Wilkins.

Schuster, P.M. (2000). *Communication: The key to the therapeutic relationship.* Philadelphia: F.A. Davis.

Classical References

Coltrane, F., & Pugh, C. (1978). Danger signals in staff/patient relationships. *Journal of Psychiatric Nursing & Mental Health Services, 16*(6), 34-36. doi:10.3928/0279-3695-19780601-06

Luft, J. (1970). *Group processes: An introduction to group dynamics* (3rd ed.). Palo Alto, CA: Mayfield Publishing.

Peplau, H.E. (1962). Interpersonal techniques: The crux of psychiatric nursing. *American Journal of Nursing, 62*(6), 50-54. doi:10.1007/978-1-349-13441-0_13

Peplau, H.E. (1991). *Interpersonal relations in nursing.* New York: Springer.

Raths, L., Harmin, M., & Simon, S. (1978). *Values and teaching: Working with values in the classroom* (2nd ed.). Columbus, OH: Merrill.

Sullivan, H.S. (1953). *The interpersonal theory of psychiatry.* New York: W.W. Norton.

Travelbee, J. (1971). *Interpersonal aspects of nursing* (2nd ed.). Philadelphia: F.A. Davis.

Therapeutic Communication

8

CORE CONCEPTS

Communication

Therapeutic Communication

KEY TERMS

density	motivational interviewing	public distance
distance	paralanguage	social distance
intimate distance	personal distance	territoriality

OBJECTIVES

After reading this chapter, the student will be able to:

1. Discuss the transactional model of communication.
2. Identify types of preexisting conditions that influence the outcome of the communication process.
3. Define *territoriality*, *density*, and *distance* as components of the environment.
4. Identify components of nonverbal expression.
5. Describe therapeutic and nontherapeutic verbal communication techniques.
6. Describe motivational interviewing as a communication strategy.
7. Describe active listening.
8. Discuss therapeutic feedback.

HOMEWORK ASSIGNMENT

Please read the chapter and answer the following questions:

1. A client asks the nurse for advice about a personal situation, and the nurse responds, "What do *you* think you should do?" This is an example of what technique? Is it therapeutic or nontherapeutic?
2. "Just hang in there. Everything will be all right." If the nurse makes this statement to a client, it is an example of what technique? Is it therapeutic or nontherapeutic?
3. Why might it be more appropriate to conduct a client interview in a conference room or interview room rather than in the client's room or nurse's office?
4. Name the five elements of constructive feedback.
5. Write a one-page journal entry reflecting on things that friends or close relatives have told you characterize your style of communicating with others. How can you use this self-awareness to promote the development of therapeutic communication?

Development of the *therapeutic interpersonal relationship* was described in Chapter 7, Relationship Development, as the process by which nurses provide care for clients in need of psychosocial intervention. *Therapeutic use of self* was identified as the instrument for delivery of care. The focus of this chapter is on *techniques*—or, more specifically, *interpersonal communication techniques*—to facilitate the delivery of that care.

In their classic work on therapeutic communication, Hays and Larson (1963) stated, "To relate therapeutically with a patient it is necessary for the nurse to understand his or her role and its relationship to the patient's illness" (p. 1). They describe the role of the nurse as providing the client with the opportunity to accomplish the following:

1. Identify and explore problems in relating to others.
2. Discover healthy ways of meeting emotional needs.
3. Experience a satisfying interpersonal relationship.

These goals are achieved through use of interpersonal communication techniques (both verbal and nonverbal). The nurse must be aware of the therapeutic or nontherapeutic value of the communication techniques used with the client because they are the tools of psychosocial intervention.

CORE CONCEPT

Communication

An interactive process of transmitting information between two or more entities.

What Is Communication?

It has been said that individuals "cannot *not* communicate." Every word spoken, every movement made, and every action taken or not taken gives a message to someone. Interpersonal communication is a *transaction* between the sender and the receiver. In the transactional model of communication, both participants simultaneously perceive each other, listen to each other, and are mutually involved in creating meaning in a relationship. The transactional model is illustrated in Figure 8–1.

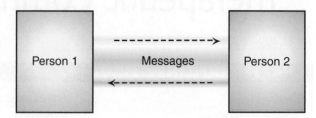

FIGURE 8–1 The Transactional Model of Communication.

The Impact of Preexisting Conditions

In all interpersonal transactions, the sender and receiver each bring certain preexisting conditions to the exchange that influence both the intended message and the way in which it is interpreted. Examples of these conditions include one's value system, internalized attitudes and beliefs, culture and religion, social status, gender, background knowledge and experience, and age or developmental level. The type of environment in which the communication takes place may also influence the outcome of the transaction. Figure 8–2 shows how these influencing factors are positioned on the transactional model.

Values, Attitudes, and Beliefs

Values, attitudes, and beliefs are learned ways of thinking. Children generally adopt the value systems and internalize the attitudes and beliefs of their parents. Children may retain this way of thinking into adulthood or develop a different set of attitudes and values as they mature.

Values, attitudes, and beliefs can influence communication in numerous ways. For example, prejudice is expressed verbally through negative stereotyping.

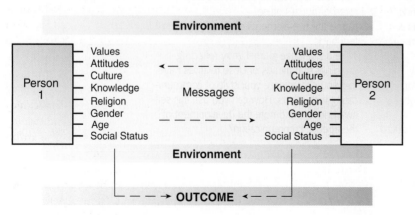

FIGURE 8–2 Factors influencing the Transactional Model of Communication.

One's value system may be communicated with behaviors that are symbolic in nature. For example, an individual who values youth may dress and behave in a manner that is characteristic of one who is much younger. Persons who value freedom and the American way of life may fly the U.S. flag in front of their homes each day. In each of these situations, a message is being communicated.

Culture and Religion

Communication has its roots in culture. Cultural mores, norms, ideas, and customs provide the basis for our way of thinking. Cultural values are learned and differ from society to society. For example, in some European countries (e.g., Italy, Spain, and France), men may greet each other with hugs and kisses. These behaviors are appropriate in those cultures but may communicate a different message in the United States or England.

Religion can influence communication as well. Priests and ministers who wear clerical collars publicly communicate their mission in life. The collar may also influence the way in which others relate to them, either positively or negatively. Other symbolic gestures, such as wearing a cross around the neck or hanging a crucifix on the wall, communicate an individual's religious beliefs.

Social Status

Studies of nonverbal indicators of social status or power have suggested that high-status persons are associated with gestures that communicate their higher-power position. For example, they use less eye contact, have a more relaxed posture, use louder voice pitch, place hands on hips more frequently, are "power dressers," have greater height, and maintain more distance when communicating with individuals considered to be of lower social status.

Gender

Gender influences the manner in which individuals communicate. Most cultures have *gender signals* that are recognized as either masculine or feminine and provide a basis for distinguishing between members of each gender. Examples include differences in posture, both standing and sitting, between men and women in the United States. Men usually stand with thighs 10 to 15 degrees apart, the pelvis rolled back, and the arms slightly away from the body. Women often stand with legs close together, the pelvis tipped forward, and the arms close to the body. When sitting, men may lean back in the chair with legs apart or may rest the ankle of one leg over the knee of the other. Women tend to sit more upright in the chair with legs together, perhaps crossed at the ankles, or one leg crossed over the other at thigh level.

Roles have historically been identified as either male or female. For example, in the United States masculinity typically was communicated through such roles as husband, father, breadwinner, doctor, lawyer, or engineer. Traditional female roles included those of wife, mother, homemaker, nurse, teacher, or secretary.

Gender signals are changing in U.S. society as sexual roles become less distinct. Behaviors that had been considered typically masculine or feminine in the past may now be generally accepted in members of both genders. Words such as *unisex* communicate a desire by some individuals to diminish the distinction between genders and minimize the discrimination of either. Gender roles are changing as both women and men enter professions that were once dominated by members of the opposite gender.

Age or Developmental Level

Age influences communication, which is never more evident than during adolescence. In their struggle to separate from parental confines and establish their own identity, adolescents generate a unique pattern of communication that changes from generation to generation. Words such as *dude, groovy, clueless, awesome, cool,* and *wasted* have had special meaning for certain generations of adolescents. The technological age has produced a whole new language for today's teenagers. Communication by text messaging includes such acronyms as BRB ("be right back"), BFF ("best friends forever"), and MOS ("mom over shoulder").

Developmental influences on communication may relate to physiological alterations. One example is American Sign Language, the system of unique gestures used by many people who are deaf or hearing impaired. Individuals who are blind at birth never learn the subtle nonverbal gesticulations that accompany language, which can totally change the meaning of the spoken word.

Environment in Which the Transaction Takes Place

The place where communication occurs influences the outcome of the interaction. Some individuals who feel uncomfortable and refuse to speak during a group therapy session may be willing to discuss problems privately on a one-to-one basis with the nurse.

Territoriality, density, and **distance** are aspects of environment that communicate messages. *Territoriality* is the innate tendency to own space. Individuals lay claim to areas around them as their own. This influences communication when an interaction takes place in the territory "owned" by one or the other. Interpersonal communication can be more successful if the interaction takes place in a "neutral" area. For example, with the concept of territoriality in mind, the nurse may choose to conduct the psychosocial assessment in an interview room rather than in his or her office or in the client's room.

Density refers to the number of people within a given environmental space. It has been shown to influence interpersonal interaction. Some studies indicate that a correlation exists between prolonged high-density situations and certain behaviors, such as aggression, stress, criminal activity, hostility toward others, and a deterioration of mental and physical health.

Distance is the means by which various cultures use space to communicate. Hall (1966) identified four kinds of spatial interaction, or distances, that people maintain from each other in their interpersonal interactions and the kinds of activities in which people engage at these various distances. **Intimate distance** is the closest distance that individuals will allow between themselves and others. In mainstream American culture, this distance, which is restricted to interactions of an intimate nature, is 0 to 18 inches. **Personal distance** is approximately 18 to 40 inches and reserved for interactions that are personal in nature, such as close conversations with friends or colleagues. **Social distance** is about 4 to 12 feet away from the body. Interactions at this distance include conversations with strangers or acquaintances, such as at a cocktail party or in a public building. A **public distance** is one that exceeds 12 feet. Examples include speaking in public or yelling to someone some distance away. This distance is considered public space, and communicants are free to move about in it during the interaction.

Nonverbal Communication

About 70 to 80 percent of all effective communication is nonverbal (Khan, 2014). Some aspects of nonverbal expression were discussed in the previous section on preexisting conditions that influence communication. Other components of nonverbal communication include physical appearance and dress, body movement and posture, touch, facial expressions, eye behavior, and vocal cues or paralanguage. These nonverbal messages vary from culture to culture.

Physical Appearance and Dress

Physical appearance and dress are part of the total nonverbal stimuli that influence interpersonal responses, and under some conditions, they are the primary determinants of such responses. Body coverings—both dress and hair—are manipulated by the wearer in a manner that conveys a distinct message to the receiver. Dress can be formal or casual, stylish or unkempt. Hair can be long or short, and even the presence or absence

of hair conveys a message about the person. Other body adornments that are also considered potential communicative stimuli include tattoos, masks, cosmetics, badges, jewelry, and eyeglasses. Some jewelry worn in specific ways can give special messages (e.g., a gold band or diamond ring worn on the third finger of the left hand, a pin bearing Greek letters worn on the lapel, or the wearing of a ring that is inscribed with the insignia of a college or university). Some individuals convey a specific message with the total absence of any type of body adornment.

Body Movement and Posture

The way in which an individual positions his or her body communicates messages regarding self-esteem, gender identity, status, and interpersonal warmth or coldness. The individual whose posture is slumped, with head and eyes pointed downward, conveys a message of low self-esteem. Specific ways of standing or sitting are considered to be either feminine or masculine within a defined culture. In the United States, to stand straight and tall with head high and hands on hips indicates a superior status over the person being addressed.

Reece and Whitman (1962) identified response behaviors that were used to designate individuals as either "warm" or "cold" persons. Individuals who were perceived as warm responded to others with a shift of posture toward the other person, a smile, direct eye contact, and hands that remained still. Individuals who responded to others with a slumped posture, by looking around the room, drumming fingers on the desk, and not smiling were perceived as cold.

Touch

Touch is a powerful communication tool. It can elicit both negative and positive reactions, depending on the people involved and the circumstances of the interaction. It is a very basic and primitive form of communication, and the appropriateness of its use is culturally determined.

Touch can be categorized according to the message communicated (Knapp & Hall, 2014):

Functional-professional: This type of touch is impersonal and businesslike. It is used to accomplish a task.

EXAMPLE

A tailor measuring a customer for a suit or a physician examining a client

Social-polite: This type of touch is still rather impersonal, but it conveys an affirmation or acceptance of the other person.

EXAMPLE

A handshake

Friendship-warmth: Touch at this level indicates a strong liking for the other person, a feeling that he or she is a friend.

EXAMPLE

Laying one's hand on the shoulder of another

Love-intimacy: This type of touch conveys an emotional attachment or attraction for another person.

EXAMPLE

Engaging in a strong, mutual embrace

Sexual arousal: Touch at this level is an expression of physical attraction only.

EXAMPLE

Touching another in the genital region

Some cultures encourage more touching of various types than do others. "Contact cultures" (e.g., France, Latin America, Italy) use a greater frequency of touch cues than do those in "noncontact cultures" (e.g., Germany, United States, Canada) (Givens, 2013c). The nurse should understand the cultural meaning of touch before using this method of communication in specific situations.

Facial Expressions

Next to human speech, facial expression is the primary source of communication. Facial expressions reveal an individual's emotional state, such as happiness, sadness, anger, surprise, and fear. The face is a complex multimessage system. Facial expressions serve to complement and qualify other communication behaviors and at times even take the place of verbal messages. A summary of feelings associated with various facial expressions is presented in Table 8–1.

Eye Behavior

Eyes have been called the "windows of the soul." It is through eye contact that individuals view and are viewed by others in a revealing way, creating an interpersonal connection. In American culture, eye contact conveys a personal interest in the other person. Eye contact indicates that the communication channel is open, and it is often the initiating factor in verbal interaction between two people.

Eye behavior is regulated by social rules. These rules dictate where, when, for how long, and at whom we can look. Staring is often used to register disapproval of the behavior of another. People are extremely sensitive to being looked at, and if the gazing or staring behavior violates social rules, they often assign meaning to it, such as the following statement implies: "He kept staring at me, and I began to wonder if I was dressed inappropriately or had mustard on my face!"

TABLE 8–1 **Summary of Facial Expressions**

FACIAL EXPRESSION	ASSOCIATED FEELINGS
NOSE	
Nostril flare	Anger; arousal
Wrinkling up	Dislike; disgust
LIPS	
Grin; smile	Happiness; contentment
Grimace	Fear; pain
Compressed	Anger; frustration
Canine-type snarl	Disgust
Pouted; frown	Unhappiness; discontented; disapproval
Pursing	Disagreement
Sneer	Contempt; disdain
BROWS	
Frown	Anger; unhappiness; concentration
Raised	Surprise; enthusiasm
TONGUE	
Stick out	Dislike; disagree
EYES	
Widened	Surprise; excitement
Narrowed; lids squeezed shut	Threat; fear
Stare	Threat
Stare, blink, then look away	Dislike; disinterest
Eyes downcast; lack of eye contact	Submission; low self-esteem
Eye contact (generally intermittent as opposed to a stare)	Self-confidence; interest

SOURCES: Givens, D.B. (2013b). Facial expression. In *The Nonverbal Dictionary of Gestures, Signs, and Body Language Cues.* Retrieved from http://www.nonverbal-dictionary.org/2012/12/facial-expression.html; Hughey, J.D. (1990). *Speech communication.* Stillwater: Oklahoma State University; Simon, M. (2005). *Facial expressions: A visual reference for artists.* New York: Watson-Guptill.

Gazing at another's eyes arouses strong emotions. Thus, eye contact rarely lasts longer than 3 seconds before one or both viewers experience a powerful urge to glance away. Breaking eye contact lowers stress levels (Givens, 2013a).

Vocal Cues or Paralanguage

Paralanguage is the gestural component of the spoken word. It consists of pitch, tone, and loudness of spoken messages; the rate of speaking; expressively placed pauses; and emphasis assigned to certain words. These vocal cues greatly influence the way individuals interpret verbal messages. A normally soft-spoken individual whose pitch and rate of speaking increases may be perceived as being anxious or tense.

Different vocal emphases can alter interpretation of the message. Three examples follow:

1. "I felt **SURE** you would notice the change."
   Interpretation: I was **SURE** you would, but you didn't.
2. "I felt sure **YOU** would notice the change."
   Interpretation: I thought **YOU** would, even if nobody else did.
3. "I felt sure you would notice the **CHANGE**."
   Interpretation: Even if you didn't notice anything else, I thought you would notice the **CHANGE**.

Verbal cues play a major role in determining responses in human communication situations. *How* a message is verbalized can be as important as *what* is verbalized.

CORE CONCEPT
Therapeutic Communication
Caregiver verbal and nonverbal techniques that focus on the care receiver's needs and advance the promotion of healing and change. Therapeutic communication encourages exploration of feelings and fosters understanding of behavioral motivation. It is nonjudgmental, discourages defensiveness, and promotes trust.

Therapeutic Communication Techniques

Hays and Larson (1963) identified a number of techniques to assist the nurse in interacting more therapeutically with clients. These are important "technical procedures" carried out by the nurse working in psychiatry, and they should serve to enhance development of a therapeutic nurse-client relationship. Table 8–2 includes a list of these techniques, a short explanation of their usefulness, and examples of each.

TABLE 8–2 Therapeutic Communication Techniques

TECHNIQUE	EXPLANATION/RATIONALE	EXAMPLES
Using silence	Silence gives the client the opportunity to collect and organize thoughts, to think through a point, or to consider introducing a topic of greater concern than the one being discussed.	The client pauses midsentence in answering a question. The nurse remains quiet, does not "rescue" the client with prompts or by moving on to another question, and ensures that his or her body language and facial expression project interest in and willingness to wait for the client to answer.
Accepting	Conveys an attitude of reception and regard.	"Yes, I understand what you said." Eye contact; nodding.
Giving recognition	Acknowledging and indicating awareness is better than complimenting, which reflects the nurse's judgment.	"Hello, Mr. J. I notice that you made a ceramic ash tray in OT." "I see you made your bed."
Offering self	Making oneself available on an unconditional basis helps to increase the client's feelings of self-worth.	"I'll stay with you awhile." "We can eat our lunch together." "I'm interested in talking with you."
Giving broad openings	Allowing the client to take the initiative in introducing the topic emphasizes the importance of the client's role in the interaction.	"What would you like to talk about today?" "Tell me what you are thinking."
Offering general leads	General leads, or prompts, offer the client encouragement to continue.	"Yes, I see." "Go on." "And after that?"
Placing the event in time or sequence	Clarifying the relationship of events in time enables the nurse and client to view them in perspective.	"What seemed to lead up to . . . ?" "Was this before or after . . . ?" "When did this happen?"
Making observations	Verbalizing what is observed or perceived encourages the client to recognize specific behaviors and compare perceptions with the nurse.	"You seem tense." "I notice you are pacing a lot." "You seem uncomfortable when you. . . ."

TABLE 8–2 Therapeutic Communication Techniques–cont'd

TECHNIQUE	EXPLANATION/RATIONALE	EXAMPLES
Encouraging description of perceptions	Asking the client to verbalize what is being perceived is often used with clients experiencing hallucinations.	"Tell me what is happening now." "Are you hearing the voices again?" "What do the voices seem to be saying?"
Encouraging comparison	Asking the client to compare similarities and differences in ideas, experiences, or interpersonal relationships helps the client recognize life experiences that tend to recur as well as those aspects of life that are changeable.	"Was this something like . . . ?" "How does this compare with the time when . . . ?" "What was your response the last time this situation occurred?"
Restating	Repeating the main idea of what the client has said lets the client know whether an expressed statement has been understood and gives him or her the chance to continue or to clarify if necessary.	Cl: "I can't study. My mind keeps wandering." Ns: "You have trouble concentrating." Cl: "I can't take that new job. What if I can't do it?" Ns: "You're afraid you will fail in this new position."
Reflecting	Questions and feelings are referred back to the client so that they may be recognized and accepted and so that the client may recognize that his or her point of view has value—a good technique to use when the client asks the nurse for advice.	Cl: "What do you think I should do about my wife's drinking problem?" Ns: "What do *you* think you should do?" Cl: "My sister won't help a bit with my mother's care. I have to do it all!" Ns: "You feel angry when she doesn't help."
Focusing	Taking notice of a single idea or even a single word works especially well with a client who is moving rapidly from one thought to another. This technique is *not* therapeutic, however, with the client who is very anxious. Focusing should not be pursued until the anxiety level has subsided.	"This point seems worth looking at more closely. Perhaps you and I can discuss it together."
Exploring	Delving further into a subject, idea, experience, or relationship is especially helpful with clients who tend to remain on a superficial level of communication. However, if the client chooses not to disclose further information, the nurse should refrain from pushing or probing in an area that obviously creates discomfort.	"Please explain that situation in more detail." "Tell me more about that particular situation."
Seeking clarification and validation	Striving to explain that which is vague or incomprehensible and searching for mutual understanding of what has been said facilitates and increases understanding for both client and nurse.	"I'm not sure that I understand. Would you please explain?" "Tell me if my understanding agrees with yours." "Do I understand correctly that you said . . . ?"
Presenting reality	When the client has a misperception of the environment, the nurse defines reality or indicates his or her perception of the situation for the client.	"I understand that the voices seem real to you, but I do not hear any voices." "There is no one else in the room but you and me."
Voicing doubt	Expressing uncertainty as to the reality of the client's perceptions is a technique often used with clients experiencing delusional thinking.	"I understand that you believe that to be true, but I see the situation differently." "I find that hard to believe (or accept)." "That seems rather doubtful to me."

Continued

TABLE 8–2 **Therapeutic Communication Techniques–cont'd**

TECHNIQUE	EXPLANATION/RATIONALE	EXAMPLES
Verbalizing the implied	Putting into words what the client has only implied or said indirectly is a helpful technique to use with clients who are reticent to speak as well as with clients who are mute or are otherwise experiencing impaired verbal communication. This clarifies that which is *implicit* rather than *explicit*.	Cl: "It's a waste of time to be here. I can't talk to you or anyone." Ns: "Are you feeling that no one understands?" Cl: (Mute) Ns: "It must have been very difficult for you when your husband died in the fire."
Attempting to translate words into feelings	When feelings are expressed indirectly, the nurse tries to "desymbolize" what has been said and to find clues to the underlying true feelings.	Cl: "I'm way out in the ocean." Ns: "You must be feeling very lonely right now."
Formulating a plan of action	When a client has a plan in mind for dealing with what is considered to be a stressful situation, it may serve to prevent anger or anxiety from escalating to an unmanageable level.	"What could you do to let your anger out harmlessly?" "Next time this comes up, what might you do to handle it more appropriately?"

SOURCE: Adapted from Hays, J.S., & Larson, K.H. (1963). *Interacting with patients.* New York: Macmillan.

Nontherapeutic Communication Techniques

Several approaches are considered to be barriers to open communication between the nurse and client. Hays and Larson (1963) identified a number of these techniques, which are presented in Table 8–3. Nurses should recognize and eliminate the use of these patterns in their relationships with clients. Avoiding these communication barriers will maximize the effectiveness of communication and enhance the nurse-client relationship.

Active Listening

To listen actively is to be attentive and really desire to hear and understand what the client is saying, both verbally and nonverbally. Attentive listening creates a climate in which the client can communicate. With active listening, the nurse communicates acceptance and respect for the client, and trust is enhanced. A climate is established within the relationship that promotes openness and honest expression.

TABLE 8–3 **Nontherapeutic Communication Techniques**

TECHNIQUE	EXPLANATION/RATIONALE	EXAMPLES
Giving reassurance	Indicating to the client that there is no cause for anxiety devalues the client's feelings and may discourage the client from further expression of feelings if he or she believes they will only be downplayed or ridiculed.	"I wouldn't worry about that if I were you." "Everything will be all right." Better to say: "We will work on that together."
Rejecting	Refusing to consider or showing contempt for the client's ideas or behavior may cause the client to discontinue interaction with the nurse for fear of further rejection.	"Let's not discuss. . . ." "I don't want to hear about. . . ." Better to say: "Let's look at that a little closer."
Approving or disapproving	Sanctioning or denouncing the client's ideas or behavior implies that the nurse has the right to pass judgment on whether the client's ideas or behaviors are "good" or "bad" and that the client is expected to please the nurse. The nurse's acceptance of the client is then seen as conditional depending on the client's behavior.	"That's good. I'm glad that you. . . ." "That's bad. I'd rather you wouldn't. . . ." Better to say: "Let's talk about how your behavior invoked anger in the other clients at dinner."

TABLE 8-3 Nontherapeutic Communication Techniques—cont'd

TECHNIQUE	EXPLANATION/RATIONALE	EXAMPLES
Agreeing or disagreeing	Indicating accord with or opposition to the client's ideas or opinions implies that the nurse has the right to pass judgment on whether the client's ideas or opinions are "right" or "wrong." Agreement prevents the client from later modifying his or her point of view without admitting error. Disagreement implies inaccuracy, provoking the need for defensiveness on the part of the client.	"That's right. I agree." "That's wrong. I disagree." "I don't believe that." Better to say: "Let's discuss what you feel is unfair about the new community rules."
Giving advice	Telling the client what to do or how to behave implies that the nurse knows what is best and that the client is incapable of any self-direction. It nurtures the client in the dependent role by discouraging independent thinking.	"I think you should. . . ." "Why don't you. . . ." Better to say: "What do *you* think you should do?" or "What do *you* think would be the best way to solve this problem?
Probing	Persistent questioning of the client and pushing for answers to issues the client does not wish to discuss causes the client to feel used and valued only for what is shared with the nurse and places the client on the defensive.	"Tell me how your mother abused you when you were a child." "Tell me how you feel toward your mother now that she is dead." "Now tell me about. . . ." Better technique: The nurse should be aware of the client's response and discontinue the interaction at the first sign of discomfort.
Defending	Attempting to protect someone or something from verbal attack, or defending what the client has criticized, implies that he or she has no right to express ideas, opinions, or feelings. Defending does not change the client's feelings and may cause the client to think the nurse is taking sides against the client.	"No one here would lie to you." "You have a very capable physician. I'm sure he has only your best interests in mind." Better to say: "I will try to answer your questions and clarify some issues regarding your treatment."
Requesting an explanation	Asking the client to provide the reasons for thoughts, feelings, behavior, and events— asking "why" a client did something or feels a certain way—can be very intimidating and implies that the client must defend his or her behavior or feelings.	"Why do you think that?" "Why do you feel this way?" "Why did you do that?" Better to say: "Describe what you were feeling just before that happened."
Indicating the existence of an external source of power	Attributing the source of thoughts, feelings, and behavior to others or to outside influences encourages the client to project blame for his or her thoughts or behaviors on others rather than accepting the responsibility personally.	"What makes you say that?" "What made you do that?" "What made you so angry last night?" Better to say: "You became angry when your brother insulted your wife."
Belittling feelings expressed	When the nurse misjudges the degree of the client's discomfort, a lack of empathy and understanding may be conveyed. Telling the client to "perk up" or "snap out of it" causes the client to feel insignificant or unimportant. When one is experiencing discomfort, it is no relief to hear that others are or have been in similar situations.	Cl: "I have nothing to live for. I wish I were dead." Ns: "Everybody gets down in the dumps at times. I feel that way myself sometimes." Better to say: "You must be very upset. Tell me what you are feeling right now."

Continued

TABLE 8–3 Nontherapeutic Communication Techniques—cont'd

TECHNIQUE	EXPLANATION/RATIONALE	EXAMPLES
Making stereotyped comments	Clichés and trite expressions are meaningless in a nurse-client relationship. When the nurse makes empty conversation, it encourages a like response from the client.	"I'm fine, and how are you?" "Hang in there. It's for your own good." "Keep your chin up." Better to say: "The therapy must be difficult for you at times. How do you feel about your progress at this point?"
Using denial	Denying that a problem exists blocks discussion with the client and precludes helping the client identify and explore areas of difficulty.	Cl: "I'm nothing." Ns: "Of course you're something. Everybody is somebody." Better to say: "You're feeling like no one cares about you right now."
Interpreting	With this technique, the therapist seeks to make conscious that which is unconscious, to tell the client the meaning of his or her experience.	"What you really mean is. . . ." "Unconsciously you're saying. . . ." Better technique: The nurse must leave interpretation of the client's behavior to the psychiatrist. The nurse has not been prepared to perform this technique, and in attempting to do so, may endanger other nursing roles with the client.
Introducing an unrelated topic	Changing the subject causes the nurse to take over the direction of the discussion. This may occur in order to get to something that the nurse wants to discuss with the client or to get away from a topic that he or she prefers not to discuss.	Cl: "I don't have anything to live for." Ns: "Did you have visitors this weekend?" Better technique: The nurse must remain open and free to hear the client and to take in all that is being conveyed, both verbally and nonverbally.

SOURCE: Adapted from Hays, J.S., & Larson, K.H. (1963). *Interacting with patients*. New York: Macmillan.

Several nonverbal behaviors have been designated as facilitative skills for attentive listening. Those listed here can be identified by the acronym SOLER:

S—Sit squarely facing the client. This nonverbal cue gives the message that the nurse is there to listen and is interested in what the client has to say.

O—Observe an open posture. Posture is considered "open" when arms and legs remain uncrossed. This nonverbal cue suggests that the nurse is open to what the client has to say. With a closed position, the nurse can convey a somewhat defensive stance, possibly invoking a similar response in the client.

L—Lean forward toward the client. Leaning forward conveys to the client that the nurse is involved in the interaction, interested in what is being said, and making a sincere effort to be attentive.

E—Establish eye contact. Eye contact, intermittently directed, is another behavior that conveys the nurse's involvement and willingness to listen to what the client has to say. The absence of eye "contact or the constant shifting of eye contact elsewhere in the environment gives the message that the nurse is not really interested in what is being said.

> **CLINICAL PEARL** Ensure that eye contact conveys warmth and is accompanied by smiling and intermittent nodding of the head and does not come across as staring or glaring, which can create intense discomfort in the client.

R—Relax. Whether sitting or standing during the interaction, the nurse should communicate a sense of being relaxed and comfortable with the client. Restlessness and fidgetiness communicate a lack of interest and may convey a feeling of discomfort that is likely to be transferred to the client.

Motivational Interviewing

Patient-centered care has been identified as an important focus in the quest to improve the quality of nurse communication and therapeutic relationships with clients (Institute of Medicine, 2003). **Motivational interviewing** is an evidence-based, patient-centered style of communicating that promotes behavior change by guiding clients to explore their own motivation for change and the advantages and disadvantages of their decisions. This style of communication incorporates active listening and verbal therapeutic communication techniques, but it is focused on what the client wants rather than on what the nurse thinks *should* be the next steps in behavior change. Motivational interviewing was originally developed for use with clients who were struggling with substance use disorders, primarily because this style of communication may decrease defensive client responses. It has since gained widespread acceptance as a patient-centered communication strategy that promotes behavior change for clients with many different health-care issues. See the "Real People, Real Stories" box for an example of motivational interviewing described in a process recording format.

Process Recordings

Process recordings are written reports of verbal interactions with clients. They are verbatim accounts recorded by the nurse or student as a tool for improving interpersonal communication techniques. Process recording can take many forms but usually includes the verbal and nonverbal communication of both nurse and client. The exercise provides a means for the nurse to analyze both the content and pattern of the interaction. Process recording, which is not considered documentation, is intended to be used as a learning tool for professional development. An example of one type of process recording is presented in Table 8–4.

Real People, Real Stories: A Sample of Motivational Interviewing in a Process Recording Format

The following is part of an interaction with Alan, incorporating motivational interviewing communication strategies in a process recording format. Learn more about Alan's story in the chapter on substance use disorders.

Interaction	Nurse's Thoughts and Feelings	Communication Technique/Evaluation
Karyn: You mentioned that you were at an event and you commented that you "needed a drink." Tell me more about what was happening. (SOLER)	I wasn't sure if Alan was willing to talk about this, but I thought it was important to facilitate his looking at his behavior in response to this experience.	Technique: **Exploring** Evaluation: This approach was effective. Alan talked more about the event and was able to articulate some thoughts and feelings as well.
Alan: (nodding) I was perturbed. I felt like I was stuck at this event. There was supposed to be entertainment but it got cancelled due to rain, and suddenly I noticed people were drinking and smoking. It brought back a lot of memories. (looks down)	I was glad that Alan was open to discussing this experience, but he said so many things in this short statement that I had to be thoughtful about what to follow up on.	

Karyn: So you felt perturbed and stuck. . . . (looking up, not making direct eye contact)	I was thinking that I don't usually explore feelings right off the bat because I believe it's better to help someone fully describe events and thoughts first (or at least it's less threatening), but I've interacted with Alan many times, he's been through rehab, sober for seven years, and he's pretty comfortable talking about feelings	Technique: **Reflecting**
		    Evaluation: This technique was effective. Alan began to process his thoughts about why he might be feeling perturbed and stuck.
		    I think I may have been not making direct eye contact because of my perception that feelings can be a little more threatening for some people to talk about.

Alan: Yeah, but it didn't last long. Maybe it had something to do with the fact that there was nothing else going on and it seemed like the whole thing became about drinking. But then I just blacked it out.	My immediate thought was that I want to tell him to go to an AA meeting or call his sponsor, but I was trying to incorporate a motivational interviewing strategy, and that meant it would be better to help him explore his motivation for how to respond to this experience. I didn't know what he meant by "blacked it out," but I felt uncomfortable when he said that.	

Continued

Real People, Real Stories: A Sample of Motivational Interviewing in a Process Recording Format—cont'd

Interaction	Nurse's Thoughts and Feelings	Communication Technique/Evaluation
Karyn: What do you mean when you say you blacked it out? (SOLER)	I thought this was an important statement to clarify, since it might help him explore how he behaved in response to this event.	Technique: **Clarifying** Evaluation: Asking this question was effective. Alan talked at length about his thoughts and feelings.
Alan: (silent for several seconds) I do need to go back to an AA meeting. I mean, am I different than other people? I know there are other people out there that have to be struggling with the same kind of things. When I was in rehab, my mom and her boyfriend were always there taking me to meetings. My sister went, too. . . . (silent for several more seconds) I know it's important (silence) . . . about 75 percent of the people I went to rehab with are back out there using again.	Alan seemed to be thinking a lot about this and was responding with several different thoughts, so I felt like it was important to just use silence and facilitate his reflection. I thought Alan seemed to be genuinely considering a behavior change.	
Karyn: You said that you need to go back to a meeting and that they are important. Is it more helpful to go to meetings when you just start thinking about needing a drink, or do you think that meetings are only necessary after you actually take a drink?	I knew that Alan had not been going to meetings regularly for the last couple of years, even though he acknowledges their importance, so I wanted to know more about whether he thought behavior change (such as going to AA meetings) was necessary at this point.	Technique: **Restating, focusing** Evaluation: Restatement was effective. The way I chose to focus was probably leading Alan to choose the "right" answer, and that makes it harder to evaluate whether he is just telling me what I want to hear or is really motivated. It might have been better to use the technique of formulating a plan of action.
Alan: Oh no, you've got to go long before you take that first drink. (silence) People told me when I was in rehab that they could tell I was really listening in meetings . . . the meetings were helpful (silence), and I just reconnected with my sponsor on Facebook, so I need to get back to a meeting to see him.	Alan seemed like he was thinking about what is important to him, so I continued to remain silent to facilitate that process.	
Karyn: You've identified three reasons why you believe you need to go to a meeting: because they are helpful to you, because you want to find out if others are struggling with the same kinds of thoughts that you are, and because you need to reconnect with your sponsor. Do you have a plan in mind for how to follow through with that?	I was thinking that he talks about needing to go to AA, and I was feeling anxious about wanting him to commit to that, but at the same time, I recognized that the motivation for change and commitment to a plan of action has to come from him.	Technique: **Summarizing, formulating a plan of action** Evaluation: I think the techniques were effective, although Alan may not be ready to formulate an action plan at present.
Alan: Well, I haven't done it yet. I guess I'm still just thinking about it.	I was appreciating his honesty and thinking that this is the challenge of motivational interviewing: accepting where the client is at while continuing to explore and facilitate his or her motivations for behavior change.	

TABLE 8–4 Sample Process Recording

NURSE VERBAL (NONVERBAL)	CLIENT VERBAL (NONVERBAL)	NURSE'S THOUGHTS AND FEELINGS CONCERNING THE INTERACTION	ANALYSIS OF THE INTERACTION
Do you still have thoughts about harming yourself? (Sitting facing the client; looking directly at client.)	Not really. I still feel sad, but I don't want to die. (Looking at hands in lap.)	Felt a little uncomfortable. Always a hard question to ask.	**Therapeutic.** Asking a direct, closed-ended question about suicidal intent to elicit specific information.
Tell me what you were feeling before you took all the pills the other night. (Using SOLER techniques of active listening.)	I was just so angry! To think that my husband wants a divorce now that he has a good job. I worked hard to put him through college. (Fists clenched. Face and neck reddened.)	Beginning to feel more comfortable. Client seems willing to talk, and I think she trusts me.	**Therapeutic.** Exploring. Delving further into client's feelings to help her better understand her experience.
You wanted to hurt him because you felt betrayed. (SOLER)	Yes! If I died, maybe he'd realize that he loved me more than that other woman. (Tears starting to well up in her eyes.)	Starting to feel sorry for her.	**Therapeutic.** Attempting to translate words into feelings to convey active listening.
Seems like a pretty drastic way to get your point across. (Small frown.)	I know. It was a stupid thing to do. (Wiping eyes.)	Trying hard to remain objective.	**Nontherapeutic.** Sounds disapproving. Better to have pursued client's feelings.
How are you feeling about the situation now? (SOLER)	I don't know. I still love him. I want him to come home. I don't want him to marry her. (Starting to cry again)	Wishing there was an easy way to help relieve some of her pain.	**Therapeutic.** Focusing on client's current feelings to assess current mental status.
Yes, I can understand that you would like things to be the way they were before. (Offer client a tissue.)	(Silence. Continues to cry softly.)	I'm starting to feel some anger toward her husband. Sometimes it's so hard to remain objective!	**Therapeutic.** Conveying empathy to support caring and connectedness.
What do you think are the chances of your getting back together? (SOLER)	None. He's refused marriage counseling. He's already moved in with her. He says it's over. (Wipes tears. Looks directly at nurse.)	Relieved to know that she isn't using denial about the reality of the situation.	**Therapeutic.** Reflecting on the client's expressed feelings to encourage client to recognize and clarify their perceptions.
So how are you preparing to deal with this inevitable outcome? (SOLER)	I'm going to do the things we talked about: join a divorced women's support group, increase my job hours to full time, do some volunteer work, and call the suicide hotline if I feel like taking pills again. (Looks directly at nurse. Smiles.)	Positive feeling to know that she remembers what we discussed earlier and plans to follow through.	**Therapeutic.** Formulating a plan of action to set the foundation for problem-solving.
It won't be easy. But you have come a long way, and I feel you have gained strength in your ability to cope. (Standing. Looking at client. Smiling.)	Yes, I know I will have hard times. But I also know I have support, and I want to go on with my life and be happy again. (Standing, smiling at nurse.)	Feeling confident that the session has gone well; hopeful that the client will succeed in what she wants to do with her life.	**Therapeutic.** Presenting reality, making observations, and giving recognition to support client's progress in problem solving.

Feedback

Feedback is a method of communication for helping the client consider behavior modification by providing information about how he or she is perceived by others. Feedback can be useful to the client if presented with objectivity by a trusted individual in a manner that discourages defensiveness.

Characteristics of useful feedback include the following:

■ Feedback is descriptive rather than evaluative and focuses on the behavior rather than on the client. Avoiding evaluative language reduces the need for the client to react defensively. Objective descriptions allow clients to use the information in whatever way they choose. When the focus of feedback is on the client, the nurse makes judgments about the client.

EXAMPLE

Descriptive and focused on behavior	"Jessica was very upset in group today when you called her 'a cow' and laughed at her in front of the others."
Evaluative	"You were very rude and inconsiderate to Jessica in group today."
Focus on client	"You are a very insensitive person."

■ Feedback should be specific rather than general. Information that gives details about the client's behavior is more effective than a generalized description in promoting behavior change.

EXAMPLE

Specific	"You were talking to Joe when we were deciding on the issue. Now you want to argue about the outcome."
General	"You just don't pay attention."

■ Feedback should be directed toward behavior that the client has the capacity to modify. To provide feedback about a characteristic or situation that the client cannot change only provokes frustration.

EXAMPLE

Can modify	"I noticed that you did not want to hold your baby when the nurse brought her to you."
Cannot modify	"Your baby daughter is mentally retarded because you took drugs when you were pregnant."

■ Feedback should impart information rather than offer advice. Giving advice fosters dependence and may convey the message to the client that he or she is not capable of making decisions and solving problems independently. It is the client's right and privilege to be as self-sufficient as possible.

EXAMPLE

Imparting information	"There are various methods of assistance for people who want to lose weight, such as Overeaters Anonymous, Weight Watchers, regular visits to a dietitian, and the Physician's Weight Loss Program. You can decide what is best for you."
Giving advice	"You obviously need to lose a great deal of weight. I think the Physician's Weight Loss Program would be best for you."

■ Feedback should be well-timed. Feedback is most useful when given at the earliest appropriate opportunity following the specific behavior.

EXAMPLE

Prompt response	"I saw you hit the wall with your fist just now when you hung up the phone after talking to your mother."
Delayed response	"You need to learn some more appropriate ways of dealing with your anger. Last week after group I saw you pounding your fist against the wall."

Summary and Key Points

■ Interpersonal communication is a transaction between the sender and the receiver.
■ In all interpersonal transactions, the sender and receiver each bring certain preexisting conditions to the exchange that influence both the intended message and the way in which it is interpreted.
■ Examples of these preexisting conditions include one's value system, internalized attitudes and beliefs, culture and religion, social status, gender, background knowledge and experience, age or developmental level, and the type of environment in which the communication takes place.
■ Nonverbal expression is a primary communication system in which meaning is assigned to various gestures and patterns of behavior.
■ Some components of nonverbal communication include physical appearance and dress, body movement and posture, touch, facial expressions, eye behavior, and vocal cues or paralanguage.
■ Meaning of the nonverbal components of communication is culturally determined.
■ Therapeutic communication is an intentional process that applies both verbal and nonverbal techniques to focus on the care *receiver's* needs and advance the promotion of healing and change.
■ Motivational interviewing is an evidence-based, patient-centered style of therapeutic communication

that facilitates clients' exploration of their own motivations for behavior change and guides the client to explore the advantages and disadvantages of their decisions.

■ Nurses must be aware of and avoid techniques that are considered barriers to effective communication.

■ Active listening is described as attentiveness to what the client is saying through both verbal and nonverbal cues. Skills associated with active listening include sitting squarely facing the client, observing an open posture, leaning forward toward the client, establishing eye contact, and being relaxed.

■ Process recordings are written reports of verbal interactions with clients. They are used as learning tools for professional development.

■ Feedback is a method of communication for helping the client consider a modification of behavior.

■ The nurse must be aware of the therapeutic or nontherapeutic value of the communication techniques used with the client because they are the tools of psychosocial intervention.

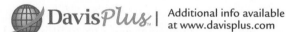
DavisPlus | Additional info available at www.davisplus.com

Review Questions
Self-Examination/Learning Exercise

Select the answer that is most appropriate for each of the following questions.

1. A client states, "I refuse to shower in this room. I must be very cautious. The FBI has placed a camera in here to monitor my every move." Which of the following is the most therapeutic response?
   a. "That's not true."
   b. "I have a hard time believing that is true."
   c. "Surely you don't really believe that."
   d. "I will help you search this room so that you can see there is no camera."

2. Simone, a depressed client who has been unkempt and untidy for weeks, today comes to group therapy wearing makeup and a clean dress with hair washed and combed. Which of the following responses by the nurse is most appropriate?
   a. "Simone, I see you have put on a clean dress and combed your hair."
   b. "Simone, you look wonderful today!"
   c. "Simone, I'm sure everyone will appreciate that you have cleaned up for the group today."
   d. "Now that you see how important it is, I hope you will do this every day."

3. Dorothy was involved in an automobile accident while under the influence of alcohol. She swerved her car into a tree and narrowly missed hitting a child on a bicycle. She is in the hospital with multiple abrasions and contusions. She is talking about the accident with the nurse. Which of the following statements by the nurse is most appropriate?
   a. "Now that you know what can happen when you drink and drive, I'm sure you won't let it happen again."
   b. "You know that was a terrible thing you did. That child could have been killed."
   c. "I'm sure everything is going to be okay now that you understand the possible consequences of such behavior."
   d. "How are you feeling about what happened?"

4. Judy has been in the hospital for 3 weeks. She has used Valium "to settle her nerves" for the past 15 years. She was admitted by her psychiatrist for safe withdrawal from the drug. She has passed the physical symptoms of withdrawal at this time but states to the nurse, "I don't know if I will be able to make it without Valium after I go home. I'm already starting to feel nervous. I have so many personal problems." Which is the most appropriate response by the nurse?
   a. "Why do you think you need drugs to deal with your problems?"
   b. "Everybody has problems, but not everybody uses drugs to deal with them. You'll just have to do the best that you can."
   c. "Let's explore some things you can do to decrease your anxiety without resorting to drugs."
   d. "Just hang in there. I'm sure everything is going to be okay."

Continued

Review Questions—cont'd
Self-Examination/Learning Exercise

5. Mrs. S. asks the nurse, "Do you think I should tell my husband about my affair with my boss?" Which is the most appropriate response by the nurse?
   a. "What do you think would be best for you to do?"
   b. "Of course you should. Marriage has to be based on truth."
   c. "Of course not. That would only make things worse."
   d. "I can't tell you what to do. You have to decide for yourself."

6. Abby, an adolescent, just returned from group therapy and is crying. She says to the nurse, "All the other kids laughed at me! I try to fit in, but I always seem to say the wrong thing. I've never had a close friend. I guess I never will." Which is the most appropriate response by the nurse?
   a. "What makes you think you will never have any friends?"
   b. "You're feeling pretty down on yourself right now."
   c. "I'm sure they didn't mean to hurt your feelings."
   d. "Why do you feel this way about yourself?"

7. Walter is angry with his psychiatrist and says to the nurse, "He doesn't know what he is doing. That medication isn't helping a thing!" The nurse responds, "He has been a doctor for many years and has helped many people." This is an example of what nontherapeutic technique?
   a. Rejecting
   b. Disapproving
   c. Probing
   d. Defending

8. The client says to the nurse, "I've been offered a promotion, but I don't know if I can handle it." The nurse replies, "You're afraid you may fail in the new position." This is an example of which therapeutic technique?
   a. Restating
   b. Making observations
   c. Focusing
   d. Verbalizing the implied

9. The environment in which the communication takes place influences the outcome of the interaction. Which of the following are aspects of the environment that influence communication? (Select all that apply.)
   a. Territoriality
   b. Density
   c. Dimension
   d. Distance
   e. Intensity

10. The nurse says to a client, "You are being readmitted to the hospital. Why did you stop taking your medication?" What communication technique does this represent?
   a. Disapproving
   b. Requesting an explanation
   c. Disagreeing
   d. Probing

Review Questions—cont'd
Self-Examination/Learning Exercise

11. Joe has been in rehabilitation for alcohol dependence. When he returns from a visit to his home, he tells the nurse, "We were having a celebration and I did have one drink, but it really wasn't a problem." The nurse notices that his breath smells of alcohol. Which of the following responses by the nurse demonstrates a motivational interviewing style of communication?
    a. "You are obviously not motivated to change, so perhaps we should discuss your discharge from the treatment program."
    b. "You need to abstain from alcohol in order to recover, so let me talk to the doctor about the consequences of your behavior."
    c. "Why would you destroy everything you've worked so hard to achieve?"
    d. "What do you mean when you say, 'It really wasn't a problem'?"

12. Bill, who has been diagnosed with schizophrenia and has been on medication for several months, states, "I'm not taking that stupid medication anymore." Which of the following responses by the nurse demonstrates a motivational interviewing style of communication?
    a. "Don't you know that if you don't take your medication you will never recover?"
    b. "Why won't you cooperate with the treatment your doctor prescribed?"
    c. "Bill, the medication is not stupid."
    d. "Tell me more about why you don't want to take the medication."

References

Givens, D.B. (2013a). Eye contact. In *The Nonverbal Dictionary of Gestures, Signs, and Body Language Cues*. Retrieved from: http://www.nonverbal-dictionary.org/2012/12/eyes-contact.html

Givens, D.B. (2013b). Facial expression. In *The Nonverbal Dictionary of Gestures, Signs, and Body Language Cues*. Retrieved from: http://www.nonverbal-dictionary.org/2012/12/facial-expression.html

Givens, D.B. (2006c). Touch cue. In *The Nonverbal Dictionary of Gestures, Signs, and Body Language Cues*. Retrieved from http://web.archive.org/web/20060627081330/members.aol.com/doder1/touch1.htm

Institute of Medicine. (2003). *Health professions education: A bridge to quality*. Washington, DC: Institute of Medicine.

Hughey, J.D. (1990). *Speech communication*. Stillwater: Oklahoma State University.

Khan, A. (2014). *Principles for personal growth*. Bellevue, WA: YouMe Works.

Knapp, M.L., & Hall, J.A. (2014). *Nonverbal communication in human interaction* (8th ed.). Belmont, CA: Wadsworth.

Simon, M. (2005). *Facial expressions: A visual reference for artists*. New York: Watson-Guptill.

Classical References

Hall, E.T. (1966). *The hidden dimension*. Garden City, NY: Doubleday.

Hays, J.S., & Larson, K.H. (1963). *Interacting with patients*. New York: Macmillan.

Reece, M., & Whitman, R. (1962). Expressive movements, warmth, and verbal reinforcement. *Journal of Abnormal and Social Psychology, 64,* 234-236. doi:http://dx.doi.org/10.1037/h0039792

9

The Nursing Process in Psychiatric-Mental Health Nursing

CORE CONCEPTS

Assessment

Evaluation

Nursing Diagnosis

Outcomes

CHAPTER OUTLINE

Objectives

Homework Assignment

The Nursing Process

Why Nursing Diagnosis?

Nursing Case Management

Applying the Nursing Process in the Psychiatric Setting

Concept Mapping

Documentation of the Nursing Process

Summary and Key Points

Review Questions

KEY TERMS

case management

case manager

concept mapping

critical pathways of care

Focus Charting®

interdisciplinary

managed care

Nursing Interventions Classification (NIC)

Nursing Outcomes Classification (NOC)

nursing process

PIE charting

problem-oriented recording

OBJECTIVES

After reading this chapter, the student will be able to:

1. Define *nursing process*.
2. Identify six steps of the nursing process, and describe nursing actions associated with each.
3. Describe the benefits of using nursing diagnosis.
4. Discuss the list of nursing diagnoses approved by NANDA International for clinical use and testing.
5. Define and discuss the use of case management and critical pathways of care in the clinical setting.
6. Apply the six steps of the nursing process in caring for a client in the psychiatric setting.
7. Document client care that validates use of the nursing process.

HOMEWORK ASSIGNMENT

Please read the chapter and answer the following questions:

1. Nursing outcomes (sometimes referred to as *goals*) are derived from the nursing diagnosis. Name two essential aspects of an acceptable outcome or goal.
2. Define *managed care.*
3. The American Nurses Association identifies certain interventions that may be performed only by psychiatric nurses in advanced practice. What are they?
4. In Focus Charting®, one item cannot be used as the focus for documentation. What is this item?

For many years, the **nursing process** has provided a systematic framework for the delivery of nursing care. This framework fulfills the requirement for a *scientific methodology* in order for nursing to be considered a profession.

This chapter examines the steps of the nursing process as they are set forth by the American Nurses Association (ANA) in *Nursing: Scope and Standards of Practice* (ANA, 2015). An explanation is provided for the implementation of case management and the critical pathways of care tool used with this methodology. A description of concept mapping is included, and documentation that validates the use of the nursing process is discussed.

The Nursing Process

Definition

The nursing process consists of six steps and uses a problem-solving approach that has come to be accepted as nursing's scientific methodology. It is goal-directed with the objective of quality client care delivery.

The nursing process is dynamic, not static. It is an ongoing process that continues for as long as the nurse and client have interactions directed toward change in the client's physical or behavioral responses. Figure 9–1 presents a schematic of the ongoing nursing process.

Standards of Practice

The ANA, in collaboration with the American Psychiatric Nurses Association (APNA) and the International Society of Psychiatric-Mental Health Nurses

(ISPN) (2014) has delineated a set of standards that psychiatric-mental health nurses are expected to follow as they provide care for their clients. The ANA (2015) describes a standard of practice as an authoritative statement that is defined and promoted by the profession and that provides the foundation for evaluating quality of nursing practice. The nursing process is a critical thinking model that integrates professional standards of practice to assess, diagnose, identify outcomes, plan, implement, and evaluate nursing care.

Following is a discussion of the standards of practice for psychiatric-mental health nurses as set forth by the ANA, APNA, and ISPN (2014). Many of these standards outline the registered nurse's role in each step of the nursing process and apply them to the psychiatric-mental health nurse. Three changes in the current standards of practice reflect issues and trends that have evolved more recently.

 First, patients are now referred to as *health-care consumers*. This term reflects the trend toward patient-centered care and conceptualizing that relationship as a collaborative partnership.

Second, counseling interventions (performed by psychiatric-mental health registered nurses) are now differentiated from psychotherapy (performed by psychiatric-mental health *advanced practice* registered nurses). The third change, in Standard 5G. Therapeutic Relationship and Counseling, adds the phrase "assisting healthcare consumers in their individual recovery journeys." This language supports the recovery model of intervention, a current trend toward focus on a collaborative recovery process rather than health-care provider–prescribed treatment alone. (See Chapter 21, The Recovery Model, for more information.)

> ## CORE CONCEPT
> **Assessment**
> A systematic, dynamic process by which the registered nurse, through interaction with the patient, family, groups, communities, populations, and healthcare providers, collects and analyzes data. Assessment may include the following dimensions: physical, psychological, sociocultural, spiritual, cognitive, functional abilities, developmental, economic, and lifestyle (ANA et al., 2014, p. 87).

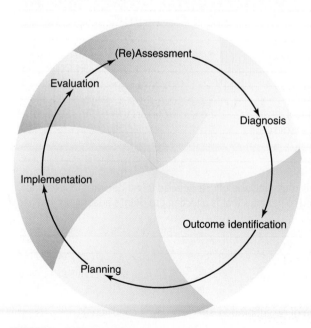

FIGURE 9–1 The ongoing nursing process.

Standard 1. Assessment

The psychiatric-mental health registered nurse collects and synthesizes comprehensive health data that are pertinent to the healthcare consumer's health and/or situation (ANA et al., 2014. p. 44).

In this first step, a database to determine the best possible client care is established. Information for this database is gathered from a variety of sources, including interviews with the client and/or family, observation of the client and his or her environment, consultation with other health team members, review of the client's records, and a nursing physical examination. A biopsychosocial assessment tool based on the stress-adaptation framework is included in Box 9–1.

(Text continued on page 172)

BOX 9–1 **Nursing History and Assessment Tool**

I. General Information
Client name: _____
Room number: _____
Doctor: _____
Age: _____
Sex: _____ Name and phone no. of significant other: _____
Race: _____
Dominant language: _____
Marital status: _____
Chief complaint: _____
_____

Allergies: _____
Diet: _____
Height/weight: _____
Vital signs: TPR/BP _____

City of residence: _____
Diagnosis (admitting & current): _____

Conditions of admission:
Date: _____ Time: _____
Accompanied by: _____
Route of admission (wheelchair; ambulatory; cart): _____
Admitted from: _____

II. Predisposing Factors
A. *Genetic Influences*
1. Family configuration (use genograms):
      Family of origin: Present family:

   Family dynamics (describe significant relationships between family members): _____
   _____
   _____
   _____
   _____

2. Medical/psychiatric history:
   a. Client: _____
   _____
   _____
   _____

   b. Family members: _____
   _____
   _____
   _____

3. Other genetic influences affecting present adaptation. This might include effects specific to gender, race, appearance, such as genetic physical defects, or any other factor related to genetics that is affecting the client's adaptation that has not been mentioned elsewhere in this assessment.
   _____
   _____

B. *Past Experiences*
1. Cultural and social history:
   a. Environmental factors (family living arrangements, type of neighborhood, special working conditions):
   _____
   _____
   _____

BOX 9–1 **Nursing History and Assessment Tool–cont'd**

    b. Health beliefs and practices (personal responsibility for health; special self-care practices):
_____
_____

    c. Religious beliefs and practices: _____
_____

    d. Educational background: _____
_____

    e. Significant losses/changes (include dates): _____
_____
_____

    f. Peer/friendship relationships: _____
_____
_____

    g. Occupational history: _____
_____
_____

    h. Previous pattern of coping with stress: _____
_____
_____

    i. Other lifestyle factors contributing to present adaptation: _____
_____
_____

C. *Existing Conditions*
1. Stage of development (Erikson):
    a. Theoretically: _____
    b. Behaviorally: _____
    c. Rationale: _____
_____
_____

2. Support systems: _____
_____

3. Economic security: _____
_____

4. Avenues of productivity/contribution:
    a. Current job status: _____
_____

    b. Role contributions and responsibility for others: _____
_____

III. Precipitating Event
    Describe the situation or events that precipitated this illness/hospitalization: _____
_____
_____

Continued

BOX 9–1 **Nursing History and Assessment Tool–cont'd**

IV. Client's Perception of the Stressor
   Client's or family member's understanding or description of stressor/illness and expectations of hospitalization:
   _____
   _____
   _____

V. Adaptation Responses
   A. *Psychosocial*
   1. Anxiety level (circle one of the 4 levels and check the behaviors that apply):   Mild   Moderate Severe Panic
      calm _____ friendly _____ passive _____ alert _____ perceives environment correctly _____ cooperative _____
      impaired attention _____ "jittery" _____ unable to concentrate _____ hypervigilant _____ tremors _____ rapid
      speech _____ withdrawn _____ confused _____ disoriented _____ fearful _____ hyperventilating _____ misinterpreting
      the environment (hallucinations or delusions) _____ depersonalization _____ obsessions _____ compulsions _____
      somatic complaints _____ excessive hyperactivity _____ other _____
      _____

   2. Mood/affect (circle as many as apply): happiness   sadness   dejection   despair   elation   euphoria   suspi-
      ciousness   apathy (little emotional tone)   anger/hostility

   3. Ego defense mechanisms (describe how used by client):
      Projection _____
      Suppression _____
      Undoing _____
      Displacement _____
      Intellectualization _____
      Rationalization _____
      Denial _____
      Repression _____
      Isolation _____
      Regression _____
      Reaction Formation _____
      Splitting _____
      Religiosity _____
      Sublimation _____
      Compensation _____

   4. Level of self-esteem (circle one):   low   moderate   high
      Things client likes about self _____
      _____
      Things client would like to change about self _____
      _____
      Objective assessment of self-esteem:
      Eye contact _____
      General appearance _____
      _____
      Personal hygiene _____
      Participation in group activities and interactions with others _____
      _____

   5. Stage and manifestations of grief (circle one):
               Denial   Anger   Bargaining   Depression   Acceptance
      Describe the client's behaviors that are associated with this stage of grieving in response to loss or change.
      _____
      _____
      _____

BOX 9–1 **Nursing History and Assessment Tool–cont'd**

6. Thought processes (circle as many as apply):   clear   logical   easy to follow   relevant   confused   blocking   delusional   rapid flow of thoughts   slowness in thought   suspicious
   Recent memory (circle one):   loss   intact   Remote memory (circle one):   loss   intact
   Other: _____
   _____

7. Communication patterns (circle as many as apply):   clear   coherent   slurred speech   incoherent   neologisms   loose associations   flight of ideas   aphasic   perseveration   rumination   tangential speech   loquaciousness   slow, impoverished speech   speech impediment (describe) _____
   Other _____
   _____

8. Interaction patterns (describe client's pattern of interpersonal interactions with staff and peers on the unit, e.g., manipulative, withdrawn, isolated, verbally or physically hostile, argumentative, passive, assertive, aggressive, passive-aggressive, other): _____
   _____
   _____
   _____

9. Reality orientation (check those that apply):
   Oriented to: Time _____   Person _____
   Place _____   Situation _____

10. Ideas of destruction to self/others?   Yes   No
    If yes, consider plan; available means _____
    _____
    _____
    _____

B. *Physiological*
1. Psychosomatic manifestations (describe any somatic complaints that may be stress-related): _____
   _____
   _____
   _____

2. Drug history and assessment:
   Use of prescribed drugs:

Name	Dosage	Prescribed for	Results

Use of over-the-counter drugs:

Name	Dosage	Used for	Results

Continued

BOX 9–1 **Nursing History and Assessment Tool–cont'd**

Use of street drugs or alcohol:

Name	Amount Used	How Often Used	When Last Used	Effects Produced
_____	_____	_____	_____	_____
_____	_____	_____	_____	_____
_____	_____	_____	_____	_____
_____	_____	_____	_____	_____

3. Pertinent physical assessments:
   a. Respirations: normal _____ labored _____
      Rate _____ Rhythm _____

   b. Skin: warm _____ dry _____ moist _____ cool _____ clammy _____ pink _____
      cyanotic _____ poor turgor _____ edematous _____
      Evidence of: rash _____ bruising _____ needle tracks _____ hirsutism _____
      loss of hair _____ other _____
      _____

   c. Musculoskeletal status: _____ weakness _____ tremors _____
      Degree of range of motion (describe limitations) _____
      _____

      Pain (describe) _____
      _____

      Skeletal deformities (describe) _____
      Coordination (describe limitations) _____

   d. Neurological status:
      History of (check all that apply): seizures _____ (describe method of control) _____
      _____
      headaches (describe location and frequency) _____
      fainting spells _____ dizziness _____
      tingling/numbness (describe location) _____

   e. Cardiovascular: B/P _____ Pulse _____
      History of (check all that apply):
      hypertension _____ palpitations _____
      heart murmur _____ chest pain _____
      shortness of breath _____ pain in legs _____
      phlebitis _____ ankle/leg edema _____
      numbness/tingling in extremities _____
      varicose veins _____

   f. Gastrointestinal:
      Usual diet pattern: _____
      Food allergies: _____
      Dentures? Upper _____ Lower _____
      Any problems with chewing or swallowing? _____
      Any recent change in weight? _____
      Any problems with:
      Indigestion/heartburn? _____
        Relieved by _____
      Nausea/vomiting? _____
        Relieved by _____
      History of ulcers? _____
      Usual bowel pattern _____
        Constipation? _____ Diarrhea? _____
      Type of self-care assistance provided for either of the above problems _____
      _____

BOX 9-1 **Nursing History and Assessment Tool–cont'd**

g. Genitourinary/Reproductive:

Usual voiding pattern _____

Urinary hesitancy? _____ Frequency? _____

Nocturia? _____ Pain/burning? _____

Incontinence? _____

Any genital lesions? _____

  Discharge? _____ Odor? _____

History of sexually transmitted disease? _____

  If yes, please explain: _____

  _____

Any concerns about sexuality/sexual activity? _____

  _____

Method of birth control used _____

Females:

  Date of last menstrual cycle _____

  Length of cycle _____

  Problems associated with menstruation? _____

  _____

Breasts: Pain/tenderness? _____

  Swelling? _____ Discharge? _____

  Lumps? _____ Dimpling? _____

Practice breast self-examination? _____

Frequency? _____

Males:

  Penile discharge? _____

  Prostate problems? _____

h. Eyes:

	Yes	No	Explain
Glasses?			
Contacts?			
Swelling?			
Discharge?			
Itching?			
Blurring?			
Double vision?			

i. Ears

	Yes	No	Explain
Pain?			
Drainage?			
Difficulty hearing?			
Hearing aid?			
Tinnitus?			

j. Medication side effects:

What symptoms is the client experiencing that may be attributed to current medication usage?

_____

_____

k. Altered lab values and possible significance: _____

_____

_____

l. Activity/rest patterns:

Exercise (amount, type, frequency) _____

_____

Leisure time activities: _____

_____

Continued

BOX 9–1 Nursing History and Assessment Tool–cont'd

Patterns of sleep: Number of hours per night _____
Use of sleep aids? _____
Pattern of awakening during the night? _____
_____
Feel rested upon awakening? _____

m. Personal hygiene/activities of daily living:
Patterns of self-care: independent _____
Requires assistance with: mobility _____
         hygiene _____
         toileting _____
         feeding _____
         dressing _____
         other _____
Statement describing personal hygiene and general appearance _____
_____
_____
_____

n. Other pertinent physical assessments: _____
_____
_____

VI. Summary of Initial Psychosocial/Physical Assessment:

Knowledge Deficits Identified:

Nursing Diagnoses Indicated:

An example of a simple and quick mental status evaluation is presented in Table 9–1. Sometimes the term *mental status assessment* is used to describe an assessment of the cognitive aspects of functioning, as is the case with tools such as Folstein's Mini-Mental State Evaluation (Folstein, Folstein, & McHugh, 1975). Likewise, the tool in Table 9–1 focuses strictly on a brief assessment of the cognitive aspects of mental functioning. In psychiatry and psychiatric-mental health nursing, mental status assessment assumes a much broader definition and includes assessment of mood, affect, behavior, relationships, speech, perceptual disturbances, insight, and judgment in addition to cognitive function. A comprehensive mental status assessment guide, with explanations and selected sample interview questions, is provided in Appendix C, Mental Status Assessment.

CORE CONCEPT

Nursing Diagnosis
Clinical judgments about individual, family, or community experiences/responses to actual or potential health problems/life processes. A nursing diagnosis provides the basis for selection of nursing interventions to achieve outcomes for which the nurse has accountability (NANDA International [NANDA-I], 2015a).

Standard 2. Diagnosis

The psychiatric-mental health registered nurse analyzes the assessment data to determine diagnoses, problems, and areas of focus for care and treatment, including level of risk (ANA et al., 2014, p. 46).

TABLE 9–1 **Brief Mental Status Evaluation**	
AREA OF MENTAL FUNCTION EVALUATED	EVALUATION ACTIVITY
Orientation to time	"What year is it?" "What month is it?" "What day is it?" (3 points)
Orientation to place	"Where are you now?" (1 point)
Attention and immediate recall	"Repeat these words now: bell, book, & candle." (3 points) "Remember these words, and I will ask you to repeat them in a few minutes."
Abstract thinking	"What does this mean: No use crying over spilled milk." (3 points)
Recent memory	"Say the 3 words I asked you to remember earlier." (3 points)
Naming objects	Point to eyeglasses and ask, "What is this?" Repeat with 1 other item (e.g., calendar, watch, pencil). (2 points possible)
Ability to follow simple verbal command	"Tear this piece of paper in half and put it in the trash container." (2 points)
Ability to follow simple written command	Write a command on a piece of paper (e.g., TOUCH YOUR NOSE), give the paper to the client, and say, "Do what it says on this paper." (1 point for correct action)
Ability to use language correctly	Ask the patient to write a sentence. (3 points if sentence has a subject, a verb, and valid meaning)
Ability to concentrate	"Say the months of the year in reverse, starting with December." (1 point each for correct answers from November through August; 4 points possible)
Understanding spatial relationships	Instruct client to draw a clock, put in all the numbers, and set the hands on 3 o'clock. (clock circle = 1 pt; numbers in correct sequence = 1 pt; numbers placed on clock correctly = 1 pt; two hands on the clock = 1 pt; hands set at correct time = 1 pt; 5 points possible)

Scoring: 30–21 = normal; 20–11 = mild cognitive impairment; 10–0 = severe cognitive impairment (scores are not absolute and must be considered within the comprehensive diagnostic assessment).
SOURCES: Beers, M.H. (2005). *The Merck manual of health & aging.* New York: Ballentine; Kaufman, D.M., & Zun, L. (1995). A quantifiable, brief mental status examination for emergency patients. *Journal of Emergency Medicine, 13*(4), 440-456; Kokman, E., Smith, G.E., Petersen, R.C., Tangalos, E., & Ivnik, R.C. (1991). The short test of mental status: Correlations with standardized psychometric testing. *Archives of Neurology, 48*(7), 725-728; Folstein, M.F., Folstein, S.E., & McHugh, P.R. (1975). Mini-mental state: A practical method for grading the cognitive state of patients for the clinician. *Journal of Psychiatric Research, 12*(3), 189-198; Pfeiffer, E. (1975). A short portable mental status questionnaire for the assessment of organic brain deficit in elderly patients. *Journal of the American Geriatric Society, 23*(10), 433-441.

In the second step, data gathered during the assessment are analyzed. Diagnoses and potential problem statements are formulated and prioritized. Diagnoses are congruent with available and accepted classification systems (e.g., *NANDA International Nursing Diagnoses: Definitions and Classification* [see Appendix E, Assigning NANDA International Nursing Diagnoses to Client Behaviors]).

CORE CONCEPT

Outcomes

Client behaviors and responses that are collaboratively agreed upon, measurable, desired results of nursing interventions.

Standard 3. Outcomes Identification

The psychiatric-mental health registered nurse identifies expected outcomes and the healthcare consumer's goals for a plan individualized to the healthcare consumer or to the situation (ANA et al., 2014, p. 48).

Expected outcomes are derived from the diagnosis. They must be measurable and include a time estimate for attainment. They must be realistic for the client's capabilities, and they are most effective when formulated cooperatively by the interdisciplinary team members, the client, and significant others.

Nursing Outcomes Classification

The **Nursing Outcomes Classification (NOC)** is a comprehensive, standardized classification of client outcomes developed to evaluate the effects of nursing interventions (Moorhead et al., 2013). The outcomes have been linked to NANDA International (NANDA-I) diagnoses and to the **Nursing Interventions Classification (NIC).** NANDA-I, NIC, and NOC represent all domains of nursing and can be used together or separately (Moorhead & Dochterman, 2012). Each of the NOC outcomes has a label name, a definition, a list of indicators to evaluate client status in relation to the outcome, and a five-point Likert scale to measure client status (Moorhead et al., 2013).

Standard 4. Planning

The psychiatric-mental health registered nurse develops a plan that prescribes strategies and alternatives to assist the healthcare consumer in attainment of expected outcomes (ANA et al., 2014, p. 50).

The care plan is individualized to the client's mental health problems, condition, or needs and is developed in collaboration with the client, significant others, and interdisciplinary team members if possible. For each diagnosis identified, the most appropriate interventions are selected on the basis of current psychiatric-mental health nursing practice, standards, relevant statutes, and research evidence. Client education and necessary referrals are included. Priorities for delivery of nursing care are determined on the basis of safety needs and the client's risk for harm to self or others. Elements of the plan should be prioritized with input from the client, the family, and others as appropriate (ANA et al., 2014).

Nursing Interventions Classification

NIC is a comprehensive, standardized language describing treatments that nurses perform in all settings and specialties (Bulechek, Butcher, Dochterman, & Wagner, 2013). NIC includes both physiological and psychosocial interventions as well as those for illness treatment, illness prevention, and health promotion. NIC interventions are comprehensive, based on research, and reflect current clinical practice. They were developed inductively on the basis of existing practice.

Each NIC intervention has a definition and a detailed set of activities that describe what a nurse does to implement the intervention. The use of standardized language is thought to enhance continuity of care and facilitate communication among nurses and between nurses and other providers.

Standard 5. Implementation

The psychiatric-mental health registered nurse implements the identified plan (ANA et al., 2014, p. 52).

Interventions selected during the planning stage are executed, taking into consideration the nurse's level of practice, education, and certification. The care plan serves as a blueprint for delivery of safe, ethical, and appropriate interventions. Documentation

of interventions also occurs at this step in the nursing process.

Several specific interventions are included among the standards of psychiatric-mental health clinical nursing practice (ANA et al., 2014):

Standard 5A. Coordination of Care

The psychiatric-mental health registered nurse coordinates care delivery (ANA et al., 2014, p. 54).

Standard 5B. Health Teaching and Health Promotion

The psychiatric-mental health registered nurse employs strategies to promote health and a safe environment (ANA et al., 2014, p. 55).

Standard 5C. Consultation

The psychiatric-mental health advanced practice registered nurse provides consultation to influence the identified plan, enhance the abilities of other clinicians to provide services for healthcare consumers, and effect change (ANA et al., 2014, p. 57).

Standard 5D. Prescriptive Authority and Treatment

The psychiatric-mental health advanced practice registered nurse uses prescriptive authority, procedures, referrals, treatments, and therapies in accordance with state and federal laws and regulations (ANA et al., 2014, p. 58).

Standard 5E. Pharmacological, Biological, and Integrative Therapies

The psychiatric-mental health registered nurse incorporates knowledge of pharmacological, biological, and complementary interventions with applied clinical skills to restore the healthcare consumer's health and prevent further disability (ANA et al., 2014, p. 59).

Standard 5F. Milieu Therapy

The psychiatric-mental health registered nurse provides, structures, and maintains a safe, therapeutic, recovery-oriented environment in collaboration with healthcare consumers, families, and other healthcare clinicians (ANA et al., 2014, p. 60).

Several models have been developed to identify what constitutes a therapeutic environment. These are discussed further in Chapter 12, Milieu Therapy—The Therapeutic Community. Incorporation of the health-care environment and the community of clients, their families, and health-care providers is a unique aspect of treatment for the client with a psychiatric-mental health disorder.

Standard 5G. Therapeutic Relationship and Counseling

The psychiatric-mental health registered nurse (PMH-RN) uses the therapeutic relationship and counseling interventions to assist healthcare consumers in their individual recovery journeys by improving and regaining their previous coping abilities, fostering mental health, and preventing mental disorder and disability (ANA et al., 2014, p. 62).

As mentioned previously, therapeutic relationship and counseling interventions are part of the role of registered nurses practicing in psychiatric-mental health settings. These are basic psychoeducational and problem discussion interventions and are differentiated from psychotherapy that requires advanced practice education and competency.

Standard 5H. Psychotherapy

The psychiatric-mental health advanced practice registered nurse conducts individual, couples, group, and family psychotherapy using evidence-based psychotherapeutic frameworks and the nurse-client therapeutic relationship (ANA et al., 2014, p. 63).

CORE CONCEPT

Evaluation

The process of determining the healthcare consumer's progress toward attainment of expected outcomes, and the effectiveness of the registered nurse's care and interventions (ANA et al., 2014, p. 88).

Standard 6. Evaluation

The psychiatric-mental health registered nurse evaluates progress toward attainment of expected outcomes (ANA et al., 2014, p. 65).

During the evaluation step, the nurse measures the success of the interventions in meeting the outcome criteria. The client's response to treatment is documented, validating use of the nursing process in the delivery of care. The diagnoses, outcomes, and plan of care are reviewed and revised as need is determined by the evaluation.

Why Nursing Diagnosis?

The concept of nursing diagnosis is not new. For centuries, nurses have identified specific client responses for which nursing interventions were used in an effort to improve quality of life. Historically, however, the autonomy of practice to which nurses were entitled by virtue of their licensure was lacking in the provision of nursing care. Nurses assisted physicians as required and performed a group of specific tasks that were considered within their scope of responsibility.

The term *diagnosis* in relation to nursing first began to appear in the literature in the early 1950s. The formalized organization of the concept, however,

was initiated in 1973 with the convening of the First Task Force to Name and Classify Nursing Diagnoses. The Task Force of the National Conference Group on the Classification of Nursing Diagnoses was developed during this conference and charged with the task of identifying and classifying nursing diagnoses.

Also in the 1970s, the ANA began to write standards of practice around the steps of the nursing process, of which nursing diagnosis is an inherent part. This format encompassed both the general and specialty standards outlined by the ANA.

From this progression, a policy statement that includes a definition of nursing was published in 1980. The ANA defined nursing as "the diagnosis and treatment of human responses to actual or potential health problems" (ANA, 2010). This definition has been expanded to describe more appropriately nursing's commitment to society and to the profession. The ANA (2017) defines nursing as follows:

> Nursing is the protection, promotion, and optimization of health and abilities, prevention of illness and injury, alleviation of suffering through the diagnosis and treatment of human response, and advocacy in the care of individuals, families, communities, and populations.

Nursing diagnosis is an inherent component of both the original and expanded definitions.

Decisions regarding professional negligence are made on the basis of the standards of practice defined by the ANA and the individual state nurse practice acts. A number of states have incorporated the steps of the nursing process, including nursing diagnosis, into the scope of nursing practice described in their nurse practice acts. When this is the case, it is the legal duty of the nurse to show that nursing process and nursing diagnosis were accurately implemented in the delivery of nursing care.

NANDA-I evolved from the original 1973 task force to name and classify nursing diagnoses. The major purpose of NANDA-I is to "to develop, refine and promote terminology that accurately reflects nurses' clinical judgments. NANDA-I will be a global force for the development and use of nursing's standardized terminology to ensure patient safety through evidence-based care, thereby improving the health care of all people" (NANDA-I, 2015b). The list of NANDA-I-approved diagnoses is by no means all-inclusive. In an effort to maintain a common language within nursing and encourage clinical testing, most of the nursing diagnoses used in this text are taken from the 2015–2017 list approved by NANDA-I. However, in a few instances, nursing diagnoses that have been retired by NANDA-I for various reasons will continue to be used because of their appropriateness and suitability in describing specific behaviors.

The use of nursing diagnosis affords a degree of autonomy that historically has been lacking in the practice of nursing. Nursing diagnosis describes the client's condition, facilitating the prescription of interventions and establishment of parameters for outcome criteria based on unique components of the nursing profession. The ultimate benefit is to the client, who receives effective and consistent nursing care based on knowledge of the problems that he or she is experiencing and of the most beneficial nursing interventions to resolve them.

Nursing Case Management

The concept of **case management** evolved with the advent of diagnosis-related groups (DRGs) and shorter hospital stays. Case management is a model of care delivery that can result in improved client care. In this model, clients are assigned a manager who negotiates with multiple providers to obtain diverse services. This type of health-care delivery process serves to decrease fragmentation of care while striving to contain cost of services.

Case management in the acute care setting aims to organize client care through an episode of illness so that specific clinical and financial outcomes are achieved within an allotted time frame. Commonly, the allotted time frame is determined by the established protocols for length of stay as defined by the DRGs.

Case management has been shown to be an effective method of treatment for individuals with a severe and persistent mental illness. This type of care strives to improve functioning by assisting the individual to solve problems, improve work and socialization skills, promote leisure-time activities, and enhance overall independence.

Ideally, case management incorporates concepts of care at the primary, secondary, and tertiary levels of prevention. Various definitions have emerged and should be clarified, as follows.

Managed care refers to a strategy employed by purchasers of health services who make determinations about various services in order to maintain quality and control costs. In a managed care program, individuals receive health care based on need as assessed by coordinators of the providership. Managed care exists in many settings, including (but not limited to):

■ Insurance-based programs
■ Employer-based medical providerships
■ Social service programs
■ The public health sector

Managed care may exist in virtually any setting in which a private or government-based organization is responsible for payment of health-care services for a group of people. Examples of managed care are health maintenance organizations (HMOs) and preferred provider organizations (PPOs).

Case management, the method used to achieve managed care, is the actual coordination of services required to meet the needs of a client within the fragmented health-care system. Case management strives to help at-risk clients prevent avoidable episodes of illness while controlling health-care costs for the consumer and third-party payers.

Types of clients who benefit from case management include (but are not limited to):

■ The frail elderly
■ Individuals with developmental disabilities
■ Individuals with physical disabilities
■ Individuals with mental disabilities
■ Individuals with long-term, medically complex problems that require multifaceted, costly care (e.g., high-risk infants, those who are HIV positive or who have AIDS, and transplant clients)
■ Individuals who are severely compromised by an acute episode of illness or an acute exacerbation of a severe and persistent illness (e.g., schizophrenia)

The **case manager** is responsible for negotiating with multiple health-care providers to obtain a variety of services for the client. Nurses are exceptionally qualified to serve as case managers. The very nature of nursing, which incorporates knowledge about the biological, psychological, and sociocultural aspects related to human functioning, makes nurses highly appropriate for this role. Several years of experience as a registered nurse is usually required for employment as a case manager. Some case management programs prefer advanced practice registered nurses who have experience working with the specific populations for whom the service will be rendered. The American Nurses Credentialing Center (ANCC) offers an examination for nurses to become board certified in nursing case management.

Critical Pathways of Care

Critical pathways of care (CPCs) may be used as the tools for provision of care in a case management system. A critical pathway is an abbreviated care plan that provides outcome-based guidelines for goal achievement within a designated length of stay. A sample CPC is presented in Table 9–2. Only one nursing diagnosis is used in this sample, but a comprehensive CPC may have nursing diagnoses for several individual problems and incorporates responsibilities of other team members as well.

CPCs are intended to be used by the entire interdisciplinary team, which may include a nurse case

TABLE 9–2 Sample Critical Pathway of Care for Client in Alcohol Withdrawal

Estimated Length of Stay: 7 Days—Variations From Designated Pathway Should Be Documented in Progress Notes

NURSING DIAGNOSES AND CATEGORIES OF CARE	TIME DIMENSION	GOALS AND/OR ACTIONS	TIME DIMENSION	GOALS AND/OR ACTIONS	TIME DIMENSION	DISCHARGE OUTCOME
Risk for injury related to CNS agitation					Day 7	Client shows no evidence of injury obtained during ETOH withdrawal
Referrals	Day 1	Psychiatrist Assess need for: Neurologist Cardiologist Internist			Day 7	Discharge with follow-up appointments as required
Diagnostic studies	Day 1	Blood alcohol level Drug screen (urine and blood) Chemistry profile Urinalysis Chest x-ray ECG	Day 4	Repeat of selected diagnostic studies as necessary		
Additional assessments	Day 1 Day 1–5 Ongoing Ongoing	VS q4h I&O Restraints prn for client safety Assess withdrawal symptoms: tremors, nausea/vomiting, tachycardia, sweating, high blood pressure, seizures, insomnia, hallucinations	Day 2–3 Day 6 Day 4	VS q8h if stable DC I&O Marked decrease in objective withdrawal symptoms	Day 4–7 Day 7	VS bid; remain stable Discharge; absence of objective withdrawal symptoms
Medications	Day 1 Day 2 Day 1–6 Day 1–7	*Librium 200 mg in divided doses Librium 160 mg in divided doses Librium prn Maalox pc & hs *Note: Some physicians may elect to use Serax or Tegretol in the detoxification process	Day 3 Day 4	Librium 120 mg in divided doses Librium 80 mg in divided doses	Day 5 Day 6 Day 7	Librium 40 mg Discontinue Librium Discharge; no withdrawal symptoms
Client education			Day 5	Discuss goals of AA and need for outpatient therapy	Day 7	Discharge with information regarding AA attendance or outpatient treatment

AA, Alcoholics Anonymous; bid, twice a day; DC, discontinue; ECG, electrocardiogram; ETOH, alcohol; hs, bedtime; I&O, intake and output; pc, after meals; prn, as needed; q4h, every 4 hours; q8h, every 8 hours; VS, vital signs.

manager, clinical nurse specialist, social worker, psychiatrist, psychologist, dietitian, occupational therapist, recreational therapist, chaplain, and others. The team decides what categories of care are to be performed, by what date, and by whom. Each member of the team is then expected to carry out his or her functions according to the time line designated on the CPC.

> Unlike a nursing care plan, CPCs have the benefit of describing what an episode of care will look like when implemented by team members in collaboration with one another. Clarity about how team members collaborate is important not only for providing efficient patient care but also for improving quality and safety.

As case manager, the nurse is ultimately responsible for ensuring that each assignment is carried out. If variations occur in any of the categories of care, rationale must be documented in the progress notes. For example, with the sample CPC presented in Table 9–2, the nurse case manager may admit the client into the detoxification center. The nurse contacts the psychiatrist to inform him or her of the admission. The psychiatrist performs additional assessments to determine if other consultations are required and writes the orders for the initial diagnostic work-up and medication regimen. Within 24 hours, the interdisciplinary team meets to decide on other categories of care, complete the CPC, and make individual care assignments from the CPC. This particular sample CPC relies heavily on nursing care of the client through the critical withdrawal period. However, other problems for the same client, such as imbalanced nutrition, impaired physical mobility, or spiritual distress, may involve other members of the team to a greater degree. Each member of the team stays in contact with the nurse case manager regarding individual assignments. Ideally, team meetings are held daily or every other day to review progress and modify the plan as required.

CPCs can be standardized, as they are intended to be used with uncomplicated cases. A CPC can be viewed as protocol for clients who have specific problems for which a designated outcome can be predicted.

Applying the Nursing Process in the Psychiatric Setting

Based on the definition of *mental health* set forth in Chapter 2, Mental Health and Mental Illness: Historical and Theoretical Concepts, the nurse's role in psychiatry is to help the client successfully adapt to stressors in the environment. Goals are directed toward changes in thoughts, feelings, and behaviors that are age appropriate and congruent with local and cultural norms.

Therapy in the psychiatric setting is very often team oriented, or **interdisciplinary.** Therefore, it is important to delineate nursing's involvement in the treatment regimen. Nurses are valuable members of the team. Having progressed beyond the role of custodial caregiver in the psychiatric setting, they provide defined services within the scope of nursing practice. Nursing diagnosis is helping to define these nursing boundaries, providing the degree of autonomy and professionalism that has for so long been unrealized.

For example, a newly admitted client with the medical diagnosis of schizophrenia may be demonstrating the following behaviors:

- Inability to trust others
- Hearing voices
- Refusal to interact with staff and peers
- Fear of failure
- Poor personal hygiene

From these assessments, the treatment team may determine that the client has the following problems:

- Paranoid delusions
- Auditory hallucinations
- Social withdrawal
- Developmental regression

Team goals would be directed toward the following:

- Reducing suspiciousness
- Terminating auditory hallucinations
- Increasing feelings of self-worth

From this team treatment plan, nursing may identify the following nursing diagnoses:

- Disturbed sensory perception, auditory (evidenced by hearing voices)*
- Disturbed thought processes (evidenced by delusions)*
- Low self-esteem (evidenced by fear of failure and social withdrawal)
- Self-care deficit (evidenced by poor personal hygiene)

Nursing diagnoses are prioritized according to life-threatening potential. Maslow's hierarchy of needs is an appropriate model to follow when prioritizing nursing diagnoses. In this instance, Disturbed sensory perception (auditory) is identified as the priority nursing diagnosis because the client may be hearing voices that command him or her to harm self or others. Psychiatric nursing, regardless of the setting—hospital (inpatient or outpatient), office, home, community—is

---

*Disturbed sensory perception and Disturbed thought processes have been removed from the NANDA-I list of approved nursing diagnoses (NANDA-I, 2012). However, they will continue to be used in this textbook because of their appropriateness to certain behaviors.

goal-directed care. The goals (or expected outcomes) are client-oriented, measurable, and focused on problem resolution (if this is realistic) or on a more short-term outcome (if resolution is unrealistic). For example, in the previous situation, expected outcomes for the identified nursing diagnoses might be as follows:

The client:

- Demonstrates trust in one staff member within 3 days
- Verbalizes understanding that the voices are not real (not heard by others) within 5 days
- Completes one simple craft project within 5 days
- Takes responsibility for own self-care and performs activities of daily living independently by time of discharge

Nursing's contribution to the interdisciplinary treatment regimen will focus on establishing trust on a one-to-one basis (thus reducing the level of anxiety that may be promoting hallucinations), giving positive feedback for small day-to-day accomplishments in an effort to build self-esteem, and assisting with and encouraging independent self-care. These interventions describe *independent nursing* actions and goals that are evaluated apart from, while also being directed toward achievement of, the *team's* treatment goals.

In this manner of collaboration with other team members, nursing provides a unique service based on sound knowledge of psychopathology, scope of practice, and legal implications of the role. Although there is no question that implementing physician's orders is an important aspect of nursing care, nursing interventions that enhance achievement of the overall goals of treatment are important contributions as well. The nurse who administers a medication prescribed by the physician to decrease anxiety may also choose to stay with the anxious client and offer reassurance of safety and security, thereby providing an independent nursing action that is distinct from, yet complementary to, the medical treatment.

Concept Mapping*

Concept mapping is a diagrammatic teaching and learning strategy that allows students and faculty to visualize interrelationships between medical diagnoses, nursing diagnoses, assessment data, and treatments. Basically, it is a diagram of client problems and interventions. Compared to the commonly used column format care plans, concept map care plans are more succinct. They primarily serve to enhance critical-thinking skills and clinical reasoning ability by creating a holistic picture of various client problems and their interconnectedness to one another.

The nursing process is foundational to developing and using the concept map care plan, just as with all types of nursing care plans. Client data are collected and analyzed, nursing diagnoses are formulated, outcome criteria are identified, nursing actions are planned and implemented, and the success of the interventions in meeting the outcome criteria is evaluated.

The concept map care plan may be presented in its entirety on one page, or the assessment data and nursing diagnoses may appear in diagram format on one page, with outcomes, interventions, and evaluation written on a second page. Alternatively, the diagram may appear in circular format, with nursing diagnoses and interventions branching off the "client" in the center of the diagram. Or, it may begin with the "client" at the top of the diagram, with branches emanating in a linear fashion downward.

Whatever format is chosen to visualize the concept map, the diagram should reflect the nursing process in a stepwise fashion, beginning with the client and his or her reason for needing care, nursing diagnoses with subjective and objective clinical evidence for each, nursing interventions, and outcome criteria for evaluation.

Figure 9–2 presents one example of a concept map care plan. It is assembled for the hypothetical client with schizophrenia discussed in the previous section, "Applying the Nursing Process in the Psychiatric Setting." Different colors may be used in the diagram to designate various components of the care plan. Connecting lines are drawn between components to indicate any relationships that exist. For example, there may be a relationship between two nursing diagnoses (e.g., between the nursing diagnoses of Pain or Anxiety and Disturbed sleep pattern). A line between these nursing diagnoses should be drawn to show the relationship.

Concept map care plans permit viewing the "whole picture" without generating a great deal of paperwork. Because they reflect the steps of the nursing process, concept map care plans also are valuable guides for documentation of client care. Doenges, Moorhouse, and Murr (2016) note that traditional care plans fail to clarify how all the client's identified needs are related, so the user may not develop a holistic view. The concept map clarifies those linkages. Whether these care-planning strategies are used for learning or in actual practice, both the concept map and traditional care plan are useful tools for developing and visualizing the critical-thinking process that goes into planning client care.

Documentation of the Nursing Process

*Content in this section is adapted from Doenges, Moorhouse, & Murr (2016) and Schuster (2015).

Equally as important as using the nursing process in the delivery of care is documenting its use in writing.

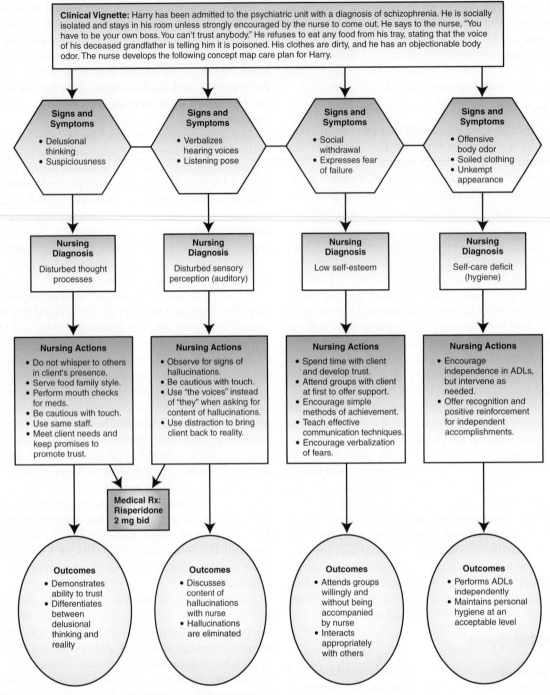

FIGURE 9–2 Example of a concept map care plan for a client with schizophrenia.

Some contemporary nursing leaders advocate that with solid standards of practice and procedures in place within the institution, nurses need only chart when there has been a deviation in the care as outlined by that standard. This method of documentation, known as *charting by exception*, is not widely accepted, as many legal decisions are still based on the precept that "if it was not charted, it was not done."

Because nursing process and diagnosis are mandated by nurse practice acts in some states, documentation of their use is considered evidence in those states when determining certain cases of negligence by nurses. Some health-care organization accrediting agencies also require that nursing process be reflected in the delivery of care.

A variety of documentation methods can be used to reflect use of the nursing process in the delivery of nursing care. Three examples are presented here: problem-oriented recording (POR); Focus Charting®; and the problem, intervention, evaluation (PIE) system of documentation.

Problem-Oriented Recording

Problem-oriented recording, based on a list of problems, follows the subjective, objective, assessment, plan, implementation, and evaluation (SOAPIE) format. When used in nursing, the problems (nursing diagnoses) are identified on a written plan of care, with appropriate nursing interventions described for each. Documentation written in the SOAPIE format includes the following:

S = Subjective data: Information gathered from what the client, family, or other source has said or reported

O = Objective data: Information gathered through direct observation by the person performing the assessment; may include a physiological measurement such as blood pressure or a behavioral response such as affect

A = Assessment: The nurse's interpretation of the subjective and objective data

P = Plan: The actions or treatments to be carried out (may be omitted in daily charting if the plan is clearly explained in the written nursing care plan and no changes are expected)

I = Intervention: Those nursing actions that were actually carried out

E = Evaluation: Evaluation of the problem following nursing intervention (some nursing interventions cannot be evaluated immediately, so this section may be optional)

Table 9–3 shows how POR corresponds to the steps of the nursing process. Following is an example of a three-column documentation in the POR format.

EXAMPLE

DATE/TIME	PROBLEM	PROGRESS NOTES
9-12-17 1000	Social isolation	**S:** States he does not want to sit with or talk to others; "they frighten me." **O:** Stays in room alone unless strongly encouraged to come out; no group involvement; at times listens to group conversations from a distance but does not interact; some hypervigilance and scanning noted **A:** Inability to trust; panic level of anxiety; delusional thinking **I:** Initiated trusting relationship by spending time alone with the client; discussed his feelings regarding interactions with others; accompanied client to group activities; provided positive feedback for voluntarily participating in assertiveness training

TABLE 9–3 Validation of the Nursing Process With Problem-Oriented Recording

PROBLEM-ORIENTED RECORDING	WHAT IS RECORDED	NURSING PROCESS
S and O (Subjective and Objective data)	Verbal reports to, and direct observation and examination by, the nurse	Assessment
A (Assessment)	Nurse's interpretation of S and O	Diagnosis and outcome identification
P (Plan) (Omitted in charting if written plan describes care to be given)	Description of appropriate nursing actions to resolve the identified problem	Planning
I (Intervention)	Description of nursing actions actually carried out	Implementation
E (Evaluation)	A reassessment of the situation to determine results of nursing actions implemented	Evaluation

Focus Charting

Another type of documentation that reflects use of the nursing process is **Focus Charting®**. Focus Charting differs from POR in that the main perspective has been changed from "problem" to "focus," and a data, action, and response (DAR) format has replaced SOAPIE.

Lampe (1985) suggested that a focus for documentation can be any of the following:

■ Nursing diagnosis
■ Current client concern or behavior
■ Significant change in the client status or behavior
■ Significant event in the client's therapy

The focus cannot be a medical diagnosis. The documentation is organized in the format of DAR. These categories are defined as follows:

D = Data: Information that supports the stated focus or describes pertinent observations about the client

A = Action: Immediate or future nursing actions that address the focus, and evaluation of the present care plan along with any changes required

R = Response: Description of client's responses to any part of the medical or nursing care

Table 9–4 shows how Focus Charting corresponds to the steps of the nursing process. Following is an example of a three-column documentation in the DAR format.

EXAMPLE

DATE/TIME	FOCUS	PROGRESS NOTES
9-12-17 1000	Social isolation related to mistrust, panic anxiety, delusions	**D:** States he does not want to sit with or talk to others; they "frighten" him; stays in room alone unless strongly encouraged to come out; no group involvement; at times listens to group conversations from a distance, but does not interact; some hypervigilance and scanning noted
		A: Initiated trusting relationship by spending time alone with client; discussed his feelings regarding interactions with others; accompanied client to group activities; provided positive feedback for voluntarily participating in assertiveness training
		R: Cooperative with therapy; still acts uncomfortable in the presence of a group of people; accepted positive feedback from nurse

TABLE 9–4 Validation of the Nursing Process With Focus Charting

FOCUS CHARTING	WHAT IS RECORDED	NURSING PROCESS
D (Data)	Information that supports the stated focus or describes pertinent observations about the client	Assessment
Focus	A nursing diagnosis; current client concern or behavior; significant change in client status; significant event in the client's therapy (*Note:* If outcome appears on written care plan, it need not be repeated in daily documentation unless a change occurs.)	Diagnosis and outcome identification
A (Action)	Immediate or future nursing actions that address the focus; appraisal of the care plan along with any changes required	Plan and implementation
R (Response)	Description of client responses to any part of the medical or nursing care	Evaluation

The PIE Method

The PIE method, or more specifically, "APIE" (assessment, problem, intervention, evaluation), is a systematic approach of documenting to nursing process and nursing diagnosis. A problem-oriented system, **PIE charting** uses accompanying flow sheets that are individualized by each institution. Criteria for documentation are organized in the following manner:

A = Assessment: A complete client assessment is conducted at the beginning of each shift. Results are documented under this section in the progress notes. Some institutions elect instead to use a daily client assessment sheet designed to meet specific needs of the unit. Explanation of any deviation from the norm is included in the progress notes.

P = Problem: A problem list, or list of nursing diagnoses, is an important part of the APIE method of charting. The name or number of the problem being addressed is documented in this section.

I = Intervention: Nursing actions are performed, directed at resolution of the problem.

E = Evaluation: Outcomes of the implemented interventions are documented, including an evaluation of client responses to determine the effectiveness of nursing interventions and the presence or absence of progress toward resolution of a problem.

Table 9–5 shows how APIE charting corresponds to the steps of the nursing process. Following is an example of a three-column documentation in the APIE format.

EXAMPLE

DATE/TIME	PROBLEM	PROGRESS NOTES
9-12-17 1000	Social isolation	A: States he does not want to sit with or talk to others; they "frighten" him; stays in room alone unless strongly encouraged to come out; no group involvement; at times listens to group conversations from a distance but does not interact; some hypervigilance and scanning noted P: Social isolation related to inability to trust, panic level of anxiety, and delusional thinking I: Initiated trusting relationship by spending time alone with client; discussed his feelings regarding interactions with others; accompanied client to group activities; provided positive feedback for voluntarily participating in assertiveness training E: Cooperative with therapy; still uncomfortable in the presence of a group of people; accepted positive feedback from nurse

TABLE 9–5 Validation of the Nursing Process With APIE Method

APIE CHARTING	WHAT IS RECORDED	NURSING PROCESS
A (Assessment)	Subjective and objective data about the client that are gathered at the beginning of each shift	Assessment
P (Problem)	Name (or number) of nursing diagnosis being addressed from written problem list, and identified outcome for that problem (*Note:* If outcome appears on written care plan, it need not be repeated in daily documentation unless a change occurs.)	Diagnosis and outcome identification
I (Intervention)	Nursing actions performed, directed at problem resolution	Plan and implementation
E (Evaluation)	Appraisal of client responses to determine effectiveness of nursing interventions	Evaluation

Electronic Documentation

Most health-care facilities have implemented an electronic health record (EHR) or electronic documentation system. Federal regulations and programs have incentivized the move to EHR systems by requiring health-care organizations to use them in order to receive Medicare and Medicaid reimbursement; as of 2015, progressive reductions in reimbursement have been initiated for health-care providers who are not demonstrating meaningful use of EHRs.

◆ The rationale for this move is that EHR systems have been shown to improve both the quality of client care and the efficiency of the health-care system (U.S. Government Accountability Office, 2010). In 2003, the U.S. Department of Health and Human Services commissioned the Institute of Medicine (IOM) to study the capabilities of an EHR system. The IOM

identified a set of eight core functions that EHR systems should perform in the delivery of safer, higher-quality, and more efficient health care (Institute of Medicine, 2003):

1. **Health information and data:** EHRs would provide more rapid access to important patient information (e.g., allergies, laboratory test results, a medication list, demographic information, and clinical narratives), thereby improving care providers' abilities to make sound clinical decisions in a timely manner.

2. **Results management:** Computerized results of all types (e.g., laboratory test results, radiology procedure result reports) can be accessed more easily by the provider at the time and place they are needed.

3. **Order entry and order management:** Computer-based order entries improve workflow processes by

eliminating lost orders and ambiguities caused by illegible handwriting, generating related orders automatically, monitoring for duplicate orders, and improving the speed with which orders are executed.

4. **Decision support:** Computerized decision support systems enhance clinical performance for many aspects of health care. Using reminders and prompts, improvement in regular screenings and other preventive practices can be accomplished. Other aspects of health-care support include identifying possible drug interactions and facilitating diagnosis and treatment.

5. **Electronic communication and connectivity:** Improved communication among care associates, such as medicine, nursing, laboratory, pharmacy, and radiology team members, can enhance client safety and quality of care. Efficient communication among providers improves continuity of care, allows for more timely interventions, and reduces the risk of adverse events.

6. **Patient support:** Computer-based interactive client education, self-testing, and self-monitoring have been shown to improve control of chronic illnesses.

7. **Administrative processes:** Electronic scheduling systems (e.g., for hospital admissions and outpatient procedures) increase the efficiency of health-care organizations and provide more timely service to patients.

8. **Reporting and population health management:** Health-care organizations are required to report health-care data to government and private sectors for patient safety and public health. Uniform electronic data standards facilitate this process at the provider level, reduce the associated costs, and increase the speed and accuracy of the data reported.

Table 9–6 lists some of the advantages and disadvantages of paper records and EHRs.

TABLE 9–6 **Advantages and Disadvantages of Paper Records and EHR Systems**	
PAPER*	**EHR SYSTEM**
ADVANTAGES ■ People know how to use it. ■ It is fast for current practice. ■ It is portable. ■ It is nonbreakable. ■ It accepts multiple data types, such as graphs, photographs, drawings, and text. ■ Legal issues and costs are understood. **DISADVANTAGES** ■ It can be lost. ■ It is often illegible and incomplete. ■ It has no remote access. ■ It can be accessed by only one person at a time. ■ It is often disorganized. ■ Information is duplicated. ■ It is hard to store. ■ It is difficult to research, and continuous quality improvement is laborious. ■ Same client has separate records at each facility (physician's office, hospital, home care). ■ Records are shared only through hard copy.	**ADVANTAGES** ■ Can be accessed by multiple providers from remote sites. ■ Facilitates communication between disciplines. ■ Provides reminders about completing information. ■ Provides warnings about incompatibilities of medications or variances from normal standards. ■ Reduces redundancy of information. ■ Requires less storage space and is more difficult to lose. ■ Easier to research for audits, quality assurance, and epidemiological surveillance. ■ Provides immediate retrieval of information (e.g., test results). ■ Provides links to multiple databases of health-care knowledge, thus providing diagnostic support. ■ Decreases charting time. ■ Reduces errors due to illegible handwriting. ■ Facilitates billing and claims procedures. **DISADVANTAGES** ■ Excessive expense to initiate the system. ■ Substantial learning curve involved for new users; training and retraining required. ■ Stringent requirements to maintain security and confidentiality. ■ Technical difficulties are possible. ■ Legal and ethical issues involving privacy and access to client information. ■ Requires consistent use of standardized terminology to support information sharing across wide networks.

*From Young, K.M., & Catalano, J. T. (2015). Nursing informatics. In J.T. Catalano (Ed.), *Nursing now! Today's issues, tomorrow's trends* (7th ed.). Philadelphia: F.A. Davis. With permission.

Summary and Key Points

- The nursing process provides a methodology by which nurses may deliver care using a systematic, scientific approach.
- The focus of the nursing process is goal directed and based on a decision-making or problem-solving model consisting of six steps: assessment, diagnosis, outcome identification, planning, implementation, and evaluation.
- Assessment is a systematic, dynamic process by which the nurse, through interaction with the client, significant others, and health-care providers, collects and analyzes data about the client.
- Nursing diagnoses are clinical judgments about individual, family, or community responses to actual or potential health problems and life processes.
- Outcomes are measurable, expected, patient-focused goals that translate into observable behaviors.
- Evaluation is the process of determining both the client's progress toward the attainment of expected outcomes and the effectiveness of nursing care.
- The psychiatric nurse uses the nursing process to assist clients to adapt successfully to stressors within the environment.
- The nurse serves as a valuable member of the interdisciplinary treatment team, working both independently and cooperatively with other team members.

- Case management is an innovative model of care delivery that serves to provide quality client care while controlling health-care costs. Critical pathways of care serve as the tools for provision of care in a case management system.
- Nurses may serve as case managers, who are responsible for negotiating with multiple health-care providers to obtain a variety of services for the client.
- Concept mapping is a diagrammatic teaching and learning strategy that allows students and faculty to visualize interrelationships between medical diagnoses, nursing diagnoses, assessment data, and treatments. The concept map care plan is an innovative approach to planning and organizing nursing care.
- Nurses must document that the nursing process has been used in the delivery of care. Three methods of documentation that reflect use of the nursing process are POR, Focus Charting, and the PIE method.
- Many health-care facilities have implemented the use of EHRs or electronic documentation systems. EHRs have been shown to improve both the quality of client care and the efficiency of the healthcare system.

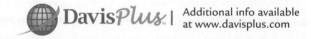

DavisPlus | Additional info available at www.davisplus.com

Review Questions
Self-Examination/Learning Exercise

Select the answer that is most appropriate for each of the following questions.

1. The nurse is using nursing process to care for a client who is suicidal. Which of the following nursing actions is a part of the assessment step of the nursing process?
   a. Identifies nursing diagnosis: Risk for suicide
   b. Notes that client's family reports recent suicide attempt
   c. Prioritizes the necessity of maintaining a safe client environment
   d. Obtains a short-term contract from the client to seek out staff if feeling suicidal

2. The nurse is using nursing process to care for a client who is suicidal. Which of the following nursing actions is a part of the diagnosis step of the nursing process?
   a. Identifies nursing diagnosis: Risk for suicide
   b. Notes that client's family reports recent suicide attempt
   c. Prioritizes the necessity for maintaining a safe environment for the client
   d. Obtains a short-term contract from the client to seek out staff if feeling suicidal

Continued

Review Questions—cont'd
Self-Examination/Learning Exercise

3. The nurse is using nursing process to care for a client who is suicidal. Which of the following nursing actions is a part of the outcome identification step of the nursing process?
   a. Prioritizes the necessity for maintaining a safe environment for the client
   b. Determines if nursing interventions have been appropriate to achieve desired results
   c. Obtains a short-term contract from the client to seek out staff if feeling suicidal
   d. Establishes goal of care: Client will not harm self during hospitalization

4. The nurse is using nursing process to care for a client who is suicidal. Which of the following nursing actions is a part of the planning step of the nursing process?
   a. Prioritizes the necessity for maintaining a safe environment for the client
   b. Determines if nursing interventions have been appropriate to achieve desired results
   c. Obtains a short-term contract from the client to seek out staff if feeling suicidal
   d. Establishes goal of care: Client will not harm self during hospitalization

5. The nurse is using nursing process to care for a client who is suicidal. Which of the following nursing actions is a part of the implementation step of the nursing process?
   a. Prioritizes the necessity for maintaining a safe environment for the client
   b. Determines if nursing interventions have been appropriate to achieve desired results
   c. Collaborates with the client to develop a plan for ongoing safety and suicide prevention
   d. Establishes goal of care: Client will not harm self during hospitalization

6. The nurse is using nursing process to care for a client who is suicidal. Which of the following nursing actions is a part of the evaluation step of the nursing process?
   a. Prioritizes the necessity for maintaining a safe environment for the client
   b. Determines if nursing interventions have been appropriate to achieve desired results
   c. Obtains a short-term contract from the client to seek out staff if feeling suicidal
   d. Establishes goal of care: Client will not harm self during hospitalization

7. S.T. is a 15-year-old girl who has just been admitted to the adolescent psychiatric unit with a diagnosis of anorexia nervosa. She is 5 feet 5 inches tall and weighs 82 pounds. She was selected to join the cheer-leading squad for the fall but states that she is not as good as the others on the squad. The treatment team has identified the following problems: refusal to eat, occasional purging, refusing to interact with staff and peers, and fear of failure. Which of the following nursing diagnoses would be appropriate for S.T.? (Select all that apply.)
   a. Social isolation
   b. Disturbed body image
   c. Low self-esteem
   d. Imbalanced nutrition: Less than body requirements

8. S.T. is a 15-year-old girl who has just been admitted to the adolescent psychiatric unit with a diagnosis of anorexia nervosa. She is 5 feet 5 inches tall and weighs 82 pounds. She was selected to join the cheer-leading squad for the fall but states that she is not as good as the others on the squad. The treatment team has identified the following problems: refusal to eat, occasional purging, refusing to interact with staff and peers, and fear of failure. Which of the following nursing diagnoses would be the priority diagnosis for S.T.?
   a. Social isolation
   b. Disturbed body image
   c. Low self-esteem
   d. Imbalanced nutrition: Less than body requirements

9. Nursing diagnoses are prioritized according to which of the following?
   a. Degree of potential for resolution
   b. Legal implications associated with nursing intervention
   c. Life-threatening potential
   d. Client and family requests

Review Questions—cont'd
Self-Examination/Learning Exercise

10. Which of the following describe advantages of electronic health records (EHRs)? (Select all that apply.)
    a. They reduce redundancy of information.
    b. They reduce privacy issues.
    c. They decrease charting time.
    d. They facilitate communication between disciplines.

References

American Nurses Association (2017). *What is nursing?* Retrieved from http://www.nursingworld.org/EspeciallyForYou/What-is-Nursing

American Nurses Association (ANA). (2015). *Nursing: Scope and standards of practice* (3rd ed.). Silver Spring, MD: ANA.

American Nurses Association (ANA). (2010). *Nursing's social policy statement: The essence of the profession* (3rd ed.). Silver Spring, MD: ANA.

American Nurses Association (ANA), American Psychiatric Nurses Association (APNA), & International Society of Psychiatric-Mental Health Nurses (ISPN). (2014). *Psychiatric-mental health nursing: Scope and standards of practice* (2nd ed.). Silver Spring, MD: ANA.

Beers, M.H. (2005). *Merck manual of health & aging.* New York: Ballentine.

Doenges, M.E., Moorhouse, M.F., & Murr, A.C. (2016). *Nursing diagnosis manual: Planning, individualizing, and documenting client care* (5th ed.). Philadelphia: F.A. Davis.

Institute of Medicine. 2003. *Key capabilities of an electronic health record system: Letter report.* Washington, DC: The National Academies Press. doi:https://doi.org/10.17226/10781.

Kaufman, D.M., & Zun, L. (1995). A quantifiable, brief mental status examination for emergency patients. *Journal of Emergency Medicine, 13*(4), 440-456. doi:10.1016/0736-4679(95)80000-X

Kokman, E., Smith, G.E., Petersen, R.C., Tangalos, E., & Ivnik, R.C. (1991). The short test of mental status: Correlations with standardized psychometric testing. *Archives of Neurology, 48*(7), 725-728. doi:10.1001/archneur.1991.00530190071018

Lampe, S.S. (1985). Focus charting: Streamlining documentation. *Nursing Management, 16*(7), 43-46.

Moorhead, S., & Dochterman, J.M. (2012). Languages and development of the linkages. In M. Johnson, S. Moorhead, G. Bulechek, M. Butcher, M. Maas, & E. Swanson, *NOC and NIC linkages to NANDA-I and clinical conditions: Supporting critical reasoning and quality care* (3rd ed., pp. 1-10). Maryland Heights, MO: Mosby.

Moorhead, S., Johnson, M., Maas, M., & Swanson, E. (2013). *Nursing Outcomes Classification (NOC)* (5th ed.). St. Louis, MO: Mosby Elsevier.

NANDA International. (2015a). *Nursing diagnoses: Definitions and classification, 2015–2017.* Hoboken, NJ: Wiley-Blackwell.

NANDA International. (2015b). *About NANDA International.* Retrieved from www.nanda.org/AboutUs.aspx

Pfeiffer, E. (1975). A short portable mental status questionnaire for the assessment of organic brain deficit in elderly patients. *Journal of the American Geriatric Society, 23*(10), 433-441. doi:10.1111/j.1532-5415.1975.tb00927.x

Schuster, P.M. (2015). *Concept mapping: A critical-thinking approach to care planning* (4th ed.). Philadelphia: F.A. Davis.

U.S. Government Accountability Office (GAO). (2010). Features of integrated systems support patient care strategies and access to care, but systems face challenges. GAO-11-49. Washington, DC: GAO.

Young, K.M., & Catalano, J. T. (2015). Nursing informatics. In J.T. Catalano (Ed.), *Nursing now! Today's issues, tomorrow's trends* (7th ed., pp. 429-451). Philadelphia: F.A. Davis.

Classical References

Folstein, M.F., Folstein, S.E., & McHugh, P.R. (1975). Mini-mental state: A practical method for grading the cognitive state of patients for the clinician. *Journal of Psychiatric Research, 12*(3), 189-198. doi:http://dx.doi.org/10.1016/0022-3956(75)90026-6

10

Therapeutic Groups

CORE CONCEPTS

Group

Group Therapy

KEY TERMS

altruism	democratic	psychodrama
autocratic	laissez-faire	universality
catharsis		

OBJECTIVES

After reading this chapter, the student will be able to:

1. Define a group.
2. Discuss eight functions of a group.
3. Identify various types of groups.
4. Describe physical conditions that influence groups.
5. Discuss therapeutic factors that occur in groups.
6. Describe the phases of group development.
7. Identify various leadership styles in groups.
8. Identify various roles that members assume within a group.
9. Discuss psychodrama as a specialized form of group therapy.
10. Describe the role of the nurse in group therapy.

HOMEWORK ASSIGNMENT
Please read the chapter and answer the following questions:

1. What is the difference between therapeutic groups and group therapy?
2. What are the expectations of the leader in the initial or orientation phase of group development?
3. How does an autocratic leadership style affect member enthusiasm and morale?
4. How does size of the group influence group dynamics?

Human beings are complex creatures who share their activities of daily living with various *groups* of people. As Forsyth (2010) stated, "The tendency to join with others in groups is perhaps the single most important characteristic of humans and the processes that unfold within these groups leave an indelible imprint on their members and on society" (p. 1).

Health-care professionals share their personal lives with groups of people and encounter multiple group situations in their professional operations. Team conferences, committee meetings, grand rounds, and inservice sessions are but a few instances in which this occurs. In psychiatry, work with clients and families often takes the form of groups. With group work, not only does the nurse have the opportunity to reach out to a greater number of people at one time, but those individuals also assist each other by sharing their feelings, opinions, ideas, and behaviors with the group. Clients learn from each other in a group setting.

This chapter explores various types and methods of therapeutic groups that can be used with psychiatric clients and the role of the nurse in group intervention.

CORE CONCEPT
Group
A *group* is a collection of individuals whose association is founded on commonalities of interest, values, norms, or purpose. Membership in a group is generally by chance (born into the group), by choice (voluntary affiliation), or by circumstance (the result of life-cycle events over which an individual may or may not have control).

Functions of a Group

Sampson and Marthas (1990) outlined the following eight functions that groups serve for their members. They contend that groups may serve more than one function and usually serve different functions for different members of the group.

1. **Socialization:** The cultural group into which individuals are born begins the process of teaching social norms. This process is continued throughout their lives by members of other groups with which they become affiliated.
2. **Support:** One's fellow group members are available in time of need. Individuals derive a feeling of security from group involvement.
3. **Task completion:** Group members provide assistance in endeavors that are beyond the capacity of one individual alone or when results can be achieved more effectively as a team.
4. **Camaraderie:** Members of a group provide the joy and pleasure that individuals seek from interactions with significant others.
5. **Information sharing:** Learning takes place within groups. Knowledge is gained when individual members learn how others in the group have resolved situations similar to those with which they are currently struggling.
6. **Normative influence:** This function relates to the ways in which groups enforce the established norms. As group members interact, they influence each other about expected norms for communication and behavior.

7. **Empowerment:** Groups help to bring about improvement in existing conditions by providing support to individual members who seek to bring about change. Groups have power that individuals alone do not.
8. **Governance:** Groups that provide governance functions oversee and direct activities often within the context of a larger group organization. "For example, groups or committees that oversee strategic planning, ensure compliance with quality standards, or establish rules and policies" within a larger organization.

Types of Groups

The functions of a group vary depending on the reason the group was formed. Clark (2009) identified three types of groups in which nurses most often participate: task, teaching, and supportive/therapeutic groups.

Task Groups

The function of a task group is to accomplish a specific outcome or task. The focus is on solving problems and making decisions to achieve this outcome. Often, a deadline is placed on completion of the task, and such importance is placed on a satisfactory outcome that conflict in the group may be smoothed over or ignored in order to focus on the priority at hand.

Teaching Groups

Teaching, or educational, groups exist to convey knowledge and information to a number of individuals. Nurses can be involved in many types of teaching groups, such as medication education, childbirth education, breast self-examination, and effective parenting classes. These groups usually have a set time frame or specified number of meetings. Members learn from each other as well as from the designated instructor. The objective of teaching groups is verbalization or demonstration by the learner of the material presented by the end of the designated period.

Supportive/Therapeutic Groups

Supportive or therapeutic groups are primarily concerned with preventing future upsets by teaching participants effective ways to deal with emotional stress arising from situational or developmental crises.

CORE CONCEPT
Group Therapy
A form of psychosocial treatment in which a number of clients meet together with a therapist for purposes of sharing, gaining personal insight, and improving interpersonal coping strategies.

For the purposes of this text, it is important to differentiate between *therapeutic groups* and *group therapy.* Leaders of group therapy generally have advanced degrees in psychology, social work, nursing, or medicine. They often have additional training or experience in conducting group psychotherapy based on various theoretical frameworks such as psychoanalytic, psychodynamic, interpersonal, or family dynamics, under the supervision of accomplished professionals. Approaches based on these theories are used by group therapy leaders to encourage improvement in group members' abilities to function on an interpersonal level.

Therapeutic groups, on the other hand, are not designed for psychotherapy. They focus instead on group relations, interactions among group members, and the consideration of selected issues. Like group therapists, individuals who lead therapeutic groups must be knowledgeable in *group process;* that is, the *way* in which group members interact with each other. Interruptions, silences, judgments, glares, and scapegoating are examples of group processes (Clark, 2009). These interactions may occur whether or not there is a designated group leader, but nurses acting as group leaders can guide the ways in which members interact to facilitate accomplishing the group's goals or tasks. This is one reason that group leaders are often referred to as *group facilitators.* They must also have thorough knowledge of *group content,* the topic or issue being discussed by the group, and the ability to present the topic in language that can be understood by all members. Many nurses who work in psychiatry lead supportive/therapeutic groups.

Self-Help Groups

Nurses may also be involved in self-help groups, a type of group that has grown in number and in credibility in recent years. They allow clients to talk about their fears and relieve feelings of isolation while receiving comfort and advice from others undergoing similar experiences. Examples of self-help groups for clients and families dealing with disorders such as Alzheimer's disease or anorexia nervosa, Weight Watchers, Alcoholics Anonymous, Reach to Recovery, Parents Without Partners, Overeaters Anonymous, Adult Children of Alcoholics, and many others related to specific needs or illnesses. These groups may or may not have a professional leader or consultant. They are run by the members, and leadership often rotates from member to member.

Nurses may become involved with self-help groups either voluntarily or because their advice or participation has been requested by the members. The nurse may function as a referral agent, resource person, member of an advisory board, or leader of the group. Self-help groups are a valuable source of referral for clients with specific problems. However, nurses must be knowledgeable about the purposes of the group, membership, leadership, benefits, and problems that might threaten the success of the group before making referrals to their clients for a specific self-help group. The nurse may find it necessary to attend several meetings of a particular group, if possible, to assess its effectiveness of purpose and appropriateness for client referral.

Physical Conditions That Influence Group Dynamics

Seating

When preparing the setting for a group, there should be no barrier between members. For example, a circle of chairs is better than chairs set around a table. Members should be encouraged to sit in different chairs at each meeting. This openness and change creates a feeling of discomfort that encourages anxious and unsettled behaviors that can then be explored within the group.

Size

Various authors have suggested different ranges of size as ideal for group interaction: 5 to 10 (Yalom & Leszcz, 2005), 2 to 15 (Sampson & Marthas, 1990), and 4 to 12 (Clark, 2009). Group size does make a difference in the interaction among members. The larger the group, the less time is available to devote to individual members. In larger groups, more aggressive individuals are most likely to be heard, whereas quieter members may be left out of the discussions altogether. Understanding this dynamic alerts the nurse group leader to this possibility and allows him or her to facilitate interaction that promotes greater involvement for all members. Conversely, larger groups provide more opportunities for individuals to learn from other members. The wider range of life experiences and knowledge provides a greater potential for effective group problem-solving. Studies have indicated that a composition of 7 or 8 members provides a favorable climate for optimal group interaction and relationship development.

Membership

Whether the group is open or closed is another condition that influences the dynamics of group process. Open groups are those in which members leave and others join at any time while the group is active. The continuous movement of members in and out of the group creates the type of discomfort described previously that encourages unsettled behaviors in individual members and fosters the exploration of feelings. These are the most common types of groups held on short-term inpatient units, although they are used in outpatient and long-term care facilities as well. Closed groups usually have a predetermined, fixed time frame. All members join at the time the group is organized and terminate at the end of the designated time period. Closed groups are often composed of individuals with common issues or problems they wish to address.

Therapeutic Factors

Why are therapeutic groups helpful? Yalom and Leszcz (2005) described 11 therapeutic factors that individuals can achieve through interpersonal interactions within the group, some of which are present in most groups in varying degrees:

1. **Instillation of hope:** By observing the progress of others in the group with similar problems, a group member garners hope that his or her problems can also be resolved.
2. **Universality:** Through **universality,** individuals come to realize that they are not alone in the problems, thoughts, and feelings they are experiencing. Anxiety is relieved by the support and understanding of others in the group who share similar (universal) experiences.
3. **Imparting of information:** Knowledge is gained through formal instruction as well as sharing of advice and suggestions among group members.
4. **Altruism: Altruism** is assimilated by group members through mutual sharing and concern for each other. Providing assistance and support to others creates a positive self-image and promotes self-growth.
5. **Corrective recapitulation of the primary family group:** Group members are able to reexperience early family conflicts that remain unresolved. Attempts at resolution are promoted through feedback and exploration.
6. **Development of socializing techniques:** Through interaction with and feedback from other members within the group, individuals are able to correct maladaptive social behaviors and learn and develop new social skills.
7. **Imitative behavior:** In this setting, one who has mastered a particular psychosocial skill or developmental task can be a valuable role model for others. Individuals may imitate selected behaviors that they wish to develop in themselves.
8. **Interpersonal learning:** The group offers many and varied opportunities for interacting with other people. Insight is gained regarding how one perceives and is being perceived by others.
9. **Group cohesiveness:** Members develop a sense of belonging that separates the individual ("I am") from the group ("we are"). Out of this alliance emerges a common feeling that both individual members and the total group are of value to each other.
10. **Catharsis:** Within the group, members are able to express both positive and negative feelings—perhaps feelings that have never been expressed before—in a nonthreatening atmosphere. This **catharsis,** or open expression of feelings, is beneficial for the individual within the group.
11. **Existential factors:** The group is able to help individual members take direction of their own lives and accept responsibility for the quality of their existence.

It may be helpful for a group leader to explain these therapeutic factors to members. Positive responses are experienced by individuals who understand and are able to recognize therapeutic factors as they occur within the group.

Phases of Group Development

Groups, like individuals, move through phases of life-cycle development. Ideally, groups progress from the phase of infancy to advanced maturity in an effort to fulfill the objectives set forth by the membership. Unfortunately, as with individuals, some groups become fixed in early developmental levels and never progress, or they experience periods of regression in the developmental process. Three phases of group development are discussed here.

Phase I. Initial or Orientation Phase
Group Activities

Leader and members work together to establish the rules that will govern the group (e.g., when and where meetings will occur, the importance of confidentiality, how meetings will be structured). Goals of the group are established. Members are introduced to each other.

Leader Expectations

The leader is expected to orient members to specific group processes, encourage members to participate without disclosing too much too soon, promote an environment of trust, and ensure that rules established by the group do not interfere with fulfillment of the goals.

Member Behaviors

In phase I, members have not yet established trust and will respond to this lack of trust by being overly polite. There is a fear of not being accepted by the group. They may try to "get on the good side" of the leader with compliments and conforming behaviors. A power struggle may ensue as members compete for their position in the "pecking order" of the group.

Phase II. Middle or Working Phase

Group Activities

Ideally, during the working phase, cohesiveness has been established within the group. This phase is when productive work toward completion of the task is undertaken. Problem-solving and decision-making occur within the group. In the mature group, cooperation prevails, and differences and disagreements are confronted and resolved.

Leader Expectations

The leader becomes less of a leader and more of a facilitator during the working phase. Some leadership functions are shared by certain members of the group as they progress toward resolution. The leader helps to resolve conflict and continues to foster cohesiveness among the members while ensuring that they do not deviate from the intended task or purpose for which the group was organized.

Member Behaviors

At this point, trust has been established among the members. They turn more often to each other and less often to the leader for guidance. They accept criticism from each other, using it in a constructive manner to create change. Occasionally, subgroups form in which two or more members conspire with each other to the exclusion of the rest of the group. To maintain group cohesion, these subgroups must be confronted and discussed by the entire membership. Conflict is managed by the group with minimal assistance from the leader.

Phase III. Final or Termination Phase

Group Activities

The longer a group has existed, the more difficult termination is likely to be for the members. Termination should be mentioned from the outset of group formation and be discussed in depth for several meetings prior to the final session. A sense of loss that precipitates the grief process may be evident, particularly in groups that have been successful in their stated purpose.

Leader Expectations

In the termination phase, the leader encourages the group members to reminisce about what has occurred within the group, review the goals and discuss the actual outcomes, and provide feedback to each other about individual progress within the group. The leader encourages members to discuss feelings of loss associated with termination of the group.

Member Behaviors

Members may express surprise over the actual materialization of the end. This represents the grief response of denial, which may then progress to anger. Anger toward other group members or toward the leader may reflect feelings of abandonment (Sampson & Marthas, 1990). These feelings may lead to individual members' discussions of previous losses for which similar emotions were experienced. Successful termination of the group may help members develop the skills needed when losses occur in other dimensions of their lives.

Leadership Styles

Lippitt and White (1958) identified three of the most common group leadership styles: autocratic, democratic, and laissez-faire. Table 10–1 outlines various similarities and differences among the three leadership styles.

Autocratic

Autocratic leaders have personal goals for the group. They withhold information from group members, particularly issues that may interfere with achievement of their own objectives. The message that is conveyed to the group is: "We will do it my way. My way is best." The focus in this style of leadership is on the leader. Members are dependent on the leader for problem-solving, decision-making, and permission to perform. The approach of the autocratic leader is one of persuasion, striving to convince others in the group that his or her ideas and methods are superior. Productivity is high with this type of leadership, but often morale within the group is low because of lack of member input and creativity.

Democratic

The **democratic** leadership style focuses on the members of the group. Information is shared with members in an effort to allow them to make decisions regarding group goals. Members are encouraged to participate fully in solving problems that affect the group, including taking action to effect change. The message that is conveyed to the group is: "Decide what must be done, consider the alternatives, make a selection, and proceed with the actions required to complete the task." The leader provides guidance and expertise as needed. Productivity is lower than it is with autocratic leadership, but morale is much higher because of the extent of input allowed all members of the group and the potential for individual creativity.

Laissez-Faire

This leadership style allows people to do as they please. There is no direction from the leader. In fact, the **laissez-faire** leader's approach is noninvolvement. Goals for the group are undefined. No decisions are made, no problems are solved, and no action is taken.

TABLE 10–1 Leadership Styles–Similarities and Differences

CHARACTERISTICS	AUTOCRATIC	DEMOCRATIC	LAISSEZ-FAIRE
Focus	Leader	Members	Undetermined
Task strategy	Members are persuaded to adopt leader's ideas	Members engage in group problem-solving	No defined strategy exists
Member participation	Limited	Unlimited	Inconsistent
Individual creativity	Stifled	Encouraged	Not addressed
Member enthusiasm and morale	Low	High	Low
Group cohesiveness	Low	High	Low
Productivity	High	High (may not be as high as autocratic)	Low
Individual motivation and commitment	Low (tend to work only when leader is present to urge them to do so)	High (satisfaction derived from personal input and participation)	Low (feelings of frustration from lack of direction or guidance)

Members become frustrated and confused, and productivity and morale are low.

Member Roles

Benne and Sheats (1948) identified three major types of roles that individuals play within the membership of the group. These are roles that serve to

1. Complete the task of the group.
2. Maintain or enhance group processes.
3. Fulfill personal or individual needs.

Task roles and maintenance roles contribute to the success or effectiveness of the group. Personal roles satisfy needs of the individual members, sometimes to the extent of interfering with the effectiveness of the group.

Table 10–2 outlines specific roles within these three major types and the behaviors associated with each.

Psychodrama

A specialized type of therapeutic group, called **psychodrama,** was introduced by Jacob L. Moreno, a Viennese psychiatrist. Moreno's method employs a dramatic approach in which clients become "actors" in life-situation scenarios.

The group leader is called the *director,* group members are the *audience,* and the *set* or *stage* may be specially designed or just a room or area selected for this purpose. Actors are members from the audience who agree to take part in the "drama" by role-playing a situation about which they have been informed by the director. Usually, the situation is an issue with which an individual client has been struggling. The client plays the role of himself or herself and is called the *protagonist.* In this role, he or she is able to express true feelings toward individuals (represented by group members) with whom unresolved conflicts exist.

TABLE 10–2 Member Roles Within Groups

ROLE	BEHAVIORS
TASK ROLES	
Coordinator	Clarifies ideas and suggestions that have been made within the group; brings relationships together to pursue common goals
Evaluator	Examines group plans and performance, measuring against group standards and goals
Elaborator	Explains and expands upon group plans and ideas
Energizer	Encourages and motivates group to perform at its maximum potential
Initiator	Outlines the task at hand for the group and proposes methods for solution
Orienter	Maintains direction within the group

Continued

TABLE 10–2 Member Roles Within Groups—cont'd

ROLE	BEHAVIORS
MAINTENANCE ROLES	
Compromiser	Relieves conflict within the group by assisting members to reach a compromise agreeable to all
Encourager	Offers recognition and acceptance of others' ideas and contributions
Follower	Listens attentively to group interaction; is a passive participant
Gatekeeper	Encourages acceptance of and participation by all members of the group
Harmonizer	Minimizes tension within the group by intervening when disagreements produce conflict
INDIVIDUAL (PERSONAL) ROLES	
Aggressor	Expresses negativism and hostility toward other members; may use sarcasm in effort to degrade the status of others
Blocker	Resists group efforts; demonstrates rigid and sometimes irrational behaviors that impede group progress
Dominator	Manipulates others to gain control; behaves in authoritarian manner
Help-seeker	Uses the group to gain sympathy from others; seeks to increase self-confidence from group feedback; lacks concern for others or for the group as a whole
Monopolizer	Maintains control of the group by dominating the conversation
Mute or silent member	Does not participate verbally; remains silent for a variety of reasons—may feel uncomfortable with self-disclosure or may be seeking attention through silence
Recognition seeker	Talks about personal accomplishments in an effort to gain attention for self
Seducer	Shares intimate details about self with group; is the least reluctant of the group to do so; may frighten others in the group and inhibit group progress with excessive premature self-disclosure

SOURCES: Benne, K.D., & Sheats, P. (1948, Spring). Functional roles of group members. *Journal of Social Issues, 4*(2), 41-49; Hobbs, D.J., & Powers, R.C. (1981). *Group member roles: For group effectiveness.* Ames: Iowa State University, Cooperative Extension Service; Larson, M.L., & Williams, R.A. (1978). How to become a better group leader? Learn to recognize the strange things that happen to some people in groups. *Nursing, 8*(8), 65-72.

In some instances, the group leader may ask for a client to volunteer as protagonist for that session. The client may choose a situation he or she wishes to enact and select the audience members to portray the roles of others in the life situation. The psychodrama setting provides the client with a safer and less-threatening atmosphere than the real situation, facilitating the expression of true feelings and resolution of interpersonal conflicts.

When the drama has been completed, group members from the audience discuss the situation they have observed, offer feedback, express their feelings, and relate their own similar experiences. In this way, all group members benefit from the session, either directly or indirectly.

Nurses often serve as actors or role players in psychodrama sessions. Leaders of psychodrama have graduate degrees in psychology, social work, nursing, or medicine with additional training in group therapy and specialty preparation to become a psychodramatist.

The Role of the Nurse in Therapeutic Groups

Nurses participate in group situations on a daily basis. In health-care settings, nurses serve on or lead task groups that create policy, describe procedures, and plan client care. They are also involved in a variety of other groups aimed at the institutional effort of serving the consumer. Nurses are encouraged to use the steps of the nursing process as a framework for task group leadership.

In psychiatry, nurses may lead various types of therapeutic groups, such as client education, assertiveness training, grief support, parenting, and transition to discharge groups, among others. To function effectively in the leadership capacity for these groups, nurses must recognize the various processes that occur in groups, such as the phases of group development, the roles that people play within groups, and the motivation behind these behaviors. They also need to be able to select the most appropriate leadership style for the type of group. Generalist nurses may develop these skills as part of their undergraduate educations, or they may pursue additional study while serving and learning as the coleader of a group with a more experienced nurse leader.

Generalist nurses in psychiatry should not serve as leaders of psychotherapy groups. The *Psychiatric-Mental Health Nursing Scope and Standards of Practice* (American Nurses Association, American Psychiatric Nurses Association, & International Society of Psychiatric Nurses, 2014) specifies that nurses who serve as group psychotherapists should have a minimum of a master's degree in psychiatric nursing. Educational preparation in group theory, extended practice as a group coleader or leader under the supervision of an experienced psychotherapist, and participation in group therapy on an experiential level are also recommended. Additional specialist training is required beyond the master's level to prepare nurses to become family therapists or psychodramatists.

Leading therapeutic groups is within the realm of nursing practice. Because group work is such a common therapeutic approach in the discipline of psychiatry, nurses working in this field must continually strive to expand their knowledge and use of group process as a significant psychiatric nursing intervention.

> **CLINICAL PEARL** Knowledge of human behavior in general and the group process in particular is essential to effective group leadership.

Summary and Key Points

- A group has been defined as a collection of individuals whose association is founded on shared commonalities of interest, values, norms, or purpose.
- Eight group functions have been identified: socialization, support, task completion, camaraderie, informational, normative, empowerment, and governance.
- The three major types of group are task groups, teaching groups, and supportive/therapeutic groups.
- The function of task groups is to solve problems, make decisions, and achieve a specific outcome.
- In teaching groups, knowledge and information are conveyed to a number of individuals.
- The function of supportive/therapeutic groups is to educate people to deal effectively with emotional stress in their lives.

- In self-help groups, members share the same type of problem and help each other to prevent decompensation related to that problem.
- Therapeutic groups differ from group therapy in that the focus is not on psychotherapy but rather on interaction and relationships among group members with regard to a selected issue. Group therapy is more focused on specific models of psychotherapy, and the leaders generally have advanced degrees in psychology, social work, nursing, or medicine. Placement of the seating and size of the group can influence group interaction.
- Groups can be open (when members leave and others join at any time while the group is active) or closed (when groups have a predetermined, fixed time frame and all members join at the same time and leave when the group disbands).
- Yalom and Leszcz (2005) describe the following therapeutic factors that individuals derive from participation in therapeutic groups: instillation of hope, universality, imparting of information, altruism, corrective recapitulation of the primary family group, development of socializing techniques, imitative behavior, interpersonal learning, group cohesiveness, catharsis, and existential factors.
- Groups progress through three phases: the initial (orientation) phase, the working phase, and the termination phase.
- Group leadership styles include autocratic, democratic, and laissez-faire.
- Members play various roles within groups. These roles are categorized as task, maintenance, and personal roles.
- Psychodrama is a specialized type of group therapy that uses a dramatic approach in which clients become "actors" in life-situation scenarios.
- The psychodrama setting provides the client with a safer and less-threatening atmosphere than the real situation in which to express and work through unresolved conflicts.
- Nurses lead various types of therapeutic groups in the psychiatric setting. Knowledge of human behavior in general and the group process in particular is essential to effective group leadership.
- Specialized training, in addition to a master's degree, is required for nurses to serve as group psychotherapists or psychodramatists.

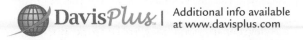

DavisPlus | Additional info available at www.davisplus.com

Review Questions
Self-Examination/Learning Exercise

Select the answer that is most appropriate for each of the following questions:

1. Nicole is the nurse leader of a childbirth preparation group. Each week she shows films and sets out reading materials. She expects the participants to utilize their time on a topic of their choice or practice skills they have observed on the films. Two couples have dropped out of the group, stating, "This is a big waste of time." Which type of group and style of leadership is described in this situation?
   a. Task group, democratic leadership
   b. Teaching group, laissez-faire leadership
   c. Self-help group, democratic leadership
   d. Supportive-therapeutic group, autocratic leadership

2. Aisha is a psychiatric nurse who has been selected to lead a group for women who desire to lose weight. The criterion for membership is that they must be at least 20 pounds overweight. All have tried to lose weight on their own many times in the past without success. At their first meeting, Aisha provides suggestions as the members determine what their goals will be and how they plan to go about achieving those goals. They decided how often they wanted to meet and what they planned to do at each meeting. Which type of group and style of leadership is described in this situation?
   a. Task group, autocratic leadership
   b. Teaching group, democratic leadership
   c. Self-help group, laissez-faire leadership
   d. Supportive-therapeutic group, democratic leadership

3. Erik is a staff nurse on a surgical unit. He has been selected as leader of a newly established group of staff nurses organized to determine ways to decrease the number of medication errors occurring on the unit. Erik has definite ideas about how to bring this about. He has also applied for the position of Head Nurse on the unit and believes that if he is successful in leading the group toward achievement of its goals, he can also facilitate his chances for promotion. At each meeting, he addresses the group in an effort to convince the members to adopt his ideas. Which type of group and style of leadership is described in this situation?
   a. Task group, autocratic leadership
   b. Teaching group, autocratic leadership
   c. Self-help group, democratic leadership
   d. Supportive-therapeutic group, laissez-faire leadership

4. The nurse leader is explaining about group "therapeutic factors" to members of the group. She tells the group that group situations are beneficial because members can see that they are not alone in their experiences. Nurse Carol appropriately identifies this as evidence of which therapeutic factor?
   a. Altruism
   b. Imitative behavior
   c. Universality
   d. Imparting of information

5. Nurse Carol is the leader of a bereavement group for widows. Elena is a new member who listens to the group and learns that Jane has been a widow for 5 years now. Jane has adjusted well and Elena thinks maybe she can too. Nurse Carol appropriately identifies this as evidence of which therapeutic factor?
   a. Universality
   b. Imitative behavior
   c. Installation of hope
   d. Imparting of information

Review Questions—cont'd
Self-Examination/Learning Exercise

6. Paul is a member of an anger management group. He knew that people did not want to be his friend because of his violent temper. In the group, he has learned to control his temper and form satisfactory interpersonal relationships with others. This is an example of which therapeutic factor?
   a. Catharsis
   b. Altruism
   c. Imparting of information
   d. Development of socializing techniques

7. Benjamin is a member of an Alcoholics Anonymous group. He learned about the effects of alcohol on the body when a nurse from the chemical dependency unit spoke to the group. This is an example of which therapeutic factor?
   a. Catharsis
   b. Altruism
   c. Imparting of information
   d. Universality

8. Sandra is the nurse leader of a supportive-therapeutic group for individuals with anxiety disorders. In this group, Helen talks incessantly. When someone else tries to make a comment, she refuses to allow him or her to speak. What type of member role is Helen assuming in this group?
   a. Aggressor
   b. Monopolizer
   c. Blocker
   d. Seducer

9. Sandra is the nurse leader of a supportive-therapeutic group for individuals with anxiety disorders. On the first day the group meets, Valerie speaks first and begins by sharing the intimate details of her incestuous relationship with her father. What type of member role is Valerie assuming in this group?
   a. Aggressor
   b. Monopolizer
   c. Blocker
   d. Seducer

10. Sandra is the nurse leader of a supportive-therapeutic group for individuals with anxiety disorders. Violet, who is beautiful but lacks self-confidence, states to the group, "Maybe if I became a blond my boyfriend would love me more." Larry responds, "Listen, dummy, you need more than blond hair to keep the guy around. A bit more in the brains department would help!" What type of member role is Larry assuming in this group?
    a. Aggressor
    b. Monopolizer
    c. Blocker
    d. Seducer

11. A nurse on the psychiatric unit is asked to lead a psychoeducational group on self-esteem for the in-patients on the unit. It is an open group, and the nurse is aware that the attendees are multicultural. Which of the following evidence-based skills are important for the nurse to possess to effectively lead this group? (Select all that apply.)
    a. Awareness that contact alone with people of different cultures will improve their intercultural communication
    b. Skills of emotional intelligence
    c. Training in culturally specific language interpretation and communication styles
    d. Recognition that people from cultures that do not value self-esteem will need to be prohibited from attending the group
    e. An attitude of willingness to identify and correct intercultural misunderstandings when they occur

IMPLICATIONS OF RESEARCH FOR EVIDENCE-BASED PRACTICE

Atieno-Okech, J.E., Pimpleton, A.M., Vannatta, R., & Champe, J. (2015). Intercultural communication: An application to group work. *Journal for Specialists in Group Work, 40*(3), 268-293. doi.org/10.1080/01933922.2015.1056568

DESCRIPTION OF THE STUDY: Interdisciplinary literature on intercultural communication was reviewed to serve as a source of evidence-based strategies for improving intercultural communication. The authors note that as the diversity of the U.S. population continues to grow, counseling and therapy groups will grow in diversity and demand attention to intercultural communication in order to remain an effective tool for support, psychoeducation, and therapy.

RESULTS OF THE STUDY: The literature supports that discrepancies in communication style, differing cultural values, and ethnocentrism have been identified as major intercultural barriers in communication. "Languaculture," a concept developed by Agar (1994), refers to culturally specific ways of interpreting language and is identified as an important knowledge base for group leaders. The case study presented by the authors describes a white female group leader who was using the communication technique of reflection with an African American male who perceived this reflection of his feelings as a taunt rather than as helpful. Attempting to "curiously and respectfully" seek understanding when these miscommunications occur is identified as a group leader's responsibility.

Other studies found that contact alone did not translate into improved communication and relationships in an intercultural group. The biggest deterrents were apathy, ethnocentrism, and inexperience. The group leader therefore must be aware of and attend to cues that may indicate a breakdown in communication between members before conflict or outright hostility arises. Studies showed that emotional intelligence is associated with the ability to read verbal and nonverbal cues, so this is an important skill for group leaders.

IMPLICATIONS FOR NURSING PRACTICE: Nurses will likely be engaged in intercultural groups among peers in the workplace as well as when leading therapeutic patient groups. The following skills are identified as important to evidence-based practice when leading groups:

1. Awareness of one's own cultural values and biases to evaluate and counter ethnocentrism as a barrier to communication
2. Training in culturally specific ways of interpreting language and communication
3. Emotional intelligence skills to recognize when communication breakdowns are surfacing
4. An attitude of wanting to understand and correct intercultural miscommunication when it occurs

References

Agar, M. (1994). *Language shock: Understanding the culture of conversation*. New York: William Morrow.

American Nurses Association (ANA), American Psychiatric Nurses Association (APNA), & International Society of Psychiatric Nurses (ISPN). (2014). *Psychiatric-mental health nursing: scope and standards of practice* (2nd ed.). Silver Spring, MD: ANA.

Atieno-Okech, J.E., Pimpleton, A.M., Vannatta, R., & Champe, J. (2015). Intercultural communication: An application to group work. *Journal for Specialists in Group Work, 40*(3), 268-293. doi.org/10.1080/01933922.2015.1056568

Clark, C.C. (2009). *Group leadership skills for nurses and health professionals* (5th ed.). New York: Springer.

Forsyth, D.R. (2010). *Group dynamics* (5th ed.). Belmont, CA: Cengage Learning.

Sampson, E.E., & Marthas, M. (1990). *Group process for the health professions* (3rd ed.). Albany, NY: Delmar Publishers.

Yalom, I.D., & Leszcz, M. (2005). *The theory and practice of group psychotherapy* (5th ed.). New York: Basic Books.

Classical References

Benne, K.D., & Sheats, P. (1948, Spring). Functional roles of group members. *Journal of Social Issues, 4*(2), 41-49. doi:10.1111/j.1540-4560.1948.tb01783.x

Hobbs, D.J., & Powers, R.C. (1981). *Group member roles: For group effectiveness*. Ames: Iowa State University, Cooperative Extension Service.

Larson, M.L., & Williams, R.A. (1978). How to become a better group leader? Learn to recognize the strange things that happen to some people in groups. *Nursing, 8*(8), 65-72. doi:10.1007/s10912-015-9346-4

Lippitt, R., & White, R.K. (1958). An experimental study of leadership and group life. In E.E. Maccoby, T.M. Newcomb, & E.L. Hartley (Eds.), *Readings in social psychology* (3rd ed.). New York: Holt, Rinehart, & Winston.

Intervention With Families

11

CORE CONCEPTS

Family

Family Therapy

KEY TERMS

boundaries	genograms	reframing
disengagement	marital schism	scapegoating
double-bind communication	marital skew	subsystems
enmeshment	paradoxical intervention	triangles
family structure	pseudohostility	
family system	pseudomutuality	

OBJECTIVES
After reading this chapter, the student will be able to:

1. Define the term *family*.
2. Identify stages of family development.
3. Describe major variations to the American middle-class family life cycle.
4. Discuss characteristics of adaptive family functioning.
5. Describe behaviors that interfere with adaptive family functioning.
6. Discuss the essential components of family systems, structural, and strategic therapies.
7. Construct a family genogram.
8. Apply the steps of the nursing process in therapeutic intervention with families.

HOMEWORK ASSIGNMENT
Please read the chapter and answer the following questions:

1. Describe the concept of reframing.
2. Describe the process of triangulation in a dysfunctional family pattern.
3. How are genograms helpful in family therapy?
4. What behaviors are indicative of a positive family climate?

What is a family? Wright and Leahey (2013) propose the following definition: a family is who they say they are. Many family structures exist within society today, such as the biological family of procreation, the nuclear family that incorporates one or more members of the extended family (family of origin), the sole-parent family, the stepfamily, the communal family, and the same-sex couple or family. Labeling individuals as "families" based on their group composition may not be the best characterization, however. Instead, family consideration may be more appropriately determined on the basis of attributes of affection, strong emotional ties, a sense of belonging, and durability of membership (Wright & Leahey, 2013).

Many nurses have interactions with family members on a daily basis. A client's illness or hospitalization affects all members of the family, and nurses must understand how to work with the family as a unit, knowing that family members can have a profound effect on the client's healing process.

Nurse generalists should be familiar with the tasks associated with adaptive family functioning. With this knowledge, they are able to assess family interaction and recognize problems when they arise. They can provide support to families with ill members and make referrals to other professionals when assistance is required to restore adaptive functioning.

Nurse specialists usually possess an advanced degree in nursing. Some nurse specialists have education or experience that qualifies them to perform family therapy. Family therapy is an approach that incorporates theories and models designed to explore family dynamics, dysfunctional patterns, and methods for adaptive change within the context of the family. This chapter explores the stages of family development and compares the "typical" family within various subcultures. Characteristics of adaptive family functioning and behaviors that interfere with this adaptation are discussed. Theoretical components of selected therapeutic approaches are described. Instructions for construction of a family genogram are included. Nursing process provides the framework for nursing intervention with families.

CORE CONCEPT

Family

Two or more individuals who depend on one another for emotional, physical, and economical support. The members of the family are self-defined (Kaakinen & Hanson, 2015, p. 5).

Stages of Family Development

McGoldrick, Garcia-Preto, and Carter (2015) discuss stages and developmental tasks that describe the traditional family life cycle and acknowledge that this is only one of many trajectories for family development in today's society. It is clear that accomplishment of these tasks would vary among diverse cultural groups and among the various forms of family structure previously described. These stages, however, provide a valuable framework from which the nurse may study families, emphasizing expansion (the addition of members), contraction (the loss of members), and realignment of relationships as members experience developmental changes. These stages of family development are described in the following paragraphs and summarized in Table 11–1.

TABLE 11-1 Stages of the Traditional Family Life Cycle

FAMILY LIFE-CYCLE STAGES	EMOTIONAL PROCESS OF TRANSITION: KEY PRINCIPLES	CHANGES REQUIRED IN FAMILY STATUS TO PROCEED DEVELOPMENTALLY
The single young adult	Accepting separation from parents and emotional and financial responsibility for self	■ Differentiation of self in relation to family of origin ■ Development of intimate peer relationships ■ Establishment of self in respect to work and financial independence ■ Establishment of self in community and larger society
The family joined through marriage/union	Commitment to new system	■ Formation of partner systems ■ Realignment of relationships with extended family, friends, and larger community and social system to include new partners
The family with young children	Accepting new members into the system	■ Adjustment of couple system to make space for children ■ Collaboration in child rearing, financial and housekeeping tasks ■ Realignment of relationships with extended family to include parenting and grandparenting roles ■ Realignment of relationships with community and larger social system to include new family structure and relationships

TABLE 11–1 **Stages of the Traditional Family Life Cycle–cont'd**		
FAMILY LIFE-CYCLE STAGES	EMOTIONAL PROCESS OF TRANSITION: KEY PRINCIPLES	CHANGES REQUIRED IN FAMILY STATUS TO PROCEED DEVELOPMENTALLY
The family with adolescents	Increasing flexibility of family boundaries to permit children's independence and grandparents' frailties	■ Shifting of parent-child relationships to permit adolescents to move in and out of system ■ Refocus on midlife couple and career issues ■ Beginning shift toward caring for older generation ■ Realignment with community and larger social system to include shifting family of emerging adolescent and parents in new formation patterns of relating
The family launching children and moving on in midlife	Accepting a multitude of exits from and entries into the family system	■ Renegotiation of couple system as a dyad ■ Development of adult-to-adult relationships between parents and grown children ■ Realignment of relationships to include in-laws and grandchildren ■ Realignment of relationships with community and larger social system to include new structure and constellation of family relationships ■ Exploration of new interests/career given the freedom from child-care responsibilities ■ Dealing with care needs, disabilities and death of parents (grandparents)
The family in later life (late middle age to end of life)	■ Accepting the shifting of generational roles ■ Accepting the realities of limitations and death	■ Maintaining own and/or couple functioning and interests in face of physiological decline; exploration of new familial and social role options ■ Supporting more central role of middle generations ■ Realignment of the system in relation to community and larger social system to acknowledge changed pattern of family relationships of this stage ■ Making room in the system for the wisdom and experience of the elders; supporting the older generation without overfunctioning for them ■ Dealing with loss of spouse, siblings, and other peers and preparation for own death; life review and integration ■ Managing reversed roles in caretaking between middle and older generations

Adapted from McGoldrick, M., Garcia-Preto, N. & Carter, B. (2015). Overview: The life cycle in its changing context. In M. McGoldrick, N. Garcia-Preto, & B. Carter. (2015). *The expanding family life cycle: Individual, family, and social perspectives* (5th ed., pp.1-19). Boston: Allyn & Bacon. Reprinted by permission.

The Single Young Adult

This model begins with the launching of the young adult from the family of origin. This is a difficult stage because young adults must decide what social standards from the family of origin will be preserved and what standards they will eventually incorporate into a new family. Tasks of this stage include forming an identity separate from the parents, establishing intimate peer relationships, and advancing toward financial independence. Problems can arise when either the young adults or the parents encounter difficulty terminating the interdependent relationship that has existed in the family of origin.

The Family Joined Through Marriage/Union

Uniting as a couple is a difficult transition that must include the integration of contrasting issues that each partner brings to the relationship and issues they may have redefined for themselves as a couple. In addition, the new couple must renegotiate relationships with parents, siblings, and other relatives in view of the new partnership. Tasks of this stage include establishing a new identity as a couple, realigning relationships with members of extended family, and making decisions about having children. Problems can arise if either partner remains too enmeshed with their family of origin or when the couple chooses to cut themselves off completely from extended family.

The Family With Young Children

Adjustments in relationships must occur with the arrival of children. The entire family system is affected, and role realignments are necessary for both new parents and new grandparents. Tasks of this stage include making adjustments within the marital system to meet the responsibilities associated with parenthood while maintaining the integrity of the couple relationship, sharing equally in the tasks of child rearing, and integrating the roles of extended family members into the newly expanded family organization. Problems can arise when parents lack knowledge about normal childhood development and adequate patience to allow children to express themselves through behavior.

The Family With Adolescents

This stage of family development is characterized by a great deal of turmoil and transition. Parents are approaching a midlife stage, and adolescents are undergoing biological, emotional, and sociocultural changes that place demands on each individual and on the family unit. Grandparents, too, may require assistance with the tasks of later life. These developments can create a "sandwich" effect for the parents, who must deal with issues confronting three generations. Tasks of this stage include redefining the level of dependence so that adolescents are provided with greater autonomy while parents remain responsive to the teenager's dependency needs. Midlife issues related to marriage, career, and aging parents must also be resolved during this period. Problems can arise when parents are unable to relinquish control and allow the adolescent greater autonomy and freedom to make independent decisions or when parents are unable to agree and support each other in this effort.

The Family With Children Leaving Home

A great deal of realignment of family roles occurs during this stage, characterized by the intermittent exiting and entering of various family members. Children leave home for further education and careers; marriages occur, and new spouses, in-laws, and children enter the system; and new grandparent roles are established. Adult-to-adult relationships among grown children and their parents are renegotiated. Tasks associated with this stage include reestablishing the bond of the dyadic marital relationship; realigning relationships to include grown children, in-laws, and new grandchildren; and accepting the additional caretaking responsibilities and eventual death of elderly parents. Problems can arise when feelings of loss and depression become overwhelming in response to the departure of children from the home, when parents are unable to accept their children as adults or cope with the disability or death of their own parents, and when the marital bond has deteriorated.

The Family in Later Life (Late Middle Age to End of Life)

This stage can begin with retirement and last until the death of both spouses (Wright & Leahey, 2013). However, many older people who have the opportunity to do so are choosing to retire early, while large numbers of those over age 65 are remaining in the workforce and delaying retirement. Thus, the beginning of this stage varies widely. Most adults in their later years are still a prominent part of the family system, and many are able to offer support to their grown children in the middle generation. Tasks traditionally associated with this stage include exploring new social roles related to retirement and possible change in socioeconomic status; accepting some decline in physiological functioning; dealing with the deaths of spouse, siblings, and friends; and confronting and preparing for one's own death. A growing trend is an increasing number of older adults living with and in many cases assuming primary responsibility for their grandchildren. Currently, 10 percent of all children under the age of 18 in the United States are living with a grandparent (U.S. Census Bureau, 2015). When older adults have failed to fulfill the tasks associated with earlier levels of development and are dissatisfied with the way their lives have gone, they may be unable to find happiness in retirement or emotional satisfaction with children and grandchildren and have difficulty accepting the deaths of loved ones or preparing for their own impending deaths.

Major Variations

Divorce

McGoldrick, Garcia-Preto, and Carter (2015) also discuss stages and tasks of families experiencing divorce and remarriage. Data on marriage, divorce, and remarriage in the United States show that about half of first marriages end in divorce (Centers for Disease Control [CDC], 2015). Whether related to single, never married, or divorced parents, the number of children who live with one parent has tripled since 1960 from 9 percent to 27 percent (U.S. Census Bureau, 2015). Stages in the family life cycle of divorce include deciding to divorce, planning the breakup of the system, separation, and divorce. Tasks include accepting one's own part in the failure of the marriage, working cooperatively on problems related to finances and child custody and visitation, realigning relationships with extended family, and mourning the loss of the marriage relationship and the intact family.

After the divorce, the custodial parent must adjust to functioning as the single leader of an ongoing family while working to rebuild a new social network. The noncustodial parent must find ways to continue to be an effective parent in a different kind of parenting role.

Remarriage

Approximately 75 percent of people who divorce eventually remarry (Stepfamily Foundation, 2016). Currently, less than half (46%) of children are living in a family with two parents in their first marriage (Pew Research Center, 2015). The challenges that face the joining of two established families are immense, and statistics reveal that the rate of divorce for remarried couples is even higher than the divorce rate following first marriages (Cory, 2013). Stages in the remarried family life cycle include entering the new relationship, planning the new marriage and family, and remarriage and reestablishment of family. Tasks include making a firm commitment to confronting the complexities of combining two families, maintaining open communication, facing fears, realigning relationships with extended family to include new spouse and children, and encouraging healthy relationships with biological (noncustodial) parents and grandparents.

Problems can arise when there is a blurring of boundaries between the custodial and noncustodial families. Children may contemplate issues such as

- Who is the boss now?
- Who is most important, the child or the new spouse?
- Mom loves her new husband more than she loves me.
- Dad lets me do more than my new stepdad does.
- I don't have to mind him; he's not my real dad.

Confusion and distress for both the children and the parents can be minimized with the establishment of clear boundaries and open communication.

Cultural Variations

It is difficult to generalize about variations in family life-cycle development according to culture. Most families have become acculturated to the U.S. society and conform to the life-cycle stages previously described. However, cultural diversity does exist, and nurses must be aware of possible differences in family expectations related to sociocultural beliefs. The following are possible variations to consider.

Marriage

A number of U.S. subcultures maintain traditional values in terms of marriage. These views, along with the influence of Roman Catholicism, exert important influences on attitudes toward marriage in many Italian American and Latino American families. Although the tradition of arranged marriages is disappearing in Asian American families, there is still frequently a strong influence by the family on mate selection in this culture. In most of these subcultures, the father is considered the authority figure and head of the household, and the mother assumes the role of homemaker and caretaker. Family loyalty is intense, and a breach of this loyalty brings considerable shame to the family.

Jewish families have traditionally valued marriage and have prohibited marriage to non-Jews, but that cultural value has shifted in recent years. Valley (2005) makes the following statement about Jewish families:

> The Jewish family today encompasses a wide variety of textures and forms. Decades of high intermarriage have diversified the customs and complexions of the family. High divorce rates, meanwhile, have altered the very definition of what is "normal." Whereas single-parent households were once a rare exception, they now account for an increasing proportion of American Jewish families. Some in the community have interpreted the changing family in strident and judgmental terms: it is a sign of rampant assimilation, loss of tradition, or moral permissiveness. But such scolding does nothing to respond to the new realities and to the changing needs of Jews today. (p. 2)

Children

In traditional Latino American and Italian American cultures, children are central to the family system. Many of these individuals have strong ties to Roman Catholicism, which historically has promoted marital relations for procreation only and encouraged families to have large numbers of children. Regarding birth control, the Catechism of the Catholic Church pronounces as immoral any means that interferes with or hinders procreation (U.S. Catholic Church, 2016).

In the traditional Jewish community, having children is seen as a scriptural and social obligation. "You shall be fruitful and multiply" is a commandment of the Torah.

In some traditional Asian American cultures, sons are more highly valued than daughters (Earp, 2017; Chang, 2017). Younger siblings are expected to follow the guidance of the oldest son throughout their lives, and when the father dies, the oldest son takes over the leadership of the family.

In all of these cultures, children are expected to be respectful of their parents and not bring shame to the family. Especially in the Asian culture, children learn a sense of obligation to their parents for bringing them into this world and caring for them when they were helpless. This is viewed as a debt that can never be truly repaid, and no matter what the parents may do, the child is still obligated to give respect and obedience.

Extended Family

The concept of extended family varies among societies (Purnell, 2013). The extended family is extremely important in the Western European, Latino, and Asian cultures, playing a central role in all aspects of life, including decision-making.

In some U.S. subcultures, such as Asian, Latino, Italian, and Iranian, it is not uncommon to find several generations living together. Older family members are valued for their experience and wisdom. Because extended families often share living quarters or at least live nearby, tasks of child rearing may be shared by several generations.

Divorce

In the Jewish community, divorce is often seen as a violation of family togetherness. Some Jewish parents take their child's divorce personally, with a response that reflects, "How could you possibly do this to me?"

Because Roman Catholicism has traditionally opposed divorce, those cultures that are largely Catholic have followed this dictate. Historically, a low divorce rate has existed among Italian Americans, Irish Americans, and Latino Americans. The number of divorces among these subcultures is on the rise, however, particularly in successive generations that have become acculturated into a society where divorce is more acceptable.

Family Functioning

Boyer and Jeffrey (1994) describe six elements on which families are assessed to be either functional or dysfunctional. Each can be viewed on a continuum, although families rarely fall at extreme ends of the continuum. Rather, they tend to be dynamic and fluctuate from one point to another within the different areas. These six elements of assessment are described below and summarized in Table 11–2.

Communication

Functional communication patterns are those in which verbal and nonverbal messages are clear, direct, and congruent between sender and intended receiver. Family members are encouraged to express honest feelings and opinions, and all members participate in decisions that affect the family system. Each member is an active listener to the other members of the family.

Behaviors that interfere with functional communication include the following:

Making Assumptions

With this behavior, one assumes that others will know what is meant by an action or an expression (or sometimes even what one is thinking); or, conversely, assumes to know what another member is thinking or feeling without checking to make certain.

> **EXAMPLE**
>
> A mother says to her teenaged daughter, "You should have known that I expected you to clean up the kitchen while I was gone!"

Belittling Feelings

This behavior involves ignoring or minimizing another's feelings when they are expressed. Belittling a

TABLE 11–2 **Family Functioning: Elements of Assessment**		
ELEMENTS OF ASSESSMENT	CONTINUUM	
	FUNCTIONAL	**DYSFUNCTIONAL**
Communication	Clear, direct, open, honest, with congruence between verbal and nonverbal	Indirect, vague, controlled, with many double-bind messages
Self-concept reinforcement	Supportive, loving, praising, approving, with behaviors that instill confidence	Unsupportive, blaming, put-downs, refusing to allow self-responsibility
Family members' expectations	Flexible, realistic, individualized	Judgmental, rigid, controlling, ignoring individuality
Handling differences	Tolerant, dynamic, negotiating	Attacking, avoiding, surrendering
Family interactional patterns	Workable, constructive, flexible, promoting the needs of all members	Contradictory, rigid, self-defeating, destructive
Family climate	Trusting, growth-promoting, caring, general feeling of well-being	Distrusting, emotionally painful, with absence of hope for improvement

SOURCE: Adapted from Boyer, P.A., & Jeffrey, R.J. (1994). *A guide for the family therapist.* Northvale, NJ: Jason Aronson.

person's feelings encourages the individual to withhold honest feelings to avoid being hurt by the negative response.

EXAMPLE

When the young woman confides to her mother that she is angry because the grandfather has touched her breast, the mother responds, "Oh, don't be angry. He doesn't mean anything by that."

Failing to Listen

With this behavior, one does not hear what the other individual is saying. Failing to listen can mean not hearing the words by "tuning out" the message, or it can be "selective" listening, in which a person hears only a selective part of the message or interprets it in a selective manner.

EXAMPLE

The father explains to Johnny, "If the contract comes through and I get this new job, we'll have a little extra money and we will consider sending you to State U." Johnny relays the message to his friend, "Dad says I can go to State U!"

Communicating Indirectly

Indirect communication usually means that an individual does not or cannot present a message to a receiver directly, so he or she seeks to communicate through a third person.

EXAMPLE

A father does not want his teenage daughter to see a certain boyfriend but wants to avoid the angry response he expects from his daughter if he tells her so. He expresses his feelings to his wife, hoping she will share them with their daughter.

Presenting Double-Bind Messages

Double-bind communication conveys a "damned if I do and damned if I don't" message. A family member may respond to a direct request by another family member, only to be rebuked when the request is fulfilled. This concept appears again in the section on the strategic model of family therapy later in this chapter.

EXAMPLE

The father tells his son he is spending too much time playing football, and as a result, his grades are falling. The son is expected to bring his grades up over the next 9 weeks or his car will be taken away. When the son tells the father he has quit the football team so he can study more, Dad responds angrily, "I won't allow any son of mine to be a quitter!"

Self-Concept Reinforcement

Functional families strive to reinforce and strengthen each member's self-concept, with the positive result that family members feel loved and valued. Boyer and Jeffrey (1994) stated:

> The manner in which children see and value themselves is influenced most significantly by the messages they receive concerning their value to other members of the family. Messages that convey praise, approval, appreciation, trust, and confidence in decisions and that allow family members to pursue individual needs and ultimately to become independent are the foundation blocks of a child's feelings of self-worth. Adults also need and depend heavily on this kind of reinforcement for their own emotional well-being. (p. 27)

Behaviors that interfere with self-concept reinforcement include the following:

Expressing Denigrating Remarks

These remarks are commonly called "put-downs." Individuals receive messages that they are worthless or unloved.

EXAMPLE

A child spills a glass of milk at the table. The mother responds, "You are hopeless! How could anybody be so clumsy?!"

Withholding Supportive Messages

Some family members find it very difficult to provide others with reinforcing and supportive messages. This difficulty may occur because they themselves have not been the recipients of reinforcement from significant others and have not learned how to provide support to others.

EXAMPLE

A 10-year-old boy playing Little League baseball retrieves the ball and throws it to second base for an out. After the game he says to his Dad, "Did you see my play on second base?" Dad responds, "Yes, I did, son, but if you had been paying better attention, you could have caught the ball for a direct and immediate out."

Taking Over

Taking over occurs when one family member fails to permit another member to develop a sense of responsibility and self-worth. Instead, the person who takes over does things for the individual and thereby prevents him or her from managing the situation independently.

EXAMPLE

Twelve-year-old Eric has a job delivering the evening paper, which he usually begins right after school. Today he must serve a 1-hour detention after school for being late to class yesterday. He tells his Mom, "Tommy said he would throw my papers for me today if I help him wash his Dad's car on Saturday." Mom responds, "Never mind. Tell Tommy to forget it. I'll take care of your paper route today."

Family Members' Expectations

All individuals have some expectations about the outcomes of the life situations they experience. These expectations are related to and significantly influenced by earlier life experiences. In functional families, expectations are realistic, thereby avoiding setting up members for failure. In functional families, expectations are also flexible. Life situations are full of extraneous and unexpected interferences. Flexibility allows for changes and interruptions to occur without creating conflict. Finally, in functional families, expectations are individualized. Each family member is different, with different strengths and limitations. The outcome of a life situation for one family member may not be realistic for another. Each member must be valued independently, and comparison among members must be avoided.

Behaviors that interfere with adaptive functioning in terms of member expectations include the following:

Ignoring Individuality

When family members are expected to perform or behave in ways that undermine their individuality or do not suit their current life situation, their individuality is being ignored. This sometimes happens when parents expect their children to fulfill the hopes and dreams the parents have failed to achieve, yet the children have their own, different hopes and dreams.

EXAMPLE

Bob, an only child, leaves for college next year. Bob's father, Robert, inherited a hardware store that was founded by Bob's great-grandfather and has been in the family for three generations. Robert expects Bob to major in business, work in the store after college, and take over the business when Robert retires. Bob, however, has a talent for writing, wants to major in communication, and wants to work in television news when he graduates. Robert sees this plan as a betrayal of the family.

Demanding Proof of Love

Boyer and Jeffrey (1994) state:

> Family members place expectations on others' behavior that are used as standards by which the expecting member determines how much the other members care for him or her. The message attached to these expectations is: "If you will not be as I wish you to be, you don't love me." (p. 32)

EXAMPLE

"If you don't take over the hardware store, you don't love me" is the message that Bob receives from his father in the previous example.

Handling Differences

It is difficult to conceive of two or more individuals living together who agree on everything all of the time. Serious problems in a family's functioning appear when differences become equated with disapproval or when disagreement is perceived as offensive. Members of a functional family understand that it is acceptable to disagree and deal with differences in an open, nonattacking manner. Members are willing to hear the other person's position, respect the other person's right to hold an opposing position, and work to modify the expectations on both sides of the issue in order to negotiate a workable solution.

Behaviors that interfere with successful family negotiations include the following:

Attacking

Personal attacks can occur when a difference of opinion deteriorates. One person may blame the other with insulting remarks, reminders of past transgressions may occur, and the situation intensifies with destructive expressions of anger and hurt.

EXAMPLE

When Nadya's husband, Denis, buys an expensive set of golf clubs, Nadya responds, "How could you do such a thing? You know we can't afford those! No wonder we don't have a nice house like all our friends. You spend all our money before we can save for a down payment. You're so selfish! We'll never have anything nice, and it's all your fault!"

Avoiding

With this tactic, differences are never acknowledged openly. The individual who disagrees avoids discussing it for fear that the other person will withdraw love or approval or become angry in response to the disagreement. Avoidance also occurs when an individual fears loss of control of his or her temper if the disagreement is brought out into the open.

EXAMPLE

Vicki and Clint have been married 6 months. This is Vicki's second marriage, and she has a 4-year-old son from her first marriage, Derek, who lives with her and Clint. Both Vicki and Clint work, and Derek goes to day care. Since the marriage 6 months ago, Derek cries every night continuously unless Vicki spends all her time with him, which she does in order to keep him quiet. Clint resents this but says nothing for fear he will come across as interfering; however, he has started going back to work in his office in the evenings to avoid the family situation.

Surrendering

The person who surrenders in the face of disagreement does so at the expense of denying his or her own needs or rights. The individual avoids expressing a difference of opinion for fear of angering another person or of losing approval and support.

EXAMPLE

Elaine is the only child of wealthy parents. She attends an exclusive private college in a small New England town, where she met Andrew, the son of a farming couple from the area. Andrew attended the local community college for 2 years but chose to work on his parents' farm rather than continue college. Elaine and Andrew love each other and want to be married, but Elaine's parents say they will disown her if she marries Andrew, who they believe is below her social status. Elaine breaks off her relationship with Andrew rather than challenge her parents' wishes.

Family Interactional Patterns

Interactional patterns have to do with the ways in which families "behave." All families develop recurring, predictable patterns of interaction over time. These are often thought of as family rules. The mentality conveys, "This is the way we have always done it," and provides a sense of security and stability for family members that comes from predictability. These interactions may have to do with communication, self-concept reinforcement, expressing expectations, and handling differences (all of the behaviors that were discussed previously), but because they are repetitive and recur over time, they become the rules that govern patterns of interaction among family members.

Family rules are functional when they are workable, constructive, and promote the needs of all family members. They are dysfunctional when they become contradictory, self-defeating, and destructive. Family therapists often find that individuals are unaware that dysfunctional family rules exist and may vehemently deny their existence even when confronted with a specific behavioral interaction. The development of dysfunctional interactional patterns occurs through a habituation process and out of fear of change or reprisal or through a lack of knowledge as to how a given situation might be handled differently. Many are derived from the parents' own childhood experiences.

Patterns of interaction that interfere with adaptive family functioning include the following:

Patterns That Cause Emotional Discomfort

Interactions can promote hurt and anger in family members. This is particularly true of emotions that individuals feel uncomfortable expressing or are not permitted (according to family rules) to express openly. These interactional patterns include behaviors such as never apologizing or never admitting that one has made a mistake, forbidding flexibility in life situations ("You must do it my way, or you will not do it at all"), making statements that devalue the worth of others, or withholding statements that promote increased self-worth.

EXAMPLE

Priscilla and Bill had been discussing buying a new car but could not agree on the make or model to buy. One day, Bill appeared at Priscilla's office over the lunch hour and said,

"Come outside and see our new car." In front of the building, Bill had parked a brand new sports car that he explained he had purchased with their combined savings. Priscilla was furious but kept quiet and proceeded to finish her workday. At home she expressed her anger to Bill for making the purchase without consulting her. Bill refused to apologize or admit to making a mistake. They both remained cool and hardly spoke to each other for weeks.

Patterns That Perpetuate or Intensify Problems

When problems go unresolved over a long period of time, it sometimes appears to be easier just to ignore them. If problems of the same nature occur, the tendency to ignore them then becomes the safe and predictable pattern of interaction for dealing with this type of situation. This may occur until the problem intensifies to a point when it can no longer be ignored.

EXAMPLE

Dan works hard in the automobile factory and demands peace and quiet from his family when he comes home from work. His children have learned over the years not to share their problems with him because they fear his explosive temper. Their mother attempts to handle unpleasant situations alone as best she can. When son Ron was expelled from school for being caught smoking pot for the third time, Dan yelled, "Why wasn't I told about this before?"

Patterns That Are in Conflict With Each Other

Some family rules may appear to be functional—very workable and constructive—on the surface, but in practice they may serve to destroy healthy interactional patterns. Boyer and Jeffrey (1994) describe the following scenario as an example.

EXAMPLE

Dad insists that all members of the family eat dinner together every evening. No one may leave the table until everyone is finished because dinnertime is one of the few times left when the family can be together. Yet Dad frequently uses the time to reprimand Bobby about his poor grades in math, to scold Ann for her sloppy room, or to make not-so-subtle gibes at Mom for "spending all day on the telephone and never getting anything accomplished."

Family Climate

The atmosphere or climate of a family is composed of a blend of the feelings and experiences that result from family members' verbal and nonverbal sharing and interacting. A positive family climate is founded on trust and reflected in open communication, joyfulness and laughter, expressions of caring and mutual respect, the valuing of each individual as unique, and a general feeling of security and well-being. In a dysfunctional family, the climate is evidenced by tension, frustration, guilt, anger and resentment, depression, and despair.

CORE CONCEPT

Family Therapy

A type of therapeutic modality in which the focus of treatment is on the family as a unit. It represents a form of intervention in which members of a family are assisted to identify and change problematic, maladaptive, self-defeating, repetitive relationship patterns (Goldenberg, Goldenberg, & Pelavin, 2013).

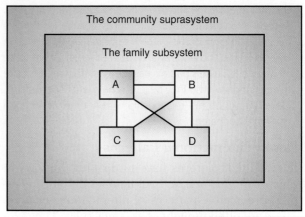

Key:

A = Father subsystem	CD = Sibling subsystem
B = Mother subsystem	AD = Parent-child subsystem
C = Child subsystem	BC = Parent-child subsystem
D = Child subsystem	AC = Parent-child subsystem
AB = Marital subsystem	BD = Parent-child subsystem

FIGURE 11–1 A hierarchy of systems.

Therapeutic Modalities With Families

While family therapy is reserved for the advanced practice psychiatric nurse, the theoretical foundations for family therapy are useful to the generalist nurse for understanding and assessing family dynamics and making appropriate referrals when family dysfunction is identified.

The Family as a System

General systems theory is a way of organizing thought according to the holistic perspective. A system is considered greater than the sum of its parts. A system is considered dynamic and ever changing. A change in one part of the system causes a change in the other parts of the system and in the system as a whole. When studying families, it is helpful to conceptualize a hierarchy of systems.

The family can be viewed as a system composed of various **subsystems,** such as the marital subsystem, parent-child subsystems, and sibling subsystems. Each of these subsystems is further divided into subsystems of individuals. The family system is also a subsystem of a larger suprasystem, such as the neighborhood or community. A schematic of a hierarchy of systems is presented in Figure 11–1.

Major Concepts

Bowen (1978) did a great deal of work with families using a systems approach. Bowen's theoretical approach to family therapy is composed of eight major concepts: (1) differentiation of self, (2) triangles, (3) nuclear family emotional process, (4) family projection process, (5) multigenerational transmission process, (6) sibling position, (7) emotional cutoff, and (8) societal emotional process.

Differentiation of Self

Differentiation of self is the ability to define oneself as a separate being. The Bowen theory suggests that "a person with a well-differentiated self recognizes his [or her] realistic dependence on others, but can stay calm and clear headed enough in the face of conflict, criticism, and rejection to distinguish thinking rooted in a careful assessment of the facts from thinking clouded by emotionality" (Bowen Center, 2016a).

The degree of differentiation of self can be viewed on a continuum from high levels, in which an individual manifests a clearly defined sense of self, to low or undifferentiated levels, in which emotional fusion exists and the individual is unable to function separately from a relationship system. Healthy families encourage differentiation, and the process of separation from the family ego mass is most pronounced during the ages of 2 to 5 and again between the ages of 13 and 15. Families that do not understand the child's need to be different during these times may perceive the child's behavior as objectionable.

Bowen (1971) used the term *stuck-togetherness* to describe the family with the fused ego mass. When family fusion occurs, none of the members has a true sense of self as an independent individual. Boundaries between members are blurred, and the family becomes enmeshed without individual distinguishing characteristics. In this situation, family members can neither gain true intimacy nor separate and become individuals.

Triangles

The concept of **triangles** refers to a three-person emotional configuration that is considered a significant element in evaluating the communication, behavior, and relationships within the family system. Bowen (1978) offers the following description of triangles:

The basic building block of any emotional system is the triangle. When emotional tension in a two-person system exceeds a certain level, it triangles in a third person, permitting the tension to shift about within the triangle. Any two in the original triangle can add a new triangle. An emotional system is composed of a series of interlocking triangles. (p. 306)

Triangles are dysfunctional in that they offer relief from anxiety through diversion rather than through resolution of the issue. To diffuse stress and conflict in a two-person relationship, one or both individuals may draw a third person into the mix either for sympathy or to deflect from the issues that are creating the stress between them (Nichols & Davis, 2017). When the dynamics within a triangle stabilize, a fourth person may be brought in to form additional triangles in an effort to reduce tension. This triangulation can continue almost indefinitely as extended family and people outside the family, including the family therapist, may become entangled in the process. The therapist working with families must strive to remain "de-triangled" from this emotional system.

Nuclear Family Emotional Process

The nuclear family emotional process describes the patterns of emotional functioning in a single generation. The nuclear family begins with a relationship between two people who form a couple. The most open relationship usually occurs during courtship, when most individuals choose partners with similar levels of differentiation. The lower the level of differentiation, the greater the possibility of problems in the future. A degree of fusion occurs with permanent commitment. This fusion results in anxiety and must be dealt with by each partner in an effort to maintain a healthy degree of differentiation.

Family Projection Process

Spouses who are unable to work through the undifferentiation or fusion that occurs with permanent commitment may project the resulting anxiety onto the children when they become parents. This occurrence is manifested as a father-mother-child triangle. These triangles are common and exist in various gradations of intensity in most families with children.

The child who becomes the target of the projection may be selected for various reasons:

- A particular child reminds one of the parents of an unresolved childhood issue.
- The child is of a particular gender or position in the family.
- The child is born with special needs.
- The parent has a negative attitude about the pregnancy.

This behavior is called **scapegoating.** It is harmful to both the child's emotional stability and his or her ability to function outside the family. A child who is scapegoated may become identified as "the problem child" and is vulnerable to accepting this label as his or her identity. The potential outcomes are risk for poor self-esteem, difficulty developing healthy relationships, and other emotional problems.

Multigenerational Transmission Process

Bowen (1978) described the multigenerational transmission process as the manner in which interactional patterns are transferred from one generation to another. Attitudes, values, beliefs, behaviors, and patterns of interaction are passed along from parents to children over many lifetimes, so that it becomes possible to show in a family assessment that a certain behavior has existed within a family through multiple generations.

Genograms A convenient way to plot a multigenerational assessment is with the use of **genograms.** Genograms offer the convenience of a great deal of information in a small amount of space. They can also be used as teaching tools with the family itself. An overall picture of the life of the family over several generations can be conveyed, including roles that various family members play as well as emotional distance between specific individuals. Areas for change can be easily identified. A sample genogram is presented in Figure 11–2.

Sibling Position

This view suggests that birth order in a family influences the development of predictable personality characteristics. For example, firstborn children are thought to be perfectionistic, reliable, and conscientious; middle children are described as independent, loyal, and intolerant of conflict; and youngest children tend to be charming, precocious, and gregarious (Leman, 2009). Bowen used this thesis to help determine levels of differentiation within a family and the possible direction of the family projection process. For example, if an oldest child exhibits characteristics more representative of a youngest child, there is evidence that this child may be the product of triangulation. Sibling position profiles are also used when studying multigenerational transmission processes and verifiable data are missing for certain family members.

Is there evidence to support profiled sibling personality traits based on birth order? The answer is complex. Hartshorne (2010) states that the majority of the 65,000 research studies on this topic are flawed and the remainder show no significant effect. Eckstein and Kaufman's work (2012) suggests that perceptions about roles and personality characteristics may be influenced by parents' expectations and stereotypes about birth-order related roles. Family size has been identified as a variable that matters; in two studies that were controlled for family size, Kristensen and Bjerkedal (2007) found a small but significant difference in IQ based on

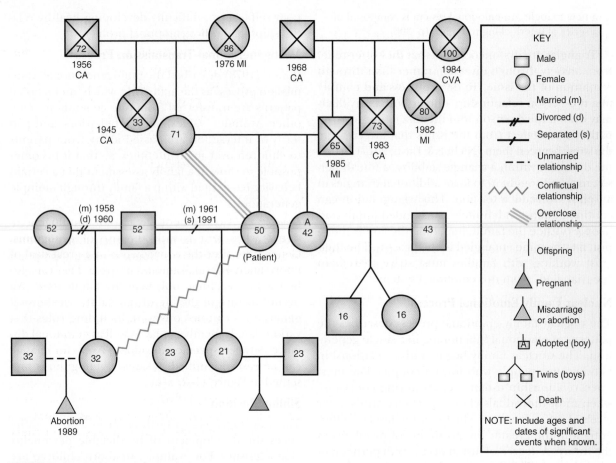

FIGURE 11–2 Sample genogram.

birth order, and Hartshorne, Salem-Hartshorne, and Hartshorne (2009) found that birth order influenced how individuals choose their friends and their spouses. When assessing a family to identify dysfunctions based on profiling sibling position, the nurse needs to consider many variables to make the best clinical judgment.

Emotional Cutoff

Emotional cutoff describes differentiation of self from the perception of the child. All individuals have some degree of unresolved emotional attachment to their parents, and the lower the level of differentiation, the greater the degree of unresolved emotional attachment.

Emotional cutoff has very little to do with how far away one lives from the family of origin. Individuals who live great distances from their parents can still be undifferentiated, whereas some individuals are emotionally cut off from their parents who live in the same town or even the same neighborhood.

Bowen (1976) suggests that emotional cutoff is the result of dysfunction within the family of origin in which fusion has occurred and that emotional cutoff promotes the same type of dysfunction in the new nuclear family. He contends that maintaining some emotional contact with the family of origin promotes healthy differentiation.

Societal Emotional Process

The Bowen theory views society as an emotional system. The concept of societal emotional process compares society's response to stress to the same type of response seen in individuals and families in response to emotional crisis: stress creates uncomfortable levels of anxiety that lead to hasty solutions, which add to the problems, and the cycle continues. This concept of Bowen's theory is explained as follows (Bowen Center, 2016b):

Human societies undergo periods of regression and progression in their history. The current regression seems related to factors such as the population explosion, a sense of diminishing frontiers, and the depletion of natural resources. The "symptoms" of societal regression include a growth of crime and violence, an increasing divorce rate, a more litigious attitude, a greater polarization between racial groups, less principled decision-making by leaders, the drug abuse epidemic, an increase in bankruptcy, and a focus on rights over responsibilities.

Goals and Techniques of Therapy

The goal of Bowen's systems approach to family therapy is to increase the level of differentiation of self while remaining in touch with the family system. The premise is that intense emotional problems within the nuclear family can be resolved only by resolving undifferentiated relationships with the family of origin. Emphasis is given to the understanding of past relationships.

The therapeutic role is that of "coach" or supervisor, and emotional involvement with the family is minimized. Therapist techniques include the following:

1. Defining and clarifying the relationship between the family members
2. Helping family members develop one-to-one relationships with each other and minimizing triangles within the system
3. Teaching family members about the functioning of emotional systems
4. Promoting differentiation by encouraging members to speak as individuals rather than as a family unit

The Structural Model

Structural family therapy is associated with a model developed by Minuchin (1974). In this model, the family is viewed as a social system within which the individual lives and to which the individual must adapt. The individual both contributes and responds to stresses within the family.

Major Concepts

Systems

The structural model views the family as a system. The structure of the **family system** is founded on a set of invisible principles that influence the interaction among family members. These principles concern how, when, and with whom to relate, and are established over time and through repeated transactions until they become rules that govern the conduct of various family members (Goldenberg, Stanton, & Goldenberg, 2016).

Transactional Patterns

Transactional patterns are the rules established over time that organize the ways in which family members relate to one another. A hierarchy of authority is one example of a transactional pattern. Usually, parents have a higher level of authority in a family than the children, so parental behavior reflects this role. A balance of authority may exist between husband and wife, or one may reflect a higher level than the other. These patterns of behavioral expectations differ from family to family and may trace their origin over generations of family negotiations.

Subsystems

Minuchin (1974) describes subsystems as smaller elements that make up the larger family system. Subsystems can be individuals or can consist of two or more persons united by gender, relationship, generation, interest, or purpose. A family member may belong to several subsystems at the same time, in which he or she may experience different levels of power and require different types of skills. For example, a young man has a different level of power and a different set of expectations in his father-son subsystem than in a subsystem with his younger brother.

Boundaries

Boundaries define the level of participation and interaction among subsystems. Boundaries are appropriate when they permit appropriate contact with others while preventing excessive interference. Clearly defined boundaries promote adaptive functioning. Maladaptive functioning can occur when boundaries are *rigid* or *diffuse*.

A rigid boundary is characterized by decreased communication and lack of support and responsiveness. Rigid boundaries prevent a subsystem (family member or subgroup) from achieving appropriate closeness or interaction with others in the system. Rigid boundaries promote **disengagement**, or extreme separateness, among family members.

A diffuse boundary is characterized by dependency and overinvolvement. Diffuse boundaries interfere with adaptive functioning because of the overinvestment, overinvolvement, and lack of differentiation between certain subsystems. Diffuse boundaries promote **enmeshment**, or exaggerated connectedness, among family members.

EXAMPLE

Sally and Jim have been married for 12 years, during which time they have tried without success to have children. Six months ago they were thrilled to have the opportunity to adopt a 5-year-old girl, Annie. Since both Sally and Jim have full-time teaching jobs, Annie stays with her maternal grandmother, Krista, during the day after she gets home from half-day kindergarten.

At first, Annie was a polite and obedient child. However, in the last few months, she has become insolent and oppositional and has temper tantrums when she cannot have her way. Sally and Krista agree that Annie should have whatever she desires and should not be punished for her behavior. Jim believes that discipline is necessary, but Sally and Krista refuse to enforce any guidelines he tries to establish. Annie is aware of this discordance and manipulates it to her full advantage.

In this situation, diffuse boundaries exist among the Sally-Krista-Annie subsystems. They have become enmeshed. They have also established a rigid boundary against Jim, disengaging him from the system.

Goal and Techniques of Therapy

The goal of structural family therapy is to facilitate change in the **family structure.** Family structure is changed with modification of the family principles, or transactional patterns, that are contributing to dysfunction within the family. The family is viewed as the unit of therapy, and all members are counseled together. Little, if any, time is spent exploring past experiences. The focus of structural therapy is on the present. Therapist techniques include the following:

■ **Joining the family:** The therapist must become a part of the family if restructuring is to occur. The therapist joins the family but maintains a leadership position. He or she may at different times join various subsystems within the family but ultimately includes the entire family system as the target of intervention.

■ **Evaluating the family structure:** Even though a family may come for therapy because of the behavior of one family member (the identified patient), the family as a unit is considered problematic. The family structure is evaluated by assessing transactional patterns, system flexibility and potential for change, boundaries, family developmental stage, and role of the identified patient within the system.

■ **Restructuring the family:** An alliance or contract for therapy is established with the family. By becoming an actual part of the family, the therapist is able to manipulate the system and facilitate the circumstances and experiences that can lead to structural change.

The Strategic Model

The strategic model of family therapy uses the interactional or communications approach. Communication theory is viewed as the foundation for this model. Communication is the actual transmission of information among individuals. All behavior sends a message, so all behavior in the presence of two or more individuals is communication. In this model, families considered to be functional are open systems where clear and precise messages, congruent with the situation, are sent and received. Healthy communication patterns promote nurturance and individual self-worth. Dysfunctional families are viewed as partially closed systems in which communication is vague and messages are often inconsistent and incongruent with the situation. Destructive patterns of communication tend to inhibit healthful nurturing and decrease individual feelings of self-worth.

Major Concepts

Double-Bind Communication

Double-bind communication occurs when a statement is made and succeeded by a contradictory statement. It also occurs when a statement is made accompanied by nonverbal expression that is inconsistent with the verbal communication. These incompatible communications can interfere with ego development in an individual and promote mistrust of all communications. Double-bind communication often results in a "damned if I do and damned if I don't" situation.

EXAMPLE

A mother freely gives and receives hugs and kisses from her 6-year-old son some of the time, while at other times she pushes him away saying, "Big boys don't act like that." The little boy receives a conflicting message and is presented with an impossible dilemma: "To please my mother I must not show her that I love her, but if I do not show her that I love her, I'm afraid I will lose her."

Pseudomutuality and Pseudohostility

A healthy, functioning individual is able to relate to other people while still maintaining a sense of separate identity. In a dysfunctional family, patterns of interaction may be reflected in the remoteness or closeness of relationships. These relationships may reflect erratic interaction (i.e., sometimes remote and sometimes close) or inappropriate interaction (i.e., excessive closeness or remoteness).

Pseudomutuality and pseudohostility are seen as collective defenses against the reality of the underlying meaning of the relationships in a dysfunctional family system. **Pseudomutuality** is characterized by a facade of mutual regard. Emotional investment is directed at maintaining outward representation of reciprocal fulfillment rather than in the relationship itself. The style of relating is fixed and rigid and allows family members to deny underlying fears of separation and hostility.

EXAMPLE

Janet, age 16, is the only child of State Senator J. and his wife. Janet was recently involved in a joyriding experience with a group of teenagers her parents call "the wrong crowd." In family therapy, Mrs. J. says, "We have always been a close family. I can't imagine why she is doing these things." Senator J. states, "I don't know another colleague who has a family that is as close as mine." Janet responds, "Yes, we are close. I just don't see my parents very much. Dad has been in politics since I was a baby, and Mom is always with him. I wish I could spend more time with them. But we are a close family."

Pseudohostility is also a fixed and rigid style of relating, but the facade being maintained is that of a state of chronic conflict and alienation among family members. This relationship pattern allows family members to deny underlying fears of tenderness and intimacy.

EXAMPLE

Jack, 14, and his sister Jill, 15, will have nothing to do with each other. When they are together, they can agree on nothing, and the barrage of put-downs is constant. This behavior reflects pseudohostility used by individuals who are afraid to reveal feelings of intimacy.

Schism and Skew

Lidz and associates (1957) observed two patterns within families that relate to a dysfunctional marital dyad. A **marital schism** is defined as "a state of severe chronic disequilibrium and discord, with recurrent threats of separation." Each partner undermines the other, mutual trust is absent, and a competition exists for closeness with the children. Often a partner establishes an alliance with his or her parent against the spouse. Children lack appropriate role models. **Marital skew** describes a relationship in which there is lack of equal partnership. One partner dominates the relationship and the other partner. The marriage remains intact as long as the passive partner allows the domination to continue. Children also lack role models when a marital skew exists.

Goal and Techniques of Therapy

The goal of strategic family therapy is to create change in destructive behavior and communication patterns among family members. The identified family *problem* is the unit of therapy, and all family members need not be counseled together. In fact, strategic therapists may prefer to see subgroups or individuals separately in an effort to achieve problem resolution. Therapy is oriented in the present, and the therapist assumes full responsibility for devising an effective strategy for family change. Therapeutic techniques include the following:

■ **Paradoxical intervention:** A paradox can be called a contradiction in therapy, or "prescribing the symptom." With **paradoxical intervention,** the therapist requests that the family continue to engage in the behavior that they are trying to change. Alternatively, specific directions may be given for continuing the defeating behavior. For example, a couple that regularly engages in insulting shouting matches is instructed to have one of these encounters on Tuesdays and Thursdays from 8:30 to 9 p.m. Boyer and Jeffrey (1994) explained this technique in the following manner:

A family using its maladaptive behavior to control or punish other people loses control of the situation when it finds itself continuing the behavior under a therapist's direction and being praised for following instructions. If the family disobeys the therapist's instruction, the price it pays is sacrificing the old behavior pattern and experiencing more satisfying ways of interacting with one another. A family that maintains

it has no control over its behavior, or whose members contend that others must change before they can themselves suddenly finds itself unable to defend such statements. (p. 125)

■ **Reframing:** Goldenberg and associates (2016) describe **reframing** as "relabeling problematic behavior by viewing it in a new, more positive light that emphasizes its good intention." Therefore, with reframing, the *behavior* may not actually change, but the *consequences* of the behavior may change because of a change in the meaning attached to the behavior. This technique is sometimes referred to as *positive reframing.*

EXAMPLE

Tom has a construction job and makes a comfortable living for his wife, Sue, and their two children. Tom and Sue have been arguing a lot and came to the therapist for counseling. Sue says Tom frequently drinks too much and is often late getting home from work. Tom counters, "I never used to drink on my way home from work, but Sue started complaining to me the minute I walked in the door about being so dirty and about tracking dirt and mud on 'her nice, clean floors.' It was the last straw when she made me undress before I came in the house and leave my dirty clothes and shoes in the garage. I thought a man's home was his castle. Well, I sure don't feel like a king. I need a few stiff drinks to face her nagging!"

The therapist used reframing to attempt change by helping Sue to view the situation in a more positive light. He suggested to Sue that she try to change her thinking by focusing on how much her husband must love her and her children to work as hard as he does. He asked her to focus on the dirty clothes and shoes as symbols of his love for them and to respond to his "dirty" arrivals home with greater affection. This positive reframing set the tone for healing and for increased intimacy within the marital relationship.

The Evolution of Family Therapy

Bowen's family theory and the structural and strategic models are sometimes referred to as basic models of family therapy.

While some family therapists adhere to a specific theoretical framework, Nichols (2017) suggested that contemporary family therapists "borrow from each other's arsenal of techniques." The basic models described here have provided a foundation for the progression and growth of the discipline of family therapy. Examples of newer models include the following:

■ **Narrative therapy:** Narrative therapy is an approach to treatment that emphasizes the role of the stories people construct about their experience (Nichols, 2016).

■ **Feminist family therapy:** This form of family therapy employs a collaborative, egalitarian, nonsexist intervention, applicable to both men and women, addressing family gender roles, patriarchal attitudes, and social and economic inequalities in male-female relationships (Goldenberg et al., 2016).

- **Social constructionist therapy:** Social constructionist therapy shifts attention away from an inspection of the origin or the exact nature of a family's presenting problems to an examination of the stories (interpretations, explanations, theories about relationships) family members have told themselves that account for how they have lived their lives. Social constructionist therapists are particularly interested in expanding clients' rigid and inflexible views of the world (Goldenberg et al., 2016).

- **Psychoeducational family therapy:** This type of family therapy emphasizes educating family members to help them understand and cope with a seriously disturbed family member While family therapists may use a psychoeducational approach in treatment, psychiatric-mental health registered nurses also use psychotherapeutic education strategies with individual clients and with families (American Nurses' Association, American Psychiatric Nurses Association, & International Society of Psychiatric-Mental Health Nurses, 2014). When provided with supportive education about mental illness and management strategies, families can have an important impact on patient recovery. In one recent 14-year follow-up study (Ran et al., 2015), researchers found that in families where psychoeducational family interventions were used for patients with schizophrenia, patient adherence to treatment and social functioning maintained enduring improvement over the course of the study.

The goal of family therapy, in general, is to promote change and improve adaptive functioning within the context of the family. Since nurses interact with families in most health-care settings, understanding these frameworks for assessing and intervening with families is an important aspect of every nurse's knowledge base.

The Nursing Process–A Case Study

Assessment

Wright and Leahey (2013) have developed the Calgary Family Assessment Model (CFAM), a multidimensional model originally adapted from a framework developed by Tomm and Sanders (1983). The CFAM consists of three major categories: structural, developmental, and functional. Wright and Leahey (2013) state:

> Each category contains several subcategories. It is important for each nurse to decide which subcategories are relevant and appropriate to explore and assess with each family at each point in time—that is, not all subcategories need to be assessed at a first

meeting with a family, and some subcategories need never be assessed. If the nurse uses too many subcategories, he or she may become overwhelmed by all the data. If the nurse and the family discuss too few subcategories, each may have a distorted view of the family's strengths or problems and the family situation. (pp. 51–52)

A diagram of the CFAM is presented in Figure 11–3. The three major categories are listed, along with the subcategories for assessment under each. This diagram is used to assess the Marino family, a case study presented in Box 11–1.

Structural Assessment

A graphic representation of the Marino family structure is presented in the genogram in Figure 11–4.

Internal Structure

The Marino family consists of a husband, wife, and their biological son and daughter who live together in the same home. They conform to the traditional gender roles. John is the eldest child from a rather large family, and Nancy has no siblings. In this family, their son, Peter, is the firstborn, and his sister, Anna, is 2 years younger. Neither spousal, sibling, nor spousal-sibling subsystems appear to be close in this family, and some are clearly conflictual. Problematic subsystems include John-Nancy, John-Nancy-children, and Nancy-Ethel. The subsystem boundaries are quite rigid, and the family members appear to be emotionally disengaged from one another.

External Structure

This family has ties to extended family, although the availability of support is questionable. Nancy's parents offered little emotional support to her as a developing child. They never approved of her marriage to John and still remain distant and cold. John's family consists of a father, mother, two brothers, and two sisters. They are warm and supportive most of the time, but cultural influences interfere with their understanding of this current situation. At this time, the Marino family is probably receiving the most support from health-care professionals who have intervened during Anna's hospitalization.

Context

John is a second-generation Italian American. His family of origin is large, warm, and supportive. However, John's parents believe that family problems should be dealt with in the family, and they disapprove of bringing "strangers" in to hear what they consider to be private information. They believe that Anna's physical condition should be stabilized, and then she should be discharged to deal with family problems at home.

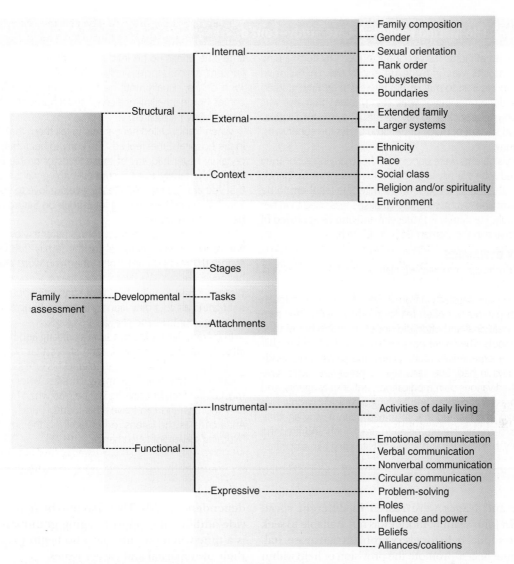

FIGURE 11–3 Branching diagram of the Calgary Family Assessment Model (CFAM). (From Wright, L. M., & Leahey, M. [2013]. *Nurses and families: A guide to family assessment and intervention* [6th ed.]. Philadelphia: F.A. Davis Company, with permission.)

BOX 11–1 **The Marino Family–A Case Study**

John and Nancy Marino have been married for 19 years. They have a 17-year-old son, Peter, and a 15-year-old daughter, Anna. Anna was recently hospitalized for taking an overdose of fluoxetine, her mother's prescription antidepressant. The family is attending family therapy sessions while Anna is in the hospital. Anna states, "I just couldn't take the fighting anymore! Our house is an awful place to be. Everyone hates each other, and everyone is unhappy. Dad drinks too much, and Mom is always sick! Peter stays away as much as he can and I don't blame him. I would too if I had someplace to stay. I just thought I'd be better off dead."

John Marino, age 44, is the oldest of five children. His father, Paulo, age 66, is a first-generation Italian American whose parents emigrated from Italy in the early 1900s. Paulo retired last year after 32 years as a cutter in a meatpacking plant.

His wife, Carla, age 64, has never worked outside the home. John and his siblings all worked at minimum-wage jobs during high school, and John and his two brothers worked their way through college. His two sisters married young, and both are housewives and mothers. John was able to go to law school with the help of loans, grants, and scholarships. He has held several positions since graduation and is currently employed as a corporate attorney for a large aircraft company.

Nancy, age 43, is the only child of Sam and Ethel Jones. Sam, age 67, inherited a great deal of money from his family who had been in the shipping business. He is currently the chief executive officer of this business. Ethel, also 67, was an aspiring concert pianist when she met Sam. She chose to give up her career for marriage and family, although Nancy believes her mother always resented doing so. Nancy was

Continued

BOX 11–1 **The Marino Family–A Case Study–cont'd**

reared in an affluent lifestyle. She attended private boarding schools as she was growing up and chose an exclusive college in the East to pursue her interest in art. She studied in Paris during her junior year. Nancy states that she was never emotionally close to her parents. They traveled a great deal, and she spent much of her time under the supervision of a nanny.

Nancy's parents were opposed to her marrying John. They perceived John's family to be below their social status. Nancy, on the other hand, loved John's family. She felt them to be very warm and loving, so unlike what she was used to in her own family. Her family is Protestant and also disapproved of her marrying in the Roman Catholic Church.

FAMILY DYNAMICS

As their marriage progressed, Nancy's health became very fragile. She had continued her artistic pursuits but seemed to achieve little satisfaction from it. She tried to keep in touch with her parents but often felt spurned by them. They traveled a great deal and often did not even inform her of their whereabouts. They were not present at the birth of her children. She experiences many aches and pains and spends many days in bed. She sees several physicians, who have prescribed various pain medications, antianxiety agents, and antidepressants but can find nothing organically wrong. Five years ago, she learned that John had been having an affair with his secretary. He promised to break it off and fired the secretary, but Nancy has had difficulty trusting him since that

time. She brings up his infidelity whenever they have an argument, which is increasingly often lately. When he is home, John drinks, usually until he falls asleep. Peter frequently comes home smelling of alcohol and a number of times has been clearly intoxicated.

When Nancy called her parents to tell them that Anna was in the hospital, Ethel replied, "I'm sorry to hear that, dear. We certainly never had any of those kinds of problems on our side of the family. But I'm sure everything will be okay now that you are getting help. Please give our love to your family. Your father and I are leaving for Europe on Saturday and will be gone for 6 weeks."

Although more supportive, John's parents view this situation as somewhat shameful for the family. John's dad responded, "We had hard times when you were growing up, but never like this. We always took care of our own problems. We never had to tell a bunch of strangers about them. It's not right to air your dirty laundry in public. Bring Anna home. Give her your love and she will be okay."

In therapy, Nancy blames John's drinking and his admitted affair for all their problems. John states that he drinks because it is the only way he can tolerate his wife's complaining about his behavior and her many illnesses. Peter is very quiet most of the time but says he will be glad when he graduates in 4 months and can leave "this looney bunch of people." Anna cries as she listens to her family in therapy and says, "Nothing's ever going to change."

John and Nancy were reared in different social classes. In John's family, money was not available to seek out professional help for every problem that arose. Italian cultural beliefs promote the provision of help within the nuclear and extended family network. If outside counseling is sought, it is often with the family priest. John and Nancy did not seek this type of counseling because they no longer attend church regularly.

In Nancy's family, money was available to obtain the very best professional help at the first sign of trouble. However, Nancy's parents refused to acknowledge, both then and now, that any difficulty ever existed in their family situation.

The Marino family lives comfortably on John's salary as a corporate attorney. They have health insurance and access to any referrals that are deemed necessary. They are well educated but have been attempting to deny the dysfunctional dynamics that exist in their family.

Developmental Assessment

The Marino family falls within the "family with adolescents" stage of McGoldrick and associates' (2015) family life cycle. In this stage, parents are expected to respond to adolescents' requests for increasing independence while being available to continue to fulfill dependency needs. They may also be required to provide additional support to aging grandparents. This is a time when parents may also begin to reexamine their own marital and career issues.

The Marino family is not fulfilling the dependency needs of its adolescents; in fact, they may be establishing premature independence. The parents are absorbed in their own personal problems to the exclusion of their children. Peter responds to this neglect by staying away as much as possible, drinking with his friends, and planning to leave home at the first opportunity. Anna's attempted suicide is a cry for help. She has needs that are unfulfilled by her parents, and this crisis situation may be required for them to recognize that a problem exists. This may be the time when they begin to reexamine their unresolved marital issues. Extended family are still self-supporting and do not require assistance from John and Nancy at this time.

Functional Assessment

Instrumental Functioning

This family has managed to adjust to the maladaptive functioning in an effort to meet physical activities of daily living. They subsist on fast food, or sometimes

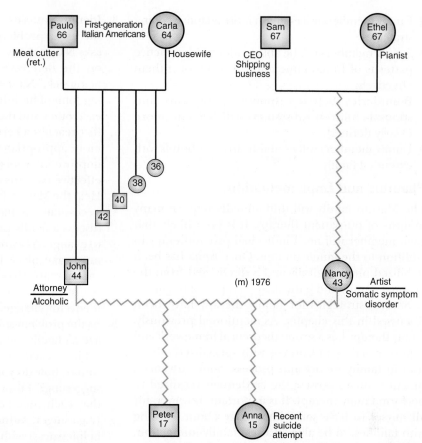

FIGURE 11–4 Genogram of the Marino family

Nancy or Anna will prepare a meal. Seldom do they sit down at table to eat together. Nancy must take pain medication or sedatives to sleep. John usually drinks himself to sleep. Anna and Peter take care of their own needs independently. Often they do not even see their parents in the evenings. Each manages to do fairly well in school. Peter says, "I don't intend to ruin my chances of getting out of this hell hole as soon as I can!"

Expressive Functioning

John and Nancy Marino argue a great deal about many topics. This family seldom shows affection to one another. Nancy and Anna express sadness with tears, whereas John and Peter have a tendency to withdraw or turn to alcohol when experiencing unhappiness. Nancy somaticizes her internal pain, and numbs this pain with medication. Anna internalized her emotional pain until it became unbearable. A notable lack of constructive communication is evident.

This family is unable to solve its problems effectively. In fact, it is unlikely that it has even identified its problems, which undoubtedly have been in existence for a long while. These problems have only recently been revealed in light of Anna's suicide attempt.

Diagnosis

The following nursing diagnoses were identified for the Marino family:

■ **Interrupted family processes** related to unsuccessful achievement of family developmental tasks and dysfunctional coping strategies evidenced by inability of family members to relate to each other in an adaptive manner; adolescents' unmet dependency needs; inability of family members to express a wide range of feelings and to send and receive clear messages.

■ **Disabled family coping** related to highly ambivalent family relationships and lack of support evidenced by inability to problem-solve; each member copes in response to dysfunctional family processes with destructive behavior (John drinks, Nancy somaticizes, Peter drinks and withdraws, and Anna attempts suicide).

Outcome Identification

The following criteria were identified as measurement of outcomes in counseling of the Marino family:

■ Family members will demonstrate effective communication patterns.

■ Family members will express feelings openly and honestly.

■ Family members will establish more adaptive coping strategies.

■ Family members will be able to identify destructive patterns of functioning and problem-solve them effectively.

■ Boundaries between spousal subsystems and spousal-children subsystems will become more clearly defined.

■ Family members will establish stronger bonds with extended family.

Planning and Implementation

The Marino family will undoubtedly require many months of outpatient therapy. It is even likely that each member will need individual psychotherapy in addition to the family therapy. Once Anna has been stabilized physiologically and is discharged from the hospital, family and individual therapy will begin.

Several strategies for family therapy have been discussed in this chapter. As mentioned previously, family therapy has a strong theoretical framework and is performed by individuals with specialized education in family theory and process. Some advanced practice nurses possess the credentials required to perform family therapy. It is important, however, for all nurses to have some knowledge about working with families, to be able to assess family interaction, and to recognize when problems exist.

Some interventions with the Marino family might include the following:

1. Create a therapeutic environment that fosters trust in which the family members can feel safe and comfortable. The nurse can promote this type of environment by being empathetic, listening actively (see Chapter 8, Therapeutic Communication), accepting feelings and attitudes, and being nonjudgmental.

2. Promote effective communication by
   a. Seeking clarification when vague and generalized statements are made (e.g., Anna states, "I just want my family to be like my friends' families." The nurse asks, "Anna, would you please explain to the group exactly what you mean by that?").
   b. Setting clear limits (e.g., "Peter, it is okay to state when you are angry about something that has been said. It is not okay to throw the chair against the wall").
   c. Being consistent and fair (e.g., "I encourage each of you to contribute to the group process and to respect one another's opportunity to contribute equally").
   d. Addressing each individual clearly and directly and encouraging family members to do the same (e.g., "Nancy, I think it would be more appropriate if you directed that statement to John instead of to me").

3. Identify patterns of interaction that interfere with successful problem resolution. For example, John asks Nancy many "Why?" questions that keep her on the defensive. He criticizes her for "always being sick." Nancy responds by frequently reminding John of his infidelity. Peter and Anna interrupt each other and their parents when the level of conflict reaches a certain point. Provide examples of more appropriate ways to communicate that can improve interpersonal relations and lead to more effective patterns of interaction.

4. Help the Marino family identify problems that may necessitate change. Encourage each member to discuss a family process that he or she would like to change. As a group, promote discussion of what must take place for change to occur and allow each member to explore whether he or she could realistically cooperate with the necessary requirements for change.

5. As the problem-solving process progresses, encourage all family members to express honest feelings. Address each one directly: "John (Nancy, Peter, Anna), how do you feel about what the others are suggesting?" Ensure that all participants understand that each member may express honest feelings (e.g., anger, sadness, fear, anxiety, guilt, disgust, helplessness) without criticism, judgment, or fear of personal reprisal.

6. Avoid becoming triangled in the family emotional system. Remain neutral and objective. Do not take sides in family disagreements; instead, provide alternative explanations and suggestions (e.g., "Perhaps we can look at that situation in a different light . . .").

7. Reframe vague problem descriptions into ones for which resolution is more realistic. For example, rather than defining the problem as "We don't love each other anymore," the problem could be defined as "We do not spend time together in family activities anymore." This definition evolves from the family members' description of what they mean by the more general problem description.

8. Discuss present coping strategies. Encourage each family member to describe how he or she copes with stress and with the adversity within the family. Explore each member's possible contribution to the family's problems. Encourage family members to discuss possible solutions among themselves.

9. Identify community resources that may assist individual family members and provide support for establishing more adaptive coping mechanisms. For example, Alcoholics Anonymous for John, Al-Anon for Nancy, and Alateen for Peter and Anna. Other groups that may be of assistance to this family include Emotions Anonymous, Parents

Support Group, Families Helping Families, Marriage Enrichment, Parents of Teenagers, and We Saved Our Marriage (WESOM). Local self-help networks often provide a directory of resources within specific communities.

10. Discuss with the family the possible need for psychotherapy for individual members. Provide names of therapists who would perform assessments to determine individual needs. Encourage follow-through with appointments.

11. Assist family members in planning leisure time activities together. This could include time to play together, exercise together, or engage in a shared project.

Evaluation

Evaluation is the final step in the nursing process. In this step, progress toward attainment of outcomes is measured.

1. Do family members demonstrate effective patterns of communication?

2. Can family members express feelings openly and honestly without fear of reprisal?

3. Can family members accept their own personal contributions to the family's problems?

4. Can individual members identify maladaptive coping methods and express a desire to improve?

5. Do family members work together to solve problems?

6. Can family members identify resources in the community from which they can seek assistance and support?

7. Do family members express a desire to form stronger bonds with the extended family?

8. Are family members willing to seek individual psychotherapy?

9. Are family members pursuing shared activities?

Summary and Key Points

■ Nurses must have sufficient knowledge of family functioning to assess family interaction and recognize when problems exist.

■ McGoldrick and associates (2015) identify the following stages that describe the family life cycle:
  ▪ The single young adult
  ▪ The family joined through marriage/union
  ▪ The family with young children
  ▪ The family with adolescents
  ▪ The family launching children and moving on in midlife
  ▪ The family in later life (late middle age to end of life)

■ Tasks of families experiencing divorce and remarriage, and those that vary according to cultural norms, are also important to understand as the demographics of family life continue to change in society.

■ Families are assessed as functional or dysfunctional on the basis of the following six elements: communication, self-concept reinforcement, family members' expectations, handling differences, family interactional patterns, and family climate.

■ Bowen viewed the family as a system that was composed of various subsystems. His theoretical approach to family therapy includes eight major concepts: differentiation of self, triangles, nuclear family emotional process, family projection process, multigenerational transmission process, sibling position, emotional cutoff, and societal emotional process.

■ In the structural model of family therapy, the family is viewed as a social system within which the individual lives and to which the individual must adapt.

■ In the strategic model of family therapy, communication is viewed as the foundation of functioning. Functional families are open systems where clear and precise messages are sent and received. Dysfunctional families are viewed as partially closed systems in which communication is vague, and messages are often inconsistent and incongruent with the situation.

■ Many family therapists today follow an eclectic approach and incorporate concepts from several models into their practices.

■ The nursing process is used as a framework for assessing, diagnosing, planning, implementing, and evaluating care to families who require assistance to maintain or regain adaptive functioning.

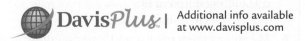 DavisPlus ™ | Additional info available at www.davisplus.com

Review Questions
Self-Examination/Learning Exercise

Select the answer that is most appropriate for each of the following questions.

1. The nurse-therapist is counseling the Smith family: Mr. and Mrs. Smith, 10-year-old Rob, and 8-year-old Lisa. When Mr. and Mrs. Smith start to argue, Rob hits Lisa and Lisa starts to cry. The Smiths then turn their attention to comforting Lisa and scolding Rob, complaining that he is "out of control and we don't know what to do about his behavior." These dynamics are an example of which of the following?
   a. Double-bind messages
   b. Triangulation
   c. Pseudohostility
   d. Multigenerational transmission

2. Using Bowen's systems approach with a family in therapy, the therapist would:
   a. Try to change family principles that may be promoting dysfunctional behavior patterns.
   b. Strive to create change in destructive behavior through improvement in communication and interaction patterns.
   c. Encourage increase in the differentiation of individual family members.
   d. Promote change in dysfunctional behavior by encouraging the formation of more diffuse boundaries between family members.

3. Using the structural approach with a family in therapy, the therapist would:
   a. Try to change family principles that may be promoting dysfunctional behavior patterns.
   b. Strive to create change in destructive behavior through improvement in communications and interaction patterns.
   c. Encourage increase in the differentiation of individual family members.
   d. Promote change in dysfunctional behavior by encouraging the formation of more diffuse boundaries between family members.

4. Using the strategic approach with a family in therapy, the therapist would:
   a. Try to change family principles that may be promoting dysfunctional behavior patterns.
   b. Strive to create change in destructive behavior through improvement in communication and interaction patterns.
   c. Encourage increase in the differentiation of individual family members.
   d. Promote change in dysfunctional behavior by encouraging the formation of more diffuse boundaries between family members.

5. Emma, a nurse in a family medicine outpatient clinic, conducts initial interviews when new families are referred. She has just finished interviewing a mother who has come to the clinic with her three children, ages 5, 7, and 11. The mother says to the oldest child, "You have been such a help to me, playing with your brothers while I talk to the nurse." In assessing family interaction, the nurse recognizes this statement as a direct indicator of which of the following?
   a. Family climate
   b. Family members' expectations
   c. Handling differences
   d. Self-concept reinforcement

6. The intermittent exiting and entering of various family members and reestablishing of the bond of the dyadic marital relationship are characteristics associated with which stage of family development?
   a. The newly married couple
   b. The family with adolescents
   c. The family launching grown children
   d. The family in later life

Review Questions—cont'd
Self-Examination/Learning Exercise

7. The nurse psychotherapist is working with the Juarez family in the outpatient mental health clinic. The husband says, "We can't agree on anything! And it seems like every time we disagree on something, it ends up in a screaming match." Which of the following prescriptions by the nurse represents a paradoxical intervention for the Jones family?
   a. Mr. and Mrs. Juarez must not have a disagreement for one full day.
   b. Mr. and Mrs. Juarez will yell at each other on Tuesdays and Thursdays from 8 p.m. until 8:10 p.m.
   c. Mr. and Mrs. Juarez must refrain from yelling at each other until the next counseling session.
   d. Mr. and Mrs. Juarez must not discuss serious issues until they can do so without yelling at each other.

8. Mr. and Mrs. Jones have been married for 21 years. Mr. Jones is the family breadwinner, and Mrs. Jones has never worked outside the home. Mr. Jones has always made all the decisions for the family, and Mrs. Jones has always been compliant. According to the strategic model of family therapy, this is an example of which of the following?
   a. Marital schism
   b. Pseudomutuality
   c. Marital skew
   d. Pseudohostility

9. Jack and Ann have come to the clinic for family therapy. They have been married for 18 years. Jack had an affair with his secretary 5 years ago. He fired the secretary and assures Ann and the nurse that he has been faithful ever since. Jack tells the nurse, "We have never been able to get along with each other. We can't talk about anything—all we do is shout at each other. And every time she gets angry with me, she brings up my infidelity. I can't even imagine how many times each of us has threatened divorce over the years. Our kids don't have any idea what it is like to have parents who get along with each other. I've really had enough!" The nurse would most likely document which of the following in her assessment of this couple?
   a. Marital skew
   b. Pseudohostility
   c. Double-bind communication
   d. Marital schism

10. Mr. and Mrs. Smith and their three children (ages 5, 8, and 10) are in therapy with the nurse psychotherapist. Mrs. Smith tells the nurse that their marriage has been "falling apart" since the birth of their youngest child, Tom. She explains that they "did not want a third child, and I became pregnant even after my husband had undergone a vasectomy. We were very angry, the pregnancy was a problematic one, and the child has been difficult since birth. We had problems before he was born, but since Tom was born, things have gone from bad to worse. No one can control him, and he is wrecking our family!" The nurse assesses that which of the following may be occurring in this family?
    a. Scapegoating
    b. Triangling
    c. Disengagement
    d. Enmeshment

References

American Nurses' Association (ANA), American Psychiatric Nurses Association, & International Society of Psychiatric-Mental Health Nurses. (2014). *Psychiatric-mental health nursing: Scope and standards of practice* (2nd ed.). Silver Spring, MD: ANA.

Bowen Center. (2016a). Bowen theory: Differentiation of self. Retrieved from www.thebowencenter.org/pages/conceptds.html

Bowen Center. (2016b). Bowen theory: Societal emotional process. Retrieved from www.thebowencenter.org/pages/conceptsep.html

Boyer, P.A., & Jeffrey, R.J. (1994). *A guide for the family therapist.* Northvale, NJ: Jason Aronson.

Centers for Disease Control and Prevention. (2015). National vital statistics system: National marriage and divorce rate trends. (United States 2000–2014). Retrieved from www.cdc.gov/nchs/nvss/marriage_divorce_tables.htm

Chang, K. (2017). Chinese Americans. In J.N. Giger (Ed.), *Transcultural nursing: Assessment and intervention* (7th ed., pp. 383-402). St. Louis, MO: Mosby.

Cory, T.L. (2013). Second marriages—Think before you leap. *HealthScope.* Retrieved from http://www.healthscopemag.com/health-scope/second-marriages-think-before-you-leap/

Earp, J.B.K. (2017). Korean Americans. In J.N. Giger (Ed.), *Transcultural nursing: Assessment and intervention* (7th ed., pp. 534-553). St. Louis, MO: Mosby.

Eckstein, D., & Kaufman, J. A. (2012). The role of birth order in personality: An enduring intellectual legacy of Alfred Adler. *Journal of Individual Psychology, 68*(1), 60-74. doi:10.1037/gpr0000013

Goldenberg, I., Stanton, M., & Goldenberg, H. (2016). *Family therapy: An overview* (9th ed.). Belmont, CA: Brooks/Cole.

Goldenberg, I., Goldenberg, H., & Pelavin, E.G. (2013). Family therapy. In D. Wedding & R.J. Corsini (Eds.), *Current Psychotherapies* (10th ed., 373-407). Belmont, CA: Brooks/Cole.

Hartshorne, J.K. (2010). How birth order affects your personality. *Scientific American.* Retrieved from www.scientificamerican.com/article/ruled-by-birth-order

Hartshorne, J.K., Salem-Hartshorne, N., & Hartshorne, T.S. (2009). Birth order effects in the formation of long-term relationships. *Journal of Individual Psychology, 65*(2),156.

Kaakinen, J.R., & Hanson, S.M.H. (2015). Family health care nursing: An introduction. In J.R. Kaakinen, D.P. Coehlo, R. Steele, A. Tabacco, & S.M.H. Hanson (Eds.), *Family health care nursing* (5th ed., pp. 3-32). Philadelphia: F.A. Davis.

Kreider, R.M., & Ellis, R. (2011). *Living arrangements of children: 2009.* Current Population Reports, p. 70-126. Washington, DC: U.S. Census Bureau.

Kristensen, P., & Bjerkedal, T. (2007). Explaining the relation between birth order and intelligence. *Science, 316*(5832), 1717. doi:10.1126/science.1141493

Leman, K. (2009). *The birth order book: Why you are the way you are.* Grand Rapids, MI: Revell.

McGoldrick, M., Garcia-Preto, N. & Carter, B. (2015). *The expanding family life cycle: Individual, family, and social perspectives* (5th ed.). Boston: Allyn & Bacon.

Nichols, M.P. & Davis, S.D. (2017). *Family therapy: Concepts and methods* (11th ed.). Boston, MA: Pearson.

Pew Research Center. (2015). *The American family today.* Retrieved from www.pewsocialtrends.org/2015/12/17/1-the-american-family-today/

Purnell, L.D. (2013). The Purnell model for cultural competence. In L.D. Purnell (Ed.), *Transcultural health care: A culturally competent approach* (4th ed., pp. 15-44). Philadelphia: F.A. Davis.

Ran, M.S., Chan, C. L.-W., Ng, S.-M., Guo, L.-T., & Xiang, M.-Z. (2015). The effectiveness of psychoeducational family intervention for patients with schizophrenia in a 14 year follow-up study in a Chinese rural area. *Psychological Medicine, 45*(10), 2197-2204. doi:10.1017/S0033291715000197

The Stepfamily Foundation. (2016). *Stepfamily statistics.* Retrieved from www.stepfamily.org/stepfamily-statistics.html

Tomm, K., & Sanders, G. (1983). Family assessment in a problem oriented record. In J.C. Hansen & B.F. Keeney (Eds.), *Diagnosis and assessment in family therapy.* London: Aspen Systems.

U.S. Catholic Church. (2016). *Catechism of the Catholic Church* (2nd ed.) Washington, DC: USCCB Publishing.

U.S. Census Bureau. (2015). *One in five children receive food stamps, census bureau reports.* Retrieved from www.census.gov/newsroom/press-releases/2015/cb15-16.html

Valley, E. (2005). The changing nature of the Jewish family. *Contact: The Journal of Jewish Life Network, 7*(3), 1-16.

Wright, L.M., and Leahey, M. (2013). *Nurses and families: A guide to family assessment and intervention* (6th ed.). Philadelphia: F.A. Davis.

Classical References

Bowen, M. (1971). The use of family theory in clinical practice. In J. Haley (Ed.), *Changing families.* New York: Grune & Stratton.

Bowen, M. (1976). Theory in the practice of psychotherapy. In P. Guerin (Ed.), *Family therapy: Theory and practice.* New York: Gardner Press.

Bowen, M. (1978). *Family therapy in clinical practice.* New York: Jason Aronson.

Lidz, T., Cornelison, A., Fleck, S., & Terry, D. (1957). The intrafamilial environment of schizophrenic patients: II. Marital schism and marital skew. *American Journal of Psychiatry, 114,* 241-248. doi:http://dx.doi.org/10.1176/ajp.114.3.241

Minuchin, S. (1974). *Families and family therapy.* Cambridge, MA: Harvard University Press.

Milieu Therapy—The Therapeutic Community

CORE CONCEPTS

Milieu Therapy

KEY TERMS

milieu   therapeutic community

OBJECTIVES

After reading this chapter, the student will be able to:

1. Define *milieu therapy*.
2. Explain the goal of therapeutic community/milieu therapy.
3. Identify seven basic assumptions of a therapeutic community.
4. Discuss conditions that characterize a therapeutic community.
5. Identify the various therapies that may be included in the program of the therapeutic community and the health-care workers that make up the interdisciplinary treatment team.
6. Describe the role of the nurse on the interdisciplinary treatment team.

HOMEWORK ASSIGNMENT

Please read the chapter and answer the following questions:

1. How are unit rules established in a therapeutic community setting?
2. Which member of the interdisciplinary treatment team has a focus on rehabilitation and vocational training?
3. How are client responsibilities assigned in the therapeutic community setting?
4. Which member of the interdisciplinary treatment team serves as leader?

Standard 5F of the *Psychiatric-Mental Health Nursing: Scope and Standards of Practice* (American Nurses Association [ANA], American Psychiatric Nurses Association, & International Society of Psychiatric Nurses, 2014) states, "The psychiatric-mental health nurse provides, structures, and maintains a safe, therapeutic, and recovery-oriented environment in collaboration with healthcare consumers, families, and other healthcare clinicians" (p. 60).

This chapter defines and explains the goal of milieu therapy. The conditions necessary for a therapeutic environment are discussed, and the roles of the various health-care workers within the interdisciplinary team are delineated. An interpretation of the nurse's role in milieu therapy is included.

Milieu, Defined

The word **milieu,** French for "middle," is translated in English as "surroundings, or environment." In psychiatry, therapy involving the milieu, or environment, may be called milieu therapy, **therapeutic community,** or the therapeutic environment. The goal of milieu therapy is to manipulate the environment so that all aspects of the client's hospital experience are considered therapeutic. Within this therapeutic community setting, the client is expected to learn adaptive coping, interaction, and relationship skills that can be adapted to other aspects of his or her life.

CORE CONCEPT

Milieu Therapy

A scientific structuring of the environment in order to effect behavioral changes and improve the psychological health and functioning of the individual (Skinner, 1979).

Current Status of the Therapeutic Community

Milieu therapy came into its own from the 1960s through early 1980s. During this period, psychiatric inpatient treatment provided sufficient time to implement programs of therapy that were aimed at social rehabilitation. Lengths of stay averaged from 28 to 30 days for acute care hospitalizations and several months or years for long-term hospitalizations. Nursing's focus of establishing interpersonal relationships with clients fit well within this concept of therapy. Patients were encouraged to be active participants in their therapy, and individual autonomy was emphasized.

The current focus of inpatient psychiatric care has changed. Acute care hospitalization lengths of stay now average 2 to 3 days. Hall (1995) stated:

> Care in inpatient psychiatric facilities can now be characterized as short and biologically based. By the time patients have stabilized enough to benefit from the socialization that would take place in a milieu as treatment program, they [often] have been discharged. (p. 51)

Although strategies for milieu therapy are still used, they have been modified to conform to the short-term approach to care or to outpatient treatment programs. Some programs (e.g., those for children and adolescents, clients with substance addictions, and geriatric clients) have successfully adapted the concepts of milieu treatment to their specialty needs (Bowler, 1991; DeSocio, Bowllan, & Staschak, 1997; Jani & Fishman, 2004; Menninger Clinic, 2012; Whall, 1991).

Echternacht (2001) suggested that more emphasis should be placed on unstructured components of milieu therapy. She described these components as a multitude of complex interactions between clients, staff, and visitors that occur around the clock. Echternacht called these interactions "fluid group work." They involve spontaneous opportunities within the milieu environment for the psychiatric nurse to provide "on-the-spot therapeutic interventions designed to enhance socialization competency and interpersonal relationship awareness. Emphasis is on social skills and activities in the context of interpersonal interactions" (p. 40). With fluid group work, the nurse applies psychotherapeutic knowledge and skills to brief clinical encounters that occur spontaneously in the therapeutic milieu setting. Echternacht believes that by using these techniques, nurses can "reclaim their milieu therapy functions in the midst of a changing health care environment" (p. 40).

Many of the original concepts of milieu therapy are presented in this chapter. It is important to remember that modifications to these concepts are applied for practice in a variety of settings.

Basic Assumptions

Skinner (1979) outlined seven basic assumptions on which a therapeutic community is based:

1. **The health in each individual is to be realized and encouraged to grow.** All individuals are considered to have strengths as well as limitations. These healthy aspects of the individual are identified and serve as a foundation for personality growth and the ability to function adaptively and productively in all aspects of life.

2. **Every interaction is an opportunity for therapeutic intervention.** Within this structured setting, it is virtually impossible to avoid interpersonal interaction. The ideal situation exists for clients to improve communication and relationship development skills. Learning occurs from immediate feedback of personal perceptions.

3. **The client owns his or her own environment.** Clients should have the opportunity to make decisions and solve problems related to the environment (milieu) of the unit. In this way, personal needs for autonomy as well as needs that pertain to the group as a whole are fulfilled.

4. **Each client owns his or her own behavior.** Each individual within the therapeutic community is expected to take responsibility for his or her own actions.
5. **Peer pressure is a useful and powerful tool.** Behavioral group norms are established through peer pressure. Feedback is direct and frequent so that behaving in a manner acceptable to the other members of the community becomes essential.
6. **Inappropriate behaviors are dealt with as they occur.** Individuals examine the significance of their behavior, look at how it affects other people, and discuss more appropriate ways of behaving in certain situations.
7. **Restrictions and punishment are to be avoided.** Destructive behaviors can usually be controlled with group discussion. However, if an individual requires external controls, temporary isolation is preferred over lengthy restriction or other harsh consequences.

Conditions That Promote a Therapeutic Community

In a therapeutic community setting, the setting is the foundation, and everything that happens to the client or within the client's environment is considered part of the treatment program. Community factors—such as social interactions, the physical structure of the treatment setting, and schedule of activities—may generate negative responses from some clients. These stressful experiences are used as examples to help the client learn how to manage stress more adaptively in real-life situations.

Under what conditions, then, is a hospital environment considered therapeutic? A number of classic criteria have been identified, some of which today are relevant only to long-term hospital treatment programs in which client stays are at least a month:

1. **Basic physiological needs are fulfilled.** As Maslow (1968) suggested, individuals do not move to higher levels of functioning until the basic biological needs for food, water, air, sleep, exercise, elimination, shelter, and sexual expression have been met. These needs, of course, are relevant in hospital stays of any length. As mentioned previously, stabilization of biological and safety needs has become a primary goal of short-term, acute care psychiatric hospitalizations.
2. **The physical facilities are conducive to achievement of the goals of therapy.** Space is provided so that each client has sufficient privacy, as well as physical space for therapeutic interaction with others. Furnishings are arranged to present a homelike atmosphere—usually in spaces that accommodate communal living, dining, and activity areas—for facilitation of interpersonal interaction and communication. Physical space considerations are relevant in the therapeutic milieu of any psychiatric treatment setting because the promotion of therapeutic interaction is at the core of this type of therapy.
3. **A democratic form of self-government exists.** In the classic therapeutic community, clients participate in the decision-making and problem-solving that affect the management of the treatment setting. This is accomplished through regular community meetings. These meetings are attended by staff and clients, and all individuals have equal input into the discussions. At these meetings, the norms rule, and behavioral limits of the treatment setting are identified and discussed. This reinforces the democratic posture of the treatment setting, because these are expectations that affect all clients equally. An example might be the rule that no client may enter a room occupied by a client of the opposite gender. Reasons for expectations and consequences of violating the rules may also be discussed.

Other issues that may be discussed at the community meetings include those with which certain clients have disagreements. A democratic decision is then made by the entire group. For example, several clients in an inpatient unit may disagree with the hours designated for watching television on a weekend night. They may elect to bring up this issue at a community meeting and suggest an extension in television-viewing time. After discussion by the group, a vote will be taken, and clients and staff agree to abide by the expressed preference of the majority. Some therapeutic communities in long-term settings elect officers (usually a president and a secretary) who serve for a specified time period. The president calls the meeting to order, conducts the business of discussing old and new issues, and asks for volunteers (or makes appointments, alternately, so that all clients have a turn) to accomplish the daily tasks associated with community living, such as cleaning the tables after each meal and watering plants in the treatment facility. New assignments are made at each meeting.

The secretary reads the minutes of the previous meeting and takes minutes of the current meeting. Minutes are important in the event that clients have a disagreement about issues that were discussed at previous meetings. Minutes provide written evidence of decisions made by the group. In treatment settings where clients have short attention spans or disorganized thinking, meetings are brief. Business is generally limited to introductions and expectations of the here and now. Discussions also may include comments about a recent occurrence in the group or an issue a member is bothered by or has questions about. These meetings are usually facilitated by staff, although all clients have equal input into the discussions.

All clients are expected to attend the meetings. Exceptions are made when aspects of an individual's therapy interfere or take precedence. An explanation is made to clients present so that false perceptions of danger are not generated by another person's absence. All staff members are expected to attend the meetings unless client care precludes their attendance. Today, a formally structured self-government is feasible only in long-term hospital treatment programs. However, encouraging clients to engage in discussion and problem-solving with staff and other clients is relevant to the therapeutic milieu in any hospital treatment program.

4. **Responsibilities are assigned according to client capabilities.** Increasing self-esteem is an ultimate goal of the therapeutic community. Therefore, a client should not be set up for failure by being assigned a responsibility beyond his or her level of ability. By assigning responsibilities that promote achievement, self-esteem is enhanced. Consideration must also be given to times during which the client will show some regression in the treatment regimen. Adjustments in assignments should be made in a way that preserves self-esteem and provides for progression to greater degrees of responsibility as the client returns to previous level of functioning.

5. **A structured program of social and work-related activities is scheduled as part of the treatment program.** Each client's therapeutic program consists of group activities in which interpersonal interaction and communication with other individuals are emphasized. Time is also devoted to personal problems. Various group activities may be selected for clients with specific needs (e.g., an exercise group for a person who expresses anger inappropriately, an assertiveness group for a person who is passive-aggressive, or a stress-management group for a person who is anxious). A structured schedule of activities is the major focus of a therapeutic community. Through these activities, change in the client's personality and behavior can be achieved. New coping strategies are learned and social skills are developed. In the group situation, the client is able to practice what he or she has learned to prepare for transition to the general community.

6. **Community and family are included in the program of therapy in an effort to facilitate discharge from treatment.** An attempt is made to include family members and the community in the treatment program with respect to the client's rights and preferences for confidentiality. It is important to retain as many links as possible to the client's life outside of therapy. Family members are invited to participate in specific therapy groups and, in some instances, to share meals with the client in the communal dining room. Connection with community life may be maintained through client group activities, such as shopping, picnicking, attending movies, bowling, and visiting the zoo. Inpatient clients may be awarded passes to visit family and may participate in work-related activities, the length of time being determined by the activity and the client's condition. These connections with family and community facilitate the discharge process and may help to prevent the client from becoming too dependent on therapy.

The Program of Therapeutic Community

Care for clients in the therapeutic community is coordinated by an interdisciplinary treatment (IDT) team. An initial assessment is made by the admitting psychiatrist, nurse, or other designated admitting agent who, in collaboration with the client, establishes priorities for care. The IDT team then develops a comprehensive treatment plan and goals of therapy and assigns intervention responsibilities. (See Box 12–1 for a QSEN Teaching Strategy on Teamwork and Collaboration within the Interdisciplinary Treatment Team.) All members sign the treatment plan and meet regularly to update the plan as needed. Depending on the size of the treatment facility and scope of the therapy program, members representing a variety of disciplines may participate in the promotion of a therapeutic community. For example, an IDT team may include a psychiatrist, clinical psychologist, psychiatric clinical nurse specialist, psychiatric nurse, mental health technician, psychiatric social worker, occupational therapist, recreational therapist, art therapist, music therapist, psychodramatist, dietitian, and chaplain.

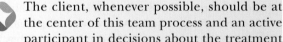 The client, whenever possible, should be at the center of this team process and an active participant in decisions about the treatment plan. The essence of patient-centered care emphasizes client involvement and decision-making authority unless the client's cognitive processes and decision-making are so impaired by illness that they are harmful to self or others. Table 12–1 provides an explanation of responsibilities and educational preparation required for professional members of the IDT team.

BOX 12–1 QSEN TEACHING STRATEGY

Assignment: Interviewing Members of the Interdisciplinary Team
The Process of Teamwork and Collaboration

Competency Domain: Teamwork and Collaboration, Safety

Learning Objectives: Student will:

• Explain the process for collaboration between nursing and other members of the interdisciplinary team.
• Identify different team members' responsibilities with regard to key safety issues such as suicide prevention, reporting to outside individuals/agencies regarding suspicions of abuse and duty to warn, and managing safety within the therapeutic milieu.
• Evaluate the contributions of each discipline within the interdisciplinary team to elements of milieu therapy.

Strategy Overview:

This assignment is meant to familiarize the student with the roles and responsibilities of various members of the interdisciplinary team and to evaluate the processes that promote teamwork and collaboration within milieu therapy. Students may be assigned to specific activities in preparation for a clinical conference discussion or asked to complete a reflective writing assignment on the function of the interdisciplinary treatment team in the provision of milieu therapy.

1. Attend an interdisciplinary treatment team meeting to evaluate individual disciplines' contributions and describe the process of collaboration.
2. Interview one or more members of the interdisciplinary team to identify their perceptions of how the process of collaboration works between their discipline and nursing. Sample questions might include the following:
   In what ways does your discipline collaborate with nursing?
   How effective is collaboration between disciplines within the IDT?
   What barriers exist to effective collaboration between disciplines?
   What is your disciplines role in
       Suicide prevention within the milieu?
       Reporting to outside individuals or agencies?
       Managing safety within the milieu?
3. Attend structured group activities to evaluate the contributions of various team members in promoting the therapeutic milieu.

TABLE 12–1 The Interdisciplinary Treatment Team in Psychiatry

TEAM MEMBER	RESPONSIBILITIES	CREDENTIALS
Psychiatrist	Serves as the leader of the team. Responsible for diagnosis and treatment of mental disorders. Performs psychotherapy; prescribes medication and other somatic therapies.	Medical degree with residency in psychiatry and license to practice medicine.
Clinical psychologist	Conducts individual, group, and family therapy. Administers, interprets, and evaluates psychological tests that assist in the diagnostic process.	Doctorate in clinical psychology with 2- to 3-year internship supervised by a licensed clinical psychologist. State license is required to practice
Psychiatric clinical nurse specialist	Conducts individual, group, and family therapy. Presents educational programs for nursing staff. Provides consultation services to nurses who require assistance in the planning and implementation of care for individual clients.	Registered nurse with minimum of a master's degree in psychiatric nursing. Some institutions require certification by national credentialing association.
Psychiatric nurse	Provides ongoing mental and physical assessment of client condition. Manages the therapeutic milieu on a 24-hour basis. Administers medications. Assists clients with all therapeutic activities as required. Focus is on one-to-one relationship development.	Registered nurse with hospital diploma, associate degree, or baccalaureate degree. Some psychiatric nurses have national certification.

Continued

TABLE 12–1 **The Interdisciplinary Treatment Team in Psychiatry—cont'd**		
TEAM MEMBER	RESPONSIBILITIES	CREDENTIALS
Mental health technician (also called psychiatric aide or assistant or psychiatric technician)	Functions under the supervision of the psychiatric nurse. Provides assistance to clients in the fulfillment of their activities of daily living. Assists activity therapists as required in conducting their groups. May also participate in one-to-one relationship development.	Varies by state. Requirements include high school education, with additional vocational education or on-the-job training. Some hospitals hire individuals with baccalaureate degree in psychology in this capacity. Some states require a licensure examination to practice.
Psychiatric social worker	Conducts individual, group, and family therapy. Is concerned with client's social needs, such as placement, financial support, and community requirements. Conducts in-depth psychosocial history on which the needs assessment is based. Works with client and family to ensure that requirements for discharge are fulfilled and needs can be met by appropriate community resources.	Minimum of a master's degree in social work. Some states require additional supervision and subsequent licensure by examination.
Occupational therapist	Works with clients to help develop (or redevelop) independence in performance of activities of daily living. Focus is on rehabilitation and vocational training in which clients learn to be productive, thereby enhancing self-esteem. Creative activities and therapeutic relationship skills are used.	Baccalaureate or master's degree in occupational therapy.
Recreational therapist	Uses recreational activities to promote clients to redirect their thinking or to rechannel destructive energy in an appropriate manner. Clients learn skills (e.g., bowling, volleyball, exercises, jogging) that can be used during leisure time and during times of stress following discharge from treatment. Some programs include activities such as picnics, swimming, and even group attendance at the state fair when it is in session.	Baccalaureate or master's degree in recreational therapy.
Music therapist	Encourages clients in self-expression through music. Clients listen to music, play instruments, sing, dance, and compose songs that help them get in touch with feelings and emotions that they may not be able to experience in any other way.	Graduate degree with specialty in music therapy.
Art therapist	Uses the client's creative abilities to encourage expression of emotions and feelings through artwork. Helps clients to analyze their own work in an effort to recognize and resolve underlying conflict.	Graduate degree with specialty in art therapy.
Psychodramatist	Directs clients in the creation of a "drama" that portrays real-life situations. Individuals select problems they wish to enact, and other clients play the roles of significant others in the situations. Some clients are able to "act out" problems that they are unable to work through in a more traditional manner. All members benefit through intensive discussion that follows.	Graduate degree in psychology, social work, nursing, or medicine with additional training in group therapy and specialty preparation to become a psychodramatist.
Dietitian	Plans nutritious meals for all clients. Consults with clients with specific eating disorders, such as anorexia nervosa, bulimia nervosa, obesity, and pica.	Baccalaureate or master's degree with specialty in dietetics.

TABLE 12–1	**The Interdisciplinary Treatment Team in Psychiatry—cont'd**	
TEAM MEMBER	RESPONSIBILITIES	CREDENTIALS
Chaplain	Assesses, identifies, and attends to the spiritual needs of clients and their family members. Provides spiritual support and comfort as requested by client or family. May provide counseling if educational background includes this type of preparation.	College degree with advanced education in theology, seminary, or rabbinical studies.

The Role of the Nurse in Milieu Therapy

One of the first nursing interventions in establishing a foundation for trust and maintaining a therapeutic milieu is orienting the new client to the environment, to his or her rights and responsibilities within the unit milieu, to the structured activities designed for personal growth, and to any limits or restrictions necessary to maintain safety. Availability to provide support and validation to clients throughout their treatment is also an essential nursing competency in milieu therapy (ANA et al., 2014), and this, too, is rooted in a trusting relationship. Active listening and inquiring about the client's expectations for treatment are key communication skills in providing support and validation and in establishing a foundation for patient-centered care.

Milieu therapy can take place in a variety of inpatient and outpatient settings. In the hospital, nurses are generally the only members of the IDT team who spend time with the clients on a 24-hour basis, and they assume responsibility for management of the therapeutic milieu. In all settings, the nursing process is used for the delivery of nursing care. In the management of the therapeutic milieu, the same model (ongoing assessment, diagnosis, outcome identification, planning, implementation, and evaluation) is necessary for effective treatment. Nurses are involved in all day-to-day activities that pertain to client care, and their suggestions and options are given serious consideration in care planning for individual clients. Information from the initial nursing assessment is used to create the IDT plan. Nurses have input into therapy goals and participate in the regular updates and modification of treatment plans.

In some treatment facilities, a separate nursing care plan is required in addition to the IDT plan. In this case, the nursing care plan must reflect diagnoses specific to nursing and include problems and interventions from the IDT plan that have been assigned to the nurse. Attention must be given to assure that the nursing care plan effectively collaborates with the IDT plan so that care is coordinated and consistent among team members.

In the therapeutic milieu, nurses are responsible for ensuring that clients' physiological needs are met. Clients must be encouraged to perform as independently as possible in fulfilling activities of daily living. However, the nurse must make ongoing assessments and provide assistance for those who require it. Assessing physical status is an important nursing responsibility that must not be overlooked in a psychiatric setting that emphasizes holistic care.

Reality orientation for clients who have disorganized thinking or who are disoriented or confused is important in the therapeutic milieu. Clocks with large hands and numbers, calendars that give the day and date in large print, and orientation boards that discuss daily activities and news happenings can help keep clients oriented to reality. Nurses should ensure that clients have written schedules of assigned activities and that they arrive at those activities on schedule. Some clients may require an identification sign on their door to remind them which room is theirs. On short-term units, nurses who are dealing with psychotic clients usually rely on a basic activity or topic that helps keep people oriented: for example, showing pictures of the hospital where they are housed, introducing people who were admitted during the night, and providing name badges with their first names.

Nurses are responsible for the management of medication administration on inpatient psychiatric units. In some treatment programs, clients are expected to accept the responsibility and request their medication at the appropriate time. Although ultimate responsibility lies with the nurse, he or she must encourage clients to be self-reliant. Nurses must work with the clients to determine methods that result in achievement and provide positive feedback for successes.

A major focus of nursing in the therapeutic milieu is the one-to-one relationship that grows out of developing trust between client and nurse. Many clients with psychiatric disorders have never achieved the ability to trust. If this can be accomplished in a relationship with the nurse, the trust may be generalized to other relationships in the client's life. Within an atmosphere of trust, the client is encouraged to express feelings and emotions and discuss unresolved issues that are creating problems in his or her life.

In acute care hospitalizations, the ability to establish trust quickly and to assess and collaborate with the client about their post-discharge needs has become an essential role for nurses, since many aspects of the recovery treatment plan will occur in treatment settings other than inpatient hospitalization. Do not underestimate the importance of these short-term relationships. Clients in outpatient treatment often identify that something a nurse said or something they learned within the hospital milieu planted the seeds for their ongoing recovery plan.

> **CLINICAL PEARL** 💬
>
> Developing trust means keeping promises that have been made. It means total acceptance of the individual as a person, separate from behavior that is unacceptable. It means responding to the client with concrete behaviors that are understandable to him or her (e.g., "If you are frightened, I will stay with you"; "If you are cold, I will bring you a blanket"; "If you are thirsty, I will bring you a drink of water").

The nurse is responsible for setting limits on unacceptable behavior in the therapeutic milieu. This requires stating to the client in understandable terminology what behaviors are not acceptable and what the consequences will be if the limits are violated. These limits must be established, written, and carried out by all staff. Consistency in enforcing the consequences of violating the established limits is essential for learning is to be reinforced.

The role of client teacher is important in the psychiatric area, as it is in all areas of nursing. Nurses must be able to assess learning readiness in individual clients. Do they want to learn? What is their level of anxiety? What is their level of ability to understand the information being presented? Topics for client education in psychiatry include information about medical diagnoses, side effects of medications, the importance of continuing to take medications, and stress management, among others. Some topics must be individualized for specific clients, whereas others may be taught in group situations. Table 12–2 outlines various topics of nursing concern for client education in psychiatry. (Sample teaching guides are online.)

Echternacht (2001) stated:

> Milieu therapy interventions are recognized as one of the basic-level functions of psychiatric-mental health nurses as addressed [in the *Psychiatric-Mental Health Nursing: Scope and Standards of Practice*, (ANA, 2014)]. Milieu therapy has been described as an

TABLE 12–2	The Therapeutic Milieu—Topics for Client Education

1. Ways to increase self-esteem
2. Ways to deal with anger appropriately
3. Stress-management techniques
4. How to recognize signs of increasing anxiety and intervene to stop progression
5. Normal stages of grieving and behaviors associated with each stage
6. Assertiveness techniques
7. Relaxation techniques
   a. Progressive relaxation
   b. Tense and relax
   c. Deep breathing
   d. Autogenics
8. Medications (specify)
   a. Reason for taking
   b. Harmless side effects
   c. Side effects to report to physician
   d. Importance of taking regularly
   e. Importance of not stopping abruptly
9. Effects of (substance) on the body
   a. Alcohol
   b. Other depressants
   c. Stimulants
   d. Hallucinogens
   e. Narcotics
   f. Cannabinols
10. Problem-solving skills
11. Thought-stopping/thought-switching techniques
12. Sex education including information about sexually transmitted infections
13. The essentials of good nutrition
14. Exploring spiritual needs
15. Management of leisure time
16. Strategies for goal setting and accomplishment
17. (For parents/guardians)
    a. Signs and symptoms of substance abuse
    b. Effective parenting techniques

excellent framework for operationalizing [Hildegard] Peplau's interpretation and extension of Harry Stack Sullivan's Interpersonal Theory for use in nursing practice. (p. 39). . . .

Now is the time to rekindle interest in the therapeutic milieu concept and to reclaim nursing's traditional milieu intervention functions. Nurses need to identify the number of registered nurses necessary to carry out structured and unstructured milieu functions consistent with their Standards of Practice. (p. 43)

Summary and Key Points

■ In psychiatry, milieu therapy (or a therapeutic community) constitutes a manipulation of the environment in an effort to create behavioral changes and to improve the psychological health and functioning of the individual.

- The goal of therapeutic community is for the client to learn adaptive coping, interaction, and relationship skills that can be generalized to other aspects of his or her life.
- The community environment itself serves as the primary tool of therapy.
- According to Skinner (1979), a therapeutic community is based on seven basic assumptions:
  - The health in each individual is to be realized and encouraged to grow.
  - Every interaction is an opportunity for therapeutic intervention.
  - The client owns his or her own environment.
  - Each client owns his or her behavior.
  - Peer pressure is a useful and a powerful tool.
  - Inappropriate behaviors are dealt with as they occur.
  - Restrictions and punishment are to be avoided.
- Because the goals of milieu therapy relate to helping the client learn to generalize that which is learned to other aspects of his or her life, the conditions that promote a therapeutic community in the psychiatric setting are similar to the types of conditions that exist in real-life situations.
- Conditions that promote a therapeutic community include the following:
  - The fulfillment of basic physiological needs
  - Physical facilities that are conducive to achievement of the goals of therapy
  - The existence of a democratic form of self-government
  - The assignment of responsibilities according to client capabilities
- A structured program of social and work-related activities
- The inclusion of community and family in the program of therapy in an effort to facilitate discharge from treatment
- The program of therapy on the milieu unit is conducted by the IDT team.
- The team centers on the patient and includes some or all of the following disciplines (and potentially others): psychiatrist, clinical psychologist, psychiatric clinical nurse specialist, psychiatric nurse, mental health technician, psychiatric social worker, occupational therapist, recreational therapist, art therapist, music therapist, psychodramatist, dietitian, and chaplain.
- Nurses play a crucial role in the management of a therapeutic milieu. They are involved in the assessment, diagnosis, outcome identification, planning, implementation, and evaluation of all treatment programs.
- Nurses have significant input into the IDT plans, which are developed for all clients. They are responsible for ensuring that clients' basic needs are fulfilled; assessing physical and psychosocial status; administering medication; helping the client develop trusting relationships; setting limits on unacceptable behaviors; educating clients; and ultimately, helping clients, within the limits of their capability, to become productive members of society.

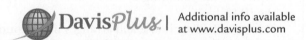 **DavisPlus** | Additional info available at www.davisplus.com

Review Questions
Self-Examination/Learning Exercise

Select the answer that is most appropriate for each of the following questions.

1. Which of the following are basic assumptions of milieu therapy? (Select all that apply.)
   a. The client owns his or her own environment.
   b. Each client owns his or her behavior.
   c. Peer pressure is a useful and powerful tool.
   d. Inappropriate behaviors are punished immediately.

2. John tells the nurse, "I think lights out at 10 o'clock on a weekend is stupid. We should be able to watch TV until midnight!" Which of the following is the most appropriate response from the nurse on the milieu unit?
   a. "John, you were told the rules when you were admitted."
   b. "You may bring it up before the others at the community meeting, John."
   c. "Some people want to go to bed early, John."
   d. "You are not the only person on this unit, John. You must think of others besides yourself."

Continued

Review Questions—cont'd
Self-Examination/Learning Exercise

3. In prioritizing care within the therapeutic environment, which of the following nursing interventions would receive the highest priority?
   a. Ensuring that the physical facilities are conducive to achievement of the goals of therapy
   b. Scheduling a community meeting for 8:30 each morning
   c. Attending to the nutritional and comfort needs of all clients
   d. Establishing contacts with community resources

4. In the community meeting, which of the following actions is most important for reinforcing the democratic posture of the therapy setting?
   a. Allowing each person a specific and equal amount of time to talk
   b. Reviewing group rules and behavioral limits that apply to all clients
   c. Reading the minutes from yesterday's meeting
   d. Waiting until all clients are present before initiating the meeting

5. One of the goals of therapeutic community is for clients to become more independent and accept self-responsibility. Which of the following approaches by staff best encourages fulfillment of this goal?
   a. Including client input and decisions into the treatment plan
   b. Insisting that each client take a turn as "president" of the community meeting
   c. Making decisions for the client regarding plans for treatment
   d. Requiring that the client be bathed, dressed, and attend breakfast on time each morning

6. Client teaching is an important nursing function in milieu therapy. Which of the following statements by the client indicates the need for knowledge and a readiness to learn?
   a. "Get away from me with that medicine! I'm not sick!"
   b. "I don't need psychiatric treatment. It's my migraine headaches that I need help with."
   c. "I've taken Valium every day of my life for the last 20 years. I'll stop when I'm good and ready!"
   d. "The doctor says I have bipolar disorder. What does that really mean?"

7. Which of the following activities would be a responsibility of the clinical psychologist member of the IDT?
   a. Locates halfway house and arranges living conditions for client being discharged from the hospital
   b. Manages the therapeutic milieu on a 24-hour basis
   c. Administers and evaluates psychological tests that assist in diagnosis
   d. Conducts psychotherapy and administers electroconvulsive therapy treatments

8. Which of the following activities would be a responsibility of the psychiatric clinical nurse specialist on the IDT team?
   a. Manages the therapeutic milieu on a 24-hour basis
   b. Conducts group therapies and provides consultation and education to staff nurses
   c. Directs a group of clients in acting out a situation that is otherwise too painful for a client to discuss openly
   d. Locates halfway house and arranges living conditions for client being discharged from the hospital

9. On the milieu unit, duties of the staff psychiatric nurse include which of the following? (Select all that apply.)
   a. Medication administration
   b. Client teaching
   c. Medical diagnosis
   d. Reality orientation
   e. Relationship development
   f. Group therapy

Review Questions—cont'd
Self-Examination/Learning Exercise

10. Lashona was sexually abused as a child. She is a client on the milieu unit with a diagnosis of Borderline Personality Disorder. She has refused to talk to anyone. Which of the following therapies might the IDT team choose for Lashona? (Select all that apply.)
  a. Music therapy
  b. Art therapy
  c. Psychodrama
  d. Electroconvulsive therapy

References

American Nurses Association (ANA), American Psychiatric Nurses Association, & International Society of Psychiatric Nurses. (2014). *Psychiatric-mental health nursing: Scope and standards of practice.* Silver Spring, MD: ANA.

Bowler, J.B. (1991). Transformation into a healing healthcare environment: Recovering the possibilities of psychiatric/mental health nursing. *Perspectives in Psychiatric Care, 27*(2), 21-25. doi:10.1111/j.1744-6163.1991.tb00339.x

DeSocio, J., Bowllan, N., & Staschak, S. (1997). Lessons learned in creating a safe and therapeutic milieu for children, adolescents, and families: Developmental considerations. *Journal of Child and Adolescent Psychiatric Nursing 10*(4), 18-26. doi:10.1111/j.1744-6171.1997.tb00418.x

Echternacht, M.R. (2001). Fluid group: Concept and clinical application in the therapeutic milieu. *Journal of the American Psychiatric Nurses Association, 7*(2), 39-44. doi:10.1067/mpn.2001.115760

Hall, B.A. (1995). Use of milieu therapy: The context and environment as therapeutic practice for psychiatric-mental health nurses. In C.A. Anderson (Ed.), *Psychiatric nursing 1974 to 1994: A report on the state of the art* (pp. 46-56). St. Louis: Mosby-Year Book.

Jani, S., & Fishman, M. (2004). Advances in milieu therapy for adolescent residential treatment. Program presented at the American Academy of Child and Adolescent Psychiatry 2004 Annual National Meeting. Retrieved from https://milieu-therapy.com/links-resources/presentations/

Menninger Clinic. (2012). Professionals in crisis program. Retrieved from www.menningerclinic.com/patient-care/inpatient-treatment/professionals-in-crisis-program/milieu-therapy

Whall, A.L. (1991). Using the environment to improve the mental health of the elderly. *Journal of Gerontological Nursing, 17*(7), 39.

Classical References

Maslow, A. (1968). *Towards a psychology of being* (2nd ed.). New York: D. Van Nostrand.

Skinner, K. (1979). The therapeutic milieu: Making it work. *Journal of Psychiatric Nursing and Mental Health Services, 17*(8), 38-44.

13

Crisis Intervention

KEY TERMS

crisis intervention   disaster

OBJECTIVES
After reading this chapter, the student will be able to:

1. Define *crisis*.
2. Describe four phases in the development of a crisis.
3. Identify types of crises that occur in people's lives.
4. Discuss the goal of crisis intervention.
5. Describe the steps in crisis intervention.
6. Identify the role of the nurse in crisis intervention.
7. Apply the nursing process to care of victims of disasters.

HOMEWORK ASSIGNMENT
Please read the chapter and answer the following questions:

1. Name the three factors that determine whether or not a person experiences a crisis in response to a stressful situation.
2. What is the goal of crisis intervention?
3. Individuals in crisis need to develop more adaptive coping strategies. How does the nurse provide assistance with this process?
4. Describe behaviors common to preschool children following a traumatic event.

Stressful situations are a part of everyday life. Any stressful situation can precipitate a crisis. Crises result in a disequilibrium from which many individuals require assistance to recover. **Crisis intervention** and resolution require problem-solving skills that are often diminished by the level of anxiety accompanying disequilibrium. Assistance with problem-solving during the crisis period preserves self-esteem and promotes growth with resolution.

In recent years, individuals in the United States have been faced with a number of catastrophic events, including natural disasters such as tornados, earthquakes, hurricanes, and floods. Man-made disasters, such as the Oklahoma City and Boston Marathon

234

bombings and the attacks on the World Trade Center and the Pentagon, have created psychological stress of astronomical proportions in populations around the world.

This chapter examines the phases in the development of a crisis and the types of crises that occur in people's lives. The methodology of crisis intervention, including the role of the nurse, is explored. A discussion of disaster nursing is also presented.

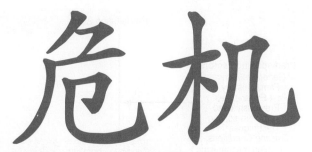

FIGURE 13–1 Chinese symbol for crisis.

> **CORE CONCEPTS**
> **Crisis**
> A sudden event in one's life that disturbs homeostasis, during which usual coping mechanisms cannot resolve the problem (Lagerquist, 2012, p. 795).

Characteristics of a Crisis

A number of characteristics have been identified that can be viewed as assumptions upon which the concept of crisis is based (Aguilera, 1998; Caplan, 1964):

1. Crisis occurs in all individuals at one time or another and is not necessarily equated with psychopathology.
2. Crises are precipitated by specific identifiable events.
3. Crises are personal by nature. What may be considered a crisis situation by one individual may not be so for another.
4. Crises are acute, not chronic, and will be resolved in one way or another within a brief period.
5. A crisis situation contains the potential for psychological growth or deterioration.

Individuals who are in crisis feel helpless to change. They do not believe they have the resources to deal with the precipitating stressor. Levels of anxiety rise to the point that the individual becomes nonfunctional, thoughts become obsessional, and all behavior is aimed at relief of the anxiety being experienced. The feeling is overwhelming and may affect the individual physically as well as psychologically.

Bateman and Peternelj-Taylor (1998) have stated:

Outside Western culture, a crisis is often viewed as a time for movement and growth. The Chinese symbol for crisis consists of the characters for *danger* and *opportunity* [Fig. 13–1]. When a crisis is viewed as an opportunity for growth, those involved are much more capable of resolving related issues and more able to move toward positive changes. When the crisis experience is overwhelming because of its scope and nature or when there has not been adequate preparation for the necessary changes, the dangers seem paramount and overshadow any potential growth. The results are maladaptive coping and dysfunctional behavior. (pp. 144–145)

Phases in the Development of a Crisis

The development of a crisis situation follows a relatively predictable course. Caplan (1964) outlined four phases through which individuals progress in response to a precipitating stressor and that culminate in the state of acute crisis.

Phase 1: *The individual is exposed to a precipitating stressor.* Anxiety increases; previous problem-solving techniques are employed.

Phase 2: *When previous problem-solving techniques do not relieve the stressor, anxiety increases further.* The individual begins to feel a great deal of discomfort at this point. Coping techniques that have worked in the past are attempted, only to create feelings of helplessness when they are not successful. Feelings of confusion and disorganization prevail.

Phase 3: *All possible resources, both internal and external, are called on to resolve the problem and relieve the discomfort.* The individual may try to view the problem from a different perspective or even to overlook certain aspects of it. New problem-solving techniques may be used, and, if effectual, resolution may occur at this phase, with the individual returning to a higher, a lower, or the previous level of precrisis functioning.

Phase 4: *If resolution does not occur in previous phases, Caplan states that "the tension mounts beyond a further threshold or its burden increases over time to a breaking point. Major disorganization of the individual with drastic results often occurs"* (p. 41). Anxiety may reach panic levels. Cognitive functions are disordered, emotions are labile, and behavior may reflect the presence of psychotic thinking.

These phases are congruent with the transactional model of stress adaptation outlined in Chapter 1, The Concept of Stress Adaptation. The relationship between the two perspectives is presented in Figure 13–2. When an individual perceives a stressor as a threat to

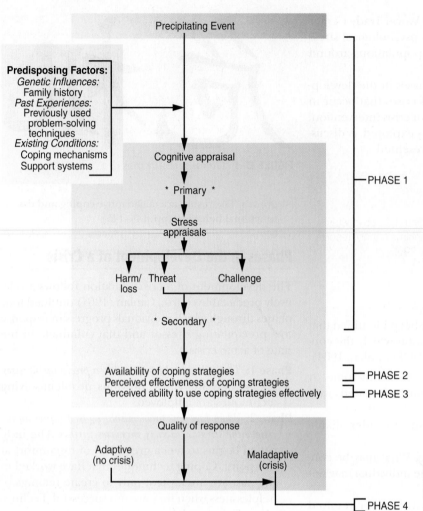

FIGURE 13–2 Relationship between transactional model of stress/adaptation and Caplan's phases in the development of a crisis.

his or her well-being and lacks adaptive coping strategies or employs maladaptive strategies, crisis ensues. Similarly, Aguilera (1998) spoke of "balancing factors" that affect the way in which an individual perceives and responds to a precipitating stressor. A schematic of these balancing factors is illustrated in Figure 13–3.

The paradigm set forth by Aguilera suggests that whether or not an individual experiences a crisis in response to a stressful situation depends on the following three factors:

1. **The individual's perception of the event:** If the event is perceived realistically, the individual is more likely to draw upon adequate resources to restore equilibrium. If the perception of the event is distorted, attempts at problem-solving are likely to be ineffective, and equilibrium is not restored.
2. **The availability of situational supports:** Aguilera stated, "Situational supports are those persons who are available in the environment and who can be depended on to help solve the problem" (p. 37).

Without adequate situational supports during a stressful situation, an individual is most likely to feel overwhelmed and alone.
3. **The availability of adequate coping mechanisms:** When a stressful situation occurs, individuals draw upon behavioral strategies that have been successful for them in the past. If these coping strategies work, a crisis may be diverted. If not, disequilibrium may continue and tension and anxiety increase.

Crises are acute, time-limited situations that will be resolved in one way or another within 1 to 3 months. Crises can become growth opportunities when individuals learn new methods of coping that can be preserved and used when similar stressors recur. However, when new coping mechanisms or balancing factors are not identified and incorporated, the crisis situation can evolve into longer-term problems and sometimes symptoms of emotional or mental illness, including depression, anxiety, and trauma/stressor-related disorders.

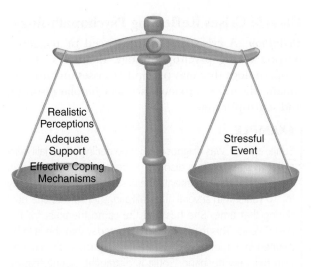

Stressful event is balanced by realistic perceptions, adequate support, effective coping mechanisms ➡ Equilibrium ➡ **No crisis**

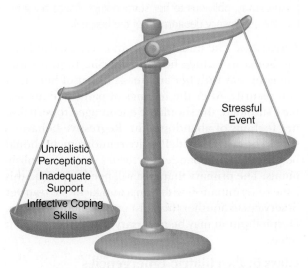

Problem unresolved ➡ Disequilibrium ➡ **Crisis**

FIGURE 13–3 The effect of balancing factors in a stressful event.

Types of Crises

Baldwin (1978) identified six classes of emotional crises, which progress by degree of severity. As the measure of psychopathology increases, the source of the stressor changes from external to internal. The type of crisis determines the method of intervention selected.

Class 1: Dispositional Crises

Definition An acute response to an external situational stressor.

EXAMPLE

Brittany and Ethan have been married for 3 years and have a 1-year-old daughter. Ethan has been having difficulty with

his boss at work. Twice during the past 6 months, he has exploded in anger at home and become abusive with Brittany. Last night he became angry that dinner was not ready when he expected. He grabbed the baby from Brittany and tossed her, screaming, into her crib. He hit and punched Brittany until she feared for her life. This morning when he left for work, she took the baby and went to the emergency department of the city hospital, not knowing what else to do.

Intervention Physical care of wounds and screening for domestic violence issues should be conducted in the emergency department. The mental health counselor can provide support and guidance in terms of presenting alternatives for managing the health and safety of herself and her child. The emergency department nurse should encourage and empower Brittany to clarify her needs and issues so referrals for agency assistance can be made.

Class 2: Crises of Anticipated Life Transitions

Definition Normal life-cycle transitions that are anticipated but over which the individual may feel a lack of control.

EXAMPLE

College student J.T. is placed on probationary status because of low grades this semester. His wife had a baby and had to quit her job. He increased his working hours from part time to full time to compensate and therefore had little time for studies. He presents himself to the student-health nurse practitioner complaining of numerous vague physical complaints.

Intervention Physical examination should be performed (physical symptoms could be caused by depression) and ventilation of feelings encouraged. Reassurance and support should be provided as needed. J.T. should be referred to services that can provide financial and other types of needed assistance. Problematic areas should be identified and approaches to change discussed.

Class 3: Crises Resulting From Traumatic Stress

Definition Crisis precipitated by an unexpected external stressor over which the individual has little or no control and as a result of which he or she feels emotionally overwhelmed and defeated.

EXAMPLE

Ava is a waitperson whose shift ended at midnight. Two weeks ago, while walking to her car in the deserted parking lot, she was abducted by two men with guns, taken to an abandoned building, and raped and beaten. Since that time, her physical wounds have nearly healed. However,

Ava cannot be alone, is constantly fearful, relives the experience in flashbacks and dreams, and is unable to eat, sleep, or work at her job in the restaurant. Her friend offers to accompany her to the mental health clinic.

Intervention The nurse should offer Ava the opportunity to talk about the experience and express her feelings about the trauma when she demonstrates readiness. The nurse should offer reassurance and support; discuss stages of grief and how rape may precipitate feelings of loss, including loss of control, loss of power, and loss of a sense of self-worth, triggering the grief response; identify support systems that can help Ava to resume her normal activities; and explore new methods of coping with emotions arising from a situation with which she has had no previous experience. These interventions should be conducted in an environment that is sensitive to the impact of trauma on a person's sense of self, and all interventions should convey dignity, respect, and hopefulness and promote the client's empowerment to make choices in her or his care (SAMHSA, 2014). See Chapter 28, Trauma- and Stressor-Related Disorders, for more information on trauma-informed care.

Class 4: Maturational/Developmental Crises

Definition Crises that occur in response to failed attempts to master developmental tasks associated with transitions in the life cycle.

EXAMPLE

Jada and Caleb have been married for 2 years, and their firstborn child is 4 months old. Jada's mother was recently diagnosed with cancer, and the prognosis is unclear. Over the past 3 weeks, Jada has become increasingly anxious and disorganized, calling the nurse practitioner 10 to 15 times each day with new fears that she is not addressing her child's health needs. Jada has been screaming at Caleb that he is never there when she needs help with the baby and states she is thinking of dropping their child off at the Children's Service Agency because she believes they are both unable to be effective parents. She agrees to see a counselor at Caleb's insistence.

Intervention The primary intervention is to help Jada with anxiety reduction. When individuals have intense anxiety, their ability to gain insight about contributing factors and explore options for behavior change is impaired. The safety of their child should also be carefully assessed. Referrals and guidance in parenting skills may lessen the anxiety associated with this new developmental phase. Anxiety and grief related to Jada's mother's illness could also be explored as a possible factor contributing to the current crisis.

Class 5: Crises Reflecting Psychopathology

Definition A crisis that is influenced or triggered by preexisting psychopathology. Examples of psychopathology that may precipitate crises include personality disorders, anxiety disorders, bipolar disorder, and schizophrenia.

EXAMPLE

Sonja, age 29, was diagnosed with borderline personality disorder at age 18. This disorder is believed to be rooted in deep fear of abandonment. She has been in weekly therapy for 10 years, with several hospitalizations for suicide attempts during that time. She has had the same therapist for the past 6 years. This therapist told Sonja today that she is to be married in 1 month and will be moving across the country with her new husband. Sonja is distraught, stating that no one cares about her and that she would be better off dead. She is found wandering in and out of traffic on a busy expressway, oblivious to her surroundings. Police bring her to the emergency department of the hospital.

Intervention The initial intervention is aimed at helping Sonja to reduce her anxiety. She requires that someone stay with her and reassure her of her safety and security. After the feelings of panic and anxiety have subsided, she should be encouraged to verbalize her feelings of abandonment. Regressive behaviors should be discouraged. Positive reinforcement should be given for independent activities and accomplishments. The primary therapist will need to pursue this issue of termination with Sonja and facilitate transfer of services to another therapist or treatment program. Hospitalization may be necessary to maintain patient safety.

Class 6: Psychiatric Emergencies

Definition Crisis situations in which general functioning has been severely impaired and the individual rendered incompetent or unable to assume personal responsibility for his or her behavior. Examples include acute suicide risk, drug overdose, reactions to hallucinogenic drugs, acute psychoses, uncontrollable anger, and alcohol intoxication.

EXAMPLE

Jennifer, age 16, had been dating Joe, the star high school football player, for 6 months. After the game on Friday night, Jennifer and Joe went to Jackie's house, where a number of high school students had gathered for an after-game party. No adults were present. About midnight, Joe told Jennifer that he did not want to date her anymore. Jennifer became hysterical, and Jackie was frightened by her behavior. She took Jennifer to her parent's bedroom and gave her a Valium from a bottle in her mother's medicine cabinet. She left Jennifer lying on her parent's bed and returned to the party downstairs. About an hour later, she returned to her parent's bedroom and found that Jennifer had removed the bottle of Valium from the cabinet and swallowed all of the tablets. Jennifer was unconscious and Jackie could not awaken her. An ambulance was called and Jennifer was transported to the local hospital.

Intervention Emergency medical care, including monitoring vital signs, ensuring maintenance of adequate airway, and initiating gastric lavage and/or activated charcoal, is the priority in this case. Jennifer is a minor, so notifying the parents is essential as well. Inpatient hospitalization is justifiable to assure patient safety. Discussing feelings about self-esteem, rejection, and loss will help Jennifer explore more adaptive methods of dealing with stressful situations.

Crisis Intervention

Individuals experiencing crises have an urgent need for assistance. In **crisis intervention,** the therapist or other intervener becomes part of the individual's life situation. Because of the individual's emotional state, he or she is unable to problem-solve and consequently requires guidance and support from another to help mobilize the resources needed to resolve the crisis.

Lengthy psychological interpretations are not appropriate for crisis intervention. It is a time for doing what is needed to help the individual get relief and for calling into action all the people and resources required to do so. Aguilera (1998) has stated:

> The goal of crisis intervention is the resolution of an immediate crisis. Its focus is on the supportive, with the restoration of the individual to his precrisis level of functioning or possibly to a higher level of functioning. The therapist's role is direct, supportive, and that of an active participant. (p. 24)

Crisis intervention takes place in inpatient settings, outpatient settings, and the community. In the past few decades, people with mental illness have been increasingly involved with criminal justice personnel as first responders to manage mental health crisis situations. In 1988, the fatal shooting by police officers of a man with mental illness prompted the development of the *crisis intervention team (CIT) model* to assure that select police officers are trained to identify mental illness and substance abuse, use de-escalation techniques, and divert individuals from criminal justice systems to mental health professionals (Watson & Fulambarker, 2012). Not all states have developed CIT training programs, but several studies have demonstrated improved safety outcomes for patients with mental illness where CIT-trained officers are available. Other resources that may be available for patients with mental illness who are experiencing an acute crisis include 24-hour crisis phone lines, walk-in crisis centers, mobile crisis teams, respite and residential services, and hospital services, including 23-hour observation beds (National Alliance on Mental Illness [NAMI], 2015). Nurses have a responsibility to know what resources exist in their community of practice. They can then become an important advocate for crisis intervention training in communities and can also be a support to families by encouraging them to ask for CIT-trained officers (where available) when faced with a family member's psychiatric crisis.

A more recent trend in some states, counties, and mental health facilities is to utilize *peer support specialists.* These individuals have personal experience with mental illness and are trained and/or credentialed to help clients navigate everyday challenges of living with a mental illness. Evidence has demonstrated their effectiveness in diffusing psychiatric crises (NAMI, 2014).

The basic methodology for crisis intervention work by health-care professionals relies heavily on orderly problem-solving techniques and structured activities focused on change. Through adaptive change, crises are resolved and growth occurs. Because of the time limitation of crisis intervention, the individual must experience some degree of relief almost from the first interaction. Crisis intervention, then, is not aimed at major personality change or reconstruction (as may be the case in long-term psychotherapy), but rather at using a given crisis situation at the very least to restore functioning and at most to enhance personal growth.

Phases of Crisis Intervention: The Role of the Nurse

Nurses respond to crisis situations on a daily basis. Crises can occur on every unit in the general hospital, in the home setting, in the community health-care setting, in schools and offices, and in private practice. Nurses may be called on to function as crisis helpers in virtually any setting committed to the practice of nursing.

Roberts and Ottens (2005) describe the clinical application of Robert's seven-stage model of crisis intervention. This model is summarized in Table 13–1. Aguilera (1998) described four phases in the technique of crisis intervention that are clearly comparable to the steps of the nursing process. These phases are discussed in the following paragraphs.

Phase 1. Assessment

In this phase, the nurse gathers information regarding the precipitating stressor and the resulting crisis

TABLE 13–1 Roberts' Seven-Stage Crisis Intervention Model

STAGE	INTERVENTIONS
Stage I. Psychosocial and Lethality Assessment	■ Conduct a rapid but thorough biopsychosocial assessment.
Stage II. Rapidly Establish Rapport	■ The counselor uses genuineness, respect, and unconditional acceptance to establish rapport with the client. ■ Skills such as good eye contact, a nonjudgmental attitude, flexibility, and maintaining a positive mental attitude are important.
Stage III. Identify the Major Problems or Crisis Precipitants	■ Identify the precipitating event that has led the client to seek help at the present time. ■ Identify other situations that led up to the precipitating event. ■ Prioritize major problems with which the client needs help. ■ Discuss client's current style of coping, and offer assistance in areas where modification would be helpful in resolving the present crisis and preventing future crises.
Stage IV. Deal With Feelings and Emotions	■ Encourage the client to vent feelings. Provide validation. ■ Use therapeutic communication techniques to help the client explain his or her story about the current crisis situation. ■ Eventually, and cautiously, begin to challenge maladaptive beliefs and behaviors, and help the client adopt more rational and adaptive options.
Stage V. Generate and Explore Alternatives	■ Collaboratively explore options with the client. ■ Identify coping strategies that have been successful for the client in the past. ■ Help the client problem-solve strategies for confronting current crisis adaptively.
Stage VI. Implement an Action Plan	■ There is a shift at this stage from crisis to resolution. ■ Develop a concrete plan of action to deal directly with the current crisis. ■ Having a concrete plan restores the client's equilibrium and psychological balance. ■ Work through the meaning of the event that precipitated the crisis. How could it have been prevented? What responses may have aggravated the situation?
Stage VII. Follow-Up	■ Plan a follow-up visit with the client to evaluate the postcrisis status of the client. ■ Beneficial scheduling of follow-up visits include 1-month and 1-year anniversaries of the crisis event.

Adapted from Roberts, A.R., & Ottens, A.J. (2005). The seven-stage crisis intervention model: A road map to goal attainment, problem solving, and crisis resolution. *Brief Treatment and Crisis Intervention, 5*(4), 329-339.

that prompted the individual to seek professional help. A nurse in crisis intervention might perform some of the following assessments:

■ Ask the individual to describe the event that precipitated this crisis.
■ Determine when it occurred.
■ Assess the individual's mental *and* physical status.
■ Determine if the individual has experienced this stressor before. If so, what method of coping was used? Have these methods been tried this time?
■ If previous coping methods were tried, what was the result?

■ If new coping methods were tried, what was the result?
■ Assess suicide or homicide potential, plan, and means.
■ Assess the adequacy of support systems.
■ Determine level of precrisis functioning. Assess the usual coping methods, available support systems, and ability to problem-solve.
■ Assess the individual's perception of personal strengths and limitations.
■ Assess the individual's use of substances.

Information from the comprehensive assessment is then analyzed, and appropriate nursing diagnoses reflecting the immediacy of the crisis situation are identified. Some nursing diagnoses that may be relevant include the following:

- Ineffective coping
- Anxiety (severe to panic)
- Disturbed thought processes (resigned from the NANDA-I list of approved diagnoses but used for purposes of this textbook)
- Risk for self- or other-directed violence
- Rape-trauma syndrome
- Posttrauma syndrome
- Fear

Phase 2. Planning of Therapeutic Intervention

In the planning phase of crisis intervention, the nurse selects the appropriate nursing actions for the identified nursing diagnoses. In planning the interventions, the type of crisis, as well as the individual's strengths, desired choices, and available resources for support, are taken into consideration. Goals are established for crisis resolution and a return to or increase in the precrisis level of functioning.

Phase 3. Intervention

During phase 3, the actions identified in phase 2 are implemented. The following interventions are the focus of nursing in crisis intervention:

- Use a reality-oriented approach. The focus of the problem is on the here and now.
- Remain with the individual experiencing panic anxiety.
- Establish a rapid working relationship by showing unconditional acceptance, by active listening, and by attending to immediate needs.
- Discourage lengthy explanations or rationalizations of the situation; promote an atmosphere for verbalization of true feelings.
- Set firm limits on aggressive, destructive behaviors. At high levels of anxiety, behavior is likely to be impulsive and regressive. Establish at the outset what is acceptable and what is not, and maintain consistency.
- Clarify the problem the individual is facing. The nurse does this by describing his or her perception of the problem and comparing it with the individual's perception of the problem.
- Help the individual determine what he or she believes precipitated the crisis.
- Acknowledge feelings of anger, guilt, helplessness, and powerlessness without judgment.
- Guide the individual through a problem-solving process by which he or she may move in the direction of positive life change.

- Help the individual confront the factors that are contributing to the experience of crisis.
- Encourage the individual to discuss changes he or she would like to make. Jointly determine whether or not desired changes are realistic.
- Encourage exploration of feelings about aspects of the situation that cannot be changed, and explore alternative ways of coping more adaptively in these situations.
- Discuss alternative strategies for creating changes that are realistically possible.
- Weigh benefits and consequences of each alternative.
- Assist the individual to select alternative coping strategies that will help alleviate future crisis situations.
- Identify external support systems and new social networks from which the individual may seek assistance in times of stress.

> **CLINICAL PEARL** Coping mechanisms are highly individual, and the choice ultimately must be made by the client. The nurse may offer suggestions and provide guidance to help the client identify realistic coping mechanisms that can promote positive outcomes in a crisis situation.

Phase 4. Evaluation of Crisis Resolution and Anticipatory Planning

To evaluate the outcome of crisis intervention, a reassessment is made to determine if the stated objective was achieved:

- Have positive behavioral changes occurred?
- Has the individual developed more adaptive coping strategies? Have they been effective?
- Has the individual grown from the experience by gaining insight into his or her responses to crisis situations?
- Does the individual believe that he or she could respond with healthy adaptation in future stressful situations to prevent crisis development?
- Can the individual describe a plan of action for dealing with stressors similar to the one that precipitated this crisis?

During the evaluation period, the nurse and client summarize what has occurred during the intervention. They review what the individual has learned and anticipate how he or she will respond in the future. A determination is made regarding follow-up therapy; if needed, the nurse provides referral information.

Disaster Nursing

Although there are many definitions of **disaster,** a common feature is that the event overwhelms local resources and threatens the function and safety of the community (Norwood, Ursano, & Fullerton, 2000). A violent disaster, whether natural or man-made, may cause devastation to property or life. Such tragedies leave victims with a damaged sense of safety and well-being and varying degrees of emotional trauma. Spiritual distress often occurs as victims question, "How could this have happened?" and "What is most important in life?" A care plan for responding to spiritual distress is included in Table 13–2. Children, who lack life experiences and coping skills, are particularly vulnerable. Their sense of order and security has been seriously disrupted, and they are unable to understand that the disruption is time-limited and that their world will eventually return to normal.

Application of the Nursing Process to Disaster Nursing

Background Assessment Data

Individuals respond to traumatic events in many ways. Grieving is a natural response following any loss, and it may be more extreme if the disaster is directly experienced or witnessed. The emotional effects of loss and disruption may show up immediately or appear weeks or months later.

Psychological and behavioral responses common in adults following trauma and disaster include anger; disbelief; sadness; anxiety; fear; irritability; arousal; numbing; sleep disturbance; and increases in alcohol, caffeine, and tobacco use (Norwood et al., 2000). Preschool children commonly experience separation anxiety, regressive behaviors, nightmares, and hyperactive or withdrawn behaviors. Older children may have difficulty concentrating, somatic complaints, sleep disturbances, and concerns about safety. Adolescents' responses are often similar to those of adults.

Norwood and associates (2000) stated:

> Traumatic bereavement is recognized as posing special challenges to survivors. While the death of loved ones is always painful, an unexpected and violent death can be more difficult to assimilate. Family members may develop intrusive images of the death based on information gleaned from authorities or the media. Witnessing or learning of violence to a loved one also increases vulnerability to psychiatric disorders. The knowledge that one has been exposed to toxins is a potent traumatic stressor . . . and the focus of much concern in the medical community preparing for responses to terrorist attacks using biological, chemical, or nuclear agents. (p. 214)

Nursing Diagnoses and Outcome Identification

Information from the assessment is analyzed, and appropriate nursing diagnoses reflecting the immediacy of the situation are identified. Some nursing diagnoses that may be relevant include the following:

■ Risk for injury (trauma, suffocation, poisoning)
■ Risk for infection
■ Anxiety (panic)
■ Fear
■ Spiritual distress
■ Risk for post-trauma syndrome
■ Ineffective community coping

The following criteria may be used for measurement of outcomes in the care of the client having experienced a traumatic event. Time lines are individually determined.

The client:

■ Demonstrates behaviors necessary to protect self from further injury
■ Identifies interventions to prevent/reduce risk of infection
■ Is free of infection and/or physical injury
■ Maintains anxiety at manageable level
■ Expresses beliefs and values about spiritual issues
■ Demonstrates ability to deal with emotional reactions in an individually appropriate manner
■ Demonstrates an increase in activities to improve community functioning

Planning and Implementation

Table 13–2 provides a plan of care for the client who has experienced a traumatic event. Selected nursing diagnoses are presented, along with outcome criteria, appropriate nursing interventions, and rationales for each.

Evaluation

In the final step of the nursing process, a reassessment is conducted to determine if the nursing actions have been successful in achieving the objectives of care. Evaluation of the nursing actions for the client who has experienced a traumatic event may be facilitated by gathering information utilizing the following types of questions:

■ Has the client escaped serious injury, or have injuries been resolved?
■ Have infections been prevented or resolved?
■ Is the client able to maintain anxiety at manageable level?
■ Does he or she demonstrate appropriate problem-solving skills?

(Text continued on page 249)

Table 13–2 | CARE PLAN FOR THE CLIENT WHO HAS EXPERIENCED A TRAUMATIC EVENT

NURSING DIAGNOSIS: ANXIETY (PANIC)/FEAR

RELATED TO: Real or perceived threat to physical well-being; threat of death; situational crisis; exposure to toxins; unmet needs

EVIDENCED BY: Persistent feelings of apprehension and uneasiness; sense of impending doom; impaired functioning; verbal expressions of having no control or influence over situation, outcome, or self-care; sympathetic stimulation; extraneous physical movements

OUTCOME CRITERIA	NURSING INTERVENTIONS	RATIONALE
Client demonstrates that anxiety is at a manageable level. Client demonstrates use of positive coping mechanisms to manage anxiety.	1. Determine degree of anxiety/fear present, associated behaviors (e.g., laughter, crying, calm or agitation, excited or hysterical behavior, expressions of disbelief and/or self-blame), and reality of perceived threat.	1. Clearly understanding client's perception is pivotal to providing appropriate assistance in overcoming the fear. Individual may be agitated or totally overwhelmed. Panic state increases risk for client's own safety and the safety of others in the environment.
	2. Note degree of disorganization.	2. Client may be unable to handle activities of daily living or work requirements and need more intensive intervention.
	3. Create as quiet an area as possible. Maintain a calm confident manner. Speak in even tone using short, simple sentences.	3. Decreases sense of confusion or overstimulation; enhances sense of safety. Helps client focus on what is said and reduces transmission of anxiety.
	4. Develop trusting relationship with client.	4. Trust is the basis of a therapeutic nurse-client relationship and enables them to work effectively together.
	5. Identify whether incident has reactivated preexisting or coexisting situations (physical or psychological).	5. Concerns and psychological issues may be recycled every time trauma is reexperienced and affect how client views the current situation.
	6. Determine presence of physical symptoms (e.g., numbness, headache, tightness in chest, nausea, and pounding heart).	6. Physical problems need to be differentiated from anxiety symptoms so appropriate treatment can be given.
	7. Identify psychological responses (e.g., anger, shock, acute anxiety, panic, confusion, denial). Record emotional changes.	7. Although these are normal responses at the time of the trauma, they will recycle repeatedly until they are dealt with adequately.
	8. Discuss with client the perception of what is causing the anxiety.	8. Increases the ability to connect symptoms to subjective feeling of anxiety, providing opportunity to gain insight/control and make desired changes.
	9. Assist client to correct any distortions being experienced. Share perceptions with client.	9. Perceptions based on reality will help to decrease fearfulness. How the nurse views the situation may help client to see it differently.

Continued

Table 13–2 | CARE PLAN FOR THE CLIENT WHO HAS EXPERIENCED A TRAUMATIC EVENT–cont'd

OUTCOME CRITERIA	NURSING INTERVENTIONS	RATIONALE
	10. Explore with client or significant other the manner in which client has previously coped with anxiety-producing events.	10. May help client regain sense of control and recognize significance of trauma.
	11. Engage client in learning new coping behaviors (e.g., progressive muscle relaxation, thought-stopping).	11. Replacing maladaptive behaviors can enhance ability to manage and deal with stress. Interrupting obsessive thinking allows client to use energy to address underlying anxiety, whereas continued rumination about the incident can retard recovery.
	12. Encourage use of techniques to manage stress and vent emotions such as anger and hostility.	12. Reduces the likelihood of eruptions that can result in abusive behavior.
	13. Give positive feedback when client demonstrates better ways to manage anxiety and is able to calmly and realistically appraise the situation.	13. Provides acknowledgment and reinforcement, encouraging use of new coping strategies. Enhances ability to deal with fearful feelings and gain control over situation, promoting future successes.
	14. Administer medications as indicated: antianxiety: diazepam, alprazolam, oxazepam; or antidepressants: fluoxetine, paroxetine, bupropion.	14. Antianxiety medication provides temporary relief of anxiety symptoms, enhancing ability to cope with situation. Antidepressants lift mood and help suppress intrusive thoughts and explosive anger.

NURSING DIAGNOSIS: SPIRITUAL DISTRESS

RELATED TO: Physical or psychological stress; energy-consuming anxiety; loss(es), intense suffering; separation from religious or cultural ties; challenged belief and value system

EVIDENCED BY: Expressions of concern about disaster and the meaning of life and death or belief systems; inner conflict about current loss of normality and effects of the disaster; anger directed at deity; engaging in self-blame; seeking spiritual assistance

OUTCOME CRITERIA	NURSING INTERVENTIONS	RATIONALE
Client expresses beliefs and values about spiritual issues.	1. Determine client's religious/spiritual orientation, current involvement, and presence of conflicts.	1. Provides baseline for planning care and accessing appropriate resources.
	2. Establish environment that promotes free expression of feelings and concerns. Provide calm, peaceful setting when possible.	2. Promotes awareness and identification of feelings so they can be dealt with.

Table 13–2 | CARE PLAN FOR THE CLIENT WHO HAS EXPERIENCED A TRAUMATIC EVENT–cont'd

OUTCOME CRITERIA	NURSING INTERVENTIONS	RATIONALE
	3. Listen to client's and significant others' expressions of anger, concern, alienation from God, belief that situation is a punishment for wrongdoing, and so on.	3. It is helpful to understand client's and significant others' points of view and how they are questioning their faith in the face of tragedy.
	4. Note sense of futility, feelings of hopelessness and helplessness, lack of motivation to help self.	4. These thoughts and feelings can result in client feeling paralyzed and unable to move forward to resolve the situation.
	5. Listen to expressions of inability to find meaning in life and reason for living. Evaluate for suicidal ideation.	5. May indicate need for further intervention to prevent suicide attempt.
	6. Determine support systems available to client.	6. Presence or lack of support systems can affect client's recovery.
	7. Ask how you can be most helpful. Convey acceptance of client's spiritual beliefs and concerns.	7. Promotes trust and comfort, encouraging client to be open about sensitive matters.
	8. Make time for nonjudgmental discussion of philosophic issues and questions about spiritual impact of current situation.	8. Helps client to begin to look at basis for spiritual confusion. *Note:* There is a potential for care provider's belief system to interfere with client finding own way. Therefore, it is most beneficial to remain neutral and not espouse own beliefs.
	9. Discuss difference between grief and guilt and help client to identify and deal with each, assuming responsibility for own actions, expressing awareness of the consequences of acting out of false guilt.	9. Blaming self for what has happened impedes dealing with the grief process and needs to be discussed and dealt with.
	10. Use therapeutic communication skills of reflection and active-listening.	10. Helps client find own solutions to concerns.
	11. Encourage client to experience meditation, prayer, and forgiveness. Provide information that anger with God is a normal part of the grieving process.	11. This can help to heal past and present pain.
	12. Assist client to develop goals for dealing with life situation.	12. Enhances commitment to goal, optimizing outcomes and promoting sense of hope.

Continued

Table 13–2 | CARE PLAN FOR THE CLIENT WHO HAS EXPERIENCED A TRAUMATIC EVENT–cont'd

OUTCOME CRITERIA	NURSING INTERVENTIONS	RATIONALE
	13. Identify and refer to resources that can be helpful (e.g., pastoral/parish nurse or religious counselor, crisis counselor, psychotherapy, Alcoholics/Narcotics Anonymous).	13. Specific assistance may be helpful to recovery (e.g., relationship problems, substance abuse, suicidal ideation).
	14. Encourage participation in support groups.	14. Discussing concerns and questions with others can help client resolve feelings.

NURSING DIAGNOSIS: RISK FOR POST-TRAUMA SYNDROME

RELATED TO: Events outside the range of usual human experience; serious threat or injury to self or loved ones; witnessing violent or tragic events; exaggerated sense of responsibility; survivor's guilt or role in the event; inadequate social support

OUTCOME CRITERIA	NURSING INTERVENTIONS	RATIONALE
Client demonstrates ability to deal with emotional reactions in an individually appropriate manner.	1. Determine involvement in event (e.g., survivor, significant other, rescue/aid worker, health-care provider, family member).	1. All those concerned with a traumatic event are at risk for emotional trauma and have needs related to their involvement in the event. *Note:* Close involvement with victims affects individual responses and may prolong emotional suffering.
	2. Evaluate current factors associated with the event, such as displacement from home due to illness or injury, natural disaster, or terrorist attack. Identify how client's past experiences may affect current situation.	2. Affects client's reaction to current event and is basis for planning care and identifying appropriate support systems and resources.
	3. Listen for comments of taking on responsibility (e.g., "I should have been more careful or gone back to get her").	3. Statements such as these are indicators of "survivor's guilt" and blaming self for actions.
	4. Identify client's current coping mechanisms.	4. Noting positive or negative coping skills provides direction for care.
	5. Determine availability and usefulness of client's support systems, family, social contacts, and community resources.	5. Family and others close to client may also be at risk and require assistance to cope with the trauma.
	6. Provide information about signs and symptoms of posttrauma response, especially if individual is involved in a high-risk occupation.	6. Awareness of these factors helps individual identify need for assistance when signs and symptoms occur.

Table 13–2 | CARE PLAN FOR THE CLIENT WHO HAS EXPERIENCED A TRAUMATIC EVENT—cont'd

OUTCOME CRITERIA	NURSING INTERVENTIONS	RATIONALE
	7. Identify and discuss client's strengths as well as vulnerabilities.	7. Provides information to build on for coping with traumatic experience.
	8. Evaluate individual's perceptions of events and personal significance (e.g., rescue worker trained to provide lifesaving assistance but recovering only dead bodies).	8. Events that trigger feelings of despair and hopelessness may be more difficult to deal with, and require long-term interventions.
	9. Provide emotional and physical presence by sitting with client/significant other and offering solace.	9. Strengthens coping abilities.
	10. Encourage expression of feelings. Note whether feelings expressed appear congruent with events experienced.	10. It is important to talk about the incident repeatedly. Incongruencies may indicate deeper conflict and can impede resolution.
	11. Note presence of nightmares, reliving the incident, loss of appetite, irritability, numbness and crying, and family or relationship disruption.	11. These responses are normal in the early postincident time frame. If prolonged and persistent, they may indicate need for more intensive therapy.
	12. Provide a calm, safe environment.	12. Helps client deal with the disruption in his or her life.
	13. Encourage and assist client in learning stress-management techniques.	13. Promotes relaxation and helps individual exercise control over self and what has happened.
	14. Recommend participation in debriefing sessions that may be provided following major disaster events.	14. Dealing with the stresses promptly may facilitate recovery from the event or prevent exacerbation.
	15. Identify employment, community resource groups.	15. Provides opportunity for ongoing support to deal with recurrent feelings related to the trauma.
	16. Administer medications as indicated, such as antipsychotics (e.g., chlorpromazine, haloperidol, olanzapine, or quetiapine) or carbamazepine (Tegretol).	16. Low doses of antipsychotics may be used for reduction of psychotic symptoms when loss of contact with reality occurs, usually for clients with especially disturbing flashbacks. Carbamazepine may be used to alleviate intrusive recollections or flashbacks, impulsivity, and violent behavior.

Continued

Table 13–2 | CARE PLAN FOR THE CLIENT WHO HAS EXPERIENCED A TRAUMATIC EVENT—cont'd

NURSING DIAGNOSIS: INEFFECTIVE COMMUNITY COPING

RELATED TO: History of exposure to disasters (earthquakes, tornados, floods, reemerging infectious agents, terrorist activity); ineffective or nonexistent community resources (e.g., lack of or inadequate emergency medical system, transportation system, or disaster planning systems), inadequate resources for problem-solving

EVIDENCED BY: Deficits of community participation; community does not meet expectations of its members; expressed perception of vulnerability and powerlessness; stressors perceived as excessive; excessive community conflicts or problems (vandalism, robbery, unemployment, homicides, terrorism, poverty); high illness rates

OUTCOME CRITERIA	NURSING INTERVENTIONS	RATIONALE
Client demonstrates an increase in activities to improve community functioning.	1. Evaluate community activities that are related to meeting collective needs within the community and between the community and the larger society. Note immediate needs, such as health care, food, shelter, funds.	1. Provides a baseline to determine community needs in relation to current concerns or threats.
	2. Note community reports of functioning, including areas of weakness or conflict.	2. Provides a view of how the community sees these areas.
	3. Identify effects of related factors on community activities.	3. In the face of a current threat, local or national, community resources need to be evaluated, updated, and given priority to meet the identified need.
	4. Determine availability and use of resources. Identify unmet demands or needs of the community.	4. Information necessary to identify what else is needed to meet the current situation.
	5. Determine community strengths.	5. Promotes understanding of the ways in which the community is already meeting the identified needs.
	6. Encourage community members/groups to engage in problem-solving activities.	6. Promotes a sense of working together to meet the needs.
	7. Develop a plan jointly with the members of the community to address immediate needs.	7. Deals with deficits in support of identified goals.
	8. Create plans managing interactions within the community and between the community and the larger society.	8. Meets collective needs when the concerns/threats are shared beyond a local community.
	9. Make information accessible to the public. Provide channels for dissemination of information to the community as a whole (e.g., print media, radio/television reports and community bulletin boards; Internet sites; speaker's bureau; reports to committees, councils, advisory boards).	9. Readily available accurate information can help citizens deal with the situation.

Table 13–2 | CARE PLAN FOR THE CLIENT WHO HAS EXPERIENCED A TRAUMATIC EVENT—cont'd

OUTCOME CRITERIA	NURSING INTERVENTIONS	RATIONALE
	10. Make information available in different modalities and geared to differing educational levels and cultures of the community.	10. Using languages other than English and making written materials accessible to all members of the community promotes understanding.
	11. Seek out and evaluate needs of underserved populations.	11. Homeless and those residing in lower income areas may have special requirements that need to be addressed with additional resources.

SOURCE: Doenges, M.E., Moorhouse, M.F., & Murr, A.C. (2016). *Nurse's pocket guide: Diagnoses, prioritized interventions, and rationales* (14th ed.). Philadelphia: F.A. Davis. With permission.

■ Is the client able to discuss his or her beliefs about spiritual issues?

■ Does the client demonstrate the ability to deal with emotional reactions in an individually appropriate manner?

■ Does he or she verbalize a subsiding of the physical manifestations (e.g., pain, nightmares, flashbacks, fatigue) associated with the traumatic event?

■ Has there been recognition of factors affecting the community's ability to meet its own demands or needs?

■ Has there been a demonstration of increased activities to improve community functioning?

■ Has a plan been established and put in place to deal with future contingencies?

When acute crises are not resolved, an individual may be vulnerable to acute stress disorders and trauma-related disorders. See Chapter 28 for more information on these topics.

Summary and Key Points

■ A *crisis* is defined as "a sudden event in one's life that disturbs homeostasis, during which usual coping mechanisms cannot resolve the problem" (Lagerquist, 2012, p. 795).

■ All individuals experience crises at one time or another. This does not necessarily indicate psychopathology. However, individuals with psychopathology are also vulnerable to crisis and may experience an exacerbation of psychiatric symptoms when in crisis.

■ Crises are precipitated by specific identifiable events and are determined by an individual's personal perception of the situation.

■ Crises are acute rather than chronic and generally last no more than a few weeks to a few months.

■ Crises occur when an individual is exposed to a stressor and previous problem-solving techniques are ineffective. This causes the level of anxiety to rise. Panic may ensue when new techniques are tried and resolution fails to occur.

■ Six types of crises have been identified: dispositional crises, crises of anticipated life transitions, crises resulting from traumatic stress, maturation/developmental crises, crises reflecting psychopathology, and psychiatric emergencies. The type of crisis determines the method of intervention selected.

■ Crisis intervention is designed to provide rapid assistance for individuals who have an urgent need.

■ The minimum therapeutic goal of crisis intervention is psychological resolution of the individual's immediate crisis and restoration to at least the level of functioning that existed before the crisis period. A maximum goal is improvement in functioning above the precrisis level.

■ Nurses regularly respond to individuals in crisis in all types of settings. Nursing process is the vehicle by which nurses assist individuals in crisis with a short-term problem-solving approach to change.

■ A four-phase technique of crisis intervention includes assessment/analysis, planning of therapeutic intervention, intervention, and evaluation of crisis resolution and anticipatory planning.

■ Through this structured method of assistance, nurses help individuals in crisis to develop more adaptive coping strategies for dealing with stressful situations in the future.

■ Nurses have many important skills that can assist individuals and communities in the wake of traumatic events. Nursing interventions presented in this chapter were developed for the nursing diagnoses of panic anxiety/fear, spiritual distress, risk for posttrauma syndrome, and ineffective community coping.

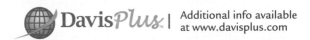 DavisPlus | Additional info available at www.davisplus.com

Review Questions
Self-Examination/Learning Exercise

Select the best response to each of the following questions.

1. Which of the following is a correct assumption regarding the concept of crisis?
   a. Crises occur only in individuals with psychopathology.
   b. The stressful event that precipitates crisis is seldom identifiable.
   c. A crisis situation contains the potential for psychological growth or deterioration.
   d. Crises are chronic situations that recur many times during an individual's life.

2. Crises occur when an individual:
   a. Is exposed to a precipitating stressor.
   b. Perceives a stressor to be threatening.
   c. Has no support systems.
   d. Experiences a stressor and perceives coping strategies to be ineffective.

3. Amanda's mobile home was destroyed by a tornado. Amanda received only minor injuries but is experiencing disabling anxiety in the aftermath of the event. What is this type of crisis called?
   a. Crisis resulting from traumatic stress
   b. Maturational/developmental crisis
   c. Dispositional crisis
   d. Crisis of anticipated life transitions

4. The most appropriate crisis intervention with Amanda (from question 3) would be to:
   a. Encourage her to recognize how lucky she is to be alive.
   b. Discuss stages of grief and feelings associated with each.
   c. Identify community resources that can help Amanda.
   d. Suggest that she find a place to live that provides a storm shelter.

5. Jenny reported to the high school nurse that her mother drinks too much. She is drunk every afternoon when Jenny gets home from school. Jenny is afraid to invite friends over because of her mother's behavior. What is this type of crisis called?
   a. Crisis resulting from traumatic stress
   b. Maturational/developmental crisis
   c. Dispositional crisis
   d. Crisis reflecting psychopathology

6. The most appropriate nursing intervention with Jenny (from question 5) would be to:
   a. Facilitate arrangements for her to start attending Alateen meetings.
   b. Help her identify the positive things in her life and recognize that her situation could be a lot worse than it is.
   c. Teach her about the effects of alcohol on the body and that it can be hereditary.
   d. Refer her to a psychiatrist for private therapy to learn to deal with her home situation.

7. Ginger, age 19 and an only child, left 3 months ago to attend a college of her choice 500 miles away from her parents. It is Ginger's first time away from home. She has difficulty making decisions and will not undertake anything new without first consulting her mother. They talk on the phone almost every day. Ginger has recently started having anxiety attacks. She consults the nurse practitioner in the student health center. What is this type of crisis called?
   a. Crisis resulting from traumatic stress
   b. Dispositional crisis
   c. Psychiatric emergency
   d. Maturational/developmental crisis

Review Questions—cont'd
Self-Examination/Learning Exercise

8. The most appropriate nursing intervention with Ginger (from question 7) would be to:
   a. Suggest she move to a college closer to home.
   b. Work with Ginger on unresolved dependency issues.
   c. Help her find someone in the college town from whom she could seek assistance rather than calling her mother regularly.
   d. Recommend that the college physician prescribe an antianxiety medication for Ginger.

9. Marie, age 56, is the mother of five children. Her youngest child, who had been living at home and attending the local college, recently graduated and accepted a job in another state. Marie has never worked outside the home and has devoted her life to satisfying the needs of her husband and children. Since the departure of her last child from home, Marie has become increasingly despondent. Her husband has become very concerned and takes her to the local mental health center. What is this type of crisis called?
   a. Dispositional crisis
   b. Crisis of anticipated life transitions
   c. Psychiatric emergency
   d. Crisis resulting from traumatic stress

10. The most appropriate nursing intervention with Marie (from question 9) would be to:
   a. Refer her to her family physician for a complete physical examination.
   b. Suggest she seek outside employment now that her children have left home.
   c. Identify convenient support systems for times when she is feeling particularly despondent.
   d. Begin grief work and assist her to recognize areas of self-worth separate and apart from her children.

11. Which of the following is a desired outcome of working with an individual who has witnessed a traumatic event and is now experiencing panic anxiety?
   a. The individual will experience no anxiety.
   b. The individual will demonstrate hope for the future.
   c. The individual will identify that anxiety is at a manageable level.
   d. The individual will verbalize acceptance of self as worthy.

12. Andrew, a New York City firefighter, and his entire unit responded to the terrorist attacks at the World Trade Center. Working as a team, he and his best friend, Carlo, entered the area together. Carlo was killed when the building collapsed. Andrew was injured but survived. Since that time, Andrew has had frequent nightmares and anxiety attacks. He says to the mental health worker, "I don't know why Carlo had to die and I didn't!" This statement by Andrew suggests that he is experiencing:
   a. Spiritual distress.
   b. Night terrors.
   c. Survivor's guilt.
   d. Suicidal ideation.

13. Intervention with Andrew (from question 15) would include:
   a. Encouraging expression of feelings.
   b. Antianxiety medications.
   c. Participation in a support group.
   d. a and c.
   e. All of the above.

Communication Exercises

1. A client you have been working with for several days approaches you with apparent signs of agitation and yells in a loud voice, "I want out of this hospital right now! You don't listen to a thing I say, and my doctor just wants my money." How will you respond?

2. Shelley enters the emergency room accompanied by a friend who reports that Shelley was raped after leaving a college campus party the night before. Shelley is staring off into space, exhibits a closed posture, and is mumbling inaudibly. How will you introduce yourself and begin to intervene in this crisis situation?

3. Thomas was secluded and restrained after punching another patient on the inpatient psychiatric unit. The next day he asks you what happened last night, stating he does not remember, and says he wants to know why he was arrested and tied up like an animal. What will you communicate to Thomas about the prior events and the crisis intervention process?

References

Aguilera, D.C. (1998). *Crisis intervention: Theory and methodology* (8th ed.). St. Louis, MO: Mosby.

Bateman, A., & Peternelj-Taylor, C. (1998). Crisis intervention. In C.A. Glod (Ed.), *Contemporary psychiatric-mental health nursing: The brain-behavior connection*. Philadelphia: F.A. Davis.

Doenges, M.E., Moorhouse, M.F., & Murr, A.C. (2016). *Nurse's pocket guide: Diagnoses, prioritized interventions, and rationales* (14th ed.). Philadelphia: F.A. Davis.

Lagerquist, S.L. (2012). *Davis's NCLEX-RN success* (3rd ed.). Philadelphia: F.A. Davis.

National Alliance on Mental Illness. (2015). Crisis services. Retrieved from www.nami.org/NAMI/media/NAMI-Media/Images/FactSheets/Crisis-Service-FS.pdf

National Alliance on Mental Illness. (2014). *State mental health legislation 2014: Trends, themes, and effective practices*. Retrieved from www.nami.org/legreport2014

Norwood, A.E., Ursano, R.J., & Fullerton, C.S. (2000). Disaster psychiatry: Principles and practice. *Psychiatric Quarterly, 71*(3), 207-226. doi:10.1023/A:1004678010161

Roberts, A.R., & Ottens, A.J. (2005). The seven-stage crisis intervention model: A road map to goal attainment, problem solving, and crisis resolution. *Brief Treatment and Crisis Intervention, 5*(4), 329-339. doi:http://dx.doi.org/10.1093/brief-treatment/mhi030

SAMHSA. (2014). *SAMHSA's concept of trauma and guidance for a trauma-informed approach*. Retrieved from https://store.samhsa.gov/shin/content//SMA14-4884/SMA14-4884.pdf

Watson, A.C., & Fulambarker, A.J. (2012). The crisis intervention team model of police response to mental health crisis: A primer for mental health practitioners. *Best Practices in Mental Health, 8*(2), 71-81.

Classical References

Baldwin, B.A. (1978, July). A paradigm for the classification of emotional crises: Implications for crisis intervention. *American Journal of Orthopsychiatry, 48*(3), 538-551. doi:10.1111/j.1939-0025.1978.tb01342.x

Caplan, G. (1964). *Principles of preventive psychiatry*. New York: Basic Books.

Assertiveness Training

14

CORE CONCEPTS

Assertive Behavior

KEY TERMS

aggressive	emotional intelligence	passive-aggressive
assertive	nonassertive	thought-stopping

OBJECTIVES
After reading this chapter, the student will be able to:

1. Define *assertive behavior*.
2. Discuss basic human rights.
3. Differentiate among nonassertive, assertive, aggressive, and passive-aggressive behaviors.
4. Describe techniques that promote assertive behavior.

5. Demonstrate thought-stopping techniques.
6. Discuss the role of the nurse in assertiveness training.

HOMEWORK ASSIGNMENT
Please read the chapter and answer the following quetions

1. What is the goal of assertive behavior?
2. Assertive individuals accept negative aspects about themselves and admit when they have made a mistake. What is this technique called?

3. What technique may be used to rid the mind of negative thoughts with which an individual may be obsessed? Give an example.
4. Why are "I" statements an effective communication technique?

Alberti and Emmons (2008) have proposed the following questions:

Are you able to express warm, positive feelings to another person? Are you comfortable starting a conversation with strangers at a party? Do you sometimes feel ineffective in making your desires clear to others? Do you have difficulty saying no to persuasive people?

Are you often at the bottom of the "pecking order," pushed around by others? Or maybe you're the one who pushes others around to get your way? (p. 5)

Assertive behavior promotes a feeling of personal power and self-confidence. These two components are commonly lacking in clients with emotional disorders. Becoming more assertive empowers individuals by promoting self-esteem without diminishing the esteem of others.

This chapter describes a number of rights that are considered basic to human beings. Various kinds of behaviors are explored, including assertive, nonassertive, aggressive, and passive-aggressive. Techniques that promote assertive behavior and the nurse's role in assertiveness training are presented.

CORE CONCEPT

Assertive Behavior

Assertive behavior promotes equality in human relationships, enabling us to act in our own best interests, to stand up for ourselves without undue anxiety, to express honest feelings comfortably, to exercise personal rights without denying the rights of others (Alberti & Emmons, 2008, p. 8).

Assertive Communication

Assertive behavior helps us feel good about ourselves and increases our self-esteem. It helps us feel good about other people and increases our ability to develop satisfying relationships. Assertive communication is characterized by honesty, directness, appropriateness, and respect for one's own basic rights as well as the rights of others.

Honesty is basic to assertive behavior. Assertive honesty is not an outspoken declaration of everything that is on one's mind. It is instead an accurate representation of feelings, opinions, or preferences expressed in a manner that promotes self-respect and respect for others.

Direct communication is stating what one wants to convey with clarity and candor. Hinting and "beating around the bush" are indirect forms of communication.

Communication must occur in an appropriate context to be considered assertive. The location and timing, as well as the manner (tone of voice, nonverbal gestures) in which the communication is presented, must be correct for the situation.

Basic Human Rights

A number of authors have identified "assertive rights" (Bishop, 2013; Davis, Eshelman, & McKay, 2008; Lloyd, 2002; Schuster, 2000; Sobel & Ornstein, 1996). Following is a composite of 10 basic assertive human rights adapted from an aggregation of sources:

1. The right to be treated with respect
2. The right to express feelings, opinions, and beliefs
3. The right to say "no" without feeling guilty
4. The right to make and accept responsibility for mistakes
5. The right to be listened to and taken seriously
6. The right to change your mind
7. The right to ask for what you want
8. The right to put yourself first, sometimes
9. The right to set your own priorities
10. The right to refuse justification for your feelings or behavior

In accepting these rights, an individual also accepts the responsibilities that accompany them. Rights and responsibilities are reciprocal entities. To experience one without the other is inherently destructive to an individual. Some responsibilities associated with basic assertive human rights are presented in Table 14–1.

Response Patterns

Individuals develop patterns of responding to others. Some of these patterns have developed through

■ Watching other people (role modeling).
■ Being positively reinforced or punished for a certain response.
■ Inventing an individual response style.
■ Not being able to think of different or better ways to respond.
■ Not developing the proper skills for a better response.
■ Consciously and intentionally choosing a response style.

The nurse should be able to recognize his or her own pattern of responding as well as that of others. Four common response patterns are discussed here: nonassertive, assertive, aggressive, and passive-aggressive.

Nonassertive Behavior

Individuals who behave in a **nonassertive** (sometimes called *passive*) manner seek to please others at the expense of their own basic human rights. They seldom let their true feelings show and often feel hurt and anxious because they allow others to choose for them. They seldom achieve their own desired goals. They come across as very apologetic and tend to be self-deprecating. They use actions instead of words and hope someone will "guess" what they want. Their voices are hesitant, weak, and expressed in a monotone. Their eyes are usually downcast. They feel uncomfortable in interpersonal interactions. All they want is to please and to be liked by others. Their behavior helps them avoid unpleasant situations and confrontations with others; however, they often harbor anger and resentment.

TABLE 14–1 Assertive Rights and Responsibilities

RIGHTS	RESPONSIBILITIES
1. To be treated with respect	To treat others in a way that recognizes their human dignity
2. To express feelings, opinions, and beliefs	To accept ownership of our feelings and show respect for those that differ from our own
3. To say "no"	To analyze each situation individually, recognizing all human rights as equal (others have the right to say "no," too)
4. To make mistakes	To accept responsibility for own mistakes and try to correct them
5. To be listened to	To listen to others
6. To change your mind	To accept the possible consequences that the change may incur; to accept the same flexibility in others
7. To ask for what you want	To accept others' right to refuse your request
8. To put yourself first, sometimes	To put others first, sometimes
9. To set your own priorities	To consider one's limitations as well as strengths in directing independent activities, to be a dependable person
10. To refuse to justify feelings or behavior	To accept ownership of own feelings and behavior, to accept others without requiring justification for their feelings and behavior

Assertive Behavior

Individuals who demonstrate **assertive** behavior stand up for their own rights while protecting the rights of others. Feelings are expressed openly and honestly. They assume responsibility for their own choices and allow others to choose for themselves. They maintain self-respect and respect for others by treating everyone equally and with human dignity. They communicate tactfully, using lots of "I" statements. Their voices are warm and expressive, and eye contact is intermittent but direct. These individuals desire to communicate effectively with and be respected by others. They are self-confident and experience satisfactory and pleasurable relationships with others.

Aggressive Behavior

Individuals who use **aggressive** response patterns defend their own basic rights by violating the basic rights of others. Feelings are often expressed dishonestly and inappropriately. They say what is on their mind, often at the expense of others. Aggressive behavior commonly results in *put-downs,* leaving the receiver feeling hurt, defensive, and humiliated. Individuals responding aggressively devalue the self-worth of those on whom they impose their choices. They typically express an air of superiority, and their voices are often loud, demanding, angry, or cold and emotionless. Eye contact may be an attempt to intimidate others by "staring them down." They want to increase their feelings of power by dominating or humiliating others. Aggressive behavior hinders interpersonal relationships.

Passive-Aggressive Behavior

Individuals using **passive-aggressive** behavior *respond* to others by appearing passive and accepting of other's demands while *behaving* in ways that suggest anger and resentment are their true feelings. This kind of behavior is sometimes referred to as *indirect,* or *covert, aggression* and takes the form of passive, nonconfrontational action. This pattern of communication is dishonest, manipulative, and sly, and it undermines others with behavior that expresses the opposite of what they are feeling. It is critical and sometimes sarcastic. Individuals employing passive-aggressive behavior allow others to make choices for them, then resist by using passive behaviors such as procrastination, dawdling, stubbornness, and "forgetfulness." They use actions instead of words to convey their messages, and the actions express covert aggression. They become sulky, irritable, or argumentative when asked to do something they do not want to do. They may protest to others about the demand but will not confront the person who has made the demand. The goal is domination through retaliation. This behavior offers a feeling of control and power, although the individual actually feels resentment. This style of communication is associated with extremely low self-confidence.

A comparison of these four behavior patterns is presented in Table 14–2.

TABLE 14–2 **Comparison of Behavioral Response Patterns**

	NONASSERTIVE	ASSERTIVE	AGGRESSIVE	PASSIVE-AGGRESSIVE
BEHAVIORAL CHARACTERISTICS	Passive, does not express true feelings, self-deprecating, denies own rights	Stands up for own rights, protects rights of others, honest, direct, appropriate	Violates rights of others, expresses feelings dishonestly and inappropriately	Defends own rights with passive resistance, is critical and sarcastic; often expresses opposite of true feelings
EXAMPLES	"Uh, well, uh, sure, I'll be glad to stay and work an extra shift."	"I don't want to stay and work an extra shift today. I stayed over yesterday. It's someone else's turn today."	"You've got to be kidding!"	"Okay, I'll stay and work an extra shift." (Then to peer: "How dare she ask me to work over again! Well, we'll just see how much work she gets out of me!")
GOALS	To please others; to be liked by others	To communicate effectively; to be respected by others	To dominate or humiliate others	To dominate through retaliation
FEELINGS	Anxious, hurt, disappointed with self, angry, resentful	Confident, successful, proud, self-respecting	Self-righteous, controlling, superior	Anger, resentment, manipulated, controlled
COMPENSATION	Is able to avoid unpleasant situations and confrontations with others	Increased self-confidence, self-respect, respect for others, satisfying interpersonal relationships	Anger is released, increasing feeling of power and superiority	Feels self-righteous and in control
OUTCOMES	Goals not met; others meet *their* goals at nonassertive person's expense; anger and resentment grow; feels violated and manipulated	Goals met; desires most often fulfilled while defending own rights as well as rights of others	Goals may be met but at the expense of others; they feel hurt and vengeful	Goals not met, nor are the goals of others met due to retaliatory nature of the interaction

SOURCES: Alberti, R.E., & Emmons, M.L. (2008). *Your perfect right* (9th ed.). Atascadero, CA: Impact Publishers; Bishop, S. (2013). *Develop your assertiveness*. Philadelphia: Kogan Page; Davis, M., Eshelman, E.R., & McKay, M. (2008). *The relaxation and stress reduction workbook* (6th ed.). Oakland, CA: New Harbinger Publications; Lloyd, S.R. (2002). *Developing positive assertiveness* (3rd ed.). Menlo Park, CA: Crisp Publications; and Powell, T.J., & Enright, S.J. (1990). *Anxiety and stress management.* London: Routledge.

Behavioral Components of Assertive Behavior

Alberti and Emmons (2008) have identified several defining characteristics of assertive behavior:

■ **Eye contact:** Eye contact is considered appropriate when intermittent (i.e., looking directly at the person to whom one is speaking but looking away now and then). Individuals feel uncomfortable when someone stares at them continuously and intently. Intermittent eye contact conveys the message that one is interested in what is being said.

■ **Body posture:** Sitting and leaning slightly toward the other person in a conversation suggests an active interest in what is being said. Emphasis on an assertive stance can be achieved by standing with an erect posture squarely facing the other person. A slumped posture conveys passivity or nonassertiveness.

■ **Distance/physical contact:** The distance between two individuals in an interaction or the physical contact between them has a strong cultural influence. For example, mainstream culture of the United States considers intimate distance as approximately 18 inches from the body. Invasion of this space may be interpreted by some individuals as very aggressive.

■ **Gestures:** Nonverbal gestures also are variable among different cultures. In assertive communication, gestures add emphasis, warmth, depth, or power to the spoken word with awareness of and sensitivity to the impact on the receiver .

■ **Facial expression:** Various facial expressions convey different messages (e.g., surprise, anger, fear). It is difficult to "fake" these messages. In assertive communication, the facial expression is congruent with the verbal message.

■ **Voice:** The voice conveys a message by its loudness, softness, degree and placement of emphasis, and evidence of emotional tone. In assertive communication, the voice conveys an acceptable volume to communicate confidence without being too loud or forceful.

■ **Fluency:** The ability to discuss a subject with ease and obvious knowledge conveys assertiveness and self-confidence. This message is impeded by numerous pauses or filler words such as "and, uh . . ." or "you know. . . ."

■ **Timing:** Assertive responses are most effective when they are spontaneous and immediate. However, most people have experienced times when it was inappropriate to respond (e.g., in front of a group of people) or times when an appropriate response is generated only after the fact ("If only I had said . . ."). Alberti and Emmons (2008, p. 77) stated that "it is never too late to be assertive!" It is correct and worthwhile to seek out the individual at a later time and express the assertive response.

■ **Listening:** Assertive listening means giving the other individual full attention by making eye contact, nodding to indicate acceptance of what is said, and taking time to understand the message before responding.

■ **Thoughts:** Cognitive processes affect one's assertive behavior. Two such processes are an individual's attitudes about the appropriateness of assertive behavior in general and the appropriateness of assertive behavior for oneself specifically. Assertive communication is supported by a belief that being assertive is a reasonable, appropriate, and healthy way to communicate.

■ **Content:** The content of assertive communication includes "I" statements to describe one's feelings and needs. "You" statements, such as "You never listen to me" or "You don't respect my parenting decisions," tend to put others on the defensive. Instead, "I" statements such as "I'm upset because I don't feel like you're hearing me" or "I need you to respect my decision on this parenting issue," tend to lessen defensiveness and increase the likelihood that the message will be received and heard.

■ **Persistence:** This element of assertive behavior involves maintaining confidence in and commitment to one's needs and feelings even when someone is pressuring the individual to cave in to demands. It often means repeating a stated feeling or need in an effort to be heard and respected. Persistence, as with other aspects of assertive behavior, employs "I" communication statements. For example, when someone is trying to pressure another person to drink alcohol, a persistent response might be "As I already told you, I am not interested in drinking alcohol, and I need for you to stop pressuring me."

Techniques That Promote Assertive Behavior

The following techniques have been shown to be effective in responding to criticism and avoiding manipulation by others:

1. **Standing up for one's basic human rights**

EXAMPLE

"I have the right to express my opinion."

2. **Assuming responsibility for one's own statements**

EXAMPLE

"I *don't want* to go out with you tonight," instead of "I *can't* go out with you tonight." The latter implies a lack of power or ability.

3. **Responding as a broken record;** that is, persistently repeating in a calm voice what is wanted

EXAMPLE

Telephone salesperson: I want to help you save money by changing long-distance services.

Assertive response: I don't want to change my long-distance service.

Telephone salesperson: I can't believe you don't want to save money!

Assertive response: I don't want to change my long-distance service.

4. **Agreeing assertively;** that is, assertively accepting negative aspects about oneself and admitting when an error has been made

EXAMPLE

Ms. Jones: You sure let that meeting get out of hand. What a waste of time.

Ms. Smith: Yes, I didn't do a very good job of conducting the meeting today.

5. **Inquiring assertively;** that is, seeking additional information about critical statements

EXAMPLE

Male board member: You made a real fool of yourself at the board meeting last night.

Female board member: Oh, really? Just what about my behavior offended you?

Male board member: You were so damned pushy!

Female board member: Were you offended that I spoke up for my beliefs, or was it because my beliefs are in direct opposition to yours?

6. **Shifting from content to process;** that is, changing the focus of the communication from discussing the topic at hand to analyzing what is actually going on in the interaction

EXAMPLE

Wife: Would you please call me if you will be late for dinner?

Husband: Why don't you just get off my back! I always have to account for every minute of my time with you!

Wife: Sounds to me like we need to discuss some other things here. What are you *really* angry about?

7. **Clouding or fogging;** that is, concurring with the critic's argument without becoming defensive and without agreeing to change

EXAMPLE

Nurse 1: You never come to the Nurses Association meetings. I don't know why you even belong!

Nurse 2: You're right. I haven't attended very many of the meetings.

8. **Defusing;** that is, putting off further discussion with an angry individual until he or she is calmer

EXAMPLE

"You are very angry right now. I don't want to discuss this matter with you while you are so upset. I will discuss it with you in my office at 3 o'clock this afternoon."

9. **Delaying assertively;** that is, putting off further discussion with another individual until one is calmer

EXAMPLE

"That's a very challenging position you have taken, Mr. Brown. I'll need time to give it some thought. I'll call you later this afternoon."

10. **Responding assertively with irony**

EXAMPLE

Man: I bet you're one of them so-called women's libbers, aren't you?

Woman: Why, yes. Thank you for noticing.

11. **Using "I" statements,** which allow an individual to take ownership for his or her feelings rather than saying they are caused by another person

"I" statements are sometimes called "feeling" statements. They express directly what an individual is

feeling. "You" statements are accusatory and put the receiver on the defensive. "I" statements have four parts:

1. How I feel: *These are my feelings and I accept ownership of them.*
2. When: *Describe in a neutral manner the behavior that is the problem.*
3. Why: *Describe what it is about the behavior that is objectionable.*
4. What I need (suggesting change): *Offer a preferred alternative to the behavior using "I" statements.*

EXAMPLE

John has just returned from a hunting trip and walked into the living room in his muddy boots, leaving a trail of mud on the carpet. His wife, Mary, may respond as follows:

With a "you" statement: "You are such a jerk! Can't you see the trail of mud you are leaving on the carpet? I just cleaned this carpet. You make me so angry!"

With an "I" statement: "I feel so angry when you walk on the carpet in your muddy boots. I just cleaned it, and now I will have to clean it again. I would appreciate it if you would remove your boots on the porch before you come in the house."

"You" statements are negative and focus on what the person has done wrong. They do not explain what is being requested of the person. "I" statements are more positive. They explain *how* one is feeling, *why* he or she is feeling that way, and *what* the individual wants instead. Hopkins (2013) stated the following about the importance of "I" statements:

> Part of being assertive involves the ability to appropriately express your needs and feelings. You accomplish this by using "I" statements. These [statements] indicate ownership, do not attribute blame, focus on behavior, identify the effect of the behavior, are direct and honest, and contribute to the growth of your relationship with each other. (p. 2)

Thought-Stopping Techniques

Assertive thinking is sometimes inhibited by repetitive, negative thoughts of which the mind refuses to let go. Individuals with low self-worth may be obsessed with thoughts such as, "I know he'd never want to go out with me. I'm too ugly (or plain, or fat, or dumb)" or "I just know I'll never be able to do this job well" or "I just can't seem to do anything right." This type of thinking fosters the belief that one's individual rights do not deserve the same consideration as those of others and reflects nonassertive communication and behavioral response patterns.

Thought-stopping techniques, as described here, were developed by psychiatrist Joseph Wolpe (1990) and are intended to eliminate intrusive, unwanted thoughts.

Method

In a practice setting, with eyes closed, the individual concentrates on an unwanted recurring thought. Once the thought is clearly established in the mind, he or she shouts aloud: "STOP!" This action interrupts the thought, and it is actually removed from one's awareness. The individual then immediately shifts his or her thoughts to one that is considered pleasant and desirable.

It is possible that the unwanted thought may soon recur, but with practice, the length of time between recurrences will increase until the unwanted thought is no longer intrusive.

Obviously, one cannot go about his or her daily life shouting, "STOP!" in public places. After a number of practice sessions, the technique is equally effective if "stop!" is used silently in the mind.

Role of the Nurse in Assertiveness Training

It is important for nurses to become aware of and recognize their own behavioral responses. Common questions used to assess and develop self-awareness include: Are my behaviors mostly nonassertive? Assertive? Aggressive? Passive-aggressive? Do I consider my behavioral responses effective? Do I wish to change? Remember, all individuals have the right to choose whether or not they want to be assertive. A self-assessment of assertiveness is found in Box 14–1.

Assertive communication is part of a larger set of competencies referred to as **emotional intelligence (EI).** This concept, first developed by Salovey and Mayer (1990) and elaborated by Goleman (2006), includes four sets of competencies: self-awareness (of emotions and behavior), social awareness (awareness of other's feelings, or empathy), self-management (which includes self-control), and relationship management (which includes skills in teamwork and collaboration). Each of these competencies is relevant to developing skill in assertive communication. To communicate assertively, individuals must be aware of their own feelings and the feelings of others; they must be aware of and develop skill in their ability to control their emotions and behavior; and they must respond in ways

---

BOX 14–1 An Assertiveness Quiz

Assign a number to each item using the following scale: 1 = Never; 3 = Sometimes; 5 = Always

_____ 1. I ask others to do things without feeling guilty or anxious.
_____ 2. When someone asks me to do something I don't want to do, I say no without feeling guilty or anxious.
_____ 3. I am comfortable when speaking to a large group of people.
_____ 4. I confidently express my honest opinions to authority figures (such as my boss).
_____ 5. When I experience powerful feelings (anger, frustration, disappointment, and so on), I verbalize them easily.
_____ 6. When I express anger, I do so without blaming others for "making me mad."
_____ 7. I am comfortable speaking up in a group situation.
_____ 8. If I disagree with the majority opinion in a meeting, I can "stick to my guns" without feeling uncomfortable or being abrasive.
_____ 9. When I make a mistake, I acknowledge it.
_____ 10. I tell others when their behavior creates a problem for me.
_____ 11. Meeting new people in social situations is something I do with ease and comfort.
_____ 12. When discussing my beliefs, I do so without labeling the opinions of others as "crazy," "stupid," "ridiculous," or "irrational."
_____ 13. I assume that most people are competent and trustworthy, and I do not have difficulty delegating tasks to others.
_____ 14. When considering doing something I have never done, I feel confident I can learn to do it.
_____ 15. I believe that my needs are as important as those of others, and I am entitled to have my needs satisfied.
_____ TOTAL SCORE

SCORING:
1. If your total score is 60 or higher, you have a consistently assertive philosophy and probably handle most situations well.
2. If your total score is 45 to 59, you have a fairly assertive outlook but may benefit from some assertiveness training.
3. If your total score is 30 to 44, you may be assertive in some situations, but your natural response is either nonassertive or aggressive. Assertiveness training is suggested.
4. If your total score is 15 to 29, you have considerable difficulty being assertive. Assertiveness training is recommended.

SOURCE: Lloyd, S.R. (2002). Developing positive assertiveness (3rd ed.). Menlo Park, CA: Crisp Publications. With permission.

that effectively manage relationships, including skills that resolve conflicts rather than escalate them.

 In professional roles, assertive communication and EI are important competencies for effective teamwork and collaboration.

The ability to respond assertively is especially important to nurses who are committed to further development of the profession. Assertiveness skills facilitate the implementation of change—change that is required if the image of nursing is to be upheld to the level of professionalism that most nurses desire. Assertive communication is useful in the political arena for nurses who choose to become involved at state and national levels in striving to influence legislation and ultimately improve our country's system of health-care provision.

Nurses who understand and use assertiveness skills themselves can in turn assist clients who wish to effect behavioral change in an effort to increase self-esteem and improve interpersonal relationships. When using assertive communication and teaching clients about assertiveness, it is important to be clear that assertive communication does not necessarily assure a particular response. For example, a spouse may assertively communicate that she or he feels overwhelmed and needs more help with the housework, but the other spouse still has control over whether or not to respect those wishes. Instead, assertive communication is a way to communicate one's feelings and needs in a manner that is less likely to generate defensiveness from the receiver and more likely to allow the message to be heard. Evidence supports that assertiveness skills training is beneficial in reducing symptoms of depression

and interpersonal difficulties and for improving one's self-esteem, even among individuals with severe mental illness such as schizophrenia (Maaly, Merfat, & Faten, 2016; Shean, 2013; Tavakoli et al., 2014).

The nursing process is a useful tool for nurses who are involved in helping clients increase their assertiveness.

Assessment

Nurses can help clients become more aware of their behavioral responses. Many tools exist for assessing the level of assertiveness, but it is difficult to *generalize* when attempting to measure assertive behaviors. Box 14–2 and Figure 14–1 represent examples of assertiveness inventories that could be personalized to explore life situations of individual clients more specifically. Obviously, the everyday situations that require assertiveness are not the same for all individuals.

Diagnosis

Possible nursing diagnoses for individuals needing assistance with assertiveness include the following:

- Coping, defensive
- Coping, ineffective
- Decisional conflict
- Denial
- Personal identity, disturbed
- Powerlessness
- Rape-trauma syndrome
- Self-esteem, low
- Social interaction, impaired
- Social isolation

BOX 14–2 Everyday Situations That May Require Assertiveness

AT WORK
How do you respond when:

1. You receive a compliment on your appearance or someone praises your work?
2. You are criticized unfairly?
3. You are criticized legitimately by a superior?
4. You have to confront a subordinate for continual lateness or sloppy work?
5. Your boss makes a sexual innuendo or makes a pass at you?

IN PUBLIC
How do you respond when:

1. In a restaurant, the food you ordered arrives cold or overcooked?
2. A fellow passenger in a no-smoking compartment lights a cigarette?
3. You are faced with an unhelpful shop assistant?
4. Somebody barges in front of you in a waiting line?
5. You take an inferior article back to a shop?

AMONG FRIENDS
How do you respond when:

1. You feel angry with the way a friend has treated you?
2. A friend makes what you consider to be an unreasonable request?
3. You want to ask a friend for a favor?
4. You ask a friend for repayment of a loan of money?
5. You have to negotiate with a friend on which film to see or where to meet?

AT HOME
How do you respond when:

1. One of your parents criticizes you?
2. You are irritated by a persistent habit in someone you love?
3. Everybody leaves the cleaning-up chores to you?
4. You want to say "no" to a proposed visit to a relative?
5. Your partner feels amorous but you are not in the mood?

SOURCE: From Powell, T.J., & Enright, S.J. (1990). Anxiety and stress management. London: Routledge. With permission.

DIRECTIONS: Fill in each block with a rating of your assertiveness on a 5-point scale. A rating of 0 means you have no difficulty asserting yourself. A rating of 5 means that you are completely unable to assert yourself. Evaluation can be made by analyzing the scores:

1. Totally by activity, including all of the different people categories
2. Totally by people, including all of the different activity categories
3. On an individual basis, considering specific people and specific activities

PEOPLE / ACTIVITY	Friends of the same sex	Friends of the opposite sex	Intimate relations or spouse	Authority figures	Relatives/ family members	Colleagues and sub-ordinates	Strangers	Service workers: waiters, shop assistants, etc.
Giving and receiving compliments								
Asking for favors/help								
Initiating and maintaining conversation								
Refusing requests								
Expressing personal opinions								
Expressing anger/dis-pleasure								
Expressing liking, love, affection								
Stating your rights and needs								

FIGURE 14–1 Rating your assertiveness. (From Powell, T.J., & Enright, S.J. [1990]. *Anxiety and stress management.* London: Routledge, with permission.)

Outcome Identification and Implementation

The goal for nurses working with individuals needing assistance with assertiveness is to help them develop more satisfying interpersonal relationships. Individuals who do not feel good about themselves either allow others to violate their rights or cover up their low self-esteem by being overtly or covertly aggressive. Individuals should be given information regarding their individual human rights. They must know these rights before they can assert them.

Outcome criteria are derived from specific nursing diagnoses. Time lines are individually determined. Examples include the following:

■ The client verbalizes and accepts responsibility for his or her own behavior.
■ The client is able to express opinions and disagree with the opinions of others in a socially acceptable manner without feeling guilty.
■ The client is able to verbalize positive aspects about self.

■ The client verbalizes choices made in a plan to maintain control over his or her life situation.
■ The client approaches others in an appropriate manner for one-to-one interaction.

In a clinical setting, nurses can teach clients techniques to increase their assertive responses. This can be done on a one-to-one basis or in group situations. Once these techniques have been discussed, nurses can assist clients to practice them through role-playing. Each client should compose a list of specific personal examples of situations that create difficulties for him or her. These situations will then be simulated in the therapy setting so that the client may practice assertive responses in a nonthreatening environment. In a group situation, feedback from peers can provide valuable insight about the effectiveness of the response.

> **CLINICAL PEARL** An important part of this type of intervention is to ensure that clients are aware of the differences among assertive, nonassertive, aggressive, and passive-aggressive

behaviors in the same situation. When discussion is held about what the best (assertive) response would be, it is also important to discuss the other types of responses as well so that clients can begin to recognize their pattern of response and make changes accordingly.

CLINICAL EXAMPLE

Linda comes to day hospital once a week to attend group therapy and assertiveness training. She has had problems with depression and low self-esteem and is married to a man who is verbally abusive. He is highly critical, is seldom satisfied with anything Linda does, and blames her for negative consequences that occur in their lives whether or not she is involved.

Since the beginning of the assertiveness training group, the nurse who leads the group has taught the participants about basic human rights and the various types of response patterns. When the nurse asks for client situations to be presented in group, Linda volunteers to discuss an incident that occurred in her home this week. She related that she had just put some chicken on the stove to cook for supper when her 7-year-old son came running in the house yelling that he had been hurt. Linda went to him and observed that he had blood dripping down the side of his head from his forehead. He said he and some friends had been playing on the jungle gym in the schoolyard down the street and he had fallen and hit his head. Linda went with him to the bathroom to clean the wound and apply some medication. Her husband, Joe, was reading the newspaper in the living room. By the time she got back to the chicken on the stove, it was burned and inedible. Her husband shouted, "You stupid woman! You can't do anything right!" Linda did not respond but burst into tears.

The nurse asked the other members in the group to present some ideas about how Linda could have responded to Joe's criticism. After some discussion, they agreed that Linda might have stated, "I made a mistake. I am not stupid and I do lots of things right." They also discussed other types of responses and why they were less acceptable. They recognized that Linda's lack of verbal response and bursting into tears was a nonassertive response. They also agreed on other examples, such as the following:

1. An aggressive response might be, "Cook your own supper!" and toss the skillet out the back door.
2. A passive-aggressive response might be to fix sandwiches for supper and not speak to Joe for 3 days.

Practice on the assertive response began, with the nurse and various members of the group playing the role of Joe so that Linda could practice until she felt comfortable with the response. She participated in the group for 6 months, regularly submitting situations with which she needed help. She also learned from the situations presented by other members of the group. These weekly sessions gave Linda the self-confidence that she needed to stand up to Joe's criticism. She became aware of her basic human rights and, with practice, was able to protect her rights by communicating them assertively. She was happy to report to the group after a few months that Joe seemed to be less critical and that their relationship was improving.

Evaluation

Evaluation requires that the nurse and client assess whether or not these techniques are achieving the desired outcomes. Reassessment might include the following questions:

■ Is the client able to accept criticism without becoming defensive?
■ Can the client express true feelings to (spouse, friend, boss, and others) when his or her basic human rights are violated?
■ Is the client able to decline a request without feeling guilty?
■ Can the client verbalize positive qualities about himself or herself?
■ Does the client verbalize improvement in interpersonal relationships?

Assertiveness training serves to extend and create more flexibility in an individual's communication style so that he or she has a greater choice of responses in various situations. Although change does not come easily, assertiveness training can be an effective way of changing behavior. Nurses can assist individuals to become more assertive, thereby encouraging them to become what they want to be, promoting an improvement in self-esteem, and fostering a respect for their own rights and the rights of others.

Summary and Key Points

■ Assertive behavior helps individuals feel better about themselves by encouraging them to stand up for their own basic human rights.
■ Basic human rights have equal representation for all individuals.
■ Along with rights comes an equal number of responsibilities. Part of being assertive includes living up to these responsibilities.
■ Assertive behavior increases self-esteem and the ability to develop satisfying interpersonal relationships. This is accomplished through honesty, directness, appropriateness, and respecting one's own rights and the rights of others.
■ Individuals develop patterns of responding in various ways, such as role modeling, by receiving positive or negative reinforcement, or by conscious choice.
■ Patterns of responding can take the form of nonassertiveness, assertiveness, aggressiveness, or passive-aggressiveness.

- Individuals who communicate in a *nonassertive* manner seek to please others at the expense of denying their own basic human rights.
- Individuals who communicate in an *assertive* manner stand up for their own rights while protecting the rights of others.
- Those who respond *aggressively* defend their own rights by violating the basic rights of others.
- Individuals who respond in a *passive-aggressive* manner defend their own rights by expressing resistance to social and occupational demands.
- Some important behavioral considerations of assertive behavior include eye contact, body posture, distance/physical contact, gestures, facial expression, voice, fluency, timing, listening, thoughts, content, and persistence.
- Using "I" statements is an important technique of assertive communication.

- Competency in the skills of emotional intelligence is foundational to effective assertive communication and behavior.
- Negative thinking can sometimes interfere with one's ability to respond assertively. Thought-stopping techniques help individuals remove negative, unwanted thoughts from awareness and promote the development of a more assertive attitude.
- Nurses can assist individuals to learn and practice assertiveness techniques.
- The nursing process is an effective vehicle for providing the information and support to clients as they strive to create positive change in their lives.

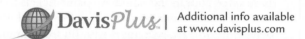

DavisPlus | Additional info available at www.davisplus.com

Review Questions
Self-Examination/Learning Exercise

Select the answer that is most appropriate for each of the following questions.

1. Your husband says, "You're crazy to think about going to college! You're not smart enough to handle the studies and the housework, too." Which of the following is an example of a nonassertive response?
   a. "I will do what I can and the best that I can."
   b. (Thinking to yourself): "We'll see how *he* likes cooking dinner for a change."
   c. "You're probably right. Maybe I should reconsider."
   d. "I'm going to do what I want to do, when I want to do it, and you can't stop me!"

2. You are having company for dinner, and they are due to arrive in 20 minutes. You are about to finish cooking and still have to shower and dress. The doorbell rings and it is a man selling a new product for cleaning windows. Which of the following is an example of an aggressive response?
   a. "I don't do windows!" and slam the door in his face.
   b. "I'll take a case," and write him a check.
   c. "Sure, I'll take three bottles." Then to yourself you think: "I'm calling this company tomorrow and complaining to the manager about their salespeople coming around at dinnertime!"
   d. "I'm very busy at the moment. I don't wish to purchase any of your product. Thank you."

3. You are in a movie theater that prohibits smoking. The person in the seat next to you just lit a cigarette and the smoke is very irritating. Which of the following is an example of an assertive response?
   a. You say nothing.
   b. "Please put your cigarette out. Smoking is prohibited."
   c. You say nothing but begin to frantically fan the air in front of you and cough loudly and convulsively.
   d. "Put your cigarette out, you slob! Can't you read the 'no smoking' sign?"

Continued

Review Questions—cont'd
Self-Examination/Learning Exercise

4. You have been studying for a nursing exam all afternoon and lost track of time. Your husband expects dinner on the table when he gets home from work. You have not started cooking yet when he walks in the door and shouts, "Why the heck isn't dinner ready?" Which of the following is an example of a passive-aggressive response?
   a. "I'm sorry. I'll have it done in no time, honey." But then you move very slowly and take a long time to cook the meal.
   b. "I'm tired from studying all afternoon. Make your own dinner, you bum! I'm tired of being your slave!"
   c. "I haven't started dinner yet. I'd like some help from you."
   d. "I'm so sorry. I know you're tired and hungry. It's all my fault. I'm such a terrible wife!"

5. You and your best friend, Jill, have had plans for 6 months to go on vacation together to Hawaii. You have saved your money and have plane tickets to leave in 3 weeks. She has just called you and reported that she is not going. She has a new boyfriend, they are moving in together, and she does not want to leave him. You are very angry with Jill for changing your plans. Which of the following is an example of an assertive response?
   a. "I'm very disappointed and very angry. I'd like to talk to you about this later. I'll call you."
   b. "I'm very happy for you, Jill. I think it's wonderful that you and Jack are moving in together."
   c. You tell Jill that you are very happy for her, but then say to another friend, "Well, that's the end of my friendship with Jill!"
   d. "What? You can't do that to me! We've had plans! You're acting like a real slut!"

6. A typewritten report for your psychiatric nursing class is due tomorrow at 8 a.m. The assignment was made 4 weeks ago, and yours is ready to turn in. Your roommate says, "I finally finished writing my report, but now I have to go to work, and I don't have time to type it. Please be a dear and type it for me. Otherwise, I'll fail!" You have a date with your boyfriend. Which of the following is an example of an aggressive response?
   a. "Okay, I'll call Ken and cancel our date."
   b. "I don't want to stay here and type your report. I'm going out with Ken."
   c. "You've got to be kidding! What kind of a fool do you take me for, anyway?"
   d. "Okay, I'll do it." However, when your roommate returns from work at midnight, you are asleep and the report has not been typed.

7. You are asked to serve on a committee on which you do not wish to serve. Which of the following is an example of a nonassertive response?
   a. "Thank you, but I don't wish to be a member of that committee."
   b. "I'll be happy to serve." But then you don't show up for any of the meetings.
   c. "I'd rather have my teeth pulled!"
   d. "Okay, if I'm really needed, I'll serve."

8. You're on your way to the laundry room when you encounter a fellow dorm tenant who often asks you to "throw a few of my things in with yours." You view this as an imposition. He asks you where you're going. Which of the following is an example of a passive-aggressive response?
   a. "I'm on my way to the Celtics game. Where do you think I'm going?"
   b. "I'm on my way to do some laundry. Do you have anything you want me to wash with mine?"
   c. "It's none of your damn business!"
   d. "I'm going to the laundry room. Please don't ask me to do some of yours. I resent being taken advantage of in that way."

Review Questions—cont'd
Self-Examination/Learning Exercise

9. At a hospital committee meeting, a fellow nurse who is the chairperson has interrupted you each time you have tried to make a statement. The next time it happens, you intend to respond assertively. Which of the following is an example of an assertive response?
   a. "You make a lousy leader! You won't even let me finish what I'm trying to say!"
   b. You say nothing.
   c. "Excuse me. I would like to finish my statement."
   d. You say nothing, but you fail to complete your assignment and do not show up for the next meeting.

10. A fellow worker often borrows small amounts of money from you with the promise that she will pay you back "tomorrow." She currently owes you $15 and has not yet paid back any that she has borrowed. She asks if she can borrow a couple of dollars for lunch. Which of the following is an example of a nonassertive response?
   a. "I've decided not to loan you any more money until you pay me back what you already borrowed."
   b. "I'm so sorry. I only have enough to pay for my own lunch today."
   c. "Get a life, will you? I'm tired of you sponging off me all the time!"
   d. "Sure, here's two dollars." Then to the other workers in the office: "Be sure you never lend Cindy any money. She never pays her debts. I'd be sure never to go to lunch with her if I were you!"

References

Alberti, R.E., & Emmons, M.L. (2008). *Your perfect right* (9th ed.). Atascadero, CA: Impact Publishers.

Bishop, S. (2013). *Develop your assertiveness.* Philadelphia: Kogan Page.

Davis, M., Eshelman, E.R., & McKay, M. (2008). *The relaxation and stress reduction workbook* (6th ed.). Oakland, CA: New Harbinger Publications.

Goleman, D. (2006). *Working with emotional intelligence.* New York: Bantam.

Hopkins, L. (2013). Assertive communication: Six tips for effective use. *EzineArticles.* Retrieved from http://ezinearticles.com/?Assertive-Communication-6-Tips-For-Effective-Use&id=10259

Lloyd, S.R. (2002). *Developing positive assertiveness* (3rd ed.). Menlo Park, CA: Crisp Publications.

Maaly, I.E.M, Merfat, A.M., & Faten, A.H. (2016). The effectiveness of social skill training on depressive symptoms, self-esteem, and interpersonal difficulties among schizophrenic patients. *International Journal of Advanced Nursing Studies,* 5 (1), 43-50. doi:10.14419/ijans.v5i1.5386

Powell, T.J., & Enright, S.J. (1990). *Anxiety and stress management.* London: Routledge.

Salovey, P., & Mayer, J.D. (1990). Emotional intelligence. *Imagination, Cognition, and Personality, 9,* 185-211. doi:0.2190/DUGG-P24E-52WK-6CDG

Schuster, P.M. (2000). Communication: The key to the therapeutic relationship. Philadelphia: F.A. Davis.

Shean, G.D. (2013). Empirically based psychosocial therapies for schizophrenia. The disconnection between science and practice. *Schizophrenia Research and Treatment.* Retrieved from https://www.hindawi.com/journals/schizort/2013/792769

Sobel, D.S., & Ornstein, R. (1996). *The healthy mind/healthy body handbook.* New York: Patient Education Media.

Tavakoli, P., Setoodeh, G., Dashtbozorgi, B., Komili-Sani, H., & Pakseresht, S. (2014). The influence of assertiveness training on self-esteem in female students of government high schools of Shiraz, Iran: A randomized controlled trial. *Nursing Practice Today 2014, 1*(1), 17-23.

Wolpe, J. (1990). *The practice of behavior therapy* (4th ed.) Elmsford, NY: Pergamon Press.

15

Promoting Self-Esteem

CHAPTER OUTLINE

KEY TERMS

body image

boundaries

contextual stimuli

enmeshed boundaries

flexible boundaries

focal stimuli

moral-ethical self

residual stimuli

rigid boundaries

self-consistency

self-ideal

OBJECTIVES

After reading this chapter, the student will be able to:

1. Identify and define components of the self-concept.
2. Discuss influencing factors in the development of self-esteem and its progression through the life span.
3. Describe the verbal and nonverbal manifestations of low self-esteem.
4. Discuss the concept of boundaries and its relationship to self-esteem.
5. Apply the nursing process with clients who are experiencing disturbances in self-esteem.

HOMEWORK ASSIGNMENT

Please read the chapter and answer the following questions:

1. Children need unconditional love to promote positive self-esteem. How do parents demonstrate unconditional love?
2. Since her parents' divorce, 10-year-old Juliet and her mother have become inseparable. They spend all their spare time together, and Juliet has become her mother's confidant. This is an example of what type of boundary?
3. How does fulfillment of the developmental tasks described by Erikson promote a healthy self-esteem?
4. Name the three components of self-concept and the meaning that individuals attach to each.

Whereas self-concept describes individuals' *thoughts and beliefs* about themselves, self-esteem describes how individuals *feel* about themselves. Hosogi and associates (2012) describe self-esteem as a feeling of self-appreciation that is indispensable for adaptation in society. The awareness of self (i.e., the ability to form an identity and then attach a value to it) is an important differentiating factor between humans and other animals. This capacity for judgment becomes a contributing factor in disturbances of self-esteem.

The promotion of self-esteem is about stopping irrational self-judgments. It is about helping individuals change how they perceive and feel about themselves. A healthy self-esteem means having a balanced, accurate view of oneself which includes being able to recognize one's flaws while maintaining a good opinion of one's abilities (Mayo Clinic, 2014). This chapter describes the developmental progression and the verbal and behavioral manifestations of self-esteem. The concept of **boundaries** and its relationship to self-esteem is explored. Nursing care of clients with disturbances in self-esteem is described in the context of the nursing process.

CORE CONCEPT

Self-Concept

Self-concept is the cognitive or thinking component of the self that evolves through dynamic interaction in the environment and personal reflection to develop a set of beliefs about oneself (Huitt, 2011).

Components of Self-Concept

Body Image

An individual's **body image** is a subjective perception of one's physical appearance based on self-evaluation and on reactions and feedback from others. Gorman and Sultan (2008) state:

> Body image is the mental picture a person has of his or her own body. It significantly influences the way a person thinks and feels about his or her body as a whole, about its functions, and about the internal and external sensations associated with it. It also includes perceptions of the way others see the person's body and is central to self-concept and self-esteem. (p. 9)

An individual's body image may not necessarily coincide with his or her actual appearance. For example, individuals who have been overweight for many years and then lose weight often have difficulty perceiving of themselves as thin. They may even continue to choose clothing in the size they were before they lost weight.

A disturbance in one's body image may occur with changes in structure or function. Examples of changes in bodily structure include amputations, mastectomy, and facial disfigurements. Functional alterations are conditions such as colostomy, paralysis, and impotence. Alterations in body image are often experienced as losses.

Personal Identity

This component of self-concept is composed of the moral-ethical self, self-consistency, and self-ideal.

The **moral-ethical self** is that aspect of the personal identity that evaluates who the individual says he or she is. This component of the personal self observes, compares, sets standards, and makes judgments that influence an individual's self-evaluation.

Self-consistency is the component of the personal identity that strives to maintain a stable self-image. Even if the self-image is negative, because of this need for stability and self-consistency, the individual resists letting go of the image from which he or she has achieved a measure of constancy.

Self-ideal relates to an individual's perception of what he or she wants to be, to do, or to become. The concept of the ideal self arises out of the perception one has of the expectations of others. Disturbances in self-concept can occur when individuals are unable to achieve their ideals and self-expectations.

CORE CONCEPT

Self-Esteem

Self-esteem is the degree of regard or respect that individuals have for themselves and is a measure of worth that they place on their abilities and judgments.

Self-Esteem

Warren (1991) stated:

> Self-esteem breaks down into two components: (1) the ability to say that "I am important," "I matter," and (2) the ability to say "I am competent," "I have something to offer to others and the world. (p. 1)

Maslow (1970) postulated that individuals must achieve positive self-esteem before they can achieve self-actualization (see Chapter 2, Mental Health and Mental Illness: Historical and Theoretical Concepts). On a day-to-day basis, one's self-value is challenged by changes within the environment. With a positive self-worth, individuals are able to adapt successfully to the demands associated with situational and maturational stressors that occur. The ability to adapt to these environmental changes is impaired when individuals hold themselves in low esteem.

Self-esteem is very closely related to the other components of the self-concept. Just as with body image and personal identity, the development of self-esteem is largely influenced by perceptions about how one is viewed by significant others. It begins in early childhood and vacillates throughout the life span.

Development of Self-Esteem

How self-esteem is established has been the topic of investigation for a number of theorists and clinicians. In a longitudinal study of self-esteem development (Erol & Orth, 2011), several factors were consistently correlated with higher self-esteem:

■ **Emotional stability:** At each age, individuals who had emotional stability had higher self-esteem than those who had unstable emotions.
■ **Extraversion:** The personality trait of extroversion, which includes a social, outgoing personality, was consistently associated with higher self-esteem than was the trait of introversion.
■ **Conscientiousness:** At each age, the personality trait of conscientiousness, which includes a desire to be thoughtful, careful, and to do the right thing, was associated with higher self-esteem.
■ **A high sense of mastery:** The sense that one has control over the forces affecting one's life or that one is able to be effective was consistently associated with higher self-esteem. Part of developing a sense of mastery involves clear differentiation of those things over which a person has control and those things that are beyond a person's ability to control. For example, individuals can choose how they communicate with another person, but they do not have control over how the other person responds. Clarity about these differences supports a person's sense of mastery. In contrast, becoming overly concerned with what someone else's responses and opinions (something one has no control over) say about their worth may contribute to a person devaluing himself or herself, which is the foundation for low self-esteem.
■ **Low risk taking:** At any age, proneness to engage in risky behavior was associated with lower self-esteem, and low risk taking was correlated with higher self-esteem.
■ **Being healthy:** At any age, the perception of being healthy was associated with higher self-esteem.

Warren (1991) outlined the following focus areas to be emphasized by parents and others who work with children when encouraging the growth and development of positive self-esteem:

■ **A sense of competence:** Everyone needs to feel skilled at something. Warren (1991) stated, "Children do not necessarily need to be THE best at a skill in order to have positive self-esteem; what they need to feel is that they have accomplished their PERSONAL best effort" (p. 1).
■ **Unconditional love:** Children need to know that they are loved and accepted by family and friends regardless of success or failure. Unconditional love is demonstrated by expressive touch, realistic praise, and separation of criticism of the person from criticism of the behavior.
■ **A sense of survival:** Everyone fails at something from time to time. Self-esteem is enhanced when individuals learn from failure and grow in the knowledge that they are stronger for having experienced it.
■ **Realistic goals:** Low self-esteem can be the result of not being able to achieve established goals. Individuals may set themselves up for failure by setting goals that are unattainable. Goals can be unrealistic when they are beyond a child's capability to achieve, require an inordinate amount of effort to accomplish, and are based on exaggerated fantasy.
■ **A sense of responsibility:** Children gain positive self-worth when they are assigned areas of responsibility or are expected to complete tasks that they perceive are valued by others.
■ **Reality orientation:** Personal limitations abound within our world, and it is important for children to recognize and achieve a healthy balance between what they can possess and achieve and what is beyond their capability or control.

Other factors have been found to be influential in the development of self-esteem:

■ **The responses of others:** The development of self-esteem can be positively or negatively influenced by the responses of others, particularly significant others, and by how individuals perceive those responses. Role modeling and teaching children strategies for evaluating and keeping in perspective the responses of others contributes to their ability to develop self-esteem.
■ **Hereditary factors:** Factors that are genetically determined, such as physical appearance, size, or inherited infirmity, can affect the development of self-esteem. Reinforcing a child's strengths and helping the child to differentiate factors over which her or she has control or the ability to change contributes to a sense of mastery and self-esteem.
■ **Environmental conditions:** The development of self-esteem can be influenced by demands from the environment. For example, intellectual prowess

may be incorporated into the self-worth of an individual who is reared in an academic environment.

Developmental Progression of Self-Esteem Through the Life Span

The development of self-esteem progresses throughout the life span. Erikson's (1963) theory of personality development provides a useful framework for illustration. Erikson describes eight transitional or maturational crises, the resolution of which can have a profound influence on self-esteem. If a crisis is successfully resolved at one stage, the individual develops healthy coping strategies that he or she can draw on to help fulfill tasks of subsequent stages. When an individual fails to achieve the tasks associated with a developmental stage, emotional growth is inhibited, and he or she is less able to cope with subsequent maturational or situational crises.

Trust versus Mistrust (Birth to 18 Months)

The development of trust results in a feeling of confidence in the predictability of the environment. Achievement of trust results in positive self-esteem through the instillation of self-confidence, optimism, and faith in the gratification of needs.

Unsuccessful resolution results in the individual experiencing emotional dissatisfaction with the self and suspiciousness of others, thereby promoting negative self-esteem.

Autonomy versus Shame and Doubt (18 Months to 3 Years)

With motor and mental development come greater movement and independence within the environment. The child begins active exploration and experimentation. Achievement of the task results in a sense of self-control and the ability to delay gratification, as well as a feeling of self-confidence in one's ability to perform.

This task remains unresolved when the child's independent behaviors are restricted or when the child fails because of unrealistic expectations. Negative self-esteem is promoted by a lack of self-confidence, a lack of pride in the ability to perform, and a sense of being controlled by others.

Initiative versus Guilt (3 to 6 Years)

Positive self-esteem is gained through initiative when creativity is encouraged and performance is recognized and positively reinforced. In this stage, children strive to develop a sense of purpose and the ability to initiate and direct their own activities.

This is the stage during which the child begins to develop a conscience. He or she becomes vulnerable to the labeling of behaviors as "good" or "bad." Guidance and discipline that rely heavily on shaming the child creates guilt and results in a decrease in self-esteem.

Industry versus Inferiority (6 to 12 Years)

Self-confidence is gained at this stage through learning, competing, performing successfully, and receiving recognition from significant others, peers, and acquaintances.

Negative self-esteem is the result of nonachievement, unrealistic expectations, or when accomplishments are consistently met with negative feedback. The child develops a sense of personal inadequacy.

Identity versus Role Confusion (12 to 20 Years)

During adolescence, the individual is striving to redefine the sense of self. Positive self-esteem occurs when individuals are allowed to experience independence by making decisions that influence their lives.

Failure to develop a new self-definition results in a sense of self-consciousness, doubt, and confusion about one's role in life. This can occur when adolescents are encouraged to remain in the dependent position; when discipline in the home has been overly harsh, inconsistent, or absent; and when parental support has been lacking. These conditions are influential in the development of low self-esteem.

Intimacy versus Isolation (20 to 30 Years)

Intimacy is achieved when one is able to form a lasting relationship or a commitment to another person, a cause, an institution, or a creative effort (Murray, Zentner, & Yakimo, 2009). Positive self-esteem is promoted through this capacity for giving of oneself to another.

Failure to achieve intimacy results in behaviors such as withdrawal, social isolation, aloneness, and the inability to form lasting intimate relationships. Isolation occurs when love in the home has been deprived or distorted through the younger years, causing a severe impairment in self-esteem.

Generativity versus Stagnation (30 to 65 Years)

Generativity promotes positive self-esteem through gratification from personal and professional achievements and from meaningful contributions to others.

Failure to achieve generativity occurs when earlier developmental tasks are not fulfilled and the individual does not achieve the degree of maturity required to derive gratification out of a personal concern for the welfare of others. He or she lacks self-worth and becomes withdrawn and isolated.

Ego Integrity versus Despair (65 Years and older)

Ego integrity results in a sense of self-worth and self-acceptance as one reviews life goals, accepting that some were achieved and some were not. The individual has little desire to make major changes in how his or her life has progressed. Positive self-esteem is evident.

Individuals in despair possess a sense of self-contempt and disgust with how life has progressed. They feel worthless and helpless and would like to have a second chance at life. Earlier developmental tasks of self-confidence, self-identity, and concern for others remain unfulfilled. Negative self-esteem prevails.

In the late 1990s, Erikson advanced the concept of transcendence as an additional stage that occurs after the stage of integrity versus despair (Erikson & Erikson, 1997). This stage incorporates the tasks of broadening personal boundaries and developing an increased sense of meaning in life. Accomplishment of these tasks in the life span of 80 years and beyond contributes to one's sense of self-worth and satisfaction with life.

Manifestations of Low Self-Esteem

Individuals with low self-esteem perceive themselves to be incompetent, unlovable, insecure, and unworthy and manifest behaviors that demonstrate their feelings about themselves. The number of manifestations

exhibited is influenced by the degree to which an individual experiences low self-esteem. Nursing theorist Roy (1976, 2009) categorized these behaviors according to the type of stimuli that give rise to manifestations of low self-esteem and affirmed the importance of collecting this type of information in the nursing assessment. Stimulus categories are identified as *focal*, *contextual*, and *residual*. A summary of these types of influencing factors is presented in Table 15–1.

Focal Stimuli

A **focal stimulus** is the *immediate* concern that is causing the threat to self-esteem and the stimulus that is engendering the current behavior. Examples of focal stimuli include termination of a significant relationship or loss of employment.

Contextual Stimuli

Contextual stimuli are all of the other stimuli present in the person's environment that *contribute* to the behavior being caused by the focal stimulus. Examples

TABLE 15–1 **Factors That Influence Manifestations of Low Self-Esteem**		
FOCAL	**CONTEXTUAL**	**RESIDUAL**
Any experience or situation causing the individual to question or decrease his or her value of self; experiences of loss are particularly significant.	1. Body changes experienced because of growth or illness 2. Maturational crises associated with developmental stages 3. Situational crises and the individual's ability to cope 4. The individual's perceptions of feedback from significant others 5. Ability to meet expectations of self and others 6. The feeling of control one has over life situation 7. One's self-definition and the use of it to measure self-worth 8. How one copes with feelings of guilt, shame, and powerlessness 9. How one copes with the required changes in self-perception 10. Awareness of what affects self-concept and the manner with which these stimuli are dealt 11. The number of failures experienced before judging self as worthless 12. The degree of self-esteem one possesses 13. How one copes with limits within the environment 14. The type of support from significant others and how one responds to it 15. One's awareness of and ability to express feelings 16. One's current feeling of hope and comfort with the self	1. Age and coping mechanisms one has developed 2. Stressful situations previously experienced and how well one coped with them 3. Previous feedback from significant others that contributed to self-worth 4. Coping strategies developed through experiences with previous developmental crises 5. Previous experiences with powerlessness and hopelessness and how one coped with them 6. Coping with previous losses 7. Coping with previous failures 8. Previous experiences meeting expectations of self and others 9. Previous experiences with control of self and the environment and quality of coping response 10. Previous experience with decision-making and subsequent consequences 11. Previous experience with childhood limits and whether those limits were clear, defined, and enforced

SOURCE: From Driever, M.J. (1976). Problem of low self-esteem. In C. Roy (Ed.), *Introduction to nursing: An adaptation model* (pp. 232-242). Englewood Cliffs, NJ: Prentice-Hall, with permission.

of contextual stimuli (related to the previously mentioned focal stimuli) might be preoccupation with guilt about the effects a divorce may have on one's children or the perception that advanced age will interfere with obtaining employment.

Residual Stimuli

Residual stimuli are previous experiences that influence one's maladaptive behavior in response to focal and contextual stimuli. For example, being reared in an atmosphere of ridicule and deprecation may affect current adaptation to divorce. Previous experiences with multiple job losses may affect one's current perceptions about self-efficacy in acquiring a new job.

Symptoms of Low Self-Esteem

Driever (1976) identified a number of behaviors manifested by the individual with low self-esteem. It is clear that low self-esteem and depression share many of the same symptoms. Indeed, low self-esteem is an underlying feature in many types of depressive disorders. These behaviors are presented in Box 15–1.

Boundaries

The word *boundary* is used to denote the personal space, both physical and psychological, that individuals identify as their own. Boundaries are sometimes referred to as *limits:* the limit or degree to which individuals feel comfortable in a relationship. Boundaries define and differentiate an individual's physical and psychological space from the physical and psychological space of others.

Boundaries help individuals define the self and are part of the individuation process. More important, boundaries are a measure of self-esteem; healthy boundaries communicate self-respect and an expectation to be treated well in interpersonal relationships (Collingwood, 2016). Types of physical boundaries include physical closeness, touching, sexual behavior, eye contact, privacy (e.g., mail, diary, doors, nudity, bathroom, telephone), and pollution (e.g., noise and smoke), among others. Examples of invasions of physical boundaries are reading someone else's diary, smoking in a nonsmoking public area, and touching someone who does not wish to be touched.

Types of psychological boundaries include beliefs, feelings, choices, needs, time alone, interests, confidences, individual differences, and spirituality, among others. Examples of invasions of psychological boundaries are being criticized for doing something differently than others; having personal information shared in confidence told to others; and being told one "should" believe, feel, decide, choose, or think in a certain way.

BOX 15–1 Manifestations of Low Self-Esteem

1. Loss of appetite/weight loss
2. Overeating
3. Constipation or diarrhea
4. Sleep disturbances (insomnia or difficulty falling or staying asleep)
5. Hypersomnia
6. Complaints of fatigue
7. Poor posture
8. Withdrawal from activities
9. Difficulty initiating new activities
10. Decreased libido
11. Decrease in spontaneous behavior
12. Expression of sadness, anxiety, or discouragement
13. Expression of feeling of isolation, being unlovable, unable to express or defend oneself, and too weak to confront or overcome difficulties
14. Fearful of angering others
15. Avoidance of situations of self-disclosure or public exposure
16. Tendency to stay in background, be a listener rather than a participant
17. Sensitivity to criticism; self-conscious
18. Expression of feelings of helplessness
19. Various complaints of aches and pains
20. Expression of being unable to do anything "good" or productive; expression of feelings of worthlessness and inadequacy
21. Expressions of self-deprecation, self-dislike, and unhappiness with self
22. Denial of past successes and accomplishments and of possibility for success with current activities
23. Feeling that anything one does will fail or be meaningless
24. Ruminating about problems
25. Seeking reinforcement from others; making efforts to gain favors but failing to reciprocate such behavior
26. Seeing self as a burden to others
27. Alienation from others by clinging and self-preoccupation
28. Self-accusatory
29. Demanding reassurance but not accepting it
30. Hostile behavior
31. Angry at self and others but unable to express these feelings directly
32. Decreased ability to meet responsibilities
33. Decreased interest, motivation, concentration
34. Decrease in self-care, hygiene

Adapted from Lloyd, S. R. (2002). Developing positive assertiveness (3rd ed.). Menlo Park, CA: Crisp Learning.

Boundary Pliancy

Boundaries can be rigid, flexible, or enmeshed. The behavior of dogs and cats can be a good illustration of **rigid boundaries** and **flexible boundaries.** Most dogs want to be as close to people as possible. When "their people" walk into the room, the dog is likely to be all over them. They want to be where their people are and do what they are doing. Dogs have very flexible boundaries.

Cats, on the other hand, have very distinct boundaries. They do what they want, when they want. They decide how close they will be to their people, and when. Cats take notice when their people enter a room but may not even acknowledge their presence (until the cat decides the time is right). Their boundaries are less flexible than those of dogs.

Rigid Boundaries

Individuals who have rigid boundaries often have a hard time trusting others. They keep others at a distance and are difficult to communicate with. They reject new ideas or experiences and often withdraw, both emotionally and physically.

EXAMPLE

Brent and Meghan were seeing a marriage counselor because they were unable to agree on many aspects of raising their children, and it was beginning to interfere with their relationship. Meghan runs a day-care service out of their home, and Brent is an accountant. Meghan states, "He never once changed a diaper or got up at night with a child. Now that they are older, he refuses to discipline them in any way." Brent responds, "In my family, my Mom took care of the house and kids and my Dad kept us clothed and fed. That's the way it should be. It's Meghan's job to raise the kids. It's my job to make the money." Brent's boundaries are considered rigid because he refuses to consider the ideas of others or to experience alternative ways of doing things.

Flexible Boundaries

Healthy boundaries are flexible. That is, individuals must be able to let go of their boundaries and limits *when appropriate.* In order to have flexible boundaries, individuals must be aware of who is considered safe and when it is safe to let others invade their personal space.

EXAMPLE

Kristen always takes the hour from 4 to 5 p.m. for her own. She takes no phone calls and tells the children that she is not to be disturbed during that hour. She reads or takes a long leisurely bath and relaxes before it is time to start dinner. Today her private time was interrupted when her 15-year-old daughter came home from school crying because she had not made the cheerleading squad. Kristen used her private time to comfort her daughter who was experiencing a traumatic response to the failure.

Sometimes boundaries can be too flexible. Individuals with boundaries that are too loose are like chameleons. They take their "colors" from whomever they happen to be with at the time. That is, they allow others to make their choices and direct their behavior.

EXAMPLE

At a cocktail party, Diane agreed with one person that the winter had been so unbearable she had hardly been out of the house. Later, at the same party, she agreed with another person that the winter had seemed milder than usual.

Enmeshed Boundaries

Enmeshed boundaries occur when two people's boundaries are so blended together that neither can be sure where one stops and the other begins, or one individual's boundaries may be blurred with another's. The individual with enmeshed boundaries may be unable to differentiate his or her feelings, wants, and needs from the other person's.

EXAMPLES

1. Fran's parents are in town for a visit. They say to Fran, "Dear, we want to take you and Dave out to dinner tonight. What is your favorite restaurant?" Fran automatically responds, "Villa Roma," knowing that the Italian restaurant is Dave's favorite.
2. If a mother has difficulty allowing her daughter to individuate, the mother may perceive the daughter's experiences as happening to her. For example, Aileen got her hair cut without her mother's knowledge. It was styled with spikes across the top of her head. When her mother saw it, she said, "How dare you go around looking like that! What will people think of me?"

Establishing Boundaries

Boundaries are established in childhood. Unhealthy boundaries are the products of unhealthy, troubled, or dysfunctional families. The boundaries enclose painful feelings that have their origin in the dysfunctional family and that have not been dealt with. McKay and Fanning (2000) explain the correlation between unhealthy boundaries and self-esteem disturbances and how they can arise out of negative role models:

> Modeling self-esteem means valuing oneself enough to take care of one's own basic needs. When parents put themselves last or chronically sacrifice for their kids, they teach them that a person is only worthy insofar as he or she is of service to others. When parents set consistent, supportive limits and protect themselves from overbearing demands, they send a message to their children that both are important and both have legitimate needs. (p. 312)

In addition to the lack of positive role models, unhealthy boundaries may also be the result of abuse or neglect. These circumstances can cause a delay in psychosocial development. Individuals must then resume the grief process as an adult in order to continue the developmental progression. They learn to recognize feelings, work through core issues, and tolerate emotional pain as their own. They complete the individuation process, go on to develop healthy boundaries, and learn to appreciate their self-worth.

The Nursing Process

Assessment

Clients with self-esteem problems may manifest any of the symptoms presented in Box 15–1. Some clients with disturbances in self-esteem make direct statements that reflect guilt, shame, or negative self-appraisal, but often it is necessary for the nurse to ask specific questions to obtain this type of information. In particular,

clients who have experienced abuse or other severe trauma often have kept feelings and fears buried for years, and behavioral manifestations of low self-esteem may not be readily evident.

Various tools for measuring self-esteem exist. One is presented in Box 15–2. This particular tool can be used as a self-inventory by the client, or it can be adapted and used by the nurse to format questions for assessing level of self-esteem in the client.

Diagnosis and Outcome Identification

NANDA International has accepted, for use and testing, four nursing diagnoses that relate to self-esteem. These diagnoses are chronic low self-esteem, situational low self-esteem, risk for chronic low self-esteem, and risk for situational low self-esteem (Herdman & Kamitsuru, 2014). Each is described here with its definitions and defining characteristics.

BOX 15–2 Self-Esteem Inventory

Place a check mark in the column that most closely describes your answer to each statement. Each check is worth the number of points listed above each column.

	3 Often or a Great Deal	2 Sometimes	1 Seldom or Occasionally	0 Never or Not at All
1. I become angry or hurt when criticized.				
2. I am afraid to try new things.				
3. I feel stupid when I make a mistake.				
4. I have difficulty looking people in the eye.				
5. I have difficulty making small talk.				
6. I feel uncomfortable in the presence of strangers.				
7. I am embarrassed when people compliment me.				
8. I am dissatisfied with the way I look.				
9. I am afraid to express my opinions in a group.				
10. I prefer staying home alone to participating in group social situations.				
11. I have trouble accepting teasing.				
12. I feel guilty when I say "no" to people.				
13. I am afraid to make a commitment to a relationship for fear of rejection.				
14. I believe that most people are more competent than I.				
15. I feel resentment toward people who are attractive and successful.				
16. I have trouble thinking of any positive aspects about my life.				
17. I feel inadequate in the presence of authority figures.				
18. I have trouble making decisions.				
19. I fear the disapproval of others.				
20. I feel tense, stressed out, or uptight.				

Problems with low self-esteem are indicated by items scored with a 3 or by a total score higher than 46.

Chronic Low Self-Esteem

Definition Long-standing negative self-evaluating and/or negative feelings about self or self-capabilities.

Defining characteristics

- Dependent on others' opinions
- Hesitant to try new situations
- Underestimates ability to deal with situations
- Hesitant to try new things
- Indecisive behavior
- Exaggerates negative feedback about self
- Guilt
- Nonassertive behavior
- Excessively seeks reassurance
- Overly conforming
- Shame
- Passive
- Frequent lack of success in life events
- Rejection of positive feedback

Situational Low Self-Esteem

Definition Development of a negative perception of self-worth in response to a current situation.

Defining characteristics

- Helplessness
- Indecisive behavior
- Nonassertive behavior
- Purposelessness
- Self-negating verbalizations
- Situational challenges to self-worth
- Underestimates ability to deal with the situation

Risk for Chronic Low Self-Esteem

Definition Vulnerable to long-standing negative self-evaluating and/or negative feelings about self or self-capabilities, which may compromise health.

Risk factors

- Cultural incongruence
- Exposure to traumatic situation
- Inadequate affection received
- Inadequate group membership
- Inadequate respect from others
- Ineffective coping with loss
- Insufficient feeling of belonging
- Psychiatric disorder
- Spiritual incongruence
- Repeated failures
- Repeated negative reinforcement

Risk for Situational Low Self-Esteem

Definition Vulnerable to developing negative perception of self-worth in response to a current situation, which may compromise health.

Risk factors

- Alterations in body image
- Alteration in social role
- Behavior inconsistent with values
- Decrease in control over environment
- Developmental transition
- Functional impairment
- History of abandonment
- History of abuse
- History of loss
- History of neglect
- History of rejection
- Inadequate recognition
- Pattern of failure
- Pattern of helplessness
- Physical illness
- Unrealistic self-expectations

Outcome Criteria

Outcome criteria include short- and long-term goals. Time lines for achievement are individually determined. The following criteria may be used for measurement of outcomes in the care of the client with disturbances of self-esteem.

The client:

- Is able to express positive aspects about self and life situation
- Is able to accept positive feedback from others
- Is able to attempt new experiences
- Is able to accept personal responsibility for own problems
- Is able to accept constructive criticism without becoming defensive
- Is able to make independent decisions about life situation
- Uses intermittent, appropriate eye contact
- Is able to develop positive interpersonal relationships
- Is able to communicate needs and wants to others assertively

Planning and Implementation

In Table 15–2, a plan of care using selected self-esteem diagnoses accepted by NANDA International is presented. Outcome criteria, appropriate nursing interventions, and rationales are included for each diagnosis.

> **CLINICAL PEARL** Ensure that client goals are realistic. Unrealistic goals set up the client for failure. Provide encouragement and positive reinforcement for attempts at change. Give recognition of accomplishments, however small.

Evaluation

Reassessment is conducted to determine if the nursing actions have been successful in achieving the objectives

Table 15–2 | CARE PLAN FOR THE CLIENT WITH PROBLEMS RELATED TO SELF-ESTEEM

NURSING DIAGNOSIS: CHRONIC LOW SELF-ESTEEM

RELATED TO: Lack of affection/approval; repeated failures; repeated negative reinforcement

EVIDENCED BY: Exaggerates negative feedback about self and expressions of shame and guilt

OUTCOME CRITERIA	NURSING INTERVENTIONS	RATIONALE
Client verbalizes positive aspects of self and abandons irrational, negative self-judgments.	1. Be supportive, accepting, and respectful without invading client's personal space.	1. Individuals who have had long-standing feelings of low self-worth may be uncomfortable with personal attentiveness.
	2. Explore inaccuracies in self-perception with client.	2. Client may not see positive aspects of self that others see, and bringing it to awareness may help change perception.
	3. Have client list successes and strengths. Provide positive feedback.	3. Helps client to develop internal self-worth and new coping behaviors.
	4. Assess content of negative self-talk and educate client about the impact of cognitive distortions (irrational thinking) on self-esteem.	4. Self-blame, shame, and guilt promote feelings of low self-worth. Depending on chronicity and severity of the problem, this is likely to be the focus of long-term psychotherapy with client. Assisting client to recognize the impact of negative cognition on self-esteem lays the foundation for referral to longer-term treatment such as cognitive therapies (see Chapter 19, Cognitive Therapy).

NURSING DIAGNOSIS: SITUATIONAL LOW SELF-ESTEEM

RELATED TO: Failure (either real or perceived) in a situation of importance to the individual or loss (either real or perceived) of a concept of value to the individual

EVIDENCED BY: Indecisive behavior and expressions of helplessness and uselessness

OUTCOME CRITERIA	NURSING INTERVENTIONS	RATIONALE
Client identifies source of threat to self-esteem and works through the stages of the grief process to resolve the loss or failure.	1. Convey an accepting attitude; encourage client to express self openly.	1. An accepting attitude enhances trust and communicates to client that the nurse believes he or she is a worthwhile person, regardless of what is expressed.
	2. Encourage client to express anger. Do not become defensive if initial expression of anger is displaced on nurse/therapist. Assist client to explore angry feelings and direct them toward the intended object/person or other loss.	2. Verbalization of feelings in a nonthreatening environment may help client come to terms with unresolved issues related to the loss.

Continued

Table 15–2 | CARE PLAN FOR THE CLIENT WITH PROBLEMS RELATED TO SELF-ESTEEM–cont'd

OUTCOME CRITERIA	NURSING INTERVENTIONS	RATIONALE
	3. Assist client to avoid ruminating about past failures. Withdraw attention if client persists.	3. Lack of attention to these undesirable behaviors may discourage their repetition.
	4. Educate client about the importance of focusing on positive attributes if self-esteem is to be enhanced. Encourage discussion of past accomplishments and offer support in undertaking new tasks. Offer recognition of successful endeavors and positive reinforcement of attempts made.	4. Recognition and positive reinforcement enhance self-esteem and encourage repetition of desirable behaviors.

NURSING DIAGNOSIS: RISK FOR SITUATIONAL LOW SELF-ESTEEM

RISK FACTORS: Developmental changes; functional impairment; disturbed body image; loss; history of abuse or neglect; unrealistic self-expectations; physical illness; failures/rejections

OUTCOME CRITERIA	NURSING INTERVENTIONS	RATIONALE
Client's self-esteem is preserved.	1. Provide an open environment and trusting relationship.	1. Facilitates client's ability to deal with current situation.
	2. Determine client's perception of the loss/failure and the meaning of it to him or her.	2. Assessment of the cause or contributing factor is necessary to provide assistance to client.
	3. Identify response of family or significant others to client's current situation.	3. Provides additional background assessment data with which to plan client's care.
	4. Permit appropriate expressions of anger.	4. Anger is a stage in the normal grieving process and must be dealt with for progression to occur.
	5. Provide information about normalcy of individual grief reaction.	5. Individuals who are unaware of normal feelings associated with grief may feel guilty and try to deny certain feelings.
	6. Discuss and assist with planning for the future. Communicate hope, but avoid giving false reassurance.	6. In a state of anxiety and grief, individuals need assistance with decision-making and problem-solving. They may find it difficult or impossible to envision any hope for the future.

of care. Evaluation of the nursing actions for the client with self-esteem disturbances may be facilitated by gathering information using the following types of questions:

■ Is the client able to discuss past accomplishments and other positive aspects about his or her life?
■ Does the client accept praise and recognition from others in a gracious manner?

■ Is the client able to try new experiences without extreme fear of failure?
■ Can he or she accept constructive criticism now without becoming overly defensive and shifting the blame to others?
■ Does the client accept personal responsibility for problems rather than attributing feelings and behaviors to others?

■ Does the client participate in decisions that affect his or her life?

■ Can the client make rational decisions independently?

■ Has he or she become more assertive in interpersonal relations?

■ Is improvement observed in the physical presentation of self-esteem, such as eye contact, posture, changes in eating and sleeping, fatigue, libido, elimination patterns, self-care, and complaints of aches and pains?

Summary and Key Points

■ Emotional wellness requires that an individual have some degree of self-worth—a perception that he or she possesses a measure of value to self and others.

■ Self-concept is a cognitive component of the self that includes a set of beliefs about oneself.

■ Body image encompasses one's appraisal of physical attributes, functioning, sexuality, wellness-illness state, and appearance.

■ The personal identity component of self-concept is composed of the moral-ethical self, the self-consistency, and the self-ideal.

■ Self-consistency is the component of the personal identity that strives to maintain a stable self-image.

■ Self-ideal relates to an individual's perception of what he or she wants to be, do, or become.

■ Self-esteem refers to the degree of regard or respect that individuals have for themselves and is a measure of worth that they place on their abilities and judgments. It is largely influenced by the perceptions of how one is viewed by significant others.

■ High self-esteem is associated with emotional stability, extroversion, conscientiousness, a sense of mastery, low risk taking, and better health. Genetics and environmental conditions may also be influencing factors.

■ The development of self-esteem progresses throughout the life span. Erikson's theory of personality development elaborates on the importance of accomplishing developmental tasks in self-esteem. The behaviors associated with low self-esteem are numerous and correlated with signs and symptoms of depression.

■ Stimuli that trigger behaviors associated with low self-esteem may include focal, contextual, and/or residual stimuli.

■ Boundaries, or personal limits, help individuals define the self and are part of the individuation process.

■ Boundaries are a measure of self-esteem.

■ Boundaries are physical and psychological and may be rigid, flexible, or enmeshed.

■ Unhealthy boundaries are often the result of dysfunctional family systems.

■ The nursing process is the vehicle for delivery of care to clients needing assistance with self-esteem disturbances.

■ The four nursing diagnoses relating to self-esteem that have been accepted by NANDA International include chronic low self-esteem, situational low self-esteem, risk for chronic low self-esteem, and risk for situational low self-esteem.

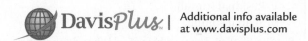

DavisPlus | Additional info available at www.davisplus.com

Review Questions
Self-Examination/Learning Exercise

Select the answer that is most appropriate for each of the following questions.

1. Kaylee, age 26, graduated from law school with a 3.2/4.0 grade point average. She recently took the bar exam and did not pass. Because of this, she had to give up her job at a law firm. She became very depressed and sought counseling at the mental health clinic. During the intake assessment, Kaylee says to the psychiatric nurse, "I am a complete failure. I'm so dumb, I can't do anything right." What is the most appropriate nursing diagnosis for Kaylee?
   a. Chronic low self-esteem
   b. Situational low self-esteem
   c. Defensive coping
   d. Risk for situational low self-esteem

Continued

Review Questions—cont'd
Self-Examination/Learning Exercise

2. Which of the following outcome criteria would be most appropriate for the client described in question 1?
   a. Kaylee is able to express positive aspects about herself and her life situation.
   b. Kaylee is able to accept constructive criticism without becoming defensive.
   c. Kaylee is able to develop positive interpersonal relationships.
   d. Kaylee is able to accept positive feedback from others.

3. Amanda tried out for the cheerleading squad in junior high but was rejected. At age 15, she had looked forward to trying out for the cheerleading squad in high school. She took cheerleading classes and practiced for many hours every day. However, when tryouts were held, she was not selected. She has become despondent, and her mother takes her to the mental health clinic for counseling. Amanda tells the nurse, "What's the use of trying? I'm not good at anything!" Which of the following nursing interventions is best for Amanda's specific problem?
   a. Encourage Amanda to talk about her feeling of shame over the second failure.
   b. Assist Amanda to problem-solve her reasons for not making the team.
   c. Help Amanda understand the importance of good self-care and personal hygiene in the maintenance of self-esteem.
   d. Explore with Amanda her past successes and accomplishments.

4. The psychiatric nurse encourages Amanda (the client in question 3) to express her anger. Why is this an appropriate nursing intervention?
   a. Anger is the basis for self-esteem problems.
   b. The nurse suspects that Amanda was abused as a child.
   c. The nurse is attempting to guide Amanda through the grief process.
   d. The nurse recognizes that Amanda has long-standing repressed anger.

5. A law school graduate failing the bar exam and a 15-year-old high school girl not being selected for the cheerleading squad are examples of which of the following?
   a. Focal stimuli
   b. Contextual stimuli
   c. Residual stimuli
   d. Spatial stimuli

6. The husband says to his wife, "What do you want to do tonight?" and his wife responds, "Whatever you want to do." This is an example of which of the following?
   a. Extremely rigid boundaries
   b. A boundary violation
   c. Extremely flexible boundaries
   d. Showing respect for the boundary of another

7. Twins Jan and Jean still dress alike even though they are grown and married. This is an example of which of the following?
   a. Rigid boundary
   b. Enmeshed boundary
   c. A boundary violation
   d. Boundary pliancy

8. Karen's counselor asked her if she would like a hug. This is an example of which of the following?
   a. Rigid boundary
   b. A boundary violation
   c. Enmeshed boundary
   d. Showing respect for the boundary of another

Review Questions—cont'd
Self-Examination/Learning Exercise

9. Jessica told Andrea a secret that Eva had told her. This is an example of which of the following?
   a. Too flexible a boundary
   b. A boundary violation
   c. Too rigid a boundary
   d. An enmeshed boundary

10. Tommy says to his friend, "I can't ever talk to my Daddy until after he has read his newspaper." This is an example of which of the following?
   a. A rigid boundary
   b. A boundary violation
   c. An enmeshed boundary
   d. A flexible boundary

11. A nurse is engaging in psychoeducation about improving self-esteem with Shelley, who has depression and low self-esteem. Which of the following are important for the nurse to assess? (Select all that apply.)
   a. Shelley's focal, contextual, and residual stimuli
   b. Shelley's abilities with regard to establishment of boundaries
   c. Shelley's age and whether or not she is married
   d. The nurse's awareness of his or her own ability to establish appropriate boundaries
   e. Shelley's predominant communication style and her understanding of assertiveness

References

Collingwood, J. (2016). The importance of personal boundaries. *PsychCentral*. Retrieved from http://psychcentral.com/lib/the-importance-of-personal-boundaries

Erol, R.Y., & Orth, U. (2011). Self-esteem development from age 14 to 30 years: A longitudinal study. *Journal of Personality and Social Psychology, 101*(3), 607-619. doi:http://dx.doi.org/10.1037/a0024299

Gorman, L.M., & Sultan, D.F. (2008). *Psychosocial nursing for general patient care* (3rd ed.). Philadelphia: F.A. Davis.

Herdman, T.H., & Kamitsuru, S. (Eds.). (2014). *NANDA-I nursing diagnoses: Definitions and classification, 2015–2017*. Oxford: Wiley Blackwell.

Hosogi, M., Okada, A., Fujii, C., Noguchi, K., & Watanabe, K. (2012). Importance and usefulness of evaluating self-esteem in children. *Biopsychosocial Medicine, 6*(9). doi:10.1186/1751-0759-6-9

Huitt, W. (2011). Self and self-views. *Educational Psychology Interactive*. Valdosta, GA: Valdosta State University. Retrieved from www.edpsycinteractive.org/topics/self/self.html

Lloyd, S.R. (2002). *Developing Positive Assertiveness* (3rd ed.), Menlo Park, CA: Crisp Learning.

Mayo Clinic. (2014). Self-esteem check: Too low or just right? Retrieved from www.mayoclinic.org/healthy-lifestyle/adult-health/in-depth/self-esteem/art-20047976

McKay, M., & Fanning, P. (2000). *Self-esteem: A proven program of cognitive techniques for assessing, improving, and maintaining your self-esteem* (3rd ed.). Oakland, CA: New Harbinger Publications.

Murray, R.B., Zentner, J.P., & Yakimo, R. (2009). *Health promotion strategies through the life span* (8th ed.). Upper Saddle River, NJ: Prentice Hall.

Roy, C. (2009). *The Roy adaptation model* (3rd ed.). Upper Saddle River, NJ: Pearson Education.

Warren, J. (1991). Your child and self-esteem. *The Prairie View, 30*(2), 1.

Classical References

Driever, M.J. (1976). Problem of low self-esteem. In C. Roy (Ed.), *Introduction to nursing: An adaptation model* (pp. 232-242). Englewood Cliffs, N.J.: Prentice-Hall.

Erikson, E.H. (1963). *Childhood and society* (2nd ed.). New York: W.W. Norton.

Erikson, E.H. & Erikson, J.M. (1997). *The life cycle completed: Extended version with new chapters on the ninth stage of development*. New York: W.W. Norton.

Maslow, A. (1970). *Motivation and personality* (2nd ed.). New York: Harper & Row.

Roy, C. (1976). *Introduction to nursing: An adaptation model*. Englewood Cliffs, N.J.: Prentice Hall.

16 Anger and Aggression Management

KEY TERMS

modeling   operant conditioning   prodromal syndrome

OBJECTIVES

After reading this chapter, the student will be able to:

1. Define and differentiate between *anger* and *aggression*.
2. Identify when the expression of anger becomes a problem.
3. Discuss predisposing factors to the maladaptive expression of anger.
4. Apply the nursing process to clients expressing anger or aggression.
   a. **Assessment:** Describe physical and psychological responses to anger.

b. **Diagnosis/Outcome Identification:** Formulate nursing diagnoses and outcome criteria for clients expressing anger and aggression.
c. **Planning/Intervention:** Describe nursing interventions for clients demonstrating maladaptive expressions of anger.
d. **Evaluation:** Evaluate achievement of the projected outcomes in the intervention with clients demonstrating maladaptive expression of anger.

HOMEWORK ASSIGNMENT

Please read the chapter and answer the following questions:

1. What symptoms often precede violent behavior?
2. What is the goal of anger management?
3. What psychiatric diagnoses are correlated with increased risk of violence?

4. Under what conditions might a nurse determine that a client should be placed in restraints?

Anger need not be a negative expression. It is a normal human emotion that, when handled appropriately and expressed assertively, can provide an individual with a positive force to solve problems and make decisions concerning life situations. Anger becomes a problem when it is not expressed or when it is expressed aggressively. Violence occurs when individuals lose control of their anger. Violent acts are becoming commonplace in the United States. In 2015, according to Bureau of

Justice statistics, 2.7 million people experienced at least one violent victimization (Truman & Morgan, 2016). Violent crimes are reported daily by the news media, and health-care workers see the results each day in the emergency departments of general hospitals.

This chapter addresses the concepts of anger and aggression. Predisposing factors to the maladaptive expression of anger are discussed, and the nursing process as a vehicle for delivery of care to assist clients in the management of anger and aggression is described.

Anger and Aggression, Defined

> ### CORE CONCEPTS
> **Anger**
> Anger is "an emotional state that varies in intensity from mild irritation to intense fury and rage," according to Charles Spielberger, a clinical psychologist best known for developing the State/Trait Anxiety Inventory. Anger is accompanied by physiological and biological changes, such as increases in heart rate, blood pressure, and levels of the energy hormones adrenaline and noradrenaline (American Psychological Association [APA], 2017).

Anger is a normal, healthy emotion that serves as a warning signal and alerts us to potential threat or trauma. It triggers energy that sets us up for a good fight or quick flight and can range from mild irritation to rage. Warren (1993) outlines some fundamental points about anger:

■ Anger is not a primary emotion, but it is typically experienced as an almost automatic inner response to hurt, frustration, or fear.
■ Anger is physiological arousal. It instills feelings of power and generates preparedness.
■ Anger and aggression are significantly different.
■ The expression of anger is learned.
■ The expression of anger can come under personal control.

Anger is a very powerful emotion. When it is denied or buried, it can precipitate a number of physical problems such as migraine headaches, ulcers, colitis, and even coronary heart disease. When turned inward on oneself, anger can result in depression and low self-esteem. When it is expressed inappropriately, it commonly interferes with relationships. When suppressed, anger may turn into resentment, which often manifests in negative, passive-aggressive behavior.

Anger creates a state of preparedness by arousing the sympathetic nervous system. The activation of this system results in increased heart rate and blood pressure, increased secretion of epinephrine (resulting in additional physiological arousal), and increased levels of serum glucose, among others. Anger prepares the body, physiologically, to fight. When anger goes unresolved, this physiological arousal can be the predisposing factor to a number of health problems. Even if the situation that created the anger is removed by miles or years, it can be replayed through the memory, reactivating the sympathetic arousal when this occurs.

Table 16–1 lists positive and negative functions of anger.

> ### CORE CONCEPT
> **Aggression**
> *Aggression* has many different definitions depending on the context in which it is described. When describing aggression as a behavioral response to anger, aggression has been defined as a behavior intended to threaten or injure the victim's security or self-esteem. It means "to go against," "to assault," or "to attack." It is a response that aims at inflicting pain or injury on objects or persons (Warren, 1993, pp. 119–120). Aggression may include verbal and physical attacks that intend harm to another and often reflect a desire for dominance and control (Kassinove, 2016). Aggression, in general, may range from a self-protective response to a destructive, violent act (Perry, 2016).

The term *anger* often takes on a negative connotation because of its link with aggression. Aggression is one way individuals express anger. It is sometimes used to try to force someone into compliance with the aggressor's wishes, but at other times, the only objective seems to be the infliction of punishment and pain. In virtually all instances, aggression is a negative function or destructive use of anger.

Predisposing Factors to Anger and Aggression

A number of factors have been implicated in the way an individual expresses anger. Some theorists view aggression as purely biological, and some suggest that it results from individuals' interactions with their environments. It is likely a combination of both.

Modeling

Role **modeling** is one of the strongest forms of learning. Children model their behavior at a very early age after their primary caregivers, usually parents. How parents or significant others express anger becomes the child's method of anger expression.

Whether role modeling is positive or negative depends on the behavior of the models. Much has been written about the abused child becoming physically abusive as an adult, which may be connected to a learned response.

Role models are not always in the home, however. Evidence supports the role of television and video violence as a predisposing factor to later aggressive behavior (American Psychological Association, 2013). Whether modeling occurs in the home, the community,

TABLE 16–1 **The Functions of Anger**

POSITIVE FUNCTIONS OR CONSTRUCTIVE USES	NEGATIVE FUNCTIONS OR DESTRUCTIVE USES
Anger energizes and mobilizes the body for self-defense.	Without cognitive input, anger may result in impulsive behavior, disregarding possible negative consequences.
Communicated assertively, anger can promote conflict resolution.	Communicated passive-aggressively or aggressively, conflict escalates, and the problem that created the conflict goes unresolved.
Anger arousal is a personal signal of threat or injustice against the self. The signal elicits coping responses to deal with the distress.	Anger can lead to aggression when the coping response is displacement. Anger can be destructive if it is discharged against an object or person unrelated to the true target of the anger.
Anger is constructive when it provides a feeling of control over a situation and the individual is able to assertively take charge of a situation.	Anger can be destructive when the feeling of control is exaggerated and the individual uses the power to intimidate others.
Anger is constructive when it is expressed assertively, serves to increase self-esteem, and leads to mutual understanding and forgiveness.	Anger can be destructive when it masks honest feelings, weakens self-esteem, and leads to hostility and rage.

SOURCES: Adapted from Gorman, L.M., & Sultan, D.F. (2008). *Psychosocial nursing for general patient care* (3rd ed.). Philadelphia: F.A. Davis; Waughfield, C.G. (2002). *Mental health concepts* (5th ed.). Albany, NY: Delmar.

or popular media, its role in the development of aggression has been well supported.

Operant Conditioning

Operant conditioning occurs when a specific behavior is reinforced. A positive reinforcement is a response to specific behavior that is pleasurable or offers a reward. A negative reinforcement is a response to specific behavior that prevents an undesirable result from occurring.

Anger responses can be learned through operant conditioning. For example, when a child wants something and has been told no by a parent, he or she might have a temper tantrum. If the parent then gives the child an ice cream cone, the anger displayed during the temper tantrum has been positively reinforced (or rewarded).

An example of learning by negative reinforcement follows: A mother asks the child to pick up her toys, and the child becomes angry and has a temper tantrum. If, when the temper tantrum begins, the mother thinks, "Oh, it's not worth all this!" and picks up the toys herself, the anger has been negatively reinforced (the child was rewarded by not having to pick up her toys).

Neurophysiological Factors

The neurophysiology of aggression is extremely complex and only partially understood despite years of research. Perry (2016) describes the findings as such: "Any factors which increase the activity or reactivity of the brainstem (e.g., chronic traumatic stress, testosterone, dysregulated serotonin or norepinephrine systems) or decrease the moderating capacity of the limbic or cortical areas (e.g., neglect) will increase an individual's aggressivity, impulsivity, and capacity to display violence." Loss of function in the cortex (and subsequently decreased moderating capacity) can also occur as a result of many pathological processes, including stroke, dementia, alcohol intoxication, and traumatic brain injuries. Tumors in the brain, particularly in the areas of the limbic system and the temporal lobes; trauma to the brain resulting in cerebral changes; and diseases such as encephalitis (or medications that may effect this syndrome), have all been implicated in the predisposition to aggression and violent behavior.

Individuals may be genetically predisposed to aggression attributable to the effects of genetic variants of the serotoninergic systems that control levels of serotonin in the central and peripheral nervous systems, its biological effects, its rate of production, and synaptic release (Pavlov, Chistiakov, & Chekhonin, 2012).

Biochemical Factors

The impact of hormones, particularly testosterone, in aggression has been the focus of animal research, and although it has been associated with increased aggression in animals and in correlation studies in humans, the effects of testosterone administration have yielded mixed results (Sadock, Sadock, & Ruiz, 2015). For example, in one controlled study where anabolic-androgenic steroids were given to normal subjects, the participants reported both positive and negative mood symptoms; the latter included anger, hostility, and violent feelings (Sadock et al., 2015). Although aggression is modulated by several hormonal systems, testosterone is identified as playing a key role, while deficits in serotonin have been associated with an increase in impulsivity (Vetulani, 2013).

Socioeconomic Factors

High rates of violence exist within the subculture of poverty in the United States. Exposure to violence has been identified as having an impact on future tendencies toward aggression. An ongoing controversy exists as to whether economic inequality or absolute poverty is most responsible for aggressive and violent behavior within this subculture. That is, does violence occur because individuals perceive themselves as disadvantaged relative to other persons, or does violence occur because of the deprivation itself? These concepts are not easily understood and are still under investigation.

Environmental Factors

Three environmental factors that have been shown to increase risks for aggression are crowding, temperature, and noise (Archer, 2012). All three of these environmental factors increase stress, which has a multitude of effects on mood and behavior. Current behavior and past experiences are also environmental factors that influence aggressive expression. The three best predictors of violent behavior in this context are alcohol intake, a history of childhood abuse, and a history of violent acts with criminal activity or arrests (Sadock et al., 2015). Numerous other substances of abuse have been associated with aggression, including cocaine, methamphetamines and amphetamines, bath salts, anabolic steroids, synthetic marijuana, PCP, and alpha PVP (also known as *flakka*).

The Nursing Process

CORE CONCEPT

Anger Management

The use of various techniques and strategies to control responses to anger-provoking situations. The goal of anger management is to reduce both the emotional feelings and the physiological arousal that anger engenders.

Assessment

Nurses must be aware of the risk factors and symptoms associated with anger and aggression in order to make an accurate assessment. In a meta-analysis of prevalence and risk factors for violence by psychiatric acute inpatients (Iozzino et al., 2015), the researchers found that close to 1 in 5 patients may commit an act of violence. The highest risk factors were male gender, a diagnosis of schizophrenia, substance use, and a

history of violence. The best intervention is prevention, so risk factors for assessing violence potential are also presented.

Anger

Anger is often manifested in the following ways:

- Frowning facial expression
- Clenched fists
- Low-pitched verbalizations forced through clenched teeth
- Yelling and shouting
- Intense eye contact or avoidance of eye contact
- Hypersensitivity, easily offended
- Defensive response to criticism
- Passive-aggressive behaviors
- Lack of control or overcontrolled emotions
- Intense discomfort; continuous state of tension
- Flushed face
- Anxious, tense, angry facial expression (affect)

Anger is often described as a secondary emotion. For example, it may be a response to unresolved grief, depression, fear, anxiety, or unresolved posttraumatic stress. Anger is also one of the stages of the normal grief process and thus is an expected emotion. Because of the negative connotation of the word *anger,* some clients will not acknowledge that they are feeling angry. These individuals need assistance to recognize their true feelings and understand that anger is a perfectly acceptable emotion; it is one's *behavior* in response to anger that may be unacceptable, such as when it results in aggression.

Aggression

Aggression can arise from a number of feeling states, including anger, anxiety, guilt, frustration, or suspiciousness. Aggressive behaviors can be classified as mild (e.g., sarcasm), moderate (e.g., slamming doors), severe (e.g., threats of physical violence against others), or extreme (e.g., physical acts of violence against others). Aggression may be associated with (but not limited to) the following defining characteristics:

- Pacing, restlessness
- Threatening body language
- Verbal or physical threats
- Loud voice, shouting, use of obscenities, argumentative
- Threats of homicide or suicide
- Increase in agitation, with overreaction to environmental stimuli
- Panic anxiety, leading to misinterpretation of the environment
- Suspiciousness and defensive posturing
- Angry mood, often disproportionate to the situation
- Destruction of property
- Acts of physical harm toward another person

Aggression is often differentiated as reactive versus proactive. Reactive aggression is defined as fear based and impulsive; proactive aggression is described as predatory and calculated. In both cases, there is intent to harm another, but the motives differ. *Intent* is a requisite in the definition of aggression. It refers to behavior that is *intended* to inflict harm or destruction. Accidents that lead to *unintentional* harm or destruction are not considered aggression.

Assessing Risk Factors

Prevention is the key issue in managing aggressive or violent behavior. The individual who becomes violent usually feels an underlying helplessness. The following three factors have been identified as important considerations in assessing for potential violence:

1. Past history of violence
2. Client diagnosis
3. Current behavior

Past history of violence is widely recognized as a major risk factor for violence in a treatment setting. Also highly correlated with assaultive behavior is diagnosis. Diagnoses such as schizophrenia, major depression, bipolar disorder, and substance use disorders have a strong correlation with violent behavior (Friedman, 2006). Substance abuse, in addition to mental illness, compounds the increased risk of violence. Neurocognitive disorders and antisocial, borderline, and intermittent explosive personality disorders have also been associated with a risk for violent behavior.

Novitsky, Julius, and Dubin (2009) state:

The successful management of violence is predicated on an understanding of the dynamics of violence. A patient's threatening behavior is commonly an overreaction to feelings of impotence, helplessness, and perceived or actual humiliation. Aggression rarely occurs suddenly and unexpectedly. (p. 50)

Novitsky and associates describe a **prodromal syndrome** characterized by anxiety and tension, verbal abuse and profanity, and increasing hyperactivity. These escalating behaviors usually do not occur in stages but most often overlap and sometimes occur simultaneously. Behaviors associated with this prodromal stage include rigid posture; clenched fists and jaws; grim, defiant affect; talking in a rapid, raised voice; arguing and demanding; using profanity and threatening verbalizations; agitation and pacing; and pounding and slamming.

Most assaultive behavior is preceded by a period of increasing hyperactivity. Behaviors associated with the prodromal syndrome should be considered emergent and demand immediate attention. Keen observation skills and background knowledge for accurate assessment are critical factors in predicting potential for violent behavior. The Brøset Violence Checklist is presented in Box 16–1. It is a quick, simple, and reliable checklist that can be used as a risk assessment for potential violence. Testing has shown a 63 percent accuracy for prediction of violence at a score of 2 and above (Almvik, Woods, & Rasmussen, 2000). De-escalation techniques are also included.

Diagnosis and Outcome Identification

NANDA International does not include a separate nursing diagnosis for anger. The nursing diagnosis of complicated grieving may be used when anger is expressed inappropriately and the etiology is related to a loss.

The following nursing diagnoses may be considered for clients demonstrating inappropriate expression of anger or aggression:

■ Ineffective coping related to negative role modeling and dysfunctional family system, evidenced by

---

BOX 16–1 The Brøset Violence Checklist

Score 1 point for each behavior observed. At a score of ≥ 2, begin de-escalation techniques.

Behaviors	Score
Confusion	
Irritability	
Boisterousness	
Physical threats	
Verbal threats	
Attacks on objects	
TOTAL SCORE	

DE-ESCALATION TECHNIQUES

Calm voice	Helpful attitude
Walk outdoors or fresh air	Reduction in demands
Identify consequences	Decrease waiting times and request refusals
Group participation	
Open hands and nonthreatening posture	Verbal redirection and limit setting
Relaxation techniques	Distract with a more positive activity (e.g., soft music or a quiet room)
Allow phone call	
Express concern	Time-out/quiet time/open seclusion
Offer food or drink	
Reduce stimulation and loud noise	Offer prn medication

If de-escalation techniques fail:

1. Suggest prn medications
2. Time-out or unlocked seclusion, which can progress to locked seclusion

SOURCE: From Almvik, R., Woods, P., & Rasmussen, K. (2000). The Brøset violence checklist: Sensitivity, specificity, and interrater reliability. Journal of Interpersonal Violence, 15(12), 1284-1296, with permission. De-escalation techniques reprinted with permission from Barbara Barnes, Milwaukee County Behavioral Health Division.

yelling, name calling, hitting others, and temper tantrums as expressions of anger

■ Risk for self-directed or other-directed violence related to having been nurtured in an atmosphere of violence; history of violence

Outcome Criteria

Outcome criteria include short- and long-term goals. Time lines are individually determined. The following criteria may be used for measurement of outcomes in the care of the client needing assistance with management of anger and aggression.

The client:

■ Is able to recognize when he or she is angry and seeks out staff/support person to talk about his or her feelings

■ Is able to take responsibility for own feelings of anger

■ Demonstrates the ability to exert internal control over feelings of anger

■ Is able to diffuse anger before losing control

■ Uses the tension generated by the anger in a constructive manner

■ Does not cause harm to self or others

■ Is able to use steps of the problem-solving process rather than becoming violent as a means of seeking solutions

Planning and Implementation

In Table 16–2, a plan of care is presented for the client who expresses anger inappropriately. Outcome criteria, appropriate nursing interventions, and rationales are included for each diagnosis. Cognitive-behavioral therapy (CBT) as a strategy for anger management and aggression reduction is an evidence-based treatment that, especially when incorporated in treatment for children and adolescents, has demonstrated effectiveness in reducing maladaptive aggression (Smeets et al., 2015). While CBT is typically conducted by advanced practice nurses and other trained specialists, the generalist psychiatric nurse can incorporate principles of this modality in psychoeducation, which provides a foundation for referral to longer-term CBT.

Table 16–2 | CARE PLAN FOR THE INDIVIDUAL WHO EXPRESSES ANGER INAPPROPRIATELY

NURSING DIAGNOSIS: INEFFECTIVE COPING

RELATED TO: Negative role modeling and dysfunctional family system

EVIDENCED BY: Yelling, name calling, hitting others, and temper tantrums as expressions of anger

OUTCOME CRITERIA	NURSING INTERVENTIONS	RATIONALE
Client is able to recognize anger in self and take responsibility before losing control.	1. Remain calm when dealing with an angry client.	1. Anger expressed by the nurse will most likely incite increased anger in client.
	2. Set verbal limits on behavior. Clearly delineate the consequences of inappropriate expression of anger and always follow through.	2. Consistency in enforcing the consequences is essential if positive outcomes are to be achieved. Inconsistency creates confusion and encourages testing of limits.
	3. Have client keep a diary of angry thoughts and feelings, what triggered them, and how they were handled.	3. This provides a more objective measure of the problem. Introducing client to some basic principles of cognitive reflection not only encourages problem-solving in the short term but lays the groundwork for referral to longer-term CBT if this is identified as desirable.
	4. Avoid touching client when he or she becomes angry.	4. Client may view touch as threatening and could become violent.

Continued

Table 16–2 | CARE PLAN FOR THE INDIVIDUAL WHO EXPRESSES ANGER INAPPROPRIATELY–cont'd

OUTCOME CRITERIA	NURSING INTERVENTIONS	RATIONALE
	5. Help client determine the true source of the anger.	5. Many times, anger is being displaced onto a safer object or person. If resolution is to occur, the first step is to identify the source of the problem.
	6. Help client find alternative ways of releasing tension, such as physical outlets, and more appropriate ways of expressing anger, such as seeking out staff when feelings emerge.	6. Client will likely need assistance to problem-solve more appropriate ways of behaving.
	7. Role-model appropriate ways of expressing anger assertively, such as, "I dislike being called names. I get angry when I hear you saying those things about me."	7. Role modeling is one of the strongest methods of learning.

NURSING DIAGNOSIS: RISK FOR SELF-DIRECTED OR OTHER-DIRECTED VIOLENCE

RISK FACTORS: Having been nurtured in an atmosphere of violence; history of violence

OUTCOME CRITERIA	NURSING INTERVENTIONS	RATIONALE
Client will not harm self or others. Client verbalizes anger rather than hit others.	1. Observe client for escalation of anger (called the *prodromal syndrome*): increased motor activity, pounding, slamming, tense posture, defiant affect, clenched teeth and fists, arguing, demanding, and challenging or threatening staff.	1. Violence may be prevented if risks are identified in time.
	2. When these behaviors are observed, first ensure that sufficient staff are available to help with a potentially violent situation. Attempt to defuse the anger beginning with the least restrictive means.	2. The initial consideration must be having enough help to diffuse a potentially violent situation. Client rights must be honored, while preventing harm to client and others.
	3. Techniques for dealing with aggression:	3. Aggression control techniques promote safety and reduce risk of harm to client and others:
	a. Talking down. Say, "John, you seem very angry. Let's sit down and talk about it." (Be attentive to safe physical distance from the patient and the nurse's ability to exit [i.e., ensure that client does not position self between a door and nurse].)	a. Promotes a trusting relationship and may prevent client's anxiety from escalating while attending to the safety needs of the nurse as well.
	b. Physical outlets. "such as exercise, using a punching bag, or engaging in another activity that provides an acceptable outlet for	b. Provides effective way for client to release tension associated with high levels of anger. Staying with the client offers an opportunity to

Table 16–2 | CARE PLAN FOR THE INDIVIDUAL WHO EXPRESSES ANGER INAPPROPRIATELY—cont'd

OUTCOME CRITERIA	NURSING INTERVENTIONS	RATIONALE
	energy. Offer to stay with the client during this activity."	provide support and to assess the client's perception of the activity's effectiveness.
	c. Medication. If agitation continues to escalate, offer client choice of taking medication voluntarily. If he or she refuses, reassess the situation to determine if harm to self or others is imminent.	c. Tranquilizing medication may calm client and prevent violence from escalating.
	d. Call for assistance. Remove self and other clients from the immediate area. Call violence code, push panic button, call for assault team, and follow other measures established by the institution. Sufficient staff to indicate a show of strength may be enough to de-escalate the situation, and client may agree to take the medication.	d. Client and staff safety are of primary concern. Many states, accrediting bodies (such as The Joint Commission), and/or facilities require that staff members working with hospitalized psychiatric patients be trained and/or certified in psychiatric emergency interventions to assure that the strategies used are in the best interest of staff and patient safety.
	e. Seclusion or restraints. If client is not calmed by talking down or by medication, use of mechanical restraints and/or seclusion may be necessary. Be sure to have sufficient staff available to assist and appropriately deal with an out-of-control client. Follow protocol for restraints/seclusion established by the institution. Restraints should be used as a last resort, after all other interventions have been unsuccessful and client is clearly at risk of harm to self or others.	e. Clients who do not have internal control over their own behavior may require external controls, such as seclusion and/or mechanical restraints, in order to prevent harm to self or others, but since they are a more restrictive measure, they should be used only as a last resort after all other measures have been attempted and have failed.
	f. Observation and documentation. Hospital policy typically dictates the requirements for observation of client in restraints. Basic safety principles include that client in restraints should be observed throughout the period of restraint. Every 15 minutes, client should be monitored to ensure that circulation to extremities is not compromised (check temperature, color, pulses). Assist client	f. Client safety and well-being are nursing priorities.

Continued

Table 16–2 | CARE PLAN FOR THE INDIVIDUAL WHO EXPRESSES ANGER INAPPROPRIATELY—cont'd

OUTCOME CRITERIA	NURSING INTERVENTIONS	RATIONALE
	with needs related to nutrition, hydration, and elimination. Position client so that comfort is facilitated, breathing is unobstructed, and aspiration prevented. Clients should not be restrained in the prone position.	
	g. Ongoing assessment. As agitation decreases, assess client's readiness for restraint removal or reduction. With assistance from other staff members, remove one restraint at a time, while assessing client's response. This minimizes the risk of injury to client and staff.	g. Gradual removal of the restraints allows for testing of the client's self-control. Client and staff safety are of primary concern.
	h. Debriefing. It is important, when a client loses control, for staff to follow up with a discussion about the situation. This discussion should occur among staff and with client (when client has regained control). The staff should discuss factors that necessitated the crisis intervention, factors that contributed to the failure of less restrictive interventions, and staff's thoughts about the safety and effectiveness of the intervention. When client has regained control, a debriefing should occur in which client is encouraged to discuss thoughts about what contributed to the crisis situation and about staff interventions and to explore strategies to avert a crisis situation in the future. It is also important to discuss the situation with other clients who witnessed the episode so they understand and process what happened. Some clients may fear that they could be at risk for experiencing a crisis or that they might be in danger when someone else's behavior becomes aggressive.	h. Debriefing helps to diminish the emotional impact of the intervention. Mutual feedback is shared, and staff has an opportunity to process and learn from the event.

Evaluation

Evaluation consists of reassessment to determine if the nursing interventions have been successful in achieving the objectives of care. The following type of information may be gathered to determine the success of working with a client exhibiting inappropriate expression of anger:

- Is the client able to recognize when he or she is angry now?
- Can the client take responsibility for these feelings and keep them in check without losing control?
- Does the client seek out staff/support person to talk about feelings of anger when they occur?
- Is the client able to transfer tension generated by the anger into constructive activities?
- Has harm to client and others been avoided?
- Is the client able to solve problems adaptively without undue frustration and without becoming violent?

Summary and Key Points

- Anger, a normal human emotion, is not necessarily a negative response.
- When used appropriately, anger can provide positive assistance with problem-solving and decision-making in everyday life situations.
- Violence occurs when individuals lose control of their anger.
- Anger is viewed as the emotional response to one's perception of a situation.
- When denied or buried, anger can precipitate a number of psychophysiological disorders.
- When anger is turned inward on the self, it can result in depression.
- When expressed inappropriately, anger commonly interferes with interpersonal relationships.
- When anger is suppressed, it often turns to resentment.
- Anger generates a physiological arousal comparable to the stress response discussed in Chapter 1, The Concept of Stress Adaptation.

- Aggression is one way in which individuals express anger.
- Aggression is behavior intended to threaten or injure the victim's security or self-esteem.
- Aggression can be physical or verbal, but it is virtually always designed to punish.
- Aggression is a negative function or destructive use of anger.
- Various predisposing factors to the way individuals express anger have been implicated. Some theorists suggest that the etiology is purely biological, whereas others believe it depends on psychological and environmental factors.
- Some possible predisposing factors include role modeling, operant conditioning, neurophysiological disorders (e.g., brain tumors, trauma, or diseases), biochemical factors (e.g., increased levels of androgens or other alterations in hormone levels and neurotransmitter involvement), socioeconomic factors (e.g., living in poverty), and environmental factors (e.g., physical crowding, uncomfortable temperature, use of alcohol or drugs).
- Nurses must be aware of the symptoms associated with anger and aggression in order to make an accurate assessment.
- Prevention is the key issue in the management of aggressive or violent behavior.
- Elements identified as key risk factors in the potential for violence among acute psychiatric inpatients include (1) male gender, (2) substance use, (3) past history of violence, and (4) a diagnosis of schizophrenia.
- CBT is an evidence-based treatment strategy for reducing maladaptive aggression, especially in the treatment of aggression in children and adolescents.

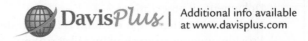

DavisPlus | Additional info available at www.davisplus.com

Review Questions
Self-Examination/Learning Exercise

Select the answer that is most appropriate for each of the following questions.

1. John, age 27, was brought to the emergency department by two police officers. He smelled strongly of alcohol and was combative. His blood alcohol level was measured at 293 mg/dL. His girlfriend reports that he drinks excessively every day and is verbally and physically abusive. The nurses give John the nursing diagnosis of Risk for other-directed violence. What would be appropriate outcome objectives for this diagnosis? (Select all that apply.)
   a. The client will not verbalize anger or hit anyone.
   b. The client will verbalize anger rather than hit others.
   c. The client will not harm self or others.
   d. The client will be restrained if he becomes verbally or physically abusive.

2. John, who was hospitalized with alcohol intoxication and violent behavior, is sitting in the dayroom watching TV with the other clients when the nurse approaches with his 5 p.m. dose of haloperidol. John says, "I feel in control now. I don't need any drugs." The nurse's best response is based on which of the following statements?
   a. John must have the medication, or he will become violent.
   b. John knows that if he will not take the medication orally, he will be restrained and given an intramuscular injection.
   c. John has the right to refuse the medication provided there is no immediate danger to self or others.
   d. John must take the medication at this time in order to maintain adequate blood levels.

3. The nurse hears John, a client with a history of violence, yelling in the dayroom. The nurse observes his increased agitation, clenched fists, and loud, demanding voice. He is challenging and threatening staff and the other clients. The nurse's *priority* intervention would be to:
   a. Call for assistance.
   b. Draw up a syringe of prn haloperidol.
   c. Ask John if he would like to talk about his anger.
   d. Tell John if he does not calm down he will have to be restrained.

4. John, a client with a history of violence, has been hospitalized on the psychiatric unit. He becomes agitated and begins to threaten the staff and other clients. When all other interventions fail, John is placed in restraints in the seclusion room for his and others' protection. Which of the following are interventions for the client in restraints? (Select all that apply.)
   a. Check temperature and pulse of extremities.
   b. Document all observations.
   c. Explain to the client that restraint is his punishment for violent behavior.
   d. Provide ongoing assessment and observation.
   e. Withhold food and fluid until client is calm and can be released from restraints.

5. When it has been assessed that a client is in control and no longer requires restraining, how does the nurse proceed?
   a. The nurse removes the restraints.
   b. The nurse calls for assistance to remove the restraints.
   c. With assistance, the nurse removes one restraint.
   d. The nurse tells the client he will have to wait until the doctor comes in.

6. Which of these procedures is important immediately following an episode of violence on the unit? (Select all that apply.)
   a. Document all observations and occurrences.
   b. Conduct a debriefing with staff.
   c. Discuss what occurred with other clients who witnessed the incident.
   d. Warn the client that it could happen again if he becomes violent.

Review Questions—cont'd
Self-Examination/Learning Exercise

7. A client who has been in restraints is now calm. He apologizes to the nurse and says, "I hope I didn't hurt anyone." The nurse's best response is:
   a. "This is our job. We know how to handle violent clients."
   b. "We understand you were out of control and didn't really mean to hurt anyone."
   c. "It is fortunate that no one was hurt. You will not be placed in restraints as long as you can control your behavior."
   d. "It is an unpleasant situation to have to restrain someone, but we have to think of the other clients. We can't have you causing injury to others. I just hope it won't happen again."

8. John and his girlfriend had an argument during her visit. Which behavior by John would indicate he is learning to adaptively problem-solve his frustrations?
   a. John says to the nurse, "Give me some of that medication before I end up in restraints!"
   b. When his girlfriend leaves, John goes to the exercise room and punches on the punching bag.
   c. John says to the nurse, "I guess I'm going to have to dump that broad!"
   d. John says to his girlfriend, "You'd better leave before I do something I'm sorry for."

9. Which of the following assessment data would the nurse consider as risk factors for possible violence in a client? (Select all that apply.)
   a. A diagnosis of somatization disorder
   b. A diagnosis of schizophrenia or bipolar disorder
   c. Substance intoxication
   d. Argumentative and demanding behavior
   e. Past history of violence

10. Which of the following is true about *aggression*? (Select all that apply.)
    a. It is goal directed.
    b. Its aim is to do harm to a person or object.
    c. It has a requisite of *intent*.
    d. It energizes and mobilizes the body for self-defense.

References

Almvik, R., Woods, P., & Rasmussen, K. (2000). The Brøset Violence Checklist: Sensitivity, specificity, and interrater reliability. *Journal of Interpersonal Violence, 15*(12), 1284-1296. doi:10.1034/j.1600-0447.106.s412.22.x

American Psychological Association. (2013). Violence in the media: Psychologists study TV and video game violence for potential harmful effects. Retrieved from www.apa.org/action/resources/research-in-action/protect.aspx

American Psychological Association. (2017). Controlling anger before it controls you. Retrieved from www.apa.org/topics/anger/control.aspx

Archer, D. (2012). Environmental stressors and violence. *Psychology Today.* Retrieved from https://www.psychologytoday.com/blog/reading-between-the-headlines/201206/environmental-stressors-and-violence

Friedman, R.A. (2006). Violence and mental illness—How strong is the link? *New England Journal of Medicine, 355*(20), 2064-2066. doi:10.1056/NEJMp068229

Gorman, L.M., & Sultan, D.F. (2008). *Psychosocial nursing for general patient care* (3rd ed.). Philadelphia: F.A. Davis.

Iozzino, L., Ferrari, C., Large, M., Nielssen, O., & Girolamo, G. (2015). Prevalence and risk factors of violence by psychiatric acute inpatients: A systematic review and meta-analysis. *PLoS ONE, 10*(6). doi:10.1371/journal.pone.0128536

Kassinove, H. (2016). How to recognize and deal with anger. Retrieved from www.apa.org/helpcenter/recognize-anger.aspx

Novitsky, M.A., Julius, R.J., & Dubin, W.R. (2009). Non-pharmacologic management of violence in psychiatric emergencies. *Primary Psychiatry, 16*(9), 49-53.

Pavlov, K.A., Chistiakov, D.A., & Chekhonin, V. P. (2012). Genetic determinants of aggression and impulsivity in humans. *Journal of Applied Genetics, 53*(1), 61-82. doi:10.1007/s13353-011-0069-6.

Perry, B. (2016). Aggression and violence: The neurobiology of experience. Retrieved from http://teacher.scholastic.com/professional/bruceperry/aggression_violence.htm

Sadock, B.J., Sadock, V.A., & Ruiz, P. (2015). *Synopsis of psychiatry: Behavioral sciences/clinical psychiatry* (11th ed.). Philadelphia: Lippincott Williams & Wilkins.

Smeets, K.C., Leeijen, A., Van Der Molen, M.J., Scheepers, F.E., Buitelaar, J.K., & Rommelse, N. (2015). Treatment moderators of cognitive behavior therapy to reduce aggressive behavior: A meta-analysis. *European Child Adolescent Psychiatry*, 24, 255-264. doi:10.1007/s00787-014-0592-1

Truman, J. L., & Morgan, R.E. (2016). Criminal victimization, 2015. *Bureau of Justice Statistics*. Retrieved from www.bjs.gov/index.cfm?ty=pbdetail&iid=5804

Vetulani, J. (2013). Neurochemistry of impulsiveness and aggression. *Psychiatria Polska*, *47*(1), 103-115.

Classical References

Warren, N.C. (1993). *Make anger your ally* (3rd ed.). Wheaton, IL: Tyndale House Publishers.

Waughfield, C.G. (2002). *Mental health concepts* (5th ed.). Albany, NY: Delmar.

Suicide Prevention

17

CORE CONCEPTS

Suicide
Suicide Risk Assessment
Suicide Prevention

KEY TERMS

altruistic suicide
anomic suicide
collaborative safety plan

egoistic suicide
suicide risk factors
suicide warning signs

OBJECTIVES
After reading this chapter, the student will be able to:

1. Discuss epidemiological statistics and risk factors related to suicide.
2. Describe predisposing factors implicated in the etiology of suicide.
3. Differentiate between facts and myths regarding suicide.
4. Apply the nursing process to individuals exhibiting suicidal behavior.

HOMEWORK ASSIGNMENT
Please read the chapter and answer the following questions:

1. How are age, race, and gender associated with suicide risk?
2. Your neighbor tells you he is going to visit his sister-in-law in the hospital. The sister-in-law has been hospitalized after attempting suicide. Your neighbor asks, "What should I say when I go to visit Jane?" What suggestions might you give him?
3. John's father died by suicide when John was a teenager. John's wife, Mary, tells the mental health nurse that she is afraid John "inherited" that predisposition from his father. How should the nurse respond to Mary?
4. The nurse notes that the mood of a client being treated for depression and suicidal ideation suddenly brightens, and the client states, "I feel fine now. I don't feel depressed anymore." Why would this statement alert the nurse of a potential problem?
5. Write a one- to two-page journal reflecting on your previous experiences with suicide, examining your thoughts and feelings and their potential impact on your nursing practice. (Note: Self-awareness on the issue of suicide is identified as an essential competency for psychiatric nurses [American Psychiatric Nurses Association (APNA), 2015] and is relevant to all nurses in developing skills necessary for this aspect of nursing assessment and intervention).

Suicide is not a diagnosis or a disorder; it is a behavior. Specifically, it is the act of taking one's own life, and it derives from the Latin words for "one's own killing." Many religions hold that suicide is a sin that is strictly forbidden. Canetto (American Psychiatric Association, 2010) states, "Everywhere, suicidal behavior is culturally scripted. Women and men adopt the self-destructive behaviors that are expected of them within their cultures." A recent, more secular view has influenced how some individuals view suicide in our society. Growing support for an individual's right to choose death over pain has been evidenced by an increasing number of states that are considering or have adopted physician-assisted suicide laws. Some individuals are striving to advance the cause of physician-assisted suicides for the terminally ill. In 2008, Oregon was the only state in which physician-assisted suicide was legal. Since then, Montana, Vermont, Washington, and most recently, California, adopted similar laws. New Mexico did so as well, but it was overturned on appeal in August 2015. Can suicide be a rational act? Most people in our society do not yet believe that it can.

In the field of psychiatry, suicide is considered an irrational act associated with mental illness and most commonly, but not exclusively, with depression. More than 90 percent of all persons who attempt or die by suicide have a diagnosed mental disorder (National Institute of Mental Health [NIMH], 2015). However, since this phenomenon does not capture all of those who take their own lives, we must not ignore individuals in the community and in nonpsychiatric healthcare settings who may be at risk. This chapter explores suicide from an epidemiological and etiological perspective. Care of the suicidal client is presented in the context of the nursing process.

Historical Perspectives

In ancient Greece, individuals were said to have "committed" suicide because it was an offense against the state, and individuals who committed suicide were denied burial in community sites (Minois, 2001). In the culture of the imperial Roman army, individuals sometimes resorted to suicide to escape humiliation or abuse. In the Middle Ages, suicide was viewed as a selfish or criminal act (Minois, 2001). Individuals who "committed" suicide were often denied cemetery burial, and their property was confiscated and shared by the crown and the courts (MacDonald & Murphy, 1991).

The issue of suicide changed during the Renaissance period. Although condemnation was still expected, the view became philosophical, allowing intellectuals to discuss the issue more freely. Most philosophers of the 17th and 18th centuries condemned suicide, but some writers recognized a connection between suicide and melancholy or other severe mental disturbances (Minois, 2001). Suicide was illegal in England until 1961, and only in 1993 was it decriminalized in Ireland.

Most religions consider suicide as a sin against God. Judaism, Christianity, Islam, Hinduism, and Buddhism all condemn suicide. The Catholic church today still teaches that suicide is wrong, that it is in opposition to proper love of self and love of God, and that it wrongs others through the experience of loss and grief (Byron, 2016). But as Byron (2016) points out, some of the church's condemnation may have been rooted in a "denial of the responsibility to understand the pain that produces such an act," and he stresses the importance of encouraging those who "are hurting to open up," which, it is hoped, will remove some of the taboos of discussing suicide within the church. Replacing the term *committed* suicide (which has persisted in use long since its decriminalization) may also help to reduce the stigma and taboo that has historically been associated with open conversation about suicide.

Epidemiological Factors

In 2014, the most recent year for which statistics have been recorded, 42,773 people died by suicide (American Foundation for Suicide Prevention [AFSP], 2016). This is the highest rate of suicide in more than 15 years. These statistics have established suicide as the second-leading cause of death (behind unintentional injuries) among young Americans aged 10 to 34 years, the fourth-leading cause of death for individuals aged 35 to 54, the eighth-leading cause of death for individuals aged 55 to 64, and the tenth-leading cause of death overall (Centers for Disease Control and Prevention [CDC], 2016). Many more people attempt suicide than die by suicide (about 12:1), and countless others seriously contemplate the act without carrying it out. Since statistics about numbers of suicide attempts reflect only those who have entered a treatment setting, the numbers could be much higher. With a steady incline in suicide rates from 2000 to 2014, suicide has become a major health-care problem in the United States. Not only are the number of suicides on the incline, but the demographics have changed. Historically, the highest rates of suicide were among the elderly, but currently the highest rate of suicide occurs among middle-aged individuals and those ages 85 and older. Historically, the suicide rate has been lower among military personnel than among the general population. However, in some time periods since the Iraq War began—including in 2010 and 2011—more soldiers died by suicide than died in combat (Nock et al., 2013). See Chapter 38, Military Families, for further discussion.

A wealth of research is being conducted to better understand the best strategies for prevention, the best methods for assessment of suicide risk, what differentiates those with suicidal ideation from those who attempt, and what kind of treatments and interventions are supported by evidence. The federal government, through the Substance Abuse and Mental Health Services Administration, has endorsed the Zero Suicide movement (National Action Alliance for Suicide Prevention, 2015), an effort to identify evidence-based strategies for suicide prevention, so there is a great deal of national attention to this issue. Within the next several years, our understanding of and approaches to treatment may dramatically change. We are certainly beginning to recognize that, with suicide rates on the rise, our conventional interventions have not adequately addressed the complex needs of this population.

Confusion exists over the reality of various notions regarding suicide. Some currently accepted facts and myths relating to suicide are presented in Table 17–1.

TABLE 17–1 Facts and Myths About Suicide

MYTHS	FACTS
People who talk about suicide do not act on their ideas. Suicide happens without warning.	Eight out of 10 people who kill themselves have given definite clues and warnings about their suicidal intentions. Very subtle clues may be ignored or disregarded by others.
You cannot stop a suicidal person. He or she is fully intent on dying.	Most suicidal people are very ambivalent about their feelings regarding living or dying. Most are "gambling with death" and see it as a cry for someone to save them.
Once a person is suicidal, he or she is suicidal forever.	Suicidal ideation and risk fluctuate over time and may be time-limited. If provided adequate support and resources, a suicidal person can go on to lead a normal life. However, multiple suicide attempts may reflect greater chronicity of suicidal ideation. Reassessment over time is important to identify current risks.
Improvement after severe depression means that the suicidal risk is over.	Most suicides occur within about 3 months after the beginning of "improvement," when the individual has the energy to carry out suicidal intentions.
Suicide is inherited, or "runs in families."	Suicide is not inherited. It is an individual matter and can be prevented. However, suicide by a close family member increases an individual's risk factor for suicide.
All suicidal individuals are mentally ill, and suicide is the act of a psychotic person.	Although a majority of people who attempt suicide are extremely unhappy or clinically depressed, they are not necessarily psychotic. They are merely unable at that point in time to see an alternative solution to what they consider an unbearable problem.
Suicidal thoughts and attempts should be considered manipulative or attention-seeking behavior and should not be taken seriously.	All suicidal behavior must be approached with the gravity of the potential act in mind. Attention should be given to the possibility that the individual is issuing a cry for help.
People usually take their own lives by overdosing on drugs.	Gunshot wounds are the leading cause of death among suicide victims.
If an individual has attempted suicide, he or she will not do it again.	Between 50% and 80% of all people who ultimately kill themselves have at least one previous attempt.
Suicide always happens in an impulsive moment.	People often contemplate, imagine, plan strategies, write notes, post things on the Web. The importance of in-depth exploration and assessment cannot be overstated.
Young children (aged 5–12) can't be suicidal.	Annually, 30 to 35 children under the age of 12 take their own lives and not all are clinically depressed.

SOURCES: Cardoza, K. (2016). 6 myths about suicide that every parent and educator should know. Retrieved from www.npr.org/sections/ed/2016/09/02/478835539; National Alliance on Mental Illness. (2015). Risks of suicide. Retrieved from www.nami.org/Learn-More/Mental-Health-Conditions/Related-Conditions/Risk-of-Suicide; The Samaritans. (2015). Suicide myths and misconceptions. Retrieved from http://samaritansnyc.org/myths-about-suicide.

Risk Factors

Suicide risk factors are identified as factors that have statistically been correlated with a higher incidence of suicide. They should be differentiated from **suicide warning signs** which are identified as factors suggesting a more immediate concern. Both are included as part of a comprehensive assessment of overall risk for suicide.

Marital Status

Some evidence has suggested that the suicide rate for single, never-married persons is twice that for married persons and that divorce increases risk for suicide particularly among men, who are three times more likely than divorced women to take their own lives (Sadock, Sadock, & Ruiz, 2015). Widows and widowers have also been identified at higher risk, but a longitudinal study (Kposowa, 2000) found being single or widowed had no effect on suicide rates. However, their evidence supported that divorced men are twice as likely as married men to die by suicide. Among women, the study showed no significant difference in risk of suicide by marital categories. The authors highlight that the evidence is difficult to sort out and can be misleading if data is not stratified over several variables, including age, socioeconomic status, and other factors.

For those who are divorced and widowed, the stresses associated with major life changes and loss are influential. Evidence has demonstrated that *change* in marital status increases risk for suicidal behavior, particularly in the first year after the change and particularly among older people (Roškar et al., 2011; Yamauchi et al., 2013). Again, it should be noted that demographics such as marital status, age, and gender may inform about populations that are statistically at higher risk, but none of these factors are predictive of immediate risk. A thorough assessment of variables, including risk factors, warning signs, and a host of other data, are essential to identifying individuals at acute risk for attempting suicide.

Gender

More women than men attempt suicide, but men succeed more often. Successful suicides number about 70 percent for men and 30 percent for women. This success rate has to do with the lethality of the means. Women tend to overdose; men use more lethal means, such as firearms. These differences between men and women may also reflect differing societal expectations; women are more likely than men to seek and accept help from friends or professionals.

Age

Suicide risk and age are, in general, positively correlated, particularly with men. Although rates among women remain fairly constant throughout life, rates among men increase with age. The most recent statistics, according to the American Foundation for Suicide Prevention, revealed that in 2013, the highest rate of suicide occurred in the 45- to 64-year-old age group and among those 85 or older (AFSP, 2016). A consistent high rate of suicide in both age groups was shown for the period 2000 to 2014, but the 45 to 64 age group showed a steady incline in suicide rates over the same period.

Although adolescents may statistically have a lower rate of suicide than some other age groups, it is still important to note that suicide has been the third-leading cause of death in this population over several years, and in 2013 jumped to the second-leading cause of death where it remained in 2014 (CDC, 2016). Several factors put adolescents at risk for suicide, including impulsive and high-risk behaviors, untreated mood disorders (e.g., major depression and bipolar disorder), access to lethal means (e.g., firearms), and substance abuse. One recent study (Reyes et al., 2015) found a link between some modes of anger expression in adolescents and suicide risk; in particular, hopelessness and hostility modes of anger expression were associated with an increase in suicidal tendency. The latest statistics from the Centers for Disease Control and Prevention (CDC) indicate that the most common method of completed suicide for adolescent males is firearms; for adolescent females, it is suffocation (CDC, 2015a).

Among children younger than age 10, the statistics demonstrate a low number of suicides, and some have argued that younger children do not have the capacity to intentionally consider and follow through with a suicide attempt. Anecdotal evidence has shown this is not always the case, with some therapists identifying 5- to 9-year-old children actively talking about suicide (Jobes, 2015). Research is beginning to emerge that supports real risk in young children (Duran & McGuinness, 2016). Bridge and associates (2015) studied a large sample of children aged 5 to 11 and found that an average of 33 children per year die by suicide within this age group in the United States, predominately from suffocation and hanging. These researchers also noted that suicide was never coded as a cause of death for children under 5 years of age. But when Whalen and associates (2015) studied children in the 3 to 7 age group, they found about 11 percent with suicidal ideation. This risk was correlated with male gender, psychiatric illness in their mothers, and psychiatric illness in the child. Duran and McGuinness (2016) stress that the implications for nursing are clear; direct inquiry about suicide ideas is a "necessary component in healthcare encounters with children," including those in primary care, emergency departments, and with the school nurse.

Although the elderly comprise just over 13 percent of the population, they account for almost 15 percent of all suicides. In general, 70 percent of all suicides are among white males, but white males over the age of 80 are at the greatest risk of all age, gender, and race groups. Almost 84 percent of elderly suicides are male, which is about five times greater than for females, and firearms are the most common means of taking one's own life (American Association of Suicidology, 2015). The overall rate of suicide for females declines after age 65.

Religion

Historically, suicide rates among Protestants and Jews have been higher than among Roman Catholic or Muslim populations, but the degree of orthodoxy and affiliation with one's religion may be an important variable (Sadock et al., 2015). One study revealed that men and women who consider themselves affiliated with a religion are less likely than their nonreligious counterparts to attempt suicide (Rasic et al., 2009). The authors found that religious affiliation is associated with decreased suicide attempts in both the general population and in those with a mental illness, independent of the availability of social support systems.

Socioeconomic Status

Individuals in the very highest and lowest social classes have higher suicide rates than those in the middle classes (Sadock et al., 2015). With regard to occupation, suicide rates are higher among physicians, artists, dentists, law enforcement officers, lawyers, and insurance agents. There are more suicides among the unemployed than among the employed, and suicide rates increase during economic recessions and depressions.

Ethnicity

With regard to ethnicity, statistics show that whites are at highest risk for suicide (14.7%), followed by American Indian and Alaska Natives (10.9%), Hispanic Americans (6.3%), Asian Americans (5.9%), and African Americans (5.5%) (CDC, 2016). Recent research has highlighted two trends that illuminate issues of concern within specific groups. First, although suicide rates among whites are higher in adults and the elderly, within the American Indian community, young adults have a higher risk for suicide than in any other ethnic group, and the rate is higher than that of the general population (Almendrala, 2015). Almendrala relays the story of a psychiatrist called to a reservation where there had been 17 suicides in the previous 8 months, and the community members described themselves as "grieved out." The second trend of concern, as Almendrala reports, is that the rates of suicide may be underestimated in this population because death certificates do not always report accurately regarding ethnicity.

Another recent study examined suicide trends among school-aged children younger than 12 (Bridge et al., 2015). A significant finding was that suicide rates for black children 5 to 11 years of age nearly doubled over the period from 1993 to 2012, while the overall suicide rate in this age group remained relatively stable during the same time period. The use of hanging and/or suffocation as a means of taking one's own life also significantly increased in this population. It is hard to imagine what causes children so young to take their own lives. The contributing factors to these recent trends are not well understood and will require further research, including a review of the impact of healthcare disparities for select communities and populations.

Other Risk Factors

As previously stated, more than 90 percent of people who kill themselves have a diagnosable mental disorder, most commonly a mood disorder or a substance abuse disorder (NIMH, 2015). Individuals who have been hospitalized for a psychiatric illness have a 5 to 10 times greater suicide risk than those with psychiatric illness in the general population (Sadock et al., 2015). This higher risk may be a reflection of the severity of their mental illness. Other recent research supports an increased risk of suicide in the period following discharge from psychiatric hospitalization, especially for those not connected to a system of care (Olfson et al., 2016). Suicide risk may increase early in treatment with antidepressants. One possible reason is that as an individual's energy returns, he or she may have an increased ability to act out self-destructive wishes. Although suicide is often thought of as strictly related to depression, there is also a recognized risk of suicide among people with schizophrenia, bipolar disorders, personality disorders, eating disorders, anxiety disorders, and substance use disorders. The importance of thorough suicide risk assessment for anyone seeking mental health services cannot be overstated.

Severe insomnia is associated with increased suicide risk even in the absence of depression. Use of alcohol, and particularly a combination of alcohol and barbiturates, increases the risk of suicide. Withdrawal from stimulants increases suicide risk as the person begins to "crash." Psychosis, especially with command hallucinations (hearing voices telling one to harm or kill oneself), increases risk, as does affliction with a chronic, painful, and/or disabling illness.

Several studies have indicated a higher risk factor for suicide among gay men, lesbians, and transgender (LGBT) individuals (Cassels, 2011; Cochran & Mays, 2000; Eisenberg & Resnick, 2006; King et al., 2008; Plöderl, 2013). This increased risk may be a function of the social stigma and discrimination associated with being part of a marginalized group. Additional personal stressors, including isolation, victimization, and stressful interpersonal relationships with family, peers, and community, are not uncommon. A report from the CDC (2015b) identified that in a study of youth in grades 7 to 12, lesbian, gay, and bisexual youth were twice as likely as their heterosexual peers to attempt suicide (this study did not address the risk for transgender individuals). Another study, however, found that transgender individuals are also a high-risk population for suicide, with an alarming 41 percent lifetime prevalence (Stroumsa, 2014). See Chapter 30, Issues Related to Human Sexuality and Gender Dysphoria, for further discussion on this topic.

Higher risk is also associated with a family history of suicide, especially in a same-gender parent, and with individuals who have made previous suicide attempts. About half of individuals who kill themselves have previously attempted suicide. Loss of a loved one through death or separation and lack of employment or increased financial burden also increase risk.

In recent years, a number of suicides have been reported in the media among young people who are the victims of bullying. Zweig and Dank (2013) reported that 41 percent of youth are victims of physical bullying (most often boys), 17 percent are victims of cyberbullying, and girls are more likely to be victims of psychological bullying. Clearly, bullying is a prevalent concern among youth. Klomek, Sourander, and Gould (2011) report:

> Studies among middle school and high school students show an increased risk of suicidal behavior among bullies and victims. Both perpetrators and victims are at the highest risk for suicidal ideation.

Being bullied via the Internet or e-mail (called *cyberbullying*) has also been associated with increased risk of depression and suicidal behavior among young people. Researchers found that both perpetrators and victims of cyberbullying had more suicidal ideation and were more likely to attempt suicide than those who had not experienced such forms of peer aggression (Bauman, Toomey, & Walker, 2013; Hinduja & Patchin, 2010). Edgerton and Limber (2013), in a research brief on suicide and bullying, caution that although research does show that those who are bullied have high levels of suicidal thoughts and attempts, there is not enough research to identify a cause-and-effect relationship. Other risk factors such as mental health problems appear to play a larger role.

Predisposing Factors: Theories of Suicide

Psychological Theories

Anger Turned Inward

Freud (1957) believed that suicide was a response to intense self-hatred. The anger originated toward a love object but was ultimately turned inward against the self. In other words, Freud thought that suicide occurred as a result of an earlier repressed desire to kill someone else.

Hopelessness and Other Symptoms of Depression

Hopelessness has long been identified as a symptom of depression and an underlying factor in the predisposition to suicide. Although the many symptoms identified in suicide assessment tools attempt to assess for seriousness of suicide ideation, current research is attempting to glean which symptoms might be more predictive of the move from ideation to attempts. In addition to hopelessness, the strength of the person's intention to die has also been identified as significant (Jobes, 2015).

History of Aggression and Violence

A history of violent behavior or impulsive acts has been associated with increased risk for suicide (Sadock et al., 2015), although recent evidence suggests that impulsive traits are higher in individuals with suicide ideation but not necessarily associated with more attempts (Klonsky & May, 2015b).

Shame and Humiliation

Some individuals have viewed suicide as a "face-saving" mechanism—a way to prevent public humiliation following a social defeat such as a sudden loss of status or income. Often, these individuals are too embarrassed to seek treatment or other support systems.

Sociological Theories

Durkheim's Theory

Durkheim's classic work (1951) studied the individual's interaction with the society in which he or she lived. He believed that the more cohesive the society and the more that the individual felt an integrated part of society, the less likely he or she was to carry out suicide. Durkheim described three social categories of suicide:

1. **Egoistic suicide** is the response of the individual who feels separate from the mainstream of society. Integration is lacking, and the individual does not feel a part of any cohesive group (such as a family or a church).
2. **Altruistic suicide** is the opposite of egoistic suicide. The individual who is prone to altruistic suicide is excessively integrated into the group. The group is often governed by cultural, religious, or political ties, and allegiance is so strong that the individual will sacrifice his or her life for the group.
3. **Anomic suicide** occurs in response to changes in an individual's life (e.g., divorce, loss of job) that

disrupt feelings of relatedness to the group. An interruption in the customary norms of behavior instills feelings of separateness and fears of being without support from the formerly cohesive group.

Interpersonal Theory of Suicide

Thomas Joiner's (2005) interpersonal theory of suicide supports some of the same principles advanced by Durkheim associating lack of a feeling of belonging with suicide risk. But Joiner's theory introduces the concept that suicide ideation and suicide attempts need to be understood as distinct processes. He proposed that low connectedness and a high sense of burden interact with each other to increase suicide thoughts and desires, but those features in the presence of high capability for suicide are strongly associated with the move from ideation to lethal attempts.

The Three-Step Theory

Klonsky and May (2015a), inspired by Joiner's theory and based on their research finding that impulsivity is elevated in people who have made suicide attempts and those who have thoughts and have never made an attempt, sought to identify the factors that elevate suicide ideation to an active risk for attempts. Their research supported the following three-step trajectory:

1. Pain (usually psychological pain) when combined with hopelessness significantly increases suicide ideation (for both men and women and across age groups).
2. Connectedness prevents suicide ideation from escalating in those at risk, but when pain and hopelessness exceed one's sense of connectedness to others, suicide ideation becomes active.
3. When strong, active suicide ideation is present, it leads to an attempt only if one has the capacity to make an attempt.

Biological Theories

Genetics

Twin studies have shown a much higher concordance rate for monozygotic twins than for dizygotic twins. Some studies with people who have attempted suicide have focused on the genotypic variations in the gene for tryptophan hydroxylase, with results indicating significant association to suicidality (Sadock et al., 2015). Tryptophan hydroxylase is an enzyme associated with the synthesis of serotonin, and diminished serotonin has implications for both depression and suicidal behavior. These findings suggest the potential for genetic predisposition toward suicidal behavior.

Neurochemical Factors

A number of studies have revealed a deficiency of serotonin (measured as a decrease in the levels of 5-hydroxyindole acetic acid [5-HIAA] in the cerebrospinal fluid) in depressed clients who attempted suicide (Sadock et al., 2015). These studies, as well as postmortem studies, have supported the hypothesis that deficiencies in central nervous system serotonin are associated with suicide.

However, a recent meta-analysis examining biological factors found that they are, in general, weak predictors of a future suicide attempt or death by suicide (Chang et al., 2016). The only two biological factors that had statistical significance in this analysis were cytokines (anti-inflammatory response chemicals) and low levels of fish oil nutrients (including omega-3).

Application of the Nursing Process With the Suicidal Client

A multitude of research studies are being published that explore suicide from many different vantage points to identify demographics, risk factors, predictors of risk for suicide attempts, and strategies for prevention. Many of these studies are helping nurses become more aware of the phenomenon of suicide and understand the limitations of research in making a clinical judgment about a patient's actual risks versus statistical risks.

Influential organizations across the nation are advancing the importance of improving the quality of care, documentation, and reporting of details around sentinel events related to acts of or deaths by suicide. In addition to government-initiated national strategies for suicide prevention, The Joint Commission (2016) has advanced standards that include requiring hospitals to conduct risk assessments "identifying specific patient characteristics and environmental features that may increase or decrease the risk of suicide." The American Psychiatric Nurses Association (APNA, 2015; Puntil et al., 2013) has taken a leadership role in identifying psychiatric-mental health nurse essential competencies for assessment and management of individuals at risk for suicide. The CDC (2011) has advanced strategies for uniform definition and reporting about acts of self-directed violence to improve data collection and ultimately improve our understanding and prevention of suicide.

At the heart of this wealth of information is the necessity for accurate, comprehensive assessment that includes collaboration with the patient and other clinicians and is rooted in strategies to form a therapeutic relationship of trust and open communication.

Assessment

When nurses assess a client's suicide ideation, it is important to identify and distinguish ideas (thoughts), plans (intentions), and attempts (behavior). Each of these assessment factors can provide information about level of risk. When the client has attempted self-injury, it is important to distinguish between *suicidal self-injury* and *nonsuicidal self-injury*. The latter injury is often used as a method to release emotions, but it may also be a way of communicating the severity of distress that the client is experiencing (Nock et al., 2013).

The following basic items should be considered when conducting a suicidal assessment: demographics; presenting symptoms and medical-psychiatric diagnoses; suicidal ideas or acts; interpersonal support system; analysis of the suicidal crisis; psychiatric, medical, and family history; and coping strategies. Dr. David Satcher, as Surgeon General of the United States, spoke of risk factors and protective factors in his "Call to Action to Prevent Suicide" (U.S. Public Health Service, 1999). This report initiated a national movement toward research designed to better understand predictors of suicide risk and develop more effective evidence-based interventions. Current models have clarified risk factors as different from warning signs that are associated with a greater potential for suicide and suicidal behavior. Protective factors have been identified that are associated with reduced potential for suicide. Examples of protective factors are outlined in Box 17–1. Figure 17–1 presents a model for differentiating low, high, and imminent

---

BOX 17–1 Examples of Protective Factors

Resilient temperament

Social competency

Skills in problem-solving, coping, and conflict resolution

Perception of social support from adults and peers

Positive expectations, optimism for the future; identification of future goals

Connectedness to family, school, community

Presence and involvement of caring adults (for adolescents)

Integration in social networks

Cultural and religious beliefs that discourage suicide and encourage preservation of life

Access to quality social services and clinical health care for mental, physical, and substance use disorders

Support through ongoing medical and mental health-care relationships

Restricted access to highly lethal means of suicide

SOURCE: Crosby, A.E., Ortega, L., & Melanson, C. (2011). Self-directed Violence Surveillance: Uniform definitions and recommended data elements, Version 1.0. Atlanta (GA): Centers for Disease Control and Prevention, National Center for Injury Prevention and Control. Retrieved from www.cdc.gov/violenceprevention/pdf/Self-Directed-Violence-a.pdf

---

suicide risk. The goal of such models is not to predict a suicide attempt but to identify the level of intervention needed to prevent an attempt.

Demographics

The following demographics are identified when evaluating a client for suicide risk. Although demographics alone do not directly translate into an individual's risk, they provide information as part of a comprehensive assessment of proximal or potentiating risk factors.

■ **Age:** Adolescents and the elderly have been generally identified as high-risk groups, but recent statistics demonstrating the highest incidence in the 45- to 64-years age group suggests that nurses should pay close attention to assessing for suicide risk in all age groups.

■ **Gender:** Males are at higher risk for suicide than females, but females attempt suicide more frequently.

■ **Ethnicity/race:** The CDC reports highest rates of suicide among Caucasians followed by American Indians (CDC, 2015a).

■ **Marital status:** Single, divorced, and widowed individuals are at higher risk for suicide than are married people particularly during periods of change in status.

■ **Socioeconomic status:** Individuals in the highest and lowest socioeconomic classes are at higher risk than those in the middle classes.

■ **Occupation:** Health-care professionals (especially physicians), law enforcement officers, dentists, artists, mechanics, lawyers, and insurance agents have all been identified as occupational groups incurring greater risks for suicide (Sadock et al., 2015).

■ **Religion:** People with close religious affiliations may be at lower risk for attempting suicide if they believe, for example, that suicide is an unforgivable sin that is strictly forbidden within the religion. Conversely, people without close affiliations that impose restrictions about suicide may be at greater risk.

■ **Family history:** A family history of suicide increases an individual's risk for suicide.

■ **Military history:** Suicide rates among military personnel now exceed those of the general population (Nock et al., 2013).

Presenting Symptoms and Medical-Psychiatric Diagnosis

Assessment data must be gathered regarding any psychiatric or physical condition for which a client is being treated. Mood disorders (major depression and bipolar disorders) are the disorders most commonly

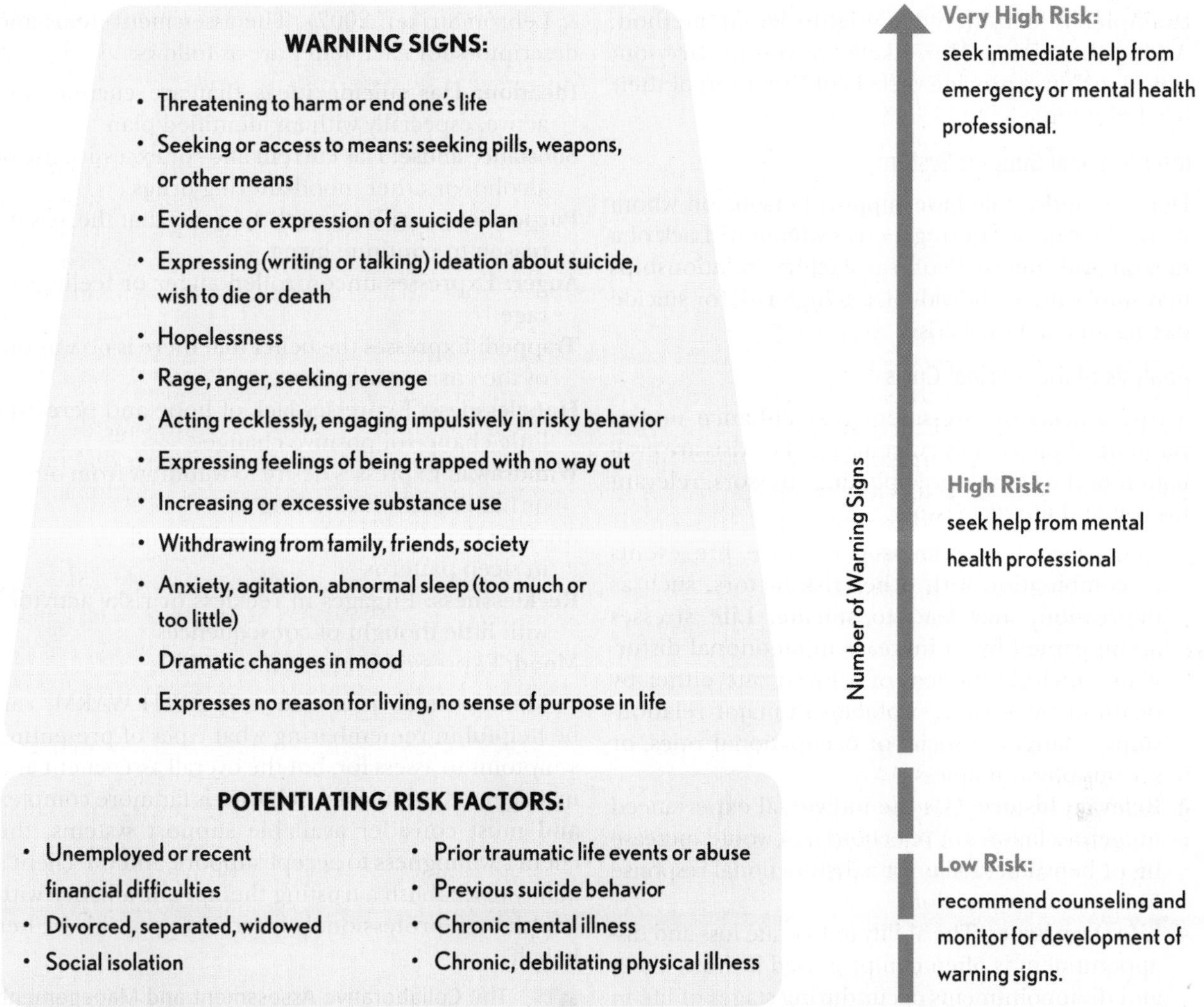

WARNING SIGNS:

- Threatening to harm or end one's life
- Seeking or access to means: seeking pills, weapons, or other means
- Evidence or expression of a suicide plan
- Expressing (writing or talking) ideation about suicide, wish to die or death
- Hopelessness
- Rage, anger, seeking revenge
- Acting recklessly, engaging impulsively in risky behavior
- Expressing feelings of being trapped with no way out
- Increasing or excessive substance use
- Withdrawing from family, friends, society
- Anxiety, agitation, abnormal sleep (too much or too little)
- Dramatic changes in mood
- Expresses no reason for living, no sense of purpose in life

POTENTIATING RISK FACTORS:

- Unemployed or recent financial difficulties
- Divorced, separated, widowed
- Social isolation
- Prior traumatic life events or abuse
- Previous suicide behavior
- Chronic mental illness
- Chronic, debilitating physical illness

Number of Warning Signs

Very High Risk: seek immediate help from emergency or mental health professional.

High Risk: seek help from mental health professional

Low Risk: recommend counseling and monitor for development of warning signs.

FIGURE 17–1 Risk factors and warning signs for suicide. Reprinted with permission from the Ontario Hospital Association.

associated with suicide. Substance use disorders are also associated with risk for suicide attempts. Other psychiatric disorders in which suicide risks have been identified include anxiety disorders, schizophrenia, anorexia nervosa, and borderline and antisocial personality disorders. Chronic and terminal physical illnesses have also been identified as potentiating risk factors.

Suicidal Ideas or Acts

How serious is the client's intent to die by suicide? Does the person have a plan? If so, does he or she have the means? How lethal are the means? Does he or she intend to carry out this plan? Has the individual ever attempted suicide before? These questions must be asked by the person conducting the assessment of the client who is suicidal.

Individuals may provide both behavioral and verbal clues as to the intent of their act. Examples of behavioral clues that may indicate a decision to carry out

suicidal intent include giving away prized possessions, getting financial affairs in order, writing suicide notes, and sudden lift in mood.

Verbal clues may be both direct and indirect. Examples of direct statements include "I want to die" or "I'm going to kill myself." Examples of indirect statements include "This is the last time you'll see me," "I won't be around much longer for the doctor to worry about," or "I don't have anything worth living for anymore."

Other assessments include determining whether the individual has a plan, and if so, whether he or she has the means to carry out that plan. If the person states the suicide will be carried out with a gun, does he or she have access to a gun? Bullets? If pills are planned, what kind of pills? Are they accessible? The lethality of the method identified by an individual with suicide ideation or by one who has already made an attempt provides meaningful information about the client's intent to die. Use of firearms, for example, is considered a highly lethal method. Asking the client, "How likely are you to carry out this plan?" may provide verbal confirmation of their level of intent.

Interpersonal Support System

Does the individual have support persons on whom he or she can rely during a crisis situation? Lack of a meaningful network of satisfactory relationships may implicate an individual as a high risk for suicide during an emotional crisis.

Analysis of the Suicidal Crisis

Three aspects of assessment that enhance understanding of the client's current suicidal crisis are evaluation of the client's precipitating stressors, relevant history, and life stage issues.

■ **The precipitating stressor:** Adverse life events in combination with other risk factors, such as depression, may lead to suicide. Life stresses accompanied by an increase in emotional disturbance include the loss of a loved one either by death or by divorce, problems in major relationships, changes in social or occupational roles, or serious physical illness.

■ **Relevant history:** Has the individual experienced numerous failures or rejections that would increase his or her vulnerability for a dysfunctional response to the current situation?

■ **Life stage issues:** The ability to tolerate loss and disappointment is often compromised if those losses and disappointments occur during stages of life in which the individual struggles with developmental issues (e.g., adolescence, midlife).

Psychiatric, Medical, and Family History

The individual should be assessed with regard to previous psychiatric treatment for depression, alcoholism, or previous suicide attempts. Medical history should be obtained to determine the presence of chronic, debilitating, or terminal illness. Is there a history of depressive disorder in the family, and has a close relative committed suicide in the past?

Coping Strategies

How has the individual handled previous crisis situations? How does this situation differ from previous ones?

Presenting Symptoms

Several acronyms have been developed as mnemonic devices to summarize important factors that may increase a person's risk for suicidal behavior. One of these is the acronym IS PATH WARM? (American Association of Suicidology, 2015; Juhnke, Granello, & Lebrón-Striker, 2007). The assessment items and descriptors for each letter are as follows:

Ideation: Has suicide ideas that are current and active, especially with an identified plan

Substance abuse: Has current and/or excessive use of alcohol or other mood-altering drugs

Purposelessness: Expresses thoughts that there is no reason to continue living

Anger: Expresses uncontrolled anger or feelings of rage

Trapped: Expresses the belief that there is no way out of the current situation

Hopelessness: Expresses lack of hope and perceives little chance of positive change

Withdrawal: Expresses desire to withdraw from others or has begun withdrawing

Anxiety: Expresses anxiety, agitation, and/or changes in sleep patterns

Recklessness: Engages in reckless or risky activities with little thought of consequences

Mood: Expresses dramatic mood shifts

Mnemonic devices such as IS PATH WARM? can be helpful in remembering what types of presenting symptoms to assess for, but the overall assessment and management of suicidal behavior is far more complex and must consider available support systems, the client's willingness to accept support, and the client's ability to establish a trusting therapeutic alliance with health-care professionals intervening on his or her behalf.

 The Collaborative Assessment and Management of Suicidality (CAMS) model is an evidence-based approach that focuses on the importance of patient-centered, problem-focused intervention to build an alliance with patients for collaboration in reducing risk for suicidal behavior (Jobes, 2012). This model focuses on assessment, which necessarily includes asking the patient to identify what is driving the desire to take his or her own life so that alternatives (identifying and capitalizing on motivations to live) can be explored. For all health-care professionals, this work begins with developing skill in asking basic and direct questions such as "Are you having thoughts of hurting or killing yourself?"

Beyond the basic questions of whether or not a person has suicidal ideas, a plan, and access to means, there must be recognition that patients are not always forthcoming or truthful in their answers to such questions. Several strategies for enhancing a collaborative, therapeutic relationship and communication about suicide assessment have been elaborated. Since nurses are often at the front line of this assessment in medical-surgical, emergency department, outpatient care, schools, and other health-care settings, they must be thoughtful, comprehensive, and conscientious in this pursuit regardless of the practice setting and whether or not the patient has been identified as having mental health issues. Shea (2009) states that nurses need to assess not only what the client is directly stating about his or her suicidal intent (stated intent) but also the amount of thinking, planning, and behaviors associated with suicide ideation (reflected intent) and the suicide intent that is withheld from the nurse (withheld intent). A summary of guiding principles in suicide risk assessment are included in Table 17–2.

One model for enhancing communication in suicide assessment is the CASE (Chronological Assessment of Suicide Events) approach. It is described as a flexible guide for interviewing that includes communication techniques designed to elicit and enhance detailed, valid feedback from clients about sensitive topics such as suicide. Several examples, as elaborated by Shea (2009), follow:

■ *Normalizing* communicates that the client is not the only one who experiences suicidal ideation. Example: "Sometimes when people are in a lot of emotional pain, they have thoughts of killing themselves. Have you had any thoughts like that?"

TABLE 17–2 Guiding Principles for Suicide Risk Assessment

PRINCIPLES	EXPLANATION
Screening for suicide risk should be conducted as an essential component of health assessment, and risk factors, warning signs, and threats should be taken seriously.	This includes identifying through detailed assessment the individual's unique situation to discern additional resources, consults, and interventions needed to ensure patient safety.
Establishment of a therapeutic relationship is foundational to effective suicide risk assessment.	This includes establishing trust through empathy and respect, which provides a safe environment for the client to tell his or her story.
Suicide risk assessment is complex and challenges the nurse to use many different communication strategies.	This includes exploring the client's thoughts, feelings, and behaviors from a variety of perspectives.
Suicide risk assessment is an ongoing process, and level of risk can increase or decrease over time.	This includes assessing over time for fluctuations in risk factors, changes in stress level, changes in intensity of ideation, changes in intention to act on suicide ideation, and changes in support systems.
Collaboration with the client and other sources of information facilitates confidence in clinical judgments.	This includes information provided by other people who are familiar with the client from home, work, or school and other clinical team members. Collaboration also implies that all those involved in the client's care are working together.
Suicide risk assessment uses direct rather than indirect language.	This includes using terminology such as "suicide" and "death" rather than "not happy with living" or other indirect statements. It also communicates to the client that these are acceptable topics to discuss.
Suicide risk assessment attempts to discern the underlying message.	This includes attempting to discern when the patient is communicating unbearable distress, feeling trapped, feeling hopeless, and/or feeling driven to avoid additional emotional or physical pain.
Suicide risk assessment considers cultural context.	This includes recognizing that anyone regardless of race, religion, or culture may be at risk for suicide. Some cultural or religious prohibitions may influence someone's willingness to openly discuss personal feelings.
Suicide risk assessment is documented in detail.	This includes risk factors, warning signs, underlying themes, level of risk, clinical judgments, and recommended interventions.

SOURCE: Adapted from Perlman, C.M., Neufeld, E., Martin, L., Goy, M., & Hirdes, J.P. (2011). Risk Assessment Inventory: A resource guide for Canadian healthcare organizations. Toronto: Ontario Hospital Association and Canadian Patient Safety Institute.

- Asking about behavioral events rather than the client's opinions may elicit more concrete information. Example: "What did you do when you had those thoughts?" "How many pills did you take?" "What happened next?"
- Gentle assumptions encourage further discussion by assuming there is more to tell. Example: "What other times have you attempted suicide?"
- Denial of the specific is helpful when a client generally denies suicidal ideation. This strategy encourages more in-depth thought and response by asking questions that might trigger memories of specific events. Example: After the client denies suicidal ideation in response to a general question, the nurse asks more specifically, "Have you ever had thoughts of overdosing?" "Have you ever had thoughts about shooting yourself?"
- Chronologically exploring the presenting suicide event, recent suicide events, past suicide events, and finally the immediate suicide events can broaden the nurse's understanding of the client's immediate suicidal intent in the context of his or her behavior over time.

Diagnosis and Outcome Identification

Nursing diagnoses for the suicidal client may include the following:

- Risk for suicide related to feelings of hopelessness and desperation
- Hopelessness related to absence of support systems and perception of worthlessness

Outcome Criteria

Outcome criteria include short- and long-term goals. Time lines are individually determined. The criteria that follow may be used for measurement of outcomes in the care of the suicidal client.

The client:

1. Has experienced no physical harm to self
2. Develops a safety plan and sets realistic goals for self
3. Expresses some optimism and hope for the future

Planning and Implementation

Table 17–3 provides a plan of care for the hospitalized client who is suicidal. Nursing diagnoses are presented, along with outcome criteria, appropriate nursing interventions, and rationales for each.

Intervention With the Client Who Is Suicidal Following Discharge or in an Outpatient Setting

In some instances, it may be determined that suicidal intent is low and that hospitalization is not required. Instead, the client with suicidal ideation may be treated in an outpatient setting. Guidelines for treatment of such clients on an outpatient basis include the following:

- The person should have immediate access to support systems and be tied in to a system of care, as the term following hospital discharge is a high-risk period. Arrangements must be made for the client to stay with family or friends.

Table 17–3 | CARE PLAN FOR THE SUICIDAL CLIENT

NURSING DIAGNOSIS: RISK FOR SUICIDE
RELATED TO: Feelings of hopelessness and desperation

OUTCOME CRITERIA	NURSING INTERVENTIONS	RATIONALES
Client will not harm self.	1. Ask client directly: "Have you thought about harming yourself in any way? If so, what do you plan to do? Do you have the means to carry out this plan? How strong are your intentions to die?"	1. The risk of suicide is greatly increased if client has developed a plan with lethal means and particularly if means are accessible for client to execute the plan.
	2. Create a safe environment for client. Remove all potentially harmful objects from client's access (sharp objects, straps, belts, ties, glass items, alcohol). Supervise closely during meals and medication administration. Perform room searches as deemed necessary.	2. Client safety is a nursing priority.

Table 17-3 | CARE PLAN FOR THE SUICIDAL CLIENT—cont'd

OUTCOME CRITERIA	NURSING INTERVENTIONS	RATIONALES
	3. Maintain close observation of client. Depending on level of suicide precaution, provide one-to-one contact, constant visual observation, or every-15-minute checks. Place in room close to nurse's station; do not assign to private room. Accompany to off-unit activities if attendance is indicated. May need to accompany to bathroom.	3. Close observation is necessary to ensure that client does not harm self in any way. Being alert for suicidal and escape attempts facilitates prevention or interruption of harmful behavior.
	4. Maintain special care in administration of medications.	4. Prevents saving up to overdose or discarding and not taking.
	5. Make rounds at frequent, *irregular* intervals (especially at night, toward early morning, at change of shift, or other predictably busy times for staff).	5. Prevents staff surveillance from becoming predictable. To be aware of client's location is important, especially when staff is busy and least available and observable.
	6. Encourage client to express honest feelings, including anger. Provide hostility release if needed.	6. Depression and suicidal behaviors may be viewed as anger turned inward on the self. If this anger can be verbalized in a nonthreatening environment, client may be able to eventually resolve these feelings.
Client develops a safety plan for management of suicidal thoughts and urges.	1. Establish a trusting, therapeutic relationship to encourage open discussion of suicide.	1. Establishing trust and open communications encourages client to share thoughts and feelings.
	2. Collaborate with client to develop a safety plan that includes recognition of warning signs, coping strategies, supportive people and places, resources and contact information for crisis management, and plans to restrict access to lethal means.	2. Development of a comprehensive **collaborative safety plan** concretizes resources and management strategies. Actively engaging the client in collaboration on the development of a safety plan promotes client ownership and investment in the process.
	3. Assess verbal and nonverbal clues to identify the likelihood that client intends to follow through with the established safety plan and evaluate client's follow-through with safety plan measures while still hospitalized.	3. Assessment of client safety includes analyzing congruence of verbal communication, nonverbal communication, and behavior.

Continued

Table 17–3 | CARE PLAN FOR THE SUICIDAL CLIENT—cont'd

NURSING DIAGNOSIS: HOPELESSNESS

RELATED TO: Absence of support systems and perception of worthlessness

EVIDENCED BY: Verbal cues (despondent content, "I can't"); decreased affect; lack of initiative; suicidal ideas or attempts

OUTCOME CRITERIA	NURSING INTERVENTIONS	RATIONALES
Client verbalizes a measure of hope and acceptance of life and situations over which he or she has no control.	1. Identify stressors in client's life that precipitated current crisis. Include assessing degree of emotional pain and hopelessness in relationship to feelings of connectedness or lack of connectedness with others.	1. It is important to identify causative or contributing factors in order to plan appropriate assistance.
	2. Determine coping behaviors previously used and client's perception of effectiveness then and now.	2. It is important to identify client's strengths and encourage their use in current crisis situation.
	3. Encourage client to explore and verbalize feelings and perceptions related to reasons for wanting to die as well as reasons for wanting to live.	3. Identification of feelings underlying behaviors helps client to begin process of taking control of own life and enables the nurse to help client focus on maximizing his or her reasons for wanting to live.
	4. 💬 Provide expressions of hope to client in positive, low-key manner (e.g., "I know you feel you cannot go on, but I believe that things can get better for you. What you are feeling is temporary. It is okay if you don't see it just now.").	4. Even though client feels hopeless, it is helpful to hear positive expressions from others. Client's current state of mind may prevent him or her from identifying anything positive in life. It is important to accept client's feelings nonjudgmentally and to affirm his or her personal worth and value.
	5. Help client identify areas of life situation that are under his or her own control.	5. Client's emotional condition may interfere with ability to problem solve. Assistance may be required to perceive benefits and consequences of available alternatives accurately.
	6. Identify sources that client may use after discharge when crises occur or feelings of hopelessness and possible suicidal ideation prevail.	6. Client should be informed of local suicide hotlines or other local support services from which he or she may seek assistance following discharge from hospital. A concrete plan provides hope in the face of a crisis situation.

If this is not possible, hospitalization should be reconsidered.

■ A detailed safety plan should be developed that is an outgrowth of a comprehensive risk assessment and a collaborative, problem-solving discussion with the client. This intervention explores with the client what he or she will do to stay safe if there is a repeat or increase in suicidal thoughts or urges.

See Box 17–2 for more on the essential components of a safety plan.

■ A safety plan should not be confused with a no-suicide contract. See Box 17–3 to learn about issues associated with this type of document.

■ Enlist the help of family or friends to ensure that the home environment is safe from dangerous items, such as firearms or stockpiled drugs. Give

---

BOX 17–2 Essential Components of a Safety Plan

According to Stanley and Brown (2008, pp. 3–4), the essential components of a safety plan include nursing support and assistance for the following:

1. Recognizing warning signs that precede suicide crises
2. Identifying and employing internal coping strategies that the client can implement without needing to contact additional support people
3. Identifying supportive family members and friends with whom he or she can discuss suicide and who may help resolve a potential crisis
4. Identifying people and healthy social settings that he or she can use for general support and distraction from suicidal thoughts and urges
5. Identifying resources and contact information for mental health professionals and agencies when needed in an escalating crisis situation
6. Problem-solving with the client ways to reduce the potential for access to and use of lethal means

Once the safety plan is elaborated with the client, an evaluation of the appropriateness of the plan and a collaborative assessment of the likelihood that the client will implement this plan should be conducted.

Assessment for suicidal risk and responsive intervention must be ongoing, as suicidal ideas and intent may change over hours, days, or longer time periods. The need for revision of the safety plan may become evident. Critical times for reassessment of risk and reevaluation of the safety plan (Hoffman, 2013) include the following:

1. When there is a change in the client's clinical presentation or worsening of symptoms
2. When medications or treatments are changed
3. When significant others identify an increase in concern
4. When a client stops treatment

BOX 17–3 The Issue of No-Suicide Contracts

A critical issue that needs to be understood is that of no-suicide contracts, sometimes called *safety contracts,* a strategy used by some clinicians in the context of a long-term, therapeutic relationship in which the client "promises" to contact the clinician before acting on suicidal ideation. No-suicide contracts are not the same as the development of a thorough safety plan. Contracting with a client is a controversial and often misused strategy (Hoffman, 2013; Shea, 2009). Evidence has not supported the efficacy of this method as a primary intervention (Drew, 2001; Freedenthal, 2013; Rudd, Mandrusiak, & Joiner, 2006). In fact, it may even be counterproductive in clients with borderline or passive-aggressive pathology (Shea, 2009). Such contracts should *never* be used in short-term encounters with clients, such as in emergency departments or during brief hospital stays, or with clients who are unknown, agitated, psychotic, impulsive, or under the influence of drugs and alcohol (Hoffman, 2013). They should never be used with the presumption that they will deter a client from attempting

suicide. Shea adds that if clinicians use a safety contract with the belief that it will be a deterrent to suicide, they should understand that it not only "guarantees nothing [but also] may yield a false sense of security" among clinicians (2009, p. 21). The consequential danger is that clinicians may become less watchful or feel less need to reassess the client, thus missing critical signs of increasing suicide risk. Outside of practicing therapy in an advanced practice role, nurses should avoid no-suicide contracting altogether. Even in the conduct of therapy, it should be used with great caution and for limited, specific assessment purposes.

In general, it is important to recognize that not all suicidal individuals are alike, so interventions should be multifaceted, and suicide prevention plans should be comprehensive. Many models and tools for suicide assessment have been developed. One such model, SAFE-T (**S**uicide **A**ssessment **F**ive-step **E**valuation and **T**riage), summarizes the key elements in suicide assessment (see Box 17–4).

support persons the telephone number of the counselor or an emergency contact person in the event that the counselor is not available.

■ Appointments may need to be scheduled daily or every other day at first until the immediate suicidal crisis has subsided.

■ Establish rapport and promote a trusting relationship. It is important for the suicide counselor to become a key person in the client's support system at this time.

■ Accept the client's feelings in a nonjudgmental manner.

> **CLINICAL PEARL** Be direct. Talk openly and matter-of-factly about suicide. Listen actively and encourage expression of feelings, including anger.

■ Discuss the current crisis situation in the client's life using the problem-solving approach. Offer alternatives to suicide while at the same time empathizing with the client's pain that led to viewing suicide as an option (Jobes, 2012). An example of this kind of communication might be:

💬 "I understand how this emotional pain you've been experiencing led you to consider suicide, but I'd like to explore with you some alternative ways to decrease your pain and to identify some reasons for continuing to live."

■ Help the client identify areas of life that are within his or her control and those that cannot be controlled. Discuss feelings associated with these control issues. It is important for the client to feel some control over his or her life situation in order to perceive a measure of self-worth.

■ The physician or nurse practitioner may prescribe antidepressants for an individual who is experiencing suicidal depression. It is wise to prescribe no more than a three-day supply of the medication with no refills. The prescription can then be renewed at the client's next counseling session.

NOTE: Sadock and associates (2015) have stated:

Patients with depressive disorders are at increased risk of suicide as they begin to improve and regain the energy needed to plan and carry out a suicide (paradoxical suicide). It is usually unwise to give a depressed patient a prescription for a large number of antidepressants, especially tricyclic drugs, at the time of hospital discharge. (p. 366)

■ Psychological interventions that have demonstrated effectiveness in reducing suicidal behavior include dialectical behavior therapy, cognitive-behavioral therapy, and CAMS (Jobes, 2015).

Single interventions, including hospitalization, medication alone, and no-suicide contracts, are not supported by evidence as effective in reducing suicides (Jobes, 2015). Clients need to be actively engaged as partners in each step of the assessment and intervention process.

Information for Family and Friends of the Suicidal Client

The following suggestions are recommended for family and friends of an individual who is suicidal:

■ Take any hint of suicide seriously. Anyone expressing suicidal feelings needs immediate attention.

■ Do not keep secrets. If a suicidal person says, "Promise you won't tell anyone," do not make that promise. Suicidal individuals are ambivalent about dying, and suicidal behavior is a cry for help. It is that ambivalence that leads the person to confide to you the suicidal thoughts. Get help for the person and for yourself. 1-800-SUICIDE is a national hotline that is available 24 hours a day.

■ Be a good listener. If a person expresses suicidal thoughts or feels depressed, hopeless, or worthless, be supportive. Let the person know you are there for him or her and are willing to help the person seek professional help.

■ Many people find it awkward to put into words how another person's life is important for their own well-being, but it is important to stress that the person's life is important to you and to others. Emphasize in specific terms the ways in which the person's suicide would be devastating to you and to others.

■ Express concern for an individual who expresses thoughts about suicide. The individual may make veiled comments or comments that sound as if he or she is joking, or the person may be withdrawn and reluctant to discuss his or her thoughts and feelings. In each case, ask questions, acknowledge the person's pain and feelings of hopelessness, and encourage the individual to talk to someone else if he or she does not feel comfortable talking with you.

■ Familiarize yourself with suicide intervention resources, such as mental health centers and suicide hotlines.

■ Ensure that access to firearms or other means of self-harm is restricted.

■ Communicate caring and commitment to provide support. Fleener (2013) offers the following specific suggestions for families and friends when interacting with someone who is suicidal.

　■ Acknowledge and accept the person's feelings, and be an active listener.

　■ Try to give the person hope, and remind the person that what he or she is feeling is temporary.

- Stay with the person. Do not leave the person alone. Go to where he or she is, if necessary.
- Show love and encouragement. Hold the person, hug him or her, touch him or her. Allow the person to cry and express anger.
- Help the person seek professional help.
- Remove any items from the home with which the person may harm himself or herself.
- If there are children present, try to remove them from the home. Perhaps a friend or relative can assist by taking the children to their home. This type of situation can be extremely traumatic for children.
- DO NOT judge suicidal people, show anger toward them, provoke guilt in them, discount their feelings, or tell them to "snap out of it." This is a very real and serious situation to individuals experiencing suicidal ideation. They are in real pain. They feel the situation is hopeless and that there is no other way to resolve it aside from suicide.

Intervention With Families and Friends of Suicide Victims

Suicide of a family member can induce a whole gamut of feelings in the survivors. It has long been recognized that the bereavement process for families in which a member has taken his or her own life is complicated and requires an understanding by health-care providers of the unique burdens of this type of loss. Macnab (1993) identified the following symptoms that may be evident after the suicide of a loved one:

- A sense of guilt and responsibility
- Anger, resentment, and rage that can never find its "object"

BOX 17–4 SAFE-T: Suicide Assessment Five-Step Evaluation and Triage

1. Identify risk factors
   Note those that can be modified to reduce risk.
2. Identify protective factors
   Note those that can be enhanced.
3. Conduct suicide inquiry
   Evaluate suicidal thoughts, plans, behavior, and intent.
4. Determine risk level and intervention
   Choose appropriate intervention to address and reduce level of risk.
5. Document
   Record assessment of risk, rationale, intervention, and follow-up.

SOURCE: Reprinted from U.S. Department of Health and Human Services, Substance Abuse and Mental Health Services Administration, www.samhsa.gov.

- A heightened sense of emotionality, helplessness, failure, and despair
- A recurring self-searching: "If only I had done something," "If only I had not done something," "If only . . ."
- A sense of confusion and search for an explanation: "Why did this happen?" "What does it mean?" "What could have stopped it?" "What will people think?"
- A sense of inner injury; the family feels wounded and does not know how they will ever get over it and get on with life
- A severe strain placed on relationships; a sense of impatience, irritability, and anger among family members
- A heightened feeling of vulnerability to illness and disease with this added burden of emotional stress

Read "Real People, Real Stories" for a better understanding of one person's lived experience of losing a child to suicide. Strategies for assisting survivors of suicide victims include the following:

- Encourage the clients to talk about the suicide, each responding to the others' viewpoints and reconstructing of events. Share memories.
- Be aware of any blaming or scapegoating of specific family members. Discuss how each person fits into the family situation, both before and after the suicide.
- Listen to feelings of guilt and self-persecution. Gently move the individuals toward the reality of the situation.
- Encourage the family members to discuss individual relationships with the lost loved one. Focus on both positive and negative aspects of the relationships. Gradually point out the irrationality of any idealized concepts of the deceased person. The family must be able to recognize both positive and negative aspects about the person before grief can be resolved.
- No two people grieve in the same way. It may appear that some family members are overcoming the grief faster than others. All family members must be made to understand that if this occurs, it is not because those family members care less—it is just that they grieve differently. Variables that enter into this phenomenon include individual past experiences, personal relationship with the deceased person, and individual temperament and coping abilities.
- Recognize how the suicide has caused disorganization in family coping. Reassess interpersonal relationships in the context of the event. Discuss coping strategies that have been successful in times of stress in the past, and work to reestablish these strategies within the family. Identify new adaptive coping strategies that can be incorporated.

Real People, Real Stories: Surviving the Loss of a Loved One to Suicide

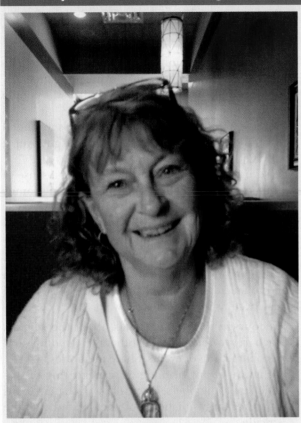

Losing a loved one to suicide results in a grief process often complicated by stigma, misinformation, lack of information, and sometimes a sense of alienation from others. Emmy's story describes her ongoing journey to grapple with the loss of her son to suicide.

Karyn: We've talked before, but tell me more about your journey since Paul's death.

Emmy: My son Paul died in 1986 at age 17. The thing I remember most is that no one was talking about it. There were 10 students who died in his high school. Two others were known to be suicides.

Karyn: Do you mean no one was talking about it in the school system?

Emmy: Well, the students in Paul's class took up a collection that was for Paul, but the school couldn't decide how to use it, so it just sat there for the longest time. My other son heard they were going to use the money for supplies, so I went and talked to them to make sure that didn't happen. The school eventually built a memorial garden that became dedicated to all of the students who had died.

Paul died in June, and in August, when all the other students were returning to school, I got a call from a community suicide survivors counselor who told me she was holding a high school assembly to discuss suicide. I wanted her to talk to the ninth and tenth graders, but they wouldn't permit it. I thought the younger kids needed to talk about and learn about this too—they had been my younger son's classmates, and they were affected by it as well. When the suicide counselor intervened, the teachers were told to watch Paul's friends for any evidence of "copycat" behavior, but that was all. I felt the school administration thought there was a stigma in talking about the cause of his death. I found out later that the seniors were talking about and memorializing Paul in their study halls. They were remembering him as a friend who was missed.

Karyn: How has your family coped with Paul's death?

Emmy: We didn't talk about Paul for the longest time; it was as if he didn't exist. We were very separate; we all went in our own directions. My husband started taking long bicycle trips, and he worked on a suicide hotline. I got very involved with offering a program for high school students called Listening POST (people offering students time), which allowed students to talk about anything they wanted to.

Karyn: I know you've told me that you're still close to several of Paul's peers.

Emmy: Oh yes, and their children too. But our family just became very separate. I don't even know how my other son got through his freshman year of high school. We went to a suicide survivors group as a family, and it was important to me as an outlet to talk, but we didn't talk as a family . . . and then we just stopped going, and the people who knew Paul didn't talk to us. I *so* wanted to talk to people who knew Paul.

After we stopped going to the survivors group, I started going to CoDA [Co-Dependents Anonymous] meetings, even though I don't think I'm codependent. It was more because I needed to talk . . . to understand how this happened. I felt like I wasn't there for him. . . . I was busy with my job and maybe I wasn't tuned in to his moods. I was always taught that boys don't like to talk about feelings.

Karyn: Yes, I guess I've been taught that, too.

Emmy: I just remember that night he told his dad and I that he loved us, he went to bed, and the next morning we found him. I just couldn't make sense of it. Years later, one of Paul's peers, who now has a teenage son, said he could finally tell me what he remembered. And there were signs. Apparently, he had said to some friends (while they were drinking alcohol), "Have you ever thought of killing yourself?" and they all laughed about it and nothing more was said. I also found out that he told an older peer, whom he had met at church camp, that he didn't want to live. The peer smacked him and told him if he ever had thoughts like that again that

---

Real People, Real Stories: Surviving the Loss of a Loved One to Suicide–cont'd

he [Paul] needed to come talk to him first. But they never told anyone else; they kept it among their peers. They thought they were all-knowing, and never told an adult. He was hysterical when he found out what happened.

On that last weekend, he had been partying with his friends . . . there was alcohol involved . . . and the friend that was with him told me that someday he would tell me what went down that day. But it's 30 years later, and I still don't know. I know he was at the party with a girl, but I've never been able to find her or talk with her. She went to a different school.

Karyn: And much of this information that you do know came 10 or more years after his death?

Emmy: Yes.

Karyn: What a long journey you've been on trying to put all the pieces together

Emmy: (tearful) That's exactly it. Trying to put the pieces together, sort it out . . . but it never gets solved. . . . It's like being in a maze and you can't get out, and I had a lot of guilt. . . . Now I recognize that he just made some tragic bad choices.

Karyn: Appreciating that we don't "get over" such tremendous loss but rather amend our lives with some different understanding of love and loss, what has been most helpful in your healing?

Emmy: Yes, I think there was a point when I realized it was okay to feel some happiness. Being with people who don't know me makes it easier. My faith and fellowship group has been an important part of healing. CoDA was helpful because we talked about how different people process things, and I could understand better how

people can get stuck. I used to say that my other son had lost his brother. I couldn't say that I had lost a son. When I had to fill out a health assessment at one point, and I had to respond to the question of how many pregnancies I'd had, that was the most difficult question . . . because I had to acknowledge . . . the reality. And I involved myself with all the boys who were on the track team with Paul and the Listening POST and just talked about everything.

Karyn: What is the most important thing that nurses need to know?

Emmy: By the time we would have had any contact with nurses, it was too late. There were no ER, medical, or mental health visits prior to that. If they were to have an impact, it would have been in prevention in the schools. For example, I didn't know at that time to ask questions like, "Are you having thoughts of hurting yourself?" and "Do you have a plan in mind?" And Paul put on a different face for me. He wasn't solitary; he had lots of friends; he was active on the track team. . . .

Karyn: I think you're not alone with not having been taught about things like suicide assessment. Because, as you've said, historically people haven't talked about it. There is an organization called Red Flags National that promotes mental health education for students, parents, and teachers as a standard part of health education in schools.

Emmy: Yes. It needs to be talked about. It's been helpful for me to talk about it even now. I've never had to try to explain the story before.

To learn more about Red Flags National, go to www.redflags.org.

■ Identify resources that provide support: religious beliefs and spiritual counselors, close friends and relatives, support groups for survivors of suicide. One online connection that puts individuals in contact with survivors' groups specific to each state is the American Foundation for Suicide Prevention at www.afsp.org. A list of resources that provide information and help for issues regarding suicide is presented in Box 17–5.

Evaluation

Evaluation of the client who is suicidal is an ongoing process accomplished through continuous reassessment and determination of goal achievement. Once

the immediate crisis has been resolved, extended psychotherapy may be indicated. The long-term goals of individual or group psychotherapy for the client would be for him or her to:

■ Develop and maintain a more positive self-concept.
■ Learn more effective ways to express feelings to others.
■ Achieve successful interpersonal relationships.
■ Feel accepted by others and achieve a sense of belonging.

A person contemplating suicide feels worthless and hopeless. These goals serve to instill a sense of self-worth while offering a measure of hope and a meaning for living.

BOX 17-5 Resources Related to Suicide Prevention

National Suicide Hotline
1-800-SUICIDE (24/7)

National Suicide Prevention Lifeline
www.suicidepreventionlifeline.org
1-800-273-TALK (24/7)

American Association of Suicidology
www.suicidology.org
1-202-237-2280

Depression and Bipolar Support Alliance (DBSA)
www.dbsalliance.org
1-800-826-3632

American Foundation for Suicide Prevention
www.afsp.org
1-888-333-AFSP (2377)

National Institute of Mental Health
www.nimh.nih.gov
1-866-615-6464

American Psychiatric Association
www.psych.org
1-703-907-7300

Mental Health America
www.nmha.org
1-703-684-7722
1-800-969-6642

American Psychological Association
www.apa.org
1-800-374-2721

Screening for Mental Health Stop a Suicide Today!
www.stopasuicide.org
1-781-239-0071

Boys Town
Cares for troubled boys and girls and families in crisis. Staff
is trained to handle calls related to violence and suicide.
www.boystown.org
1-800-448-3000 (24/7 national hotline)

Centre for Suicide Prevention
www.suicideinfo.ca
1-403-245-3900

Centers for Disease Control and Prevention
National Center for Injury Prevention and Control
Division of Violence Prevention
www.cdc.gov/injury/index.html
1-800-CDC-INFO
1-403-266-HELP (Hotline in Calgary)

National Alliance on Mental Illness
www.nami.org
1-800-950-NAMI

Summary and Key Points

■ More than 90 percent of all persons who attempt or die by suicide have a diagnosed mental disorder.

■ Suicide is the second-leading cause of death among young Americans aged 15 to 34 years, the fourth-leading cause of death for those aged 35 to 44, and the fifth-leading cause of death for individuals aged 45 to 64. Based on recent statistics, the highest rates of suicide among all age groups occurred among those 45 to 64 years of age followed by those 85 years of age and older.

■ Single (never married), divorced, and widowed people may be at greater risk for suicide than married people, but evidence supports that recent change in status is a proximal risk factor

■ More women than men attempt suicide, but men succeed more often.

■ Depressed men and women who consider themselves affiliated with a religion are less likely than their nonreligious counterparts to attempt suicide.

■ Individuals in the very highest and lowest social classes have higher suicide rates than those in the middle classes.

■ Whites are at highest risk for suicide, followed by American Indians and Alaska Natives, Hispanic Americans, Asian Americans, and African Americans.

■ Psychiatric disorders that predispose individuals to suicide include mood disorders, substance use disorders, schizophrenia, anorexia nervosa, borderline and antisocial personality disorders, and anxiety disorders.

■ Predisposing factors include internalized anger, hopelessness and other symptoms of severe depression, history of aggression and violence, shame and humiliation, developmental stressors, sociological influences, genetics, and neurochemical factors.

■ Suicide risk assessment should be a patient-centered, collaborative process in the context of a therapeutic relationship and should chronologically explore presenting suicide events, recent events, past events, and immediate intentions.

■ Assessment of the level of intervention needed includes identifying the number of proximal or potentiating risks as well as the number of warning signs.

■ It is important for the nurse to determine the seriousness of the client's suicidal intentions, the existence of a plan, and the availability and lethality of the method.

■ The suicidal person should not be left alone.

■ A safety plan is developed with the client following a comprehensive suicide risk assessment and includes assisting the client to recognize warning signs, identify and employ internal coping strategies, engage family members and friends as available support persons, identify people and social settings that can be used to distract from suicidal thoughts or urges, identify resources and contact information for crisis

intervention, and problem-solve ways to restrict access to lethal means.

■ Once the crisis intervention is complete, the individual may require long-term psychotherapy, during which he or she works to:
  ■ Develop and maintain a more positive self-concept.
  ■ Learn more effective ways to express feelings.
  ■ Improve interpersonal relationships.
  ■ Achieve a sense of belonging and a measure of hope for living.

■ Evidence-based psychological interventions include dialectical behavior therapy, cognitive-behavioral therapy, and the CAMS approach.

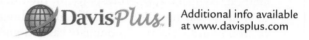 **DavisPlus** | Additional info available at www.davisplus.com

Review Questions
Self-Examination/Learning Exercise

Select the answer that is most appropriate for each of the following questions.

1. Which of the following individuals is at highest risk for a suicide attempt?
   a. John, who reports he is in deep emotional pain, feels hopeless, and says "No one is there for me."
   b. Kelly, who has been seeing a doctor for chronic, intractable pain and is taking pain medication.
   c. Jim, an American Indian who just graduated from high school with honors.
   d. Mike, a physician who reports feeling "burnt out" and is considering retirement.

2. The nurse in the emergency department encounters a patient, Niko, who is expressing suicide ideation. The nurse recognizes that which of the following considerations are important to good suicide risk assessment? (Select all that apply.)
   a. Collaborating with the patient
   b. Asking specific questions about leisure activities
   c. Establishing trust and open communication with the patient
   d. Asking the patient specific questions about the strength of his intention to die
   e. Identifying whether the patient has thought about a plan for trying to kill himself

3. Theresa, age 27, was admitted to the psychiatric unit from the medical intensive care unit where she was treated for taking a deliberate overdose of her antidepressant medication, trazodone (Desyrel). She says to the nurse, "My boyfriend broke up with me. We had been together for six years. I love him so much. I know I'll never get over him." Which is the best response by the nurse?
   a. "You'll get over him in time, Theresa."
   b. "Forget him. There are other fish in the sea."
   c. "You must be feeling very sad about your loss."
   d. "Why do you think he broke up with you, Theresa?"

4. The nurse identifies the primary nursing diagnosis for Theresa as Risk for suicide related to feelings of hopelessness from loss of relationship. Which is the outcome criterion that would be most appropriate for this diagnosis?
   a. The client has experienced no physical harm to herself.
   b. The client sets realistic goals for herself.
   c. The client expresses some optimism and hope for the future.
   d. The client has reached a stage of acceptance in the loss of the relationship with her boyfriend.

Continued

Review Questions—cont'd
Self-Examination/Learning Exercise

5. Theresa is hospitalized following a suicide attempt after breaking up with her boyfriend. Freudian psychoanalytic theory would explain Theresa's suicide attempt in which of the following ways?
   a. She feels hopeless about her future without her boyfriend.
   b. Without her boyfriend, she feels like an outsider with her peers.
   c. She is feeling intense guilt because her boyfriend broke up with her.
   d. She is angry at her boyfriend for breaking up with her and has turned the anger inward on herself.

6. Theresa is hospitalized following a suicide attempt after breaking up with her boyfriend. Theresa says to the nurse, "When I get out of here, I'm going to try this again, and next time I'll choose a no-fail method." Which is the best response by the nurse?
   a. "You are safe here. We will make sure nothing happens to you."
   b. "You're just lucky your roommate came home when she did."
   c. "What exactly do you plan to do?"
   d. "I don't understand. You have so much to live for."

7. In determining degree of suicidal risk with a client, the nurse assesses the following behavioral manifestations: severely depressed, withdrawn, statements of worthlessness, difficulty accomplishing activities of daily living, no close support systems. The nurse identifies the client's risk for suicide as which of the following?
   a. Low risk
   b. High risk
   c. Imminent risk
   d. Unable to be determined

8. Theresa, who has been hospitalized following a suicide attempt, is placed on suicide precautions on the psychiatric unit. She admits that she is still feeling suicidal. Which of the following interventions are most appropriate in this instance? (Select all that apply.)
   a. Restrict access to any item that might be harmful by placing the client in a seclusion room.
   b. Check on Theresa every 15 minutes at irregular intervals, or assign a staff person to stay with her on a one-to-one basis.
   c. Obtain an order from the physician to give Theresa a sedative to calm her and reduce suicide ideas.
   d. Do not allow Theresa to participate in any unit activities while she is on suicide precautions.
   e. Ask Theresa specific questions about her thoughts, plans, and intentions related to suicide.

9. Which of the following interventions are appropriate for a client on suicide precautions? (Select all that apply.)
   a. Remove all sharp objects, belts, and other potentially dangerous articles from the client's environment.
   b. Accompany the client to off-unit activities.
   c. Reassess intensity of suicidal thoughts and urges on a regular basis.
   d. Put all of the client's possessions in storage and explain to her that she may have them back when she is off suicide precautions.

10. Success of long-term psychotherapy with Theresa (who attempted suicide following a break-up with her boyfriend) could be measured by which of the following behaviors?
   a. Theresa has a new boyfriend.
   b. Theresa has an increased sense of self-worth.
   c. Theresa does not take antidepressants anymore.
   d. Theresa told her old boyfriend how angry she was with him for breaking up with her.

Communication Exercises

1. Mr. J. was brought to the emergency department by his brother, who is concerned about Mr. J.'s worsening depression. During the assessment, Mr. J. tells the nurse, "None of this matters. There's nothing that can make this any better." What would be an appropriate response by the nurse?

2. Mr. J. admits to the nurse that he has had suicidal ideas for the last couple of weeks. How would the nurse intervene with Mr. J. at this point?

3. Mr. J. tells the nurse that ever since his wife died 3 months ago, he does not want to go on living. What would be an example of empathic communication in response to this statement by Mr. J.?

References

Almendrala, A. (2015). Native American youth suicide rates are at crisis levels. Retrieved from www.huffingtonpost.com/entry/native-american-youth-suicide-rates-are-at-crisis-levels_us_560c3084e4b0768127005591

American Association of Suicidology. (2015). Know the warning signs. Retrieved from www.suicidology.org/resources/warning-signs

American Foundation for Suicide Prevention. (2016). Suicide statistics. Retrieved from https://afsp.org/about-suicide/suicide-statistics

American Psychiatric Association. (2010). Culture matters in suicidal behavior patterns and prevention, psychologist says. Retrieved from www.apa.org/news/press/releases/2010/08/suicidal-behavior-patterns.aspx

American Psychiatric Nurse's Association. (2015). Psychiatric-mental health nursing essential competencies for the assessment and management of individuals at risk for suicide. Retrieved from www.apna.org/i4a/pages/index.cfm?pageID=5684

Bauman, S., Toomey, R.B., & Walker, J.L. (2013). Associations among bullying, cyberbullying, and suicide in high school students. *Journal of Adolescence, 36*(2), 341-350. doi:10.1016/j.adolescence.2012.12.001

Bridge, J.A., Asti, L., Horowitz, L.M., Greenhouse, J.B., Fontanella, C.A., Sheftall, A.H., & Campo, J.V. (2015). Suicide trends among elementary school–aged children in the United States from 1993 to 2012. *JAMA Pediatrics, 169*(7), 673-677. doi:10.1001/jamapediatrics.2015.0465

Byron, W.J. (2016). Do people who commit suicide go to hell? *Catholic Digest.* Retrieved from www.catholicdigest.com/articles/faith/knowledge/2007/04-01/do-people-who-commit-suicide-go-to-hell

Cardoza, K. (2016). 6 myths about suicide that every parent and educator should know. Retrieved from www.npr.org/sections/ed/2016/09/02/478835539

Cassels, C. (2011). "Striking" risk for suicidality, depression in gay teens. *Medscape Medical News.* Retrieved from www.medscape.com/viewarticle/740429

Centers for Disease Control and Prevention. (2016). Leading causes of death, national and regional, 1999–2014. Retrieved from http://webappa.cdc.gov/sasweb/ncipc/leadcaus10_us.html htp://webappa.cdc.gov/sasweb/ncipc/leadcaus10_us.html

Centers for Disease Control and Prevention. (2015a). Suicide facts at a glance, 2015. Retrieved from https://www.cdc.gov/violenceprevention/pdf/suicide-datasheet-a.pdf

Centers for Disease Control and Prevention. (2015b). Gay and bisexual men's health. Retrieved from www.cdc.gov/msmhealth/suicide-violence-prevention.htm

Centers for Disease Control and Prevention. (2011). Self-directed violence surveillance: Uniform definitions and recommended data elements. Retrieved from www.cdc.gov/violenceprevention/pdf/Self-Directed-Violence-a.pdf

Chang, B.P., Franklin, J.C., Ribeiro, J.D., Fox, K.R., Bentley, K.H., Kleiman, E.M., & Nock, M.K. (2016). Biological risk factors for suicidal behaviors: A meta-analysis. *Translational Psychiatry, 6*(9), e887. doi:10.1038/tp.2016.165

Cochran, S.D., & Mays, V.M. (2000). Lifetime prevalence of suicide symptoms and affective disorders among men reporting same-sex sexual partners: Results from NHANES III. *American Journal of Public Health, 90*(4), 573-578. doi:10.2105/AJPH.90.4.573

Crosby, A.E., Ortega, L., & Melanson, C. (2011). Self-directed Violence Surveillance: Uniform definitions and recommended data elements, version 1.0. Atlanta, GA: Centers for Disease Control and Prevention, National Center for Injury Prevention and Control. Retrieved from www.cdc.gov/violenceprevention/pdf/Self-Directed-Violence-a.pdf

Drew, B. (2001). Self-harm and no-suicide contract in psychiatric inpatient settings. *Archives of Psychiatric Nursing, 15*(3), 99-106. doi:10.1053/apnu.2001.23748

Duran, S., & McGuinness, T.M. (2016). Suicide in childhood. *Journal of Psychosocial Nursing, 54*(10), 27-30.

Edgerton, E., & Limber, S. (2013). Research brief: Suicide and bullying. Retrieved from https://www.stopbullying.gov/blog/2013/02/27/research-brief-suicide-and-bullying

Eisenberg, M.E., & Resnick, M.D. (2006). Suicidality among gay, lesbian and bisexual youth: The role of protective factors. *Journal of Adolescent Health, 39*(5), 662-668. doi:http://dx.doi.org/10.1016/j.jadohealth.2006.04.024

Fleener, P. (2013). How to help a suicidal person. *Mental Health Today.* Retrieved from www.mental-health-today.com/suicide/sui2.htm

Freedenthal, S. (2013). The use of no-suicide contracts. Retrieved from www.speakingofsuicide.com/2013/05/15/no-suicide-contracts

Hinduja, S., & Patchin, J.W. (2010). Bullying, cyberbullying, and suicide. *Archives of Suicide Research, 14*(3), 206-221. doi:10.1080/13811118.2010.494133

Hoffman, R. (2013). Contracting for safety: A misused tool. *Pennsylvania Patient Safety Advisory, 10*(2), 82-84

Jobes, D.A. (2015, September). Clinical suicidology: Innovations in assessment treatment of suicidal risk. Presentation at Psychiatric Grand Rounds, Summa Health Systems, Akron, OH.

Jobes, D.A. (2012). The Collaborative Assessment and Management of Suicidality (CAMS): An evolving evidence-based clinical approach to suicide risk. *Suicide and Life Threatening Behavior, 42*(6), 640-653. doi:10.1111/j.1943-278X.2012.00119.x

Joiner, T.E. (2005). *Why people die by suicide.* Cambridge, MA: Harvard University Press.

Juhnke, G.A., Granello, P.F., & Lebrón-Striker, M. (2007). IS PATH WARM? A suicide assessment mnemonic for counselors. *ACA Professional Counseling Digest.* Retrieved from www.counseling.org/resources/library/ACA%20Digests/ACAPCD-03.pdf

King, M., Semlyen, J., Tai, S.S., Killaspy, H., Osborn, D., Popelyuk, D., & Nazareth, I. (2008). A systematic review of mental disorder, suicide, and deliberate self harm in lesbian, gay, and bisexual people. *BMC Psychiatry, 8*(70). doi:10.1186/1471-244X-8-70

Klomek, A.B., Sourander, A., & Gould, M.S. (2011). Bullying and suicide: Detection and intervention. *Psychiatric Times, 28*(2). Retrieved from www.psychiatrictimes.com/suicide/content/article/10168/1795797#

Klonsky, D.E., & May, A.M. (2015a). The three-step theory (3ST): A new theory of suicide rooted in the "ideation-to-action" framework. *International Journal of Cognitive Therapy, 8*(2), 114–129. doi:10.1521/ijct.2015.8.2.114

Klonsky, D.E., & May, A.M. (2015b). Impulsivity and suicide risk: Review and clinical implications. *Psychiatric Times, 32* (8). Retrieved from http://www.psychiatrictimes.com/special-reports/impulsivity-and-suicide-risk-review-and-clinical-implications/page/0/2

Kposowa, A. (2000). Marital status and suicide in the National Longitudinal Mortality Study. *Journal of Epidemiology and Community Health, 54*(4), 254-261. doi:http://dx.doi.org/10.1136/jech.54.4.254

National Action Alliance for Suicide Prevention. (2015). What is Zero Suicide? Retrieved from http://actionallianceforsuicideprevention.org/sites/actionallianceforsuicideprevention.org/files/zero_suicide_final6.pdf

National Alliance on Mental Illness. (2015). Risks of suicide. Retrieved from www.nami.org/Learn-More/Mental-Health-Conditions/Related-Conditions/Risk-of-Suicide

National Institute of Mental Health. (2015). Director's blog: The under-recognized public health crisis of suicide. Retrieved from www.nimh.nihgov/about/director/2010/the-under-recognized-public-health-crisis-of-suicide.shtml

Nock, M.K., Deming, C.A., Fullerton, C.S., Gilman, S.E., Goldenberg, M., Kessler, R. C., McCarroll, J. E., & Ursan, R. J. (2013). Suicide among soldiers: A review of psychosocial risk and protective factors. *Psychiatry, 76*(2), 97-125. doi: 10.1521/psyc.2013.76.2.97

Olfson, M., Wall, M., Wang, S., Crystal, S., Shang-Min Liu. S.-M., Gerhard, T., & Blanco, C. (2016) Short-term suicide risk after psychiatric hospital discharge. *JAMA Psychiatry, 73*(11), 1119-1126. doi:10.1001/jamapsychiatry.2016.2035

Perlman, C.M., Neufeld, E., Martin, L., Goy, M., & Hirdes, J.P. (2011). Risk Assessment Inventory: A resource guide for Canadian healthcare organizations. Toronto: Ontario Hospital Association and Canadian Patient Safety Institute.

Plöderl, M., Wagenmakers, E.J., Tremblay, P., Ramsay, R., Kralovek, K., Fartacek, C., & Fartacek, R. (2013). Suicide risk and sexual orientation: A critical review. *Archives of Sexual Behavior, 42*(5), 715-727. doi:10.1007/s10508-012-0056-y

Puntil, C., York, J., Limandri, B., Greene, P., Arauz, E., & Hobbs, D. (2013). Competency-based training for PMH nurse generalists: Inpatient intervention and prevention of suicide. *Journal of the American Psychiatric Nurses Association, 19*(4), 205-210. doi:10.1177/1078390313496275

Rasic, D.T., Belik, S.L., Elias, B., Katz, L.Y., Enns, M., & Sareen, J. (2009). Spirituality, religion, and suicidal behavior in a nationally representative sample. *Journal of Affective Disorders, 114*(1), 32-40. doi:10.1016/j.jad.2008.08.007

Reyes, M.S., Cayubit, F.O., Angala, M. H., Bries, S.C., Capalungan, J. T., & McCutcheon, L.E. (2015). Exploring the link between adolescent anger expression and tendencies for suicide: A brief report. *North American Journal of Psychology 17*(1), 113-118.

Roškar, S., Podlesek, A., Kuzmanič, M., Demšar, L.O., Zaletel, M., & Marušič, A. (2011). Suicide risk and its relationship to change in marital status. *Crisis, 32*(1), 24-30. doi:10.1027/0227-5910/a000054

Rudd, D.M., Mandrusiak, M., & Joiner, T.E. (2006). The case against no-suicide contract: The commitment to treatment statement as a practice alternative. *Journal of Clinical Psychology, 62*(2), 243–251. doi:10.1002/jclp.20227

Sadock, B.J., Sadock, V.A., & Ruiz, P. (2015). *Synopsis of psychiatry: Behavioral sciences/clinical psychiatry* (11th ed.). Philadelphia: Lippincott Williams & Wilkins.

Shea, S.C. (2009). Suicide assessment: Part 1: Uncovering suicidal intent: A sophisticated art; Part 2: Uncovering suicidal intent using the chronological assessment of suicide events. *Psychiatric Times, 26*(12), 1-26. Retrieved from www.psychiatric times.com/display/article/10168/1491291

Stanley, B., & Brown, G.K. (2008). *The safety plan treatment manual to reduce suicide risk: Veteran version.* Washington, DC: U.S. Department of Veterans Affairs.

Stroumsa, D. (2014). The state of transgender health care: Policy, law, and medical frameworks. *American Journal of Public Health, 104*(3), 31-37. doi:10.2105/AJPH.2013.301789

The Joint Commission. (2016). Sentinel Event Alert 56: Detecting and treating suicide ideation in all settings. Retrieved from https://www.jointcommission.org/sea_issue_56

The Samaritans. (2015). Suicide myths and misconceptions. Retrieved from http://samaritansnyc.org/myths-about-suicide

Whalen, D., Dixon-Gordon, K., Belden, A., Barch, D., & Luby, J. (2015). Correlates and consequences of suicidal cognitions and behaviors in children ages 3 to 7 years. *Journal of the American Academy of Child & Adolescent Psychiatry, 54*(11), 926-937. doi:10.1016/j.jaac.2015.08.009

Yamauchi, T. Fujita, T., Tachimori, H., Takeshima, T., Inagaki, M., & Sudo, A. (2013). Age-adjusted relative suicide risk by marital and employment status over the past 25 years in Japan. *Journal of Public Health, 35*(1), 49-56. doi:10.1093/pubmed/fds054

Zweig, J., & Dank, M. (2013). Technology, teen dating, violence and abuse, and bullying. *The Urban Institute.* Retrieved from www.urban.org/sites/default/files/alfresco/publication-pdfs/412891

Classical References

Durkheim, E. (1951). *Suicide: A study of sociology.* Glencoe, IL: Free Press.

Freud, S. (1957). *Mourning and melancholia, Vol. 14* (standard ed.) London: Hogarth Press. (Original work published 1917.)

MacDonald, M., & Murphy, T. R. (1991). *Sleepless souls: Suicide in early modern England.* New York: Oxford University Press.

Macnab, F. (1993). *Brief psychotherapy: An integrative approach in clinical practice.* West Sussex, England: Wiley.

Minois, G. (2001). *History of suicide: Voluntary death in Western culture.* Baltimore: Johns Hopkins University Press.

U.S. Public Health Service (USPHS). (1999). The Surgeon General's call to action to prevent suicide. Washington, DC: USPHS.

18

Behavior Therapy

CORE CONCEPTS

Behavior Therapy

Stimulus

KEY TERMS

aversive stimulus

classical conditioning

conditioned response

conditioned stimulus

contingency contracting

covert sensitization

discriminative stimuli

extinction

flooding

modeling

negative reinforcement

operant conditioning

overt sensitization

positive reinforcement

Premack principle

reciprocal inhibition

shaping

stimulus generalization

systematic desensitization

time-out

token economy

unconditioned response

unconditioned stimulus

OBJECTIVES

After reading this chapter, the student will be able to:

1. Discuss the principles of classical and operant conditioning as foundations for behavior therapy.
2. Identify various techniques used in the modification of client behavior.
3. Implement the principles of behavior therapy using the steps of the nursing process.

HOMEWORK ASSIGNMENT

Please read the chapter and answer the following questions:

1. A mother is teaching her young child how to dress himself. Each time he makes an attempt, she praises him profusely, even though he has made several mistakes. She does this until he is able to dress himself appropriately. What is this technique called?
2. Flooding (implosive therapy) is used to desensitize individuals to phobic stimuli. When is this technique contraindicated?
3. A nurse is working with parents of a toddler whom they say falls to the ground, screams, and kicks his legs whenever he does not get his way. They usually just give in to his wishes to keep him from behaving this way. The nurse decides to teach the parents about the technique of extinction. What would this entail?

A behavior is considered maladaptive when it is age inappropriate, interferes with adaptive functioning, or is misunderstood by others in terms of cultural inappropriateness. In the behavioral approach to therapy, behavior and personality develop through learning processes or, more correctly, through the interaction of the environment with an individual's genetic endowment. The basic assumption of this approach is that problematic behaviors occur when there has been inadequate learning and therefore can be corrected through the provision of appropriate learning experiences. The principles of behavior therapy as we know it today are based on the early studies of **classical conditioning** by Pavlov (1927) and **operant conditioning** by Skinner (1938). Although in this text the concepts are presented separately for reasons of clarification, behavioral change procedures are often combined with cognitive procedures *(cognitive behavior therapy)* and with issues related to emotional regulation *(dialectical behavior therapy)*. Concepts of cognitive therapy are presented in Chapter 19, Cognitive Therapy.

Classical Conditioning

Classical conditioning is a process of learning introduced by the Russian physiologist Ivan Pavlov. In his experiments with dogs, during which he hoped to learn more about the digestive process, he inadvertently discovered that organisms can learn to respond in specific ways if they are conditioned to do so. Pavlov found that, as expected, the dogs salivated when they began to eat the food offered to them, a reflexive response that Pavlov called an **unconditioned response.** However, he also noticed that with time, the dogs began to salivate when the food came into their range of view, before it was even presented to them for consumption. Pavlov, concluding that this response was not reflexive but had been learned, called it a **conditioned response.** He carried the experiments even further by introducing an unrelated stimulus, one that had had no previous connection to the animal's food. He simultaneously presented the food with the sound of a bell. The animal responded with the expected reflexive salivation to the food. After a number of trials with the combined stimuli (food and bell), Pavlov found that the reflexive salivation began to occur when the dog was presented with the sound of the bell in the absence of food.

CORE CONCEPT
Stimulus
A stimulus is an environmental event that interacts with and influences an individual's behavior.

Pavlov's discovery was important in terms of how learning can occur. Pavlov found that unconditioned responses (salivation) occur in response to unconditioned stimuli (eating food). He also found that, over time, an unrelated stimulus (sound of the bell) introduced with the **unconditioned stimulus** can elicit the same response alone—that is, the conditioned response. The unrelated stimulus is called the **conditioned stimulus.** A graphic of Pavlov's classical conditioning model is presented in Figure 18–1. An example of the application of Pavlov's classical conditioning model to humans is shown in Figure 18–2. The process by which the fear response is elicited from similar stimuli (all individuals in white uniforms) is called **stimulus generalization.**

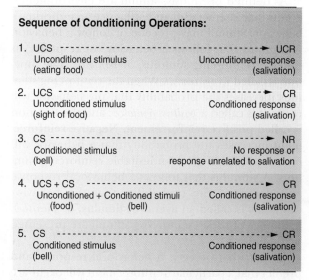

FIGURE 18–1 Pavlov's model of classic conditioning.

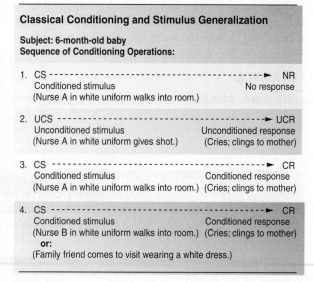

FIGURE 18–2 Example: Classical conditioning and stimulus generalization.

Operant Conditioning

The focus of operant conditioning differs from that of classical conditioning. With classical conditioning, the focus is on behavioral responses elicited by specific objects or events. With operant conditioning, additional attention is given to the consequences of the behavioral response.

Operant conditioning was introduced by B. F. Skinner (1953), an American psychologist whose work was largely influenced by Edward Thorndike's (1911) law of effect—that is, that the connection between a stimulus and a response is strengthened or weakened by the consequences of the response. A number of terms must be defined in order to understand the concept of operant conditioning.

As defined previously, stimuli are environmental events that interact with and influence an individual's behavior. Stimuli may precede or follow a behavior. A stimulus that follows a behavior (or response) is called a reinforcing stimulus, or *reinforcer*. The function is called *reinforcement*. When the reinforcing stimulus increases the probability that the behavior will recur, it is called a *positive reinforcer*, and the function is called **positive reinforcement. Negative reinforcement** increases the probability that a behavior will recur by removal of an undesirable reinforcing stimulus. A stimulus that follows a behavioral response and decreases the probability that the behavior will recur is called an **aversive stimulus,** or *punisher*. Examples of these reinforcing stimuli are presented in Table 18–1.

Stimuli that precede a behavioral response and predict that a particular reinforcement will occur are called **discriminative stimuli.** Discriminative stimuli are under an individual's control. He or she is able to *discriminate* between stimuli and *choose* according to the type of reinforcement he or she has come to associate with a specific stimulus. The following is an example of the concept of discrimination:

EXAMPLE

Mrs. M. was admitted to the hospital from a nursing home 2 weeks ago. She has no family, and no one visits her. She is very lonely. Nurse A and Nurse B have taken care of Mrs. M. on a regular basis during her hospital stay. When she is feeling particularly lonely, Mrs. M. calls Nurse A to her room, for she has learned that Nurse A will stay and talk to her for a while, but Nurse B only takes care of her physical needs and leaves. She no longer seeks out Nurse B for emotional support and comfort.

After several attempts, Mrs. M. is able to discriminate between stimuli. She can predict with assurance that calling Nurse A (and not Nurse B) will result in the reinforcement she desires.

CORE CONCEPT

Behavior Therapy

A form of psychotherapy that aims to modify maladaptive behavior patterns by reinforcing more adaptive behaviors.

Techniques for Modifying Client Behavior

Shaping

In **shaping** the behavior of another, reinforcements are given for increasingly closer approximations to the desired response. For example, in eliciting speech from an autistic child, the teacher may first reward the child for (a) watching the teacher's lips, then (b) making any sound in imitation of the teacher, then (c) forming sounds similar to the word uttered by the teacher. Shaping has been shown to be an effective way of modifying behavior for tasks that a child has not mastered on command or are not in the child's repertoire (Souders et al., 2002).

Modeling

Modeling refers to the learning of new behaviors by imitating the behavior in others. Role models are individuals who have qualities or skills that a person admires and wishes to imitate. Modeling occurs in various ways. Children imitate the behavior patterns of their parents, teachers, friends, and others. Adults and children alike model many of their behaviors after individuals observed on television and in movies. Unfortunately, modeling can result in maladaptive behaviors as well as adaptive ones.

TABLE 18–1 **Examples of Reinforcing Stimuli**			
TYPE	STIMULUS	BEHAVIORAL RESPONSE	REINFORCING STIMULUS
Positive	Messy room	Child cleans her messy room.	Child gets allowance for cleaning room.
Negative	Messy room	Child cleans her messy room.	Child does not receive scolding from the mother.
Aversive	Messy room	Child does not clean her messy room.	Child receives scolding from the mother.

In the practice setting, clients may imitate the behaviors of practitioners who are charged with their care. This can occur naturally in the therapeutic community environment. It can also occur in a therapy session in which the client watches a model demonstrate appropriate behaviors in a role-play of the client's problem. The client is then instructed to imitate the model's behaviors in a similar role-play and is positively reinforced for appropriate imitation.

Premack Principle

This technique, named for its originator, states that a frequently occurring response (R_1) can serve as a positive reinforcement for a response (R_2) that occurs less frequently (Premack, 1959). The **Premack principle** is applied by allowing R_1 to occur only after R_2 has been performed. That is, to encourage more of a particular behavior that an individual is not doing very often, a situation is created in which the person must perform that behavior *before* being permitted to do the "fun stuff" that he or she prefers to do. The person's preferred behavior becomes a reinforcement for accomplishing the desired behavior change. For example, 13-year-old Jennie has been neglecting her homework for the past few weeks. She spends a lot of time on her cell phone talking to her friends. Applying the Premack principle, being allowed to talk on the cell phone to her friends could serve as a positive reinforcement for completing her homework. A schematic of the Premack principle for this situation is presented in Figure 18–3.

Extinction

Extinction is the gradual decrease in frequency or disappearance of a response when the positive reinforcement is withheld. A classic example of this technique is its use with children who have temper tantrums. The tantrum behaviors continue as long as the parent gives attention to them but decrease and often disappear when the parent simply walks away from the child and ignores the behavior.

Contingency Contracting

In **contingency contracting,** a contract is drawn up among all parties involved. The desired behavior change and specified reinforcers for performing this behavior are stated explicitly in writing. The negative consequences, or punishers, that will be rendered for not fulfilling the terms of the contract are also delineated. The contract is specific about how reinforcers and punishment will be presented; however, flexibility is important so that renegotiations can occur if necessary.

Token Economy

Token economy is a type of contingency contracting in which the reinforcers for desired behaviors are presented in the form of *tokens*. Essential to this technique is the prior determination of items and situations of significance to the client that can be employed as reinforcements. With this therapy, tokens are awarded when desired behaviors are performed and may be exchanged for designated privileges. For example, a client may be able to "buy" a snack or cigarettes for 2 tokens, a trip to the coffee shop or library for 5 tokens, or even a trip outside the hospital (if that is a realistic possibility) for another designated number of tokens. The use of token economies was developed in the 1950s as a strategy for reinforcing desirable behaviors in long-term hospitalized patients with schizophrenia and, despite studies demonstrating their effectiveness in reinforcing adaptive behaviors, they have fallen out of favor over time (Dickerson, Tenhula, & Green-Paden, 2005). A recent review of token economy (Doll, McLaughlin, & Barretto, 2013) as a behavior modification strategy points out that most of the research predates the 1990s and that it may have meaningful current application with the advent of more research on its use in contemporary settings and therapies.

Time-Out

Time-out is an aversive stimulus or punishment during which the client is removed from the environment where the unacceptable behavior is being exhibited. The client is usually isolated so that reinforcement from the attention of others is absent.

Reciprocal Inhibition

Also called *counterconditioning*, **reciprocal inhibition** decreases or eliminates a behavior by introducing a more adaptive behavior, but one that is incompatible with the unacceptable behavior (Wolpe, 1958). An example is the introduction of relaxation exercises to an individual who is phobic. Relaxation is practiced in the presence of anxiety so that in time the individual is able to manage the anxiety in the presence of the phobic stimulus by engaging in

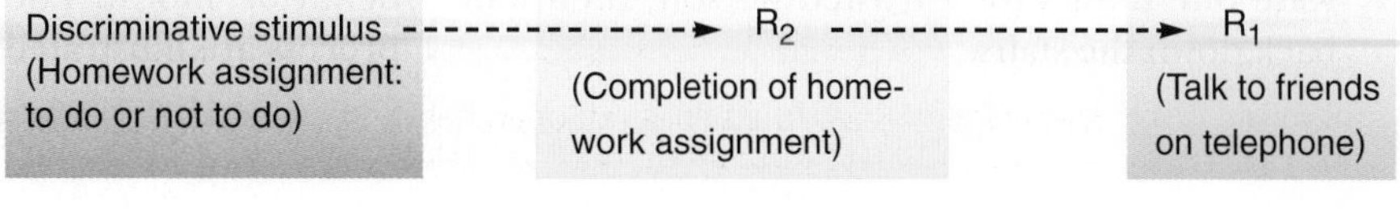

FIGURE 18–3 Example: Premack principle.

Discriminative stimulus (Homework assignment: to do or not to do) ------------> R_2 (Completion of homework assignment) ------------> R_1 (Talk to friends on telephone)

relaxation exercises. Relaxation and anxiety are incompatible behaviors.

Overt Sensitization

Overt sensitization is a type of aversion therapy that produces unpleasant consequences for undesirable behavior. For example, disulfiram (Antabuse) is a drug given to individuals who wish to stop drinking alcohol. If an individual consumes alcohol while on Antabuse therapy, symptoms of severe nausea and vomiting, dyspnea, palpitations, and headache will occur. Instead of the euphoric feeling normally experienced from the alcohol (the positive reinforcement for drinking), the individual receives a severe punishment that is intended to extinguish the unacceptable behavior (drinking alcohol).

Covert Sensitization

Covert sensitization relies on the individual's imagination rather than on medication to produce unpleasant symptoms. The technique is under the client's control and can be used whenever and wherever it is required. The individual learns to visualize nauseating scenes and even to induce a mild feeling of nausea through mental imagery. This mental image is visualized when the individual is about to succumb to an attractive but undesirable behavior. It is most effective when paired with relaxation exercises that are performed instead of the undesirable behavior. The primary advantage of covert sensitization is that the individual does not have to perform the undesired behaviors but simply imagine them.

Systematic Desensitization

Systematic desensitization is a technique for assisting individuals to overcome their fear of a phobic stimulus. It is "systematic" in that there is a hierarchy of anxiety-producing events through which the individual progresses during therapy. An example of a hierarchy of events associated with a fear of elevators may be as follows:

1. Discuss riding an elevator with the therapist.
2. Look at a picture of an elevator.
3. Walk into the lobby of a building and see the elevators.
4. Push the button for the elevator.
5. Walk into an elevator with a trusted person; disembark before the doors close.
6. Walk into an elevator with a trusted person. Allow doors to close, then open the doors and walk out.
7. Ride one floor with a trusted person, then walk back down the stairs.
8. Ride one floor with a trusted person and ride the elevator back down.
9. Ride the elevator alone.

As each of these steps is attempted, it is paired with relaxation exercises as an antagonistic behavior to anxiety. Generally, the desensitization procedures occur in the therapy setting, where the client is instructed to engage in relaxation exercises. When relaxation has been achieved, the client uses mental imagery to visualize the hierarchical step described by the therapist. If the client becomes anxious, the therapist suggests relaxation exercises again, and presents a scene that is lower in the hierarchy. Therapy continues until the individual is able to progress through the entire hierarchy with manageable anxiety. The effects of relaxation in the presence of imagined anxiety-producing stimuli transfer to the real situation once the client has achieved relaxation capable of suppressing or inhibiting anxiety responses (Ford-Martin, 2005). However, some clients are not successful in extinguishing phobic reactions through imagery. For these clients, *real-life desensitization* may be required. In these instances, the therapist may arrange for the client to be exposed to the hierarchy of steps in the desensitization process, but in real-life situations. Relaxation exercises may or may not be a part of real-life desensitization.

Flooding

This technique, sometimes called *implosive therapy,* is also used to desensitize individuals to phobic stimuli. It differs from systematic desensitization in that, instead of working up a hierarchy of anxiety-producing stimuli, the individual is "flooded" with a continuous presentation (through mental imagery) of the phobic stimulus until it no longer elicits anxiety. **Flooding** is believed to produce results faster than systematic desensitization; however, some therapists report more lasting behavioral changes with systematic desensitization. Some questions have also been raised about the ethics of encouraging a patient to endure prolonged fear and psychological discomfort, and clients may avoid this type of therapy for that reason. Flooding is contraindicated with clients for whom intense anxiety would be hazardous, such as individuals with heart disease or fragile psychological adaptation (Sadock, Sadock, & Ruiz, 2015).

Role of the Nurse in Behavior Therapy

The nursing process is the vehicle for delivery of nursing care with the client requiring assistance with behavior modification. The steps of the nursing process are illustrated in the following case study.

CASE STUDY

This example focuses on inpatient care, but these interventions can be modified and are applicable to various healthcare settings, including partial hospitalization, community outpatient clinic, home health, and private practice.

ASSESSMENT

Zach, age 8, has been admitted to the child psychiatric unit of a university medical center following evaluation by a child psychiatrist. His parents, Tom and Deborah, are at an impasse, and their marriage is suffering because of constant conflict over their son's behavior at home and at school. Tom complains bitterly that Deborah is overly permissive with their son. Tom reports that Zach argues and has temper tantrums and insists on continuing games, books, and TV whenever Deborah puts him to bed, so that an 8:30 p.m. bedtime regularly is delayed until 10:30 or later every night. Also, Deborah often cooks four or five different meals for her son's dinner if Zach stubbornly insists that he will not eat what has been prepared. At school, several teachers have complained that the child is stubborn and argumentative, is often disruptive in the classroom, and refuses to follow established rules.

When asked by the psychiatric nurse about other maladaptive behaviors, such as destruction of property, stealing, lying, or setting fires, the parents denied that these had been a problem. During the interview, Zach sat quietly without interrupting. He answered questions that were directed to him with brief responses and made light of the problems described by his parents and reported by his teachers. The nurse conducted an assessment to rule out history of trauma as an alternate explanation for his behavior, and there was no evidence of trauma in Zach's history.

During his first 3 days on the unit, the following assessments were made:

1. Zach loses his temper when he cannot have his way. He screams, stomps his feet, and sometimes kicks the furniture.
2. Zach refuses to follow directions given by staff. He merely responds, "No, I won't."
3. Zach likes to engage in behaviors that annoy the staff and other children: belching loudly, scraping his fingernails across the blackboard, making loud noises when the other children are trying to watch television, opening his mouth when it is full of food.
4. Zach blames others when he makes a mistake. He spilled his milk at lunchtime while racing to get to a specific seat he knew Tony wanted. He blamed the accident on Tony, saying, "He made me do it! He tripped me!"

Upon completion of the initial assessments, the psychiatrist diagnosed Zach with oppositional defiant disorder.

DIAGNOSIS/OUTCOME IDENTIFICATION

Nursing diagnoses and outcome criteria for Zach include the following:

NURSING DIAGNOSES	OUTCOME CRITERIA
Noncompliance with therapy	Zach participates in and cooperates during therapeutic activities.
Defensive coping	Zach accepts responsibility for own behaviors and interacts with others without becoming defensive.
Impaired social interaction	Zach interacts with staff and peers using age-appropriate, acceptable behaviors.

PLANNING/IMPLEMENTATION

A contract for Zach's care was drawn up by the admitting nurse and others on the treatment team. Zach's contract was based on a system of token economies. He discussed with the nurse the kinds of privileges he would like to earn:

■ Having a can of pop for a snack (2 tokens)
■ Getting to watch 30 minutes of TV (5 tokens)
■ Getting to stay up later on Friday nights with the other clients (7 tokens)
■ Getting to play the video games (3 tokens)
■ Getting to walk with the nurse to the gift shop to spend some of his money (8 tokens)
■ Getting to go on the outside therapeutic recreation activities such as movies, the zoo, and picnics (10 tokens)

Tokens were awarded for appropriate behaviors:

■ Gets out of bed when the nurse calls him (1 token)
■ Gets dressed for breakfast (1 token)
■ Presents himself for *all* meals in an appropriate manner: no screaming, no belching, no opening his mouth when it is full of food, no throwing of food, staying in his chair during the meal, putting his tray away in the appropriate place when he is finished (2 tokens × 3 meals = 6 tokens)
■ Completes hygiene activities (1 token)
■ Accepts blame for own mistakes (1 token)
■ Does not fight; uses no obscene language; does not "sass" staff (1 token)
■ Remains quiet while others are watching TV (1 token)
■ Participates and is not disruptive in unit meetings and group therapy sessions (2 tokens)
■ Displays no temper tantrums (1 token)
■ Follows unit rules (1 token)
■ Goes to bed at designated hour without opposition (1 token)

Tokens are awarded at bedtime for absence of inappropriate behaviors during the day. For example, if Zach has

Continued

CASE STUDY—cont'd

no temper tantrums during the day, he is awarded 1 token. Likewise, if Zach has a temper tantrum (or exhibits other inappropriate behavior), he must pay back the token amount designated for that behavior. No other attention is given to inappropriate behaviors other than withholding and payback of tokens.

EXCEPTION: If Zach is receiving reinforcement from peers for inappropriate behaviors, staff has the option of imposing time-out or isolation until the behavior is extinguished.

The contract may be renegotiated at any time between Zach and staff. Additional privileges or responsibilities may be added as they develop and are deemed appropriate.

All staff members are consistent with the terms of the contract and do not allow Zach to manipulate. There are no exceptions without renegotiation of the contract.

NOTE: Parents meet regularly with the case manager from the treatment team. Effective parenting techniques are discussed, as are other problems identified within the marriage relationship. Parenting instruction coordinates with the pattern of behavior modification Zach is receiving on the psychiatric unit. The importance of follow-through is emphasized, along with strong encouragement that the parents maintain a united front in disciplining Zach. Oppositional behaviors are nurtured by divided management.

EVALUATION

Reassessment is conducted to determine if the nursing actions have been successful in achieving the objectives of Zach care. Evaluation can be facilitated by gathering information using the following questions:

■ Does Zach participate in and cooperate during therapeutic activities?
■ Does he follow the rules of the unit (including mealtimes, hygiene, and bedtime) without opposition?
■ Does Zach accept responsibility for his own mistakes?
■ Is he able to complete a task without becoming defensive?
■ Does he refrain from interrupting when others are talking and from making noise in situations where quiet is in order?
■ Does he refrain from attempts to manipulate the staff?
■ Is he able to express anger appropriately without tantrum behaviors?
■ Does he demonstrate acceptable behavior in interactions with peers?

Summary and Key Points

■ The basic assumption of behavior therapy is that problematic behaviors occur when there has been inadequate learning and, therefore, can be corrected through the provision of appropriate learning experiences.

■ The antecedents of today's principles of behavior therapy are largely the products of laboratory efforts by Pavlov and Skinner.

■ Pavlov introduced a process that came to be known as *classical conditioning*.

■ Pavlov demonstrated in his trials with laboratory animals that a neutral stimulus could acquire the ability to elicit a conditioned response through pairing with an unconditioned stimulus. He considered the conditioned response to be a new, learned response.

■ Skinner, in his model of operant conditioning, gave additional attention to the consequences of the response as an approach to learning new behaviors.

■ Skinner believed that the connection between a stimulus and a response is strengthened or weakened by the consequences of the response.

■ Various techniques for modifying client behavior include the following:
  ■ Shaping: A technique in which reinforcements are given for increasingly closer approximations to the desired response
  ■ Modeling: The learning of new behaviors by imitating the behavior of others
  ■ Premack principle: The concept that a frequently occurring response can serve as a positive reinforcement for a response that occurs less frequently
  ■ Extinction: The gradual decrease in frequency or disappearance of a response when the positive reinforcement is withheld
  ■ Contingency contracting: A contract specifying a specific behavior change and the reinforcers to be given for performing the desired behaviors
  ■ Token economy: A type of contingency contracting in which the reinforcers for desired behaviors are presented in the form of tokens
  ■ Time-out: An aversive stimulus or punishment during which the client is removed from the environment where the unacceptable behavior is being exhibited
  ■ Reciprocal inhibition: A technique that decreases or eliminates a behavior by introducing

a more adaptive behavior that is incompatible with the unacceptable behavior
- Overt sensitization: A type of aversion therapy that produces unpleasant consequences for undesirable behavior
- Covert sensitization: Relies on an individual's imagination to produce unpleasant consequences for undesirable behaviors
- Systematic desensitization: A technique for overcoming phobias in which there is a hierarchy of anxiety-producing events through which the individual progresses
- Flooding (also called *implosion therapy*): Desensitizes individuals to phobic stimuli by "flooding" them with a continuous presentation (through mental imagery) of the phobic stimulus until it no longer elicits anxiety

- Nurses can implement behavior therapy techniques to help clients modify maladaptive behavior patterns.
- The nursing process is a systematic method of directing care for clients who require this type of assistance.

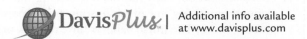 Additional info available at www.davisplus.com

Review Questions
Self-Examination/Learning Exercise

Select the answer that is most appropriate for each of the following questions.

1. A positive reinforcer:
   a. Increases the probability that a behavior will recur.
   b. Decreases the probability that a behavior will recur.
   c. Has nothing to do with modifying behavior.
   d. Always results in positive behavior.

2. A negative reinforcer:
   a. Increases the probability that a behavior will recur.
   b. Decreases the probability that a behavior will recur.
   c. Has nothing to do with modifying behavior.
   d. Always results in unacceptable behavior.

3. An aversive stimulus or punisher:
   a. Increases the probability that a behavior will recur.
   b. Decreases the probability that a behavior will recur.
   c. Has nothing to do with modifying behavior.
   d. Always results in unacceptable behavior.

Situation: B.J. has been out with his friends. He is late getting home. He knows his wife will be angry and will yell at him for being late. He stops at the florist and buys a dozen red roses for her. Questions 4, 5, and 6 are related to this situation.

4. Which of the following behaviors represents positive reinforcement on the part of the wife?
   a. She meets him at the door, accepts the roses, and says nothing further about his being late.
   b. She meets him at the door, yelling that he is late, and makes him spend the night on the couch.
   c. She meets him at the door, expresses delight with the roses, and kisses him on the cheek.
   d. She meets him at the door and says, "How could you? You know I'm allergic to roses!"

5. Which of the following behaviors represents negative reinforcement on the part of the wife?
   a. She meets him at the door, accepts the roses, and says nothing further about his being late.
   b. She meets him at the door, yelling that he is late, and makes him spend the night on the couch.
   c. She meets him at the door, expresses delight with the roses, and kisses him on the cheek.
   d. She meets him at the door and says, "How could you? You know I'm allergic to roses!"

Continued

Review Questions—cont'd
Self-Examination/Learning Exercise

6. Which of the following behaviors represents an aversive stimulus on the part of the wife?
   a. She meets him at the door, accepts the roses, and says nothing further about his being late.
   b. She meets him at the door, yelling that he is late, and makes him spend the night on the couch.
   c. She meets him at the door, expresses delight with the roses, and kisses him on the cheek.
   d. She meets him at the door and says, "How could you? You know I'm allergic to roses!"

7. Fourteen-year-old Sally has been spending many hours after school watching TV. She has virtually stopped practicing her piano lessons. Sally's parents ask for advice about how to encourage Sally to practice more. The nurse believes the Premack principle may be helpful. Which of the following does she suggest to Sally's parents?
   a. She tells Sally's parents to reward Sally each time she practices the piano, even if it is only for 5 minutes.
   b. She tells Sally's parents to ignore this behavior and eventually she will start practicing on her own.
   c. She tells Sally's parents to draw up a contract with Sally stating what the consequences will be if she does not practice the piano.
   d. She tells Sally's parents to explain to Sally that she may watch TV only after she has practiced the piano for 1 hour.

8. Jill has a fear of dogs. In helping her overcome this fear, the therapist is using systematic desensitization. List the following steps in the order in which the therapist would proceed.
   Have Jill:
   a. Look at a real dog.
   b. Look at a stuffed toy dog.
   c. Pet a real dog.
   d. Pet the stuffed toy dog.
   e. Walk past a real dog.
   f. Look at a picture of a dog.

References

Dickerson, F.B., Tenhula, W.N., & Green-Paden. (2005). The token economy for schizophrenia: Review of the literature and recommendations for future research. *Schizophrenia Research, 75*(2-3), 405-416. doi:10.1016/j.schres.2004.08.026

Doll, C., McLaughlin, T. F., & Barretto, A. (2013). The token economy: A recent review and evaluation. *International Journal of Basic and Applied Science, 2*(1), 131-149.

Ford-Martin, P.A. (2005). Behavioral therapy. *Gale Encyclopedia of Public Health.* Retrieved from www.healthline.com/galecontent/behavioral-therapy

Sadock, B.J., Sadock, V.A., & Ruiz, (2015). *Synopsis of psychiatry: Behavioral sciences/clinical psychiatry* (11th ed.). Philadelphia: Wolters Kluwer.

Souders, M.C., DePaul, D., Freeman, K.G., & Levy, S.E. (2002). Caring for children and adolescents with autism who require challenging procedures. *Pediatric Nursing, 28*(6), 555-564.

Classical References

Pavlov, I.P. (1927). *Conditioned reflexes.* London: Oxford University Press.

Premack, D. (1959). Toward empirical behavior laws: I. Positive reinforcement. *Psychological Review, 66*(4), 219-233. doi:http://dx.doi.org/10.1037/h0040891

Skinner, B.F. (1938). *The behavior of organisms.* New York: Appleton-Century-Crofts.

Skinner, B.F. (1953). *Science and human behavior.* New York: Macmillan.

Thorndike, E.L. (1911). *Animal intelligence.* New York: Macmillan.

Wolpe, J. (1958). *Psychotherapy by reciprocal inhibition.* Stanford, CA: Stanford University Press.

Cognitive Therapy

19

CORE CONCEPTS

Cognitive

Cognitive Therapy

KEY TERMS

arbitrary inference

automatic thoughts

catastrophic thinking

decatastrophizing

dichotomous thinking

distraction

magnification

minimization

overgeneralizations

personalization

schemas

selective abstraction

Socratic dialogue

OBJECTIVES
After reading this chapter, the student will be able to:

1. Discuss historical perspectives associated with cognitive therapy.
2. Identify various indications for cognitive therapy.
3. Describe goals, principles, and basic concepts of cognitive therapy.
4. Discuss a variety of cognitive therapy techniques.
5. Apply techniques of cognitive therapy within the context of the nursing process.

HOMEWORK ASSIGNMENT
Please read the chapter and answer the following questions:

1. Define *automatic thoughts*.
2. Why are automatic thoughts problematic for some people?
3. What are the three major components of cognitive therapy?
4. John submits his design of a house to some prospective clients. They ask for a few changes to be made. John thinks, "I'm a terrible architect!" What automatic thought does this statement represent?

Wright, Thase, and Beck (2008) stated:

> The writing of Epictetus in the *Enchiridion, "Men are disturbed not by things, but by the views which they take of them,"* captures the essence of the perspective that our ideas or thoughts are a controlling factor in our emotional lives. (p. 1212)

This concept provides a foundation on which the cognitive model is established. In cognitive therapy, the therapist uses various methods to create change in the client's thinking and belief system in an effort to bring about lasting emotional and behavioral change (Beck, 1995). Distorted cognitions are at the foundation of many emotional, mental, and behavioral disorders: clients with depression often seem to be consumed by negative thoughts about themselves and about how others see them, clients with anxiety disorders often have worried thoughts about past and future events, clients with personality disorders often struggle with maladaptive thoughts about their relationships with others, and so on. Could helping clients change the way they think actually improve their mood and their behavior? There is much evidence to support that it can (Brenes et al., 2015; Brent et al., 2015; Guille et al., 2015; Rohan et al., 2015; Weck & Neng, 2015).

This chapter examines the historical development of the cognitive model, defines the goals of therapy, and describes various techniques of the cognitive approach. A discussion of the role of the nurse in the implementation of cognitive behavioral techniques with clients is presented.

NOTE: Although in this text the concepts are presented separately for reasons of clarification, cognitive therapy procedures are often combined with behavioral modification techniques and are referred to as *cognitive-behavioral therapy* (CBT).

CORE CONCEPT

Cognitive

Relating to the mental processes of thinking and reasoning.

Historical Background

Cognitive therapy has its roots in the early 1960s research on depression conducted by Aaron Beck (1963, 1964). Beck was trained in the Freudian psychoanalytic view of depression as "anger turned inward." In his clinical research, he began to observe a common theme of negative cognitive processing in the thoughts and dreams of his depressed clients (Beck & Weishaar, 2011).

A number of theorists have taken from and expanded upon Beck's original concept. The common theme is the rejection of the passive listening used in psychoanalysis in favor of active, direct dialogues with clients (Beck & Weishaar, 2011). The work of contemporary behavioral therapists has also influenced the evolution of cognitive therapy. Behavioral techniques such as expectancy of reinforcement and modeling are based in cognitive processes. Lazarus and Folkman (1984), whose premises about *personal appraisal* and *coping* shape the conceptual framework of this book, have also substantially contributed to the cognitive approach to therapy. The model for cognitive therapy is based

on an individual's cognition, or more specifically, an individual's personal cognitive appraisal of an event and the resulting emotions or behaviors. Personality—which undoubtedly influences our cognitive appraisal of an event—is viewed as shaped by the interaction between innate predisposition and the environment (Beck, Davis, & Freeman, 2015). Whereas some types of therapy may be directed toward improvement in coping strategies or adaptiveness of behavioral response, cognitive therapy is aimed at modifying distorted cognitions about a situation. Since behavior and emotions are intimately linked to thoughts, this approach assumes that behavior and emotions will change as a result of changing one's thinking.

CORE CONCEPT

Cognitive Therapy

Cognitive therapy is a type of psychotherapy based on the concept of pathological mental processing. The focus of treatment is on the modification of distorted cognitions and maladaptive behaviors.

Indications for Cognitive Therapy

Cognitive therapy was originally developed for use with depression and is now used to treat a broad range of emotional disorders. In addition to depression, cognitive therapy may be used with the following clinical conditions: panic disorder, generalized anxiety disorder, social phobias, obsessive-compulsive disorder, posttraumatic stress disorder, eating disorders, substance abuse, personality disorders, schizophrenia, couples' problems, bipolar disorder, illness anxiety disorder, and somatic symptom disorder. The proponents of cognitive therapy suggest that the emphasis of therapy must be varied and individualized for clients according to their specific diagnosis, symptoms, and level of functioning (Beck, 1995; Sadock, Sadock, & Ruiz, 2015; Wright et al., 2008).

Goals and Principles of Cognitive Therapy

Beck and associates (1987) defined the goals of cognitive therapy as follows.

The client will:

1. Monitor his or her negative, automatic thoughts.
2. Recognize the connections between cognition, affect, and behavior.
3. Examine the evidence for and against distorted automatic thoughts.
4. Substitute more realistic interpretations for these biased cognitions.

5. Learn to identify and alter the dysfunctional beliefs that predispose him or her to distort experiences.

Cognitive therapy is highly structured and short-term, lasting from 12 to 16 weeks (Beck & Weishaar, 2011). Sadock and associates (2015) suggested that if a client does not improve within 25 weeks of therapy, a reevaluation of the diagnosis should be made. Although therapy must be tailored to the individual, the following principles underlie cognitive therapy for all clients (Beck, 1995).

Principle 1. Cognitive therapy is based on an ever-evolving formulation of the client and his or her problems in cognitive terms. The therapist identifies the event that precipitated the distorted cognition. Current thinking patterns that serve to maintain the problematic behaviors are reviewed. The therapist then hypothesizes about certain developmental events and enduring patterns of cognitive appraisal that may have predisposed the client to specific emotional and behavioral responses.

Principle 2. Cognitive therapy requires a sound therapeutic alliance. A trusting relationship between therapist and client must exist for cognitive therapy to succeed. The therapist must convey warmth, empathy, caring, and genuine positive regard. Development of a working relationship between therapist and client is an individual process, and clients with various disorders will require varying degrees of effort to achieve this therapeutic alliance.

Principle 3. Cognitive therapy emphasizes collaboration and active participation. Teamwork between therapist and client is emphasized. They decide together what to work on during each session, how often they should meet, and what homework assignments should be completed between sessions.

Principle 4. Cognitive therapy is goal oriented and problem focused. At the beginning of therapy, the client is encouraged to identify what he or she perceives to be the problem or problems. With guidance from the therapist, goals are established as outcomes of therapy. Assistance in problem-solving is provided as required as the client comes to recognize and correct distortions in thinking.

Principle 5. Cognitive therapy initially emphasizes the present. Resolution of distressing situations that are based in the present usually leads to symptom reduction. It is therefore more beneficial to begin with current problems and delay shifting attention to the past until (1) the client expresses a desire to do so, (2) the work on current problems produces little or no change, or (3) the therapist decides it is important to determine how dysfunctional ideas affecting the client's current thinking originated.

Principle 6. Cognitive therapy is educative, aims to teach the client to be his or her own therapist, and emphasizes relapse prevention. From the beginning of therapy, the client is taught about the nature and course of his or her disorder, about the cognitive model (i.e., how thoughts influence emotions and behavior), and about the process of cognitive therapy. The client is taught how to set goals, plan behavioral change, and intervene on his or her own behalf.

Principle 7. Cognitive therapy aims to be time limited. Clients often are seen weekly for a couple of months, followed by a number of biweekly sessions, then possibly a few monthly sessions. Some clients want periodic "booster" sessions every few months.

Principle 8. Cognitive therapy sessions are structured. Each session has a set structure which includes (1) reviewing the client's week, (2) collaboratively setting the agenda for this session, (3) reviewing the previous week's session, (4) reviewing the previous week's homework, (5) discussing this week's agenda items, (6) establishing homework for next week, and (7) summarizing this week's session. This format focuses attention on important items to maximize the use of therapy time.

Principle 9. Cognitive therapy teaches clients to identify, evaluate, and respond to their dysfunctional thoughts and beliefs. Through gentle questioning and review of data, the therapist helps the client identify his or her dysfunctional thinking, evaluate the validity of the thoughts, and devise a plan of action. This is done by helping the client examine evidence that supports or contradicts the accuracy of the thought rather than directly challenging or confronting the belief.

Principle 10. Cognitive therapy uses a variety of techniques to change thinking, mood, and behavior. Techniques from various therapies may be used within the cognitive framework. Emphasis in treatment is guided by the client's particular disorder and directed toward modification of the dysfunctional cognitions that contribute to the maladaptive behavior associated with his or her disorder. Examples of disorders and the dysfunctional thinking for which cognitive therapy may be of benefit are discussed later in this chapter.

Basic Concepts

Wright and associates (2008) stated, "The general thrust of cognitive therapy is that emotional responses are largely dependent upon cognitive appraisals of the significance of environmental cues" (p. 1213). Basic concepts include **automatic thoughts** and **schemas,** or core beliefs.

Automatic Thoughts

Automatic thoughts are those that occur rapidly in response to a situation and without rational analysis.

These thoughts are often negative and based on erroneous logic. Beck and associates (1987) called these thoughts *cognitive errors*. Following are some examples of common cognitive errors:

Arbitrary Inference In a type of thinking error known as **arbitrary inference,** the individual automatically comes to a conclusion about an incident without the facts to support it or even despite contradictory evidence.

EXAMPLE

Two months ago, Mrs. B. sent a wedding gift to the daughter of an old friend. She has not yet received acknowledgment of the gift. Mrs. B. thinks, "They obviously think I have poor taste."

Overgeneralization (Absolutistic Thinking) Sweeping conclusions are **overgeneralizations** made on the basis of one incident—an "all-or-nothing" kind of thinking.

EXAMPLE

Frank submitted an article to a nursing journal, and it was rejected. Frank thinks, "No journal will ever be interested in anything I write."

Dichotomous Thinking An individual who is using **dichotomous thinking** views situations in terms of all-or-nothing, black-or-white, or good-or-bad.

EXAMPLE

Frank submits an article to a nursing journal, and the editor returns it and asks Frank to rewrite parts of it. Frank thinks, "I'm a bad writer," instead of recognizing that revision is a common part of the publication process.

Selective Abstraction A **selective abstraction** (sometimes referred to as a *mental filter*) is a conclusion that is based on only a selected portion of the evidence. The selected portion is usually the negative evidence or what the individual views as a failure, rather than any successes that have occurred.

EXAMPLE

Jackie just graduated from high school with a 3.98/4.00 grade point average. She won a scholarship to the large state university near her home. She was active in sports and activities in high school and well liked by her peers. However, she is very depressed and dwells on the fact that she did not earn a scholarship to a prestigious Ivy League college to which she had applied.

Magnification Exaggerating the negative significance of an event is known as **magnification.**

EXAMPLE

Nancy hears that her colleague at work is having a cocktail party over the weekend, and she is not invited. Nancy thinks, "She doesn't like me."

Minimization Undervaluing the positive significance of an event is called **minimization.**

EXAMPLE

Mrs. M. is feeling lonely. She telephones her granddaughter Amy, who lives in a nearby town, and invites her to visit. Amy apologizes that she must go out of town on business and would not be able to visit at that time. While Amy is out of town, she calls Mrs. M. twice, but Mrs. M. still feels unloved by her granddaughter.

Catastrophic Thinking Always thinking that the worst will occur without considering the possibility of more likely positive outcomes is considered **catastrophic thinking.**

EXAMPLE

On Janet's first day in her secretarial job, her boss asked her to write a letter to another firm and put it on his desk for his signature. She did so and left for lunch. When she returned, the letter was on her desk with a typographical error circled in red and a note from her boss to redo the letter. Janet thinks, "This is it! I will surely be fired now!"

Personalization With **personalization,** the person takes complete responsibility for situations without considering that other circumstances may have contributed to the outcome.

EXAMPLE

Jack, who sells vacuum cleaners door-to-door, has just given a 2-hour demonstration to Mrs. W. At the end of the demonstration, Mrs. W tells Jack that she appreciates his demonstration, but she won't be purchasing a vacuum cleaner from him. Jack thinks, "I'm a lousy salesman" (when in fact, Mrs. W.'s husband lost his job last week, and they have no extra money to buy a new vacuum cleaner at this time).

Schemas (Core Beliefs)

Beck and Weishaar (2011) defined cognitive schemas as:

> Structures that contain the individual's fundamental beliefs and assumptions. Schemas develop early in life from personal experience and identification with significant others. These concepts are reinforced by further learning experiences and, in turn, influence the formation of beliefs, values, and attitudes. (p. 284)

These schemas, or core beliefs, may be adaptive or maladaptive. They may be general or specific, and they may be latent, becoming evident only when triggered by a specific stressful stimulus. Schemas differ from automatic thoughts in that they are deeper cognitive structures that serve to screen information from the environment. For this reason, they are often more difficult to modify than automatic thoughts.

However, the same techniques used for automatic thoughts can be used at the schema level. Schemas can be positive or negative and generally fall into two broad categories: those associated with *helplessness* and those associated with *unlovability* (Beck, 1995). Some examples of types of schemas are presented in Table 19–1.

Techniques of Cognitive Therapy

The three major components of cognitive therapy are didactic aspects, cognitive techniques, and behavioral interventions (Sadock et al., 2015).

Didactic (Educational) Aspects

A basic principle of cognitive therapy is to prepare the client to eventually become his or her own cognitive therapist. The therapist provides information to the client about what cognitive therapy is, how it works, and the structure of the cognitive process. Explanation about expectations of both client and therapist is provided. Reading assignments are given to reinforce learning. Some therapists use audiotape or videotape sessions to teach clients about cognitive therapy. A full explanation about the relationship between depression (or anxiety, or whatever maladaptive response the client is experiencing) and distorted thinking patterns is an essential part of cognitive therapy.

Cognitive Strategies

Strategies used in cognitive therapy include recognizing and modifying automatic thoughts and recognizing and modifying schemas. Several techniques of cognitive therapy have been elaborated (Freeman-Clevenger, 2014; Wright et al., 2008) and are described in the following sections.

Recognizing Automatic Thoughts and Schemas
Socratic Dialogue

In **Socratic dialogue** (also called *guided discovery*), the therapist questions the client to elaborate the "who, what, when, where, why, and how" of his or her situation The client is asked to describe feelings associated with specific scenarios. Questions are primarily restatements of the client's own words in a way that may stimulate insight into possible dysfunctional thinking and produce dissonance about the validity of the thoughts.

Guided Relaxation and Behavioral Rehearsal

Guided relaxation is aimed at reducing autonomic response to anxiety. Techniques may include deep breathing, imagery, mindfulness meditation, and other exercises. These techniques also increase awareness of conscious control over breathing, anxiety symptoms, and thoughts.

Behavioral rehearsal, often accomplished through role-play, affords the client an opportunity to practice a new way of responding to distressing situations and explore possible outcomes with the counselor before trying out the behavior in real-life situations. *Role-play* is a technique that should be used only when the relationship between client and therapist is exceptionally strong and there is little likelihood of maladaptive transference occurring. With role-play, the therapist assumes the role of an individual in a situation that produces a maladaptive response in the client. The situation is played out in an effort to elicit recognition of automatic thinking on the part of the client.

Automatic Thought Records

This technique, one of the most frequently used methods of recognizing automatic thoughts, is taught to and discussed with the client in the therapy session. Thought recording is assigned as homework for the client outside of therapy. The client is asked to keep a written record of situations that occur and the automatic thoughts elicited by the situation. This is called a *two-column thought recording*. Some therapists ask their clients to keep a three-column recording, which includes a description of the emotional response also associated with the situation, as illustrated in Table 19–2.

Modifying Automatic Thoughts and Schemas
Questioning the Evidence

With this technique, the client and therapist set forth the automatic thought as the hypothesis, and the

TABLE 19–1 **Examples of Types of Schemas**		
SCHEMA CATEGORY	MALADAPTIVE/NEGATIVE	ADAPTIVE/POSITIVE
Helplessness	No matter what I do, I will fail. I must be perfect. If I make one mistake, I will lose everything.	If I try and work very hard, I will succeed. I am not afraid of a challenge. If I make a mistake, I will try again.
Unlovability	I'm stupid. No one would love me. I'm nobody without a man.	I'm a lovable person. People respect me for myself.

TABLE 19–2 **Three-Column Thought Recording**		
SITUATION	AUTOMATIC THOUGHTS	EMOTIONAL RESPONSE
My girlfriend broke up with me.	I'm a stupid person. No one would ever want to marry me.	Sadness; depression
I was turned down for a promotion.	Stupid boss! He doesn't know how to manage people. It's not fair!	Anger

client is assisted to question the facts associated with their cognitions.

Examining Options and Alternatives

To help the client see a broader range of possibilities than originally considered, the therapist guides the client in learning how to generate alternatives.

Decatastrophizing

With the technique of **decatastrophizing,** the therapist assists the client to examine the validity of a negative automatic thought. The client is assisted to examine "what is the worst thing that could happen?" and then to develop a plan of action. Even if some validity exists, the client is encouraged to review ways to cope adaptively and move beyond the current crisis situation.

Reattribution

Through Socratic questioning and testing of automatic thoughts, this technique aims to reverse negative attribution of clients from self-blame (common in depression) or placing blame solely on others (common in

some personality disorders) to a more balanced attribution of responsibility.

Daily Record of Dysfunctional Thoughts (DRDT)

The DRDT is a tool commonly used in cognitive therapy to help clients identify and modify automatic thoughts. Two more columns are added to the three-column thought record presented earlier. Clients are then asked to rate the intensity of the thoughts and emotions on a 0 percent to 100 percent scale. The fourth column of the DRDT asks the client to describe a more rational cognition than the automatic thought identified in the second column and rate the intensity of the belief in the rational thought. In the fifth column, the client records any changes that have occurred as a result of modifying the automatic thought and the new rate of intensity associated with it. With this tool, the client is able to modify automatic thoughts by identifying them and actually formulating a more rational alternative. Table 19–3 presents an example of a DRDT as an extension to the three-column thought recording presented in Table 19–2.

TABLE 19–3 **Sample Daily Record of Dysfunctional Thoughts (DRDT)**				
SITUATION	AUTOMATIC THOUGHT	EMOTIONAL RESPONSE	RATIONAL RESPONSE	OUTCOME: EMOTIONAL RESPONSE
My girlfriend broke up with me.	I'm a stupid person. No one would ever want to marry me. (95%)	Sadness; depression (90%)	I'm not stupid. Lots of people like me. Just because one person doesn't want to date me doesn't mean that no one would want to. (75%)	Sadness; depression (50%)
I was turned down for a promotion.	Stupid boss! He doesn't know how to manage people. It's not fair! (90%)	Anger (95%)	I guess I have to admit the other guy's education and experience fit the position better than mine. The boss was being fair because he filled the position based on qualifications. I'll try for the next promotion that fits my qualifications better. (70%)	Anger (20%) Disappointment (80%) Hope (80%)

Cognitive Rehearsal

This technique uses mental imagery to uncover potential automatic thoughts in advance of their occurrence in a stressful situation. A discussion is held to identify ways to modify these dysfunctional cognitions. The client is then given "homework" assignments to try these newly learned methods in real situations.

Behavioral Interventions

It is believed that in cognitive therapy, an interactive relationship exists between cognitions and behavior; that is, that cognitions affect behavior and behavior influences cognitions. With this concept in mind, a number of interventions are structured for the client to assist him or her to identify and modify maladaptive cognitions and behaviors.

The following procedures, which are behavior oriented, are directed to help clients learn more adaptive behavioral strategies that will in turn have a positive effect on cognitions (Basco et al., 2004; Freeman-Clevenger, 2014; Sadock et al., 2015; Wright et al., 2008):

1. **Activity scheduling:** With this intervention, clients are asked to keep a daily log of their activities on an hourly basis and rate each activity, for mastery and pleasure, on a 0-to-10 scale. The schedule is then shared with the therapist and used to identify important areas needing concentration during therapy.

2. **Graded task assignments:** This intervention is used with clients who are facing a situation that they perceive as overwhelming. The task is broken down into subtasks that clients can complete one step at a time. Each subtask has a goal and a time interval attached to it. Successful completion of each subtask helps to increase self-esteem and decrease feelings of helplessness.

3. **Distraction:** When dysfunctional cognitions have been recognized, **distraction** can occur by engaging in activities that redirect the client's thinking and divert him or her from the intrusive thoughts or depressive ruminations that are contributing to the maladaptive responses.

4. **Miscellaneous techniques:** Relaxation exercises, assertiveness training, role modeling, social skills training, and contingency management contracts are all types of behavioral interventions used in cognitive therapy to help clients modify dysfunctional cognitions. Thought-stopping techniques (described in Chapter 14, Assertiveness Training) may also be used to restructure dysfunctional thinking patterns.

Role of the Nurse in Cognitive Therapy

Many of the techniques used in cognitive therapy are well within the scope of nursing practice, from generalist through specialist levels. Cognitive therapy requires an understanding of educational principles and the ability to use problem-solving skills to guide clients' thinking through a reframing process. The scope of contemporary psychiatric nursing practice is expanding, and although psychiatric nurses have been using some of these techniques in various degrees within their practices for years, it is important that knowledge and skills related to this type of therapy be promoted further. The value of cognitive therapy as a useful and cost-effective tool has been observed in a number of inpatient and community outpatient mental health settings.

The following case study presents the role of the nurse in cognitive therapy in the context of the nursing process.

CASE STUDY

ASSESSMENT

Brian is a 45-year-old white male admitted to the psychiatric unit of a general medical center by his family physician, Dr. Jones, who reported that Brian has become increasingly despondent over the last month. His wife reported that he has made statements such as, "Life is not worth living," and "I think I could just take all those pills Dr. Jones prescribed at one time; then it would all be over." He was admitted at 6:40 p.m., via wheelchair from admissions, accompanied by his wife. He reports no known allergies. Vital signs upon admission were temperature, 97.9°F; pulse, 80; respirations, 16; and blood pressure, 132/77. He is 5 feet 11 inches tall and weighs 160 pounds. He was referred to the psychiatrist on call, Dr. Smith. Orders include suicide precautions, level I; regular diet; chemistry profile and routine urinalysis in a.m.; Desyrel, 200 mg tid; Dalmane, 30 mg HS prn for sleep.

FAMILY DYNAMICS

Brian says he loves his wife and children and does not want to hurt them, but he feels they no longer need him. He states, "They would probably be better off without me." His wife appears to be very concerned about his condition, although in his despondency, he seems oblivious to her feelings. His mother lives in a neighboring state, and he sees her infrequently. He admits that he is somewhat bitter toward her for allowing him and his siblings to "suffer from the physical and emotional brutality of their father." His siblings and their families live in distant states, and he sees them rarely,

Continued

CASE STUDY—cont'd

during holiday gatherings. He feels closest to the older of the two brothers.

MEDICAL/PSYCHIATRIC HISTORY

Brian's father died 5 years ago at age 65 of a myocardial infarction. Brian and both his brothers have a history of high cholesterol and triglycerides from approximately age 30. During his regular physical examination 1 month ago, Brian's family doctor recognized symptoms of depression and prescribed fluoxetine. Brian's mother has a history of depressive episodes. She was hospitalized once about 7 years ago for depression, and she has taken various antidepressant medications over the years. Her family physician has also prescribed Valium for her on numerous occasions for her "nerves." No other family members have a history of psychiatric problems.

PAST EXPERIENCES

Brian was the first child in a family of four. He is 2 years older than his sister and 4 years older than the third child, a brother. He was 6 years old when his youngest sibling, also a boy, was born. Brian's father was a career Army man who moved his family many times during Brian's childhood years. Brian attended 15 schools from the time he entered kindergarten until he graduated from high school.

Brian reports that his father was very autocratic and had many rules that he expected his children to obey without question. Infraction resulted in harsh discipline. Because Brian was the oldest child, his father believed he should assume responsibility for the behavior of his siblings. Brian describes the severe physical punishment he received from his father when he or his siblings allegedly violated one of the rules. It was particularly intense when Brian's father had been drinking, which he did most evenings and weekends.

Brian's mother was very passive. Brian believes she was afraid of his father, particularly when he was drinking, so she quietly conformed to his lifestyle and offered no resistance, even though she did not agree with his disciplining of the children. Brian reports that he observed his father physically abusing his mother on a number of occasions, most often when he had been drinking.

Brian states that he had very few friends when he was growing up. With all the family moves, he gave up trying to make new friends because it became too painful to give them up when it was time to leave. He took a paper route when he was 13 years old and then worked in fast-food restaurants from age 15 on. He was a hard worker and never seemed to have difficulty finding work in any of the places where the family relocated. He states that he appreciated the independence and the opportunity of being away from home as much as his job would allow. "I guess I can honestly say I hated my father, and working was my way of getting away from all the stress that was going on in that house. I guess my dad hated me, too, because he never was satisfied with anything I did. I never did well enough for him in school, on the job, or even at home. When I think of my dad now, the memories I have are of being criticized and beaten with a belt."

On graduation from high school, Brian joined the Navy, where he learned a skill that he used after discharge to obtain a job in a large aircraft plant. He also attended the local university at night, where he earned his accounting degree. When he completed his degree, he was reassigned to the administration department of the aircraft company, and he has been in the same position for 12 years without a promotion.

PRECIPITATING EVENT

Over the last 12 years, Brian has watched while a number of his peers were promoted to management positions. Brian has been considered for several of these positions but never has been selected. Last month, a management position became available for which Brian felt he was qualified. He applied for this position, believing he had a good chance of being promoted. However, when the announcement was made, the position had been given to a younger man who had been with the company only 5 years. Brian seemed to accept the decision, but over the last few weeks he has become increasingly withdrawn. He speaks to very few people at the office and is becoming seriously behind in his work. At home, he eats very little, talks to family members only when they ask a direct question, withdraws to his bedroom very early in the evening, and does not come out until it is time to leave for work the next morning. Today, he refused to get out of bed or to go to work. His wife convinced him to talk to their family doctor, who admitted him to the hospital.

CLIENT'S PERCEPTION OF THE STRESSOR

Brian states that all his life he has "not been good enough at anything. I could never please my father. Now I can't seem to please my boss. What's the use of trying? I came to the hospital because my wife and my doctor are afraid I might try to kill myself. I must admit the thought has crossed my mind more than once. I seem to have very little motivation for living. I just don't care anymore."

DIAGNOSES AND OUTCOME IDENTIFICATION

The following nursing diagnoses were formulated for Sam:

1. Risk for suicide related to depressed mood and expression of having nothing to live for
2. Chronic low self-esteem related to lack of positive feedback and learned helplessness evidenced by a sense of worthlessness, lack of eye contact, social isolation, and negative/pessimistic outlook

The following may be used as criteria for measurement of outcomes in the planning of care for Brian:

THE CLIENT WILL:
1. Not harm self
2. Express hope for the future
3. Demonstrate increased self-esteem and perception of self as a worthwhile person

CASE STUDY—cont'd

PLANNING AND IMPLEMENTATION

Table 19–4 presents a nursing care plan for Brian employing techniques associated with cognitive therapy that are within the scope of psychiatric nursing practice. These include providing psychoeducation, use of the therapeutic relationship, and counseling interventions (American Nurses' Association, American Psychiatric Nurses Association, & International Society of Psychiatric-Mental Health Nurses, 2014). Rationales are presented for each intervention.

EVALUATION

Reassessment is conducted to determine if the nursing interventions have been successful in achieving the objectives of Brian's care. Evaluation can be facilitated by gathering information using the following questions:

1. Has self-harm to Brian been avoided?
2. Have Brian's suicidal ideations subsided?
3. Does Brian know where to seek help in a crisis situation?
4. Has Brian discussed the recent loss with staff and family?
5. Is Brian able to verbalize personal hope for the future?
6. Can Brian identify positive attributes about himself?
7. Does Brian demonstrate motivation to move on with his life without a fear of failure?

Table 19–4 | CARE PLAN FOR "BRIAN" (AN EXAMPLE OF INTERVENTION WITH COGNITIVE THERAPY)

NURSING DIAGNOSIS: RISK FOR SUICIDE

RELATED TO: Depressed mood

OUTCOME CRITERIA	NURSING INTERVENTIONS*	RATIONALE*
Brian will not harm himself.	1. Acknowledge Brian's feelings of despair.	1. Cognitive therapy focuses on pursuing client's point of view.
	2. Convey warmth, accurate empathy, and genuineness.	2. Establishing a therapeutic alliance is foundational to a therapeutic, problem-solving relationship
	3. Collaborate with the client in conducting a thorough assessment of suicide risk. (See Chapter 17, Suicide Prevention, for more information.)	3. Developing a collaborative assessment and plan for suicide prevention is foundational to working with any client at risk for suicide.
	4. Through Socratic questioning, challenge irrational pessimism. Ask Brian to discuss what problems suicide would solve. Then try to get him to think of reasons for *not* attempting suicide.	4. These techniques help the suicidal client think beyond the immediate cognition.
	5. Begin a serious discussion of alternatives.	5. Exploring alternatives initiates the process of cognitive reevaluation by looking at all possible alternatives.

NURSING DIAGNOSIS: CHRONIC LOW SELF-ESTEEM

RELATED TO: Lack of positive feedback and learned helplessness

EVIDENCED BY: A sense of worthlessness, lack of eye contact, social isolation, and negative/pessimistic outlook

OUTCOME CRITERIA	NURSING INTERVENTIONS*	RATIONALE*
Brian demonstrates increased self-esteem and perception of	1. Ask Brian to keep a three-column automatic thought recording.	1. This technique encourages clients to develop insight into their cognitive responses.

Continued

Table 19–4 | CARE PLAN FOR "BRIAN" (AN EXAMPLE OF INTERVENTION WITH COGNITIVE THERAPY)—cont'd

OUTCOME CRITERIA	NURSING INTERVENTIONS*	RATIONALE*
himself as a worthwhile person.	2. Help Brian to recognize that his worth as a person is not tied to his promotion at work. The world will go on and he can survive this loss.	2. The technique of decatastrophizing is designed to help clients put cognitions into a more balanced perspective.
	3. Help Brian to identify ways in which he could feel better about himself. For example, Sam states that he would like to update his computer skills, but he is afraid he is too old. Challenge his negative thinking about his age by incorporating the technique of "examining the evidence."	3. Generating alternatives helps clients recognize that a broader range of possibilities may exist than may be evident at the moment. Examining the evidence may help Brian understand that self-improvement is worthwhile at any age.
	4. Ask Brian to expand on his three-column automatic thought recording and make a daily record of dysfunctional thoughts (DRDT).	4. Cognitive therapists use this tool to help clients identify their automatic thoughts and modify them by coming up with more rational responses.
	5. Discourage Brian's ruminating about his failures. May need to withdraw attention if he persists. Focus on past accomplishments and offer support in undertaking new tasks. Offer recognition of successful endeavors and positive reinforcement of attempts made.	5. Lack of attention to undesirable behavior may discourage its repetition. Recognition and positive reinforcement enhance self-esteem and encourage repetition of desirable behaviors.

*Interventions and rationale for the diagnosis Risk for suicide are adapted from Beck, A.T., & Weishaar, M.E. (2011). Cognitive therapy. In R.J. Corsini and D. Wedding (Eds.), *Current psychotherapies* (9th ed., pp. 276-309). Belmont, CA: Brooks/Cole; Harvard Medical School. (2003). Confronting suicide—part II. *Harvard Mental Health Letter, 19*(12), 1-5.

Summary and Key Points

■ Cognitive therapy is founded on the premise that how people think significantly influences their feelings and behavior.

■ The concept was initiated in the 1960s by Aaron Beck in his work with depressed clients. Since that time, it has been expanded for use with a number of emotional illnesses.

■ Cognitive therapy is short-term, highly structured, and goal-oriented therapy that consists of three major components: didactic, or educational, aspects; cognitive techniques; and behavioral interventions.

■ The therapist teaches the client about the relationship between his or her illness and the distorted thinking patterns. Explanation about cognitive therapy and how it works is provided.

■ The therapist helps the client to recognize his or her negative automatic thoughts (sometimes called *cognitive errors*).

■ Once these automatic thoughts have been identified, various cognitive and behavioral techniques are used to assist the client to modify the dysfunctional thinking patterns.

■ Independent homework assignments are an important part of the cognitive therapist's strategy.

■ Many of the cognitive therapy techniques are within the scope of psychiatric-mental health nursing practice.

■ As the role of the psychiatric nurse continues to expand, the knowledge and skills associated with a variety of therapies will need to be broadened. Cognitive therapy is likely to be one in which nurses will become more involved.

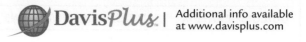 **DavisPlus** | Additional info available at www.davisplus.com

Review Questions
Self-Examination/Learning Exercise

Select the answer that is most appropriate for each of the following questions.

1. Janet failed her first test in nursing school. She thinks, "Well, that's it! I'll never be a nurse." What automatic thought does this statement represent?
   a. Overgeneralization
   b. Magnification
   c. Catastrophic thinking
   d. Personalization

2. When Jack is not accepted at the law school of his choice, he thinks, "I'm so stupid. No law school will ever accept me." What automatic thought does this statement represent?
   a. Overgeneralization
   b. Magnification
   c. Selective abstraction
   d. Minimization

3. Nancy's new in-laws came to dinner for the first time. When Nancy's mother-in-law left some food on her plate, Nancy thought, "I must be a lousy cook." What automatic thought does this statement represent?
   a. Dichotomous thinking
   b. Overgeneralization
   c. Minimization
   d. Personalization

4. Barbara burned the toast. She thinks, "I'm a totally incompetent person." What automatic thought does this statement represent?
   a. Selective abstraction
   b. Magnification
   c. Minimization
   d. Personalization

5. Opal is a 43-year-old woman who is suffering from depression and suicidal ideation. Opal says, "I'm such a worthless person. I don't deserve to live." The therapist responds, "I would like for you to think about what problems committing suicide would solve." The therapist is using which of the following cognitive therapy techniques?
   a. Imagery
   b. Role play
   c. Problem-solving
   d. Thought recording

6. The thought recording (two-column and three-column) cognitive therapy techniques help clients:
   a. Identify automatic thoughts.
   b. Modify automatic thoughts.
   c. Identify rational alternatives.
   d. All of the above.

7. The daily record of dysfunctional thoughts (DRDT) is used in cognitive therapy to help clients:
   a. Identify automatic thoughts.
   b. Modify automatic thoughts.
   c. Identify rational alternatives.
   d. All of the above.

Continued

Review Questions—cont'd
Self-Examination/Learning Exercise

8. A client tells the therapist, "I thought I would just die when my husband told me he was leaving me. If I had been a better wife, he wouldn't have fallen in love with another woman. It's all my fault." The therapist asks the client to explore what responsibilities the husband may have in the breakup. What cognitive therapy technique is the therapist using?
   a. Reattribution
   b. Role-play
   c. Decatastrophizing
   d. Thought recording

9. A client tells the therapist, "I thought I would just die when my husband told me he was leaving me. If I had been a better wife, he wouldn't have fallen in love with another woman. It's all my fault." The therapist wants to use the technique of "examining the evidence." Which of the following statements reflects this technique?
   a. "How do you think you could have been a better wife?"
   b. "Okay, you say it's all your fault. Let's discuss why it might be your fault, and then we will look at why it may not be."
   c. "Let's talk about what would make you a happier person."
   d. "Would you have wanted him to stay if he didn't really want to?"

10. The therapist teaches a client that when the idea of herself as a worthless person starts to form in her mind, she should immediately start to whistle the tune of "Dixie." What cognitive therapy technique is the therapist using?
    a. Behavioral rehearsal
    b. Social skills training
    c. Distraction
    d. Generating alternatives

References

American Nurses Association (ANA), American Psychiatric Nurses Association, & International Society of Psychiatric-Mental Health Nurses. (2014). *Psychiatric-mental health nursing: Scope and standards of practice* (2nd ed.). Silver Spring, MD: ANA.

Basco, M.R., McDonald, N., Merlock, M., & Rush, A.J. (2004). A cognitive-behavioral approach to treatment of bipolar I disorder. In J.H. Wright (Ed.), *Cognitive-behavioral therapy* (pp. 25-53). Washington, DC: American Psychiatric Publishing.

Beck, A.T., Davis, D.D., & Freeman, A. (2015). *Cognitive therapy of personality disorders* (3rd ed.). New York: Guilford Press.

Beck, A.T., Rush, A.H., Shaw, B.F., & Emery, G. (1987). *Cognitive therapy of depression.* New York: Guilford Press.

Beck, A.T., & Weishaar, M.E. (2011). Cognitive therapy. In R.J. Corsini and D. Wedding (Eds.), *Current psychotherapies* (9th ed., pp. 276-309). Belmont, CA: Brooks/Cole.

Beck, J.S. (1995). *Cognitive therapy: Basics and beyond.* New York: Guilford Press.

Brenes, G.A., Danhauer, S.C., Lyles, M.F., Hogan, P.E., & Miller, M.E. (2015). Telephone-delivered cognitive behavioral therapy and telephone-delivered nondirective supportive therapy for rural older adults with generalized anxiety disorder: A randomized clinical trial. *JAMA Psychiatry, 72*(10), 1012-1020. doi: 10.1001/jamapsychiatry.2015.1154

Brent, D.A., Brunwasser, S.M., Hollon, S.D., Weersing, V.R., Clarke, G.N., Dickerson, J.F. . . . Garber, J. (2015). Effect of a cognitive-behavioral prevention program on depression 6 years after implementation among at-risk adolescents: A randomized clinical trial. *JAMA Psychiatry, 72*(11), 1110-1118. doi:10.1001/jamapsychiatry.2015.1559

Freeman-Clevenger, S.M. (2014). Cognitive behavioral therapy. In K. Wheeler (Ed.) *Psychotherapy for the advanced practice psychiatric nurse: A how-to guide for evidence-based practice* (2nd ed., pp. 313-345). New York: Springer.

Harvard Medical School. (2003). Confronting suicide—Part II. *Harvard Mental Health Letter, 19*(12), 1-5.

Guille, C., Zhao, Z., Krystal, J., Nichols, B., Brady, K., & Sen, S. (2015). Web-based cognitive behavioral therapy intervention for the prevention of suicidal ideation in medical interns: A randomized controlled trial. *JAMA Psychiatry, 72*(12), 1192-1198. doi:10.1001/jamapsychiatry.2015.1880

Rohan, K.J., Mahon, J.N., Evans, M., Ho, S.Y., Meyerhoff, J., Postolache, T.T., &Vacek, P.M. (2015). Randomized trial of cognitive-behavioral therapy versus light therapy for seasonal affective disorder: Acute outcomes. *American Journal of Psychiatry. 172*(9), 862-869. doi:10.1176/appi.ajp.2015.14101293

Sadock, B.J., Sadock, V.A., & Ruiz, P. (2015). *Synopsis of psychiatry: Behavioral sciences/clinical psychiatry* (11th ed.). Philadelphia: Lippincott Williams & Wilkins.

Wright, J.H., Thase, M.E., & Beck, A.T. (2008). Cognitive therapy. In R.E. Hales, S.C. Yudofsky, & G.O. Gabbard (Eds.), *Textbook of psychiatry* (5th ed., pp. 1211-1256). Washington, DC: American Psychiatric Publishing.

Weck, F., & Neng, J.M. (2015). Response and remission after cognitive and exposure therapy for hypochondriasis. *Journal of Nervous and Mental Disorders, 203*(11), 883-885. doi:10.1097/NMD.0000000000000385

Classical References

Beck, A.T. (1963). Thinking and depression, I. Idiosyncratic content and cognitive distortions. *Archives of General Psychiatry, 9*(4), 324-333. doi:10.1001/archpsyc.1963.01720160014002

Beck, A.T. (1964). Thinking and depression, II. Theory and therapy. *Archives of General Psychiatry, 10*(6), 561-571. doi:10.1001/archpsyc.1964.01720240015003

Lazarus, R.S., & Folkman, S. (1984). *Stress, appraisal, and coping.* New York: Springer.

20

Electroconvulsive Therapy

KEY TERMS

insulin coma therapy   pharmacoconvulsive therapy

OBJECTIVES
After reading this chapter, the student will be able to:

1. Define *electroconvulsive therapy*.
2. Discuss historical perspectives related to electroconvulsive therapy.
3. Discuss indications, contraindications, mechanism of action, and side effects of electroconvulsive therapy.
4. Identify risks associated with electroconvulsive therapy.
5. Describe the role of the nurse in the administration of electroconvulsive therapy.

HOMEWORK ASSIGNMENT
Please read the chapter and answer the following questions:

1. Mr. J. says to the nurse, "This consent form says there is a possibility of permanent memory loss with ECT. I don't want to lose my memory!" How should the nurse respond to Mr. J.?
2. What medication is commonly given before the ECT treatment to decrease secretions?
3. Why is the client given oxygen during the procedure?

Electroconvulsive therapy (ECT) has long had a negative reputation. In the iconic depiction of this treatment in the movie *One Flew Over the Cuckoo's Nest*, it is a physically and emotionally brutal procedure imposed on unwilling clients in order to calm them. Today, ECT remains one of the most controversial treatments for psychological disorders and remains the subject of impassioned debate among various factions within both the professional and lay communities. One of the most recent debates stems from the U.S. Food and Drug Administration (FDA)'s (2016) proposed rule that categorizes ECT machines as low risk, a downgrade from their long-held high-risk classification. Critics of the procedure take offense to this proposal, with some even threatening to sue the FDA.

Despite its controversial image, ECT has been used continuously for more than 50 years, longer than any other physical treatment for mental illness. Kellner (2010) identifies that it has achieved this longevity because, when administered properly for the right illness, it can help as much as or more than any other treatment (Kellner, 2010).

This chapter explores the historical perspectives, indications and contraindications, mechanism of action, side effects, and risks associated with ECT. The role of the nurse in the care of the client receiving ECT is presented in the context of the nursing process.

Electroconvulsive Therapy, Defined

CORE CONCEPT

Electroconvulsive Therapy
The induction of a grand mal (generalized) seizure through the application of electrical current to the brain.

With ECT, seizure is induced by administering a dose of electrical current through electrodes placed either bilaterally (in the bifrontal or bifrontotemporal areas) or unilaterally on the right side of the frontotemporal area. Right unilateral ECT is associated with fewer cognitive side effects, and its efficacy can be ensured with adequate dosing strategies (Sadock, Sadock, & Ruiz, 2015). Although unilateral treatments were once conducted on the hemisphere of the nondominant hand, Sadock and associates (2015) note that the right hemisphere is involved in sustaining depressed mood regardless of handedness. The dose of electrical current is carefully controlled through the use of an ECT machine.

The amount of electrical stimulus applied is a point of controversy among clinicians. The dose of electrical stimulation must be strong enough to reach the patient's seizure threshold, but this threshold is highly variable among individuals. Further, a patient's seizure threshold may increase 25 to 200 percent during the course of ECT treatments. In this mechanism of action, ECT itself acts as an anticonvulsant because the seizure threshold increases as treatment progresses (Sadock et al., 2015).

Observing the patient for seizure activity is not always the best indicator. Movements are minimal because of the administration of a muscle relaxant before treatment. The tonic phase of the seizure usually lasts 10 to 15 seconds and may be identified by a rigid plantar extension of the feet. The clonic phase follows and is usually characterized by rhythmic movements of the muscles that decrease in frequency and finally disappear. Because of the muscle relaxant, movements may be observed merely as a rhythmic twitching of the toes. Monitoring EEG activity during the treatment provides evidence of grand mal seizure activity.

Most clients require an average of 6 to 12 treatments, but some may require up to 20 treatments (Sadock et al., 2015). Treatments are usually administered every other day, three times per week. Treatments are performed on an inpatient basis for those who require close observation and care (e.g., clients who are suicidal, agitated, delusional, catatonic, or acutely manic). Those at less risk may receive therapy at an outpatient treatment facility.

Historical Perspectives

Inducing convulsions to treat psychiatric illness was reported as early as the 16th century, although the mechanism of induction at that time was the administration of camphor. In the early 1900s, Hungarian neuropsychiatrist Ladislas Meduna observed that individuals with epilepsy had more than the average number of glial cells and that people with schizophrenia had fewer than average, sparking interest and further study into the clinical benefits of seizure induction. The first electroconvulsive therapy treatment was performed in April 1938 by Italian psychiatrists Ugo Cerletti and Lucio Bini in Rome. Other somatic therapies were tried before that time, including **insulin coma therapy** and **pharmacoconvulsive therapy.**

Insulin coma therapy was introduced by the German psychiatrist Manfred Sakel in 1933. His therapy was used for clients with schizophrenia. The insulin injection treatments induced a hypoglycemic coma, which Sakel claimed was effective in alleviating schizophrenic symptoms. This therapy required vigorous medical and nursing intervention through the stages of induced coma. Some fatalities occurred when clients failed to respond to efforts directed at termination of the coma. The efficacy of insulin coma therapy has been questioned, and its use has been discontinued in the treatment of mental illness.

Pharmacoconvulsive therapy was introduced in Budapest in 1934 by Ladislas Meduna (Fink, 2009). He induced convulsions with intramuscular injections of camphor in oil in clients with schizophrenia. He based his treatment on clinical observation and theorized the existence of a biological antagonism between schizophrenia and epilepsy. Thus, by inducing seizures he hoped to reduce schizophrenic symptoms. Because he discovered that camphor was unreliable for inducing seizures, he began using pentylenetetrazol (Metrazol). Some successes were reported in terms of reduction of psychotic symptoms, and until the advent of ECT in 1938, pentylenetetrazol was the most frequently used method for producing seizures in clients with psychosis. There was a brief resurgence of pharmacoconvulsive therapy in the late 1950s, when flurothyl (Indoklon), a potent inhalant convulsant, was introduced as an alternative for individuals who were unwilling to consent to ECT for the treatment of depression and schizophrenia. Pharmacoconvulsive therapy is no longer used in psychiatry.

Periodic recognition of the important contribution of ECT in the treatment of mental illness has been evident in the United States. An initial acceptance was observed from 1940 to 1960, followed by a 20-year period during which ECT was considered objectionable by both the psychiatric profession and the public. A second wave of acceptance began around 1980 and has been increasing to the present. The period of nonacceptability coincided with the introduction of tricyclic and monoamine oxidase inhibitor antidepressant drugs and ended with the realization among many psychiatrists that the widely heralded replacement of ECT with these chemical agents had failed to materialize (Abrams, 2002). Some individuals showed improvement with ECT after failing to respond to other forms of therapy.

Currently, an estimated 100,000 people in the United States and about 2 million people worldwide receive ECT treatments each year (Kalapatapu, 2015; Mathew, Amiel, & Sackeim, 2013). The typical client is white, female, middle aged, and from a middle- to upper-income background, receiving treatment in a private or university hospital for major depression, usually after drug therapy has proved ineffective. Largely because of the expense involved and the need for a team of highly skilled medical specialists, many public hospitals are unable to offer this service to their clients.

Indications

Major Depression

ECT has been shown to be effective in the treatment of severe depression, particularly among depressed clients who are also experiencing psychotic symptoms, catatonia, psychomotor retardation, and neurovegetative changes, such as disturbances in sleep, appetite, and energy. ECT is typically considered only after a trial of therapy with antidepressant medication has proved ineffective. It may be considered the treatment of choice when the need for treatment response is urgent, such as in patients who are extremely suicidal or are refusing food and are nutritionally compromised (Kalapatapu, 2015).

Mania

ECT is indicated in the treatment of acute manic episodes and is at least as effective as lithium (Sadock et al., 2015). At present, it is rarely used for this purpose because lithium and other pharmacotherapies are so effective in the short and long term. However, ECT has been shown to be effective in the treatment of manic clients who do not tolerate or fail to respond to lithium or other drug treatment or when life is threatened by dangerous behavior or exhaustion. ECT should not be used while a patient is receiving lithium because lithium lowers the seizure threshold and may cause prolonged seizures when combined with ECT (Sadock et al., 2015).

Recent evidence has supported the use of ECT in the treatment of bipolar disorders with mixed states (concurrent depressive and manic features). This is especially beneficial, since this type of bipolar disorder is often more severe than other types, with lower interepisode remission and higher risk for suicide (Palma et al., 2016). Nonetheless, it is still used only when the patient has failed to respond to medication.

Schizophrenia

ECT can induce a remission in some clients who present with acute schizophrenia, particularly those who have marked positive, catatonic, or affective (depression or mania) symptomatology (Sadock et al., 2015). It does not appear to be of value to individuals with chronic schizophrenic illness.

Other Conditions

ECT has been reported as useful in episodic psychosis, atypical psychosis, obsessive-compulsive disorder, delirium, and medical conditions such as neuroleptic malignant syndrome, hypopituitarism, intractable seizure disorders, and Parkinson's disease, particularly when there is comorbid depression (Kalapatapu, 2015; Sadock et al., 2015). For pregnant women and elderly individuals who are unable to take medication, ECT may be a safer alternative. Oztav and associates (2015) reported that although the literature on safety of ECT in pregnancy is scarce, their research supported others' findings that it can be used safely. They also note that 40 percent of pregnant patients treated with ECT in their study demonstrated full recovery. ECT is not effective in somatization disorders (unless there is comorbid depression), personality disorders, and anxiety disorders (Sadock et al., 2015).

Contraindications

There are no absolute contraindications for ECT. However, some patients may be considered at higher risk for adverse events that require attention and closer monitoring (Black & Andreasen, 2014; Eisendrath &

Lichtmacher, 2013; Sadock et al., 2015). High-risk conditions are largely cardiovascular and include myocardial infarction or cerebrovascular accident within the preceding 3 to 6 months, aortic or cerebral aneurysm, severe underlying hypertension, and congestive heart failure. Clients with cardiovascular problems are placed at risk because of the body's response to the seizure itself. The initial vagal response results in a sinus bradycardia and drop in blood pressure. This is followed immediately by tachycardia and a hypertensive response. These changes can be life threatening to an individual with an already compromised cardiovascular system.

Patients with intracranial lesions may be at risk for edema or brain herniation after ECT, but these risks can be decreased by pretreatment with dexamethasone in cases in which the lesion is small (Sadock et al., 2015). Patients with increased intracranial pressure are at increased risk related to increased cerebral blood flow during seizures, but Sadock and associates (2015) note that risk can be lessened by controlling the patient's blood pressure during the treatment.

Other factors that place clients at risk during ECT include severe osteoporosis, acute and chronic pulmonary disorders, and high-risk or complicated pregnancy. Because oxytocin levels increase after ECT, there is an increased risk of intrauterine contractions and premature birth with an incidence of around 3 to 6 percent (Oztav et al., 2015).

Mechanism of Action

Both therapeutic and adverse effects may result from inducing a bilateral generalized seizure, but the exact mechanism by which ECT effects a therapeutic response is unknown. Many parts of the central nervous system are affected by ECT, including hormones, neuropeptides, neurotrophic factors, and nearly every neurotransmitter (Kalapatapu, 2015). Affected neurotransmitters include serotonin, norepinephrine, and dopamine, the same biogenic amines that are affected by antidepressant drugs. Research studies on serotonin, however, have yielded such mixed results that their impact in the efficacy of ECT remains controversial (Sadock et al., 2015). Other possible mechanisms of action, based on changes that occur during ECT, include an increase of GABA transmission and an increase of endogenous opioids, both of which may raise the seizure threshold (Kalapatapu, 2015).

Several recent studies have identified an increase in gray matter, particularly in the hippocampal and amygdala areas, following ECT (Depping et al., 2016; Pirnia et al., 2016; Sartorius et al., 2015). Because these areas of the brain show a decrease in volume in major depression, the study findings are being looked at with interest as an indication of neuroplasticity and the neurorestorative effects of ECT.

One recent study revealed that the therapeutic response from ECT may be related to the modulation of white matter microstructure in pathways connecting frontal and limbic areas, which are altered in major depression (Lyden et al., 2014). The results of studies relating to the mechanism underlying the effectiveness of ECT are still ongoing and continue to bear mixed results. It may be a complex dynamic of several effects interacting with one another.

Side Effects

The most common side effects of ECT are temporary memory loss and confusion. Critics of the therapy argue that these changes represent irreversible brain damage. Proponents insist they are temporary and reversible. In one recent study that looked at long-term outcomes of ECT in clients with bipolar I disorder (Haghighi et al., 2016), the evidence supported that 2 years following ECT, cognitive skills and short-term memory were not impaired, while mood symptom recurrence had improved regardless of the level of mania. It has been argued that bilateral electrode placement may be more effective than right unilateral (RUL) placement but is associated with more cognitive side effects. However, evidence supports that a more aggressive stimulus in RUL placement improves its efficacy (Pulia et al., 2013).

Risks Associated With Electroconvulsive Therapy

Mortality

In 2011, the American Psychiatric Nurses Association (APNA) advanced a position statement in support of ECT for "severe depression that has been shown to be refractory to medication administration" (American Psychiatric Nurses Association, 2015). The APNA cites a mortality rate less than that of childbirth. Studies indicate that the mortality rate from ECT is about 0.002 percent per treatment and 0.01 percent for each patient (Sadock et al., 2015). Although the occurrence is rare, the major cause of death with ECT is from cardiovascular complications (e.g., acute myocardial infarction or cerebrovascular accident), usually in individuals with previously compromised cardiac status. Assessment and management of cardiovascular disease *prior* to treatment is vital in the reduction of morbidity and mortality rates associated with ECT.

Memory Loss

Memory impairment almost always occurs to some degree during the course of ECT treatments, but follow-up studies indicate that most patients return to their cognitive baselines after 6 months (Sadock et al., 2015). Some clients do report persistent memory impairment, and in most cases, this impairment occurs among patients who showed little improvement with ECT (Sadock et al., 2015).

Sackeim and associates (2007) reported on the results of a longitudinal study of clinical and cognitive outcomes in patients with major depression treated with ECT at seven facilities in the New York City metropolitan area. Participants were evaluated shortly following the ECT course and 6 months later. Data revealed that cognitive deficits at the 6-month interval were directly related to type of electrode placement and electrical waveform used. Bilateral electrode placement resulted in more severe and persisting (as evaluated at the 6-month follow-up) retrograde amnesia than unilateral placement. The extent of the amnesia was directly related to the number of ECT treatments received. The researchers also found that stimulation produced by sine wave (continuous) current resulted in greater short- and long-term deficits than that produced by short-pulse wave (intermittent) current.

Black and Andreasen (2014) suggested that all clients receiving ECT should be informed of the possibility for some degree of permanent memory loss. Although the potential for these effects appears to be minimal, the client must be made aware of the risks involved before consenting to treatment.

Brain Damage

The question of brain damage secondary to ECT treatments has been advanced as a concern by critics of the procedure. The subject has been studied using a variety of brain imaging modalities, and virtually all conclude there is no evidence of brain damage caused by ECT treatments (McClintock & Husain, 2011; Sadock et al., 2015). Previously cited studies on the neurorestorative effects of ECT have argued that this, too, is evidence in contradiction to ideas about brain-damaging effects of ECT.

The Role of the Nurse in Electroconvulsive Therapy

Nurses play an integral role in education and preparation for and administration of ECT. They provide support before, during, and after the treatment to the client and family and assist the medical professionals who are conducting the therapy. The nursing process provides a systematic approach to the provision of care for the client receiving ECT.

Assessment

A complete physical examination must be conducted by the appropriate medical professional prior to the initiation of ECT. This evaluation should include a thorough assessment of cardiovascular and pulmonary status as well as laboratory blood and urine studies. A skeletal history and x-ray assessment should also be considered.

The nurse may be responsible for ensuring that informed consent has been obtained from the client. "No patient who has the capacity to give voluntary consent should be given ECT without his or her written consent" and clinicians should be aware of local, state, and federal laws governing the use of ECT (Kalapatapu, 2015). If the depression is severe, the client is clearly unable to consent to the procedure, and relevant laws allow it, permission may be obtained from family or another legally responsible individual. Consent is secured only after the client or responsible individual acknowledges understanding of the procedure, including possible side effects and potential risks involved.

 Client and family must also understand that ECT is voluntary and that consent may be withdrawn at any time (American Psychiatric Association, 2001; Fetterman & Ying, 2011; Vera, 2012). This kind of education supports patient-centered care.

Nurses may also be required to assess the following:

- The client's mood and level of interaction with others
- Evidence of suicidal ideation, plan, and means
- Level of anxiety and fears associated with receiving ECT
- Thought and communication patterns
- Baseline memory for short- and long-term events
- Client and family knowledge of indications for, side effects of, and potential risks associated with ECT
- Current and past use of medications
- Baseline vital signs and history of allergies
- The client's ability to carry out activities of daily living

Diagnosis and Outcome Identification

Selection of appropriate nursing diagnoses for the client undergoing ECT is based on continual assessment before, during, and after treatment. Selected potential nursing diagnoses with outcome criteria for evaluation are presented in Table 20–1.

Planning and Implementation

ECT treatments are usually performed in the morning. The client is given nothing by mouth (NPO) for 6 to 8 hours before the treatment. Some institutional policies require that the client be placed on NPO status at midnight prior to the treatment day. The treatment team routinely consists of the psychiatrist, anesthesiologist, and two or more nurses.

Nursing interventions before the treatment include

- Ensuring that the physician and the anesthesiologist have obtained informed consent and that a signed permission form is on the chart.

TABLE 20–1 **Potential Nursing Diagnoses and Outcome Criteria for Client Receiving ECT**	
NURSING DIAGNOSES	OUTCOME CRITERIA
Anxiety (moderate to severe) related to impending therapy	Client verbalizes a decrease in anxiety following explanation of procedure and expression of fears.
Deficient knowledge related to necessity for and side effects or risks of ECT	Client verbalizes understanding of need for and side effects/risks of ECT following explanation.
Risk for injury related to risks associated with ECT	Client undergoes treatment without sustaining injury.
Risk for aspiration related to altered level of consciousness immediately following treatment	Client experiences no aspiration during ECT.
Decreased cardiac output related to vagal stimulation occurring during the ECT	Client demonstrates adequate tissue perfusion during and after treatment (absence of cyanosis or severe change in mental status).
Impaired memory/acute confusion related to side effects of ECT	Client maintains reality orientation following ECT treatment.
Self-care deficit related to incapacitation during postictal stage	Client's self-care needs are fulfilled at all times.
Risk for activity intolerance related to post-ECT confusion and memory loss	Client gradually increases participation in therapeutic activities to the highest level of personal capability.

■ Ensuring that the most recent laboratory reports (complete blood count, urinalysis) and results of electrocardiogram (ECG) and x-ray examination are available.

■ Approximately 1 hour before treatment is scheduled, taking and recording vital signs. Have the client void and remove dentures, eyeglasses or contact lenses, jewelry, and hairpins. Following institutional requirements, the client should change into hospital gown or, if permitted, into his or her own loose clothing or pajamas. At this point, it is best for the client to remain in bed. Side rails may be raised unless prohibited by institutional policy or assessed as unsafe for the individual client.

■ Approximately 30 minutes before treatment, administering the pretreatment medication as prescribed by the physician. The usual order is for atropine sulfate or glycopyrrolate (Robinul) given intramuscularly. Either of these medications may be ordered to decrease secretions (to prevent aspiration) and counteract the effects of vagal stimulation (bradycardia) induced by the ECT.

■ Staying with the client to help allay fears and anxiety. Maintain a positive attitude about the procedure, and encourage the client to verbalize feelings.

In the treatment room, the client is placed on the treatment table in a supine position, and the anesthesiologist intravenously administers a short-acting anesthetic. The two most commonly used anesthetic agents for ECT in the United States are methohexital and propofol (Kellner & Bryson, 2012). Some studies have identified methohexital (Brevital) as preferable because it increases the duration of the seizure (Pulia et al., 2013) and because of its established safety record, effectiveness, and low cost (Kalapatapu, 2015). The duration of the seizure is significant only in the sense that if it is less than 20 seconds, restimulation may be required to achieve a fully generalized seizure. Restimulation may be associated with an increase in cognitive side effects (Pulia et al., 2013). A muscle relaxant, usually succinylcholine chloride, is given intravenously to prevent severe muscle contractions during the seizure, thereby reducing the possibility of fractured or dislocated bones. Because succinylcholine paralyzes respiratory muscles as well, the client is oxygenated with pure oxygen during and after the treatment, except for the brief interval of electrical stimulation, until spontaneous respirations return (Kellner & Bryson, 2012). A blood pressure cuff may be placed on the lower leg and inflated above systolic pressure prior to the injection of the succinylcholine. This is to ensure that the seizure activity can be observed in one limb that is unaffected by the muscle relaxant.

An airway/bite block is placed in the client's mouth, and he or she is positioned to facilitate airway patency. Electrodes are placed (either bilaterally or unilaterally) on the temples to deliver the electrical stimulation.

Nursing interventions during the treatment include

■ Ensuring patency of airway. Provide suctioning if needed.

■ Assisting anesthesiologist with oxygenation as required.

- Observing readouts on machines monitoring vital signs and cardiac functioning.
- Providing support to the client's arms and legs during the seizure.
- Observing and recording the type and amount of movement induced by the seizure.

After the treatment, the anesthesiologist continues to oxygenate the client with pure oxygen until spontaneous respirations return. Most clients awaken within 10 or 15 minutes of the treatment and are confused and disoriented; however, some clients will sleep for 1 to 2 hours following the treatment. All clients require close observation in this immediate posttreatment period.

Nursing interventions in the posttreatment period include

- Monitoring pulse, respirations, and blood pressure every 15 minutes for the first hour, during which time the client should remain in bed.
- Positioning the client on side to prevent aspiration.
- Orienting the client to time and place.
- Describing what has occurred.
- Providing reassurance that confusion and memory loss will subside and memories should return following the course of ECT therapy.
- Allowing the client to verbalize fears and anxieties related to receiving ECT.
- Staying with the client until he or she is fully awake, oriented, and able to perform self-care activities without assistance.
- Providing the client with a highly structured schedule of routine activities in order to minimize confusion.

Evaluation

Evaluation of the effectiveness of nursing interventions is based on the achievement of the projected outcomes. Reassessment may be based on answers to the following questions:

- Was the client's anxiety maintained at a manageable level?
- Was the client/family teaching completed satisfactorily?
- Did the client/family verbalize understanding of the procedure, its side effects, and risks involved?
- Did the client undergo treatment without experiencing injury or aspiration?
- Has the client maintained adequate tissue perfusion during and following treatment? Have vital signs remained stable?
- With consideration to the individual client's condition and response to treatment, is the client reoriented to time, place, and situation?
- Have all of the client's self-care needs been fulfilled?

- Is the client participating in therapeutic activities to his or her maximum potential?
- What is the client's level of social interaction?

Careful documentation is an important part of the evaluation process. Some routine observations may be evaluated on flow sheets specifically identified for ECT. However, progress notes with detailed descriptions of client behavioral changes are essential to evaluate improvement and help determine the number of treatments that will be administered. Continual reassessment, planning, and evaluation ensure that the client receives adequate and appropriate nursing care throughout the course of therapy. In some cases, maintenance ECT (either weekly, biweekly, or monthly) is recommended and has been reported as effective for relapse prevention, although more evidence is needed to support the benefits of this practice (Sadock et al., 2015). Other brain stimulation treatments, such as transcranial magnetic stimulation, cranial electrical stimulation, magnetic seizure therapy, and vagal nerve stimulation, provide alternatives that may also be beneficial in treatment-resistant cases, but more research is needed to clearly identify effectiveness and best practices for their use.

 Studies such as one previously cited (Pulia et al., 2013) found that changes in anesthetic agent (from propofol to methohexital) and increasing the dose of electric stimulus demonstrated improvements in the quality of their ECT procedures and efficacy. Pulia, the nurse involved in the research, highlights the active role that nurses can play when collaborating with other members of the health-care team to pursue quality improvement.

Summary and Key Points

- ECT is the induction of a grand mal seizure through the application of electrical current to the brain.
- ECT is a safe and effective treatment alternative for individuals with depression, mania, or schizoaffective disorder who do not respond to other forms of therapy.
- There are no absolute contraindications for ECT, but some conditions have associated increased risks and require close monitoring and attention. Individuals with cardiovascular problems are at high risk for complications from ECT. Increased intracranial pressure and intracranial lesions impose higher risks for adverse events.
- Other factors that place clients at risk include severe osteoporosis, acute and chronic pulmonary disorders, and high-risk or complicated pregnancy.
- The exact mechanism of action of ECT is unknown, but there are multiple effects on central

nervous system activity, including hormones, neuropeptides, neurotrophic factors, and nearly every neurotransmitter. Studies demonstrating an increase in gray matter, particularly in the hippocampal and amygdala areas, suggest neuroplasticity and a possibly neurorestorative effect of ECT.

■ The most common side effects with ECT are temporary memory loss and confusion.

■ Although it is rare, death must be considered a risk associated with ECT. When it does occur, the most common cause is cardiovascular complications.

■ There is virtually no evidence supporting the idea that ECT causes permanent brain damage.

■ The nurse assists with ECT using the steps of the nursing process before, during, and after treatment.

■ Important nursing interventions include ensuring client safety, managing client anxiety, and providing adequate client education.

■ Nursing input into the ongoing evaluation of client behavior is an important factor in determining the therapeutic effectiveness of ECT.

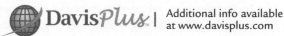

DavisPlus | Additional info available at www.davisplus.com

Review Questions
Self-Examination/Learning Exercise

Select the answer that is most appropriate for each of the following questions.

1. Electroconvulsive therapy is most commonly prescribed for which of the following?
   a. Bipolar disorder, manic
   b. Paranoid schizophrenia
   c. Major depression
   d. Obsessive-compulsive disorder

2. Which of the following best describes the average number of ECT treatments given and the timing of administration?
   a. One treatment per month for 6 to 12 months
   b. One treatment every other day, three times a week for a total of 6 to 12 treatments
   c. One treatment three times per week for 6 to 12 months
   d. One treatment every day for a total of 10 to 20 treatments

3. Which of the following conditions increases the risk of adverse events associated with ECT? (Select all that apply.)
   a. Increased intracranial pressure
   b. Recent myocardial infarction
   c. Severe underlying hypertension
   d. Congestive heart failure
   e. Breast cancer

4. A patient has been ordered ECT and asks the nurse, "Exactly how does ECT work?" Which of the following is the most accurate response by the nurse?
   a. "I'm not allowed to tell you that because that would be informed consent."
   b. "The exact mechanism is unknown, but there are several ways that ECT may have antidepressant effects."
   c. "The administration of a shock to the brain induces memory loss, which will make you forget you are depressed."
   d. "The neuroplasticity affected by seizure activity prevents further brain damage."

5. The most common side effects of ECT are:
   a. Permanent memory loss and brain damage.
   b. Fractured and dislocated bones.
   c. Myocardial infarction and cardiac arrest.
   d. Temporary memory loss and confusion.

Continued

Review Questions—cont'd
Self-Examination/Learning Exercise

6. Sam has a diagnosis of major depression. After an unsuccessful trial of antidepressant medication, Sam's physician has hospitalized him for a course of ECT treatments. Sam says to the nurse on admission, "I don't want to end up like McMurphy in *One Flew Over the Cuckoo's Nest!* I'm scared!" What is Sam's priority nursing diagnosis at this time?
   a. Anxiety related to deficient knowledge about ECT
   b. Risk for injury related to risks associated with ECT
   c. Deficient knowledge related to negative media presentation of ECT
   d. Acute confusion related to side effects of ECT

7. Sam, who has been hospitalized for ECT treatments, says to the nurse on admission, "I don't want to end up like McMurphy in *One Flew Over the Cuckoo's Nest!* I'm scared!" Which of the following statements would be most appropriate by the nurse in response to Sam's expression of concern?
   a. "I guarantee you won't end up like McMurphy, Sam."
   b. "The doctor knows what he is doing. There's nothing to worry about."
   c. "I know you are scared, Sam, and we're going to talk about what you can expect from the therapy."
   d. "I'm going to stay with you as long as you are scared."

8. What is the priority nursing intervention before starting ECT therapy?
   a. Take vital signs and record.
   b. Have the patient void.
   c. Administer succinylcholine.
   d. Ensure that the consent form has been signed.

9. Atropine sulfate is administered to a client receiving ECT for what purpose?
   a. To alleviate anxiety
   b. To decrease secretions
   c. To relax muscles
   d. As a short-acting anesthetic

10. Succinylcholine is administered to a client receiving ECT for what purpose?
    a. To alleviate anxiety
    b. To decrease secretions
    c. To relax muscles
    d. As a short-acting anesthetic

References

Abrams, R. (2002). *Electroconvulsive therapy* (4th ed.). New York: Oxford University Press.

American Psychiatric Association (APA). (2001). *The practice of electroconvulsive therapy: Recommendations for treatment, training, and privileging* (2nd ed.). Washington, DC: APA.

American Psychiatric Nurses Association. (2015). *APNA position statement: Electroconvulsive therapy.* Retrieved from www.apna. org/i4a/pages/index.cfm?pageid=4448

Black, D.W., & Andreasen, N.C. (2014). *Introductory textbook of psychiatry* (6th ed.). Washington, DC: American Psychiatric Publishing.

Depping, M.S., Nolte, H.M., Hirjak, D., & Thoman, P.A. (2016). Cerebellar volume change in response to electroconvulsive therapy in patients with major depression. *Progress in Neuro-Psychopharmacology and Biological Psychiatry.* doi:10.1016/j.pnpbp.2016.09.007

Eisendrath, S.J., & Lichtmacher, J.E. (2013). Psychiatric disorders. In M.A. Papadakis & S.J. McPhee (Eds.), *Current medical diagnosis & treatment* (52nd ed., pp. 1038-1092). New York: McGraw-Hill.

Fetterman, T.C., & Ying, P. (2011). Informed consent and electroconvulsive therapy. *Journal of the American Psychiatric Nurses Association, 17*(3), 219-222. doi:10.1177/1078390311408604

Food and Drug Administration (FDA). (2016). *Electroconvulsive therapy (ECT) devices for class II intended uses: Draft guidance for industry, clinicians and food and drug administration staff.* Retrieved from https://www.fda.gov/downloads/MedicalDevices/.../UCM478942.pdf

Fink, M. (2009). *Electroconvulsive therapy.* New York: Oxford University Press.

Haghighi, M., Barikani, R., Jahangarda, L., Ahmeadpanaha, M., Bajoghli, H., Sadeghi Bahmani, D. . . . Brand, S. (2016). Levels of mania and cognitive performance two years after ECT in patients with bipolar I disorder—Results from a follow-up study. *Comprehensive Psychiatry, 69*(2016), 71-77. doi:http://dx.doi.org/10.1016/j.comppsych.2016.05.009

Kalapatapu, R. K. (2015). Electroconvulsive therapy. *Medscape.* Retrieved from http://emedicine.medscape.com/article/1525957-overview#a1

Kellner, C.H. (2010). Speed of response to ECT. *Psychiatric Times, 27*(5). Retrieved from www.psychiatrictimes.com/display/article/10168/1567001

Kellner, C.H., & Bryson, E.O. (2012). Anesthesia advances add to safety of ECT. *Psychiatric Times, 29*(1). Retrieved from www.psychiatrictimes.com/display/article/10168/2013636

Lyden, H., Espinoza, R.T., Pirnia, T., Clark, K., Joshi, S.H., Leaver, A.M., Woods, R.P., & Narr, K.L. (2014). Electroconvulsive therapy mediates neuroplasticity of white matter microstructure in major depression. *Translational Psychiatry, 4*(4), e380. doi:10.1038/tp.2014.21

Mathew, S.J., Amiel, J.M., & Sackeim, H.A. (2013). Electroconvulsive therapy in treatment-resistant depression. *Psychiatry Weekly.* Retrieved from www.psychweekly.com/aspx/article/article_pf.aspx?articleid=52

McClintock, S.M., & Husain, M.M. (2011). Electroconvulsive therapy does not damage the brain. *Journal of the American Psychiatric Nurses Association, 17*(3), 212-213. doi:10.1177/1078390311407667

Oztav, T., Arslan, M., Corekcioglu, S., Oflezer, C., Canbek, O., & Kurt, E. (2015). Safety of electroconvulsive therapy in pregnancy. *Journal of Mood Disorders, 5*(2), 47-52. doi:10.5455/jmood.20140811124733

Palma, M., Ferreira, B., Borja-Santos, N., Trancas, B., Monteiro, C., & Cardoso, G. (2016). Efficacy of electroconvulsive therapy in bipolar disorder with mixed features. *Depression Research and Treatment, 2016.* doi:http://dx.doi.org/10.1155/2016/8306071

Pirnia, T., Josh, S.H., Leaver, A., & Narr, K. (2016). Electroconvulsive therapy and structural neuroplasticity in neocortical, limbic and paralimbic cortex. *Translational Psychiatry, 6*(6). doi:10.1038/tp.2016.102

Pulia, K., Vaidya, P., Jayaram, G., Hayat, M.J., & Reti, I.M. (2013). ECT treatment outcomes following performance improvement changes. *Journal of Psychosocial Nursing and Mental Health Services, 51*(11), 20-25. doi:10.3928/02793695-20130628-02

Sackeim, H.A., Prudic, J., Fuller, R., Keilp, J., Lavori, P.W., & Olfson, M. (2007). The cognitive effects of electroconvulsive therapy in community settings. *Neuropsychopharmacology, 32*(1), 244-254. doi:10.1038/sj.npp.1301180

Sadock, B.J., Sadock, V.A., & Ruiz, P. (2015). *Synopsis of psychiatry: Behavioral sciences/clinical psychiatry* (11th ed.). Philadelphia: Lippincott Williams & Wilkins.

Sartorius, A., Boehringer, A., Demirakca, J., & Ende, G. (2015). Electroconvulsive therapy increases temporal gray matter volume and cortical thickness. *European Neuropsychopharmacology, 26*(3), 506-517. doi:10.1016/j.euroneuro.2015.12.036

Vera, M. (2012). Nursing notes: Electroconvulsive therapy. Retrieved from http://nurseslabs.com/electroconvulsive-therapy-nursing-care

21 The Recovery Model

KEY TERMS

hope   Tidal Model   Psychological Recovery Model
purpose   WRAP Model

OBJECTIVES
After reading this chapter, the student will be able to:

1. Define *recovery*.
2. Discuss the 10 guiding principles of recovery as delineated by the Substance Abuse and Mental Health Services Administration.
3. Describe three models of recovery: Tidal Model, WRAP Model, and Psychological Recovery Model.
4. Identify nursing interventions to assist individuals with mental illness in the process of recovery.

HOMEWORK ASSIGNMENT
Please read the chapter and answer the following questions:

1. What is the basic concept of a recovery model?
2. How is recovery supported by peer groups?
3. What is the focus of the Tidal Model of Recovery?
4. What is the intended outcome in the Psychological Recovery Model?

For many years, the belief was that individuals with mental illnesses do not recover. Optimistically, the course of the illness was viewed in terms of maintenance, and pessimistically, with the expectation for deterioration. The medical model has primarily focused on treatment of symptoms, largely with psychotropic medications, but as Jacobs (2015) notes, in spite of these available treatments, people with severe mental illness "continue to have residual positive symptoms, negative symptoms and marked cognitive deficits" and as a result have difficulty "getting their lives back on track." But research suggests that striving for and achieving recovery is in fact realistic for many individuals. While critics of the recovery model argue that it is in contradiction to the scientific medical model, other literature highlights the complementary and integrative potential of both models working collaboratively (Duckworth, 2015; Jacobs, 2015).

The concept of recovery is not new. It originally began in the addictions field, referring to a person recovering from a substance-related disorder. The term has more recently been adopted by mental health professionals who believe that recovery from mental illness is also possible.

CORE CONCEPT

Recovery

A process of movement toward improvement in health and quality of life.

What Is Recovery?

A number of definitions of recovery as it applies to mental illness have been proposed. The Substance Abuse and Mental Health Services Administration (SAMHSA, 2012) suggests the following:

> Recovery from mental health disorders and substance use disorders is a process of change through which individuals improve their health and wellness, live a self-directed life, and strive to reach their full potential.

Essential to understanding recovery definitions and models is the focus on recovery as an ongoing process rather than a set of interventions with a distinct endpoint.

SAMHSA suggests that a life in recovery is supported by four major dimensions:

1. **Health:** Overcoming or managing one's disease as well as living in a physically and emotionally healthy way
2. **Home:** A stable and safe place to live
3. **Purpose:** Meaningful daily activities, such as a job, school, volunteerism, family caretaking, or creative endeavors, and the independence, income, and resources to participate in society
4. **Community:** Relationships and social networks that provide support, friendship, love, and **hope.**

William A. Anthony (1993), executive director of the Center for Psychiatric Rehabilitation at Boston University, offers this definition:

> Recovery is described as a deeply personal, unique process of changing one's attitudes, values, feelings, goals, skills, and/or roles. It is a way of living a satisfying, hopeful, and contributing life even with limitations caused by illness. Recovery involves the development of new meaning and purpose in one's life as one grows beyond the catastrophic effects of mental illness. (p. 13)

The President's New Freedom Commission on Mental Health (2003) proposed to transform the mental health system by shifting the paradigm of care of persons with serious mental illness from traditional medical psychiatric treatment toward the concept of recovery, and the American Psychiatric Association has endorsed a recovery model from a psychiatric services perspective (Sharfstein, 2005).

In a systematic review and synthesis of the various approaches to what has become known as the recovery model, Leamy and associates (2011) identified five recovery processes that form a common foundation for this model: connectedness, hope, optimism about the future, identity, meaning in life, and empowerment. The consumer is empowered to take primary control over decisions about his or her own care. The National Association of Social Workers (NASW, 2006) states, "Consumers need to be as fully informed as possible about the potential benefits and consequences of each decision. They also need to know the possible results if they become a danger to themselves or others."

Guiding Principles of Recovery

As part of its Recovery Support Strategic Initiative, a year-long effort by SAMHSA and a wide range of partners in the behavioral health-care community and other fields, a working definition of recovery from mental health and substance use disorders (previously stated) was developed. In addition, guiding principles that support the recovery definition were delineated. These principles include the following (SAMHSA, 2012):

■ **Recovery emerges from hope:** The belief that recovery is real provides the essential and motivating message of a better future—that people can and do overcome the internal and external challenges, barriers, and obstacles that confront them. Hope is internalized and can be fostered by peers, families, providers, allies, and others. Hope is the catalyst of the recovery process.

■ **Recovery is person driven:** Self-determination and self-direction are the foundations for recovery as individuals define their own life goals and design their unique paths toward those goals. Individuals optimize their autonomy and independence to the greatest extent possible by leading, controlling, and exercising choice over the services and supports that assist their recovery and resilience. In so doing, they are empowered and provided the resources to make informed decisions, initiate recovery, build on their strengths, and gain or regain control over their lives.

■ **Recovery occurs via many pathways:** Individuals are unique with distinct needs, strengths, preferences, goals, culture, and backgrounds (including trauma experiences) that affect and determine their pathways to recovery. Recovery is built on the multiple capacities, strengths, talents, coping abilities, resources, and inherent value of each individual. Recovery pathways are highly personalized. They may include professional clinical treatment, use of medications, support from families and in schools, faith-based approaches, peer support, and other approaches. Recovery is nonlinear, characterized by continual growth and improved functioning that may involve setbacks. Because setbacks are a natural, though not inevitable, part of the recovery process, it is essential to foster resilience for all individuals and families. Abstinence is the safest approach for those with substance use disorders. Use of tobacco and nonprescribed or illicit drugs is not safe for anyone. In some cases, recovery pathways can be enabled by creating a supportive environment. This is especially true for children, who may not have the legal or developmental capacity to set their own course.

■ **Recovery is holistic:** Recovery encompasses an individual's whole life, including mind, body, spirit, and community. This holistic view includes addressing self-care practices, family, housing, employment, education, clinical treatment for mental and substance use disorders, services and supports, primary health care, dental care, complementary and alternative services, faith, spirituality, creativity, social networks, transportation, and community participation. The array of services and supports available should be integrated and coordinated.

■ **Recovery is supported by peers and allies:** Mutual support and mutual aid groups, including the sharing of experiential knowledge and skills as well as social learning, play an invaluable role in recovery. Peers encourage and engage other peers and provide each other with a vital sense of belonging, supportive relationships, valued roles, and community. Through helping others and giving back to the community, one helps oneself, too. Peer-operated supports and services provide important resources to assist people along their journeys of recovery and wellness. In addictions recovery, peer support has long been recognized as foundational, especially in 12-step programs such as Alcoholics Anonymous. In mental health treatment, although formal peer support is a newer approach, the premises are similar. These individuals, sometimes called *peer support specialists,* may be trained and/or certified in supportive skills but all share the experience of living with mental illness and, as such, can provide a unique perspective for support and trust in ongoing relationships. In a fully implemented recovery model, peer support specialists should be considered equal members of the treatment team (Getty, 2015). Professionals can also play an important role in the recovery process by providing clinical treatment and other services that support individuals in their chosen recovery paths. While peers and allies play an important role for many in recovery, their role for children and youth may be slightly different. Peer supports for families are very important for children with behavioral health problems and can also play a supportive role for youth in recovery.

■ **Recovery is supported through relationships and social networks:** An important factor in the recovery process is the presence and involvement of people who believe in the person's ability to recover; who offer hope, support, and encouragement; and who suggest strategies and resources for change. Family members, peers, providers, faith groups, community members, and other allies form vital support networks. Through these relationships, people leave unhealthy and/or unfulfilling life roles behind and engage in new roles (e.g., partner, caregiver, friend, student, employee) that lead to a greater sense of belonging, personhood, empowerment, autonomy, social inclusion, and community participation.

■ **Recovery is culturally based and influenced:** "Characteristics such as race or ethnicity, religion, low socioeconomic status, gender, age, mental health, disability, sexual orientation or gender identity, geographic location, or other characteristics historically linked to exclusion or discrimination are known to influence health status" (SAMHSA, 2015). The diverse representations of culture and cultural background (including values, traditions, and beliefs) are keys to determining a person's journey and unique pathway to recovery. Further, SAMHSA (2015) clarifies that "what may work for adults in recovery may be very different for youth or older adults in recovery. For example, the promotion of resiliency in young people, and the nature of social supports, peer mentors, and recovery coaching for adolescents and transitional age youth are different than recovery support services for adults and older adults." Services should be culturally grounded, attuned, sensitive, congruent, and competent, as well as personalized to meet each individual's unique needs.

■ **Recovery is supported by addressing trauma:** The experience of trauma (such as physical or sexual abuse, domestic violence, war, disaster, and other events) is often a precursor to or associated with alcohol and drug use, mental health problems, and related issues. Services and supports should be trauma informed to foster safety (physical and emotional) and trust and should promote choice, empowerment, and collaboration.

■ **Recovery involves individual, family, and community strengths and responsibility:** Individuals, families, and communities have strengths and resources that serve as a foundation for recovery. In addition, individuals have personal responsibility for their own self-care and journeys of recovery and should be supported in speaking for themselves. Families and significant others have responsibilities to support their loved ones, especially children and youth in recovery. Communities have responsibilities to provide opportunities and resources to address discrimination and to foster social inclusion and recovery. Individuals in recovery also have a social responsibility and should have the ability to join with peers to speak collectively about their strengths, needs, wants, desires, and aspirations.

■ **Recovery is based on respect:** Community, systems, and societal acceptance and appreciation for people affected by mental health and substance use problems—including protecting their rights and eliminating discrimination—are crucial in achieving recovery. There is a need to acknowledge that taking steps toward recovery may require great courage. Self-acceptance, developing a positive and meaningful sense of identity, and regaining belief in one's self are particularly important.

The recovery model integrates services provided by professionals (e.g., medication, therapy, case management), services provided by consumers (e.g., advocacy, peer support programs, hotlines, mentoring), and services provided in collaboration (e.g., recovery education, crisis planning, community integration, consumer rights education) (Jacobson & Greenley, 2001). Jacobson and Greenley state:

> Although many of these services may sound similar to services currently being offered in many mental health systems, it is important to recognize that no service is recovery-oriented unless it incorporates the attitude that recovery is possible and has the goal of promoting hope, healing, empowerment, and connection. (p. 485)

The concepts of consumer-driven care and empowerment are closely related to the concept of patient-centered care that has been advanced by the Institute of Medicine (2003) (now the National Academy of Medicine) as one of the key elements to improving the quality of health care in the future. As this cultural shift evolves, nurses will need to be thoughtful about language and attitudes that support patient-centered recovery models. For example, a traditional goal for a patient has been described as, "Patient will comply with prescribed medication regime." In a patient-centered

recovery model, a more appropriate goal might be stated as, "Patient will discuss preferences, advantages, and disadvantages of psychotropic medication in the management of his or her illness."

Models of Recovery

There are many evidence-based models of recovery. SAMHSA lists these in a database at the National Registry for Evidence-Based Programs and Practices (www.nrepp.samhsa.gov). Three of these models, the Tidal Model, the Wellness Action Recovery Plan (WRAP), and the Psychological Recovery Model, are discussed in this chapter.

The Tidal Model

The **Tidal Model** was developed in the late 1990s by Phil Barker and Poppy Buchanan-Barker of Newcastle, United Kingdom. It is a mental health nursing recovery model that may be used as the basis for interdisciplinary mental health care (Barker & Buchanan-Barker, 2012). The authors use the power of metaphor to engage with the person in distress. The metaphor of *water* is used to describe how individuals in distress can become emotionally, physically, and spiritually *shipwrecked* (Barker & Buchanan-Barker, 2005). The Tidal Model was the first recovery model to be developed by nurses in practice, drawing largely on nursing research, and in collaboration with users and consumers of mental health services (Barker & Buchanan-Barker, 2005; Brookes, 2006).

The Tidal Model uses a person-centered approach to help people deal with their problems of human living. Focus is on the individual's personal story, which is where his or her problems first appeared and where any growth, benefit, or recovery will be found (Barker & Buchanan-Barker, 2000).

Barker and Buchanan-Barker (2005) developed a set of essential values upon which the model is based. These values, which they call the *10 Tidal Commitments,* provide practitioners with a philosophical focus for empowering people to make their own life changes rather than health-care professionals trying to manage or control "patient symptoms" (Buchanan-Barker & Barker, 2008). From these commitments, the authors developed the following Tidal Competencies, which reflect the ways the commitments are practiced in the clinical setting:

1. **Value the voice:** The person is encouraged to tell his or her story. "The person's story represents the beginning and endpoint of the helping encounter, embracing not only an account of the person's distress, but also the hope for its resolution" (p. 95). Practitioner competencies include a capacity to actively listen to the person's story

and to help the person record the story in his or her own words.

2. **Respect the language:** Individuals are encouraged to speak their own words in their own unique way. "The language of the story—complete with its unusual grammar and personal metaphors—is the ideal medium for illuminating the way to recovery. We encourage people to speak their own words in their distinctive voice" (pp. 95–96). Practitioner competencies include helping individuals express in their own language their understanding of personal experiences through use of stories, anecdotes, and metaphors.

3. **Develop genuine curiosity:** Nurses and other caregivers "need to express genuine interest in the story so that they can better understand the storyteller and the story. Genuine curiosity reflects an interest in the person and the person's unique experience" (p. 96). Practitioner competencies include showing interest in the person's story, asking for clarification of certain points, and assisting the person to unfold the story at his or her own pace.

4. **Become the apprentice:** The individual is the expert on his or her life story, and he or she must be the leader in deciding what needs to be done. "Professionals may learn something of the power of that story, but only if they apply themselves diligently and respectfully to the task by becoming apprentice-minded" (p. 96). Practitioner competencies include developing a plan of care for the individual based on his or her expressed needs or wishes and helping the individual identify specific problems and ways to address them.

5. **Use the available toolkit:** Concentration is given to the individual's strengths, which are the major tools in the recovery process. "The story contains examples of 'what has worked' for the person in the past or beliefs about 'what might work' for this person in the future. These represent the main tools that need to be used to unlock or build the story of recovery" (p. 96). Practitioner competencies include helping individuals identify what efforts may be successful in relation to solving identified problems and which persons in the individual's life may be able to provide assistance.

6. **Craft the step beyond:** The individual and the practitioner decide together what needs to be done immediately. "Any 'first step' is a crucial step, revealing the power of change and potentially pointing towards the ultimate goal of recovery" (p. 96). Practitioner competencies include helping the individual determine what kind of change would represent a step toward recovery and what he or she needs to do to take that first step in the progress toward that goal.

7. **Give the gift of time:** Change happens when the individual and practitioner spend quality time in a therapeutic relationship. "The challenge is using time for things that are important" (Young, 2010, p. 573). Practitioner competencies include acknowledging (and helping the individual understand) the importance of time dedicated to addressing the needs of the individual and the planning and implementing of care.

8. **Reveal personal wisdom:** People often do not realize their own personal wisdom, strengths, and abilities. "A key task for the professional is to help the person reveal and come to value that wisdom, so that it might be used to sustain the person throughout the voyage of recovery" (Buchanan-Barker & Barker, 2008, p. 97). Practitioner competencies include helping individuals identify personal strengths and weaknesses and develop self-confidence in their ability to help themselves.

9. **Know that change is constant:** Because change is a constant in everyone's life, important decisions and choices must be made along the path to recovery in order for growth to occur. Professional competencies include helping the individual develop awareness of the changes that are occurring and how he or she has influenced these changes. "The task of the professional helper is to develop awareness of how change is happening and to support the person in making decisions regarding the course of the recovery voyage" (p. 97).

10. **Be transparent:** Transparency is important in the teambuilding process between the individual and the professional helper. "Professionals are in a privileged position and should model confidence by being transparent at all times, helping the person understand exactly what is being done and why" (p. 97). Professional competencies include ensuring that the individual is aware of the significance of all interventions and that he or she receives copies of all documents related to the plan of care.

Young (2010) states:

> The Tidal Model is not a typical boxes-and-arrows diagram to use and follow. Instead, it is way of thinking, a paradigm for giving person-centered care that is strength-based, empowering, and relational. (p. 574)

The Wellness Recovery Action Plan (WRAP)

The **WRAP Model** was developed in 1997 by a group of 30 individuals attending a mental health recovery skills seminar conducted by Mary Ellen Copeland in Vermont. This group (which included persons with psychiatric symptoms, family members, and care providers) determined the need for a system to incorporate the skills and strategies they were learning in the seminar into their everyday lives. Copeland (2001) states:

> [WRAP] is a structured system for monitoring uncomfortable and distressing symptoms and, through planned responses, reducing, modifying or eliminating those symptoms. It also includes plans for responses from others when a person's symptoms have made it impossible to continue to make decisions, take care of him/herself and keep him/herself safe. (p. 129)

Copeland suggests that all a person needs to begin the program is a system for storing information (e.g., a notebook, computer, or tape recorder), and possibly a friend, health-care provider, or other supporter to give assistance and feedback. The program is a stepwise process through which an individual is able to monitor and manage distressing symptoms that occur in daily life. Individuals may be assisted in the process by others (e.g., health-care professionals, significant others, friends), "but to be effective and empowering, the person experiencing the symptoms must develop the plan for himself/herself" (p. 129). Steps of the WRAP process are described in the following sections.

Step 1. Developing a Wellness Toolbox

In this first step, the individual creates a list of tools, strategies, and skills that he or she has used in the past (or has heard of in the past that he or she would like to try) to assist in relieving disturbing symptoms. Copeland (2001) offers a number of examples:

■ Talking to a friend or health-care professional
■ Peer counseling or exchange listening
■ Relaxation and stress reduction exercises
■ Guided imagery
■ Journaling
■ Physical exercise
■ Attending a support group
■ Doing something special for someone else
■ Listening to music

Step 2. Daily Maintenance List

This list is divided into three parts. In part 1, the individual writes a description of how he or she feels (or would like to feel) when experiencing wellness (e.g., bright, cheerful, talkative, happy, optimistic, capable). This information is used as a reference point. In part 2, using the wellness toolbox as a reference, the individual makes a list of things he or she needs to do every day to maintain wellness. This is an important part of the plan and must be realistic so as not to set the individual up for failure or create additional frustration.

Example items for part 2 may include the following (Copeland, 2001):

■ Eat three healthy meals and three healthy snacks
■ Drink at least six 8-ounce glasses of water
■ Avoid caffeine, sugar, junk foods, and alcohol
■ Exercise for at least 30 minutes
■ Have 20 minutes of relaxation or meditation time
■ Write in my journal for at least 15 minutes
■ Take medications and vitamin supplements
■ Spend at least 30 minutes enjoying a fun, affirming, and/or creative activity

In part 3 of this step, the individual keeps a list of things that need to be done. The individual reads this list daily as a reminder, and items may be considered for accomplishment on any given day at the individual's discretion. For part 3, Copeland (2001) suggests items such as the following:

■ Spend time with counselor or case manager
■ Make an appointment with health-care professional
■ Spend time with friend or partner
■ Be in touch with my family
■ Spend time with children or pets
■ Buy groceries
■ Do the laundry
■ Write some letters
■ Remember someone's birthday or anniversary

Step 3. Triggers

This step is divided into two parts. In part 1, the individual lists events or circumstances that, should they occur, would cause distress or discomfort. These triggers are situations to which the individual is susceptible or that have triggered or increased symptoms in the past. Copeland (2001) lists the following examples:

■ The anniversary dates of losses or trauma
■ Being exhausted
■ Work stress
■ Family friction
■ A relationship ending
■ Being judged, criticized, or teased
■ Financial problems
■ Physical illness
■ Sexual harassment or inappropriate sexual behavior
■ Substance abuse

In part 2, the individual uses items from the wellness toolbox to develop a plan for what to do if triggers interfere with wellness.

Step 4. Early Warning Signs

This step is divided into two parts. Part 1 involves identification of subtle signs that indicate a possible worsening of the situation. Copeland (2001) states, "Recognizing early warning signs and reviewing them regularly will help the person to become more aware of these early warning signs, allowing the person to take action before the signs worsen" (p. 136). Some types of early warning signs include anxiety, forgetfulness, lack of motivation, avoiding others or isolating, increased irritability, increase in smoking, using substances, or feeling worthless and inadequate. In part 2, the individual develops a plan for responding to the early warning signs that result in relief or in preventing them from escalating. The plan may include items such as consulting a supporter or counselor, increasing focus on peer counseling, increasing time spent in relaxation exercises, or utilizing other interventions from the wellness toolbox until warning signs diminish.

Step 5. Things Are Breaking Down or Getting Worse

This step is divided into two parts. In part 1, the individual lists symptoms that indicate that the situation has worsened. In this stage, the symptoms are producing great discomfort, but the individual is still able to take some action on his or her own behalf. Immediate action is required to prevent a crisis from developing. Symptoms at this stage differ greatly from person to person, and Copeland (2001) states, "What may mean 'things are breaking down' to one person may mean 'crisis' to another" (p. 137). She lists a number of examples of symptoms, which may include the following:

■ Irrational responses to events and the actions of others
■ Inability to sleep or sleeping all the time
■ Headaches
■ Not eating or overeating
■ Social isolation
■ Thoughts of self-harm
■ Substance abuse or chain smoking
■ Bizarre behaviors
■ Seeing things that are not there
■ Paranoia

In part 2, the individual makes a plan that he or she thinks will help when the symptoms have worsened to this degree. The plan must be very specific and direct, with clear instructions. Some examples include the following (Copeland, 2001):

■ Call my health-care professional; ask for and follow directions.
■ Arrange for someone to stay with me around the clock until my symptoms subside.
■ Take action so that I cannot hurt myself if my symptoms get worse, such as giving my medication, checkbook, credit cards, and car keys to a previously designated friend for safe keeping.
■ Make sure I do everything on my daily check list.
■ Have at least two peer counseling sessions daily.

■ Increase use of items from wellness toolbox (e.g., relaxation exercises, physical exercises, creative activities).

Step 6. Crisis Planning

This stage identifies symptoms indicating that individuals can no longer care for themselves, make independent decisions, or keep themselves safe. This stage is multifaceted and meant for use by caregivers on behalf of the individual who developed the plan. It is composed of the following parts (Copeland, 2001, p. 130):

■ Part 1: Gathers information that describes what the person is like when well.
■ Part 2: Identifies the symptoms that indicate when others need to take responsibility for the person's care.
■ Part 3: Provides names of supporters previously identified by the individual to speak on his or her behalf.
■ Part 4: Includes the name of health-care providers and phone numbers; medications currently using; allergies to medications; medications the individual would prefer to take, if additional medication is necessary; medications that the individual refuses to take.
■ Part 5: Includes the individual's preferred treatments and treatments that he or she wishes to avoid.
■ Part 6: Identifies the individual's preferences in treatment facilities (e.g., home, community care, respite center).
■ Part 7: Identifies acceptable facilities if previous preferences cannot be executed. Facilities to avoid are also indicated.
■ Part 8: Includes an extensive description of what the individual expects from identified supporters who are acting on his or her behalf during a crisis situation.
■ Part 9: Consists of a list of indicators, developed by the individual, that communicates to supporters when their services are no longer required. The individual should update this plan periodically when he or she learns new information or changes his or her mind about certain situations. Assurance of the use of the crisis plan may be increased if it is notarized and signed in the presence of two witnesses. To further increase its potential for use, the person may appoint a durable power of attorney, although because of the variability of the legality of these documents from state to state, there is no guarantee that the plan will be followed.

Copeland states:

WRAP is a systematic method for developing skills in self-management and empowerment. It provides a means for individuals with a mental illness to work more collaboratively with healthcare providers. It is highly individualized and addresses the unique needs of the person and his/her situation. It is applicable to most any long-term illness/disability or problem situation. These benefits suggest that it can be used more widely and should be introduced as an option for individuals in need of a self-management system. (p. 149)

The Psychological Recovery Model

Andresen, Oades, and Caputi (2011) define psychological recovery as "the establishment of a fulfilling, meaningful life and a positive sense of identity founded on hopefulness and self-determination. Psychological recovery is necessary whether mental illness is biologically based or the result of the exacerbation of emotional problems caused by stress" (p. 40). The **Psychological Recovery Model** does not emphasize the absence of symptoms but focuses on the person's self-determination in the course of his or her recovery process.

In examining a number of studies, Andresen and associates (2011) identified four components that were consistently evident in the recovery process:

- **Hope:** Finding and maintaining hope that recovery can occur
- **Responsibility:** Taking responsibility for one's life and well-being
- **Self and identity:** Renewing the sense of self and building a positive identity
- **Meaning and purpose:** Finding purpose and meaning in life

Andresen and associates (2011) conceptualized a five-stage model of recovery, which they define by integrating into each stage the four components of the recovery process. An explanation of these stages is presented in the following paragraphs.

Stage 1. Moratorium

This stage is identified by dark despair and confusion. "It is called moratorium, because it seems 'life is on hold'" (p. 47).

- **Hope:** In the moratorium stage, hopelessness prevails. Consumers may even perceive feelings of hopelessness from practitioners when treatment plans emphasize stabilization and maintenance, thereby conveying messages of no hope for recovery.
- **Responsibility:** In the moratorium stage, the individual feels out of control and powerless to change.
- **Self and identity:** In the moratorium stage, individuals feel "as though they no longer know who they are as a person" (p. 59). An individual's sense of identity as a valuable and functional member of society can be lost with a diagnosis of mental illness.

- **Meaning and purpose:** The diagnosis of severe mental illness is a traumatic event that can challenge an individual's fundamental beliefs, creating a loss of meaning and purpose in life.

Stage 2. Awareness

In this stage, the individual comes to a realization that a possibility for recovery exists. Andresen and associates state, "It involves an awareness of a possible self other than that of 'sick person': a self that is capable of recovery" (p. 47).

- **Hope:** In the awareness stage, there is a dawn of hope that indeed "life is not over." This feeling of hope may emanate from significant others, professionals, or family members. Individuals may also be inspired by others who have recovered. Hope may also be derived from strong inner determination and from personal faith and spirituality.
- **Responsibility:** In this stage, the individual develops an awareness of the need to take control of his or her life. Feelings of control and responsibility lead to a sense of personal empowerment that paves the way for recovery.
- **Self and identity:** In the awareness stage, the individual comes to realize that he or she is a person independent of the illness. "The person realizes that there still exists an 'intact self' capable of taking action on one's own behalf" (p. 72).
- **Meaning and purpose:** In the awareness stage, the individual strives for a personal comprehension of the illness, why it occurred, and what the implications of the illness are for his or her future. "Seeking a meaning of the illness can be explained by theories of cognitive control, in which one tries to understand unexplainable negative events by finding a reason for them" (p. 74).

Stage 3. Preparation

This stage begins with the individual's resolve to begin the work of recovery.

- **Hope:** In the preparation stage, hope is manifested in the mobilization of personal and external resources to foster self-care and find pathways to goals. This includes identifying strengths and weaknesses, gathering knowledge and information, and seeking out available support systems.
- **Responsibility:** Taking responsibility in the preparation stage involves learning about the effects of the illness and how to recognize, monitor, and manage symptoms. Taking charge of one's life also includes the ability to be independent and take care of basic needs.
- **Self and identity:** Andresen and associates state, "During the preparation stage, the person takes

stock of his or her skills and strengths in order to build on them to rediscover a positive sense of identity" (p. 81). The person is willing to take risks and try new activities to reestablish a sense of self. Lost aspects of self are rediscovered, new aspects are identified, and both are incorporated into a new self-identity.

■ **Meaning and purpose:** The basis for a meaningful life lies in solid core values. "Living according to one's valued directions gives meaning to the work of recovery, and for this reason, some people hold on tenaciously to their goals" (p. 83). Each individual must live by certain tenets that make life personally valuable and enriching. Individuals living with a severe mental illness may require a reordering of priorities and setting of new goals as part of their recovery.

Rebuilding

The hard work of recovery takes place in the rebuilding stage. The individual "takes the necessary steps to work towards his or her goals in rebuilding a meaningful life" (p. 87).

■ **Hope:** In the rebuilding stage, the individual has hope for and looks forward to a more fulfilling life. Realistic goals are set, and the individual is encouraged to pursue the recovery process at his or her own pace. With each success, hope is renewed.

■ **Responsibility:** "Through setting and working towards goals, the person begins to actively take control of his or her life; not only management of symptoms, but also enlisting social support, improvement of self-image, handling social pressures, and building social competence" (p. 90). Assuming control of treatment decisions and illness management is an essential part of the recovery process.

■ **Self and identity:** The individual elaborates and enhances his or her sense of identity, having succeeded in previous stages in developing a positive self-identity separate from the illness and a new sense of self-confidence by succeeding at new activities. In the rebuilding stage, the work of examining core values and working toward value-congruent goals reinforces a positive sense of identity and a commitment to recovery.

■ **Meaning and purpose:** Having realistic goals and a positive sense of identity provides a sense of purpose in life. Individuals need a reason to start each day. Andresen and associates state, "Finding meaning [in life] is more than finding a valued occupation, but rather is more akin to finding a way to live. This may include, but is not limited to, vocational goals. It includes examining one's spirituality or philosophy of life. The journey is, in itself, a source of meaning for many" (p. 99).

Growth

The outcome of the psychological recovery process is growth. Although it is called the *final* stage of the psychological recovery model, it is important to remember that this is a dynamic stage and that personal growth is a continuing life process.

■ **Hope:** In the growth stage, the individual feels a sense of optimism and hope of a rewarding future. Skills that have been nurtured in the previous stages are applied with confidence, and the individual strives for higher levels of well-being.

■ **Responsibility:** "Achieving control requires sustained commitment in the face of set-backs" (p. 106). In the growth phase, individuals exhibit confidence in managing their illnesses and are resilient when relapses occur. They are empowered by personal input and decision-making regarding their treatment.

■ **Self and identity:** The individual in the growth stage has developed a strong, positive sense of self and identity. Andresen and associates state, "Many consumers have reported feeling that they are a better person as a result of their struggle with the illness. [In one research study] participants reported developing personal qualities, including strength and courage; more confidence in the self; resourcefulness and responsibility; a new philosophy of life; compassion and empathy; a sense of self-worth; and being happier and more carefree" (pp. 108–109).

■ **Meaning and purpose:** Individuals who have reached the growth stage often report a more profound sense of meaning. Some describe having achieved a sense of serenity and peace, and for others it takes the form of a spiritual awakening. Some individuals find reward in educating others about the experience of mental illness and recovery.

Andresen and associates (2011) state:

Recovery from serious mental illness is more than staying out of the hospital or a return to some arbitrary level of functioning. It is more than merely coping with the illness. In [the growth] stage, the notion of wellbeing replaces that of wellness. While wellness implies the absence of illness, wellbeing refers to a more holistic psychological experience of fulfilling life. Although we may not expect everyone (including those who do not have a mental illness) to reach the highest levels of self-actualization, we can expect that all people have the opportunity to develop a positive sense of self and identity and to live a meaningful life filled with purpose and hope for the future. (p. 113)

Nursing Interventions That Assist With Recovery

It is within the scope of nursing to assist individuals in many aspects of the mental health recovery process. Caldwell and associates (2010) state:

> Professional nurses must play an active role in client recovery because they are employed in all aspects of service delivery systems, and most times professional nurses are responsible for the delivery and coordination of care. The professional nurse must be center stage in the development and implementation of any action plan involving client recovery. (p. 44)

Nurses have historically held the promotion of wellness within a collaborative nurse-client relationship as a primary goal. Peplau (1991) described nursing as "a human relationship between an individual who is sick, or in need of health services, and a nurse especially educated to recognize and to respond to the need for help" (pp. 5–6). As previously noted, recovery models are inherently collaborative in that services are provided by professionals, by consumers, and cooperatively by both. Examples of interventions and activities in which nurses and consumers may collaborate in the client's journey to recovery are outlined in Table 21–1.

TABLE 21–1	Nurse-Client Collaboration in the Mental Health Recovery Process		
	THE TIDAL MODEL	THE WRAP MODEL	PSYCHOLOGICAL RECOVERY MODEL
Assessment	■ Client tells his or her personal story ■ Nurse actively listens and expresses interest in the story ■ Nurse helps client record story in client's own language ■ Client identifies specific problems he or she wishes to address ■ Nurse and client identify client's strengths and weaknesses	■ Client develops a wellness toolbox by creating a list of tools, strategies, and skills that have been helpful in the past ■ Client identifies strengths and weaknesses ■ Nurse provides assistance and feedback	■ Client is feeling hopeless and powerless ■ Client seeks meaning of the illness ■ Nurse helps by offering hope ■ Client begins to develop an awareness of the need to take control of and responsibility for his or her life

Interventions	■ Nurse and client determine what has worked in the past
	■ Client suggests new tools he or she would like to try
	■ Client decides what changes he or she would like to make and sets realistic goals
	■ Nurse and client decide what must be done as the first step
	■ Nurse gives positive feedback for client's efforts to make life changes and for successes achieved
	■ Nurse encourages client to be as independent as possible but offers assistance when required
	■ Nurse gives the "gift of time"
		■ Client creates a daily maintenance list:
		  ■ How he or she feels at best
		  ■ What must be done daily to maintain wellness
		  ■ Reminder list of other things that need to be accomplished
		■ Client identifies triggers that cause distress or discomfort and identifies what to do if triggers interfere with wellness
		■ Client identifies signs of worsening of symptoms and develops a plan to prevent escalation
		■ Client identifies when symptoms have worsened and help is needed
		■ Client identifies when he or she can no longer care for self and makes decisions (in writing) about treatment issues (what type, who will provide, who will represent client's interests)
		■ Nurse offers support and provides feedback and assistance when needed
			■ Client resolves to begin work of recovery
			■ Client and nurse identify strengths and weaknesses
			■ Nurse assists client to learn about effects of the illness and how to recognize, monitor, and manage symptoms
			■ Client identifies changes he or she wishes to occur and sets realistic goals to rebuild a meaningful life
			■ Client examines personal spirituality and philosophy of life in search of a meaning and purpose—one that gives him or her a "reason to start each day"

Continued

TABLE 21–1	**Nurse-Client Collaboration in the Mental Health Recovery Process—cont'd**		
	THE TIDAL MODEL	THE WRAP MODEL	PSYCHOLOGICAL RECOVERY MODEL
Outcomes	■ Client acknowledges that change has occurred and is ongoing ■ Client feels empowered to manage own self-care ■ Nurse is available for support	■ Client develops skills in self-management ■ Client develops self-confidence and hope for a brighter future	■ Client develops a positive self-identity separate from the illness ■ Client maintains commitment to recovery in the face of setbacks ■ Client feels a sense of optimism and hope of a rewarding future

If the proposals from the President's New Freedom Commission on Mental Health become fully realized, it would mean improvement in the promotion of mental health and the care of individuals with mental illness. Many nurse leaders see this period of health-care reform as an opportunity for nurses to expand their roles and assume key positions in education, prevention, assessment, and referral. Nurses are and will continue to be paramount in helping individuals with mental illness remain as independent as possible, manage their illnesses within the community setting, and strive to minimize the number of hospitalizations required. A vision of recovery from mental illness exists, and hope, trust, and self-determination should be incorporated into all treatment models.

Summary and Key Points

- Recovery is the restoration to a former and/or better state or condition.
- SAMHSA identifies four major dimensions that support a life in recovery: health, home, purpose, and community.
- The President's New Freedom Commission on Mental Health proposes to transform the mental health system by shifting the paradigm of care of persons with serious mental illness from traditional medical psychiatric treatment toward the concept of recovery.
- SAMHSA outlines 10 guiding principles that support recovery:
  - Recovery emerges from hope
  - Recovery is person driven
  - Recovery occurs via many pathways
  - Recovery is holistic
  - Recovery is supported by peers and allies

  - Recovery is supported through relationship and social networks
  - Recovery is culturally based and influenced
  - Recovery is supported by addressing trauma
  - Recovery involves individual, family, and community strengths and responsibility
  - Recovery is based on respect
- Many models of recovery exist. Three models were discussed in this chapter: the Tidal Model, the Wellness Recovery Action Plan (WRAP) Model, and the Psychological Recovery Model.
- Nurses work in key positions to assist individuals with mental illness in the recovery process. Interventions based on the three previously mentioned recovery models were included in this chapter.

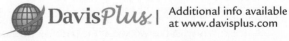
DavisPlus | Additional info available at www.davisplus.com

Communication Exercises

1. Joshua comes to his appointment at the mental health clinic and states, "I can't sit still when I take those medications, so I don't want to take them anymore." Using principles of the recovery model, what are some options for responding to this client?

2. Kelly is a war veteran who was admitted to inpatient hospitalization with depression, alcohol addiction, and complaints of troubling nightmares. She states, at the admission assessment, "I don't trust any 'mental health gurus.' You can't possibly understand what I've been through." How will you respond, and what principles of the recovery model will guide your response?

Review Questions
Self-Examination/Learning Exercise

Select the answer that is most appropriate for each of the following questions.

1. Which of the following is a true statement about mental health recovery? (Select all that apply.)
   a. Mental health recovery applies only to severe and persistent mental illnesses.
   b. Mental health recovery serves to provide empowerment to the consumer.
   c. Mental health recovery is based on the medical model.
   d. Mental health recovery is a collaborative process.

2. A nurse is assisting an individual with mental illness recovery using the Tidal Model. Which of the following is a component of this model?
   a. The wellness toolbox
   b. The daily maintenance list
   c. The individual's personal story
   d. Triggers

3. A nurse is assisting an individual with mental illness recovery using the Psychological Recovery Model. The client says to the nurse, "I have schizophrenia. Nothing can be done. I might as well die." In which stage of the Psychological Recovery Model would the nurse assess this individual to be?
   a. The awareness stage
   b. The preparation stage
   c. The rebuilding stage
   d. The moratorium stage

4. A nurse who is helping a client in the preparation stage of the Psychological Recovery Model might include which of the following interventions?
   a. Teach about effects of the illness and how to recognize, monitor, and manage symptoms.
   b. Help the client identify triggers that cause distress or discomfort.
   c. Help the client establish a daily maintenance list.
   d. Listen actively while the client composes his or her personal story.

5. A nurse who is helping a client with mental illness recovery using the WRAP Model says to the client, "First you must create a wellness toolbox." She explains to the client that a wellness toolbox is which of the following?
   a. A list of words that describe how the individual feels when he or she is feeling well
   b. A list of things the client needs to do every day to maintain wellness
   c. A list of strategies the client has used in the past that help relieve disturbing symptoms
   d. A list of the client's favorite health-care providers and phone numbers

References

Andresen, R., Oades, L.G., & Caputi, P. (2011). *Psychological recovery: Beyond mental illness.* West Sussex, UK: Wiley.

Anthony, W.A. (1993). Recovery from mental illness: The guiding vision of the mental health service system in the 1990s. *Psychosocial Rehabilitation Journal, 16*(4), 11-23. doi:http://dx.doi.org/10.1037/h0095655

Barker, P.J., & Buchanan-Barker, P. (2000). The tidal model: Reclaiming stories, recovering lives. Retrieved from www.tidal-model.com

Barker, P.J., & Buchanan-Barker, P. (2005). *The tidal model: A guide for mental health professionals.* London: Brunner-Routledge.

Barker, P.J., & Buchanan-Barker, P. (2012). Tidal model of mental health nursing. *Current Nursing.* Retrieved from currentnursing.com/nursing_theory/Tidal_Model.html

Brookes, N. (2006). Phil Barker: The tidal model of mental health recovery. In A.M. Tomey & M.R. Alligood (Eds.), *Nursing theorists and their work* (6th ed., pp. 696-725). New York: Elsevier.

Buchanan-Barker, P., & Barker, P.J. (2008). The tidal commitments: Extending the value base of mental health recovery. *Journal of Psychiatric and Mental Health Nursing, 15*(2), 93-100. doi:10.1111/j.1365-2850.2007.01209.x

Caldwell, B.A., Sclafani, M., Swarbrick, M., & Piren, K. (2010). Psychiatric nursing practice and the recovery model of care. *Journal of Psychosocial Nursing, 48*(7), 42-48. doi:10.3928/02793695-20100504-03

Copeland, M.E. (2001). Wellness recovery action plan: A system for monitoring, reducing and eliminating uncomfortable or dangerous physical symptoms and emotional feelings. In C. Brown (Ed.), *Recovery and wellness: Models of hope and empower-*

ment for people with mental illness (pp. 127-150). New York: Haworth Press.

Duckworth, K. (2015). Science meets the human experience: Integrating the medical and recovery models. Retrieved from https://www.nami.org/Blogs/NAMI-Blog/April-2015/Science-Meets-the-Human-Experience-Integrating-th#

Getty, S.M., (2015). Implementing a mental health program using the recovery model. *OT Practice 20*(3), 1-8.

Institute of Medicine. (2003). *Health professions education: A bridge to quality.* Washington, DC: Institute of Medicine.

Jacobs, K.S. (2015). Recovery model of mental illness: A complementary approach to psychiatric care. *Indian Journal of Psychological Medicine. 37*(2): 117–119. doi:10.4103/0253-7176.155605

Jacobson, N., & Greenley, D. (2001). What is recovery? A conceptual model and explication. *Psychiatric Services, 52*(4), 482-485. doi:http://dx.doi.org/10.1176/appi.ps.52.4.482

Leamy, M., Bird, V., LeBoutillier, C., Williams, J., & Slade, M. (2011). Conceptual framework for personal recovery in mental health: Systematic review and narrative synthesis. *British Journal of Psychiatry 199,* 445-452. doi:10.1192/bjp.bp.110.083733

National Association of Social Workers (NASW). (2006). NASW Practice snapshot: The mental health recovery model. Retrieved from www.socialworkers.org/practice/behavioral_health/0206snapshot.asp?

Peplau, H.E. (1991). *Interpersonal relations in nursing: A conceptual frame of reference for psychodynamic nursing.* New York: Springer.

President's New Freedom Commission on Mental Health. (2003). Achieving the promise: Transforming mental health care in America. Retrieved from govinfo.library.unt.edu/mentalhealthcommission/index.htm

Sharfstein, S. (2005). Recovery model will strengthen psychiatrist-patient relationship. *Psychiatric News, 40*(20), 3. doi:10.1176/pn.40.20.00400003

Substance Abuse and Mental Health Services Administration (SAMHSA). (2012). SAMHSA's working definition of recovery: 10 guiding principles of recovery. [Brochure]. Rockville, MD: SAMHSA.

Substance Abuse and Mental Health Services Administration (SAMHSA). (2015). Recovery and recovery support. Retrieved from www.samhsa.gov/recovery

Young, B.B. (2010). Using the tidal model of mental health recovery to plan primary health care for women in residential substance abuse recovery. *Issues in Mental Health Nursing, 31*(9), 569-575. doi:10.3109/01612840.2010.487969

4

Nursing Care of Clients With Alterations in Psychosocial Adaptation

22 Neurocognitive Disorders

KEY TERMS

aphasia	ataxia	pseudodementia
apraxia	confabulation	sundowning

OBJECTIVES
After reading this chapter, the student will be able to:

1. Define and differentiate among various neurocognitive disorders (NCDs).
2. Discuss predisposing factors implicated in the etiology of NCDs.
3. Describe clinical symptoms and use the information to assess clients with NCDs.
4. Identify nursing diagnoses common to clients with NCDs and select appropriate nursing interventions for each.
5. Identify topics for client and family teaching relevant to NCDs.
6. Discuss criteria for evaluating nursing care of clients with NCDs.
7. Describe various treatment modalities relevant to care of clients with NCDs.

HOMEWORK ASSIGNMENT
Please read the chapter and answer the following questions:

1. An alteration in which neurotransmitter is most closely associated with the etiology of Alzheimer's disease?
2. How does vascular neurocognitive disorder differ from NCD caused by Alzheimer's disease?
3. What is pseudodementia?
4. What is the primary concern for nurses working with clients with NCDs?

Neurocognitive disorders (NCDs) include those in which a clinically significant deficit in cognition or memory exists, representing a significant change from a previous level of functioning. These disorders were previously identified in the *Diagnostic and Statistical Manual of Mental Disorders, Fourth Edition, Text Revision (DSM-IV-TR)* (American Psychiatric Association [APA], 2000) as "Dementia, Delirium, Amnestic, and Other Cognitive Disorders." In the *DSM-5*, NCDs include delirium and the syndromes called major NCD or minor NCD which are then specified according to the underlying cause (such as Alzheimer's disease, Parkinson's disease or others).

This chapter presents predisposing factors, clinical symptoms, and nursing interventions for care of clients with NCDs. The objective is to provide quality care, respect the client's dignity, and promote quality of life while offering guidance and support to their families or primary caregivers.

Delirium

Clinical Findings and Course

Delirium is characterized by a disturbance in attention and awareness and a change in cognition that develop rapidly over a short period (APA, 2013). Symptoms of delirium include difficulty sustaining and shifting attention. The person is extremely distractible and must be repeatedly reminded to focus attention. Disorganized thinking prevails and is reflected by speech that is rambling, irrelevant, pressured, and incoherent, unpredictably switching from subject to subject. Reasoning ability and goal-directed behavior are impaired. Disorientation to time and place is common, and impairment of recent memory is invariably evident. Misperceptions of the environment (illusions) and false perceptions (hallucinations) prevail. Disturbances in the sleep–wake cycle occur.

The state of awareness may range from that of hypervigilance (heightened awareness to environmental stimuli) to stupor or semicoma. Sleep may fluctuate between hypersomnolence (excessive sleepiness) and insomnia. Vivid dreams and nightmares are common.

Psychomotor activity may fluctuate between agitated, purposeless movements (e.g., restlessness, hyperactivity, striking out at nonexistent objects) and a vegetative state resembling catatonic stupor. Various forms of tremor are frequently present.

Emotional instability may be manifested by fear, anxiety, depression, irritability, anger, euphoria, or apathy. These emotions may be evidenced by crying, calls for help, cursing, muttering, moaning, acts of self-destruction, fearful attempts to flee, or attacks on others who are falsely viewed as threatening. Autonomic manifestations, such as tachycardia, sweating, flushed face, dilated pupils, and elevated blood pressure, are common.

The symptoms of delirium usually begin quite abruptly (e.g., following a head injury or seizure). At other times, they may be preceded by several hours or days of prodromal symptoms (e.g., restlessness, difficulty thinking clearly, insomnia or hypersomnolence, and nightmares). The slower onset is more common if the underlying cause is systemic illness or metabolic imbalance.

The duration of delirium is usually brief (e.g., 1 week; rarely more than 1 month) and, upon elimination of the underlying causes, symptoms usually diminish over a 3- to 7-day period but in some instances may take as long as 2 weeks (Sadock, Sadock, & Ruiz, 2015). The age of the client and duration of the delirium influence rate of symptom resolution. Delirium may transition into a more permanent cognitive disorder (e.g., major NCD) and is associated with a high mortality rate because of the seriousness of the medical conditions that precipitate delirium.

Predisposing Factors
Delirium

Individuals most predisposed to delirium include those with serious medical, surgical, or neurological conditions. People older than age 65 are considered a high-risk group, and geriatric syndromes such as dementia, depression, falls, and elder abuse are often precipitating factors (Kalish, Gillham, & Unwin, 2014). Some examples of conditions known to precipitate delirium include the following (Black & Andreasen, 2014; Sadock et al., 2015):

■ Systemic infections
■ Febrile illness
■ Metabolic disorders, such as electrolyte imbalances, hypercarbia, or hypoglycemia
■ Hypoxia and chronic obstructive pulmonary disease
■ Hepatic failure or renal failure
■ Head trauma
■ Seizures
■ Migraine headaches
■ Brain abscess or brain neoplasms
■ Stroke
■ Nutritional deficiency
■ Uncontrolled pain
■ Burns
■ Heat stroke
■ Orthopedic and cardiac surgeries
■ Social isolation

Other Etiological Implications
Substance Intoxication Delirium

In this subtype, the symptoms of delirium are attributed to intoxication from certain substances, such as alcohol, amphetamines, cannabis, cocaine, hallucinogens, inhalants, opioids, phencyclidine, sedative, hypnotic, and anxiolytics, or other or unknown substances (APA, 2013).

Substance Withdrawal Delirium

Withdrawal from certain substances can precipitate symptoms of delirium that are sufficiently severe to warrant clinical attention. These substances include alcohol; opioids; sedatives, hypnotics, or anxiolytics; and others.

Medication-Induced Delirium

Medications that have been known to precipitate delirium include anticholinergics, antihypertensives, corticosteroids, anticonvulsants, cardiac glycosides, analgesics, anesthetics, antineoplastic agents, antiparkinson drugs, H_2-receptor antagonists (e.g., cimetidine), and others (Puri & Treasaden, 2012; Sadock et al., 2015).

Delirium Due to Another Medical Condition or to Multiple Etiologies

There may be evidence from the history, physical examination, or laboratory findings that symptoms of delirium are associated with another medical condition or can be attributable to more than one cause. The current evidence supports that delirium is usually the result of many factors rather than one (Kalish et al., 2014).

Neurocognitive Disorder

NCD is classified in the *DSM-5* (APA, 2013) as either mild or major, distinguished primarily by severity of symptomatology. Mild NCD has been known in some settings as mild cognitive impairment and is particularly critical because it can be a focus of early intervention to prevent or slow progression of the disorder. Major NCD constitutes what was previously described as dementia in the *DSM-IV-TR* (APA, 2000). In progressive neurodegenerative conditions, these two diagnoses may identify earlier and later stages of the same disorder. Either diagnosis may be appropriate (depending on severity of symptoms) for certain other NCDs that are the result of reversible or temporary conditions. *DSM-5* criteria for these disorders are presented in Box 22–1.

> ### CORE CONCEPT
> **Neurocognitive**
> Cognitive functions closely linked to particular areas of the brain that have to do with thinking, reasoning, memory, learning, and speaking.

> ### CORE CONCEPT
> **Dementia (Major Neurocognitive Disorder)**
> A disease process in which there is progressive decline in cognitive ability in the presence of clear consciousness. It involves many cognitive deficits and significantly impairs social and occupational functioning (Sadock et al., 2015).

BOX 22–1 A Comparison of Diagnostic Criteria

Mild Neurocognitive Disorder

A. Evidence of modest cognitive decline from a previous level of performance in one or more cognitive domains (complex attention, executive function, learning and memory, language, perceptual-motor, or social cognition) based on:
1. Concern of the individual, a knowledgeable informant, or the clinician that there has been a mild decline in cognitive function; and
2. A modest impairment in cognitive performance, preferably documented by standardized neuropsychological testing, or, in its absence, another quantified clinical assessment.

B. The cognitive deficits do not interfere with capacity for independence in everyday activities (i.e., complex instrumental activities of daily living such as paying bills or managing medications are preserved, but greater effort, compensatory strategies, or accommodation may be required).

C. The cognitive deficits do not occur exclusively in the context of a delirium.

D. The cognitive deficits are not better explained by another mental disorder (e.g., major depressive disorder, schizophrenia).

Major Neurocognitive Disorder

A. Evidence of significant cognitive decline from a previous level of performance in one or more cognitive domains (complex attention, executive function, learning and memory, language, perceptual-motor, or social cognition) based on:
1. Concern of the individual, a knowledgeable informant, or the clinician that there has been a significant decline in cognitive function; and
2. A substantial impairment in cognitive performance, preferably documented by standardized neuropsychological testing, or, in its absence, another quantified clinical assessment.

B. The cognitive deficits interfere with independence in everyday activities (i.e., at a minimum, requiring assistance with complex instrumental activities of daily living such as paying bills or managing medications).

C. The cognitive deficits do not occur exclusively in the context of a delirium.

D. The cognitive deficits are not better explained by another mental disorder (e.g., major depressive disorder, schizophrenia).

BOX 22–1 A Comparison of Diagnostic Criteria–cont'd

Specify whether due to:

- Alzheimer's disease
- Frontotemporal lobar degeneration
- Lewy body disease
- Vascular disease
- Traumatic brain injury
- Substance/medication use
- HIV infection
- Prion disease
- Parkinson's disease
- Huntington's disease
- Another medical condition
- Multiple etiologies
- Unspecified

Specify:

Without behavioral disturbance: If the cognitive disturbance is not accompanied by any clinically significant behavioral disturbance.

With behavioral disturbance *(specify disturbance):* If the cognitive disturbance is accompanied by a clinically significant behavioral disturbance (e.g., psychotic symptoms, mood disturbance, agitation, apathy, or other behavioral symptoms).

Specify whether due to:

- Alzheimer's disease
- Frontotemporal lobar degeneration
- Lewy body disease
- Vascular disease
- Traumatic brain injury
- Substance/medication use
- HIV infection
- Prion disease
- Parkinson's disease
- Huntington's disease
- Another medical condition
- Multiple etiologies
- Unspecified

Specify:

Without behavioral disturbance: If the cognitive disturbance is not accompanied by any clinically significant behavioral disturbance.

With behavioral disturbance *(specify disturbance):* If the cognitive disturbance is accompanied by a clinically significant behavioral disturbance (e.g., psychotic symptoms, mood disturbance, agitation, apathy, or other behavioral symptoms).

Specify current severity:

Mild: Difficulties with instrumental activities of daily living (e.g., housework, managing money)

Moderate: Difficulties with basic activities of daily living (e.g., feeding, dressing)

Severe: Fully dependent

SOURCE: *Reprinted with permission from the* Diagnostic and Statistical Manual of Mental Disorders, Fifth Edition *(Copyright 2013). American Psychiatric Association.*

Clinical Findings, Epidemiology, and Course

NCD constitutes a large and growing public health problem. A meta-analysis conducted in 2010 identified 35.6 million people worldwide living with some form of dementia (major NCD) (National Institute on Aging [NIA], 2015a). An estimated 5.1 million people older than age 65 (81 percent of whom are older than 75) in the United States currently have Alzheimer's disease (AD), the most common form of NCD. The prevalence of the disease doubles for every 5-year age group beyond age 65 with one of three seniors eventually dying from Alzheimer's or another form of dementia (Alzheimer's Association, 2016; NIA, 2015a). The Alzheimer's Association (2015a) reports that of those with AD, an estimated 200,000 are younger than age 65 and almost two-thirds are women. By 2050, the number of individuals aged 65 and older with AD is projected to nearly triple if current population trends continue and no preventive

treatments become available (Alzheimer's Association, 2015a). Health-care costs for end-stage patients with dementia have now been identified as greater than the costs for any other disease, including cancer and heart disease (NIA, 2015b).

This proliferation is not the result of an "epidemic." The greatest risk factor for AD is age, and the population of older adults in the United States continues to grow. Survival after diagnosis typically ranges from 3 to 12 years with most of that time spent in the severest stage of the disease (Mitchell, 2015). In spite of these alarming statistics about AD, recent studies have indicated that dementia in general has been on the decline in the United States over the past few years. This trend could be a temporary change or may be related to improved treatment and education for risk factors associated with heart disease and stroke (NIA, 2015a).

NCDs can be classified as either primary or secondary. Primary NCDs are those such as AD, in which the

NCD itself is the major sign of an organic brain disease not directly related to any other organic illness. Secondary NCDs are caused by or related to another disease or condition, such as HIV disease or a cerebral trauma.

In NCD, impairment is evident in abstract thinking, judgment, and impulse control. The conventional rules of social conduct are often disregarded. Behavior may be uninhibited and inappropriate. Personal appearance and hygiene are often neglected.

Language may or may not be affected. Some individuals may have difficulty naming objects, or the language may seem vague and imprecise. In severe forms of NCD, the individual may not speak at all **(aphasia).** The client may know his or her needs but may not know how to communicate those needs to a caregiver.

Personality change is common in NCD and may be manifested by either an alteration or accentuation of premorbid characteristics. For example, an individual who was previously very socially active may become apathetic and socially isolated. A previously neat person may become markedly untidy in his or her appearance. Conversely, an individual who had difficulty trusting others prior to the illness may exhibit extreme fear and paranoia as manifestations of the disorder.

The reversibility of NCD is dependent on the basic etiology of the disorder. Truly reversible NCD occurs in only a small percentage of cases and might be more appropriately termed *temporary*. Reversible causes of NCD (dementia or dementia-like symptoms) include some brain tumors, subdural hematomas, depression, medication reactions, normal pressure hydrocephalus, vitamin/nutritional deficiencies (especially B_6 and B_{12}), central nervous system (CNS) infections, thyroid disorders, and metabolic disorders (hypoglycemia) (Mayo Clinic, 2016a). In most clients, NCD runs a progressive, irreversible course.

As the disease progresses, **apraxia,** the inability to carry out motor activities despite intact motor function, may develop. The individual may be irritable, moody, or exhibit sudden outbursts over trivial issues. The ability to work or care for personal needs independently will no longer be possible. These individuals can no longer be left alone because they do not comprehend their limitations and are therefore at serious risk for accidents. Wandering away from the home or care setting often becomes a problem. In advanced dementia, clinical features include profound memory deficits, minimal verbal communication, loss of ambulatory ability, inability to perform activities of daily living (ADLs), and incontinence. The most common clinical complications are eating problems and infections (Mitchell, 2015).

Several causes have been described for NCD (see section "Predisposing Factors"), but AD accounts for 50 to 60 percent of all cases (Black & Andreasen, 2014). The progressive nature of symptoms associated with AD has been described according to stages (Alzheimer's Association, 2015a; NIA, 2013; Stanley, Blair, & Beare, 2005):

Stage 1. No apparent symptoms: In the first stage of the illness, there is no apparent decline in memory despite changes that are beginning to occur in the brain.

Stage 2. Forgetfulness: The individual begins to lose things or forget names of people. Losses in short-term memory are common. The individual is aware of the intellectual decline and may feel ashamed, becoming anxious and depressed, which in turn may worsen the symptoms. Maintaining organization with lists and a structured routine provide some compensation. These symptoms often are not observed by others.

Stage 3. Mild cognitive decline: In this stage, interference with work performance becomes noticeable to coworkers. The individual may get lost when driving his or her car. Concentration may be interrupted. Difficulty recalling names or words becomes noticeable to family and close associates. A decline occurs in the ability to plan or organize.

Stage 4. Mild to moderate cognitive decline: At this stage, the individual may forget major events in personal history, such as his or her own child's birthday; experience declining ability to perform tasks, such as shopping and managing personal finances; or be unable to understand current news events. He or she may deny that a problem exists by covering up memory loss with **confabulation** (creating imaginary events to fill in memory gaps). Depression and social withdrawal are common.

Stage 5. Moderate cognitive decline: At this stage, individuals lose the ability to independently perform some ADLs, such as hygiene, dressing, and grooming, and require some assistance to manage these on an ongoing basis. They may forget addresses, phone numbers, and names of close relatives. They may become disoriented about place and time, but they maintain knowledge about themselves. Frustration, withdrawal, and self-absorption are common.

Stage 6. Moderate to severe cognitive decline: At this stage, the individual may be unable to recall recent major life events or even the name of his or her spouse. Disorientation to surroundings is common, and the person may be unable to recall the day, season, or year. The person is unable to manage ADLs without assistance. Urinary and fecal incontinence are common. Sleeping becomes a problem. Psychomotor symptoms include wandering, obsessiveness, agitation, and aggression. Symptoms seem to worsen in the late afternoon and evening—a phenomenon termed **sundowning.** Communication becomes more difficult, with increasing loss of language skills. Institutional care is usually required at this stage.

Stage 7. Severe cognitive decline: In the end stages of AD, the individual is unable to recognize family members. He or she most commonly is bedfast and aphasic. Problems of immobility, such as decubiti and contractures, may occur.

Stanley and associates (2005) have described the late stages of the disorder as follows:

> During late-stage [NCD], the person becomes more chairbound or bedbound. Muscles are rigid, contractures may develop, and primitive reflexes may be present. The person may have very active hands and repetitive movements, grunting, or other vocalizations. There is depressed immune system function, and this impairment coupled with immobility may lead to the development of pneumonia, urinary tract infections, sepsis, and pressure ulcers. Appetite decreases and dysphagia is present; aspiration is common. Weight loss generally occurs. Speech and language are severely impaired, with greatly decreased verbal communication. The person may no longer recognize any family members. Bowel and bladder incontinence are present and caregivers need to complete most ADLs for the person. The sleep-wake cycle is greatly altered, and the person spends a lot of time dozing and appears socially withdrawn and more unaware of the environment or surroundings. Death may be caused by infection, sepsis, or aspiration, although there are not many studies examining cause of death. (p. 358)

Predisposing Factors

NCDs are differentiated by their etiology, although they share common symptom presentation.

Categories include NCDs due to:

- Alzheimer's disease
- Frontotemporal lobar degeneration
- Lewy body disease
- Vascular disease
- Traumatic brain injury
- Substance/medication use
- HIV infection
- Prion disease
- Parkinson's disease
- Huntington's disease
- Another medical condition
- Multiple etiologies
- Unspecified

Neurocognitive Disorder Due to Alzheimer's Disease

AD is characterized by the syndrome of symptoms identified as mild or major NCD and in the seven stages described previously. The onset of symptoms is slow and insidious, and the course of the disorder is generally progressive and deteriorating. Memory impairment is an early and prominent feature.

Refinement of diagnostic criteria now enables clinicians to use specific clinical features to identify the disease with considerable accuracy. Examination by computerized tomography (CT) scan or magnetic resonance imagery (MRI) reveals a degenerative pathology of the brain that includes atrophy, widened cortical sulci, and enlarged cerebral ventricles (Figs. 22–1 and 22–2). Microscopic examinations reveal numerous neurofibrillary tangles and senile plaques in the brains of clients with AD. These changes occur as a part of the normal aging process. However, in clients with AD, they are found in dramatically increased numbers, and their profusion is concentrated in the hippocampus and certain parts of the cerebral cortex.

Etiology

The exact cause of AD is unknown, but experts believe that with the exception of rare cases in which

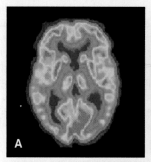
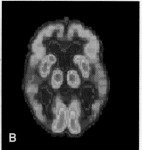

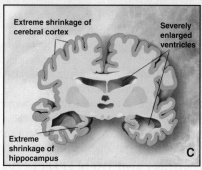

FIGURE 22–1 Changes in the Alzheimer's brain. *A.* Metabolic activity in a normal brain. *B.* Diminished metabolic activity in the Alzheimer's diseased brain. *C.* Late-stage Alzheimer's disease with generalized atrophy and enlargement of the ventricles and sulci. (Source: Alzheimer's Disease Education & Referral Center, A Service of the National Institute on Aging.)

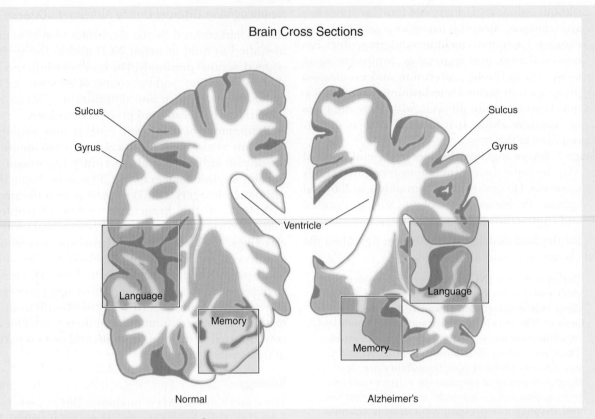

FIGURE 22–2 Neurobiology of Alzheimer's disease. (Source: American Health Assistance Foundation [2012]. www.ahaf.org/alzdis/about/BrainAlzheimer.htm, with permission.)

NEUROTRANSMITTERS

A decrease in the neurotransmitter acetylcholine has been implicated in the etiology of Alzheimer's disease. Cholinergic sources arise from the brainstem and the basal forebrain to supply areas of the basal ganglia, thalamus, limbic structures, hippocampus, and cerebral cortex.

Cell bodies of origin for the serotonin pathways lie within the raphe nuclei located in the brainstem. Those for norepinephrine originate in the locus ceruleus. Projections for both neurotransmitters extend throughout the forebrain, prefrontal cortex, cerebellum, and limbic system. Dopamine pathways arise from areas in the midbrain and project to the frontal cortex, limbic system, basal ganglia, and thalamus. Dopamine neurons in the hypothalamus innervate the posterior pituitary.

Glutamate, an excitatory neurotransmitter, has largely descending pathways with highest concentrations in the cerebral cortex. It is also found in the hippocampus, thalamus, hypothalamus, cerebellum, and spinal cord.

AREAS OF THE BRAIN AFFECTED

Areas of the brain affected by Alzheimer's disease and associated symptoms include the following:

- Frontal lobe: Impaired reasoning ability; inability to solve problems and perform familiar tasks; poor judgment; inability to evaluate the appropriateness of behavior; aggressiveness.
- Parietal lobe: Impaired orientation ability; impaired visuospatial skills (unable to remain oriented within own environment).
- Occipital lobe: Impaired language interpretation; inability to recognize familiar objects.
- Temporal lobe: Inability to recall words; inability to use words correctly (language comprehension). In late stages, some clients experience delusions and hallucinations.
- Hippocampus: Impaired memory. Short-term memory is affected initially. Later, the individual is unable to form new memories.
- Amygdala: Impaired emotions–depression, anxiety, fear, personality changes, apathy, paranoia.
- Neurotransmitters: Alterations in acetylcholine, dopamine, norepinephrine, serotonin, and others may play a role in behaviors such as restlessness, sleep impairment, mood, and agitation.

MEDICATIONS AND THEIR EFFECTS ON THE BRAIN

1. Cholinesterase inhibitors (e.g., donepezil, rivastigmine, and galantamine) act by inhibiting acetylcholinesterase, which slows the degradation of acetylcholine, thereby increasing concentrations of the neurotransmitter in the brain. Most common side effects include dizziness, gastrointestinal upset, fatigue, and headache.
2. N-methyl-D-aspartate (NMDA) receptor antagonists (e.g., memantine) act by blocking NMDA receptors from excessive glutamate, preventing continuous influx of calcium into the cells and ultimately slowing down neuronal degradation. Possible side effects include dizziness, headache, and constipation.

genetic mutations cause AD, multiple factors rather than a single cause influence the development of this illness (Alzheimer's Association, 2015a). These may include a combination of genetic predisposition, lifestyle, and environmental factors that influence changes in the brain over time (Mayo Clinic, 2016b). Several findings in research studies have led to hypotheses about contributing or causative factors:

■ **Neurotransmitter alterations:** Research has indicated that in the brains of those with AD, the enzyme required to produce acetylcholine is dramatically reduced. The reduction seems to be greatest in the nucleus basalis of the inferior medial forebrain area (Sadock et al., 2015). The decrease in production of acetylcholine reduces the amount of the neurotransmitter that is released to cells in the cortex and hippocampus, resulting in cognitive process disturbances. Other neurotransmitters believed to be disrupted in AD include norepinephrine, serotonin, dopamine, and the amino acid glutamate. It has been proposed that in NCD, excess glutamate leads to overstimulation of the *N*-methyl-D-aspartate (NMDA) receptors, causing increased intracellular calcium and subsequent neuronal degeneration and cell death. Decreased levels of somatostatin and corticotropin have also been found in individuals with AD.

■ **Plaques and tangles:** As mentioned previously, an overabundance of structures called *plaques* and *tangles* appear in the brains of individuals with AD. The plaques are made of a peptide called amyloid beta (Aβ), derived from a larger protein called amyloid precursor protein (APP) (NIA, 2011). Plaques are formed when Aβ peptides clump together and mix with molecules and other cellular matter. Tangles are formed from a special kind of cellular protein called *tau protein* that provides stability to the neuron. In AD, the tau protein is chemically altered (NIA, 2011). Strands of the protein become tangled together, interfering with the neuronal transport system. It is unknown whether the plaques and tangles cause AD or are a consequence of the disease; it should be noted that both are seen in other disorders as well as in the normal brain with age (Sadock et al., 2015). Plaques and tangles are thought to contribute to the destruction and death of neurons, leading to memory failure, personality changes, inability to carry out ADLs, and other features of the disease. The number and density of senile plaques (also called *amyloid plaques*) found in postmortem studies have been correlated with the disease severity (Sadock et al., 2015).

■ **Head trauma:** Individuals who have a history of head trauma are at risk for AD (Black & Andreasen, 2014). Studies have shown that some individuals who experienced head trauma subsequently (after years) developed AD. This hypothesis is being investigated as a possible cause. The greatest risks are among those who experience traumatic head injury and have other risk factors for AD (Smith, 2014).

■ **Genetic factors:** As many as 40 percent of clients with AD have a family history of the disease, and some families exhibit a pattern of inheritance that suggests possible autosomal-dominant gene transmission (Sadock et al., 2015). Some studies indicate that early-onset cases are more likely than late-onset cases to be familial and that between one-third and one-half of those cases may be the genetic form. Some research indicates a link between AD and gene mutations found on chromosomes 21, 14, and 1 (Alzheimer's Disease Education & Referral [ADEAR], 2015a). Mutations on chromosome 21 cause the formation of abnormal APP. Mutations on chromosome 14 cause abnormal presenilin 1 *(PS-1)* to be made, and mutations on chromosome 1 leads to the formation of abnormal presenilin 2 *(PS-2)*. Each of these mutations results in an increased amount of the Aβ protein that is a major component of the plaques associated with AD. Individuals with Down syndrome (who carry an extra copy of chromosome 21) also have an overabundance of amyloid plaques and have been found to develop a clinical syndrome of dementia almost identical to AD (Alvarez, 2016).

Two genetic variants have been identified as risk factors for late-onset AD. The apolipoprotein E epsilon 4 *(ApoE ε4)* gene, found on chromosome 19, was identified in 1993. Its exact role in the development of AD is not yet clear (ADEAR, 2015a), but it has been associated with an increase in amyloid plaques, which, as previously discussed, may contribute to neuron death and progressive symptoms of the disease (NIH, 2016). A second genetic variant, the *SORL1* gene, was identified in 2007 (Rogaeva et al., 2007). The researchers believe that the altered gene function results in increasing production of the toxic Aβ protein and subsequently the plaques associated with AD.

While much of the research has focused on toxic amyloid and tau proteins as correlated with AD, current research is exploring other molecular and cellular pathways that may be involved in the development of this disease, including glial cell activation, inflammation, glucose transport systems, and abnormal neuronal circuit activity. Since previous research has demonstrated that ketone bodies have a protective effect on neurons, some studies are focused on the impact of ketones in improving memory and learning. One recent study demonstrated that ketone-rich diets were accompanied by a reduction in toxic proteins that have been associated with development of AD (ADEAR, 2015b).

Vascular Neurocognitive Disorder

In vascular NCD, cognitive symptoms are caused by significant cerebrovascular disease. When blood flow in the brain is impaired, progressive intellectual deterioration occurs. Impairment may be located in large vessels or microvascular networks, so symptoms vary depending on the type, extent, and location of vascular lesion (APA, 2013). Vascular NCD is the second-most common form of NCD after AD (Sadock et al., 2015).

Vascular NCD differs from AD in that it has a more abrupt onset and runs a highly variable course. In vascular NCD, progression of the symptoms occurs in steps rather than as a gradual deterioration; at times, the symptoms seem to subside and the individual exhibits fairly lucid thinking. Memory may seem better and the client may become optimistic that improvement is occurring, only to experience further decline of functioning in a fluctuating pattern of progression. This irregular pattern of decline appears to be an intense source of anxiety for the client with this disorder.

In vascular NCD, clients suffer the equivalent of small strokes that destroy many areas of the brain. The pattern of deficits is variable depending on which regions of the brain have been affected. Certain focal neurological signs commonly seen with vascular NCD include weaknesses of the limbs, small-stepped gait, and difficulty with speech. The disorder is more common in men than in women.

Etiology

Vascular NCD is directly related to an interruption of blood flow to the brain. Symptoms result from death of nerve cells in regions nourished by diseased vessels. Various diseases and conditions that interfere with blood circulation have been implicated.

High blood pressure is thought to be one of the most significant factors in the etiology of multiple small strokes or cerebral infarcts. Hypertension leads to damage to the lining of blood vessels, which can result in rupture of the blood vessel with subsequent hemorrhage or an accumulation of fibrin in the vessel with intravascular clotting and inhibited blood flow. NCD also can result from infarcts related to occlusion of blood vessels by particulate matter that travels through the bloodstream to the brain. These emboli may be solid (e.g., clots, cellular debris, platelet aggregates), gaseous (e.g., air, nitrogen), or liquid (e.g., fat, following soft tissue trauma or fracture of long bones).

Cognitive impairment can occur with multiple small infarcts (sometimes called *silent strokes*) over time or with a single cerebrovascular event in a strategic area of the brain. An individual may have both vascular NCD and AD simultaneously. This is referred to as a *mixed* disorder, the prevalence of which is likely to increase as the population ages.

Frontotemporal Neurocognitive Disorder

Symptoms of frontotemporal NCD occur as a result of shrinking of the frontal and temporal anterior lobes of the brain (National Institute of Neurological Disorders and Stroke [NINDS], 2015). This type of NCD was identified as Pick's disease in the *DSM-IV-TR*. The cause of frontotemporal NCD is unknown, but a genetic factor appears to be involved. Symptoms tend to fall into two clinical patterns: (1) behavioral and personality changes and (2) speech and language problems. Common behavioral changes include increasingly inappropriate actions, lack of judgment and inhibition, and repetitive compulsive behavior. There may be a marked impairment or loss of speech or increasing difficulty in using and understanding written and spoken language (Mayo Clinic, 2014). Because of the several behavioral and personality symptoms, it may be misdiagnosed as a different mental illness. The disease progresses steadily and often rapidly, ranging from less than 2 years in some individuals to more than 10 years in others (NINDS, 2015).

Neurocognitive Disorder Due to Traumatic Brain Injury

DSM-5 criteria state that this disorder "is caused by an impact to the head or other mechanisms of rapid movement or displacement of the brain within the skull, with one or more of the following: loss of consciousness, posttraumatic amnesia, disorientation and confusion, or neurological signs (e.g., positive neuroimaging demonstrating injury, a new onset of seizures or a marked worsening of a preexisting seizure disorder, visual field cuts, anosmia, hemiparesis)" (APA, 2013). Amnesia is the most common neurobehavioral symptom following head trauma. Other symptoms may include confusion and changes in speech, vision, and personality. Depending on the severity of the injury, these symptoms may eventually subside or may become permanent (Smith, 2014). Repeated head trauma, such as the type experienced by boxers, can result in *dementia pugilistica,* a syndrome characterized by emotional lability, dysarthria, ataxia, and impulsivity (Sadock et al., 2015).

Neurocognitive Disorder Due to Lewy Body Dementia

Clinically, Lewy body NCD is fairly similar to AD; however, it tends to progress more rapidly, with earlier appearance of visual hallucinations and Parkinsonian features. Depression and delusions are also common symptoms in this population. Lewy body dementia recently gained public attention when an autopsy of famous comedian Robin Williams revealed that he was suffering from this disease. His widow reported that he had been seeking neurocognitive testing because he was aware of a decline in his mental capacities. He was also manifesting symptoms of depression and ultimately took his own life.

This disorder is distinguished by the presence of Lewy bodies—eosinophilic inclusion bodies—seen in the cerebral cortex and brainstem (Black & Andreasen, 2014). Acetylcholinesterase (ACh) concentrations are reduced in the brains of people with Lewy body NCD, and consequently, cholinesterase inhibitors are likely to be more effective for this population than for those with Alzheimer's dementia (Crystal & Jacobs, 2014). These patients are highly sensitive to extrapyramidal effects of antipsychotic medications. The disease is progressive and irreversible and may account for as many as 25 percent of all NCD cases.

Neurocognitive Disorder Due to Parkinson's Disease

NCD is observed in as many as 75 percent of clients with Parkinson's disease (APA, 2013). This disease is characterized by a loss of nerve cells in the substantia nigra and diminished dopamine activity, resulting in involuntary muscle movements, slowness, and rigidity along with tremor in the upper extremities. In some instances, the cerebral changes that occur in NCD due to Parkinson's disease closely resemble those of AD.

Neurocognitive Disorder Due to HIV Infection

Infection with the human immunodeficiency virus-type 1 (HIV-1) can result in an NCD called *HIV-1-associated cognitive/motor complex.* A less severe form, known as *HIV-1-associated minor cognitive/motor disorder,* also occurs. The severity of symptoms is correlated to the extent of brain pathology. The immune dysfunction associated with HIV disease can lead to brain infections by other organisms, and HIV-1 also appears to cause NCD directly. In the early stages, neuropsychiatric symptoms may be manifested by barely perceptible changes in a person's normal psychological presentation. Severe cognitive changes, particularly confusion, changes in behavior, and sometimes psychoses, are not uncommon in the later stages.

With the advent of the highly active antiretroviral therapies (HAART), incidence rates of NCD due to HIV infection have been on the decline. However, it is possible that the prolonged life span of HIV-infected patients taking medications may actually increase the number of individuals living with HIV-associated NCD.

Substance/Medication-Induced Neurocognitive Disorder

NCD can occur as the result of substance reactions, overuse, or abuse (Hale & Frank, 2015). Symptoms are consistent with major or mild neurocognitive disorder and persist beyond the usual duration of intoxication and acute withdrawal (APA, 2013). Substances that have been associated with the development of NCDs include alcohol, sedatives, hypnotics, anxiolytics, and inhalants. Drugs that cause anticholinergic side effects and toxins such as lead and mercury have also been implicated.

Neurocognitive Disorder Due to Huntington's Disease

Huntington's disease is transmitted as a Mendelian dominant gene. Damage is seen in the areas of the basal ganglia and the cerebral cortex. The onset of symptoms (i.e., involuntary twitching of the limbs or facial muscles, mild cognitive changes, depression, and apathy) usually occurs between age 30 and 50 years. The client usually declines into a profound state of cognitive impairment and **ataxia** (muscular incoordination). The average duration of the disease is 10 to 20 years depending on the severity of symptoms. (Huntington's Disease Society of America [HDSA], 2016).

Neurocognitive Disorder Due to Prion Disease

Prion disease is a group of disorders caused by infectious agents called *prions* and characterized by its insidious onset and rapid progression. Manifestations include problems with coordination and other movement disturbances along with rapidly progressing dementia. This type of NCD is diagnosed when there is evidence of characteristic biomarkers, including recognized lesions in the brain, specific types of proteins in the cerebrospinal fluid, and distinctive triphasic waves on electroencephalograms (APA, 2013). Five to 15 percent of cases of prion disease have a genetic component. Symptoms may develop at any age in adults but typically occur between ages 40 and 60 years.

The clinical course is extremely rapid, with the progression from diagnosis to death in less than 2 years (Rentz, 2008). The most common form of prion disease in humans is Creutzfeldt-Jakob's disease (Johns Hopkins Medicine, no date).

Neurocognitive Disorder Due to Another Medical Condition

A number of other medical conditions can cause NCD, including hypothyroidism, hyperparathyroidism, pituitary insufficiency, uremia, encephalitis, brain tumor, pernicious anemia, thiamine deficiency, pellagra, uncontrolled epilepsy, cardiopulmonary insufficiency, fluid and electrolyte imbalances, CNS and systemic infections, systemic lupus erythematosus, and multiple sclerosis (Black & Andreasen, 2014; Puri & Treasaden, 2012). The etiological factors associated with delirium and NCD are summarized in Box 22–2.

Application of the Nursing Process

Assessment

Nursing assessment of the client with delirium or mild or major NCD is based on knowledge of the symptomatology associated with the disorders previously described in this chapter. Subjective and objective data are gathered by various members of the health-care team. Clinicians report use of a variety of methods for obtaining assessment information.

Client History

Nurses play a significant role in acquiring the client history, including the specific mental and physical changes that have occurred and the age at which the changes began. If the client is unable to relate information adequately, the data should be obtained from family members or others who would be aware of the client's physical and psychosocial history.

From the client history, nurses should assess the following areas of concern: (1) type, frequency, and severity of mood swings, personality and behavioral changes, and catastrophic emotional reactions; (2) cognitive changes, such as problems with attention span, thinking process, problem-solving, and memory (recent and remote); (3) language difficulties; (4) orientation to person, place, time, and situation; and (5) appropriateness of social behavior.

The nurse also should obtain information regarding current and past medication usage, history of other drug and alcohol use, and possible exposure to toxins. Knowledge regarding the history of related symptoms or specific illnesses (e.g., Huntington's disease, AD, Pick's disease, or Parkinson's disease) in other family members might be useful.

BOX 22–2 Etiological Factors Implicated in the Development of Delirium and/or Mild or Major Neurocognitive Disorder

Biological Factors

Hypoxia: Any condition leading to a deficiency of oxygen to the brain

Nutritional deficiencies: Vitamins (particularly B and C); protein; fluid and electrolyte imbalances

Metabolic disturbances: Porphyria; encephalopathies related to hepatic, renal, pancreatic, or pulmonary insufficiencies; hypoglycemia

Endocrine dysfunction: Thyroid, parathyroid, adrenal, pancreas, pituitary

Cardiovascular disease: Stroke, cardiac insufficiency, atherosclerosis

Primary brain disorders: Epilepsy, Alzheimer's disease, Pick's disease, Huntington's chorea, multiple sclerosis, Parkinson's disease

Infections: Encephalitis, meningitis, pneumonia, septicemia, neurosyphilis (dementia paralytica), HIV disease, acute rheumatic fever, Creutzfeldt-Jakob disease

Intracranial neoplasms

Congenital defects: Prenatal infections, such as first-trimester maternal rubella

Exogenous Factors

Birth trauma: Prolonged labor, damage from use of forceps, other obstetric complications

Cranial trauma: Concussion, contusions, hemorrhage, hematomas

Volatile inhalant compounds: Gasoline, glue, paint, paint thinners, spray paints, cleaning fluids, typewriter correction fluid, varnishes, and lacquers

Heavy metals: Lead, mercury, manganese

Other metallic elements: Aluminum

Organic phosphates: Various insecticides

Substance abuse/dependence: Alcohol, amphetamines, caffeine, cannabis, cocaine, hallucinogens, inhalants, nicotine, opioids, phencyclidine, sedatives, hypnotics, anxiolytics

Other medications: Anticholinergics, antihistamines, antidepressants, antipsychotics, antiparkinsonians, antihypertensives, steroids, digitalis

Physical Assessment

Assessment of physical systems by both the nurse and the physician has two main emphases: signs of damage to the nervous system and evidence of diseases of other organs that could affect mental function. Diseases of various organ systems can induce confusion, loss of memory, and behavioral changes. These causes must be considered in diagnosing cognitive disorders. In the neurological examination, the client is asked to perform maneuvers or answer questions

that are designed to elicit information about the condition of specific parts of the brain or peripheral nerves. Testing will assess mental status and alertness, muscle strength, reflexes, sensory perception, proprioception, language skills, and coordination. Physical assessment should include looking for signs of abuse or neglect, screening for hearing or vision impairments, and conducting a mental status examination (Moussa, 2016). An example of a mental status examination for a client with NCD is presented in Box 22–3.

BOX 22–3 Mental Status Examination for Neurocognitive Disorder

Patient Name_____ Date_____
Age_____ Sex_____ Diagnosis_____

	Maximum	Client's Score
1. VERBAL FLUENCY Ask client to name as many animals as he/she can. (Time: 60 seconds) (Score 1 point/2 animals)	10 points	_____
2. COMPREHENSION		
a. Point to the ceiling	1 point	_____
b. Point to your nose and the window	1 point	_____
c. Point to your foot, the door, and ceiling	1 point	_____
d. Point to the window, your leg, the door, and your thumb	1 point	_____
3. NAMING AND WORD FINDING Ask the client to name the following as you point to them:		
a. Watch stem (winder)	1 point	_____
b. Teeth	1 point	_____
c. Sole of shoe	1 point	_____
d. Buckle of belt	1 point	_____
e. Knuckles	1 point	_____
4. ORIENTATION		
a. Date	2 points	_____
b. Day of week	2 points	_____
c. Month	1 point	_____
d. Year	1 point	_____

5. NEW LEARNING ABILITY
Tell the client: "I'm going to tell you four words, which I want you to remember." Have the client repeat the four words after they are initially presented, and then say that you will ask him/her to remember the words later. Continue with the examination, and at intervals of 5 and 10 minutes, ask the client to recall the words. Three different sets of words are provided here.

		5 min.	10 min.
a. Brown (Fun) (Grape)	2 points each:	_____	_____
b. Honesty (Loyalty) (Happiness)	2 points each:	_____	_____
c. Tulip (Carrot) (Stocking)	2 points each:	_____	_____
d. Eyedropper (Ankle) (Toothbrush)	2 points each:	_____	_____

6. VERBAL STORY FOR IMMEDIATE RECALL
Tell the client: "I'm going to read you a short story, which I want you to remember. Listen closely to what I read because I will ask you to tell me the story when I finish." Read the story slowly and carefully, but without pausing at the slash marks. After completing the paragraph, tell the client to retell the story as accurately as possible. Record the number of correct   13 points   _____

Continued

BOX 22–3 Mental Status Examination for Neurocognitive Disorder–cont'd

memories (information within the slashes) and describe confabulation if it is present. (1 point = 1 remembered item [13 maximum points])

It was July / and the Rogers family, mom, dad, and four children / were packing up their station wagon / to go on vacation.
They were taking their yearly trip / to the beach at Gulf Shores.
This year they were making a special 1-day stop / at The Aquarium in New Orleans. After a long day's drive they arrived at the motel / only to discover that in their excitement / they had left the twins / and their suitcases / in the front yard.

7. VISUAL MEMORY (HIDDEN OBJECTS)
Tell the client that you are going to hide some objects around the office (desk, bed) and that you want him/her to remember where they are. Hide four or five common objects (e.g., keys, pen, reflex hammer) in various places in the client's sight. After a delay of several minutes, ask the client to find the objects. (1 point per item found)

a. Coin	1 point	_____
b. Pen	1 point	_____
c. Comb	1 point	_____
d. Keys	1 point	_____
e. Fork	1 point	_____

8. PAIRED ASSOCIATE LEARNING
Tell the client that you are going to read a list of words two at a time. The client will be expected to remember the words that go together (e.g., big–little). When he/she is clear on the directions, read the first list of words at the rate of one pair per second. After reading the first list, test for recall by presenting the first recall list. Give the first word of a pair and ask for the word that was paired with it. Correct incorrect responses and proceed to the next pair. After the first recall has been completed, allow a 10-second delay and continue with the second presentation and recall lists.

Presentation Lists

1	2
a. High–Low	a. Good–Bad
b. House–Income	b. Book–Page
c. Good–Bad	c. High–Low
d. Book–Page	d. House–Income

Recall Lists

1	2		
a. House _____	a. High _____	2 points	_____
b. Book _____	b. Good _____	2 points	_____
c. High _____	c. House _____	2 points	_____
d. Good _____	d. Book _____	2 points	_____

9. CONSTRUCTIONAL ABILITY
Ask client to reconstruct this drawing and to draw the other 2 items: 3 points   _____

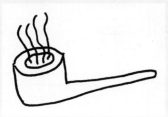

BOX 22–3 Mental Status Examination for Neurocognitive Disorder—cont'd

Draw a daisy in a flowerpot   3 points _____

Draw a clock with all the numbers and set the clock at 2:30.   3 points _____

10. WRITTEN COMPLEX CALCULATIONS

a. Addition   108
                          + 79   1 point   _____

b. Subtraction   605
                          − 86   1 point   _____

c. Multiplication   108
                          × 36   1 point   _____

d. Division   559 ÷ 43   1 point   _____

11. PROVERB INTERPRETATION

Tell the client to explain the following sayings. Record the answers.

a. Don't cry over spilled milk.   2 points _____

_____

b. Rome wasn't built in a day.   2 points _____

_____

c. A drowning man will clutch at a straw.   2 points _____

_____

d. A golden hammer can break down an iron door.   2 points _____

_____

e. The hot coal burns, the cold one blackens.   2 points _____

_____

12. SIMILARITIES

Ask the client to name the similarity or relationship between each of the two items.

a. Turnip.. Cauliflower   2 points _____
b. Car.. Airplane   2 points _____
c. Desk.. Bookcase   2 points _____
d. Poem.. Novel   2 points _____
e. Horse.. Apple   2 points _____

                                                          Maximum: 100 points _____

Normal Individuals		Clients with Alzheimer's Disease	
Age Group	Mean Score (standard deviation)	Stage	Mean Score (standard deviation)
40-49	80.9 (9.7)	I	57.2 (9.1)
50-59	82.3 (8.6)	II	37.0 (7.8)
60-69	75.5 (10.5)	III	13.4 (8.1)
70-79	66.9 (9.1)		
80-89	67.9 (11.0)		

Adapted from Strub, R.L., & Black, F. W. (2000). The mental status examination in neurology, 4th ed., Philadelphia: F.A. Davis. With permission.

A battery of psychological tests may be ordered as part of the diagnostic examination. The results of these tests may be used to make a differential diagnosis between NCD and **pseudodementia** (depression). Depression is one of the most common mental illnesses in the elderly, but it is often misdiagnosed and treated inadequately. Cognitive symptoms of depression may mimic NCD, and because of the prevalence of NCD in the elderly, providers are often too eager to make this diagnosis. A comparison of symptoms of NCD and pseudodementia (depression) is presented in Table 22–1. Nurses can assist in this assessment by carefully observing and documenting these sometimes subtle differences.

Diagnostic Laboratory Evaluations

The nurse also may be required to help the client fulfill the physician's orders for special diagnostic laboratory evaluations. Many of these tests are conducted to rule out other factors associated with dementia, such as evaluation of blood and urine samples to test for various infections, liver function studies to rule out hepatic disease, glucose tests to rule out diabetes or hypoglycemia, electrolytes to rule out imbalances, thyroid tests to rule out hypothyroidism, vitamin B_{12} test to rule out nutritional deficiencies, and drug and alcohol screening to rule out the presence of toxic substances. A rapid plasma reagin (RPR) test for syphilis and HIV testing should be included if the patient is at higher risk for these conditions (Moussa, 2016). CT scanning produces an image of the size and shape of the brain, and MRI produces a computerized image of soft tissue in the brain. Both CT and MRI scans are useful in identifying areas of atrophy such as those seen in AD and may identify other pathological processes needed for differential diagnosis. A lumbar puncture may be performed to examine the cerebrospinal fluid for evidence of CNS infection or hemorrhage if this is suspected. Positron emission tomography (PET) is used to reveal the metabolic activity of the brain, an evaluation some researchers believe is important for early diagnosis of AD. Moussa (2016) cautions that routine brain imaging is controversial and some believe it is overutilized. He adds that while there are genotyping tests that identify genetic markers for apolipoprotein E (which could suggest risk for development of AD), these tests are not indicated for clinical use.

Nursing Diagnosis and Outcome Identification

Using information collected during the assessment, the nurse completes the client database, from which the selection of appropriate nursing diagnoses is determined. Table 22–2 presents a list of client behaviors and the NANDA-I nursing diagnoses that correspond to those behaviors, which may be used in planning care for the client with an NCD.

Outcome Criteria

The following criteria may be used for measurement of outcomes in the care of the client with an NCD.

TABLE 22–1 A Comparison of Neurocognitive Disorder (NCD) and Pseudodementia (Depression)		
SYMPTOM ELEMENT	NCD	PSEUDODEMENTIA (DEPRESSION)
Progression of symptoms	Slow	Rapid
Memory	Progressive deficits; recent memory loss greater than remote; may confabulate for memory "gaps"; no complaints of loss	More like forgetfulness; no evidence of progressive deficit; recent and remote loss equal; complaints of deficits; no confabulation (will more likely answer "I don't know")
Orientation	Disoriented to time and place; may wander in search of the familiar	Oriented to time and place; no wandering
Task performance	Consistently poor performance but struggles to perform	Performance is variable; little effort is put forth
Symptom severity	Worse as the day progresses	Better as the day progresses
Affective distress	Appears unconcerned	Communicates severe distress
Appetite	Unchanged	Diminished
Attention and concentration	Impaired	Intact

TABLE 22–2 **Assigning Nursing Diagnoses to Behaviors Commonly Associated With Neurocognitive Disorders**

BEHAVIORS	NURSING DIAGNOSES
Falls, wandering, poor coordination, confusion, misinterpretation of the environment (illusions, hallucinations), lack of understanding of environmental hazards, memory deficits	Risk for trauma
Disorientation, confusion, memory deficits, inaccurate interpretation of the environment, suspiciousness, paranoia	Disturbed thought processes;* Impaired memory
Having hallucinations (hears voices, sees visions, feels crawling sensation on skin)	Disturbed sensory perception*
Aggressiveness, assaultiveness (hitting, scratching, or kicking)	Risk for other-directed violence
Inability to name objects/people, loss of memory for words, difficulty finding the right word, confabulation, incoherent, screaming and demanding verbalizations	Impaired verbal communication
Inability to perform activities of daily living: feeding, dressing, hygiene, toileting	Self-care deficit (specify)
Expressions of shame and self-degradation, progressive social isolation, apathy, decreased activity, withdrawal, depressed mood	Situational low self-esteem; Grieving

*These nursing diagnoses have been resigned from the NANDA-I list of approved diagnoses, but are used for purposes of this text.

The client:

- Has not experienced physical injury
- Has not harmed self or others
- Has maintained reality orientation to the best of his or her capability
- Is able to communicate with consistent caregiver
- Fulfills ADLs with assistance (or for client who is unable, has needs met as anticipated by caregiver)
- Discusses positive aspects about self and life

Planning and Implementation

Care for an individual with an NCD must focus on immediate needs and keeping the individual safe from harm.

Risk for Trauma

Because the individual has impairments in cognitive and psychomotor functioning, it is important to ensure that the environment is as safe as possible to prevent injury. NANDA-I defines *Risk for trauma* as "vulnerable to accidental tissue injury (e.g., wound, burn, fracture) which may compromise health" (Herdman & Kamitsuru, 2014). Table 22–3 presents this nursing diagnosis in care plan format.

Client Goals

Outcome criteria include short- and long-term goals. Time lines are individually determined.

Short-term goals

- Client will call for assistance when ambulating or conducting other activities (if it is within his or her cognitive ability).

- Client will maintain a calm demeanor, with minimal agitated behavior.
- Client will not experience physical injury.

Long-term goal

- Client will not experience physical injury.

Interventions

Interventions for preventing injury in the cognitively impaired client include the following:

- Arrange the furniture and other items in the room to accommodate the client's disabilities. Ensure that frequently used items are stored within easy access.
- Keep the bed in its lowest position. If allowed by hospital regulation or accrediting body, limited use of bedrails may provide a measure of safety.
- A room near the nurse's station may be helpful to ensure that the client has close observation. In some instances, one-to-one observation may be necessary, particularly for the delirious client.
- If the client is a smoker, ensure that cigarettes and lighter are kept at the nurse's station and dispensed only when someone is available to stay with the client while he or she is smoking.
- Assist the client with ambulation. Provide cane or walker for balance and instruct client in its proper use. Transport client in wheelchair when longer excursions are necessary.
- Teach client to hold on to hand railing if one is available or to call for assistance when ambulating if he or she is cognitively able.

Table 22–3 | CARE PLAN FOR THE CLIENT WITH A NEUROCOGNITIVE DISORDER

NURSING DIAGNOSIS: RISK FOR TRAUMA

RELATED TO: Impairments in cognitive and psychomotor functioning

OUTCOME CRITERIA	NURSING INTERVENTIONS	RATIONALE
Short-Term Goals • Client calls for assistance when ambulating or carrying out other activities (if it is within his or her cognitive ability). • Client maintains a calm demeanor, with minimal agitated behavior. • Client does not experience physical injury. Long-Term Goal • Client does not experience physical injury.	The following measures may be instituted: a. Arrange furniture and other items in the room to accommodate client's disabilities. b. Store frequently used items within easy access. c. Keep the bed in the lowest position from the floor when the client is not being immediately attended to. Pad siderails and headboard if client has history of seizures. Keep bedrails up when client is in bed (if regulations permit). d. Assign room near nurses' station; observe frequently. e. Assist client with ambulation. f. Keep a dim light on at night. g. If client is a smoker, cigarettes and lighter or matches should be kept at the nurses' station and dispensed only when someone is available to stay with client while he or she is smoking. h. Frequently orient client to place, time, and situation. i. If client is prone to wander, provide an area within which wandering can be carried out safely. j. Soft restraints may be required if client is very disoriented and hyperactive.	To ensure client safety

For the Agitated Client

■ Maintain an environment of low stimulation for an individual with disruptions in cognitive processes. Irritability, hostility, aggression, and psychotic behaviors are troublesome symptoms that require management in individuals with cognitive disorders. These behaviors often make it difficult for family to care for their loved ones and is a common cause for placement in an institution. In the United States, 16 percent of patients with dementia die in hospitals, and the majority die in nursing homes

(Mitchell, 2015). This issue requires further exploration, since many families struggle with the idea of institutionalization but are not equipped to deal with the overwhelming burden of caring for a client with an NCD.

■ Antipsychotics have historically been used to help manage behavioral symptoms in patients with NCD. Treatment of nonpsychotic behavior with antipsychotics, however, is an off-label use and could have legal implications; this is a difficult treatment issue because behavioral symptoms occur in 90 percent of patients with NCD at some point during progression of the illness (Rice & Humphries, 2014). The conventional antipsychotics are also problematic because of their tendency to induce extrapyramidal side effects. The newer atypical antipsychotics have shown some effectiveness in treating these symptoms. Although antipsychotic medications are still used for this purpose by some physicians, the U.S. Food and Drug Administration (FDA) has issued black-box warnings against their use in elderly patients with NCD-related psychosis. They have been associated with increased mortality in this patient population.

■ Remain calm and undemanding, and avoid pressing the individual to perform activities that he or she is refusing. Reasoning with some clients with NCDs may only increase the possibility for agitation. Practicing relaxation exercises and walking with the client may be of some help.

■ Recent nursing literature has highlighted novel, evidence-based interventions to reduce anxiety and agitation, including dance and other rhythmic movement therapy (Lapum & Bar, 2016) and doll therapy (Shin, 2015).

For the Client Who Wanders

A number of reasons have been proposed as to why individuals with NCD wander. Some clinicians associate wandering behavior with increased stress and anxiety or restless agitation. Others relate the behavior to stages of cognitive decline. When memory diminishes and fear sets in, individuals may wander in search of something that seems familiar to them. Increased walking at night corresponds with disruption of diurnal rhythm. In any event, wandering behavior in NCD can cause great problems for caregivers. Wandering is often a problem in midstage NCD and less so in later stages. Clients new to a nursing home may wander in an attempt to become oriented to new surroundings. Wandering behavior can also be attributed to physical causes, such as hunger, thirst, and urinary or fecal urgency. When the wandering behavior begins after a long period of stability, it is likely that a new complication may be occurring—medical, psychiatric, or cognitive. Delirium may produce the abrupt onset of wandering behavior. The goals of wandering therapy are to keep the individual safe, to prevent intrusion into others' rooms, and to try to determine contributing factors to the behavior. When caring for a client who wanders, it is important to keep the following interventions in mind:

■ Keep the individual on a structured schedule of recreational activities and a strict feeding and toileting schedule.

■ Provide a safe, enclosed place for pacing and wandering.

■ Walk with the individual for a while and gently redirect him or her back to the care unit.

■ Ensure that outdoor exits are electronically controlled.

Disturbed Thought Processes/Impaired Memory and Disturbed Sensory Perception

Disturbed thought processes and sensory perception have been resigned as nursing diagnoses by NANDA-I, but they are retained in this text because of their appropriateness in describing specific behaviors. In this instance, they are evidenced by disorientation, confusion, and inaccurate interpretation of the environment, including illusions, delusions, and hallucinations. *Disturbed thought processes* has been defined as disruptions in cognitive operations and activities. *Disturbed sensory perception* is defined as a "change in the amount or patterning of incoming stimuli accompanied by a diminished, exaggerated, distorted, or impaired response to such stimuli" (NANDA-I, 2012, p. 490). *Impaired memory* is defined as the "inability to remember or recall bits of information or behavioral skills" (Herdman & Kamitsuru, 2014, p. 259).

Client Goals

Outcome criteria include short- and long-term goals. Time lines are individually determined.

Short-term goals

■ Client utilizes measures provided (e.g., clocks, calendars, room identification) to maintain reality orientation.

■ Client experiences fewer episodes of acute confusion.

Long-term goal

■ Client maintains reality orientation to the best of his or her cognitive ability.

Interventions

For the Client Who Is Disoriented

■ Try to keep the client as oriented to reality as possible.

■ Use clocks and calendars with large numbers that are easy to read.

■ Place large, colorful signs on the doors to identify clients' rooms, bathrooms, activity rooms, dining rooms, and chapel.

■ Allow the client to have as many of his or her personal items as possible. Even an old familiar chair in the room can provide a degree of comfort.

■ If at all possible, encourage family and close friends to be a part of the client's care, to promote feelings of security and orientation.

■ Provide the client with radio, television, and music if they are diversions the client enjoys; these may add a feeling of familiarity to the environment.

■ Ensure that noise level is controlled to prevent excess stimulation. One study found that use of earplugs at night decreased risk for delirium by 53 percent and patients reported improved sleep (Van Rompaey et al., 2012)

■ Allow the client to view old photograph albums and utilize reminiscence therapy. These are excellent ways to provide orientation to reality.

■ Maintain consistency of staff and caregivers to the best extent possible. Familiarity promotes comfort and feelings of security.

■ Continuously monitor for medication side effects. Physiological changes in the elderly can alter the body's response to certain medications. Toxic effects may intensify altered cognitive processes.

■ There has been criticism about reality orientation of individuals with NCD (particularly those with moderate to severe disease process), suggesting that constant relearning of material contributes to problems with mood and self-esteem (Spector et al., 2000). See Box 22–4, Validation Therapy, for more information.

For the Client With Delusions and Hallucinations

■ Minimize focus on delusional thinking. Do not disagree with made-up stories. Instead, gently correct the client, offer reassurance that he or she is safe, and guide the conversation toward topics about real events and real people.

BOX 22–4 **Validation Therapy**

Some people believe it is not helpful (and sometimes even cruel) to try to insist that a person with moderate to severe NCD continually try to grasp what we know as the "real world." Allen (2000) states,

There is no successful alternative but to accept whatever the dementia person claims as their reality, no matter how untrue it is to us. There is no successful way to "force" a person with dementia to join the "real" world. The most frustrated caregivers are the ones who do not accept this simple fact: the world of dementia is defined by the dementia victim.

Validation therapy (VT) was originated by Naomi Feil, a gerontological social worker, who describes the process as "communicating with a disoriented elderly person by validating and respecting their feelings in whatever time or place is real to them at the time, even though this may not correspond with our 'here and now' reality" (Day, 2013). Feil suggests that the validation principle is truthful to the person with NCD because people live on several levels of awareness (Feil, 2013). She suggests that if an individual asks to see his or her spouse, and the spouse has been dead for many years, that on some level of awareness, that person knows the truth. To keep reminding the person that the spouse is dead may only serve to cause repeated episodes of grief and distress, as he or she receives the information "anew" each time it is presented (Allen, 2000).

Validation therapy validates the feelings and emotions of a person with NCD. It often also integrates redirection techniques. Allen (2000) states, "The key is to 'agree' with what they want but by conversation and 'steering' get them to do something else without them realizing they are actually being redirected. This is both validation and redirection therapy."

EXAMPLES

 Mrs. W. (agitated): That old lady stole my watch! I know she did. She goes into people's rooms and takes our things. We call her "sticky fingers"!

Nurse: That watch is very important to you. Have you looked around the room for it?

Mrs. W.: My husband gave it to me. He will be so upset that it is gone. I'm afraid to tell him.

Nurse: I'm sure you miss your husband very much. Tell me what it was like when you were together. What kinds of things did you do for fun?

Mrs. W.: We did a lot of traveling. To Italy, and England, and France. We ate wonderful food.

Nurse: Speaking of food, it is lunch time, and I will walk with you to the dining room.

Mrs. W.: Yes, I'm getting really hungry.

In this situation, the nurse validated Mrs. W.'s feelings about not being able to find her watch. She did not deny that it had been stolen, nor did she remind Mrs. W. that her husband was deceased. *(Remember: a concept of VT is that, on some level, Mrs. W. knows that her husband is dead.)* The nurse validated the emotions Mrs. W. was feeling about missing her husband. She brought up special times that Mrs. W. and her husband had spent together, which served to elevate Mrs. W.'s mood and self-esteem. Finally, she redirected Mrs. W. to the dining room to have her lunch. (The watch was eventually found in Mrs. W.'s medicine cabinet, where she had hidden it for safekeeping.)

BOX 22–4 Validation Therapy—cont'd

Feil (2013) presents another example:

When a resident asks for his wife who is dead, caregivers reply, "She'll be here to see you later." The resident may not remember much, but he clings to that statement. He continues to ask for his wife on a daily basis, and the caregivers continue to lie. Eventually, he loses trust in the caregivers, knowing that what they say is not true. With VT, the caregivers would encourage the resident to talk about his wife. They would validate his emotions and encourage him to express his needs, accepting the fact that there is a reason behind his behavior. He has not simply "forgotten that his wife died"; he needs to grieve for her. This is unfinished business. When the emotion is expressed and someone listens with empathy, it is relieved. The old man no longer needs to search for his wife. He feels safe with the caregiver, whom he trusts. He always knew on a deep level of awareness that his wife had died. (pp. 3, 4)

■ Never argue a point with the client; to do so only serves to increase his or her anxiety and agitation.

■ Do not ignore reports of hallucinations when it is clear that the client is experiencing them. It is important for the nurse to hear an explanation of the hallucination from the client. These perceptions are very real and often very frightening to the client. Unless they are appropriately managed, hallucinations can escalate into disturbing and even hostile behaviors. Visual and auditory hallucinations are the most common type in NCD. The physician may treat these manifestations with antipsychotic medication.

■ Assess for side effects of medications as a potential contributing factor to sensory perception disturbances.

■ Check to ensure that hearing aid is working properly and to ensure that faulty sounds are not being emitted.

■ Check eyeglasses to ensure that the individual is indeed wearing his or her own glasses.

■ Assess for other possible contributing factors to illusions or visual hallucination. Clients often see faces in patterns on fabrics or in pictures on the wall. A mirror can also be the culprit of false perceptions. These may need to be moved or covered.

■ Provide reassurance that the client is safe. It may be necessary to stay with the client for a while until he or she is calm.

■ Never argue that the hallucination is not real. Try to let the client know that, although you are not sharing the experience, you understand how very distressing it is for him or her.

■ Distract the client. Hallucinations are less likely to occur when the person is occupied or involved in what is going on around him or her. Focus on real situations and real people.

■ Assess whether or not the hallucinations are problematic for the patient. Not all hallucinations are upsetting.

EXAMPLE

An elderly woman approaches the nurses' station and says, "I'm so perturbed. The woman in my room refuses to turn down my bed so that I can go to sleep." The nurse may respond, "I will walk to your room with you and see that your bed is turned down." The nurse chats with the client about something that occurred during the day, and by the time they arrive at her room, there is no further mention of a woman in her room.

Impaired Verbal Communication

When individuals who are cognitively impaired begin to lose the ability to process verbal communication, the way that words are expressed becomes as important as what is said. NANDA-I defines *Impaired verbal communication* as "decreased, delayed, or absent ability to receive, process, transmit, and/or use a system of symbols" (Herdman & Kamitsuru, 2014).

Client Goals

Outcome criteria include short- and long-term goals. Time lines are individually determined.

Short-term goals

■ Client is able to make needs known to primary caregiver.

■ Client is able to understand basic communications in interactions with primary caregiver.

Long-term goal

■ In latter stages of the illness when client is unable to communicate, needs are anticipated and fulfilled by primary caregiver.

Interventions

■ Use a calm and reassuring approach when interacting with the client.

■ Use simple words, speak slowly and distinctly, and keep face-to-face contact with the client.

■ Always identify yourself to the client and call him or her by name at each meeting.

- Use nonverbal gestures to help the client understand what you want him or her to accomplish, if appropriate.
- Ask only one question (or give only one direction) at a time, and give the client plenty of time to process the information and respond. The question may need to be rephrased if it is clear that the client has not understood the meaning.
- Always try to approach the client from the front. An unexpected approach or touch from behind may startle and upset the client and may even promote aggressive behavior.
- Maintain consistency of staff and caregivers to the best extent possible. This facilitates comfort and security and promotes an effective communication process with the client.
- Should the client become verbally aggressive, remain calm and provide validation for his or her feelings: "I know this is a hard time for you. You were always so busy and so active, and you took care of so many people. Maybe you could tell me about some of those people."
- When it is clearly appropriate, use touch and affection to communicate. Sometimes clients will respond to a hug or to a hand reaching for theirs when they will respond to nothing else.

Self-Care Deficit

It is important for clients to remain as independent as possible for as long as possible. They should be encouraged to accomplish ADLs to the best of their ability. NANDA-I defines *Self-care deficit* as "impaired ability to perform or complete activities" (Herdman & Kamitsuru, 2014).

Client Goals

Outcome criteria include short- and long-term goals. Time-lines are individually determined.

Short-term goal

- Client participates in ADLs with assistance from caregiver.

Long-term goals

- Client accomplishes ADLs to the best of his or her ability.
- Unfulfilled needs are met by caregiver.

Interventions

- Provide a simple, structured environment for the client, identify self-care deficits, and offer assistance as required.
- Allow plenty of time for the client to complete tasks.
- Provide guidance and support for independent actions by talking the client through the task one step at a time.

- Provide a structured schedule of activities that does not change from day to day.
- Ensure that ADLs follow the client's usual routine as closely as possible.
- Minimize confusion by providing for consistency in assignment of daily caregivers.
- Perform an ongoing assessment of the client's ability to fulfill his or her nutritional needs, ensure personal safety, follow the medication regimen, and communicate the need for assistance with activities that he or she cannot accomplish independently. Anticipate needs that are not verbally communicated.
- If the client is to be discharged to family caregivers, assess those caregivers' ability to anticipate and fulfill client's unmet needs. Provide information to assist caregivers with this responsibility. Ensure that caregivers are aware of available community support systems from which they may seek assistance when required. Examples include adult day care centers, housekeeping and homemaker services, respite care services, and the local chapter of a national support organization. Following are two helpful resources:
  - For AD information:
    Alzheimer's Association
    225 N. Michigan Ave., Fl. 17
    Chicago, IL 60601-7633
    1-800-272-3900
    www.alz.org
  - For Parkinson's disease information:
    National Parkinson Foundation, Inc.
    200 SE 1st St, Suite 800
    Miami, FL 33131
    1-800-4PD-INFO (473-4636)
    www.parkinson.org

Concept Care Mapping

The concept map care plan (see Chapter 9, The Nursing Process in Psychiatric-Mental Health Nursing) is a diagrammatic teaching and learning strategy that allows visualization of interrelationships between medical diagnoses, nursing diagnoses, assessment data, and interventions. An example of a concept map care plan for a client with an NCD is presented in Figure 22–3.

Client and Family Education

The role of client teacher is important in the psychiatric area, as it is in all areas of nursing. A list of topics for client/family education relevant to NCDs is presented in Box 22–5.

Evaluation

In the final step of the nursing process, reassessment occurs to determine if the nursing interventions have been effective in achieving the intended goals of care. Evaluation of the client with an NCD is based on a series of short-term goals rather than on long-term

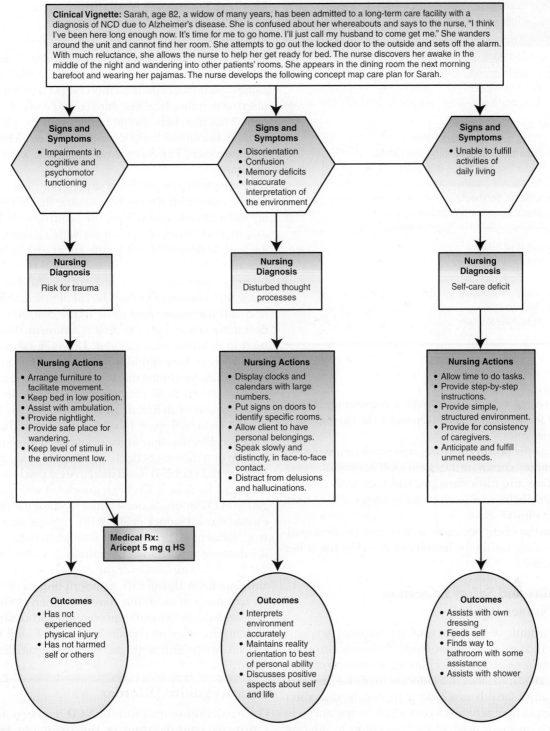

Clinical Vignette: Sarah, age 82, a widow of many years, has been admitted to a long-term care facility with a diagnosis of NCD due to Alzheimer's disease. She is confused about her whereabouts and says to the nurse, "I think I've been here long enough now. It's time for me to go home. I'll just call my husband to come get me." She wanders around the unit and cannot find her room. She attempts to go out the locked door to the outside and sets off the alarm. With much reluctance, she allows the nurse to help her get ready for bed. The nurse discovers her awake in the middle of the night and wandering into other patients' rooms. She appears in the dining room the next morning barefoot and wearing her pajamas. The nurse develops the following concept map care plan for Sarah.

Signs and Symptoms
• Impairments in cognitive and psychomotor functioning

Signs and Symptoms
• Disorientation
• Confusion
• Memory deficits
• Inaccurate interpretation of the environment

Signs and Symptoms
• Unable to fulfill activities of daily living

Nursing Diagnosis
Risk for trauma

Nursing Diagnosis
Disturbed thought processes

Nursing Diagnosis
Self-care deficit

Nursing Actions
• Arrange furniture to facilitate movement.
• Keep bed in low position.
• Assist with ambulation.
• Provide nightlight.
• Provide safe place for wandering.
• Keep level of stimuli in the environment low.

Nursing Actions
• Display clocks and calendars with large numbers.
• Put signs on doors to identify specific rooms.
• Allow client to have personal belongings.
• Speak slowly and distinctly, in face-to-face contact.
• Distract from delusions and hallucinations.

Nursing Actions
• Allow time to do tasks.
• Provide step-by-step instructions.
• Provide simple, structured environment.
• Provide for consistency of caregivers.
• Anticipate and fulfill unmet needs.

Medical Rx:
Aricept 5 mg q HS

Outcomes
• Has not experienced physical injury
• Has not harmed self or others

Outcomes
• Interprets environment accurately
• Maintains reality orientation to best of personal ability
• Discusses positive aspects about self and life

Outcomes
• Assists with own dressing
• Feeds self
• Finds way to bathroom with some assistance
• Assists with shower

FIGURE 22–3   Concept map care plan for client with major neurocognitive disorder.

goals. Outcomes are measured in terms of slowing down the process rather than stopping or curing the problem. Evaluation questions may include the following:

■ Has the client experienced injury?
■ Does the client maintain orientation to time, person, place, and situation to the best of his or her cognitive ability?

■ Is the client able to fulfill basic needs? Have those needs unmet by the client been fulfilled by caregivers?
■ Is confusion minimized by familiar objects and structured, routine schedule of activities?
■ Do the prospective caregivers have information regarding the progression of the client's illness?

BOX 22–5 Topics for Client/Family Education Related to Neurocognitive Disorders

1. Nature of the illness
   a. Possible causes
   b. What to expect
   c. Symptoms

2. Management of the illness
   a. Ways to ensure client safety
   b. How to maintain reality orientation
   c. Providing assistance with ADLs
   d. Nutritional information
   e. Difficult behaviors
   f. Medication administration
   g. Matters related to hygiene and toileting

3. Support services
   a. Financial assistance
   b. Legal assistance
   c. Caregiver support groups
   d. Respite care
   e. Home health care

■ Do caregivers have information regarding where to go for assistance and support in the care of their loved one?

■ Have the prospective caregivers received instruction in how to promote the client's safety, minimize confusion and disorientation, and cope with difficult client behaviors (e.g., hostility, anger, depression, agitation)?

■ Has the client been able to maintain the best quality of life within the limitations posed by his or her illness?

Quality and Safety Education for Nurses (QSEN)

The Institute of Medicine (now the National Academy of Medicine), in its report *Health Professions Education: A Bridge to Quality* (Greiner, Knebel, & Institute of Medicine, 2003), challenged faculties of medicine, nursing, and other health professions to ensure that their graduates have achieved a core set of competencies in order to meet the needs of the 21st-century health-care system. These competencies include *providing patient-centered care, working in interdisciplinary teams, employing evidence-based practice, applying quality improvement, maintaining safety,* and *utilizing informatics.* A QSEN teaching strategy is included in Box 22–6. The use of this type of activity is intended to arm the instructor and student with guidelines for attaining the knowledge, skills, and attitudes necessary for achievement of quality and safety competencies in nursing.

Medical Treatment Modalities

Delirium

The first step in the treatment of delirium should be the determination and correction of the underlying causes. Additional attention must be given to fluid and electrolyte status, hypoxia, anoxia, and diabetic problems. Staff members should remain with the client at all times to monitor behavior and provide reorientation and assurance. The room should maintain a low level of stimuli.

Some physicians prefer not to prescribe medications for the client with delirium, reasoning that additional agents may only compound the syndrome of brain dysfunction. However, psychosis with agitation and aggression demonstrated by the client with delirium may require chemical and/or mechanical restraint for his or her personal safety. Choice of specific therapy is made with consideration for the client's clinical condition and the underlying cause of the delirium. Low-dose antipsychotics are the most common medications used in delirium management. However, two recent meta-analyses have found mixed results. One analysis of 15 studies concluded that second-generation antipsychotics are beneficial (and preferable to haloperidol) in treatment of delirium (Kishi et al., 2015), but a second meta-analysis of 19 studies concluded that the evidence does not support use of antipsychotics for prevention or treatment of delirium (Neufeld et al., 2016). Haloperidol (Haldol) is still used to treat psychotic features, but because it has been associated with prolongation of QT intervals, nurses must monitor the client's cardiac status (Sadock et al., 2015). A benzodiazepine (e.g., lorazepam) is commonly used when the etiology is substance withdrawal (Eisendrath & Lichtmacher, 2012). Melatonin, an over-the-counter supplement, and ramelteon (Rozerem), a prescription medication for treatment of insomnia, have both been identified as potentially beneficial in prevention and treatment of delirium, since melatonin levels were found to be altered in patients with delirium (Alagiakrishnan, 2016).

Neurocognitive Disorder

Once a definitive diagnosis of NCD has been made, a primary consideration in the treatment of the disorder is the etiology. Focus must be directed to the identification and resolution of potentially reversible processes. Sadock and colleagues (2015) note that once dementia is apparent, it is essential to complete a clinical workup to identify the syndrome and its causes because "approximately 15% of people with dementia have reversible illnesses if treatment is initiated before irreversible damage takes place" (p. 704).

BOX 22–6 QSEN TEACHING STRATEGY

Assignment: Linking Evidence-Based Practice With a Nursing Procedure
Reality Orientation of Clients With Neurocognitive Disorder
Competency Domain: Evidence-Based Practice
Learning Objectives: Student will:
• Locate an evidence-based practice article on protocols for reality orientation in patients with NCDs and compare and contrast this information with the protocols established by the hospital or other assigned facility for clinical experience.
• Identify whether evidence-based practice is utilized with this protocol, and identify barriers or challenges with implementing evidence-based practice in the clinical setting.

Strategy Overview:
1. Research the nursing intervention of reality orientation of clients with NCD. Identify the pros and cons and ethical issues associated with this intervention (particularly with clients who have advanced NCD).
2. Find an evidence-based practice journal article about the intervention.
3. Locate the facility's protocol for reality orientation of clients with NCD.
4. Compare and contrast the facility's protocol with how unit staff carry out this intervention. If there are deviations from the written protocol, what are they, and why do they occur?
5. Compare and contrast the hospital's protocol with the information found in the evidence-based practice article.
6. At postconference, summarize the article on evidence-based practice to the clinical group, and report information gathered throughout the clinical day. Discuss any ethical dilemmas associated with the intervention.
7. Write a paper discussing personal reflections and feelings about this intervention.

Adapted from teaching strategy submitted by Chris Tesch, Instructor, University of South Dakota, Sioux Falls, SD. © 2009 QSEN; http://qsen.org. With permission.

The need for general supportive care with provisions for security, stimulation, patience, and nutrition, has been recognized and accepted. A number of pharmaceutical agents have been tried with varying degrees of success in the treatment of clients with NCD. Some of these drugs are described in the following sections according to symptomatology for which they are indicated. A summary of medications for clients with NCD is provided in Table 22–4.

Cognitive Impairment

Cholinesterase inhibitors are often used for treatment of mild to moderate cognitive impairment in AD and have demonstrated efficacy in treating patients

TABLE 22–4 Selected Medications Used in the Treatment of Clients With NCD

MEDICATION	CLASSIFICATION	FOR TREATMENT OF	DAILY DOSAGE RANGE (mg)	SIDE EFFECTS
Donepezil (Aricept)	Cholinesterase inhibitor	Cognitive impairment	5–10	Insomnia, dizziness, gastrointestinal (GI) upset, headache
Rivastigmine (Exelon)	Cholinesterase inhibitor	Cognitive impairment	6–12	Dizziness, headache, GI upset, fatigue
Galantamine (Razadyne)	Cholinesterase inhibitor	Cognitive impairment	8–24	Dizziness, headache, GI upset
Memantine (Namenda)	NMDA receptor antagonist	Cognitive impairment	5–20	Dizziness, headache, constipation
Memantine, extended release + donepezil (Namzaric)	Anti-Alzheimer's agent	Moderate to severe Alzheimer's type dementia	Memantine ER, 14–28 mg, and donepezil 10 mg, once daily	Headache, nausea, vomiting, dizziness, diarrhea, decreased appetite

Continued

TABLE 22–4	**Selected Medications Used in the Treatment of Clients With NCD—cont'd**			
MEDICATION	CLASSIFICATION	FOR TREATMENT OF	DAILY DOSAGE RANGE (mg)	SIDE EFFECTS
Risperidone* (Risperdal)	Antipsychotic	Agitation, aggression, hallucinations, thought disturbances, wandering	1–4 (increase dosage cautiously)	Agitation, insomnia, headache, insomnia, extrapyramidal symptoms
Olanzapine* (Zyprexa)	Antipsychotic	Agitation, aggression, hallucinations, thought disturbances, wandering	5 (increase dosage cautiously)	Hypotension, dizziness, sedation, constipation, weight gain, dry mouth
Quetiapine* (Seroquel)	Antipsychotic	Agitation, aggression, hallucinations, thought disturbances, wandering	Initial dose 25 (titrate slowly)	Hypotension, tachycardia, dizziness, drowsiness, headache, constipation, dry mouth
Haloperidol* (Haldol)	Antipsychotic	Agitation, aggression, hallucinations, thought disturbances, wandering	1–4 (increase dosage cautiously)	Dry mouth, blurred vision, orthostatic hypotension, extrapyramidal symptoms, sedation
Pimavanserin (Nuplazid)	Antipsychotic	Hallucinations and delusions specifically associated with Parkinson's disease psychosis. *Note:* Pimavanserin is not approved for dementia-related psychosis unrelated to Parkinson's disease psychosis	34 mg daily (17 mg, twice daily)	Peripheral edema, nausea, confusion, hallucinations, constipation, gait disturbance
Sertraline (Zoloft)	Antidepressant (SSRI)	Depression	50–100	Fatigue, insomnia, sedation, GI upset, headache, dizziness
Paroxetine (Paxil)	Antidepressant (SSRI)	Depression	10–40	Dizziness, headache, insomnia, somnolence, GI upset
Nortriptyline (Pamelor)	Antidepressant (tricyclic)	Depression	30–50	Anticholinergic, orthostatic hypotension, sedation, arrhythmia
Lorazepam** (Ativan)	Antianxiety (benzodiazepine)	Anxiety	1–2	Drowsiness, dizziness, GI upset, hypotension, tolerance, dependence
Oxazepam** (Serax)	Antianxiety (benzodiazepine)	Anxiety	10–30	Drowsiness, dizziness, GI upset, hypotension, tolerance, dependence
Temazepam** (Restoril)	Sedative/Hypnotic (benzodiazepine)	Insomnia	15	Drowsiness, dizziness, GI upset, hypotension, tolerance, dependence
Zolpidem (Ambien)	Sedative-hypnotic (nonbenzodiazepine)	Insomnia	5	Headache, drowsiness, dizziness, GI upset
Zaleplon (Sonata)	Sedative-hypnotic (nonbenzodiazepine)	Insomnia	5	Headache, drowsiness, dizziness, GI upset
Eszopiclone (Lunesta)	Sedative-hypnotic (nonbenzodiazepine)	Insomnia	1–2	Headache, drowsiness, dizziness, GI upset, unpleasant taste
Ramelteon (Rozerem)	Sedative-hypnotic (nonbenzodiazepine)	Insomnia	8	Dizziness, fatigue, drowsiness, GI upset

TABLE 22–4 Selected Medications Used in the Treatment of Clients With NCD–cont'd

MEDICATION	CLASSIFICATION	FOR TREATMENT OF	DAILY DOSAGE RANGE (mg)	SIDE EFFECTS
Trazodone	Antidepressant (heterocyclic)	Depression and insomnia	50	Dizziness, drowsiness, dry mouth, blurred vision, GI upset
Mirtazapine (Remeron)	Antidepressant (tetracyclic)	Depression and insomnia	7.5–15	Somnolence, dry mouth, constipation, increased appetite

*Although clinicians may still prescribe these medications in low-risk patients, no antipsychotics have been approved by the FDA for the treatment of patients with NCD-related psychosis. All antipsychotics include black-box warnings about increased risk of death in elderly patients with NCD.
**Benzodiazepines should be used only for short-term treatment.

with Lewy body dementia (Crystal & Jacobs, 2014). (Higher-dose donepezil has also been approved for moderate to severe AD.) Some of the clinical manifestations of AD are thought to result from a deficiency of the neurotransmitter acetylcholine. In the brain, acetylcholine is inactivated by the enzyme acetylcholinesterase. Donepezil (Aricept), rivastigmine (Exelon), and galantamine (Razadyne) act by inhibiting acetylcholinesterase, which slows the degradation of acetylcholine, thereby increasing concentrations of the neurotransmitter in the cerebral cortex. Because their action relies on functionally intact cholinergic neurons, the effects of these medications may lessen as the disease process advances, and there is no evidence that these medications alter the course of the underlying degenerative process.

Another medication, an NMDA receptor antagonist, was approved by the FDA in 2003. The medication, memantine (Namenda), was approved for the treatment of moderate to severe AD. Studies on the use of memantine for Parkinson's disease and dementia with Lewy bodies have been inconclusive (Schwarz, Froelich, & Burns, 2012). High levels of glutamate in the brains of AD patients are thought to contribute to the symptomatology and decline in functionality. These high levels are caused by a dysfunction in glutamate transmission. In normal neurotransmission, glutamate plays an essential role in learning and memory by triggering NMDA receptors to allow a controlled amount of calcium to flow into a nerve cell. This creates the appropriate environment for information processing. In AD, there is a sustained release of glutamate, which results in a continuous influx of calcium into the nerve cells. This increased intracellular calcium concentration ultimately leads to disruption and death of the neurons. Memantine may protect cells against excess glutamate by partially blocking NMDA receptors. Memantine has been shown in clinical trials to be effective in improving cognitive function and the ability to perform ADLs in clients with moderate to severe AD. Although it does not stop or reverse the effects of the disease, it

has been shown to slow down the progression of the decline in cognition and function (Salloway & Correia, 2009). Because memantine's action differs from that of the cholinesterase inhibitors, consideration is being given to possible coadministration of these medications. However, combination therapy with acetylcholinesterase inhibitors and memantine remains controversial because research findings have demonstrated conflicting results (Schwarz et al., 2012). In 2014, the FDA approved one such drug (Namzaric), which is a combination of memantine and donepezil.

Current drug trials are underway to test for a vaccine against AD. One study led by the Karolinska Institutet in Sweden reported positive use with CAD106, a vaccine designed to trigger the body's immune defense against Aβ (Winblad et al., 2012). So far, active vaccines have not demonstrated effectiveness in humans and in some cases have proved dangerous, so research efforts have moved to a focus on passive vaccines (McDonald, 2014). Vaccine trials have continued for the last several years without major breakthroughs. However, in 2016, a group of American and Australian researchers reported a "very promising" vaccine that they claim impacts amyloid and tau proteins, both of which are implicated in AD. It is clear that interest in such research is high, with government funding for AD research exceeding $1 billion in 2016 (LaVigne, 2016). The researchers believe that the vaccine will have both preventive and treatment benefits (Davtyan et al., 2016). They expect (pending successful clinical trials in humans) to have a treatment available within 3 to 5 years (LaVigne, 2016).

In a study funded by the National Institute on Aging and others, three drugs were evaluated in the prevention of a rare and aggressive form of autosomal-dominant AD (Bateman et al., 2012). These clinical trials included individuals who are mutation carriers and therefore genetically destined to develop AD at a young age, typically in their 30s, 40s, or 50s. To date, there have been no medications clearly identified or approved as preventive for this condition. Genotyping and genetic counseling are available options for evaluation and management (National Center for Advancing Translational Sciences, 2015). Antipsychotics have been associated with increased mortality in patients with dementia, and Moussa (2016) recommends that prescribers use low doses of quetiapine or olanzapine only "in patients with severe, disabling symptoms after informing families of the mortality risk."

Gingko biloba is a popular over-the-counter supplement advanced as having benefits for improving cognitive impairment and symptoms of dementia. Its actions include dilating blood vessels, thinning blood, modifying neurotransmitters, and reducing the density of oxygen free radicals (Birks & Grimley, 2009). But in a systematic review of 36 trials, Birks and Grimley conclude that evidence for benefits in cognitive impairment or dementia is inconsistent and unreliable.

More recent research has focused on the chemical resveratrol, found in grape skins, cacao, and other foods. It has been advanced as having anti-aging properties and neuroprotective functions, as well as possibly reducing the buildup of amyloid plaques associated with AD. The most recent of these studies (Turner et al., 2015) found promising evidence that high doses of resveratrol (up to 2000 mg daily) has CNS effects on biomarkers for AD. The researchers caution that more research is needed to fully understand the impact of these changes on the trajectory of AD.

With regard to nonpharmacologic treatments for cognitive impairment in patients with NCD, cognitive rehabilitation (which includes education about cognitive strengths and weaknesses, cognitive retraining, and compensatory strategies) has demonstrated some evidence of modest improvement in cognitive domains, although research is in the early stages (Dancis & Cotter, 2015). Recent studies have also supported that mindfulness meditation results in observable changes in brain structures related to memory and emotional responses and therefore may have benefits in the treatment of NCDs (Sorrell, 2015).

Agitation, Aggression, Hallucinations, Thought Disturbances, and Wandering

Historically, physicians have prescribed antipsychotic medications to control agitation, aggression, hallucinations, thought disturbances, and wandering in clients with NCD. The atypical antipsychotic medications, such as risperidone, olanzapine, quetiapine, and ziprasidone, were often favored because of their lessened propensity to cause anticholinergic and extrapyramidal side effects. In 2005, however, following review of a number of studies, the FDA ordered black-box warnings on drug labels of all the atypical antipsychotics, noting that the drugs are associated with an increased risk of death in elderly patients who display psychotic behaviors associated with NCD. Most of the

deaths appeared to be cardiovascular related. In July 2008, based on the results of several studies, the FDA extended this warning to include all first-generation antipsychotics as well, such as haloperidol and perphenazine. This poses a clinical dilemma for physicians who have found these medications to be helpful to their clients, and some have chosen to continue to use them in patients without significant cerebrovascular disease, in which previous behavioral programs have failed, and with consent from relatives or guardians who are clearly aware of the risks and benefits.

In 2016, a new drug, pimavanserin (Nuplazid), was approved by the FDA specifically for treatment of hallucinations and delusions in Parkinson's disease psychosis. The mechanism of action is unknown, but it is thought to provide benefit through its serotonin agonist and antagonist activities.

Anticholinergic Effects

Many antipsychotic, antidepressant, and antihistaminic medications produce anticholinergic side effects, which include confusion, blurred vision, constipation, dry mouth, dizziness, and difficulty urinating. Older people, and especially those with NCD, are particularly sensitive to these effects because of decreased cholinergic reserves. Many elderly individuals are also at increased risk for developing an anticholinergic toxicity syndrome because of the additive anticholinergic effects of multiple medications (Hall, Hall, & Chapman, 2009).

Depression

It is estimated that up to 40 percent of people with AD also suffer from major depression (Alzheimer's Association, 2015b). Recognizing the symptoms of depression in these individuals is often a challenge. Depression—which affects thinking, memory, sleep, and appetite and interferes with daily life—is sometimes difficult to distinguish from NCD. Clearly, the existence of depression in the client with NCD complicates and worsens the individual's functioning.

Antidepressant medication is sometimes used in treatment of depression in those with NCD. The selective serotonin reuptake inhibitors (SSRIs) are considered by many to be the first-line drug treatment for depression in the elderly because of their favorable side-effect profile, although patients should be assessed for hyponatremia, since this is a risk associated with SSRIs. Tricyclic antidepressants are often avoided because of cardiac and anticholinergic side effects. Trazodone may be a good choice when used at bedtime for depression and insomnia.

Not only is depression common among those with AD, but research has suggested that it may be a risk factor for the disease (Caraci et al., 2010; Geerlings et al., 2008; Wilson et al., 2014). Several theories have been advanced about the causes for this correlation, including one theory that depression directly damages the brain through the effects of stress and chronic inflammation, another that depression may decrease brain volume, and a third that depression may be an early sign of dementia (Bowers, 2014). Whatever the causes, Wilson and associates (2014) found that depression is an independent risk factor for the development of dementia. Although antidepressant medication may be prescribed for patients with dementia, a review of the research indicated that the efficacy of antidepressants in this population remains unproven (Schwarz et al., 2012).

Anxiety

The progressive loss of mental functioning is a significant source of anxiety in the early stages of NCD. It is important that clients be encouraged to verbalize their feelings and fears associated with this loss. These interventions may be useful in reducing the anxiety of clients with NCD.

Antianxiety medications may be helpful but should not be used routinely or for prolonged periods. The least toxic and most effective of the antianxiety medications are the benzodiazepines. Examples include diazepam (Valium), chlordiazepoxide (Librium), alprazolam (Xanax), lorazepam (Ativan), and oxazepam (Serax). Studies have been conducted to evaluate the concern that long-term benzodiazepine use may actually contribute to the development of dementia, but the results have been mixed (Billioti de Gage et al., 2014; Gray et al., 2016). The drugs with shorter half-lives (e.g., lorazepam and oxazepam) are preferred to longer-acting medications (e.g., diazepam), which promote a higher risk of oversedation and falls. Barbiturates are not appropriate as antianxiety agents because they frequently induce confusion and paradoxical excitement in elderly individuals.

Sleep Disturbances

Sleep problems are common in clients with NCD and often intensify as the disease progresses. Wakefulness and nighttime wandering create much distress and anguish in family members who are charged with protection of their loved one. Indeed, sleep disturbances are among the problems that most frequently initiate the need for client placement in a long-term care facility.

Some physicians treat sleep problems with sedative-hypnotic medications. The benzodiazepines may be useful for some clients but are indicated for relatively brief periods only. Examples include flurazepam (Dalmane), temazepam (Restoril), and triazolam (Halcion). Daytime sedation, cognitive impairment, risk for falls, and paradoxical agitation in elderly clients are of particular concern with these medications. The nonbenzodiazepine sedative-hypnotics zolpidem (Ambien), zaleplon (Sonata), eszopiclone (Lunesta), and ramelteon (Rozerem) and the antidepressants trazodone (Desyrel) and mirtazapine (Remeron) may also be prescribed. Daytime sedation is a potential problem with these medications, too. As previously stated, barbiturates should not be used in elderly clients. Sleep problems are usually ongoing, and most clinicians prefer to use medications only to help an individual through a short-term stressful situation. Rising at the same time each morning; minimizing daytime sleep; participating in regular physical exercise no later than 4 hours before bedtime; getting proper nutrition; avoiding alcohol, caffeine, and nicotine; and retiring at the same time each night are behavioral approaches to sleep problems that may eliminate the need for sleep aids, particularly in the early stages of NCD. Because of the tremendous potential for adverse drug reactions in the elderly, many of whom are already taking multiple medications, pharmacological treatment of insomnia should be considered only after attempts at nonpharmacological strategies have failed.

CASE STUDY AND SAMPLE CARE PLAN

NURSING HISTORY AND ASSESSMENT

Carmen is an 81-year-old widow who lives in the same small town in the same house that she shared with her husband until his death 16 years ago. She and her husband reared two daughters, Joan and Nancy, who live with their husbands in a large city about 2 hours away from Carmen. They have always visited Carmen every 1 or 2 months. She has four grown grandchildren who live in distant states and who see their grandmother on holidays.

About a year ago, Carmen's daughters began to receive reports from friends and other family members about incidents in which Carmen was becoming forgetful (e.g., forgetting to go to a cousin's birthday party, taking a wrong turn and getting lost on the way to a niece's house [where she had driven many times], returning to church to search for something she thought she had forgotten [although she could not explain what it was], sending birthday gifts to people at the wrong times). During visits, the elder daughter, Joan, found bills left

Continued

CASE STUDY AND SAMPLE CARE PLAN—cont'd

unpaid, sometimes months overdue. Housekeepers and yard workers reported to Joan that Carmen would forget she had paid them and try to pay them again, sometimes even a third time. She became very confused when she would attempt to fill her weekly pillboxes, a task she had completed in the past without difficulty. Hundreds of dollars would disappear from her wallet, and she could not tell Joan what happened to it.

Joan and her husband subsequently moved to the small town where Carmen lived. They bought a home, and Joan visited her mother every day, took care of finances, and ensured that Carmen took her daily medications, although the daughter worked in a job that required occasional out-of-town travel. As the months progressed, Carmen's cognitive abilities deteriorated. She burned food on the stove, left the house with the oven on, forgot to take her medication, got lost in her car, missed appointments, and forgot the names of neighbors she had known for many years. She began to lose weight because she was forgetting to eat her meals.

Carmen was evaluated by a neurologist, who diagnosed her with neurocognitive disorder due to Alzheimer's disease. Because they believed that Carmen needed 24-hour care, Joan and Nancy made the painful decision to place Carmen in a long-term nursing facility. In the nursing home, her condition has continued to deteriorate. Carmen wanders up and down the halls (day and night) and has fallen twice, once while attempting to get out of bed. She requires assistance to shower and dress and has become incontinent of urine. The nurses found her attempting to leave the building, saying, "I'm going across the street to visit my daughter." One morning at breakfast, she appeared in her pajamas in the communal dining room, not realizing that she had not dressed. She is unable to form new memories and sometimes uses confabulation to fill in the blanks. She asks the same questions repeatedly, sometimes struggling for the right word. She can no longer provide the correct names of items in her environment. She has no concept of time.

Joan visits Carmen daily and Nancy visits weekly, each offering support to the other in person and by phone. Carmen always seems pleased to see them but can no longer call either of them by name. They are unsure if she knows who they are.

NURSING DIAGNOSES AND OUTCOME IDENTIFICATION

From the assessment data, the nurse develops the following nursing diagnoses for Carmen:

1. **Risk for trauma** related to impairments in cognitive and psychomotor functioning; wandering; falls
   a. **Outcome criteria:** Carmen will remain injury free during her nursing home stay.
   b. **Short-term goals:**
      ■ Carmen will not fall while wandering the halls.
      ■ Carmen will not fall out of bed.

2. **Disturbed thought processes** related to cerebral degeneration evidenced by disorientation, confusion, and memory deficits
   a. **Outcome criteria:** Carmen will maintain reality orientation to the best of her cognitive ability.
   b. **Short-term goals:**
      ■ Carmen will be able to find her room.
      ■ Carman will be able to communicate her needs to staff.

3. **Self-care deficit** related to cognitive impairments, disorientation, confusion, and memory deficits
   a. **Outcome criteria:** Carmen will accomplish ADLs to the best of her ability.
   b. **Short-term goals:**
      ■ Carmen will assist with dressing herself.
      ■ Carmen will cooperate with trips to the bathroom.
      ■ Carmen will wash herself in the shower with help from the nurse.

PLANNING AND IMPLEMENTATION

RISK FOR TRAUMA

The following nursing interventions may be implemented *to ensure client safety:*

1. Arrange the furniture in Carmen's room so that it will accommodate free movement.
2. Store frequently used items within her easy reach.
3. Provide a "low bed," or possibly move her mattress from the bed to the floor, to prevent falls from bed.
4. Attach a bed alarm to alert the nurse's station when Carmen has alighted from her bed.
5. Keep a dim light on in her room at night.
6. During the day and evening, provide a well-lighted area where Carmen can safely wander.
7. Ensure that all outside doors are electronically controlled.
8. Play soft music and maintain a low level of stimuli in the environment.

DISTURBED THOUGHT PROCESSES

The following nursing interventions may be implemented *to help maintain orientation and aid in memory and recognition:*

1. Use clocks and calendars with large numbers that are easy to read.
2. Put a sign on Carmen's door with her name on it, and hang a personal item of hers on the door.
3. Ask Joan to bring some of Carmen's personal items for her room, even a favorite comfy chair if possible. Ask for some old photograph albums if they are available.
4. Keep the number of staff and caregivers to a minimum to promote familiarity.
5. Speak slowly and clearly while looking into Carmen's face.
6. Use reminiscence therapy with Carmen. Ask her to share happy times from her life with you. This technique helps decrease depression and boost self-esteem.

CASE STUDY AND SAMPLE CARE PLAN—cont'd

7. Mention the date and time in casual conversation. Refer to "spring rain," "summer flowers," "fall leaves." Emphasize holidays.
8. Correct misperceptions gently and matter-of-factly, and focus on real events and real people if false ideas should occur. Validate her feelings associated with current and past life situations.
9. Monitor for medication side effects, because toxic effects from certain medications can intensify altered thought processes.

SELF-CARE DEFICIT

The following nursing interventions may be implemented *to ensure that all Carmen's needs are fulfilled.*

1. Assess what Carmen can do independently and with which tasks she needs assistance.
2. Allow plenty of time for her to accomplish tasks that are within her ability. Clothing with easy removal or replacement, such as Velcro, facilitates independence.
3. Provide guidance and support for independent actions by talking her through tasks one step at a time.
4. Provide a structured schedule of activities that does not change from day to day.

5. Ensure that Carmen has snacks between meals.
6. Take Carmen to the bathroom regularly (according to her usual pattern, e.g., after meals, before bedtime, on arising).
7. To minimize nighttime wetness, offer fluid every 2 hours during the day and restrict fluid after 6 p.m.
8. To promote more restful nighttime sleep and less wandering at night, reduce naps during late afternoon and encourage sitting exercises, walking, and ball toss. Carbohydrate snacks at bedtime may also be helpful.

EVALUATION

The outcome criteria identified for Carmen have been met. She has experienced no injury. She has not fallen out of bed. She continues to wander in a safe area. She can find her room by herself but occasionally requires some assistance when she is anxious and confused. She has some difficulty communicating her needs to the staff, but those who work with her on a consistent basis are able to anticipate her needs. All ADLs are being fulfilled, and Carmen assists with dressing and grooming, accomplishing about half on her own. Nighttime wandering has been minimized. Soft bedtime music helps to relax her.

Summary and Key Points

- NCDs constitute a large and growing public health concern.
- Delirium is a disturbance of awareness and change in cognition that develop rapidly over a short period. Level of consciousness is often affected, and psychomotor activity may fluctuate between agitated purposeless movements and a vegetative state resembling catatonic stupor.
- The symptoms of delirium usually begin quite abruptly and often are reversible and brief.
- Delirium may be caused by a general medical condition, substance intoxication or withdrawal, or ingestion of a medication or exposure to a toxin. NCD is a syndrome of acquired, persistent intellectual impairment ranging from mild to major, with compromised function in multiple spheres of mental activity, such as memory, language, visuospatial skills, emotion or personality, and cognition.
- Dementia (also described as major NCD in the *DSM-5*) is a progressive decline of cognitive abilities in the presence of clear consciousness.
- Symptoms of NCD are insidious and develop slowly over time. In most clients, the disorder runs a progressive, irreversible course.
- NCD may be caused by genetics, cardiovascular disease, infections, neurophysiological disorders, and other medical conditions.

- Nursing care of the client with an NCD is presented around the six steps of the nursing process.
- Objectives of care for the client experiencing an acute syndrome are aimed at eliminating the etiology, promoting client safety, and facilitating a return to the highest possible level of functioning.
- Objectives of care for the client experiencing a chronic, progressive disorder are aimed at preserving the dignity of the individual, promoting deceleration of the symptoms, maximizing functional capabilities, and maintaining the best quality of life within the limitations posed by illness.
- Nursing interventions are also directed toward helping the client's family or primary caregivers learn about and cope with the changes expected in a chronic, progressive neurocognitive disorder.
- Education is provided about the disease process, expectations of client behavioral changes, methods for facilitating care, and sources of assistance and support as they struggle, both physically and emotionally, with the demands brought on by a disease process that is slowly taking their loved one away from them.

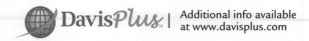
DavisPlus | Additional info available at www.davisplus.com

Review Questions
Self-Examination/Learning Exercise

Select the answer that is most appropriate for each of the following questions.

1. An example of a treatable (reversible) form of NCD is one that is caused by which of the following? (Select all that apply.)
   a. Multiple sclerosis
   b. Huntington's disease
   c. Electrolyte imbalance
   d. HIV disease
   e. Folate deficiency

2. Mrs. G. has been diagnosed with NCD due to Alzheimer's disease. The cause of this disorder is which of the following?
   a. Multiple small brain infarcts
   b. Chronic alcohol abuse
   c. Cerebral abscess
   d. Unknown

3. Mrs. G. has been diagnosed with NCD due to Alzheimer's disease. The *primary* nursing intervention in working with Mrs. G. is which of the following?
   a. Ensuring that she receives food she likes to prevent hunger
   b. Ensuring that the environment is safe to prevent injury
   c. Ensuring that she meets the other patients to prevent social isolation
   d. Ensuring that she takes care of her own ADLs to prevent dependence

4. Which of the following medications have been indicated for improvement in cognitive functioning in mild to moderate Alzheimer's disease? (Select all that apply.)
   a. Donepezil (Aricept)
   b. Rivastigmine (Exelon)
   c. Risperidone (Risperdal)
   d. Sertraline (Zoloft)
   e. Galantamine (Razadyne)

5. Mrs. G., who has NCD due to Alzheimer's disease, says to the nurse, "I have a date tonight. I always have a date on Christmas." Which of the following is the most appropriate response?
   a. "Don't be silly. It's not Christmas, Mrs. G."
   b. "Today is Tuesday, October 21, Mrs. G. We will have supper soon, and then your daughter will come to visit."
   c. "Who is your date with, Mrs. G.?"
   d. "I think you need some more medication, Mrs. G. I'll bring it to you now."

6. In addition to disturbances in cognition and orientation, individuals with Alzheimer's disease may also show changes in which of the following? (Select all that apply.)
   a. Personality
   b. Vision
   c. Speech
   d. Hearing
   e. Mobility

7. Mrs. G., who has NCD due to Alzheimer's disease, has trouble sleeping and wanders around at night. Which of the following nursing actions would be *best* to promote sleep in Mrs. G.?
   a. Ask the doctor to prescribe flurazepam (Dalmane).
   b. Ensure that Mrs. G. gets an afternoon nap so she will not be overtired at bedtime.
   c. Make Mrs. G. a cup of tea with honey before bedtime.
   d. Ensure that Mrs. G. gets regular physical exercise during the day.

Review Questions—cont'd
Self-Examination/Learning Exercise

8. The night nurse finds Mrs. G., a client with Alzheimer's disease, wandering the hallway at 4 a.m. and trying to open the door to the side yard. Which statement by the nurse probably reflects the most accurate assessment of the situation?
   a. "That door leads out to the patio, Mrs. G. It's nighttime. You don't want to go outside now."
   b. "You look confused, Mrs. G. What is bothering you?"
   c. "This is the patio door, Mrs. G. Are you looking for the bathroom?"
   d. "Are you lonely? Perhaps you'd like to go back to your room and talk for a while."

9. Which of the following factors is *not* associated with increased incidence of NCD due to Alzheimer's disease?
   a. Multiple small strokes
   b. Family history of Alzheimer's disease
   c. Head trauma
   d. Advanced age

10. Mr. Stone is a client in the hospital with a diagnosis of vascular NCD. In explaining this disorder to Mr. Stone's family, which of the following statements by the nurse is correct?
    a. "He will probably live longer than if his disorder was of the Alzheimer's type."
    b. "Vascular NCD shows stepwise progression. This is why he sometimes seems okay."
    c. "Vascular NCD is caused by plaques and tangles that form in the brain."
    d. "The cause of vascular NCD is unknown."

11. Which of the following interventions is most appropriate in helping a client with Alzheimer's disease with her ADLs? (Select all that apply.)
    a. Perform ADLs for her while she is in the hospital.
    b. Provide her with a written list of activities she is expected to perform.
    c. Assist her with step-by-step instructions.
    d. Tell her that if her morning care is not completed by 9 a.m., it will be performed for her by the nurse's aide so that she can attend group therapy.
    e. Encourage her and give her plenty of time to perform independently as many of her ADLs as possible.

TEST YOUR CRITICAL THINKING SKILLS

Joe, a 62-year-old accountant, began having difficulty remembering details necessary to perform his job. He was also having trouble at home, failing to keep his finances straight, and forgetting to pay bills. It became increasingly difficult for him to function properly at work, and eventually he was forced to retire. Cognitive deterioration continued and behavioral problems soon began. He became stubborn, verbally and physically abusive, and suspicious of most everyone in his environment. His wife and son convinced him to see a physician, who recommended hospitalization for testing.

At Joe's initial evaluation, he was fully alert and cooperative but obviously anxious and fidgety. He thought he was at his accounting office, and he could not state what year it was. He could not say the names of his parents or siblings, nor did he know who was currently the president of the United States. He could not perform simple arithmetic calculations, write a proper sentence, or copy a drawing. He interpreted proverbs concretely and had difficulty stating similarities between related objects.

Laboratory serum studies revealed no abnormalities, but a CT scan showed marked cortical atrophy. The physician's diagnosis was neurocognitive disorder due to Alzheimer's disease.

Answer the following questions related to Joe:

1. Identify the pertinent assessment data from which nursing care will be devised.
2. What is the primary nursing diagnosis for Joe?
3. How would outcomes be identified?

Communication Exercises

1. Mrs. B. is a patient on the Alzheimer's unit. The nurse hears her yelling, "Waitress! Waitress! Why can't I get some service around here?"
   - How would the nurse respond appropriately to this statement by Mrs. B.?
2. Mrs. B., who had breakfast an hour ago, says to the nurse, "I've been waiting and waiting for my breakfast. On the farm, we always had breakfast by 6 o'clock. Those were the good old days."
   - How would the nurse respond appropriately to this statement by Mrs. B?

 MOVIE CONNECTIONS

The Notebook (Alzheimer's disease)
Away From Her (Alzheimer's disease)
Iris (Alzheimer's disease)

References

Alagiakrishnan, K. (2016). Delirium medications. Retrieved from http://emedicine.medscape.com/article/288890-medication

Allen, J. (2000). Using validation therapy to manage difficult behaviors. *Prism Innovations. ElderCare Online*. Retrieved from www.ec-online.net/community/Activists/difficult behaviors.htm

Alvarez, N. (2016). Alzheimer disease in Down syndrome. Retrieved from http://emedicine.medscape.com/article/1136117-overview

Alzheimer's Association. (2015a). 2015 Alzheimer's disease facts and figures. *Alzheimer's & Dementia 2015, 11*(3). Retrieved from www.alz.org/facts/downloads/facts_figures_2015.pdf

Alzheimer's Association. (2015b). Depression and Alzheimer's. Retrieved from www.alz.org/care/alzheimers-dementia-depression.asp

Alzheimer's Association. (2016). 2016 Alzheimer's disease facts and figures. *Alzheimer's & Dementia 2016;12*(4). Retrieved from https://www.alz.org/documents_custom/2016-facts-and-figures.pdf

Alzheimer's Disease Education & Referral. (2015a). Alzheimer's disease genetics. National Institute on Aging. Retrieved from www.nia.nih.gov/alzheimers/publication/alzheimers-disease-genetics-fact-sheet

Alzheimer's Disease Education & Referral. (2015b). Translating knowledge into promising treatments. National Institute on Aging. Retrieved from https://www.nia.nih.gov/alzheimers/publication/2013-2014-alzheimers-disease-progress-report/translating-knowledge-promising

American Psychiatric Association (APA). (2000). *Diagnostic and statistical manual of mental disorders* (4th ed.) *Text revision*. Washington, DC: APA.

American Psychiatric Association (APA). (2013). *Diagnostic and statistical manual of mental Disorders* (5th ed.). Washington, DC: APA.

Bateman, R.J., Xiong, C., Benzinger, T.L.S., Fagan, A.M., Goate, A., Fox, N.C., Marcus, D.S., . . . Morris, J.C. (2012). Clinical and biomarker changes in dominantly inherited Alzheimer's disease. *New England Journal of Medicine, 367*(9), 795-804. doi:10.1056/NEJMoa1202753

Billioti de Gage, S., Moride, Y., Ducruet, T., Kurth, T., Verdoux, H., Tournier, M., . . . Bégaud, B. (2014). Benzodiazepine use and risk of Alzheimer's disease: Case-control study. *British Medical Journal, 349*, g5205. doi:http://dx.doi.org/10.1136/bmj.g5205

Birks, J., & Grimley, E. J. (2009). Ginkgo biloba for cognitive impairment and dementia. *Cochrane Database of Systematic Reviews, 21*(1), CD003120. doi:10.1002/14651858.CD003120

Black, D.W., & Andreasen, N.C. (2014). *Introductory textbook of psychiatry* (6th ed.). Washington, DC: American Psychiatric Publishing.

Bowers, E.S. (2014). Depression as a risk factor for dementia. Retrieved from www.everydayhealth.com/news/depression-risk-factor-dementia

Caraci, F., Copani, A., Nicoletti, F., & Drago, F. (2010). Depression and Alzheimer's disease: Neurobiological links and common pharmacological targets. *European Journal of Pharmacology, 626*(1), 64-71. doi:10.1016/j.ejphar.2009.10.022

Crystal, H.A., & Jacobs, D.H. (2014). Dementia with Lewy bodies: Treatment and management. *Medscape 2014*. Retrieved from emedicine.medscape.com/article/1135041-treatment

Dancis, A., & Cotter, V.T. (2015). Diagnosis and management of cognitive impairment in Parkinson's disease. *Journal for Nurse Practitioners, 11*(30), 307-313. doi:http://dx.doi.org/10.1016/j.nurpra.2014.11.023

Davtyan, H., Zagorski, K., Rajapaksha, H., Hovakimyan, A., Davtyan, A., Petrushina, I., & Ghochikyan, A. (2016). Alzheimer's disease AdvaxCpG- adjuvanted MultiTEP-based dual and single vaccines induce high-titer anti bodies against various forms of tau and Aβ pathological molecules. *Scientific Reports, 6*, 28912; doi:10.1038/srep28912.

Day, C.R. (2013). Validation therapy: A review of the literature. *Validation Training Institute*. Retrieved from www.vfvalidation.org/web.php?request=article1

Eisendrath, S.J., & Lichtmacher, J.E. (2012). Psychiatric disorders. In S.J. McPhee, M.A. Papadakis, & M.W. Rabow (Eds.), *Current medical diagnosis and treatment 2012* (pp. 1010-1064). New York: McGraw-Hill.

Feil, N. (2013). It is never good to lie to a person who has dementia. *Validation Training Institute, Inc.* Retrieved from www.vfvalidation.org//web.php?request=article5

Geerlings, M.I., den Heijer, T., Koudstaal, P.J., Hofman, A., & Breteler, M.M.B. (2008). History of depression, depressive symptoms, and medial temporal lobe atrophy and the risk of Alzheimer disease. *Neurology, 70*(15), 1258-1264. doi:10.1212/01.wnl.0000308937.30473.d1

Gray, S.L., Dublin, S., Yu, O., Walker, R., Anderson, M., Hubbard, R.A., & Larson, E.B. (2016). Benzodiazepine use and risk of incident dementia or cognitive decline: Prospective population based study. *British Medical Journal, 352*, i90. doi:http://dx.doi.org/10.1136/bmj.i90

Greiner, A., Knebel, E., & Institute of Medicine. (2003). *Health professions education: A bridge to quality*. Washington, DC: National Academies Press.

Hale, K.L., & Frank, J. (2015). Dementia causes. *eMedicineHealth.* Retrieved from www.emedicinehealth.com/script/main/art.asp?articlekey=59089&pf=3&page=2

Hall, R., Hall, R., & Chapman, M.J. (2009). Anticholinergic syndrome: Presentations, etiological agents, differential diagnosis, and treatment. *Clinical Geriatrics, 17*(11), 22-28.

Herdman, T.H., & Kamitsuru, S. (Eds.). (2014). *NANDA International nursing diagnoses: Definitions and classification 2015–2017* (10th ed.). Chichester, UK: Wiley Blackwell.

Huntington's Disease Society of America. (2016). What is Huntington's disease? Retrieved from http://hdsa.org/what-is-hd

Johns Hopkins Medicine. (No date). Prion diseases. *Health Library.* Retrieved from www.hopkinsmedicine.org/health library/conditions/nervous_system_disorders/prion_diseases_134,56

Kalish, V.B., Gillham, J. E., & Unwin, B. (2014). Delirium in older persons: Evaluation and management. *American Family Physician, 90*(3), 150-158. Retrieved from www.aafp.org/afp/2014/0801/p150.html

Kishi, T., Hirota, T., Matsunaga, S., & Iwata, N. (2015). Antipsychotic medications for the treatment of delirium: A systematic review and meta-analysis of randomised controlled trials. *Journal of Neurology, Neurosurgery, and Psychiatry, 87*(7), 767-774. doi:10.1136/jnnp-2015-311049

Lapum, J. L., & Bar, R.J. (2016). Dance for individuals with dementia. *Journal of Psychosocial Nursing, 54*(3), 31-34. doi:10.3928/02793695-20160219-05

LaVigne, P. (2016). Alzheimer's vaccine: Researchers target brain proteins in mouse study. *Vaccination Reaction.* Retrieved from www.thevaccinereaction.org/2016/08/alzheimers-vaccine-researchers-target-brain-proteins-in-mouse-study

Mayo Clinic. (2016a). Dementia: Symptoms and causes. Retrieved from www.mayoclinic.org/diseases-conditions/dementia/symptoms-causes/dxc-20198504

Mayo Clinic. (2016b). Alzheimer's disease: Symptoms and causes. Retrieved from www.mayoclinic.org/diseases-conditions/alzheimers-disease/symptoms-causes/dxc-20167103

Mayo Clinic. (2014). Frontotemporal dementia. Retrieved from www.mayoclinic.com/health/frontotemporal-dementia/DS00874

McDonald, I. (2014). Could an Alzheimer's disease vaccine be a reality? *Dementia News.* Retrieved from https://www.dementia researchfoundation.org.au/blog/could-alzheimer%E2%80%99s-disease-vaccine-be-reality

Mitchell, S. (2015). Advanced dementia. *New England Journal of Medicine, 372*(26), 2533-2540. doi:10.1056/NEJMcp1412652

Moussa, M. (2016). Alzheimer's disease. *Cardiology News.* Retrieved from http://www.mdedge.com/ecardiologynews/dsm/4936/hospital-medicine/alzheimers-disease

NANDA International (NANDA-I). (2012). *Nursing diagnoses: Definitions and classification 2012–2014.* Hoboken, NJ: Wiley-Blackwell.

National Center for Advancing Translational Sciences. (2015). Early-onset familial autosomal dominant Alzheimer disease. Retrieved from https://rarediseases.info.nih.gov/diseases/12798/early-onset-autosomal-dominant-alzheimer-disease

National Institute of Neurological Disorders and Stroke. (2015). NINDS frontotemporal dementia information page. National Institutes of Health. Retrieved from www.ninds.nih.gov/disorders/picks/picks.htm

National Institute on Aging. (2011) *Alzheimer's disease: Unraveling the mystery.* NIH Publication No. 08-3782. Washington, DC: National Institutes of Health, U.S. Department of Health and Human Services.

National Institute on Aging. (2013). About Alzheimer's disease: Symptoms. Retrieved from www.nia.nih.gov/alzheimers/topics/symptoms

National Institute on Aging. (2015a). 2014–2015 Alzheimer's disease progress report: Advancing research toward a cure. Retrieved from https://www.nia.nih.gov/alzheimers/publication/2014-2015-alzheimers-disease-progress-report/introduction

National Institute on Aging. (2015b). Health care costs for dementia found greater than for any other disease. Retrieved https://www.nia.nih.gov/newsroom/2015/10/health-care-costs-dementia-found-greater-any-other-disease

National Institutes of Health. (2016). APOE gene: Apolipoprotein E. *Genetics Home Reference.* Retrieved from https://ghr.nlm.nih.gov/gene/APOE#conditions

Neufeld, K.J., Yue, J., Robinson, T.N., Inouye, S.K., & Needham, D.M. (2016). Antipsychotic medication for prevention and treatment of delirium in hospitalized adults: A systematic review and meta-analysis. *Journal of the American Geriatrics Society, 64*(4), 705-14. doi:10.1111/jgs.14076

Puri, B.K., & Treasaden, I.H. (2012). *Textbook of psychiatry* (3rd ed.). Philadelphia: Churchill Livingstone Elsevier.

Rentz, C. (2008). Nursing care of the person with sporadic Creutzfeldt-Jakob disease. *Journal of Hospice and Palliative Nursing, 10*(5), 272-282. doi:10.1097/01

Rice, J., & Humphries, C. (2014). Off-label use of antipsychotic drugs in patients with dementia. *Journal for Nurse Practitioners, 10*(3), 200-204. doi:http://dx.doi.org/10.1016/j.nurpra.2013.11.017

Rogaeva, E., Meng. Y., Lee, J.H., Gu, Y., Kawarai, T., Zou, F., . . . St. George-Hyslop, P. (2007). The neuronal sortilin-related receptor SOR1 is genetically associated with Alzheimer disease. *Nature Genetics, 39*(2), 168-177. doi:10.1038/ng1943

Sadock, B.J., Sadock, V.A., & Ruiz, P. (2015). *Synopsis of psychiatry: behavioral sciences/clinical psychiatry* (11th ed.). Philadelphia: Lippincott Williams & Wilkins.

Salloway, S., & Correia, S. (2009). Alzheimer disease: Time to improve its diagnosis and treatment. *Cleveland Clinic Journal of Medicine, 76*(1), 49-58. doi:10.3949/ccjm.76a.072178

Schwarz, S., Froelich, L., & Burns, A. (2012). Pharmacologic treatment of dementia. *Current Opinion in Psychiatry, 25*(6), 542-550. doi:10.1097/YCO.06013e328358e4f2

Shin, J.H. (2015). Doll therapy: An intervention for nursing home residents with dementia. *Journal of Psychosocial Nursing, 53*(1), 13-18. doi:10.3928/02793695-20141218-03

Smith, G. (2014). Can a head injury cause or hasten Alzheimer's disease or other types of dementia? Mayo Clinic. Retrieved from www.mayoclinic.org/diseases-conditions/alzheimers-disease/expert-answers/alzheimers-disease/FAQ-20057837

Sorrell, J.M. (2015). Meditation for older adults. *Journal of Psychosocial Nursing, 53*(5), 15-19. doi:10.3928/02793695-20150330-01

Spector, A., Davies, S., Woods, B., & Orrell, M. (2000). Reality orientation for dementia: A systematic review of the evidence of effectiveness from randomized controlled trials. *The Gerontologist, 40*(2), 206-212. doi:https://doi.org/10.1093/geront/40.2.206

Stanley, M., Blair, K.A., & Beare, P.G. (2005). *Gerontological nursing: Promoting successful aging with older adults* (3rd ed.). Philadelphia: F.A. Davis.

Strub, R.L., & Black, F. W. (2000). *The mental status examination in neurology,* 4th ed., Philadelphia: F.A. Davis.

Turner, R.S., Thomas, R.G., Craft, S., van Dyck, C.H., Mintzer, J., Reynolds, B.A. . . . Alzheimer's Disease Cooperative Study. (2015). A randomized, double-blind, placebo-controlled trial of resveratrol for Alzheimer disease. *Neurology, 85*(16), 1383-1391. doi:10.1212/WNL.0000000000002035

Van Rompaey, B., Elseviers, M. M., Van Drom, W., Fromont, V., & Jorens, P. G. (2012). The effect of earplugs during the night on the onset of delirium and sleep perception: A randomized controlled trial in intensive care patients. *Critical Care, 16*(3), R73. doi:10.1186/cc11330

Wilson, R.S., Capuano, A.W., Boyle, P.A., Hoganson, G.M., Hizel, L.P., Shah, R.C., . . . Bennett, D.A. (2014). Clinical-pathologic study of depressive symptoms and cognitive decline in old age. *Neurology, 83*(8), 702-709. doi: http://dx.doi.org/10.1212/WNL.0000000000000715

Winblad, B., Andreasen, N., Minthon, L., Floesser, A., Imbert, G., Dumortier, T., . . . Graf, A. (2012). Safety, tolerability, and antibody response of active Aβ immuno-therapy with CAD106 in patients with Alzheimer's disease: Randomized, double-blind, placebo-controlled, first-in-human study. *The Lancet: Neurology, 11*(7), 597-604. doi:10.1016/S1474-4422(12)70140-0

Substance-Related and Addictive Disorders

23

CORE CONCEPTS

Addiction

Intoxication

Withdrawal

KEY TERMS

Alcoholics Anonymous

amphetamines

ascites

cannabis

codependency

detoxification

disulfiram

dual diagnosis

esophageal varices

Gamblers Anonymous

hepatic encephalopathy

Korsakoff's psychosis

opioids

peer assistance programs

phencyclidine

substitution therapy

Wernicke's encephalopathy

OBJECTIVES
After reading this chapter, the student will be able to:

1. Define *addiction, intoxication,* and *withdrawal*.
2. Discuss predisposing factors implicated in the etiology of substance-related and addictive disorders.
3. Identify symptomatology and use the information in assessment of clients with various substance-related and addictive disorders.
4. Identify nursing diagnoses common to clients with substance-related and addictive disorders, and select appropriate nursing interventions for each.
5. Identify topics for client and family teaching relevant to substance-related and addictive disorders.
6. Describe relevant outcome criteria for evaluating nursing care of clients with substance-related and addictive disorders.
7. Discuss the issue of substance-related and addictive disorders within the nursing profession.
8. Define *codependency,* and identify behavioral characteristics associated with the disorder.
9. Discuss treatment of codependency.
10. Describe various modalities relevant to treatment of individuals with substance-related and addictive disorders.

Substance-related disorders comprise two groups: substance-use disorders (addiction) and substance-induced disorders (intoxication, withdrawal, delirium, neurocognitive disorder, psychosis, bipolar disorder, depressive disorder, obsessive-compulsive disorder, anxiety disorder, sexual dysfunction, and sleep disorders). This chapter discusses addiction, intoxication, and withdrawal. The remainder of the substance-induced disorders are included in the chapters with which they share symptomatology (e.g., substance-induced depressive disorder is included in Chapter 25, Depressive Disorders; substance-induced anxiety disorder is included in Chapter 27, Anxiety, Obsessive-Compulsive, and Related Disorders). Also included in this chapter is a discussion of gambling disorder, a non-substance addiction disorder.

Drugs are a pervasive part of our society. Certain mood-altering substances, such as alcohol, caffeine, and nicotine, are socially acceptable and used moderately by many adult Americans. Society has even developed a relative indifference to an occasional abuse of these substances despite documentation of their negative impacts on health.

In addition, countless substances are produced for medicinal purposes. These include central nervous system (CNS) stimulants (e.g., **amphetamines**), CNS depressants (e.g., sedatives, tranquilizers), and numerous over-the-counter preparations designed to relieve nearly every kind of human ailment, real or imagined.

Some illegal substances have achieved a degree of social acceptance by certain societal subcultures. These drugs, such as marijuana and hashish, are by no means harmless, even though they are becoming legalized in some states. The long-term effects of use are still being studied, whereas the dangerous effects of other illegal substances (e.g., lysergic acid diethylamide [LSD], **phencyclidine,** cocaine, and heroin) have been well documented.

This chapter discusses the physical and behavioral manifestations and personal and social consequences related to the abuse of or addiction to alcohol, other CNS depressants, CNS stimulants, **opioids,** hallucinogens, and/or cannabis and those related to the non-substance addiction to gambling. Variations in attitudes regarding substance consumption and patterns of use are explored. For example, drinking alcohol is considered by many to be a part of the culture of college life, while at the same time, substance abuse is especially prevalent among individuals between the ages of 18 and 24. Substance-related disorders are diagnosed more commonly in men than in women, but the gender ratios vary with the class of the substance.

Codependency is described in this chapter, along with substance abuse treatment. The issue of substance impairment within the nursing profession is also explored. Nursing care for individuals with substance use and addictive disorders is presented in the context of the six steps of the nursing process. Various medical and other treatment modalities are also discussed.

Substance Use Disorder, Defined

> ### CORE CONCEPT
> **Addiction**
> A primary chronic disease of brain reward, motivation, memory, and related circuitry where a dysfunction in these circuits is connected to an individual pathologically pursuing reward and or relief by substance use and other behaviors. (American Society of Addiction Medicine [ASAM], 2015)

Substance Addiction

The *Diagnostic and Statistical Manual of Mental Disorders, Fifth Edition (DSM-5)* (American Psychiatric Association [APA], 2013) lists diagnostic criteria for addiction to specific substances, including alcohol, cannabis, hallucinogens, inhalants, opioids, sedative-hypnotics, stimulants, and tobacco. Individuals are considered to have a substance use disorder when use interferes with the ability to fulfill role obligations at work, school, or home. Often, the individual would like to control use of the substance, but attempts to do so fail and use continues to increase. Intense cravings lead to excessive time spent trying to procure more of the substance or recover from the effects of its use. Use of the substance causes problems with interpersonal relationships, and the individual may become socially isolated. Individuals with substance use disorders often participate in hazardous activities when they are impaired by the substance, and they continue to use the substance despite knowing that its use is contributing to a physical and/or psychological problem. Addiction is evident when tolerance develops and the amount required to achieve the desired effect continually increases. Symptoms characteristic of the specific substance occur when the individual with the addiction attempts to discontinue use.

Substance-Induced Disorders, Defined

CORE CONCEPT
Intoxication
A physical and mental state of exhilaration and emotional frenzy or lethargy and stupor.

Substance Intoxication

Substance intoxication is defined as the development of a reversible syndrome of symptoms following excessive use of a substance. The symptoms are drug specific and occur during or shortly after ingestion of the substance. There is a direct effect on the CNS, and disruption in physical and psychological functioning occurs. Judgment is disturbed, resulting in inappropriate and maladaptive behavior, and social and occupational functioning are impaired.

CORE CONCEPT
Withdrawal
The physiological and mental readjustment that accompanies the discontinuation of an addictive substance.

Substance Withdrawal

Substance withdrawal occurs upon abrupt reduction or discontinuation of a substance that has been used regularly over a prolonged period of time. The substance-specific syndrome includes clinically significant physical signs and symptoms as well as psychological changes such as disturbances in thinking, feeling, and behavior. Classes of psychoactive substances are defined in Box 23–1.

BOX 23–1 Classes of Psychoactive Substances

The following classes of psychoactive substances are associated with substance use and substance-induced disorders:

1. Alcohol
2. Caffeine
3. Cannabis
4. Hallucinogens
5. Inhalants
6. Opioids
7. Sedatives, hypnotics, anxiolytics
8. Stimulants
9. Tobacco

Predisposing Factors to Substance-Related Disorders

A number of factors have been implicated in the predisposition to abuse of substances. At present, no single theory can adequately explain the etiology of this problem. The interaction between various elements forms a complex collection of determinants that influence a person's susceptibility to abuse substances.

Biological Factors
Genetics

Hereditary factors appear to be involved in the development of substance use disorders, especially alcoholism. Children of alcoholics are four times more likely than other children to become alcoholics (American Academy of Child and Adolescent Psychiatry, 2015). Twin studies have demonstrated that monozygotic (one egg, genetically identical) twins have a higher rate for concordance of alcoholism than dizygotic (two eggs, genetically nonidentical) twins (Black & Andreasen, 2014). Further, biological offspring of alcoholic parents have a significantly greater incidence of alcoholism than offspring of nonalcoholic parents whether the child was reared by the biological parents or by nonalcoholic adoptive parents (Puri & Treasaden, 2011). Research continues to discover genetic influences in addiction, but currently scientists estimate that genetics account for 40 to 60 percent of a person's vulnerability (National Institute on Drug Abuse [NIDA], 2014).

Biochemistry

Although evidence shows that changes in brain structure and brain neurochemistry occur in the process of developing addiction, whether these changes wholly explain etiology remains controversial. Neurotransmitters believed to be involved in substance abuse include opioid, catecholamine (especially dopamine), and gamma-aminobutyric acid (GABA) systems (Sadock, Sadock, & Ruiz, 2015). Neuronal pathways that sense pleasure and reward, once activated, are believed responsible for pleasurable sensations associated with the substance as well as creating a "memory" that triggers desire for repeated use of the drug. These pathways are referred to as the brain-reward circuitry. Over time, the brain tries to compensate for this excessive activation by lowering levels of these neurotransmitters, resulting in the physical discomfort associated with drug withdrawal. At this point, the substance user may continue use of the substance simply to alleviate illness.

Skeptics of biochemical theories of addiction argue that since drug-dependent individuals have the capacity to change their behavior, addiction is more likely a complex interaction of several factors rather than a single biochemical process. While ongoing research will continue to shed light on specific mechanisms in addiction, both the American Society of Addiction Medicine (2015) and the Surgeon General (in a landmark report on addiction in the United States) (U.S. Department of Health and Human Services [HHS], 2016), agree that addiction is a disease of the brain.

Psychological Factors

Developmental Influences

The psychodynamic approach to the etiology of substance abuse focuses on a punitive superego and fixation at the oral stage of psychosexual development (Sadock et al., 2015). Individuals with punitive superegos turn to drugs to diminish unconscious anxiety and increase feelings of power and self-worth. Sadock and associates (2015) state, "As a form of self-medication, alcohol may be used to control panic, opioids to diminish anger, and amphetamines to alleviate depression" (pp. 619–620).

Personality Factors

Certain personality traits have been associated with an increased tendency toward addictive behavior. Some clinicians believe low self-esteem, frequent depression, passivity, antisocial personality traits, the inability to relax or to defer gratification, and the inability to communicate effectively are common in individuals who abuse substances. These personality characteristics are not necessarily *predictive* of addictive behavior, yet for reasons not completely understood, they often accompany addiction. In some cases, the substance user may be self-medicating to treat symptoms of depression or anxiety.

Cognitive Factors

Irrational thinking patterns have long been identified as a central problem in addiction. Whether these thought patterns contribute to the development of or simply perpetuate an existing addiction is unclear, but the influence they hold is widely accepted. Twerski (1997) describes these thought patterns as "addictive thinking" and suggests that when unchallenged, they may culminate in additional addictions even when a person stops using the drug to which they first became addicted. Some examples of irrational thinking patterns often associated with addiction include denial ("I'm not really addicted"), projection ("It's my wife's fault that I take drugs"), and rationalization ("I have to take drugs because I am in pain"). Exploring these thought patterns and their influence on problematic behavior, which is the basis of cognitive-behavioral therapy, has been identified as beneficial in addictions treatment (NIDA, 2012).

Sociocultural Factors

Social Learning

The effects of modeling, imitation, and identification on behavior can be observed from early childhood onward. The family appears to be an important influence in relation to substance use. Studies have shown that children and adolescents are more likely to use substances if their parents provide a model for substance use. Peers often exert substantial influence on the child or adolescent who is being encouraged to use substances for the first time. Modeling may continue to be a factor in substance use once the individual enters the workforce, particularly if the setting provides plenty of leisure time with coworkers and drinking is valued as a way to express group cohesiveness.

Conditioning

Conditioning is a term describing a learned response that occurs after repeated exposure to a stimulus. Substance abuse can become a learned response from the substance itself and from the environment where use occurs. Many substances create a pleasurable experience that encourages the user to repeat it; thus, it is the intrinsically reinforcing properties of addictive drugs that "condition" the individual to repeatedly seek out their use.

The environment in which the substance is taken also contributes to the reinforcement. If the environment is pleasurable, substance use usually increases. Further, as the substance induces a state of pleasure, the user often associates that environment with these feelings and thus with drug use. Aversive stimuli within an environment are thought to be associated with a decrease in substance use within that environment.

Cultural and Ethnic Influences

Factors within an individual's culture help establish patterns of substance use by molding attitudes, influencing patterns of consumption based on cultural acceptance, and determining the availability of the substance. For centuries, the French and Italians have considered wine an essential part of the family meal, even for children. The incidence of alcohol addiction is low, and acute intoxication from alcohol is not common. However, the possibility of chronic physiological effects associated with lifelong alcohol consumption cannot be ignored.

Historically, a high incidence of alcohol addiction has existed within the American Indian/Alaska Native (AI/AN) culture. Alcohol-related deaths among AI/AN people occur at rates 514 percent higher than that of the overall U.S. population (Purnell, 2014). Veterans Administration records show that 45 percent of AI/AN veterans are addicted to alcohol, a rate twice that of non-AI/AN veterans. Theories that attempt to explain the prevalence of alcohol abuse among this community include difficulty metabolizing alcohol, children modeling their parents' drinking habits, unemployment and poverty, and an attempt to fill the spiritual gap left by the loss of the traditional AI/AN religion.

The incidence of alcohol addiction is higher among northern Europeans than among southern Europeans. Alcohol problems in Ireland are among the highest internationally (Wilson, 2013), and drinking alcohol is a part of the social culture, as pubs are considered a hub for social activity.

Incidence of alcohol addiction among Asians is relatively low, possibly a result of genetic intolerance for the substance. Some Asians develop unpleasant symptoms when they drink alcohol, such as flushing, headaches, nausea, and palpitations. Research indicates an isoenzyme variant that quickly converts alcohol to acetaldehyde, as well as the absence of an isoenzyme that is needed to oxidize acetaldehyde, result in a rapid accumulation of acetaldehyde, which produces the unpleasant symptoms (Hanley, 2017). Some American Indians also report similar symptoms, and yet the rate of alcoholism is higher in this ethnic group (Hanley, 2017), so the role of this physical variation is unclear.

The Dynamics of Substance-Related Disorders

Alcohol Use Disorder
A Profile of the Substance

Alcohol is a natural substance formed by the reaction of fermenting sugar with yeast spores. Although there are many types of alcohol, the kind in alcoholic beverages is known scientifically as ethyl alcohol and chemically as C_2H_5OH. Its abbreviation, ETOH, is sometimes seen in medical records and other documents and publications.

By strict definition, alcohol is classified as a food because it contains calories; however, it has no nutritional value. Different alcoholic beverages are produced by using different sources of sugar for the fermentation process. For example, beer is made from malted barley, wine from grapes or berries, whiskey from malted grains, and rum from molasses. Distilled beverages (e.g., whiskey, scotch, gin, vodka, and other "hard" liquors) derive their names from further concentration of the alcohol through a process called *distillation*.

The alcohol content varies by type of beverage. For example, most American beers contain 3 to 6 percent alcohol, wines average 10 to 20 percent, and distilled beverages range from 40 to 50 percent alcohol. The average-sized drink, regardless of beverage, contains a similar amount of alcohol: 12 ounces of beer, 3 to 5 ounces of wine, and a cocktail with 1 ounce of whiskey all measure approximately 0.5 ounce. If consumed at the same rate, all would have an equal effect on the body.

Alcohol exerts a depressant effect on the CNS, resulting in behavioral and mood changes proportional to the alcoholic concentration in the blood. Most states consider legal intoxication as a blood alcohol level of 0.08 percent.

The body burns alcohol at the rate of about 0.5 ounce per hour, so behavioral changes would not be expected to occur in an individual who slowly consumed only one average-sized drink per hour. Other factors do influence these effects, however, such as an individual's physical size and whether or not the stomach contains food at the time of alcohol consumption. Alcohol is also thought to have a more profound effect when an individual is emotionally stressed or fatigued.

Historical Aspects

The use of alcohol can be traced back to the Neolithic age, with known consumption of beer and wine around 6400 BC. With the introduction of distillation by the Arabs in the Middle Ages, alchemists believed that alcohol was the answer to all of their ailments. The word *whiskey*, meaning "water of life," became widely known.

In America, AI/AN people drank beer and wine prior to the arrival of the first white immigrants. Refinement of the distillation process made beverages with high alcohol content readily available. By the early 1800s, one renowned physician of the time, Benjamin Rush, began to identify the widespread excessive, chronic alcohol consumption as a disease and an addiction. The strong religious mores on which this country was founded soon led to a driving force to prohibit the sale of alcoholic beverages. By the middle of the 19th century, 13 states had passed prohibition laws. The most notable prohibition of alcohol in the United States was from 1920 to 1933. The mandatory restrictions on national social habits resulted in the creation of profitable underground markets that led to flourishing criminal enterprises. Further, millions of dollars in federal, state, and local revenues from taxes and import duties on alcohol were lost. It is difficult to measure the value of this dollar loss against the human devastation and social costs that occur as a result of alcohol abuse in the United States today.

Patterns of Use

About two-thirds (66.6%) of Americans aged 12 years and older report being current drinkers of alcohol, and 6.4 percent met criteria for alcohol use disorder (Substance Abuse and Mental Health Services Administration [SAMHSA], 2015).

Why do people drink? In the United States, patterns show that people use alcoholic beverages to enhance the flavor of food with meals; at social gatherings to encourage relaxation and conviviality among the guests; and to promote a feeling of celebration at special occasions such as weddings, birthdays, and anniversaries. An alcoholic beverage (wine) is also used as part of the sacred ritual in some religious ceremonies. Therapeutically, alcohol is the major ingredient in many over-the-counter and prescription medicines that are prepared in concentrated form. Therefore, alcohol can be harmless and enjoyable— sometimes even beneficial—if it is used responsibly and in moderation.

Like any other mind-altering drug, however, alcohol has the potential for abuse. Indeed, it is identified as the third-largest drug problem the United States today, second only to misuse of prescription drugs followed by marijuana (SAMHSA, 2015). Annually, 88,000 deaths are related to excessive alcohol use, and it is the third-leading lifestyle-related cause of death in the United States (National Council on Alcoholism and Drug Dependence, 2017). In addition, alcohol use is a factor in more than half of all homicides, suicides, and traffic accidents. Incidents of domestic violence are commonly alcohol related. Heavy drinking contributes to illness in each of the top three causes of death: heart disease, cancer, and stroke. At any given time, up to 40 percent of hospital beds in the United States are being used to treat health conditions related to alcohol consumption. Fetal alcohol syndrome, caused by prenatal exposure to alcohol, is the leading known cause of mental retardation in the United States (Vaux, 2016).

Jellinek (1952) outlined four phases through which the alcoholic's pattern of drinking progresses. Some variability among individuals is to be expected within this model of progression.

Phase I. The Prealcoholic Phase

This phase is characterized by the use of alcohol to relieve the everyday stress and tensions of life. As a child, the individual may have observed parents or other adults drinking alcohol and enjoying the effects. The child learns that use of alcohol is an acceptable method of coping with stress. Tolerance develops, and the amount required to achieve the desired effect steadily increases.

Phase II. The Early Alcoholic Phase

This phase begins with blackouts—brief periods of amnesia that occur during or immediately following a period of drinking. Now the alcohol is no longer a source of pleasure or relief for the individual but rather a drug that is *required* by the individual. Common behaviors include sneaking drinks or secret drinking, preoccupation with drinking and maintaining the supply of alcohol, rapid gulping of drinks, and further blackouts. The individual feels enormous guilt and becomes very defensive about his or her drinking. Excessive use of denial and rationalization is evident.

Phase III. The Crucial Phase

In this phase, the individual has lost control of his or her use, and physiological addiction is clearly evident. This loss of control has been described as the inability to choose whether or not to drink. Binge drinking, lasting from a few hours to several weeks, is common. These episodes are characterized by sickness, loss of consciousness, squalor, and degradation. In this phase, the individual is extremely ill. Anger and aggression are common manifestations. Drinking is the total focus, and he or she is willing to risk losing everything that was once important in an effort to maintain the addiction. By this phase of the illness, it is not uncommon for the individual to have experienced the loss of job, marriage, family, friends, and most especially, self-respect.

Phase IV. The Chronic Phase

This phase is characterized by emotional and physical disintegration. The individual is usually intoxicated more often than he or she is sober. Emotional disintegration is evidenced by profound helplessness and self-pity. Impairment in reality testing may result in psychosis. Life-threatening physical manifestations may be evident in virtually every system of the body. Unmanaged withdrawal from alcohol results in a terrifying syndrome of symptoms that include hallucinations, tremors, convulsions, severe agitation, and panic. Depression and suicidal ideation are not uncommon. For long-term heavy drinkers, abrupt withdrawal of alcohol can be fatal.

Effects on the Body

Alcohol can induce a general, nonselective, reversible depression of the CNS. About 20 percent of the alcohol content in a single drink is absorbed directly and immediately into the bloodstream through the stomach wall. Unlike other "foods," it does not have to be digested. The blood carries the alcohol directly to the brain where it acts on the brain's central control areas, depressing brain activity. The other 80 percent of the drink's alcohol content is processed slightly more slowly through the upper intestinal tract and into the bloodstream. Only moments after alcohol is consumed, it can be found in all tissues, organs, and secretions of the body. Rapidity of absorption is influenced by various factors. For example, absorption is delayed when the drink is sipped rather than gulped, when the stomach contains food, and when the drink is wine or beer rather than a distilled beverage.

At low doses, alcohol produces relaxation, loss of inhibition, lack of concentration, drowsiness, slurred speech, and sleep. Chronic abuse results in multisystem physiological impairments. These complications include, but are not limited to, those outlined in the following sections.

Peripheral Neuropathy

Peripheral neuropathy, characterized by nerve damage, results in pain, burning, tingling, or prickly sensations of the extremities. Researchers believe it is the direct result of deficiency in the B vitamins, particularly thiamine. Nutritional deficiencies are common in chronic alcoholics because of insufficient intake of nutrients and because the toxic effect of alcohol results in malabsorption of nutrients. The process is reversible with abstinence from alcohol and restoration of required nutrients. Otherwise, permanent muscle wasting and paralysis can occur.

Alcoholic Myopathy

Alcoholic myopathy may occur as an acute or chronic condition. In the acute condition, also called *acute alcoholic necrotizing myopathy* or *alcoholic rhabdomyolysis,* the individual experiences a sudden onset of muscle pain, swelling, and weakness along with myoglobinuria, evidenced by a red tinge in the urine. Creatine kinase may be elevated before appearance of symptoms. Experimental studies have suggested that alcohol use and malnourishment are necessary to produce this syndrome (Lanska, 2016). Muscle symptoms are usually generalized, but pain and swelling may selectively involve the calves or other muscle groups. Laboratory studies show elevations of the enzymes creatine phosphokinase (CPK), lactate dehydrogenase (LDH), aldolase, and aspartate aminotransferase (AST). The symptoms of chronic alcoholic myopathy include a gradual wasting and weakness in skeletal muscles. Neither the pain and tenderness nor the elevated muscle enzymes seen in acute myopathy are evident in the chronic condition.

Alcoholic myopathy is thought to be a result of the same B vitamin deficiency that contributes to peripheral neuropathy. Improvement is observed with abstinence from alcohol and the return to a nutritious diet with vitamin supplements.

Wernicke's Encephalopathy

Wernicke's encephalopathy represents the most serious form of thiamine deficiency in alcoholics. Symptoms include paralysis of the ocular muscles, diplopia, ataxia, somnolence, and stupor. If thiamine replacement therapy is not undertaken quickly, death will ensue.

Korsakoff's Psychosis

Korsakoff's psychosis is identified by a syndrome of confusion, loss of recent memory, and confabulation in alcoholics. It is frequently encountered in clients recovering from Wernicke's encephalopathy. In the United States, the two disorders are usually considered together and are called *Wernicke-Korsakoff syndrome.* Treatment involves parenteral or oral thiamine replacement.

Alcoholic Cardiomyopathy

The effect of alcohol on the heart is an accumulation of lipids in the myocardial cells, resulting in enlargement and a weakened condition. The clinical findings of alcoholic cardiomyopathy generally relate to congestive heart failure or arrhythmia. Symptoms include decreased exercise tolerance, tachycardia, dyspnea, edema, palpitations, and nonproductive cough. Laboratory studies may show elevation of the enzymes CPK, AST, alanine aminotransferase (ALT), and LDH. Changes may be observed by electrocardiogram, and congestive heart failure may be evident on chest x-ray films.

The treatment is total permanent abstinence from alcohol. Treatment of the congestive heart failure may include rest, oxygen, digitalization, sodium restriction, and diuretics. Prognosis is encouraging if treated in the early stages. The death rate is high for individuals with advanced symptomatology.

Esophagitis

Esophagitis—inflammation and pain in the esophagus—occurs because of the toxic effects of alcohol on the esophageal mucosa and because of frequent vomiting associated with alcohol abuse.

Gastritis

The effects of alcohol on the stomach include inflammation of the stomach lining characterized by epigastric distress, nausea, vomiting, and distention. Alcohol breaks down the stomach's protective mucosal barrier, allowing hydrochloric acid to erode the stomach wall. Damage to blood vessels may result in hemorrhage.

Pancreatitis

Pancreatitis may be categorized as *acute* or *chronic*. Acute pancreatitis usually occurs a day or two after a binge of excessive alcohol consumption. Symptoms include constant, severe epigastric pain, nausea and vomiting, and abdominal distention. The chronic condition leads to pancreatic insufficiency resulting in steatorrhea, malnutrition, weight loss, and diabetes mellitus.

Alcoholic Hepatitis

Alcoholic hepatitis is inflammation of the liver caused by long-term heavy alcohol use. Clinical manifestations include an enlarged and tender liver, nausea and vomiting, lethargy, anorexia, elevated white blood cell count, fever, and jaundice. **Ascites** (fluid accumulation in the abdomen) and weight loss may be evident in more severe cases. With treatment—which includes strict abstinence from alcohol, proper nutrition, and rest—the individual can experience complete recovery. Severe cases can lead to cirrhosis or **hepatic encephalopathy.**

Cirrhosis of the Liver

Cirrhosis of the liver may be caused by anything that results in chronic injury to the liver. It is the end stage of alcoholic liver disease and results from long-term chronic alcohol abuse. There is widespread destruction of liver cells, which are replaced by fibrous (scar) tissue. Clinical manifestations include nausea and vomiting, anorexia, weight loss, abdominal pain, jaundice, edema, anemia, and blood coagulation abnormalities. Treatment includes abstention from alcohol, correction of malnutrition, and supportive care to prevent complications of the disease. Complications of cirrhosis include the following:

■ **Portal hypertension:** Elevation of blood pressure through the portal circulation results from defective blood flow through the cirrhotic liver.

■ **Ascites:** This condition, in which an excessive amount of serous fluid accumulates in the abdominal cavity, occurs in response to portal hypertension. The increased pressure results in the seepage of fluid from the surface of the liver into the abdominal cavity.

■ **Esophageal varices:** Esophageal varices are veins in the esophagus that become distended because of excessive pressure from defective blood flow through the cirrhotic liver. As this pressure increases, these varicosities can rupture, resulting in hemorrhage and sometimes death.

■ **Hepatic encephalopathy:** This serious complication occurs in response to the inability of the diseased liver to convert ammonia to urea for excretion. The continued rise in serum ammonia results in progressively impaired mental functioning, apathy, euphoria or depression, sleep disturbance, increasing confusion, and progression to coma and eventual death. Treatment includes complete abstention from alcohol, reduction of protein in the diet, and reduction of intestinal ammonia using neomycin or lactulose (National Library of Medicine, 2015).

Leukopenia

The production, function, and movement of the white blood cells are impaired in chronic alcoholics. This condition, called *leukopenia,* places the individual at high risk for contracting infectious diseases and for complicated recovery.

Thrombocytopenia

Platelet production and survival are impaired as a result of the toxic effects of alcohol. This places the alcoholic at risk for hemorrhage. Abstinence from alcohol rapidly reverses this deficiency.

Sexual Dysfunction

Alcohol interferes with the normal production and maintenance of female and male hormones, and long-term alcohol use can interfere with the liver's ability to metabolize estrogenic compounds (Sadock et al., 2015). For women, this can mean changes in the menstrual cycle and a decrease in or loss of fertility. For men, the altered hormone levels result in a diminished libido, decreased sexual performance, and impaired fertility. Gynecomastia may develop secondary to testicular atrophy.

Use During Pregnancy

Fetal Alcohol Syndrome

Prenatal exposure to alcohol can result in a broad range of disorders to the fetus, known as *fetal alcohol spectrum disorders* (FASDs), the most common of which is fetal alcohol syndrome (FAS). FAS includes physical, mental, behavioral, and/or learning disabilities with lifelong implications. There may be problems with learning, memory, attention span, communication, vision, hearing, or a combination of these (Centers for Disease Control and Prevention [CDC], 2016a). Other FASDs include alcohol-related neurodevelopmental disorder (ARND) and alcohol-related birth defects (ARBD).

There is no safe amount and no safe time to drink alcohol during pregnancy because alcohol can damage a fetus at any stage of development (CDC, 2016a; Vaux, 2016). Therefore, alcohol consumption should be avoided by women who are pregnant or trying to become pregnant. Estimates of the prevalence of FAS range from 0.2 to 1.5 per 1,000 live births (CDC, 2016a). Vaux (2016) adds that FAS crosses all racial and ethnic groups but regardless of race or ethnicity, the common feature in the development of fetal alcohol syndrome is women who drink heavily during pregnancy. Maier and West (2013) stated:

> The number of women who engage in heavy alcohol consumption during pregnancy surpasses the total number of children diagnosed with either FAS or ARND, meaning that not every child whose mother drank alcohol during pregnancy develops FAS or ARND. Moreover, the degree to which people with FAS or ARND are impaired differs from person to person. Several factors may contribute to this variation in the consequences of maternal drinking.

These factors include, but are not limited to, the following:

■ Maternal drinking pattern
■ Differences in maternal metabolism
■ Differences in genetic susceptibility
■ Timing of the alcohol consumption during pregnancy
■ Variation in the vulnerability of different brain regions

Sadock and associates (2015) report that women with alcohol-related disorders have a 35 percent risk of having a child with defects. Children with FAS may have the following characteristics or exhibit the following behaviors (CDC, 2016a):

■ Abnormal facial features (see Fig. 23–1)
■ Small head size
■ Shorter-than-average height
■ Low body weight
■ Poor coordination
■ Hyperactive behavior
■ Difficulty paying attention
■ Poor memory
■ Difficulty in school
■ Learning disabilities
■ Speech and language delays
■ Intellectual disability or low IQ
■ Poor reasoning and judgment skills
■ Sleep and sucking problems as a baby
■ Vision or hearing problems
■ Problems with the heart, kidneys, or bones

Neuroimaging of children with FAS shows abnormalities in brain size and shape. The frontal lobes and cerebellum are often smaller than normal, and the

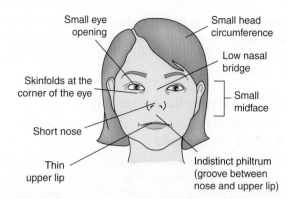

FIGURE 23–1 Facial features of fetal alcohol syndrome. (From the National Institute of Alcohol Abuse and Alcoholism of the National Institutes of Health, Washington, DC.)

corpus callosum and basal ganglia are commonly affected. Studies show that children with FAS are often at risk for psychiatric disorders, most commonly attention-deficit/hyperactivity disorder (Vaux, 2016). FAS may also co-occur with mood disorders, anxiety disorders, eating disorders, reactive attachment disorder, and conduct disorder (Elias, 2013).

Children with FAS require lifelong care and treatment. There is no cure for FAS, but it can be prevented. The Surgeon General's Advisory on Alcohol Use in Pregnancy states:

> Health professionals should inquire routinely about alcohol consumption by women of childbearing age, inform them of the risks of alcohol consumption during pregnancy, and advise them not to drink alcoholic beverages during pregnancy. (Carmona, 2005, p. 1)

Alcohol Intoxication

Symptoms of alcohol intoxication include disinhibition of sexual or aggressive impulses, mood lability, impaired judgment, impaired social or occupational functioning, slurred speech, incoordination, unsteady gait, nystagmus, and flushed face. Intoxication usually occurs at blood alcohol levels between 100 and 200 mg/dL. Death has been reported at levels ranging from 400 to 700 mg/dL.

Alcohol Withdrawal

Within 4 to 12 hours of cessation of or reduction in heavy and prolonged alcohol use (several days or longer), the following withdrawal symptoms may appear: coarse tremor of hands, tongue, or eyelids; nausea or vomiting; malaise or weakness; tachycardia; sweating; elevated blood pressure; anxiety; depressed mood or irritability; transient hallucinations or illusions; headache; and insomnia. In about 1 percent of alcoholic patients, complicated withdrawal syndrome may progress to *alcohol withdrawal delirium* (Sadock et al., 2015). Concomitant medical problems may increase this risk. Onset of delirium is usually on the second or third day following decrease or discontinuation of alcohol use. Symptoms include those described under the syndrome of delirium (Chapter 22, Neurocognitive Disorders).

Sedative, Hypnotic, or Anxiolytic Use Disorder

A Profile of the Substance

The sedative, hypnotic, anxiolytic compounds are drugs of diverse chemical structures that are capable of inducing varying degrees of CNS depression, from tranquilizing relief of anxiety to anesthesia, coma, and even death. They are generally categorized as (1) barbiturates, (2) nonbarbiturate hypnotics, and (3) antianxiety agents. Effects produced by these substances depend on size of dose and potency of drug administered.

Table 23–1 presents a selected list of drugs included in these categories. Generic names are followed in parentheses by the trade names. Common street names for each category are also included.

Several principles have been identified that are fairly typical among all CNS depressants:

1. **The effects of CNS depressants are additive with one another and with the behavioral state of the user.** For example, when these drugs are used in combination with each other or with alcohol, the depressive effects are compounded. These intense depressive effects are often unpredictable and can even be fatal. Similarly, a person who is mentally depressed or physically fatigued may have an exaggerated response to a dose of the drug that would only slightly affect a person in a normal or excited state.

2. **CNS depressants are capable of producing physiological addiction.** If large doses of CNS depressants are repeatedly administered over a prolonged duration, a period of CNS hyperexcitability occurs upon withdrawal of the drug. The response can be quite severe, even leading to convulsions and death.

3. **CNS depressants are capable of producing psychological addiction.** CNS depressants have the potential to generate a psychic drive for periodic or continuous administration of the drug to achieve maximum functioning or feeling of well-being.

4. **Cross-tolerance and cross-dependence may exist between various CNS depressants.** Cross-tolerance is exhibited when one drug results in a lessened response to another drug. Cross-dependence is a condition in which one drug can prevent withdrawal symptoms associated with physical addiction to a different drug (Julien, 2014).

TABLE 23–1 **Sedative, Hypnotic, and Anxiolytic Drugs**		
CATEGORIES	GENERIC (TRADE) NAMES	COMMON STREET NAMES
Barbiturates	Amobarbital (Amytal) Pentobarbital (Nembutal) Secobarbital (Seconal) Butabarbital (Butisol) Phenobarbital	Blue birds, blue angels (amobarbital); yellow jackets, yellow birds (pentobarbital); GBs, red birds, red devils (secobarbital)
Nonbarbiturate hypnotics	Chloral hydrate Estazolam Flurazepam Temazepam (Restoril) Triazolam (Halcion) Quazepam (Doral) Eszopiclone (Lunesta) Ramelteon (Rozerem) Zaleplon (Sonata) Zolpidem (Ambien)	Peter, Mickey (chloral hydrate); sleepers
Antianxiety agents	Alprazolam (Xanax) Chlordiazepoxide (Librium) Clonazepam (Klonopin) Clorazepate (Tranxene) Diazepam (Valium) Lorazepam (Ativan) Oxazepam (Serax) Meprobamate (Miltown)	Green and whites, roaches (Librium); candy, downers (the benzodiazepines); Vs (Valium; color designates strength); dolls, dollies (meprobamate)
Club drugs	Flunitrazepam (Rohypnol) Gamma hydroxybutyric acid (gamma hydroxybutyrate; GHB)	Date rape drug, roofies, R-2, rope (Rohypnol); G, liquid X, grievous bodily harm, easy lay (GHB)

Historical Aspects

Anxiety and insomnia, two of the most common human afflictions, were treated during the 19th century with opiates, bromide salts, chloral hydrate, paraldehyde, and alcohol (Julien, 2014). Because opiates were known to produce physical addiction, the bromides carried the risk of chronic bromide poisoning, and chloral hydrate and paraldehyde had an objectionable taste and smell, alcohol became the prescribed depressant drug of choice. However, some people refused to use alcohol either because they did not like the taste or for moral reasons, and others tended to take more than prescribed. Therefore, a search for a better sedative drug continued.

Although barbituric acid was first synthesized in 1864, it was not until 1912 that phenobarbital was introduced into medicine as a sedative drug, the first of the structurally classified group of drugs called barbiturates (Julien, 2014). Since that time, more than 2,500 barbiturate derivatives have been synthesized, but fewer than a dozen remain in medical use. Illicit use of these drugs for recreational purposes grew throughout the 1930s and 1940s.

Efforts to create depressant medications that were not barbiturate derivatives accelerated. By the mid-1950s, the market for depressants had been expanded by the appearance of the nonbarbiturates glutethimide, ethchlorvynol, methyprylon, and meprobamate. Introduction of the benzodiazepines occurred around 1960 with the marketing of chlordiazepoxide (Librium), followed shortly by its derivative diazepam (Valium). The use of these drugs and others within their group grew rapidly, and they are prescribed widely in medical practice. Their margin of safety is greater than that of barbiturates and the other nonbarbiturates. However, prolonged use of even moderate doses is likely to result in physical and psychological addiction, with a characteristic syndrome of withdrawal that can be severe.

Patterns of Use

Of all the drugs used in clinical practice, the sedative, hypnotic, anxiolytic drugs are among the most widely prescribed. Sadock and associates (2015) reported that about 15 percent of all persons in the United States have had a benzodiazepine prescribed by a physician.

Two patterns of addiction are described. The first pattern begins with an individual whose physician originally prescribed the CNS depressant as treatment for anxiety or insomnia. Independently, the individual increases the dosage or frequency from that which was prescribed. Use of the medication is justified on the basis of treating symptoms, but as tolerance grows, increasingly more drug is required to produce the desired effect. Substance-seeking behavior is evident as the individual seeks prescriptions from several physicians in order to maintain sufficient supplies.

The second pattern involves people in their teens or early 20s who use illegally obtained substances in the company of their peers. The initial objective is to achieve a feeling of euphoria. The drug is usually used intermittently during recreational gatherings. This pattern of intermittent use leads to regular use and extreme levels of tolerance. Combining use with other substances is not uncommon. Physical and psychological addiction leads to intense substance-seeking behaviors, most often through illegal channels.

Effects on the Body

The sedative, hypnotic, anxiolytic compounds depress the activity of the brain, nerves, muscles, and heart tissue. The primary action of sedatives, hypnotics, and anxiolytics is on nervous tissue. However, large doses may have an effect on other organ systems. They reduce the rate of metabolism in a variety of tissues throughout the body and depress any system that uses energy (Julien, 2014). Large doses are required to produce these effects. In lower doses, these drugs appear more selective in their depressant actions by exerting their action on the centers within the brain that are concerned with arousal (e.g., the ascending reticular activating system, in the reticular formation, and the diffuse thalamic projection system).

As stated previously, these drugs are capable of producing all levels of CNS depression—from mild sedation to death. The level is determined by dosage and potency of the drug used. In Figure 23-2, a continuum demonstrates how increasing doses of these drugs affect the level of CNS depression.

Following is a discussion of the physiological effects of these medications.

Effects on Sleep and Dreaming

Barbiturate use decreases the amount of sleep time spent dreaming. During drug withdrawal, dreaming becomes vivid and excessive. Rebound insomnia and increased dreaming (termed *REM rebound*) are not uncommon with abrupt withdrawal from long-term use of these drugs as sleeping aids (Julien, 2014).

Respiratory Depression

Barbiturates are capable of inhibiting the reticular activating system, resulting in respiratory depression that may lead to lethal overdose (Sadock et al., 2015). In addition, additive effects can occur with the concurrent use of other CNS depressants, also effecting a life-threatening situation.

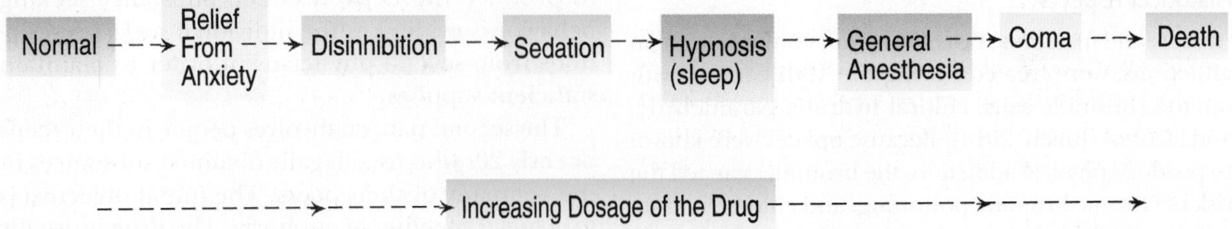

Normal – – → Relief From Anxiety – – → Disinhibition – – → Sedation – → Hypnosis (sleep) – – → General Anesthesia – – → Coma – – → Death

– – – – – – – – → – – – – – → Increasing Dosage of the Drug – – – – – – – – → – – →

FIGURE 23–2 Continuum of CNS depression with increasing doses of sedative, hypnotic, or anxiolytic drugs.

Cardiovascular Effects

Hypotension may be a problem with large doses. Only a slight decrease in blood pressure is noted with normal oral dosage. High doses of barbiturates may result in decreased cardiac output, decreased cerebral blood flow, and direct impairment of myocardial contractility (Lafferty & Abdel-Kariem, 2014).

Renal Function

In doses high enough to produce anesthesia, barbiturates may suppress urine function. At the usual sedative-hypnotic dosage, however, there is no evidence of direct action on the kidneys.

Hepatic Effects

Barbiturates may result in jaundice with doses large enough to produce acute intoxication. These drugs stimulate the production of liver enzymes, resulting in a decrease in the plasma levels of both the barbiturates and other drugs metabolized in the liver. Preexisting liver disease may predispose an individual to additional liver damage with excessive barbiturate use.

Body Temperature

High doses of barbiturates can greatly decrease body temperature. It is not significantly altered with normal dosage levels.

Sexual Function

CNS depressants tend to produce a biphasic response. There is an initial increase in libido, presumably from the primary disinhibitory effects of the drug, followed by impaired sexual pleasure. In men, this initial response is followed by decreased ability to maintain an erection.

Sedative, Hypnotic, or Anxiolytic Intoxication

The *DSM-5* (APA, 2013) describes sedative, hypnotic, or anxiolytic intoxication as the presence of clinically significant maladaptive behavioral or psychological changes that develop during, or shortly after, use of one of these substances. These maladaptive changes may include inappropriate sexual or aggressive behavior, mood lability, impaired judgment, or impaired social or occupational functioning. Other symptoms that may develop with excessive use of CNS depressants

include slurred speech, incoordination, unsteady gait, nystagmus, impairment in attention or memory, and stupor or coma.

"Club drugs" in this category include gamma hydroxybutyric acid (GHB) and flunitrazepam (Rohypnol). Like all depressants, they can produce a state of disinhibition, excitement, drunkenness, and amnesia. They have been widely implicated as "date rape" drugs, since their presence is easily disguised in drinks and they produce anterograde amnesia, the inability to remember events experienced while under their influence (Walton-Moss et al., 2013).

Sedative, Hypnotic, or Anxiolytic Withdrawal

Withdrawal from sedatives, hypnotics, or anxiolytics produces a characteristic syndrome of symptoms that develops after a marked decrease in or cessation of heavy or prolonged intake (APA, 2013). Onset of symptoms depends on the drug from which the individual is withdrawing. With short-acting sedative-hypnotics (e.g., alprazolam, lorazepam), symptoms may begin between 12 and 24 hours after the last dose, reach peak intensity between 24 and 72 hours, and subside in 5 to 10 days. Withdrawal symptoms from substances with longer half-lives (e.g., diazepam, phenobarbital, chlordiazepoxide) may begin within 2 to 7 days, peak on the fifth to eighth day, and subside in 10 to 16 days.

Severe withdrawal is most likely to occur when a substance has been used at high dosages for prolonged periods. However, withdrawal symptoms also have been reported with moderate dosages taken over a relatively short duration. Withdrawal symptoms include autonomic hyperactivity (e.g., sweating or pulse rate greater than 100), increased hand tremor, insomnia, nausea or vomiting, hallucinations, illusions, psychomotor agitation, anxiety, or grand mal seizures.

Stimulant Use Disorder

A Profile of the Substance

CNS stimulants are identified by the behavioral stimulation and psychomotor agitation they induce. They differ widely in molecular structures and mechanisms of action. The amount of CNS stimulation caused by a certain drug depends on both the area in the brain or spinal cord that is affected by the drug and the cellular mechanism fundamental to the increased excitability. The *DSM-5* (APA, 2013) categorizes caffeine-related disorders and tobacco-related disorders as separate and distinct diagnoses. For purposes of this text, these substances are discussed with the stimulant-related disorders.

Groups within this category are classified according to similarities in mechanism of action. The *psychomotor stimulants* induce stimulation by augmentation or potentiation of the neurotransmitters norepinephrine, epinephrine, or dopamine. The *general cellular stimulants* (caffeine and nicotine) exert their action directly on cellular activity. Caffeine inhibits the enzyme phosphodiesterase, allowing increased levels of adenosine 3',5'-cyclic phosphate (cAMP), a chemical substance that promotes increased rates of cellular metabolism. Nicotine stimulates ganglionic synapses. This results in increased acetylcholine, which stimulates nerve impulse transmission to the entire autonomic nervous system. A selected list of drugs included in these categories is presented in Table 23–2.

The two most prevalent and widely used stimulants are caffeine and nicotine. Caffeine is readily available in every supermarket and grocery store as a common ingredient in coffee, tea, colas, and chocolate. Nicotine is the primary psychoactive substance found in tobacco products. When used in moderation, these stimulants tend to relieve fatigue and increase alertness. They are a generally accepted part of our culture; however, with increased social awareness regarding the health risks associated with tobacco products, their use has become stigmatized in some circles.

The more potent stimulants, because of their potential for physiological addiction, are under regulation by the Controlled Substances Act. These controlled stimulants are available for therapeutic purposes by prescription only; however, they are also clandestinely manufactured and widely distributed on the illicit market. More recently, the synthetic stimulants mephedrone, 3,4-methylenedioxypyrovalerone (MDPV), methylone, and others have surfaced; because their chemical structures have been altered, they were not initially identifiable as a controlled substance or regulated by the federal government. Known as "bath salts," street names include blue silk, cloud 9, ivory wave, vanilla sky, white knight, stardust, and purple wave. In October 2011, the U.S. Drug Enforcement Administration (DEA) issued emergency scheduling of these substances to make their possession

TABLE 23–2 **CNS Stimulants**		
CATEGORIES	**GENERIC (TRADE) NAMES**	**COMMON STREET NAMES**
Amphetamines	Dextroamphetamine (Dexedrine)	Dexies, uppers, truck drivers
	Methamphetamine (Desoxyn)	Meth, speed, crystal, ice, crank, chalk fire, glass
	3,4-methylenedioxyamphetamine (MDMA)*	Adam, ecstasy, Eve, XTC
	Amphetamine + dextroamphetamine (Adderall)	Beanies, pep pills, speed, uppers, study buddies, smart pills
Synthetic stimulants	3,4-methylenedioxypyrovalerone* (MDPV) 4-methylmethcathinone (mephedrone, 4-MMC)* Methylone* Ethylone Dibutylone Alpha-PVP	Bath salts (also called blue silk, cloud 9, ivory wave, vanilla sky, white lightning, and others), flakka, gravel
Nonamphetamine stimulants	Phendimetrazine (Bontril) Benzphetamine (Didrex) Diethylpropion (Tenuate) Phentermine (Adipex-P; Ionamin) Sibutramine (Meridia)†	Diet pills
	Methylphenidate (Ritalin) Dexmethylphenidate (Focalin) Modafinil (Provigil)	Speed, uppers
Cocaine	Cocaine hydrochloride	Coke, blow, toot, snow, lady, flake, crack
Caffeine	Coffee, tea, colas, chocolate	Java, mud, brew, cocoa
Nicotine	Cigarettes, cigars, pipe tobacco, snuff	Weeds, fags, butts, chaw, cancer sticks

*Cross-listed with the hallucinogens.
†No longer marketed in the United States.

and sales illegal (except as authorized by law). They are currently designated as Schedule I substances, the most restrictive category under the Controlled Substances Act. This action was taken in response to reports of episodes of violent behavior associated with use of the substance.

Since then, yet another synthetic cathinone, alpha-PVP (α-pyrrolidinopentiophenone, commonly known as *flakka, gravel,* or *$5 insanity*), whose chemical structure is similar but not identical to bath salts, began to surface in the United States. This drug can be snorted, injected, eaten, and vaporized for inhalation in e-cigarettes. Vaporization is a particularly dangerous route because of its immediate absorption, and deaths have been reported secondary to overdose, suicide, and heart attack. But although flakka was a significant health hazard in 2014 and 2015, no deaths were reported in 2016, since China (the singular provider of this drug) banned the production and exportation of alpha-PVP (Storrs, 2016). Storrs additionally reports, however, that when one synthetic stimulant is banned, it is often replaced by another. For example, when China banned methylone (a drug similar to flakka) in 2014, it was replaced by ethylone; after ethylone was banned, a similar drug called dibutylone surfaced. This pattern creates an ongoing battle for the FDA and DEA to identify and take action on each new synthetic variant as it comes to public attention (usually through significant health consequences or deaths).

Historical Aspects

Cocaine is the most potent stimulant derived from nature. It is extracted from the leaves of the coca plant, which has been cultivated in the Andean highlands of South America since prehistoric times. Natives of the region chew the leaves of the plant for refreshment and relief from fatigue.

Coca leaves must be mixed with lime to release the cocaine alkaloid. The chemical formula for the pure form of the drug was developed in 1960. Physicians began using the drug as an anesthetic in eye, nose, and throat surgeries, and it was used in the United States in a morphine-cocaine elixir designed to relieve the suffering associated with terminal illness. These therapeutic uses are now obsolete.

Cocaine has achieved a degree of acceptability within some social circles. It is illicitly distributed as a white crystalline powder, often mixed with other ingredients to increase its volume and create more profit. The drug is most commonly "snorted," and chronic users may manifest symptoms that resemble the congested nose of a common cold. The intensely pleasurable effects of the drug create the potential for extraordinary psychological addiction.

Another form of cocaine commonly used in the United States is made by processing powdered cocaine with ammonia or sodium bicarbonate and water and heating it to remove the hydrochloride (Publishers Group, 2012). The term *crack*, the street name for this form of the drug, refers to the crackling sound heard when the mixture is smoked. Because this type of cocaine can be easily vaporized and inhaled, its effects have an extremely rapid onset. See "Real People, Real Stories" for Alan's experience with crack cocaine and alcohol addiction.

Real People, Real Stories: Alan Brunner on Substance Use Disorder

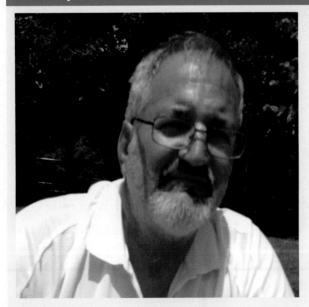

Substance use disorders often follow a progressive pattern that develops over a long period of time. Alan's story is an example of that process. See also Chapter 8, Therapeutic Communication, for an interaction with Alan that incorporates motivational interviewing. Reflect on important issues for primary prevention education. Consider examples of interventions that are ineffective or unhealthy for the user and the care provider. Incorporate an understanding of codependency in this reflection.

Karyn: Tell me about when you first used drugs or alcohol.

Alan: I was 15 years old when I first started smoking pot and 16 when I had my first drink. The pot use went from occasional use to several times a week by the time I was a senior in high school. I knew that was a problem, but the drinking progressed much more gradually. For years, I only drank on weekends. For a while, my buddy and I would share a quart on the weekend. Eventually, we each had our own quart, then two quarts each. I only drank beer. Once when I was teenager, I drank a fifth of vodka and

Real People, Real Stories: Alan Brunner on Substance Use Disorder–cont'd

I got extremely sick. My mom didn't try to rescue me or help me feel better or cover for me. I just had to live through the consequences, and that was probably a good thing; I never drank vodka again. But the beer drinking became more often and at higher amounts. Even so, it took another 35 years to recognize that it was a problem!

Karyn: Was there any history of alcoholism in your family?

Alan: Oh yeah . . . several relatives. My dad had a drinking problem, and that led to my parents divorcing when I was 14 years old. When I was 19, I moved in with my dad, and then I started drinking during the week, too—because he did. My dad always worked and had a strong work ethic, even though he was a heavy drinker, so I thought, "As long as I'm able to drink and it's not interfering with work, then it's not a problem." I also remember thinking, "It's just beer, and I would never use the 'strong' or 'bad' drugs, like cocaine—I would NEVER do that."

Karyn: So your beer drinking increased while you were living with your father?

Alan: Initially, yes, but then I was surrounding myself with people and friends who liked to drink. I moved in with a friend, and we usually drank a case of beer each night. Then I started an auto repair business with a friend who was a heavy drinker, and we had beer at the shop. Pretty soon we weren't leaving the shop until all the beer was gone. Then I got involved with auto racing, and that was an environment with lots of alcohol and cocaine.

Karyn: I remember you said you were using cocaine. Is that when the use started?

Alan: No, actually I had become friends with a deacon at my church, probably because we both liked to drink. He was the one that introduced me to cocaine.

Karyn: So you started using cocaine along with drinking?

Alan: Yeah, even though I had said I would never do that. But I discovered that if I did cocaine, I had a lot more energy and I could stay awake longer, so I could be a much "better" drinker. (chuckles)

Karyn: Tell me about when you recognized that your use was a problem.

Alan: Well, eventually, I was drinking at home because it was a waste of "good drinking time" to get together with other people. So largely, I was sitting at home in the dark drinking by myself, and the beer never even made it into the fridge. The cocaine was putting me in the company of some very bad people. I knew I had to somehow get away from that . . . and when I started using cocaine, I said, "One thing I'll never do is crack," but then I started doing that, and that's when things completely fell apart.

Karyn: Fell apart?

Alan: I was racking up a lot of legal problems. I had some DUIs and reckless operation charges before that, but now I'm getting drug possession charges, paraphernalia charges, driving with a suspended license, driving with expired license plates, more DUIs, disorderly conduct

charges. And the crack—that drug rips out your soul! You're always chasing the high that you got the first time you used it, and you never find that, so you keep using more. That's why one of my friends called crack "gotta" because you gotta have it. . . . And you don't care about ANYTHING else—you don't care if you die.

Karyn: You told me you've been clean and sober for seven years. How did you turn the corner?

Alan: I had such a huge legal mess that my lawyer was recommending I just accept the jail time (3 to 10 days) and be done with it, but the judge offered treatment in lieu of jail, and I told him that's what I wanted because I knew I needed it. I was told, though, that if I violated the treatment program, I would spend a year in jail, so I knew I was taking a big risk by going into treatment. But I knew it was the only way out—and I knew I needed it.

Karyn: So what is your relapse prevention plan?

Alan: I have an AA sponsor, and I go to meetings sometimes, but not as often as I used to. I never allow myself to become too proud about my sobriety because I know all it would take is one drink. As long as I remember that, I'm vulnerable. . . . I don't get too cocky. I've also had a lot of support from family, especially my mom. She supported me every step of the way in treatment. Having supportive people around you is essential. The relationship I had been in for many years broke up largely because she was telling my counselors that she wanted me to cut down but she wasn't in favor of abstinence—she was quite a partier, too. Staying in that relationship, I believed (and my counselors believed), was putting my sobriety at risk.

Karyn: What do you think is important for health-care providers to know or to do to help someone who has a substance use problem?

Alan: First of all, a person has to want help. You can't fix another person, and you can't help someone who doesn't want help.

Karyn: I agree, that is so important. I think health-care providers (and family caregivers) are vulnerable sometimes to thinking they can fix any health problem, which can culminate in interventions that are ineffective and unhealthy for the user and for the care provider.

Alan: Yes, and I would also say that health-care providers need to know how to recognize symptoms of problematic substance use.

Karyn: Like?

Alan: Like someone having "the shakes," someone not looking at you when they are answering questions, blaming other people for their circumstances and consequences, talking in circles. Don't ever ask someone, "Are you an alcoholic or a drug addict?" because we'll always say no unless we're in recovery—the denial is so strong. I also think not being too judgmental is important so you can find ways to open the door to discuss the issues. If someone is

Continued

too "hard-nosed" and judgmental, I think it reinforces the denial. Asking a question like "Have you ever been drinking and couldn't remember events around that time?" is good because having blackouts is a good indication of an alcohol problem. You may not be able to "fix" someone but you can "plant seeds" and hope that the information and education will have an impact at some point. I think

that's why people who are recovering themselves can be so effective as health-care providers because they can share their own story of addiction and, since most people think they are completely unique, hearing someone else's story about having been in the same place you are now may turn on a light switch and help people recognize their own need for treatment.

Amphetamine was first prepared in 1887. Various derivatives of the drug soon followed, and clinical use of the drug began in 1927. Amphetamines were used quite extensively for medical purposes through the 1960s, but recognition of their abuse potential has sharply decreased clinical use. Today, they are prescribed only to treat narcolepsy (a rare disorder resulting in an uncontrollable desire for sleep), hyperactivity disorders in children, and certain cases of obesity. Clandestine production of amphetamines for distribution on the illicit market has become a thriving business. Methamphetamine can be smoked, snorted, injected, or taken orally. The effects include an intense rush from smoking or intravenous injection and a slower onset of euphoria as a result of snorting or oral ingestion. Another form of the drug, crystal methamphetamine, is produced by slowly recrystallizing powder methamphetamine from a solvent such as methanol, ethanol, isopropanol, or acetone (Publishers Group, 2012). This colorless, odorless, large-crystal form of D-methamphetamine is commonly called *glass* or *ice* because of its appearance. Crystal meth is usually smoked in a glass pipe like crack cocaine.

The earliest history of caffeine is unknown and is shrouded by legend and myth. Caffeine was first discovered in coffee in 1820 and in tea 7 years later. Both beverages have been widely accepted and enjoyed as a "pick-me-up" by many cultures.

Tobacco use has a long history; Mayan carved drawings dated between 600 and 1000 AD are the earliest evidence that appears to depict smoking tobacco. Introduced in Europe in the mid-16th century, its use grew rapidly and soon became prevalent in the Orient. Tobacco came to America with the settlement of the earliest colonies. Today, it is grown in many countries of the world, and although smoking is decreasing in most industrialized nations, it continues to be a serious problem in developing areas.

Patterns of Use

Because of their pleasurable effects, CNS stimulants have a high abuse potential. In 2014, about 1.5 million

Americans were current cocaine users (SAMHSA, 2015). Use was highest among Americans aged 18 to 25.

Many individuals who abuse or are addicted to CNS stimulants began using the substance for the appetite-suppressant effect in an attempt at weight control. Increasingly higher doses are consumed in an effort to maintain the pleasurable effects. With continued use, these effects diminish as dysphoric effects increase. A persistent craving for the substance remains even in the face of unpleasant adverse effects from continued use.

CNS stimulant use is usually characterized by either episodic or chronic daily or near-daily use. Individuals who use the substances on an episodic basis often "binge" on the drug with consumption of very high dosages followed by a day or two of recuperation. This recuperation period is characterized by extremely intense and unpleasant symptoms and is thus often called a "crash."

The daily user may take large or small doses and may use the drug several times a day or only at a specific time during the day. The amount consumed usually increases over time as tolerance develops. Chronic users tend to rely on CNS stimulants to feel more powerful, more confident, and more decisive. They often fall into a pattern of taking "uppers" in the morning and "downers," such as alcohol or sleeping pills, at night.

The average American consumes two cups of coffee (about 200 mg of caffeine) per day. Caffeine is consumed in various amounts by about 90 percent of the population. At a level of 500 to 600 mg of daily caffeine consumption, symptoms of anxiety, insomnia, and depression are not uncommon, and caffeine dependence and withdrawal can occur. Caffeine consumption is prevalent among children as well as adults. Table 23–3 lists some common sources of caffeine.

Nicotine, an active ingredient in tobacco, is the most widely used psychoactive substance in U.S. society after caffeine. Based on 2014 statistics, 55.2 million people are current smokers of tobacco, 12 million smoke cigars, and 8.7 million use smokeless tobacco (SAMHSA, 2015). Since 1964, when the results of the first public health report on smoking were issued, the

TABLE 23–3 **Common Sources of Caffeine**	
SOURCE	CAFFEINE CONTENT (mg)
FOOD AND BEVERAGES	
5–6 oz brewed coffee	90–125
5–6 oz instant coffee	60–90
5–6 oz decaffeinated coffee	3
5–6 oz brewed tea	70
5–6 oz instant tea	45
8 oz green tea	15–30
8–12 oz cola drinks	60
12 oz Red Bull energy drink	115
2 oz high-energy drink	215–240
5–6 oz cocoa	20
8 oz chocolate milk	2–7
1 oz chocolate bar	22
PRESCRIPTION MEDICATIONS	
APCs (aspirin, phenacetin, caffeine)	32
Cafergot	100
Fiorinal	40
Migralam	100
OVER-THE-COUNTER ANALGESICS	
Anacin, Empirin, Midol, Vanquish,	32
Excedrin Migraine (aspirin, acetaminophen, caffeine)	65
OVER-THE-COUNTER STIMULANTS	
NoDoz tablets	100
Vivarin	200
Caffedrine	250

percentage of total smokers has been on the decline. However, the percentage of women and teenage smokers has declined more slowly than that of adult men. Even though tobacco use is on the decline, people with severe mental illness and those in addiction treatment continue to have higher rates of use than the general population; as many as 93 percent of people in addictions treatment and 40 percent of those with severe mental illness report using tobacco (SAMHSA, 2015).

The dangers of secondhand smoke continue to be identified as a significant health hazard. The CDC (2016b) reports that, annually, secondhand smoke claims the lives of over 49,000 nonsmokers from heart disease, stroke, and lung cancer, and 1,000 babies from the effects associated with the mother smoking during pregnancy. Additionally, smoking increases the risk of infant mortality from sudden infant death syndrome.

Effects on the Body

CNS stimulants are a group of pharmacological agents that are capable of exciting the entire nervous system. This is accomplished by increasing the activity or augmenting the capability of the neurotransmitter agents directly involved in bodily activation and behavioral stimulation. Physiological responses vary according to the potency and dosage of the drug.

Central Nervous System Effects

Stimulation of the CNS results in tremor, restlessness, anorexia, insomnia, agitation, and increased motor activity. Amphetamines, nonamphetamine stimulants, and cocaine produce increased alertness, decreased fatigue, elation and euphoria, and subjective feelings of greater mental agility and muscular power. Chronic use of these drugs may result in compulsive behavior, paranoia, hallucinations, and aggressive behavior (Publishers Group, 2012).

Cardiovascular/Pulmonary Effects

Amphetamines can induce increased systolic and diastolic blood pressure, increased heart rate, and cardiac arrhythmias (Publishers Group, 2012). These drugs also relax bronchial smooth muscle.

Cocaine intoxication typically produces a rise in myocardial demand for oxygen and an increase in heart rate. Severe vasoconstriction may occur and can result in myocardial infarction, ventricular fibrillation, and sudden death. Inhaled cocaine can cause pulmonary hemorrhage, chronic bronchiolitis, and pneumonia. Nasal rhinitis is a result of chronic cocaine snorting.

Caffeine ingestion can result in increased heart rate, palpitations, extrasystoles, and cardiac arrhythmias. Caffeine induces dilation of pulmonary and general systemic blood vessels and constriction of cerebral blood vessels.

Nicotine stimulates the sympathetic nervous system, resulting in an increase in heart rate, blood pressure, and cardiac contractility, thereby increasing myocardial oxygen consumption and demand for blood flow. Contractions of gastric smooth muscle associated with hunger are inhibited, thereby producing a mild anorectic effect.

Gastrointestinal and Renal Effects

Gastrointestinal (GI) effects of amphetamines are somewhat unpredictable; however, a decrease in GI tract motility commonly results in constipation.

Contraction of the bladder sphincter makes urination difficult. Caffeine exerts a diuretic effect on the kidneys. Nicotine stimulates the hypothalamus to release antidiuretic hormone, reducing the excretion of urine. Because nicotine increases the tone and activity of the bowel, it may occasionally cause diarrhea.

Most CNS stimulants induce a small rise in metabolic rate and various degrees of anorexia. Amphetamines and cocaine can cause a rise in body temperature.

Sexual Function

CNS stimulants appear to increase sexual urges in both men and women. Women, more frequently than men, report that stimulants make them feel sexier and have more orgasms. In fact, some men may experience sexual dysfunction with the use of stimulants. For the majority of individuals, however, these drugs exert a powerful aphrodisiac effect.

Stimulant Intoxication

Stimulant intoxication produces maladaptive behavioral and psychological changes that develop during or shortly after use of these drugs. Amphetamine and cocaine intoxication typically produces euphoria or affective blunting; changes in sociability; hypervigilance; interpersonal sensitivity; anxiety, tension, or anger; stereotyped behaviors; or impaired judgment. In severe amphetamine intoxication, symptoms may include memory loss, psychosis, and violent aggression. Physical effects include tachycardia or bradycardia, pupillary dilation, elevated or lowered blood pressure, perspiration or chills, nausea or vomiting, weight loss, psychomotor agitation or retardation, muscular weakness, respiratory depression, chest pain, cardiac arrhythmias, confusion, seizures, dyskinesias, dystonias, or coma (APA, 2013).

Intoxication from caffeine usually occurs following consumption in excess of 250 mg. Symptoms include restlessness, nervousness, excitement, insomnia, flushed face, diuresis, GI disturbance, muscle twitching, rambling flow of thought and speech, tachycardia or cardiac arrhythmia, periods of inexhaustibility, and psychomotor agitation (APA, 2013).

Stimulant Withdrawal

Stimulant withdrawal is the presence of a characteristic withdrawal syndrome that develops within a few hours to a few days after cessation of or reduction in heavy and prolonged use (APA, 2013). This syndrome is often referred to as crashing, an apt description because the symptoms include fatigue, cramps, depression, headaches, and nightmares. The dysphoria can be intense enough to result in increased risk for suicide. Peak withdrawal symptoms usually occur within 2 to 4 days of abstinence (Black & Andreasen, 2014).

The *DSM-5* (APA, 2013) states that a withdrawal syndrome can occur with abrupt cessation of caffeine intake after prolonged daily use. The symptoms begin within 24 hours after last consumption and may include headache, fatigue, drowsiness, dysphoric mood, irritability, difficulty concentrating, flu-like symptoms, nausea, vomiting, and/or muscle pain and stiffness.

Withdrawal from nicotine results in dysphoric or depressed mood; insomnia; irritability, frustration, or anger; anxiety; difficulty concentrating; restlessness; decreased heart rate; and increased appetite or weight gain (APA, 2013). A mild syndrome of nicotine withdrawal can appear when a smoker switches from regular cigarettes to low-nicotine cigarettes (Sadock et al., 2015).

Inhalant Use Disorder
Profile of the Substance

Inhalant disorders are induced by inhaling the aliphatic and aromatic hydrocarbons found in substances such as fuels, solvents, adhesives, aerosol propellants, and paint thinners. Specific examples of these substances include gasoline, varnish remover, lighter fluid, airplane glue, rubber cement, cleaning fluid, spray paint, shoe conditioner, and typewriter correction fluid. Toluene (methylbenzene, toluol, phenylmethane), a common ingredient in many inhaled substances including paints, glues, and gasoline, is responsible for the mind-altering effects that occur after inhalation.

Historical Aspects

Use of inhalants for altered consciousness or for religious rituals dates back to ancient times. In the early 19th century, ether, chloroform, and nitrous oxide were inhaled for recreational purposes. By the 1960s, the inhaling of substances for recreational effects had spread to a wide range of products, including shoe polish, paints and paint thinners, lighter fluid, and gasoline. Inhalant use among children and adolescents is widespread in the United States today.

Patterns of Use

Inhalant substances are readily available, legal, and inexpensive, three factors that make them attractive to children, teens, and young adults. Highest usage is by youths aged 12 to 17, and this is the only class of drugs used more frequently by younger than by older teens (NIDA, 2015). A national government survey of drug use in 2014 revealed that 8 percent of people in the United States aged 12 years or older acknowledged having used inhalants (NIDA, 2015). A encouraging update (NIDA, 2016) identifies a decline of drug use among teens over the past 5 years for many substances, including inhalants. Younger teens more commonly inhale glue, gasoline, and spray paints. In older teens, nitrous oxide (also known as "whippets") use is more common, and in adults, nitrites such as amyl nitrites (also called "poppers") are the most common inhalants used for mind-altering effects (NIDA, 2015).

Methods of use include "huffing"—a procedure in which a rag soaked with the substance is applied to the mouth and nose and the vapors inhaled. Another common method is called "bagging," in which the substance is placed in a paper or plastic bag from which it is inhaled by the user. The substance may also be inhaled directly from the container or sprayed in the mouth or nose.

Sadock and associates (2015) reported that

> inhalant use among adolescents may be most common in those whose parents or older siblings use illegal substances. Inhalant use among adolescents is also associated with an increased likelihood of conduct disorder or antisocial personality disorder. (p. 657)

Tolerance to inhalants has been reported with heavy use. A mild withdrawal syndrome has been documented but does not appear to be clinically significant. Among children with inhalant disorder, the products may be used several times a week, often on weekends and after school. Adults with inhalant addiction may use the substance at varying times each day or binge on the substance over a period of several days.

Effects on the Body

Inhalants are absorbed through the lungs and reach the CNS very rapidly. Inhalants generally act as CNS depressants (Black & Andreasen, 2014). The effects are relatively brief, lasting from several minutes to a few hours depending on the specific substance and amount consumed.

Central Nervous System Effects

Inhalants can cause both central and peripheral nervous system damage. Symptoms of neurological damage such as ataxia, peripheral and sensorimotor neuropathy, speech problems, and tremor can occur. Other CNS effects that have been reported with heavy inhalant use include ototoxicity, encephalopathy, parkinsonism, and damage to the protective sheath around certain nerve fibers in the brain and peripheral nervous system (Walton-Moss et al., 2013).

Respiratory Effects

Respiratory effects of inhalant use range from coughing and wheezing to dyspnea, emphysema, and pneumonia. There is increased airway resistance due to inflammation of the passages. Walton-Moss and associates (2013) note additionally that suffocation can occur as a result of inhaling substances from paper or plastic bags.

Gastrointestinal Effects

Abdominal pain, nausea, and vomiting may occur. A rash may be present around the individual's nose and mouth. Unusual breath odors are common. Long-term use has resulted in reports of liver toxicity.

Renal System Effects

Acute and chronic renal failure and hepatorenal syndrome may occur. Renal toxicity from toluene exposure has been reported, manifesting in renal tubular acidosis, hypokalemia, hypophosphatemia, hyperchloremia, azotemia, sterile pyuria, hematuria, and proteinuria (McKeown, 2015).

Inhalant Intoxication

The *DSM-5* defines inhalant intoxication as "clinically significant problematic behavioral or psychological changes that developed during or shortly after exposure to inhalants" (APA, 2013). Symptoms are similar to alcohol intoxication and may include the following (APA, 2013; Black & Andreasen, 2014):

- Dizziness; ataxia
- Euphoria; excitation; disinhibition
- Nystagmus; blurred vision; double vision
- Slurred speech
- Hypoactive reflexes
- Psychomotor retardation; lethargy
- Generalized muscle weakness
- Stupor or coma (at higher doses)

Opioid Use Disorder
Profile of the Substance

The term *opioid* refers to a group of compounds that includes opium, opium derivatives, and synthetic substitutes. Opioids exert both a sedative and an analgesic effect, and their major medical uses are pain relief, treatment of diarrhea, and relief of coughing. These drugs have addictive qualities in that they are capable of inducing tolerance and physiological and psychological addiction. The United States is currently struggling to respond to an unprecedented opiate abuse epidemic.

Opioids are popular drugs of abuse because they desensitize an individual to both psychological and physiological pain and induce a sense of euphoria. Lethargy and indifference to the environment are common manifestations.

Opioid abusers usually spend much of their time nourishing the habit. Individuals who are addicted to opioids are seldom able to hold a steady job that will support their need and must therefore secure funds from friends, relatives, or whomever they have not yet alienated with their addiction-related behavior. It is not uncommon for individuals addicted to opioids to resort to illegal means of obtaining funds, such as burglary, robbery, prostitution, or selling drugs.

Methods of administration of opioid drugs include oral ingestion; snorting; smoking; and subcutaneous, intramuscular, and intravenous injection. A selected list of opioid substances is presented in Table 23–4.

Under close supervision, opioids are indispensable in the practice of medicine. They are the most effective agents known for the relief of intense pain. However, they also induce a pleasurable effect on the CNS that promotes their abuse. The physiological and psychological addiction that occurs with opioids, as well as the development of profound tolerance, contribute to the addict's ongoing quest for more of the substance, regardless of the means.

Historical Aspects

In its crude form, opium is a brownish-black gummy substance obtained from the ripened pods of the opium poppy. References to the use of opiates have been found in the Egyptian, Greek, and Arabian cultures as early as 3000 BC. The drug became widely used both medicinally and recreationally throughout Europe during the 16th and 17th centuries. Most of the opium supply came from China, where the drug was introduced by Arab traders in the late 17th century. Morphine, the primary active ingredient of opium, was isolated in 1803 by the European chemist Friedrich Sertürner. Since that time, morphine rather than crude opium has been used throughout the world for the medical treatment of pain and diarrhea. This process was facilitated in 1853 by the development of the hypodermic syringe, which made it possible to deliver undiluted morphine quickly into the body for rapid relief from pain.

This development also created a new variety of opiate user in the United States: one who was able to self-administer the drug by injection. In addition, the large influx of Chinese immigrants into the United States during this era introduced opium smoking to this country. By the early part of the 20th century, opium addiction was widespread.

In response to the concerns over the prevalence of opium addiction, in 1914 the U.S. government passed the Harrison Narcotic Act, which created strict controls on the accessibility of opiates. Until that time, these substances were freely available to the public without a prescription. The Harrison Act banned the use of opiates for nonmedicinal purposes and drove the use of heroin underground. To this day, the beneficial uses of these substances are widely acclaimed within the medical profession, but the illicit trafficking of the drugs for recreational purposes continues to resist most efforts at control.

Patterns of Use

The development of opioid addiction may follow one of two typical behavior patterns. The first occurs in the individual who has obtained the drug by prescription from a physician for the relief of a medical problem. Abuse and addiction occur when the individual increases the amount and frequency of use, justifying the behavior as symptom treatment. He or she becomes obsessed with obtaining more and more of the substance, seeking out several physicians in order to replenish and maintain supplies.

TABLE 23–4 Opioids and Related Substances

CATEGORIES	GENERIC (TRADE) NAMES	COMMON STREET NAMES
Opioids of natural origin	Opium (ingredient in various antidiarrheal agents) Morphinan (Astramorph) Codeine (ingredient in various analgesics and cough suppressants) Kratom (opioid-like)	Black stuff, poppy, tar, big O M, white stuff, Miss Emma Terp, schoolboy, syrup, cody
Opioid derivatives	Heroin Hydromorphone (Dilaudid) Oxycodone (Percodan; OxyContin) Hydrocodone (Vicodin)	H, horse, junk, brown sugar, smack, skag, TNT, Harry DLs, 4s, lords, little D Perks, perkies, Oxy, O.C. Vike
Synthetic opiate-like drugs	Meperidine (Demerol) Methadone (Dolophine) Pentazocine (Talwin) Fentanyl (Fentora) Carfentanil Desomorphine U-47700	Doctors Dollies, done Ts Apache, China girl, China town, dance fever, goodfella, jackpot Krokodil Pink or pinky

The second pattern of behavior occurs among individuals who use the drugs for recreational purposes and obtain them from illegal sources. Opioids may be used alone to induce the euphoric effects or in combination with stimulants or other drugs to enhance the euphoria or counteract the substance's depressant effects. Tolerance develops and addiction occurs, leading the individual to procure the substance by whatever means is required to support the habit.

A recent government survey reported that there were 435,000 current heroin users aged 12 years and older in the United States in 2014 (SAMHSA, 2016). The same survey revealed an estimated 4.3 million persons who used prescription psychotherapeutic drugs nonmedically. Since 1999, prescription rates for painkillers and deaths from opiate overdoses have both quadrupled (CDC, 2016c). Efforts have been made in some states to exert stricter controls on opiate prescription practices, and 2012 marked the first year of a drop in prescription rates nationally. However, the longer-term trend has shown an increase from 76 million prescriptions for opiates in 1991 to 207 million in 2013 (NIDA, 2014). The CDC reports that 44 people die each day from prescription painkiller overdose. The most common drugs involved in prescription overdose deaths include hydrocodone (Vicodin), oxycodone (OxyContin), oxymorphone (Opana), and methadone.

One alarming trend is a significant increase in overdose deaths associated with fentanyl mixed with heroin. This frequently results in accidental overdose since fentanyl is 30 to 50 times more potent than pure heroin (CDC, 2016c). Even more recently, carfentanil (carfentanyl), a potent drug used mainly in the capture of wild animals (100 times more potent than fentanyl and 10,000 times more potent than morphine), has been responsible for rapid accidental overdose and often death when ingested along with heroin (National Institutes of Health [NIH], 2016).

Much like the trend with synthetic amphetamines discussed earlier in this chapter, a new synthetic opiate, U-47700, surfaced in 2015 and was responsible for 46 fatalities in 2016 before the substance was emergency classified as a Schedule I drug to allow the DEA more time to collect data on the substance (Duffy, 2016). Kratom, a plant from Southeast Asia that triggers opiate-like effects, surfaced in the United States and was subsequently banned; however, this decision was reversed when researchers argued that it might help them develop tools to overcome opiate and alcohol addiction as well as chronic pain (MPR, 2016). At present, the opioid epidemic remains out of control, but several national initiatives to address this public health crisis have been identified. A National Practice Guideline for use of medications to treat opioid use disorder has been established (ASAM, 2015), and for the first time in U.S. history, the Surgeon General declared illicit drug use and misuse of prescription drugs a national health-care priority and committed to the need for additional research and treatment options (HHS, 2016).

Effects on the Body

Opiates are sometimes classified as *narcotic analgesics*. They exert their major effects primarily on the CNS, the eyes, and the GI tract. Chronic morphine use or acute morphine toxicity is manifested by a syndrome of sedation, chronic constipation, decreased respiratory rate, and pinpoint pupils. Intensity of symptoms is largely dose dependent. The following physiological effects are common with opioid use.

Central Nervous System Effects

All opioids, opioid derivatives, and synthetic opioid-like drugs affect the CNS. Common manifestations include euphoria, mood changes, and mental clouding. Other common CNS effects include drowsiness and pain reduction. Pupillary constriction occurs in response to stimulation of the oculomotor nerve. CNS depression of the respiratory centers within the medulla results in respiratory depression. The antitussive response is caused by suppression of the cough center within the medulla. The nausea and vomiting commonly associated with opiate ingestion is related to the stimulation of the centers within the medulla that trigger this response.

Gastrointestinal Effects

These drugs exert a profound effect on the GI tract. Both stomach and intestinal tone increase, while peristaltic activity of the intestines is diminished. These effects lead to a marked decrease in the movement of food through the GI tract. This is a notable therapeutic effect in the treatment of severe diarrhea. In fact, no drugs have yet been developed that are more effective than the opioids for this purpose. However, constipation and even fecal impaction may be a serious problem for the chronic opioid user.

Cardiovascular Effects

In therapeutic doses, opioids have minimal effect on the action of the heart. Morphine is used extensively to relieve pulmonary edema and the pain of myocardial infarction in cardiac clients. At high doses, opioids induce hypotension, which may be caused by direct action on the heart or by opioid-induced histamine release.

Sexual Function

Opioid use causes decreased sexual function and diminished libido, and long-term use has been associated with erectile dysfunction (Deyo et al., 2013). Delayed ejaculation, impotence, and orgasm failure (in both men and women) may occur.

Opioid Intoxication

Opioid intoxication constitutes clinically significant problematic behavioral or psychological changes that develop during, or shortly after, opioid use (APA, 2013). Symptoms include initial euphoria followed by apathy, dysphoria, psychomotor agitation or retardation, and impaired judgment. Physical symptoms include pupillary constriction (or dilation due to anoxia from severe overdose), drowsiness, slurred speech, and impairment in attention or memory (APA, 2013). Symptoms are consistent with the half-life of most opioid drugs and usually last for several hours. Severe opioid intoxication can lead to respiratory depression, coma, and death.

Opioid Withdrawal

Opioid withdrawal produces a syndrome of symptoms that develops after cessation of or reduction in heavy and prolonged use of an opiate or related substance. Symptoms include dysphoric mood, nausea or vomiting, muscle aches, lacrimation or rhinorrhea, pupillary dilation, piloerection, sweating, diarrhea, yawning, fever, and insomnia (APA, 2013). With short-acting drugs such as heroin, withdrawal symptoms occur within 6 to 8 hours after the last dose, peak within 1 to 3 days, and gradually subside over a period of 5 to 10 days (Walton-Moss et al., 2013). With longer-acting drugs such as methadone, withdrawal symptoms begin within 1 to 3 days after the last dose, peak between days 4 and 6, and are complete in 14 to 21 days. Withdrawal from the ultra-short-acting meperidine begins quickly, reaches a peak in 8 to 12 hours, and is complete in 4 to 5 days (Sadock et al., 2015).

Hallucinogen Use Disorder

Profile of the Substance

Hallucinogenic substances can distort an individual's perception of reality, alter sensory perception, and induce hallucinations. For this reason, they have sometimes been referred to as "mind-expanding drugs." Some of the effects of these substances have been likened to those of a psychotic break. The hallucinations experienced by an individual with schizophrenia, however, are most often auditory, whereas substance-induced hallucinations are usually visual. Perceptual distortions have been reported by some users as spiritual, as giving a sense of depersonalization (observing oneself having the experience), or as feeling at peace with self and the universe. Others, who describe their experiences as "bad trips," report feelings of panic and a fear of dying or going insane. A

common danger reported with hallucinogenic drugs is that of flashbacks, or a spontaneous reoccurrence of the hallucinogenic state without ingestion of the drug. These can occur months after the drug was last taken.

Recurrent use can produce tolerance, encouraging users to resort to increasingly higher dosages. No evidence of physical addiction is detectable when the drug is withdrawn; however, recurrent use appears to induce a psychological addiction to the insight-inducing experiences that a user may associate with episodes of hallucinogen use (Sadock et al., 2015). This psychological addiction varies according to the drug, the dose, and the individual user. Hallucinogens are highly unpredictable in the effects they may induce each time they are used.

Many hallucinogenic substances have structural similarities. Some are produced synthetically; others are natural products of plants and fungi. A selected list of hallucinogens is presented in Table 23–5.

Historical Aspects

Hallucinogens have been used throughout history in many cultures for religious and mystical experiences, including in Aztec, Mexican Indian, and Hindu ceremonies (Parish, 2015). Use of the peyote cactus as part of religious ceremonies in the southwestern part of the United States still occurs today, although this ritual use has greatly diminished.

LSD was first synthesized in 1943 by Dr. Albert Hoffman as a clinical research tool to investigate the biochemical etiology of schizophrenia. It soon reached the illicit market, and its abuse began to overshadow the research effort.

The abuse of hallucinogens reached a peak in the late 1960s, waned during the 1970s, and returned to favor in the 1980s with the so-called designer drugs (e.g., 3,4-methylenedioxyamphetamine [MDMA], also known as "Molly" or "ecstasy," and methoxyamphetamine [MDA]). Another hallucinogen, PCP, originally was developed in the 1950s as an anesthetic, but this use was discontinued because of serious adverse effects. It continues to be used illegally and is often combined with cannabis. A number of deaths have been directly attributed to the use of PCP, and numerous accidental deaths have occurred as a result of overdose and of the behavioral changes the drug precipitates. A derivative of PCP, ketamine, is also used as a preoperative anesthetic and abused for its psychedelic properties. It produces effects similar to but somewhat less intense than those of PCP. Ketamine is also currently being studied for potential benefits in the treatment of depression and posttraumatic stress disorder.

Several therapeutic uses of LSD have been proposed, including the treatment of chronic alcoholism

TABLE 23-5 **Hallucinogens**		
CATEGORIES	GENERIC (TRADE) NAMES	COMMON STREET NAMES
Naturally occurring hallucinogens	Mescaline (the primary active ingredient of the peyote cactus)	Cactus, mesc, mescal, half moon, big chief, bad seed, peyote
	Psilocybin and psilocin (active ingredients of *Psilocybe* mushrooms)	Magic mushroom, God's flesh, shrooms
	Ololiuqui (morning glory seeds), *Salvia divinorum*	Heavenly blue, pearly gates, flying saucers, salvia
Synthetic compounds	Lysergic acid diethylamide (LSD)—synthetically produced from a fungal substance found on rye or a chemical substance found in morning glory seeds	Acid, cube, big D, California sunshine, microdots, blue dots, sugar, orange wedges, peace tablets, purple haze, cupcakes
	Dimethyltryptamine (DMT) and diethyltryptamine (DET)—chemical analogues of tryptamine	Businessman's trip
	2,5-Dimethoxy-4-methylamphetamine (DOM)	STP (serenity, tranquility, peace)
	Phencyclidine (PCP)	Angel dust, hog, peace pill, rocket fuel
	Ketamine (Ketalar)	Special K, vitamin K, kit kat
	3,4-Methylene-dioxyamphetamine (MDMA)*	XTC, ecstasy, Adam, Eve
	Methoxy-amphetamine (MDA)	Love drug
	3,4-methylenedioxypyrovalerone (MDPV)*	Bath salts (also called blue silk, cloud 9,
	4-methylmethcathinone (mephedrone, 4-MMC)*	ivory wave, vanilla sky, white knight, and
	Methylone*	others)

*Cross-listed with the CNS stimulants.

and the reduction of intractable pain such as occurs in malignant disease. A great deal more research is required regarding the therapeutic uses of LSD. At this time, there is no real evidence of the safety and efficacy of this drug in humans.

Patterns of Use

Use of hallucinogens is usually episodic. Because cognitive and perceptual abilities are so markedly affected by these substances, the user must set aside time from normal daily activities for indulgence. According to a national study in 2014, 1.2 million people reported using hallucinogens in the prior month (SAMHSA, 2015).

LSD, like other hallucinogens, does not lead to the development of physical addiction or withdrawal symptoms (Sadock et al., 2015). However, tolerance for LSD and other hallucinogens develops quickly and to a high degree. In fact, tolerance is complete after 3 to 4 consecutive days of use. Recovery from tolerance also occurs very rapidly (in 4 to 7 days), so the individual is able to achieve the desired effect from the drug repeatedly and often.

PCP is usually taken episodically, in binges that can last for several days. However, some chronic users take the substance daily. Physical addiction does not occur with PCP; however, psychological addiction characterized by craving for the drug has been reported in chronic users, as has the development of tolerance. Tolerance apparently develops quickly with frequent use.

Psilocybin is an ingredient of the *Psilocybe* mushroom indigenous to the United States and Mexico. Ingestion of these mushrooms produces an effect similar to that of LSD but of a shorter duration. This hallucinogenic chemical can now be produced synthetically.

Mescaline is the only hallucinogenic compound used legally for religious purposes today by members of the Native American Church of the United States. It is the primary active ingredient of the peyote cactus. Neither physical nor psychological addiction occurs with the use of mescaline, although as with other hallucinogens, tolerance can develop quickly with frequent use.

Salvia is an herb from the mint family that has hallucinogenic effects when dried leaves are chewed, extracted juices are consumed, or smoke from the leaves is inhaled. This particular hallucinogen is advertised and sold over the Internet, since it is not currently regulated by the Controlled Substances Act, but some states and countries have limited or banned its use (NIDA, 2015).

Among the most potent hallucinogens of the current drug culture are those categorized as amphetamine derivatives. These include 2,5-dimethoxy-4-methylamphetamine (DOM, STP), MDMA, and MDA. At lower doses, these drugs produce the "high" associated with CNS stimulants. At higher doses, hallucinogenic effects occur. These drugs have existed for many years but were rediscovered in the mid-1980s. Because of the rapid increase in recreational use, the DEA imposed an emergency classification of MDMA as a

Schedule I drug in 1985. MDMA, or ecstasy, is a synthetic drug with both stimulant and hallucinogenic qualities. It has a chemical structure similar to methamphetamine and mescaline and has become widely available throughout the world. Because of its growing popularity, the demand for this drug has led to tablets and capsules being sold as ecstasy that are not pure MDMA. Many contain drugs such as methamphetamine, PCP, amphetamine, ketamine, and *p*-methoxyamphetamine (PMA, a stimulant with hallucinogenic properties; more toxic than MDMA). This practice has increased the dangers associated with MDMA use.

Effects on the Body

The effects produced by the various hallucinogenics are highly unpredictable. The variety of effects may be related to dosage, the mental state of the individual, and the environment in which the substance is used. Some common effects have been reported (APA, 2013; Julien, 2014; Sadock et al., 2015).

Physiological Effects

- Nausea and vomiting
- Chills
- Pupil dilation
- Increased pulse, blood pressure, and temperature
- Mild dizziness
- Trembling
- Loss of appetite
- Insomnia
- Sweating
- A slowing of respirations
- Elevation in blood sugar

Psychological Effects

- Heightened response to color, texture, and sounds
- Heightened body awareness
- Distortion of vision
- Sense of slowed time
- All feelings magnified: love, lust, hate, joy, anger, pain, terror, despair
- Fear of losing control
- Paranoia, panic
- Euphoria, bliss
- Projection of self into dreamlike images
- Serenity, peace
- Depersonalization
- Derealization
- Increased libido

The effects of hallucinogens are not always pleasurable for the user. Two types of toxic reactions are known to occur. The first is the *panic reaction,* or "bad trip." Symptoms include intense anxiety, fear, and stimulation. The individual hallucinates and fears going insane. Paranoia and acute psychosis may be evident.

The second type of toxic reaction to hallucinogens is the flashback. This phenomenon refers to the transient, spontaneous repetition of a previous LSD-induced experience that occurs without taking the substance. The *DSM-5* (APA, 2013) refers to this as *Hallucinogen Persisting Perception Disorder.* Various studies have reported that 15 to 80 percent of hallucinogen users report having experienced flashbacks (Sadock et al., 2015). These episodes typically last for a few minutes or less.

Hallucinogen Intoxication

Symptoms of hallucinogen intoxication develop during or shortly after hallucinogen use. Maladaptive behavioral or psychological changes include marked anxiety or depression, ideas of reference (a type of delusional thinking that all activity within one's environment is "referred to" [about] one's self), fear of losing one's mind, paranoid ideation, and impaired judgment (APA, 2013). Perceptual changes occur while the individual is fully awake and alert and include intensification of perceptions, depersonalization, derealization, illusions, hallucinations, and synesthesias (APA, 2013). Because hallucinogens are sympathomimetics, they can cause tachycardia, hypertension, sweating, blurred vision, papillary dilation, and tremors (Black & Andreasen, 2014).

Symptoms of PCP intoxication are unpredictable. Specific symptoms are dose related and may be manifested by impulsiveness, impaired judgment, assaultiveness, and belligerence, or the individual may appear calm, stuporous, or comatose. Physical symptoms include vertical or horizontal nystagmus, hypertension, tachycardia, ataxia, diminished pain sensation, muscle rigidity, and seizures. Symptoms of ketamine intoxication appear similar to those of PCP.

General effects of MDMA (ecstasy) include increased heart rate, blood pressure, and body temperature; dehydration; confusion; insomnia; and paranoia. Overdose can result in panic attacks, hallucinations, severe hyperthermia, dehydration, and seizures. Death can occur from kidney or cardiovascular failure.

Cannabis Use Disorder

Profile of the Substance

Cannabis is the most commonly used illicit drug in the United States (NIDA, 2015) and the fourth-most commonly used psychoactive substance after caffeine, alcohol, and nicotine (Sadock et al., 2015). Cannabis has been legalized in some states for recreational and/or medicinal use. The major psychoactive ingredient of this class of substances is delta-9-tetrahydrocannabinol (THC). It occurs naturally in the plant *Cannabis sativa,* which grows readily in warm climates. Marijuana, the most prevalent type of cannabis preparation, is composed of the dried leaves, stems, and flowers of the plant. Hashish is a more potent concentrate of the resin derived from the flowering tops of the plant. Hash oil is a very concentrated form of THC made by boiling hashish in a solvent and filtering out the solid matter (Publishers Group, 2012). Cannabis products are usually smoked in the form of loosely rolled cigarettes or may be inhaled through the use of vaporizers to reduce the irritants and toxins associated with smoking. Cannabis can also be taken orally when it is prepared in food, but about two to three times the amount of cannabis must be ingested orally to equal the potency obtained by the inhalation of its smoke (Sadock et al., 2015).

At moderate dosages, cannabis produces effects resembling alcohol and other CNS depressants. By depressing higher brain centers, they release lower centers from inhibitory influences. There has been some controversy in the past over the classification of these substances. They are not narcotics, although they are legally classified as controlled substances. They are not hallucinogens, although in very high dosages they can induce hallucinations. They are not sedative-hypnotics, although they most closely resemble these substances. Like sedative-hypnotics, their action occurs in the ascending reticular activating system.

Psychological addiction has been shown to occur with cannabis, and tolerance can occur. Controversy has existed about whether physiological addiction occurs with cannabis. In the past, symptoms of cannabis withdrawal were not considered clinically significant enough for inclusion in the *DSM*. However, the *DSM-5* Substance-Related Work Group determined that subsequent research has provided significant data to support cannabis withdrawal as a valid and reliable syndrome that can negatively impact abstinence attempts of heavy cannabis users. The diagnosis of Cannabis Withdrawal has been included in the *DSM-5*.

Common cannabis preparations are presented in Table 23–6.

Historical Aspects

Products of *Cannabis sativa* have been used therapeutically for nearly 5,000 years (Julien, 2014). Cannabis was first employed in China and India as an antiseptic and an analgesic. Its use later spread to the Middle East, Africa, and Eastern Europe.

In the United States, medical interest in the use of cannabis arose during the early part of the 19th century. Many articles were published espousing its use for varied reasons. The drug was almost as commonly used for medicinal purposes as aspirin is today and could be purchased without a prescription in any

TABLE 23–6 **Cannabinoids**		
CATEGORY	COMMON PREPARATIONS	STREET NAMES
Cannabis	Marijuana	Joint, weed, pot, grass, Mary Jane, Texas tea, locoweed, MJ, hay, stick
	Hashish	Hash, bhang, ganja, charas
Synthetic Cannabinoids	NPS (new psychoactive substances) powders or liquids To be inhaled	K2, Spice, Black Mamba, Joker, Kush

drug store. It was purported to have antibacterial and anticonvulsant capabilities, to decrease intraocular pressure, decrease pain, help in the treatment of asthma, increase appetite, and generally raise one's morale.

The drug fell out of favor primarily because of the huge variation in potency within batches of medication caused by the variations in the THC content of different plants. Other medications were favored for their greater degree of solubility and faster onset of action than cannabis products. A federal law put an end to its legal use in 1937, after an association between marijuana and criminal activity became evident. In the 1960s, marijuana became the symbol of the "antiestablishment" generation and reached its peak as a drug of abuse.

Research continues in regard to the possible therapeutic uses of cannabis. It has been shown to be effective for relieving the nausea and vomiting associated with cancer chemotherapy when other antinausea medications fail. It has also been used in the treatment of chronic pain, glaucoma, multiple sclerosis, acquired immune deficiency syndrome, and epilepsy (Sadock et al., 2015).

Advocates who praise the therapeutic usefulness and support the legalization of cannabis persist within the United States today. Such groups as the Alliance for Cannabis Therapeutics (ACT) and the National Organization for the Reform of Marijuana Laws (NORML) have lobbied extensively to allow disease sufferers easier access to the drug. The medical use of marijuana has been legalized by a number of states. The U.S. Drug Enforcement Agency (2013) has stated:

The DEA supports ongoing research into potential medicinal uses of marijuana's active ingredients. As of January 2013 there are 125 researchers registered with the DEA to perform studies with marijuana, marijuana extracts, and non-tetrahydrocannabinol marijuana derivatives that exist in the plant, such as cannabidiol and cannabinol. Studies include evaluation of abuse potential, physical/psychological effects, adverse effects, therapeutic potential, and detection. Eighteen of the researchers are approved to conduct research with smoked marijuana on human subjects. At present, however, **the clear weight of the evidence is that smoked marijuana is harmful.** No matter what medical condition has been studied, other drugs already approved by the FDA have been proven to be safer and more effective than smoked marijuana. (p. 5)

Two medications that have components of the marijuana plant or related synthetic compounds are currently FDA approved. Dronabinol, a synthetic compound in the medication Marinol, is approved for nausea and vomiting associated with cancer treatment and for severe weight loss associated with AIDS. Nabilone, a chemical similar to THC and found in the medication Cesamet, is a similar FDA-approved drug. A third medication, Sativex, is an oromucosal spray containing THC and cannabidiol. It can be prescribed in the United States only with a special exemption from the FDA for use in select patients (Sadock et al., 2015).

Patterns of Use

In its 2014 National Survey on Drug Use and Health, SAMHSA (2015) reported that an estimated 22.2 million Americans aged 12 years or older were current illicit users of marijuana. This estimate represents almost 8.4 percent of the population ages 12 and older.

Many people incorrectly regard cannabis as a substance of low abuse potential. This lack of knowledge has promoted use of the substance by individuals who believe it is harmless. Tolerance, although it tends to decline rapidly, does occur with chronic use. As tolerance develops, physical addiction also occurs, resulting in a withdrawal syndrome upon cessation of drug use.

One controversy that exists regarding marijuana (particularly because of several statewide efforts toward legalization) is whether its use is a "gateway" to the use of other illicit drugs. DuPont (2016), the first director of the National Institute on Drug Abuse (NIDA), states that marijuana use is positively correlated with use of alcohol, tobacco, cocaine, and methamphetamine and that people addicted to marijuana are three times more likely to be addicted to heroin.

Effects on the Body

Following is a summary of some of the effects that have been attributed to marijuana usage. Undoubtedly, as research continues, evidence of additional physiological and psychological effects will be made available.

Cardiovascular Effects

Cannabis ingestion induces tachycardia and orthostatic hypotension (NIH, 2012). With the decrease in blood pressure, myocardial oxygen supply is decreased. Tachycardia in turn increases oxygen demand.

Respiratory Effects

Marijuana produces a greater amount of "tar" than its equivalent weight in tobacco. Because of the method by which marijuana is smoked—that is, the smoke is held in the lungs for as long as possible to achieve the desired effect—larger amounts of tar are deposited in the lungs, promoting deleterious effects.

Although the initial reaction to the inhalation of marijuana is bronchodilation, thereby facilitating respiratory function, chronic use results in obstructive airway disorders (NIH, 2012). Frequent marijuana users often have laryngitis, bronchitis, cough, and hoarseness. Cannabis smoke contains more carcinogens than tobacco smoke; therefore, lung damage and cancer are real risks for heavy users (NIH, 2012).

Reproductive Effects

Some studies have shown that with heavy marijuana use, men may have a decrease in sperm count, motility, and structure. In women, heavy marijuana use may result in a suppression of ovulation, disruption in menstrual cycles, and alteration of hormone levels.

Central Nervous System Effects

Acute CNS effects of marijuana are dose related. Many people report a feeling of being high—the equivalent of being "drunk" on alcohol. Symptoms include feelings of euphoria, relaxed inhibitions, disorientation, depersonalization, and relaxation. At higher doses, sensory alterations may occur, including impairment in judgment of time and distance, recent memory, and learning ability. Physiological symptoms may include tremors, muscle rigidity, and conjunctival redness. Toxic effects are generally characterized by panic reactions. Very heavy usage has been shown to precipitate an acute psychosis that is self-limited and short-lived once the drug is removed from the body (Julien, 2014).

Heavy long-term cannabis use is also associated with a condition called *amotivational syndrome*. Amotivational syndrome is defined as lack of motivation to persist in or complete a task that requires ongoing attention. Persons are described as "apathetic, anergic, usually gaining weight, and appearing slothful" (Sadock et al., 2015, p. 647). Evidence supports that long-term use also impairs cognitive functions of memory, attention, and organization; these impairments may also contribute to some of the symptoms apparent in amotivational syndrome.

Sexual Function

Marijuana is reported to enhance the sexual experience in both men and women. The intensified sensory awareness and the slowness of time perception are thought to increase sexual satisfaction. Marijuana also enhances sexual function by releasing inhibitions for certain activities that would normally be restrained.

Cannabis Intoxication

Cannabis intoxication is evidenced by the presence of clinically significant behavioral or psychological changes that develop during or shortly after cannabis use. Symptoms include impaired motor coordination, euphoria, anxiety, a sensation of slowed time, impaired judgment and memory, and social withdrawal. Physical symptoms include conjunctival injection (red eyes), increased appetite, dry mouth, and tachycardia (APA, 2013). The impairment of motor skills lasts for 8 to 12 hours and interferes with the operation of motor vehicles. These effects are additive to those of alcohol, which is commonly used in combination with cannabis (Sadock et al., 2015). Cannabis intoxication delirium is marked by significant cognitive impairment and difficulty performing tasks. Higher doses also impair level of consciousness.

NIDA (2015) reported a recent trend in overdoses associated with synthetic cannabinoids (such as K2, Spice, and others). These chemicals are related to THC but are significantly more powerful and dangerous than marijuana. Symptoms include agitation, high blood pressure, shaking and seizures, nausea and vomiting, hallucinations and paranoia, and violent behavior.

Cannabis Withdrawal

The *DSM-5* describes a syndrome of symptoms that occurs upon cessation of heavy, prolonged cannabis use. Symptoms occur within a week following cessation of use and may include any of the following:

■ Irritability, anger, or aggression
■ Nervousness, restlessness, or anxiety
■ Sleep difficulty (e.g., insomnia, disturbing dreams)
■ Decreased appetite or weight loss
■ Depressed mood
■ Physical symptoms, such as abdominal pain, tremors, sweating, fever, chills, or headache

Tables 23–7 and 23–8 include summaries of the psychoactive substances, including symptoms of intoxication, withdrawal, use, overdose, possible therapeutic uses, and trade and common names by which they may be referred. The dynamics of substance use disorders using the transactional model of stress and adaptation are presented in Figure 23–3.

Application of the Nursing Process

Assessment

In the pre-introductory phase of relationship development, the nurse must examine his or her feelings about working with a client who abuses substances. If these behaviors are viewed by the nurse as morally wrong and he or she has internalized these attitudes from very early in life, it may be difficult to suppress judgmental feelings. The role that alcohol or other substances has played (or plays) in the life of the nurse most certainly will affect the way in which he or she interacts with a client who has a substance use disorder.

How are attitudes examined? Some individuals may have sufficient ability for introspection to recognize whether they have unresolved issues related to substance abuse. For others, it may be more helpful to discuss these issues in a group situation, where insight may be gained from feedback regarding the perceptions of others.

Whether alone or in a group, the nurse may gain a greater understanding about attitudes and feelings related to substance abuse by responding to the following types of questions. As written here, the questions are specific to alcohol, but they could be adapted for any substance.

■ What are my drinking patterns?
■ If I drink, why do I drink? When, where, and how much?
■ If I don't drink, why do I abstain?
■ Am I comfortable with my drinking patterns?
■ If I decided not to drink any more, would that be a problem for me?
■ What did I learn from my parents about drinking?
■ Have my attitudes changed as an adult?
■ What are my feelings about people who become intoxicated?
■ Does it seem more acceptable for some individuals than for others?
■ Do I ever use terms such as "sot," "drunk," or "boozer" to describe some individuals who overindulge, yet I overlook it in others?
■ Do I ever overindulge myself?
■ Has the use of alcohol (by me or others) affected my life in any way?
■ Do I see alcohol/drug abuse as a sign of weakness? A moral problem? An illness?

Unless nurses fully understand and accept their own attitudes and feelings, they cannot be empathetic toward clients' problems. Clients in recovery need to know they are accepted for themselves, regardless of past behaviors. Nurses must be able to separate the client from the behavior and to accept that individual with unconditional positive regard.

TABLE 23-7 Psychoactive Substances: A Profile Summary

CLASS OF DRUGS	SYMPTOMS OF USE	THERAPEUTIC USES	SYMPTOMS OF OVERDOSE	TRADE NAMES	COMMON NAMES
CNS DEPRESSANTS					
Alcohol	Relaxation, loss of inhibitions, lack of concentration, drowsiness, slurred speech, sleep	Antidote for methanol consumption; ingredient in many pharmacological concentrates	Nausea, vomiting; shallow respirations; cold, clammy skin; weak, rapid pulse; coma; possible death	Ethyl alcohol, beer, gin, rum, vodka, bourbon, whiskey, liqueurs, wine, brandy, sherry, champagne	Booze, alcohol, liquor, drinks, cocktails, highballs, nightcaps, moonshine, white lightning, firewater
Other (barbiturates and nonbarbiturates)	Same as alcohol	Relief from anxiety and insomnia; as anticonvulsants and anesthetics	Anxiety, fever, agitation, hallucinations, disorientation, tremors, delirium, convulsions, possible death	Seconal, Amytal, Nembutal Valium Librium Noctec Miltown	Red birds, yellow birds, blue birds Blues/yellows Green & whites Mickies Downers
CNS STIMULANTS					
Amphetamines and related drugs	Hyperactivity, agitation, euphoria, insomnia, loss of appetite	Management of narcolepsy, hyperkinesia, and weight control	Cardiac arrhythmias, headache, convulsions, hypertension, rapid heart rate, coma, possible death	Dexedrine, Didrex, Tenuate, Bontril, Ritalin, Focalin, Meridia, Provigil	Uppers, pep pills, wakeups, bennies, eye-openers, speed, black beauties, sweet As
Cocaine	Euphoria, hyperactivity, restlessness, talkativeness, increased pulse, dilated pupils, rhinitis		Hallucinations, convulsions, pulmonary edema, respiratory failure, coma, cardiac arrest, possible death	Cocaine hydrochloride	Coke, flake, snow, dust, happy dust, gold dust, girl, Cecil, C, toot, blow, crack
Synthetic stimulants	Agitation, insomnia, irritability, dizziness, decreased ability to think clearly, increased heart rate, chest pains	Depression, paranoia, delusions, suicidal thoughts, seizures, panic attacks, nausea, vomiting, heart attack, stroke	Mephedrone, MDPV (3-4 methylenedioxypyrovalerone)	Bath salts, bliss, vanilla sky, ivory wave, purple wave	Increased heart rate, increased blood pressure, nosebleeds, hallucinations, aggressive behavior
OPIOIDS					
	Euphoria, lethargy, drowsiness, lack of motivation, constricted pupils	As analgesics; antidiarrheals, and antitussives; methadone in substitution therapy; heroin has no therapeutic use	Shallow breathing, slowed pulse, clammy skin, pulmonary edema, respiratory arrest, convulsions, coma, possible death	Heroin Morphine Codeine Dilaudid Demerol Dolophine Percodan Talwin Opium	Snow, stuff, H, harry, horse M, morph, Miss Emma Schoolboy Lords Doctors Dollies Perkies Ts Big O, black stuff

Categories of Drugs	Symptoms of Use	Therapeutic Uses	Common Names	Drugs
HALLUCINOGENS	Visual hallucinations, disorientation, confusion, paranoid delusions, euphoria, anxiety, panic, increased pulse	LSD has been proposed in the treatment of chronic alcoholism, and in the reduction of intractable pain	Acid, cube, big D	LSD
	Agitation, extreme hyperactivity, violence, hallucinations, psychosis, convulsions, possible death		Angel dust, hog, peace pill	PCP
			Mesc	Mescaline
			Businessman's trip	DMT
				STP, DOM
			Serenity and peace	MDMA
			Ecstasy, XTC	
			Special K, vitamin K, kit kat	Ketamine
			Bath salts	MDPV
CANNABINOLS	Relaxation, talkativeness, lowered inhibitions, euphoria, mood swings	Marijuana has been used for relief of nausea and vomiting associated with antineoplastic chemotherapy and to reduce eye pressure in glaucoma	Marijuana, pot, grass, joint, Mary Jane, MJ	Cannabis
	Fatigue, paranoia, delusions, hallucinations, possible psychosis		Hash, rope, Sweet Lucy	Hashish

TABLE 23-8 **Summary of Symptoms Associated With the Syndromes of Intoxication and Withdrawal**

CLASS OF DRUGS	INTOXICATION	WITHDRAWAL	COMMENTS
Alcohol	Aggressiveness, impaired judgment, impaired attention, irritability, euphoria, depression, emotional lability, slurred speech, incoordination, unsteady gait, nystagmus, flushed face	Tremors, nausea/vomiting, malaise, weakness, tachycardia, sweating, elevated blood pressure, anxiety, depressed mood, irritability, hallucinations, headache, insomnia, seizures	Alcohol withdrawal begins within 4–6 hr after last drink. May progress to delirium tremens on second or third day. Use of Librium or Serax is common for substitution therapy.
Amphetamines and related substances	Fighting, grandiosity, hypervigilance, psychomotor agitation, impaired judgment, tachycardia, pupillary dilation, elevated blood pressure, perspiration or chills, nausea and vomiting	Anxiety, depressed mood, irritability, craving for the substance, fatigue, insomnia or hypersomnia, psychomotor agitation, paranoid and suicidal ideation	Withdrawal symptoms usually peak within 2–4 days, although depression and irritability may persist for months. Antidepressants may be used.
Caffeine	Restlessness, nervousness, excitement, insomnia, flushed face, diuresis, gastrointestinal complaints, muscle twitching, rambling flow of thought and speech, cardiac arrhythmia, periods of inexhaustibility, psychomotor agitation	Headache	Caffeine is contained in coffee, tea, colas, cocoa, chocolate, some over-the-counter analgesics, "cold" preparations, and stimulants.
Cannabis	Euphoria, anxiety, suspiciousness, sensation of slowed time, impaired judgment, social withdrawal, tachycardia, conjunctival redness, increased appetite, hallucinations	Restlessness, irritability, insomnia, loss of appetite, depressed mood, tremors, fever, chills, headache, stomach pain	Intoxication occurs immediately and lasts about 3 hours. Oral ingestion is more slowly absorbed and has longer-lasting effects.
Cocaine	Euphoria, fighting, grandiosity, hypervigilance, psychomotor agitation, impaired judgment, tachycardia, elevated blood pressure, pupillary dilation, perspiration or chills, nausea/vomiting, hallucinations, delirium	Depression, anxiety, irritability, fatigue, insomnia or hypersomnia, psychomotor agitation, paranoid or suicidal ideation, apathy, social withdrawal	Large doses of the drug can result in convulsions or death from cardiac arrhythmias or respiratory paralysis.
Inhalants	Belligerence, assaultiveness, apathy, impaired judgment, dizziness, nystagmus, slurred speech, unsteady gait, lethargy, depressed reflexes, tremor, blurred vision, stupor or coma, euphoria, irritation around eyes, throat, and nose		Intoxication occurs within 5 minutes of inhalation. Symptoms last 60–90 minutes. Large doses can result in death from CNS depression or cardiac arrhythmia.
Nicotine		Craving for the drug, irritability, anger, frustration, anxiety, difficulty concentrating, restlessness, decreased heart rate, increased appetite, weight gain, tremor, headaches, insomnia	Symptoms of withdrawal begin within 24 hours of last drug use and decrease in intensity over days, weeks, or sometimes longer.
Opioids	Euphoria, lethargy, somnolence, apathy, dysphoria, impaired judgment, pupillary constriction, drowsiness, slurred speech, constipation, nausea, decreased respiratory rate and blood pressure	Craving for the drug, nausea/vomiting, muscle aches, lacrimation or rhinorrhea, pupillary dilation, piloerection or sweating, diarrhea, yawning, fever, insomnia	Withdrawal symptoms appear within 6–8 hours after last dose, reach a peak in the second or third day, and subside in 5–10 days. Times are shorter with meperidine and longer with methadone.

TABLE 23–8 Summary of Symptoms Associated With the Syndromes of Intoxication and Withdrawal—cont'd			
CLASS OF DRUGS	INTOXICATION	WITHDRAWAL	COMMENTS
Phencyclidine and related substances	Belligerence, assaultiveness, impulsiveness, psychomotor agitation, impaired judgment, nystagmus, increased heart rate and blood pressure, diminished pain response, ataxia, dysarthria, muscle rigidity, seizures, hyperacusis, delirium		Delirium can occur within 24 hours after use of phencyclidine or may occur up to a week following recovery from an overdose of the drug.
Sedatives, hypnotics, and anxiolytics	Disinhibition of sexual or aggressive impulses, mood lability, impaired judgment, slurred speech, incoordination, unsteady gait, impairment in attention or memory disorientation, confusion	Nausea/vomiting, malaise, weakness, tachycardia, sweating, anxiety, irritability, orthostatic hypotension, tremor, insomnia, seizures	Withdrawal may progress to delirium, usually within 1 week of last use. Long-acting barbiturates or benzodiazepines may be used in withdrawal substitution therapy.

Motivational Interviewing

Motivational interviewing is an approach that can be used in the assessment and intervention process for clients with any disorder, although it first gained popularity in treatment of clients with substance use disorders. It uses skills such as empathy, validation, open-ended questions, and reflection to explore the client's motivation, strengths, and readiness for change. Some of the preceding questions could easily be reframed to explore the client's attitudes and feelings. Through this process, the client is empowered to become an active partner in treatment goals while exploring reasons for resistance to behavior change. For example, rather than telling a client that he or she must abstain from alcohol and must attend 12-step meetings, the health-care professional helps the client articulate what he or she wants to achieve and then facilitates the process of exploring advantages and disadvantages of desired behavior change.

 This is a patient-centered approach that encourages empowerment and active engagement, and as such, it articulates well with two current trends in psychiatric-mental health nursing care: recognizing the importance of patient-centered care as an essential nursing competency (Institute of Medicine, 2003) and the recovery model (see Chapter 21, The Recovery Model, for further discussion of this model).

Assessment Tools

Nurses often perform the admission interview. A variety of assessment tools are appropriate for use in chemical dependency units. A nursing history and assessment tool was presented in Chapter 9, The Nursing Process in Psychiatric-Mental Health Nursing. With some adaptation, it is an appropriate instrument for creating a database on clients who abuse substances. Box 23–2 presents a drug history and assessment that could be used in conjunction with the general biopsychosocial assessment.

The Clinical Institute Withdrawal Assessment of Alcohol Scale, Revised (CIWA-Ar) is an excellent tool that is used by many hospitals to assess risk and severity of withdrawal from alcohol. It may be used for initial assessment as well as ongoing monitoring of alcohol withdrawal symptoms. A copy of the CIWA-Ar is presented in Box 23–3.

Other screening tools exist for determining whether an individual has a problem with substances. Two such tools developed by the American Psychiatric Association for the diagnosis of alcoholism include the Michigan Alcoholism Screening Test and the CAGE Questionnaire (Boxes 23–4 and 23–5). Some psychiatric units administer these surveys to all admitted clients to help determine if there is a secondary alcohol problem in addition to the psychiatric problem for which the client is being admitted (sometimes called **dual diagnosis**). These tools can be adapted to use in diagnosing problems with other drugs as well.

Dual Diagnosis

If the client is diagnosed with both mental illness and a coexisting substance disorder, he or she may be assigned to a special program that targets both problems. Traditional counseling approaches use more confrontation than is considered appropriate for clients with dual diagnoses. Most dual diagnosis programs take a supportive, less confrontational approach.

Peer support groups are an important part of the treatment program. Group members offer encouragement and practical advice to each other.

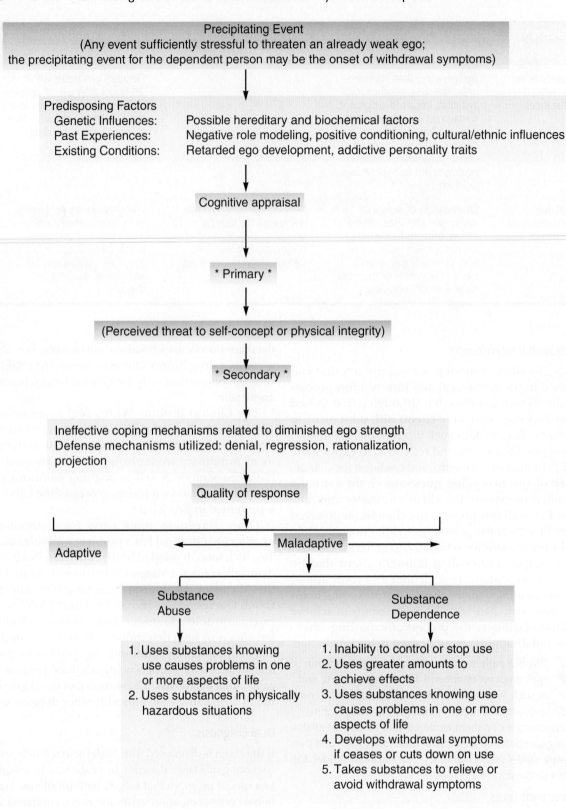

FIGURE 23–3 The dynamics of substance use disorders using the transactional model of stress and adaptation.

BOX 23-2 **Drug History and Assessment***

1. When you were growing up, did anyone in your family drink alcohol or take other kinds of drugs?
2. If so, how did the substance use affect the family situation?
3. When did you have your first drink/drugs?
4. How long have you been drinking/taking drugs on a regular basis?
5. What is your pattern of substance use?
   a. When do you use substances?
   b. What do you use?
   c. How much do you use?
   d. Where are you and with whom when you use substances?
6. When did you have your last drink/drug? What was it and how much did you consume?
7. Does using the substance(s) cause problems for you? Describe. Include family, friends, job, school, other.
8. Have you ever experienced injury as a result of substance use?
9. Have you ever been arrested or incarcerated for drinking/using drugs?
10. Have you ever tried to stop drinking/using drugs? If so, what was the result? Did you experience any physical symptoms, such as tremors, headache, insomnia, sweating, or seizures?
11. Have you ever experienced loss of memory for times when you have been drinking/using drugs?
12. Describe a typical day in your life.
13. Are there any changes you would like to make in your life? If so, what are they?
14. What plans or ideas do you have for seeing that these changes occur?

*To be used in conjunction with general biopsychosocial nursing history and assessment tool (Chapter 9, The Nursing Process in Psychiatric/Mental Health Nursing).

BOX 23-3 **Clinical Institute Withdrawal Assessment of Alcohol Scale, Revised**

Patient: Date: Time:

Pulse or heart rate, taken for one minute: Blood pressure:

NAUSEA AND VOMITING—Ask "Do you feel sick to your stomach? Have you vomited?" Observation.

0 no nausea and no vomiting
1 mild nausea with no vomiting
2
3
4 intermittent nausea with dry heaves
5
6
7 constant nausea, frequent dry heaves and vomiting

TREMOR—Arms extended and fingers spread apart. Observation.

0 no tremor
1 not visible, but can be felt fingertip to fingertip
2
3
4 moderate, with patient's arms extended
5
6
7 severe, even with arms not extended

TACTILE DISTURBANCES—Ask "Have you any itching, pins and needles sensations, any burning, any numbness, or do you feel bugs crawling on or under your skin?" Observation.

0 none
1 very mild itching, pins and needles, burning or numbness
2 mild itching, pins and needles, burning or numbness
3 moderate itching, pins and needles, burning or numbness
4 moderately severe hallucinations
5 severe hallucinations
6 extremely severe hallucinations
7 continuous hallucinations

AUDITORY DISTURBANCES—Ask "Are you more aware of sounds around you? Are they harsh? Do they frighten you? Are you hearing anything that is disturbing to you? Are you hearing things you know are not there?" Observation.

0 not present
1 very mild harshness or ability to frighten
2 mild harshness or ability to frighten
3 moderate harshness or ability to frighten
4 moderately severe hallucinations
5 severe hallucinations
6 extremely severe hallucinations
7 continuous hallucinations

Continued

BOX 23-3 Clinical Institute Withdrawal Assessment of Alcohol Scale, Revised—cont'd

PAROXYSMAL SWEATS—Observation.

0 no sweat visible
1 barely perceptible sweating, palms moist
2
3
4 beads of sweat obvious on forehead
5
6
7 drenching sweats

VISUAL DISTURBANCES—Ask "Does the light appear to be too bright? Is its color different? Does it hurt your eyes? Are you seeing anything that is disturbing to you? Are you seeing things you know are not there?" Observation.

0 not present
I very mild sensitivity
2 mild sensitivity
3 moderate sensitivity
4 moderately severe hallucinations
5 severe hallucinations
6 extremely severe hallucinations
7 continuous hallucinations

ANXIETY—Ask "Do you feel nervous?" Observation.

0 no anxiety, at ease
1 mild anxious
2
3
4 moderately anxious, or guarded, so anxiety is inferred
5
6
7 equivalent to acute panic states as seen in severe delirium or acute schizophrenic reactions

HEADACHE, FULLNESS IN HEAD—Ask "Does your head feel different? Does it feel like there is a band around your head?" Do not rate for dizziness or lightheadedness. Otherwise, rate severity.

0 not present
1 very mild
2 mild
3 moderate
4 moderately severe
5 severe
6 very severe
7 extremely severe

AGITATION—Observation

0 normal activity
1 somewhat more than normal activity
2
3
4 moderately fidgety and restless
5
6
7 paces back and forth during most of the interview, or constantly thrashes about

ORIENTATION AND CLOUDING OF SENSORIUM—Ask "What day is this? Where are you? Who am I?"

0 oriented and can do serial additions
1 cannot do serial additions or is uncertain about date
2 disoriented for date by no more than 2 calendar days
3 disoriented for date by more than 2 calendar days
4 disoriented for place/or person

The CIWA-Ar is not copyrighted and may be reproduced freely. This assessment for monitoring withdrawal symptoms requires approximately 5 minutes to administer. The maximum score is 67 (see instrument). Patients scoring less than 10 do not usually need additional medication for withdrawal. _____

Total CIWA-Ar Score _____
Rater's Initials _____
Maximum Possible Score 67

From Sullivan, J.T., Sykora, K., Schneiderman, J., Naranjo, C.A., & Sellers, E.M. (1989). Assessment of alcohol withdrawal: The revised Clinical Institute Withdrawal Assessment for Alcohol scale (CIWA-Ar). British Journal of Addiction, 84(11), 1353-1357.

Psychodynamic therapy can be useful for some individuals with dual diagnoses by delving into the personal history of how psychiatric disorders and substance abuse have reinforced one another and how the cycle can be broken. Cognitive and behavioral therapies are helpful in training clients to monitor moods and thought patterns that lead to substance abuse. Teaching clients about coping skills and stress management also promotes skills in maintaining abstinence and dealing with substance cravings.

BOX 23–4 Michigan Alcoholism Screening Test (MAST)

Answer the following questions by placing an X under yes or no.*	Yes	No
1. Do you enjoy a drink now and then?	0	0
2. Do you feel you are a normal drinker? (By normal we mean you drink less than or as much as most people.)		2
3. Have you ever awakened the morning after some drinking the night before and found that you could not remember a part of the evening?	2	
4. Does your wife, husband, parent, or other near relative ever worry or complain about your drinking?	1	
5. Can you stop drinking without a struggle after one or two drinks?		2
6. Do you ever feel guilty about your drinking?	1	
7. Do friends or relatives think you are a normal drinker?		2
8. Are you able to stop drinking when you want to?		2
9. Have you ever attended a meeting of Alcoholics Anonymous (AA)?	5	
10. Have you gotten into physical fights when drinking?	1	
11. Has your drinking ever created problems between you and your wife, husband, a parent, or other relative?	2	
12. Has your wife, husband, or another family member ever gone to anyone for help about your drinking?	2	
13. Have you ever lost friends because of your drinking?	2	
14. Have you ever gotten into trouble at work or school because of drinking?	2	
15. Have you ever lost a job because of drinking?	2	
16. Have you ever neglected your obligations, your family, or your work for 2 or more days in a row because you were drinking?	2	
17. Do you drink before noon fairly often?	1	
18. Have you ever been told you have liver trouble? Cirrhosis?	2	
19. After heavy drinking have you ever had delirium tremens (DTs) or severe shaking or heard voices or seen things that really were not there?	5	
20. Have you ever gone to anyone for help about your drinking?	5	
21. Have you ever been in a hospital because of drinking?	5	
22. Have you ever been a patient in a psychiatric hospital or on a psychiatric ward of a general hospital where drinking was part of the problem that resulted in hospitalization?	2	
23. Have you ever been seen at a psychiatric or mental health clinic or gone to any doctor, social worker, or clergyman for help with any emotional problem, where drinking was part of the problem?	2	
24. Have you ever been arrested for drunk driving, driving while intoxicated, or driving under the influence of alcoholic beverages? (If yes, how many times? _____)	2 ea	
25. Have you ever been arrested, or taken into custody, even for a few hours, because of other drunk behavior? (If yes, how many times? _____)	2 ea	

* Items are scored under the response that would indicate a problem with alcohol.
Method of scoring:
0–3 points = no problem with alcohol
4 points = possible problem with alcohol
5 or more = indicates problem with alcohol
From Selzer, M.L. (1971) The Michigan alcohol screening test: The quest for a new diagnostic instrument. American Journal of Psychiatry, 127(12), 1653-1658, with permission.

BOX 23–5 The CAGE Questionnaire

1. Have you ever felt you should **C**ut down on your drinking?
2. Have people **A**nnoyed you by criticizing your drinking?
3. Have you ever felt bad or **G**uilty about your drinking?
4. Have you ever had a drink first thing in the morning to steady your nerves or get rid of a hangover (**E**ye-opener)?

Scoring: 2 or 3 "yes" answers strongly suggests a problem with alcohol.
From Mayfield, D., McLeod, G., & Hall, P. (1974). The CAGE questionnaire: Validation of a new alcoholism screening instrument. American Journal of Psychiatry, 131(10), 1121-1123, with permission.

Individuals with dual diagnoses should be educated about 12-step recovery programs (e.g., Alcoholics Anonymous or Narcotics Anonymous). Dual diagnosis clients are sometimes resistant to attending 12-step programs, and they often do better in substance abuse support groups specifically designed for people with psychiatric disorders.

Substance-abuse groups are usually integrated into regular programming for the psychiatric client with a dual diagnosis. An individual in a psychiatric facility or day treatment program will attend a substance abuse group periodically in lieu of another scheduled activity therapy. Topics are directed toward areas that are unique to clients with mental illness, such as mixing medications with other substances, as well as topics that are common to primary substance abusers. Individuals are encouraged to discuss their personal problems.

Continued attendance at 12-step group meetings is encouraged upon discharge from treatment. Family involvement is enlisted, and preventive strategies are outlined. Individual case management is common, and success is often promoted by this close supervision.

Diagnosis and Outcome Identification

The next step in the nursing process is to identify appropriate nursing diagnoses by analyzing the data collected during the assessment phase. The individual who abuses or is dependent on substances undoubtedly has many unmet physical and emotional needs. Table 23–9 presents a list of client behaviors and the NANDA-I nursing diagnoses that correspond to those behaviors, which may be used in planning care for the client with a substance use disorder.

Outcome Criteria

The following criteria may be used for measurement of outcomes in the care of the client with substance-related disorders.

The client:

■ Has not experienced physical injury
■ Has not caused harm to self or others
■ Accepts responsibility for own behavior
■ Acknowledges association between personal problems and use of substance(s)
■ Demonstrates more adaptive coping mechanisms that can be used in stressful situations (instead of taking substances)
■ Shows no signs or symptoms of infection or malnutrition
■ Exhibits evidence of increased self-worth by attempting new projects without fear of failure and by demonstrating less defensive behavior toward others
■ Verbalizes importance of abstaining from use of substances in order to maintain optimal wellness

TABLE 23–9 Assigning Nursing Diagnoses to Behaviors Commonly Associated With Substance Use Disorders

BEHAVIORS	NURSING DIAGNOSES
Makes statements such as, "I don't have a problem with (substance). I can quit any time I want to." Delays seeking assistance; does not perceive problems related to use of substances; minimizes use of substances; unable to admit impact of disease on life pattern	Denial
Abuse of chemical agents; destructive behavior toward others and self; inability to meet basic needs; inability to meet role expectations; risk taking	Ineffective coping
Loss of weight, pale conjunctiva and mucous membranes, decreased skin turgor, electrolyte imbalance, anemia, drinks alcohol instead of eating	Imbalanced nutrition: Less than body requirements/Deficient fluid volume
Risk factors: Malnutrition, altered immune condition, failing to avoid exposure to pathogens	Risk for infection
Criticizes self and others, self-destructive behavior (abuse of substances as a coping mechanism), dysfunctional family background	Chronic low self-esteem
Denies that substance is harmful; continues to use substance in light of obvious consequences	Deficient knowledge
FOR THE CLIENT WITHDRAWING FROM CNS DEPRESSANTS: Risk factors: CNS agitation (tremors, elevated blood pressure, nausea and vomiting, hallucinations, illusions, tachycardia, anxiety, seizures)	Risk for injury
FOR THE CLIENT WITHDRAWING FROM CNS STIMULANTS: Risk factors: Intense feelings of lassitude and depression; "crashing," suicidal ideation	Risk for suicide

Planning and Implementation

Implementation with clients who abuse substances is a long-term process, often beginning with **detoxification** and progressing to total abstinence. The following sections present a group of selected nursing diagnoses, with short- and long-term goals and nursing interventions for each.

Risk for Injury

Risk for injury is defined as "vulnerable to physical damage due to environmental conditions interacting with the individual's adaptive and defensive resources, which may compromise health" (Herdman & Kamitsuru, 2014, p. 386).

Client Goals

Outcome criteria include short- and long-term goals. Time lines are individually determined.

Short-term goal

1. Client's condition will stabilize within 72 hours.

Long-term goal

2. Client will not experience physical injury.

Interventions

For the client in substance withdrawal

■ Assess the client's level of disorientation to determine specific requirements for safety.
■ Obtain a drug history, if possible. It is important to determine the type of substance(s) used, the time and amount of last use, the length and frequency of use, and the amount used on a daily basis.
■ Because subjective history is often not accurate, obtain a urine sample for laboratory analysis of substance content.

■ It is important to keep the client in as quiet an environment as possible. Excessive stimuli may increase client agitation. A private room is ideal.
■ Observe client behaviors frequently. If seriousness of the condition warrants, it may be necessary to assign a staff person on a one-to-one basis.
■ Accompany and assist the client when ambulating, and use a wheelchair for transporting the client long distances.
■ Pad the headboard and side rails of the bed with thick towels to protect the client in case of a seizure.
■ Suicide precautions may need to be instituted for the client withdrawing from CNS stimulants.
■ Ensure that smoking materials and other potentially harmful objects are stored away from the client's access.
■ Frequently orient the client to reality and the surroundings.
■ Monitor the client's vital signs every 15 minutes initially and less frequently as acute symptoms subside.
■ Follow the medication regimen as ordered by the physician. Common psychopharmacological intervention for substance intoxication and withdrawal is presented later in this chapter under the section "Treatment Modalities for Substance-Related Disorders."

Denial

Denial is defined as a "conscious or unconscious attempt to disavow the knowledge or meaning of an event to reduce anxiety and/or fear, leading to the detriment of health" (Herdman & Kamitsuru, 2014, p. 335). Table 23–10 presents this nursing diagnosis in care plan format.

Table 23–10 | CARE PLAN FOR A CLIENT WITH A SUBSTANCE USE DISORDER

NURSING DIAGNOSIS: DENIAL

RELATED TO: Lack of coping skills to manage anxiety

EVIDENCED BY: Statements indicating no problem with substance use

OUTCOME CRITERIA	NURSING INTERVENTIONS	RATIONALE
Short-Term Goal • Client diverts attention away from external issues and focuses on behavioral outcomes associated with substance use.	1. Begin by working to develop a trusting nurse-client relationship. Be honest. Keep all promises.	1. Trust is the basis of a therapeutic relationship.
	2. Convey an attitude of acceptance to client. Ensure that he or she understands "It is not *you* but your *behavior* that is unacceptable."	2. An attitude of acceptance promotes feelings of dignity and self-worth.

Continued

Table 23–10 | CARE PLAN FOR A CLIENT WITH A SUBSTANCE USE DISORDER—cont'd

OUTCOME CRITERIA	NURSING INTERVENTIONS	RATIONALE
Long-Term Goal • Client verbalizes acceptance of responsibility for own behavior and acknowledges association between substance use and personal problems.	3. Provide information to correct misconceptions about substance abuse. Client may rationalize his or her behavior with statements such as "I'm not an alcoholic. I can stop drinking any time I want. Besides, I only drink beer," or "I only smoke pot to relax before class. So what? I know lots of people who do. Besides, you can't get hooked on pot."	3. Many myths abound regarding use of specific substances. Factual information presented in a matter-of-fact, nonjudgmental way explaining what behaviors constitute substance-related disorders may help client focus on his or her own behaviors as an illness that requires help.
	4. Identify recent maladaptive behaviors or situations that have occurred in client's life, and discuss how use of substances may have been a contributing factor.	4. The first step in decreasing use of denial is for client to see the relationship between substance use and personal problems.
	5. 💬 Use confrontation with caring. Do not allow client to fantasize about his or her lifestyle (e.g., "It is my understanding that the last time you drank alcohol, you . . ." or "The lab report shows that you were under the influence of alcohol when you had the accident that injured three people").	5. Confrontation interferes with client's ability to use denial; a caring attitude preserves self-esteem and avoids putting client on the defensive.
	6. Do not accept rationalization or projection as client attempts to make excuses or blame other people or situations for his or her behavior.	6. Rationalization and projection prolong denial that problems exist in client's life because of substance use.
	7. Encourage participation in group activities.	7. Peer feedback is often more accepted than feedback from authority figures. Peer pressure can be a strong factor, as can association with individuals who are experiencing or who have experienced similar problems.
	8. Offer immediate positive recognition of client's expressions of insight gained regarding illness and acceptance of responsibility for own behavior.	8. Positive reinforcement enhances self-esteem and encourages repetition of desirable behaviors.
	9. Employ motivational interviewing techniques to begin an exploration of client's motivations and readiness for change.	9. Using a patient-centered approach that includes techniques such as reflection, open-ended questions, clarification, and validation encourages client to actively engage in problem-solving.

Client Goals

Outcome criteria include short- and long-term goals. Time lines are individually determined.

Short-term goal

■ Client will focus on behavioral outcomes associated with substance use.

Long-term goal

■ Client will verbalize acceptance of responsibility for own behavior and acknowledge association between substance use and personal problems.

Interventions

■ Begin by working to develop a trusting nurse-client relationship. Be honest and keep all promises.

■ Convey an attitude of acceptance to the client. Ensure that he or she understands "It is not *you* but your *behavior* that is unacceptable." An attitude of acceptance helps to promote the client's feelings of dignity and self-worth.

■ Provide information to correct misconceptions about substance abuse. The client may rationalize his or her behavior with statements such as, "I'm not an alcoholic. I can stop drinking any time I want. Besides, I only drink beer" or "I only smoke pot to relax before class. So what? I know lots of people who do. Besides, you can't get hooked on pot." Many myths abound regarding use of specific substances. Factual information presented in a matter-of-fact, nonjudgmental way explaining what behaviors constitute substance use disorders may help the client focus on his or her own behaviors as an illness that requires help.

■ Identify recent maladaptive behaviors or situations that have occurred in the client's life, and discuss how use of substances may have been a contributing factor. The first step in decreasing denial is for the client to see the relationship between substance use and personal problems.

■ Use confrontation with caring. Do not allow the client to fantasize about his or her lifestyle. Confrontation interferes with the client's ability to use denial; a caring attitude preserves self-esteem and avoids putting the client on the defensive.

> **CLINICAL PEARL** 💬
>
> It is important to speak objectively and nonjudgmentally to a person in denial. Examples: "It is my understanding that the last time you drank alcohol, you . . ." or "The lab report shows that your blood alcohol level was 250 when you were involved in that automobile accident."

■ Acknowledge the use of rationalization or projection as the client attempts to make excuses for or blame his or her behavior on other people or situations. Rationalization and projection prolong the client's denial that problems exist secondary to substance use.

■ Encourage participation in group activities. Peer feedback is often more accepted than feedback from authority figures. Peer pressure from individuals who are experiencing or who have experienced similar problems can be powerfully influential in confronting denial as well.

■ Offer immediate positive recognition of the client's expressions of insight regarding illness and acceptance of responsibility for own behavior. Positive reinforcement enhances self-esteem and encourages repetition of desirable behaviors.

Ineffective Coping

Ineffective coping is defined as the "inability to form a valid appraisal of the stressors, inadequate choices of practiced responses, and/or inability to use available resources" (Herdman & Kamitsuru, 2014, p. 326).

Client Goals

Outcome criteria include short- and long-term goals. Time lines are individually determined.

Short-term goal

■ Client will express true feelings about using substances as a method of coping with stress.

Long-term goal

■ Client will be able to verbalize use of adaptive coping mechanisms, instead of substance abuse, in response to stress.

Interventions

■ Spend time with the client and establish a trusting relationship.

■ Set limits on manipulative behavior. Be sure that the client knows what is acceptable, what is not, and the consequences for violating the limits set. Ensure that all staff maintain consistency with this intervention. Encourage the client to verbalize feelings, fears, and anxieties. Answer any questions he or she may have regarding the disorder. Verbalization of feelings in a nonthreatening environment may help the client come to terms with long-unresolved issues.

■ Explain the effects of substance abuse on the body. Emphasize that the prognosis is closely related to abstinence. Many clients lack knowledge about the deleterious effects of substance abuse on the body.

■ Explore with the client the options available to assist with stressful situations rather than resorting to substance use (e.g., contacting various members of Alcoholics Anonymous or Narcotics Anonymous, physical exercise, relaxation techniques, meditation).

The client may have persistently resorted to chemical use and thus possess little or no knowledge of adaptive responses to stress.

■ Provide positive reinforcement for evidence of gratification delayed appropriately. Encourage the client to be as independent as possible in performing his or her self-care. Provide positive feedback for independent decision-making and effective use of problem-solving skills.

Dysfunctional Family Processes

Dysfunctional family processes occur when "psychosocial, spiritual, and physiological functions of the family unit are chronically disorganized, which leads to conflict, denial of problems, resistance to change, ineffective problem solving, and a series of self-perpetuating crises" (Herdman & Kamitsuru, 2014, p. 290).

Client Goals

Outcome criteria include short- and long-term goals. Time lines are individually determined.

Short-term coals

■ Family members will participate in individual family programs and support groups.
■ Family members will identify ineffective coping behaviors and consequences.
■ Family will initiate and plan for necessary lifestyle changes.

Long-term goal

■ Family members will take action to change self-destructive behaviors and alter behaviors that contribute to client's addiction.

Interventions

■ Review family history; explore roles of family members, current level of functioning, circumstances involving alcohol use, strengths, and areas of growth. Explore how family members have coped with the client's addiction (e.g., denial, repression, rationalization, hurt, loneliness, projection). Persons who enable also suffer from the same feelings as the client and use ineffective methods for dealing with the situation, necessitating help in learning new and effective coping skills.

■ Determine the extent of enabling behaviors evidenced by family members; explore these behaviors with each individual and the client. Enabling behaviors are those that inhibit rather than promote change. Family and friends may enable continued substance use because the user has convinced them that this is the most helpful way to show their love. The substance abuser often relies on others to cover up for his or her inability to cope with daily responsibilities, but this scenario is less likely to promote the need for change.

■ Provide information about enabling behavior and addictive disease characteristics for both the user and nonuser. Achieving awareness and knowledge of behaviors (e.g., avoiding and shielding, taking over responsibilities, rationalizing, and subserving) provides an opportunity for individuals to begin the process of change.

■ Identify and discuss the possibility of sabotage behaviors by family members. Even though family members may verbalize a desire for the individual to become substance free, the reality of interactive dynamics is that they may unconsciously not want the individual to recover, as this would affect the family members' own role in the relationship. Additionally, they may receive sympathy or attention from others (secondary gain).

■ Assist the client's partner to understand that the client's abstinence and drug use are not the partner's responsibility and that the client's use of substances may or may not change despite involvement in treatment. Partners must come to realize and accept that the only behavior they can control is their own.

■ Involve the family in plans for discharge from treatment. Substance abuse is a family illness. Because the family has been so involved in dealing with the substance use behavior, family members need help adjusting to the new behavior of sobriety/abstinence. Encourage involvement with self-help associations, such as Alcoholics Anonymous, Al-Anon, Alateen, CoDA, and professional family therapy. These organizations put the client and family in direct contact with support systems necessary for continued sobriety and assists with problem resolution.

Concept Care Mapping

The concept map care plan (see Chapter 9) is a diagrammatic teaching and learning strategy that allows visualization of interrelationships between medical diagnoses, nursing diagnoses, assessment data, and treatments. An example of a concept map care plan for a client with a substance use disorder is presented in Figure 23–4.

Client and Family Education

The role of client teacher is important in the psychiatric area, as it is in all areas of nursing. A list of topics for client/family education relevant to substance-related disorders is presented in Box 23–6. Sample client teaching guides are available online.

Evaluation

The final step of the nursing process involves re-assessment to determine if the nursing interventions have been effective in achieving the intended goals

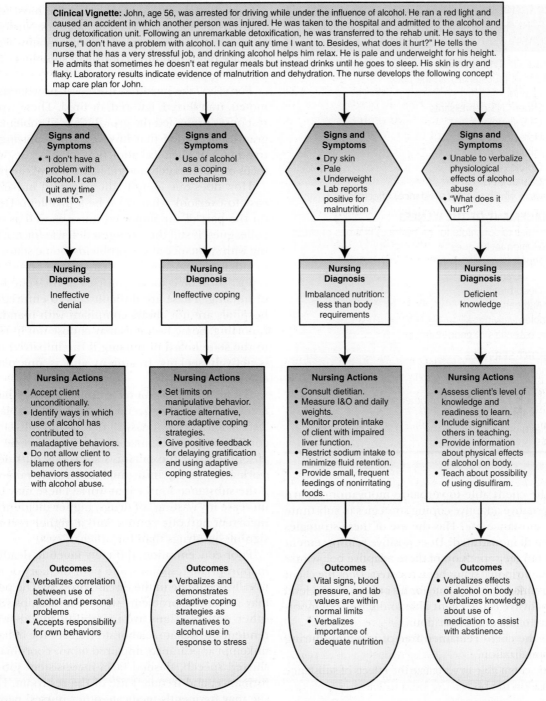

Clinical Vignette: John, age 56, was arrested for driving while under the influence of alcohol. He ran a red light and caused an accident in which another person was injured. He was taken to the hospital and admitted to the alcohol and drug detoxification unit. Following an unremarkable detoxification, he was transferred to the rehab unit. He says to the nurse, "I don't have a problem with alcohol. I can quit any time I want to. Besides, what does it hurt?" He tells the nurse that he has a very stressful job, and drinking alcohol helps him relax. He is pale and underweight for his height. He admits that sometimes he doesn't eat regular meals but instead drinks until he goes to sleep. His skin is dry and flaky. Laboratory results indicate evidence of malnutrition and dehydration. The nurse develops the following concept map care plan for John.

Signs and Symptoms
• "I don't have a problem with alcohol. I can quit any time I want to."

Signs and Symptoms
• Use of alcohol as a coping mechanism

Signs and Symptoms
• Dry skin
• Pale
• Underweight
• Lab reports positive for malnutrition

Signs and Symptoms
• Unable to verbalize physiological effects of alcohol abuse
• "What does it hurt?"

Nursing Diagnosis
Ineffective denial

Nursing Diagnosis
Ineffective coping

Nursing Diagnosis
Imbalanced nutrition: less than body requirements

Nursing Diagnosis
Deficient knowledge

Nursing Actions
• Accept client unconditionally.
• Identify ways in which use of alcohol has contributed to maladaptive behaviors.
• Do not allow client to blame others for behaviors associated with alcohol abuse.

Nursing Actions
• Set limits on manipulative behavior.
• Practice alternative, more adaptive coping strategies.
• Give positive feedback for delaying gratification and using adaptive coping strategies.

Nursing Actions
• Consult dietitian.
• Measure I&O and daily weights.
• Monitor protein intake of client with impaired liver function.
• Restrict sodium intake to minimize fluid retention.
• Provide small, frequent feedings of nonirritating foods.

Nursing Actions
• Assess client's level of knowledge and readiness to learn.
• Include significant others in teaching.
• Provide information about physical effects of alcohol on body.
• Teach about possibility of using disulfiram.

Outcomes
• Verbalizes correlation between use of alcohol and personal problems
• Accepts responsibility for own behaviors

Outcomes
• Verbalizes and demonstrates adaptive coping strategies as alternatives to alcohol use in response to stress

Outcomes
• Vital signs, blood pressure, and lab values are within normal limits
• Verbalizes importance of adequate nutrition

Outcomes
• Verbalizes effects of alcohol on body
• Verbalizes knowledge about use of medication to assist with abstinence

FIGURE 23–4 Concept map care plan for client with alcoholism.

of care. Evaluation of the client with a substance-related disorder may be accomplished by using information gathered from the following reassessment questions:

■ Has detoxification occurred without complications?
■ Is the client still in denial?
■ Does the client accept responsibility for his or her own behavior? Has he or she acknowledged a personal problem with substances?

■ Has a correlation been made between personal problems and the use of substances?
■ Does the client still make excuses or blame others for use of substances?
■ Has the client remained substance free during treatment?
■ Does the client cooperate with treatment?
■ Does the client refrain from manipulative behavior and violation of limits?

BOX 23–6 Topics for Client/Family Education Related to Substance Use Disorders

NATURE OF THE ILLNESS

1. Effects of (substance) on the body
   a. Alcohol
   b. Other CNS depressants
   c. CNS stimulants
   d. Hallucinogens
   e. Inhalants
   f. Opioids
   g. Cannabinols
2. Ways in which use of (substance) affects life.

MANAGEMENT OF THE ILLNESS

1. Activities to substitute for (substance) in times of stress
2. Relaxation techniques
   a. Progressive relaxation
   b. Tense and relax
   c. Deep breathing
   d. Autogenics
3. Problem-solving skills
4. The essentials of good nutrition

SUPPORT SERVICES

1. Financial assistance
2. Legal assistance
3. Alcoholics Anonymous (or other support group specific to another substance)
4. One-to-one support person

■ Is the client able to verbalize motivation toward alternative adaptive coping strategies to substitute for substance use? Has the use of these strategies been demonstrated? Does positive reinforcement encourage repetition of these adaptive behaviors?

■ Has nutritional status been restored? Does the client consume a diet adequate for his or her size and level of activity? Is the client able to discuss the importance of adequate nutrition?

■ Has the client remained free of infection during hospitalization?

■ Is the client able to verbalize the effects of substance abuse on the body?

The Chemically Impaired Nurse

Substance abuse and addiction has the potential for impairment in an individual's social, occupational, psychological, and physical functioning. This becomes an especially serious problem when the impaired person is responsible for the lives of others each day. Approximately 10 percent of the general population suffers from chemical addiction. In one study, researchers identified the prevalence of substance abuse among employed nurses to be 5.1 percent

(Monroe et al., 2013). Alcohol is the most widely abused drug, followed closely by narcotics. Nurses who abuse substances have an added vulnerability because they are often handling controlled substances when providing patient care.

For years, the impaired nurse was protected, promoted, transferred, ignored, or fired. These types of responses promoted the growth of the problem. Programs are needed that involve early reporting and treatment of chemical addiction as a disease, with a focus on public safety and rehabilitation of the nurse.

How does one identify the impaired nurse? It is easy to overlook what *might* be a problem. Denial, on the part of the impaired nurse as well as nurse colleagues, is still the strongest defense for not dealing with substance abuse problems. Some states have mandatory reporting laws that require observers to report substance-abusing nurses to the state board of nursing. These are difficult laws to enforce, and hospitals are not always compliant with mandatory reporting. Some hospitals may choose not to report to the state board of nursing if the impaired nurse is actively seeking treatment and is not placing clients in danger.

A number of clues for recognizing substance impairment in nurses have been identified (Ellis & Hartley, 2012). They are not easy to detect and will vary according to the substance used. There may be high absenteeism if the person's source is outside the work area, or the individual may rarely miss work if the substance source is at work. There may be an increase in "wasting" of drugs, higher incidences of incorrect narcotic counts, and a higher record of signing out drugs than for other nurses.

Poor concentration, difficulty meeting deadlines, inappropriate responses, and poor memory or recall usually occur late in the disease process. The person may also have problems with relationships. Some other possible signs are irritability, mood swings, tendency to isolate, elaborate excuses for behavior, unkempt appearance, impaired motor coordination, slurred speech, flushed face, inconsistent job performance, and frequent use of the restroom. He or she may frequently medicate other nurses' patients, and there may be patient complaints of inadequate pain control. Discrepancies in documentation may occur. Ideally, suspicious behavior is recognized by peers and intervention sought before the impaired nurse reaches late stages of the disease process. As uncomfortable as it may seem to tell a supervisor about suspected impairment in a colleague, it is in the interest of the nurse's health and critically important to ensuring patient safety.

If suspicious behavior occurs, it is important to keep careful, objective records. Confrontation with the impaired nurse will undoubtedly result in hostility and denial. Confrontation should occur in the presence of a supervisor or other nurse and should include the offer of assistance in seeking treatment. If a report is made to the state board of nursing, it should be a factual documentation of specific events and actions, not a diagnostic statement of impairment.

Each case is generally decided on an individual basis. A state board may deny, suspend, or revoke a license on the basis of a report of chemical abuse by a nurse. Several state boards of nursing have passed diversionary laws that allow impaired nurses to avoid disciplinary action by agreeing to seek treatment. Some administer the treatment programs themselves, and others refer the nurse to community resources or state nurses' association assistance programs. Treatment may entail successful completion of inpatient, outpatient, group, or individual counseling treatment program(s); evidence of regular attendance at nurse support groups or a 12-step program; random negative drug screens; and employment or volunteer activities during the suspension period. When a nurse is deemed safe to return to practice, he or she may be closely monitored for several years and required to undergo random drug screenings. The nurse also may be required to practice under specifically circumscribed conditions for a designated period of time.

In 1982, the American Nurses Association (ANA) House of Delegates adopted a national resolution to provide assistance to impaired nurses. Since that time, the majority of state nurses' associations have developed (or are developing) programs for nurses who are impaired by substances or psychiatric illness. The individuals who administer these efforts are nurse members of the state associations, as well as nurses who are in recovery themselves. For this reason, they are called **peer assistance programs.**

The peer assistance programs strive to intervene early, reduce hazards to clients, and increase prospects for the nurse's recovery. Most states provide either a hotline number that the impaired nurse or intervening colleague may call or phone numbers of peer assistance committee members. Typically, a contract is drawn up detailing the method of treatment, which may be obtained from various sources, such as employee assistance programs, Alcoholics Anonymous, Narcotics Anonymous, private counseling, or outpatient clinics. Guidelines for monitoring the course of treatment are established. Peer support is provided through regular contact with the impaired nurse, usually for a period of 2 years. Peer assistance programs serve to assist impaired nurses to recognize their impairment, obtain necessary treatment, and regain accountability within their profession.

Codependency

The concept of **codependency** arose from a need to define the dysfunctional behaviors that are evident among members of the family of a chemically addicted person. The term has been expanded to include all individuals from families that harbor secrets of physical or emotional abuse or pathological conditions. Living under these conditions results in unmet needs for autonomy and self-esteem and a profound sense of powerlessness. The codependent person is able to achieve a sense of control only through fulfilling the needs of others. Personal identity is relinquished and boundaries with the other person become blurred. The codependent person disowns his or her own needs and wants in order to respond to external demands and the demands of others. Codependence has been called "a dysfunctional relationship with oneself."

The traits associated with a codependent personality are varied. In a relationship, the codependent person derives self-worth from that of the partner, whose feelings and behaviors determine how the codependent should feel and behave. In order for the codependent to feel good, his or her partner must be happy and behave in appropriate ways. If the partner is not happy, the codependent feels responsible for *making* him or her happy. The codependent's home life is fraught with stress. Ego boundaries are weak and behaviors are often enmeshed with those of the pathological partner. Denial that problems exist is common. Feelings are kept in control, and anxiety may be released in the form of stress-related illnesses or compulsive behaviors such as eating, spending, working, or use of substances.

Wesson (2013) describes the following behaviors characteristic of codependency. She stated that codependents:

■ Have a long history of focusing thoughts and behavior on other people.
■ Are "people pleasers" and will do almost anything to get the approval of others.
■ Outwardly appear very competent, but actually feel quite needy, helpless, or perhaps nothing at all.
■ Have experienced abuse or emotional neglect as a child.
■ Are outwardly focused toward others and know very little about how to direct their own lives from their own sense of self.

The Codependent Nurse

Certain characteristics of codependence have been associated with the profession of nursing. A shortage of nurses combined with the increasing ranks of seriously ill clients may result in nurses providing care to and fulfilling everyone's needs but their own. Many health-care workers who were reared in homes with a chemically addicted person or otherwise dysfunctional family are at risk for activation of unresolved codependent tendencies. Nurses who assumed the "fixer" role in their dysfunctional families of origin during childhood may attempt to resume that role in their caregiving professions. They are attracted to a profession in which they are needed but nurture feelings of resentment for receiving so little in return. Their emotional needs go unmet, but they continue to deny that these needs exist. Instead, these unmet emotional needs may be manifested through use of compulsive behaviors, such as work or spending excessively, or addictions, such as to food or substances.

Codependent nurses have a need to be in control. They often strive for an unrealistic level of achievement. Their self-worth comes from the feeling of being needed by others and maintaining control over the environment. They nurture the dependence of others and accept the responsibility for the happiness and contentment of others. They rarely express their true feelings, and they do what is necessary to preserve harmony and maintain control. They are at high risk for physical and emotional burnout.

Treating Codependency

Cermak (1986) identified four stages in the recovery process for individuals with codependent personality:

Stage I: The Survival Stage In this first stage, codependent persons must begin to let go of the denial that problems exist or that their personal capabilities are unlimited. This initiation of abstinence from blanket denial may be a very emotional and painful period.

Stage II: The Reidentification Stage Reidentification occurs when the individuals are able to glimpse their true selves through a break in the denial system. They accept the label of codependent and take responsibility for their own dysfunctional behavior. Codependents tend to enter reidentification only after being convinced that it is more painful not to do so. They accept their limitations and are ready to face the issues of codependence.

Stage III: The Core Issues Stage In this stage, the recovering codependent must face the fact that relationships cannot be managed by force of will. Each partner must be independent and autonomous. The goal of this stage is to detach from the struggles of life that exist because of prideful and willful efforts to control things that are beyond the individual's power to control.

Stage IV: The Reintegration Stage This is a stage of self-acceptance and willingness to change when codependents relinquish the power *over others* that was not rightfully theirs but reclaim the *personal* power that

they do possess. Integrity is achieved out of awareness, honesty, and connection with one's spiritual consciousness. Control is achieved through self-discipline and self-confidence.

Self-help groups have been found helpful in the treatment of codependency. Groups developed for families of chemically addicted people, such as Al-Anon, may be of assistance. Groups specific to codependency also exist. One of these groups, which bases its philosophy on the Twelve Steps of Alcoholics Anonymous (see the section that follows) is

Co-Dependents Anonymous (CoDA)
P.O. Box 33577
Phoenix, AZ 85067-3577
888-444-2359
www.coda.org

Treatment Modalities for Substance-Related Disorders

Alcoholics Anonymous

Alcoholics Anonymous (AA) is a major self-help organization for the treatment of alcoholism. It was founded in 1935 by two alcoholics—a stockbroker, Bill Wilson, and a physician, Bob Smith—who discovered that they could remain sober through mutual support. This they accomplished not as professionals, but as peers who were able to share their common experiences. Soon they were working with other alcoholics, who in turn worked with others. The movement grew, and remarkably, individuals who had been treated unsuccessfully by professionals were able to maintain sobriety through helping one another.

Today, AA chapters exist in virtually every community in the United States. The self-help groups are based on the concept of peer support—acceptance and understanding from others who have experienced the same problems. The only requirement for membership is a desire on the part of the alcoholic person to stop drinking. Each new member is assigned a support person from whom he or she may seek assistance when the temptation to drink occurs.

A survey by the General Service Office of Alcoholics Anonymous in 2014 (Alcoholics Anonymous, 2015) revealed the following statistics: members ages 30 and younger comprised 12 percent of the membership, and the average age of AA members was 50; women comprised 38 percent; 89 percent were white, 4 percent were African American, 3 percent were Hispanic, 1 percent were Native American, and 3 percent were Asian American and other minorities. Almost half (49%) of people involved in AA were referred by a health-care professional or treatment facility. The sole purpose of AA is to help members stay sober. When sobriety has been achieved, they in turn are expected to help other alcoholic persons. The Twelve Steps that embody the philosophy of AA provide specific guidelines on how to attain and maintain sobriety (Box 23–7).

AA accepts alcoholism as an illness and promotes total abstinence as the only cure, emphasizing that the alcoholic person can never safely return to social drinking. They encourage the members to seek sobriety, taking one day at a time. The Twelve Traditions are the statements of principles that govern the organization.

AA has been the model for various self-help groups associated with addiction problems. Some of these groups and the memberships for which they are organized are listed in Table 23–11. Nurses must be fully and accurately informed about available self-help groups and their importance as a treatment resource on the health-care continuum so that they can use them as a referral source for clients with substance use disorders.

Pharmacotherapy

Disulfiram (Antabuse)

Disulfiram (Antabuse) is a drug that can be administered as a deterrent to drinking to individuals who abuse alcohol. Ingestion of alcohol while disulfiram is in the body results in a syndrome of symptoms that produce substantial discomfort for the individual and even result in death if the blood alcohol level is high. The reaction varies according to the sensitivity of the individual and how much alcohol was ingested.

BOX 23–7 **Alcoholics Anonymous**

The Twelve Steps

1. We admitted we were powerless over alcohol—that our lives have become unmanageable.
2. Came to believe that a Power greater than ourselves could restore us to sanity.
3. Made a decision to turn our will and our lives over to the care of God as we understood Him.
4. Made a searching and fearless moral inventory of ourselves.
5. Admitted to God, to ourselves, and to another human being the exact nature of our wrongs.
6. Were entirely ready to have God remove all these defects of character.
7. Humbly asked Him to remove our shortcomings.
8. Made a list of all persons we had harmed and became willing to make amends to them all.
9. Made direct amends to such people wherever possible except when to do so would injure them or others.
10. Continued to take personal inventory and when we were wrong promptly admitted it.
11. Sought through prayer and meditation to improve our conscious contact with God as we understood Him, praying only for knowledge of His will for us and the power to carry that out.
12. Having had a spiritual awakening as the result of these steps, we tried to carry this message to alcoholics and to practice these principles in all our affairs.

The Twelve Traditions

1. Our common welfare should come first; personal recovery depends upon AA unity.
2. For our group purpose there is but one ultimate authority—a loving God as He may express Himself in our group conscience. Our leaders are but trusted servants; they do not govern.
3. The one requirement for AA membership is a desire to stop drinking.
4. Each group should be autonomous except in matters affecting other groups or AA as a whole.
5. Each group has but one primary purpose—to carry its message to the alcoholic who still suffers.
6. An AA group ought never endorse, finance, or lend the AA name to any related facility or outside enterprise, lest problems of money, property, and prestige divert us from our primary purpose.
7. Every AA group ought to be fully self-supporting, declining outside contributions.
8. Alcoholics Anonymous should remain forever nonprofessional, but our service centers may employ special workers.
9. Alcoholics Anonymous, as such, ought never be organized; but we may create service boards of committees directly responsible to those they serve.
10. Alcoholics Anonymous has no opinion on outside issues; hence, the Alcoholics Anonymous name ought never be drawn into public controversy.
11. Our public relations policy is based on attraction rather than promotion; we need always maintain personal anonymity at the level of press, radio, and films.
12. Anonymity is the spiritual foundation of all our traditions, ever reminding us to place principles before personalities.

The Twelve Steps and Twelve Traditions are reprinted with permission of Alcoholics Anonymous World Services, Inc. (AAWS). Permission to reprint the Twelve Steps and Twelve Traditions does not mean that AAWS has reviewed or approved the contents of this publication, or that AA necessarily agrees with the views expressed herein. AA is a program of recovery from alcoholism only. Use of the Twelve Steps and Twelve Traditions in connection with programs and activities which are patterned after AA, but which address other problems, or in any other non-AA context, does not imply otherwise.

TABLE 23–11 Addiction Self-Help Groups

GROUP	MEMBERSHIP
Adult Children of Alcoholics (ACOA)	Adults who grew up with an alcoholic in the home
Al-Anon	Families of alcoholics
Alateen	Adolescent children of alcoholics
Children Are People	School-aged children with an alcoholic family member
Cocaine Anonymous	Cocaine addicts
Codependents Anonymous (CoDA)	Families of alcohol or other substance abusers
Families Anonymous	Parents of children who abuse substances
Fresh Start	Nicotine addicts
Gamblers Anonymous	Gambling addicts
Narcotics Anonymous	Narcotics addicts
Nar-Anon	Families of narcotics addicts
Overeaters Anonymous	Food addicts
Pills Anonymous	Polysubstance addicts
Pot Smokers Anonymous	Marijuana smokers
Smokers Anonymous	Nicotine addicts
Women for Sobriety	Female alcoholics

Disulfiram works by inhibiting the enzyme aldehyde dehydrogenase, thereby blocking the oxidation of alcohol at the stage when acetaldehyde is converted to acetate. This results in an accumulation of acetaldehyde in the blood, which is thought to produce the symptoms associated with the disulfiram-alcohol reaction. These symptoms persist as long as alcohol is being metabolized. The rate of alcohol elimination does not appear to be affected.

Symptoms of disulfiram-alcohol reaction can occur within 5 to 10 minutes of ingestion of alcohol. Mild reactions can occur at blood alcohol levels as low as 5 to 10 mg/dL. Symptoms are fully developed at approximately 50 mg/dL and may include flushed skin, throbbing in the head and neck, respiratory difficulty, dizziness, nausea and vomiting, sweating, hyperventilation, tachycardia, hypotension, weakness, blurred vision, and confusion. With a blood alcohol level of approximately 125 to 150 mg/dL, severe reactions can occur, including respiratory depression, cardiovascular collapse, arrhythmias, myocardial infarction, acute congestive heart failure, unconsciousness, convulsions, and death.

Disulfiram should not be administered until it has been ascertained that the client has abstained from alcohol for at least 12 hours. If disulfiram is discontinued, it is important for the client to understand that the sensitivity to alcohol may last for as long as 2 weeks. Consuming alcohol or alcohol-containing substances during this 2-week period could result in the disulfiram-alcohol reaction.

The client receiving disulfiram therapy should be aware of the many substances that contain alcohol. These products, such as liquid cough and cold preparations, vanilla extract, aftershave lotions, colognes, mouthwash, nail polish removers, and isopropyl alcohol, are capable of producing the symptoms described if ingested or even rubbed on the skin. The individual must read labels carefully and inform any doctor, dentist, or other health-care professional from whom assistance is sought that he or she is taking disulfiram. In addition, the client must carry a card explaining participation in disulfiram therapy, possible consequences of the therapy, and symptoms that may indicate an emergency situation.

The client must be assessed carefully before beginning disulfiram therapy. A thorough medical screening is performed before therapy commences, and written informed consent is usually required. The drug is contraindicated for clients at high risk for alcohol ingestion. It is also contraindicated for psychotic clients and clients with severe cardiac, renal, or hepatic disease.

Disulfiram therapy is not a cure for alcoholism. It provides a measure of control for the individual who desires to avoid impulse drinking. Clients receiving disulfiram therapy are encouraged to seek other assistance with their problem, such as AA or another support group, to aid in the recovery process.

Other Medications for Treatment of Alcoholism

The narcotic antagonist naltrexone (ReVia) was approved by the FDA in 1994 for the treatment of alcohol addiction. Naltrexone, which was approved in 1984 for the treatment of heroin abuse, works on the same receptors in the brain that produce the feelings of pleasure when heroin or other opiates bind to them but does not produce the same "narcotic high" and is not habit forming. Although alcohol does not bind to these brain receptors, a systematic review of the research demonstrated that naltrexone works equally well against alcohol (Garbutt et al., 1999). In comparison to the placebo-treated clients, participants on naltrexone therapy showed significantly lower overall relapse rates and fewer drinks per drinking day among those clients who did resume drinking. In another large study of veterans (mostly men), Krystal and associates (2001) concluded that evidence does not support the use of naltrexone for men with chronic severe alcohol dependence. Thus, the efficacy of selective serotonin reuptake inhibitors (SSRIs) in the decrease of alcohol craving among alcohol-dependent individuals has yielded mixed results (National Institute on Alcohol Abuse and Alcoholism, 2000). A greater degree of success was observed with moderate drinkers than with heavy drinkers.

In August 2004, the FDA approved acamprosate (Campral), which is indicated for the maintenance of abstinence from alcohol in patients with alcohol addiction who are abstinent at treatment initiation. The mechanism of action of acamprosate in maintenance of alcohol abstinence is not completely understood. It is hypothesized to restore the normal balance between neuronal excitation and inhibition by interacting with glutamate and gamma-aminobutyric acid (GABA) neurotransmitter systems. Acamprosate is ineffective in clients who have not undergone detoxification and not achieved alcohol abstinence prior to beginning treatment. It is recommended for concomitant use with psychosocial therapy.

Counseling

Counseling on a one-to-one basis is often used to help the client who abuses substances. The relationship is goal directed, and the length of the counseling may vary from weeks to years. The focus is on current reality, development of a working treatment relationship, and strengthening ego assets. The counselor must be warm, kind, and nonjudgmental yet able to set limits firmly. Research consistently demonstrates that personal characteristics of counselors are highly predictive of client outcome. In addition to technical counseling skills, many important therapeutic qualities affect the outcome of counseling, including insight, respect, genuineness, concreteness, and empathy (SAMHSA, 2014).

Counseling of the client who abuses substances passes through various phases, each of which is of indeterminate length. In the first phase, an assessment is conducted. Factual data are collected to determine whether the client does indeed have a problem with substances; that is, that substances are regularly impairing effective functioning in one or more significant life areas.

Following the assessment, in the working phase of the relationship, the counselor assists the individual to accept that the use of substances causes problems in significant life areas and that he or she is not able to prevent this from occurring. The client states a desire to make changes. The strength of the denial system is determined by the duration and extent of substance-related adverse effects in the person's life. Thus, those individuals with rather minor substance-related problems of recent origin have less difficulty with this stage than those with long-term extensive impairment. The individual also works to gain self-control and abstain from substances.

Once the problem has been identified and sobriety achieved, the client must have a concrete and workable plan for getting through the early weeks of abstinence. Anticipatory guidance through role-play helps the individual practice how he or she will respond when substances are readily obtainable and the impulse to partake is strong.

Counseling often includes the family or specific family members. In family counseling, the therapist tries to help each member see how he or she has affected, and been affected by, the substance abuse behavior. Family strengths are mobilized, and family members are encouraged to move in a positive direction. Referrals are often made to self-help groups such as Al-Anon, Nar-Anon, Alateen, Families Anonymous, and Adult Children of Alcoholics.

Group Therapy

Group therapy has long been regarded as a powerful agent of change with those who abuse substances. In groups, individuals are able to share their experiences with others going through similar problems. They are able to "see themselves in others" and thus confront their defenses about giving up the substance. They may recognize similar attitudes and defenses in others. Groups also give individuals the capacity to communicate needs and feelings directly.

In task-oriented education groups, the leader is charged with presenting material associated with substance abuse and its effects on the person's life. Other educational groups that may be effective include assertiveness techniques and relaxation training. Teaching groups differ from psychotherapy groups, whose focus is on helping individuals understand and manage difficult feelings and situations, particularly as they relate to substance use.

Therapy groups and self-help groups such as AA are complementary to each other. Whereas the self-help group focus is on achieving and maintaining sobriety, in the therapy group the individual may learn more adaptive ways of coping, how to deal with problems that may have arisen from or were exacerbated by the former substance use, and ways to improve quality of life and function more effectively without substances.

Psychopharmacology for Substance Intoxication and Substance Withdrawal

Various medications have been used to decrease the intensity of symptoms in an individual who is withdrawing from or experiencing the effects of excessive use of alcohol and other drugs. **Substitution therapy** may be required to reduce the life-threatening effects of intoxication or withdrawal from some substances. The severity of the withdrawal syndrome depends on the particular drug used, how long it has been used, the dose used, and the rate at which the drug is eliminated from the body.

Alcohol

Benzodiazepines are the most widely used group of drugs for substitution therapy in alcohol withdrawal. Chlordiazepoxide (Librium), oxazepam (Serax), lorazepam (Ativan), and diazepam (Valium) are the most common agents. The approach to treatment with benzodiazepines for alcohol withdrawal is to start with relatively high doses and reduce the dosage by 20 to 25 percent each day until withdrawal is complete. Additional doses may be given for breakthrough signs or symptoms (Black & Andreasen, 2014). In clients with liver disease, accumulation of longer-acting agents (chlordiazepoxide and diazepam) may be problematic, and use of shorter-acting benzodiazepines (lorazepam or oxazepam) is more appropriate.

Some physicians may order anticonvulsant medication (e.g., carbamazepine, valproic acid, or gabapentin) for management of withdrawal seizures. These drugs are particularly useful in individuals who undergo repeated episodes of alcohol withdrawal, which appear to "kindle" even more serious withdrawal episodes, including the production of withdrawal seizures that can result in brain damage (Julien, 2014). These anticonvulsants have been used successfully in both acute withdrawal and longer-term craving situations.

Multivitamin therapy, in combination with daily injections or oral administration of thiamine, is common protocol. Thiamine is commonly deficient in chronic alcoholics. Replacement therapy is required to prevent neuropathy, confusion, and encephalopathy.

Opioids

Examples of drugs in the opioid classification include opium, morphine, codeine, heroin, hydromorphone, oxycodone, and hydrocodone. Synthetic opiate-like narcotic analgesics include meperidine, methadone, pentazocine, and fentanyl.

Opioid intoxication is treated with narcotic antagonists such as naloxone (Narcan), naltrexone (ReVia), or nalmefene (Revex). In 2015 the FDA approved an intranasal form of naloxone hydrochloride under a fast-track approval process in response to the increase in deaths associated with drug overdose, particularly from respiratory depression and arrest. It is reported to work within 2 minutes but must be given quickly to prevent death (Brown, 2015). Naloxone nasal spray can cause severe withdrawal in patients who are opioid dependent.

Opiate withdrawal symptoms, as discussed previously, last for varying amounts of time depending on the type of opiate (see the section entitled "Opiate Withdrawal"). Withdrawal therapy includes rest, adequate nutritional support, and methadone substitution. Methadone, if ordered, is given on the first day in a dose sufficient to suppress withdrawal symptoms. The dose is then gradually tapered over a specified time. As the dose of methadone diminishes, renewed abstinence symptoms may be ameliorated by the addition of clonidine.

In October 2002, the FDA approved two forms of the drug buprenorphine for treating opiate addiction. Buprenorphine is less powerful than methadone but is considered somewhat safer and causes fewer side effects, making it especially attractive for clients who are mildly or moderately addicted. Individuals are able to access treatment with buprenorphine in office-based settings, providing an alternative to methadone clinics. Physicians are deemed qualified to prescribe buprenorphine if they hold an addiction certification from the American Society of Addiction Medicine, the American Academy of Addiction Psychiatry, the

American Psychiatric Association, or a similar association. The number of patients to whom individual physicians may provide outpatient buprenorphine treatment was previously limited to 100, but in response to the growing opioid epidemic, a new federal rule became effective in August 2016 increasing the allowable number to 275 patients, with stipulations about necessary credentialing in addictions medicine or addictions psychiatry and allowable practice settings (SAMHSA, 2016). A sublingual formulation of a combination medication with buprenorphine and naloxone (Suboxone) is also available.

Clonidine (Catapres) also has been used to suppress opiate withdrawal symptoms. As monotherapy, it is not as effective as substitution with methadone, but it is nonaddictive and serves effectively as a bridge to enable the client to stay opiate free long enough to facilitate termination of methadone maintenance.

Depressants

Substitution therapy for CNS depressant withdrawal (particularly barbiturates) is most commonly combined with the long-acting barbiturate phenobarbital (Luminal). The dosage required to suppress withdrawal symptoms is administered. When stabilization has been achieved, the dose is gradually decreased by 30 mg/day until withdrawal is complete. Long-acting benzodiazepines are commonly used for substitution therapy when the abused substance is a nonbarbiturate CNS depressant.

Stimulants

Treatment of stimulant intoxication usually begins with minor tranquilizers such as chlordiazepoxide and progresses to major tranquilizers such as haloperidol (Haldol). Antipsychotics should be administered with caution because of their propensity to lower seizure threshold. Repeated seizures are treated with intravenous diazepam.

Withdrawal from CNS stimulants is not the medical emergency observed with CNS depressants. Treatment is usually aimed at reducing drug craving and managing severe depression. The client is placed in a quiet atmosphere and allowed to sleep and eat as much as needed or desired. Suicide precautions may need to be instituted. Antidepressant therapy may be helpful in treating symptoms of depression.

Hallucinogens and Cannabinols

Substitution therapy is not required with these drugs. When adverse reactions such as anxiety or panic occur, benzodiazepines (e.g., diazepam or chlordiazepoxide) may be prescribed to prevent harm to the client or others. Psychotic reactions may be treated with antipsychotic medications.

Non-Substance Addictions

Gambling Disorder

Gambling disorder is defined by the *DSM-5* as persistent and recurrent problematic gambling behavior leading to clinically significant impairment or distress (APA, 2013). The preoccupation with and impulse to gamble often intensifies when the individual is under stress. Many impulsive gamblers describe a physical sensation of restlessness and anticipation that can be relieved only by placing a bet. Blume (2013) states:

> In some cases the initial change in gambling behavior leading to pathological gambling begins with a "big win," bringing a rapid development of preoccupation, tolerance, and loss of control. Winning brings feelings of special status, power, and omnipotence. The gambler increasingly depends on this activity to cope with disappointments, problems, and negative emotional states, pulling away from emotional attachment to family and friends.

As the need to gamble increases, the individual is forced to obtain money by any means available. This may include borrowing money from illegal sources or pawning personal items (or items that belong to others). As gambling debts accrue, or out of a need to continue gambling, the individual may desperately resort to forgery, theft, or even embezzlement. Family relationships are disrupted, and impairment in occupational functioning may occur because of absences from work in order to gamble.

Gambling behavior usually begins in adolescence; however, compulsive behaviors rarely occur before young adulthood. The disorder generally runs a chronic course, with periods of waxing and waning that are largely dependent on psychosocial stress. Prevalence estimates for problem gambling range from 3 to 5 percent, with about 1 percent meeting the criteria for a gambling disorder (Sadock et al., 2015). This condition is more common among men than women.

Various personality disorder traits have been associated with pathological gambling. In a systematic review and meta-analysis (Dowling et al., 2015), the most prevalent included narcissistic, antisocial, avoidant, obsessive-compulsive, and borderline traits. The researchers conclude that in any treatment setting for gambling disorders, screening and treatment for these common comorbid conditions must be addressed.

Gambling problems may be episodic and increase during periods of stress or depression, or the behavior may be persistent (APA, 2013). The *DSM-5* diagnostic criteria for pathological gambling are presented in Box 23–8.

Predisposing Factors to Gambling Disorder

Biological Influences

Genetic Familial and twin studies show an increased prevalence of pathological gambling in family members of individuals diagnosed with the disorder. Black and associates (2014) found that first-degree relatives of pathological gamblers were eight times more likely to develop the same condition, which suggests an underlying genetic predisposition.

Physiological Studies of dopamine receptor systems have implicated this neurotransmitter in the development of addictive personality traits, including pathological gambling (Weiss & Pontone, 2014). Support for this association comes from studies that demonstrated a correlation between the development of pathological gambling behaviors after individuals were treated with dopamine receptor agonist drugs (Moore, Glenmullen, & Mattison, 2014).

Biochemical theories suggest that, ironically, both winning and losing (perhaps related to the excitement of taking a risk) may stimulate the reward and pleasure centers of the brain. This could contribute to persistent and repeated desire to gamble even when one is not winning.

Psychosocial Influences

Sadock and associates (2015) report that the following may be predisposing factors to the development of pathological gambling: "loss of a parent by death, separation, divorce, or desertion before the child is 15 years of age; inappropriate parental discipline (absence, inconsistency, or harshness); exposure to and availability of gambling activities for the adolescent; a family emphasis on material and financial symbols; and a lack of family emphasis on saving, planning, and budgeting" (p. 691).

Treatment Modalities for Gambling Disorder

Because most pathological gamblers deny that they have a problem, treatment is difficult. In fact, most gamblers only seek treatment due to legal difficulties, family pressures, or other psychiatric complaints. Behavior therapy, cognitive-behavioral therapy, motivational interviewing, 12-step programs (Gamblers Anonymous)

BOX 23–8 Diagnostic Criteria for Gambling Disorder

A. Persistent and recurrent problematic gambling behavior leading to clinically significant impairment or distress, as indicated by the individual exhibiting four (or more) of the following in a 12-month period:

1. Needs to gamble with increasing amounts of money in order to achieve the desired excitement.
2. Is restless or irritable when attempting to cut down or stop gambling.
3. Has made repeated unsuccessful efforts to control, cut back, or stop gambling.
4. Is often preoccupied with gambling (e.g., persistent thoughts of reliving past gambling experiences, handicapping or planning the next venture, or thinking of ways to get money with which to gamble).
5. Often gambles when feeling distressed (e.g., helpless, guilty, anxious, depressed).
6. After losing money gambling, often returns another day to get even ("chasing" one's losses).
7. Lies to conceal the extent of involvement with gambling.
8. Has jeopardized or lost a significant relationship, job, or educational or career opportunity because of gambling.
9. Relies on others to provide money to relieve desperate financial situations caused by gambling.

B. The gambling behavior is not better explained by a manic episode.

Specify if:

Episodic: Meeting diagnostic criteria at more than one point in time, with symptoms subsiding between periods of gambling disorder for at least several months.

Persistent: Experiencing continuous symptoms, to meet diagnostic criteria for multiple years.

Specify if:

In early remission: After full criteria for gambling disorder were previously met, none of the criteria for gambling disorder have been met for at least 3 months but for less than 12 months.

In sustained remission: After full criteria for gambling disorder were previously met, none of the criteria for gambling disorder have been met during a period of 12 months or longer.

Specify current severity:

Mild: 4–5 criteria met.

Moderate: 6–7 criteria met.

Severe: 8–9 criteria met.

Reprinted with permission from the Diagnostic and Statistical Manual of Mental Disorders, Fifth Edition *(Copyright 2013). American Psychiatric Association.*

and self-help strategies such as bibliotherapy have all been used with pathological gambling with various degrees of success. About one-third of individuals with gambling disorders recover naturally without need for treatment (Rash, Weinstock, & Van Patten, 2016). Some medications have been used with effective results in the treatment of pathological gambling. SSRIs and clomipramine have been used to treat obsessive-compulsive disorders and may have benefits for those with gambling disorder who have comorbid obsessive-compulsive traits. Lithium, carbamazepine, and naltrexone have also been shown effective.

Possibly the most effective treatment of pathological gambling is participation by the individual in **Gamblers Anonymous** (GA). This organization of inspirational group therapy is modeled after Alcoholics Anonymous.

CASE STUDY AND SAMPLE CARE PLAN

NURSING HISTORY AND ASSESSMENT

The police bring Dan to the emergency department of the local hospital around 9 p.m. His wife, Cassandra, called 911 when Dan became violent and she began to fear for her safety. Dan was fired from his job as a foreman in a manufacturing plant for refusing to follow his supervisor's directions on a project. When cleaning up after his move, several partially used liquor bottles were found in his work area.

Cassandra reports that Dan has been drinking since he came home shortly after noon today. He bloodied her nose and punched her in the stomach when she poured the contents of a bottle he was drinking down the kitchen sink. The police responded to her call and brought Dan to the hospital in handcuffs. By the time they arrive at the hospital, Dan has calmed down and appears drugged and drowsy. His blood alcohol level measures 247 mg/dL. He is admitted to the detoxification unit of the hospital with a diagnosis of Alcohol Intoxication.

Cassandra tells the admitting nurse that she and Dan have been married for 12 years. He was a social drinker before they were married, but his drinking has increased over the years. He has been under a lot of stress at work; hates his job, his boss, and his coworkers; and is depressed a lot of the time. He never had a loving relationship with his parents, who are now deceased. For the past few years, his pattern has been to come home, start drinking immediately, and drink until he passes out for the night. She states that she has tried to get him to go for help with his drinking, but he refuses and says that he doesn't have a problem. Cassandra begins to cry and says to the nurse, "We can't go on like this. I don't know what to do!"

NURSING DIAGNOSES AND OUTCOME IDENTIFICATION

From the assessment data, the nurse develops the following nursing diagnoses for Dan:

1. **Risk for injury** related to CNS agitation from alcohol withdrawal.
   a. **Short-term goal:** Dan's condition will stabilize within 72 hours.
   b. **Long-term goal:** Dan will not experience physical injury.
2. **Ineffective denial** related to low self-esteem, weak ego development, and underlying fears and anxieties.
   a. **Short-term goal:** Dan will focus immediate attention on behavioral changes required to achieve sobriety.

   b. **Long-term goal:** Dan will accept responsibility for his drinking behaviors and acknowledge the association between his drinking and personal problems.

PLANNING AND IMPLEMENTATION

RISK FOR INJURY

The following nursing interventions may be implemented *in an effort to ensure client safety:*

1. Assess Dan's level of disorientation; frequently orient him to reality and his surroundings.
2. Obtain a drug history.
3. Obtain a urine sample for analysis.
4. Place Dan in a quiet room (private, if possible).
5. Ensure that smoking materials and other potentially harmful objects are stored away.
6. Observe Dan frequently. Take vital signs every 15 to 30 minutes.
7. Monitor for signs of withdrawal within a few hours after admission. Watch for signs of
   ■ Increased heart rate
   ■ Tremors
   ■ Headache
   ■ Diaphoresis
   ■ Agitation; restlessness
   ■ Nausea
   ■ Fever
   ■ Convulsions
8. Follow medication regimen, as ordered by physician (commonly a benzodiazepine, thiamine, multivitamin).

DENIAL

The following nursing interventions may be implemented *in an effort to help Dan accept responsibility for the behavioral consequences associated with his drinking:*

1. Develop Dan's trust by spending time with him, being honest, and keeping all promises.
2. Ensure that Dan understands that it is not *him* but his *behavior* that is unacceptable.
3. Provide Dan with accurate information about the effects of alcohol. Do this in a matter-of-fact, nonjudgmental way.
4. Point out recent negative events that have occurred in Dan's life and associate the use of alcohol with these events. Help him to see the association.
5. Use confrontation with caring: "Yes, your wife called the police. You were physically abusive. She was afraid. And

Continued

CASE STUDY AND SAMPLE CARE PLAN—cont'd

your blood alcohol level was 247 when you were brought in. You were obviously not in control of your behavior at the time."

6. Don't accept excuses for his drinking. Point out rationalization and projection behaviors. These behaviors prolong denial that he has a problem. He must directly accept responsibility for his drinking (not make excuses and blame it on the behavior of others). He must come to understand that only *he* has control of his behavior.

7. Encourage Dan to attend group therapy during treatment and Alcoholics Anonymous following treatment. Peer feedback is a strong factor in helping individuals recognize their problems and ultimately remain sober.

8. Encourage Cassandra to attend Al-Anon meetings. She can benefit from the experiences of others who have experienced and are experiencing the same types of problems as she is.

9. Help Dan to identify ways that he can cope besides using alcohol, such as exercise, sports, and relaxation. He should choose what is most appropriate for him and be given positive feedback for efforts made toward change.

EVALUATION

The outcome criteria identified for Dan have been met. He experienced an uncomplicated withdrawal from alcohol and exhibits no evidence of physical injury. He verbalizes understanding of the relationship between his personal problems and his drinking and accepts responsibility for his own behavior. He verbalizes understanding that alcohol addiction is an illness that requires ongoing support and treatment, and he regularly attends AA meetings. Cassandra regularly attends Al-Anon meetings.

Summary and Key Points

■ An individual is considered to be addicted to a substance when he or she is unable to control its use, even knowing that it interferes with normal functioning; when increasing amounts of the substance are required to produce the desired effects; and when characteristic withdrawal symptoms develop upon cessation or drastic decrease in use of the substance.

■ Substance intoxication is defined as the development of a reversible syndrome of maladaptive behavioral or psychological changes due to the direct physiological effects of a substance on the CNS and develop during or shortly after ingestion of (or exposure to) a substance.

■ Substance withdrawal is the development of a substance-specific maladaptive behavioral change, with physiological and cognitive concomitants, due to the cessation of or reduction in heavy and prolonged substance use.

■ The etiology of substance use disorders is unknown. Various contributing factors have been implicated, such as genetics, biochemical changes, developmental influences, personality factors, social learning, conditioning, and cultural and ethnic influences.

■ Seven classes of substances are presented in this chapter in terms of a profile of the substance, historical aspects, patterns of use and abuse, and effects on the body. They include alcohol, other CNS depressants, CNS stimulants, opioids, hallucinogens, inhalants, and cannabinols.

■ The nurse uses the nursing process as the vehicle for delivery of care of the client with a substance-related disorder.

■ The nurse must first examine his or her own feelings regarding personal substance use and substance use by others. Only the nurse who can be accepting and nonjudgmental of substance-use behaviors will be effective in working with these clients.

■ Special care is given to clients with dual diagnoses of mental illness and substance use disorders.

■ Addiction to substances is a problem for many members of the nursing profession. Most state boards of nursing and state nurses' associations have established avenues for peer assistance to provide help to impaired members of the profession.

■ Individuals who are reared in families with chemically addicted persons learn patterns of dysfunctional behavior that carry over into adult life. These dysfunctional behavior patterns have been termed *codependence*. Codependent persons sacrifice their own needs for the fulfillment of others' in order to achieve a sense of control. Many nurses also have codependent traits.

■ Treatment modalities for substance-related disorders include self-help groups, deterrent therapy, individual counseling, and group therapy. Substitution pharmacotherapy is frequently implemented, with clients experiencing substance intoxication or substance withdrawal. Treatment modalities are implemented on an inpatient basis or in outpatient settings, depending on the severity of the impairment.

- Gambling disorder is defined by the *DSM-5* as persistent and recurrent problematic gambling behavior leading to clinically significant impairment or distress.

- The preoccupation with and impulse to gamble intensifies when the individual is under stress. Many impulsive gamblers describe a physical sensation of restlessness and anticipation that can be relieved only by placing a bet.

- Research indicates a possible genetic component in the etiology to gambling disorder. Abnormalities in the serotonergic, noradrenergic, and dopaminergic neurotransmitter systems have also been implicated.

- A number of psychosocial influences have been implicated in the predisposition to gambling disorder, including dysfunctional family patterns.

- Behavior therapy, cognitive therapy, and psychoanalysis have been used with gambling disorder with various degrees of success. Medications such as SSRIs, clomipramine, lithium, carbamazepine, and naltrexone, have also been tried.

- Gamblers Anonymous, an organization of inspirational group therapy modeled after Alcoholics Anonymous, has been very effective in helping individuals who desire to stop gambling.

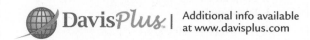

Davis*Plus* | Additional info available at www.davisplus.com

Review Questions
Self-Examination/Learning Exercise

Select the answer that is most appropriate for each of the following questions.

1. Mr. White is admitted to the hospital after an extended period of binge alcohol drinking. His wife reports that he has been a heavy drinker for a number of years. Laboratory reports reveal he has a blood alcohol level of 250 mg/dL. He is placed on the chemical addiction unit for detoxification. When would the first signs of alcohol withdrawal symptoms be expected to occur?
   a. Several hours after the last drink
   b. 2 to 3 days after the last drink
   c. 4 to 5 days after the last drink
   d. 6 to 7 days after the last drink

2. Symptoms of alcohol withdrawal include:
   a. Euphoria, hyperactivity, and insomnia.
   b. Depression, suicidal ideation, and hypersomnia.
   c. Diaphoresis, nausea and vomiting, and tremors.
   d. Unsteady gait, nystagmus, and profound disorientation.

3. Which of the following medications is the physician most likely to order for a client experiencing alcohol withdrawal syndrome?
   a. Haloperidol (Haldol)
   b. Chlordiazepoxide (Librium)
   c. Methadone (Dolophine)
   d. Phenytoin (Dilantin)

4. Dan, who has been admitted to the alcohol rehabilitation unit after being fired for drinking on the job, states to the nurse, "I don't have a problem with alcohol. I can handle my booze better than anyone I know. My boss is a jerk! I haven't missed any more days than my coworkers." What is the nurse's best response?
   a. "Maybe your boss is mistaken, Dan."
   b. "You are here because your drinking was interfering with your work, Dan."
   c. "Get real, Dan! You're a boozer and you know it!"
   d. "Why do you think your boss is a jerk, Dan?"

Continued

Review Questions—cont'd
Self-Examination/Learning Exercise

5. Dan, who has been admitted to the alcohol rehabilitation unit after being fired for drinking on the job, states to the nurse, "I don't have a problem with alcohol. I can handle my booze better than anyone I know. My boss is a jerk! I haven't missed any more days than my coworkers." Which defense mechanism is Dan using?
   a. Denial
   b. Projection
   c. Displacement
   d. Rationalization

6. Dan has been admitted to the alcohol rehabilitation unit after being fired for drinking on the job. Dan's drinking buddies come for a visit, and when they leave, the nurse smells alcohol on Dan's breath. Which of the following would be the best intervention with Dan at this time?
   a. Search his room for evidence.
   b. Ask, "Have you been drinking alcohol, Dan?"
   c. Send a urine specimen from Dan to the laboratory for drug screening.
   d. Tell Dan, "These guys cannot come to the unit to visit you again."

7. Dan begins attendance at AA meetings. Which of the statements by Dan reflects the purpose of this organization?
   a. "They claim they will help me stay sober."
   b. "I'll dry out in AA, then I can have a social drink now and then."
   c. "AA is only for people who have reached the bottom."
   d. "If I lose my job, AA will help me find another."

8. From which of the following symptoms might the nurse identify in a chronic cocaine user?
   a. Clear, constricted pupils
   b. Red, irritated nostrils
   c. Muscle aches
   d. Conjunctival redness

9. An individual who is addicted to heroin is likely to experience which of the following symptoms of withdrawal?
   a. Increased heart rate and blood pressure
   b. Tremors, insomnia, and seizures
   c. Incoordination and unsteady gait
   d. Nausea and vomiting, diarrhea, and diaphoresis

10. A polysubstance abuser makes the statement, "The green and whites do me good after speed." How might the nurse interpret the statement?
   a. The client abuses amphetamines and anxiolytics.
   b. The client abuses alcohol and cocaine.
   c. The client is psychotic.
   d. The client abuses narcotics and marijuana.

11. A client admitted to the emergency department smells strongly of alcohol, and his wife reports he has been a heavy drinker for the last 25 years. Which of the following assessment findings are consistent with long-term chronic alcohol abuse? (Select all that apply.)
   a. The client reports weak leg muscles, and his gait is unsteady.
   b. The client's abdomen is distended.
   c. The client reports he was coughing up some blood.
   d. The client reports he has double vision.
   e. Blood tests reveal a low white blood cell count.

IMPLICATIONS OF RESEARCH FOR EVIDENCE-BASED PRACTICE

Majer, J.M., Payne, J.C., & Jason, L.A. (2015). Recovery resources and psychiatric severity among persons with substance use disorders. *Community Mental Health Journal 51*(4), 437-444. doi:10.1007/s10597-014-9762-3

DESCRIPTION OF THE STUDY: This study examined social support and self-efficacy in maintaining abstinence among individuals discharged from inpatient treatment for substance use disorders. The participants ($N = 270$) were largely unemployed with an average of 6.3 prior convictions, and the majority (41.4%) reported using opiates/heroin, followed by cocaine (27.8%), alcohol (12.8%), polysubstance use (11.3%), and cannabis (6.4%).

RESULTS OF THE STUDY: The researchers found that individuals with high psychiatric severity had lower levels of self-efficacy for abstinence even though there was not a significant difference in social support. The researchers suggest that usual social support resources such as 12-step programs may not be sufficient for individuals with comorbid psychiatric illness. Abstinence self-efficacy may be inhibited by cognitive dysfunction associated with the psychiatric illness, but whatever the contributing factors, abstinence self-efficacy is highly correlated with decreasing relapse.

IMPLICATIONS FOR NURSING PRACTICE: The researchers point out that interventions related to coping skills and stress management have been shown to increase abstinence self-efficacy. Nurses play an active role in this kind of education for clients in inpatient psychiatric units. Targeting these interventions for individuals with concurrent substance abuse disorders may provide a stronger foundation for relapse prevention in this group post-discharge.

TEST YOUR CRITICAL THINKING SKILLS

Kelly, age 23, is a first-year law student engaged to a surgical resident at the local university hospital. She has been struggling to do well in law school because she wants to make her parents, two prominent local attorneys, proud of her. She had never aspired to do anything but go into law, and that is also what her parents expected her to do.

Kelly's midterm grades were not as high as she had hoped, so she increased the number of hours of study time, staying awake all night several nights a week to study. She started drinking large amounts of coffee to stay awake but still found herself falling asleep as she tried to study at the library and in her apartment. As final exams approached, she began to panic that she would not be able to continue the pace of studying she felt she needed in order to make the grades she hoped for.

One of Kelly's classmates told her that she needed some "speed" to give her that extra energy to study. Her classmate said, "All the kids do it. Hardly anyone I know gets through law school without it." She gave Kelly the name of a source.

Kelly contacted the source, who supplied her with enough amphetamines to see her through final exams. Kelly was excited, because she had so much energy, did not require sleep, and was able to study the additional hours she thought she needed for the exams. However, when the results were posted, Kelly had failed two courses and would have to repeat them in summer school if she was to continue with her class in the fall. She continued to replenish her supply of amphetamines from her contact until he told her he could not get her anymore. She became frantic and stole a prescription blank from her fiancé and forged his name for more pills.

She started taking increasing amounts of the medication in order to achieve the high she wanted to feel. Her behavior became erratic. Yesterday, her fiancé received a call from a pharmacy to clarify an order for amphetamines that Kelly had written. He insisted that she admit herself to the chemical addiction unit for detoxification.

On the unit, she appears tired and depressed, moves very slowly, and wants to sleep all the time. She keeps saying to the nurse, "I'm a real failure. I'll never be an attorney like my parents. I'm too dumb. I just wish I could die."

Answer the following questions related to Kelly:

1. What is the primary nursing diagnosis for Kelly?
2. Describe important nursing interventions to be implemented with Kelly.
3. In addition to physical safety, what would be the primary short-term goal the nurses would strive to achieve with Kelly?

💬 Communication Exercises

1. Tom is a patient on the alcohol treatment unit. He says to the nurse, "My boss and my wife ganged up on me. They think I have a drinking problem. I don't have a drinking problem! I can quit any time I want to!"
   - How would the nurse respond appropriately to this statement by Tom?
2. Tom says to the nurse, "My head hurts. I didn't sleep very well last night. I'm getting shaky and it's hot in here! I could sure use a cup of coffee and a cigarette."
   - How would the nurse respond appropriately to this statement by Tom?
3. Tom says, "Sure, I missed a couple days of work. Everyone gets sick now and then. I don't think my wife cares about what happens to me. She and my boss got together and decided I needed to be here, or I lose my job!"
   - How would the nurse respond appropriately to this statement by Tom?

MOVIE CONNECTIONS

Affliction (alcoholism)

Days of Wine and Roses (alcoholism)

I'll Cry Tomorrow (alcoholism)

When a Man Loves a Woman (alcoholism)

Clean and Sober (addiction-cocaine)

28 Days (alcoholism)

Lady Sings the Blues (addiction-heroin)

I'm Dancing as Fast as I Can (addiction-sedatives)

The Rose (polysubstance addiction)

References

Alcoholics Anonymous. (2015). Alcoholics Anonymous 2014 membership survey. Retrieved from www.aa.org/assets/en_US/p-48_membershipsurvey.pdf

American Academy of Child and Adolescent Psychiatry. (2011). *Facts for families: Children of alcoholics.* Retrieved from http://www.aacap.org/App_Themes/AACAP/docs/facts_for_families/17_children_of_alcoholics.pdf

American Psychiatric Association (APA). (2013). *Diagnostic and statistical manual of mental disorders* (5th ed.). Washington, DC: APA.

American Society of Addiction Medicine. (2015). The ASAM national practice guideline for the use of medications in the treatment of addiction involving opioid use. Retrieved from www.asam.org/docs/default-source/practice-support/guidelines-and-consensus-docs/asam-national-practice-guideline-supplement.pdf

Black, D., Coryell, W., Crowe, R., McCormick, B., Shaw, M., & Allen, J.A. (2014). Direct, controlled, blind family study of DSM-IV pathological gambling. *Journal of Clinical Psychiatry, 75*(3), 215-221. doi:10.4088/JCP.13m08566

Black, D.W., & Andreasen, N.C. (2014). *Introductory textbook of psychiatry* (6th ed.). Washington, DC: American Psychiatric Publishing.

Blume, S.G. (2013). Pathological gambling: Recognition and intervention. Retrieved from http://education.iupui.edu/soe/programs/graduate/counselor/readings_n_docs/reading4.pdf

Brown, T. (2015). FDA approves Narcan nasal spray to treat opioid overdose. Retrieved from www.medscape.com/viewarticle/854716

Carmona, R.H. (2005). *Surgeon general's advisory on alcohol use in pregnancy.* Washington, DC: U.S. Department of Health and Human Services.

Centers for Disease Control and Prevention. (2016a). Fetal alcohol spectrum disorders (FASDs). Retrieved from www.cdc.gov/ncbddd/fasd/index.html

Centers for Disease Control and Prevention. (2016b). Smoking and tobacco use. Retrieved from www.cdc.gov/tobacco/data_statistics/vital_signs/index.htm

Centers for Disease Control and Prevention. (2016c). Injury prevention and control: Prescription drug overdose. Retrieved from www.cdc.gov/drugoverdose/epidemic/index.html

Deyo, R.A., Smith, D.H., Johnson, E.S., Tillotson, C.J., Donovan, M., Yang, X., & Dobscha, S.K. (2013). Prescription opioids for back pain and use of medications for erectile dysfunction. *Spine, 38*(11), 909-915. doi:10.1097/BRS.0b013e3182830482

Dowling, N.A., Cowlishaw, S., Jackson, A.C., Merkouris, S.S., Francis, K.L., & Christensen, D.R. (2015). The prevalence of comorbid personality disorders in treatment-seeking problem gamblers: A systematic review and meta-analysis. *Journal of Personality Disorders, 29*(6):735-754. doi:10.1521/pedi_2014_28_168

Duffy, S. (2016). DEA classifies deadly synthetic opioid as schedule I. www.empr.com/news/dea-classifies-deadly-synthetic-opioid-as-schedule-i/article/572194

DuPont, R.L. (2016). Marijuana has proven to be a gateway drug. Retrieved from www.nytimes.com/roomfordebate/2016/04/26/is-marijuana-a-gateway-drug/marijuana-has-proven-to-be-a-gateway-drug

Elias, E. (2013). Improving awareness and treatment of children with fetal alcohol spectrum disorders and co-occurring psychiatric disorders. Retrieved from https://www.jbsinternational.com/sites/default/files/FASDpaperfinal_INT.pdf

Ellis, J.R., & Hartley, C.L. (2012). *Nursing in today's world: Trends, issues, and management* (10th ed.). Philadelphia: Lippincott Williams & Wilkins.

Hanley, C.E. (2017). Navajos. In J.N. Giger (Ed.), *Transcultural nursing: Assessment and intervention* (7th ed.). St. Louis, MO: Mosby.

Herdman, T.H., & Kamitsuru, S. (Eds.). (2014). *NANDA International nursing diagnoses: Definitions and classification 2015–2017* (10th ed.). Chichester, UK: Wiley Blackwell.

Institute of Medicine. (2003). *Health professions education: A bridge to quality.* Washington, DC: Institute of Medicine.

Julien, R.M. (2014). *A primer of drug action: A comprehensive guide to actions, uses and side effects of psychoactive drugs* (13th ed.). New York: Worth Publishers.

Krystal, J.H., Cramer, J.A., Krol, W.F., Kirk, G.F, & Rosenheck, R.A, for the Veterans Affairs Naltrexone Cooperative Study 425 Group. (2001). Naltrexone in the treatment of alcohol dependence. *New England Journal of Medicine, 345*(24), 1734-1739. doi:10.1056/NEJMoa011127

Lafferty, K.A., & Abdel-Kariem, R. (2014). Barbiturate toxicity. Retrieved from http://emedicine.medscape.com/article/813155-overview

Lanska, D. (2016). Alcoholic myopathy. *Medlink Neurology.* Retrieved from www.medlink.com/article/alcoholic_myopathy

Maier, S.E., & West, J.R. (2013). Drinking patterns and alcohol-related birth defects. *National Institute on Alcohol Abuse and Alcohol.* National Institutes of Health. Retrieved from http://pubs.niaaa.nih.gov/publications/arh25-3/168-174.htm

Majer, J.M., Payne, J.C., & Jason, L.A. (2015). Recovery resources and psychiatric severity among persons with substance use disorders. *Community Mental Health Journal 51*(4), 437-444. doi:10.1007/s10597-014-9762-3

McKeown, N.J. (2015). Toluene toxicity. *Medscape Reference: Drugs, diseases, and procedures.* Retrieved from http://emedicine.medscape.com/article/818939-overview

Monroe, T.B., Kenaga, H., Dietrich, M.S., Carter, M.A., & Cowan, R.L. (2013). The prevalence of employed nurses identified or enrolled in substance use monitoring programs. *Nursing Research 62*(1), 10-15. doi:10.1097/NNR.0b013e31826ba3ca

Moore, T. J., Glenmullen, J., & Mattison, D.R. (2014). Reports of pathological gambling, hypersexuality, and compulsive shopping associated with dopamine receptor agonist drugs. *JAMA Internal Medicine, 174*(12), 1930-1933. doi:10.1001/jamainternmed.2014.5262

MPR. (2016). DEA reverses decision to ban kratom. Retrieved from www.empr.com/news/dea-reverses-decision-to-ban-kratom/article/559547

National Council on Alcoholism and Drug Dependence. (2017). Facts about alcohol. Retrieved from www.ncadd.org

National Institute on Alcohol Abuse and Alcoholism. (2000). *Tenth Special Report to the U.S. Congress on Alcohol and Health.* Bethesda, MD: The Institute.

National Institute on Drug Abuse. (2012). *Principles of drug addiction treatment: A research-based guide* (3rd ed.). National Institutes of Health. Retrieved from https://www.drugabuse.gov/publications/principles-drug-addiction-treatment-research-based-guide-third-edition/evidence-based-approaches-to-drug-addiction-treatment/behavioral

National Institute on Drug Abuse. (2014). Drugs, brains, and behavior: The science of addiction. National Institutes of Health. Retrieved from www.drugabuse.gov/publications/drugs-brains-behavior-science-addiction/drug-abuse-addiction

National Institute on Drug Abuse. (2015). Trends and statistics. National Institutes of Health. Retrieved from https://www.drugabuse.gov/related-topics/trends-statistics

National Institute on Drug Abuse. (2016). Drug facts: High school and youth trends. Retrieved from https://www.drugabuse.gov/publications/drugfacts/high-school-youth-trends

National Institutes of Health. (2012). *Research report series—Marijuana abuse.* NIH Publication Number 12-3859. Revised July 2012. Washington, DC: U.S. Department of Health and Human Services.

National Institutes of Health. (2016). Carfentanil. Retrieved from https://pubchem.ncbi.nlm.nih.gov/compound/carfentanil

National Library of Medicine. (2015). Loss of brain function—Liver disease. Retrieved from www.nlm.nih.gov/medlineplus/ency/article/000302.htm

Parish, B.S. (2015). *Hallucinogen use.* Retrieved from http://emedicine.medscape.com/article/293752-overview

Publishers Group. (2012). *Streetdrugs: A drug identification guide.* Plymouth, MN: Publishers Group.

Puri, B.K., & Treasaden, I.H. (2011). *Textbook of psychiatry* (3rd ed.). Philadelphia: Churchill Livingstone Elsevier.

Purnell, L. (2014). *Culturally competent health care* (3rd ed.). Philadelphia: F.A. Davis.

Rash, C.J., Weinstock, J., & Van Patten, R. (2016). A review of gambling disorder and substance use disorders. *Dovepress 7,* 3-13. doi:https://doi.org/10.2147/SAR.S83460

Sadock, B.J., Sadock, V.A., & Ruiz, (2015). *Synopsis of psychiatry: Behavioral sciences/clinical psychiatry* (11th ed.). Philadelphia: Lippincott Williams & Wilkins.

Storrs, C. (2016). Is street drug flakka gone for good? Retrieved from www.cnn.com/2016/04/18/health/flakka-drug-disappearance/index.html

Substance Abuse and Mental Health Services Administration (SAMHSA). (2014). *Clinical supervision and professional development of the substance abuse counselor.* Treatment Improvement Protocol (TIP) Series 52, DHHS Publication No. SMA 09-4435. Rockville, MD: SAMHSA.

Substance Abuse and Mental Health Services Administration (SAMHSA). (2015). Alcohol, tobacco, and other drugs. Retrieved from www.samhsa.gov/atod

Substance Abuse and Mental Health Services Administration (SAMHSA). (2016). Medication-Assisted Treatment (MAT). Retrieved from www.samhsa.gov/medication-assisted-treatment

Twerski, A. (1997). *Addictive thinking: Understanding self-deception* (2nd ed.) Center City, MN: Hazeldon.

U.S. Department of Health and Human Services (HHS), Office of the Surgeon General. (2016). *Facing addiction in America: The surgeon general's report on alcohol, drugs, and health.* Washington, DC: HHS

U.S. Drug Enforcement Administration. (2013). The DEA position on marijuana. Retrieved from www.justice.gov/dea/docs/marijuana_position_2011.pdf

Vaux, K.K. (2016). Fetal alcohol syndrome. Retrieved from http://emedicine.medscape.com/article/974016-overview

Walton-Moss, B., Becker, K., Kub, J., & Woodruff, K. (2013). *Substance abuse: Commonly abused substances and the addiction process* (2nd ed.). Brockton, MA: Western Schools.

Weiss, H.D., & Pontone, G.M. (2014). Dopamine receptor agonist drugs and impulse control disorders. *JAMA Internal Medicine, 174*(12), 1935-1937. doi:10.1001/jamainternmed.2014.4097

Wesson, N. (2013). Codependence: What is it? How do I know if I am codependent? Retrieved from www.wespsych.com/codepend.html

Wilson, S. (2013). People of Irish heritage. In L.D. Purnell (Ed.), *Transcultural health care: A culturally competent approach* (4th ed.). Philadelphia: F.A. Davis.

Classical References

Cermak, T.L. (1986). *Diagnosing and treating co-dependence.* Center City, MN: Hazelton Publishing.

Garbutt, J.C., West, S.L., Carey, T.S., Lohr, K.N., & Crews, F.T. (1999). Pharmacological treatment of alcohol dependence: A review of the evidence. *Journal of the American Medical Association, 281*(14), 1318-1325. doi:http://dx.doi.org/10.1001/jama.281.14.1318

Jellinek, E.M. (1952). Phases of alcohol addiction. *Quarterly Journal of Studies on Alcohol, 13*(4), 673-684. doi:http://dx.doi.org/10.15288/QJSA.1952.13.673

Mayfield, D., McLeod, G., & Hall, P. (1974). The CAGE questionnaire: Validation of a new alcoholism screening instrument. *American Journal of Psychiatry, 131*(10), 1121-1123. doi:10.1176/ajp.131.10.1121

Selzer, M.L. (1971). The Michigan Alcoholism Screening Test: The quest for a new diagnostic instrument. *American Journal of Psychiatry, 127*(12), 1653-1658. doi:http://dx.doi.org/10.1176/ajp.127.12.1653

Sullivan, J.T., Sykora, K., Schneiderman, J., Naranjo, C.A., & Sellers, E.M. (1989). Assessment of alcohol withdrawal: The revised Clinical Institute Withdrawal Assessment for Alcohol scale (CIWA-Ar). *British Journal of Addiction, 84*(11), 1353-1357. doi:10.1111/j.1360-0443.1989.tb00737.x

24

Schizophrenia Spectrum and Other Psychotic Disorders

CORE CONCEPTS

Psychosis

KEY TERMS

anhedonia	echopraxia	neologism
anosognosia	extrapyramidal symptoms	paranoia
catatonia	gynecomastia	perseveration
circumstantiality	hallucinations	social skills training
clang association	illusion	tangentiality
delusions	loose association	waxy flexibility
echolalia	magical thinking	word salad

OBJECTIVES

After reading this chapter, the student will be able to:

1. Discuss the concepts of schizophrenia and other psychotic disorders.
2. Identify predisposing factors in the development of these disorders.
3. Describe various types of schizophrenia and other psychotic disorders.
4. Identify symptomatology associated with these disorders and use this information in client assessment.
5. Formulate nursing diagnoses and outcomes of care for clients with schizophrenia and other psychotic disorders.
6. Identify topics for client and family teaching relevant to schizophrenia and other psychotic disorders.
7. Describe appropriate nursing interventions for behaviors associated with these disorders.
8. Describe relevant criteria for evaluating nursing care of clients with schizophrenia and other psychotic disorders.
9. Discuss modalities relevant to treatment of schizophrenia and other psychotic disorders.

HOMEWORK ASSIGNMENT

Please read the chapter and answer the following questions:

1. Describe the neurotransmitters theorized to be involved in various symptoms of schizophrenia.
2. What is schizoaffective disorder?
3. How do delusions differ from hallucinations?
4. What was the first atypical antipsychotic to be developed? Why is it no longer considered a first-line treatment for schizophrenia?

The term *schizophrenia* was coined in 1908 by the Swiss psychiatrist Eugen Bleuler, derived from the Greek *skhizo* ("split') and *phren* ("mind").

Over the years, much debate has surrounded the concept of schizophrenia. Various definitions of the disorder have evolved, and numerous treatment strategies been proposed, but none have proven to be uniformly effective or sufficient.

Although controversy lingers, two general factors appear to be gaining acceptance among clinicians. The first is that schizophrenia is probably not a homogeneous disease entity. The *Diagnostic and Statistical Manual of Mental Disorders, Fifth Edition (DSM-5),* supports this concept by describing schizophrenia as one of the schizophrenia spectrum disorders (American Psychiatric Association [APA], 2013). While current consensus points to schizophrenia as a neurodevelopmental disorder (Álvarez et al., 2015), schizophrenia spectrum disorders may have several etiological influences, including genetic predisposition, biochemical dysfunction, physiological factors, and psychosocial stress.

The second agreed-upon factor among clinicians is that there is not now and may never be a single treatment that cures schizophrenia. Effective treatment currently requires a comprehensive, multidisciplinary effort, including pharmacotherapy and various forms of psychosocial care, such as living skills and **social skills training,** rehabilitation and recovery, and family therapy. Emerging evidence indicates that a comprehensive, patient-centered approach offers hope for a recovery process and improved quality of life in this population.

Of all the mental illnesses that cause suffering in society, schizophrenia is likely responsible for longer hospitalizations, greater chaos in family life, more exorbitant costs to individuals and governments, and more fear than any other. Because it is such an enormous threat to life and happiness and because its causes are an unsolved puzzle, it has also probably been studied more than any other mental disorder.

Risk for suicide is a major concern among patients with schizophrenia. About one-third of people with schizophrenia attempt suicide, and about 1 in 10 die from the act (Black & Andreasen, 2014). This chapter explores various theories of predisposing factors implicated in the development of schizophrenia. Symptomatology associated with different diagnostic categories of the disorder is discussed. Nursing care is presented in the context of the six steps of the nursing process. Various dimensions of medical treatment are explored.

Nature of the Disorder

CORE CONCEPT

Psychosis

A severe mental condition in which there is disorganization of the personality, deterioration in social functioning, and loss of contact with, or distortion of, reality. There may be evidence of hallucinations and delusional thinking. Psychosis can occur with or without the presence of organic impairment.

Perhaps no psychological disorder is more crippling than schizophrenia. Characteristically, disturbances in thought processes, perception, and affect invariably result in a severe deterioration of social and occupational functioning.

The lifetime prevalence of schizophrenia is about 1 percent in the general population (Sadock, Sadock, & Ruiz, 2015). Symptoms generally appear in late adolescence or early adulthood, although they may occur in middle or late adult life. Early-onset schizophrenia refers to symptoms that begin in childhood and adolescence before age 18 years. This condition, although rare, is recognized as a progressive neurodevelopmental disorder with a chronic and severely symptomatic course (Sadock et al., 2015). Some studies have indicated that symptoms occur earlier in men than in women. The pattern of development of schizophrenia may be viewed in four phases: the premorbid, prodromal, active psychotic (acute schizophrenic episode), and residual phases.

Phase I: Premorbid Phase

Premorbid signs are those that occur before there is clear evidence of illness and may include distinctive personality traits or behaviors. Premorbid personality and behavioral indications may include being very shy and withdrawn, having poor peer relationships, doing poorly in school, and demonstrating antisocial behavior. Sadock and associates (2015) stated:

In the typical, but not invariable, premorbid history of schizophrenia, patients had schizoid or schizotypal personalities characterized as quiet, passive, and introverted; as children, they had few friends. Preschizophrenic adolescents may have no close friends and no dates and may avoid team sports. They may enjoy [solitary activities] to the exclusion of social activities. (p. 311)

Current research is focused on the premorbid phase in hopes that identification of potential biomarkers and at-risk individuals may prevent transition to illness or provide early intervention (Clark et al., 2016).

Phase II: Prodromal Phase

Prodromal signs more clearly manifest as signs of developing schizophrenia than do premorbid signs. The prodromal phase of schizophrenia begins with a change from premorbid functioning and extends until the onset of frank psychotic symptoms. This phase can be as brief as a few weeks or months, but most studies indicate that the average length of the prodromal phase is between 2 and 5 years. During this phase, the individual begins to show signs of significant deterioration in function. Fifty percent complain of depressive symptoms (APA, 2013). Social withdrawal is not uncommon, and signs of cognitive impairment may begin to emerge. In addition, some adolescent patients develop sudden onset of obsessive-compulsive behavior during the prodromal phase (Sadock et al., 2015).

Recognition of the behaviors associated with the prodromal phase provides an opportunity for early intervention with a possibility for improvement in long-term outcomes. Current treatment guidelines suggest therapeutic interventions that offer support with identified problems, cognitive therapies to minimize functional impairment, family interventions to improve coping, and involvement with the schools to reduce the possibility of failure. Some controversy exists as to the benefit of pharmaceutical therapy during the prodromal phase; however, evidence supports that comprehensive treatment started at the time of the first psychotic episode is associated with better outcomes (Insel, 2015).

Phase III: Active Psychotic Phase (Acute Schizophrenic Episode)

Schizophrenia is a chronic illness but is characterized by acute episodes in which symptoms are more pronounced. In the active phase of the disorder, psychotic symptoms are typically prominent. Box 24–1 describes the *DSM-5* (APA, 2013) diagnostic criteria for schizophrenia.

Phase IV: Residual Phase

Schizophrenia is characterized by periods of remission and exacerbation and consequently is described as episodic despite being a chronic illness. A residual phase usually follows the active phase of the illness, during which symptoms of the active phase are either absent or no longer prominent. Negative symptoms

(see Box 24–3) may remain, and flat affect and impairment in role functioning are common during this phase. It has long been thought that these remaining symptoms are pervasive and stable, but current research has challenged that belief with evidence that negative symptoms can improve over time (Savill et al., 2015). Residual impairment often increases with additional episodes of active psychosis.

Prognosis

Outcomes in schizophrenia are difficult to predict, but a complete return to full premorbid functioning is uncommon. However, several factors have been associated with a more positive outcome, including high-level premorbid functioning, later age at onset, female gender, abrupt onset of symptoms with obvious precipitating factor (as opposed to gradual, insidious onset of symptoms), associated mood disturbance, rapid resolution of active-phase symptoms, minimal residual symptoms, absence of structural brain abnormalities, normal neurological functioning, and no family history of schizophrenia (Black & Andreasen, 2014; Puri & Treasaden, 2011; Sadock et al., 2015).

Predisposing Factors

The cause of schizophrenia is still uncertain. Most likely, no single factor can be implicated in the etiology; rather, the disease probably results from a combination of influences including biological, psychological, and environmental factors.

Biological Factors

In addition to the factors summarized in the following sections, Chapter 3, Concepts of Psychobiology, contains a more thorough review of the biological implications of psychiatric illness.

Genetics

The body of evidence for genetic vulnerability to schizophrenia is growing. Studies show that relatives of individuals with schizophrenia have a much higher probability of developing the disease than does the general population. Whereas the lifetime risk for developing schizophrenia is about 1 percent in most population studies, the siblings of an identified client have a 10 percent risk of developing schizophrenia, and individuals with one parent who has schizophrenia have a 5 to 6 percent chance of developing the disorder (Black & Andreasen, 2014).

How schizophrenia is inherited is uncertain. Current research is focused on determining which gene or genes are important in the vulnerability to schizophrenia and what other biomarkers may predict risk for this illness. Okazaki and associates (2016) studied

BOX 24-1 DSM-V Criteria for Schizophrenia Diagnosis

A. Two (or more) of the following, each present for a significant portion of time during a 1-month period (or less if successfully treated). At least one of these must be (1), (2), or (3):
   1. **Delusions**
   2. **Hallucinations**
   3. **Disorganized speech (e.g., frequent derailment or incoherence)**
   4. Grossly disorganized or catatonic behavior
   5. Negative symptoms (i.e., diminished emotional expression or avolition)

B. For a significant portion of the time since the onset of the disturbance, level of functioning in one or more major areas, such as work, interpersonal relations, or self-care, is markedly below the level achieved prior to the onset (or when the onset is in childhood or adolescence, there is failure to achieve expected level of interpersonal, academic, or occupational functioning).

C. Continuous signs of the disturbance persist for at least 6 months. This 6-month period must include at least 1 month of symptoms (or less if successfully treated) that meet Criterion A (i.e., active-phase symptoms) and may include periods of prodromal or residual symptoms. During these prodromal or residual periods, the signs of the disturbance may be manifested by only negative symptoms or by two or more symptoms listed in Criterion A present in an attenuated form (e.g., odd beliefs, unusual perceptual experiences).

D. Schizoaffective disorder and depressive or bipolar disorder with psychotic features have been ruled out because either (1) no major depressive or manic episodes have occurred concurrently with the active-phase symptoms; or (2) if mood episodes have occurred during active-phase symptoms, they have been present for a minority of the total duration of the active and residual periods of the illness.

E. The disturbance is not attributable to the physiological effects of a substance (e.g., a drug of abuse, a medication) or another medical condition.

F. If there is a history of autism spectrum disorder or a communication disorder of childhood onset, the additional diagnosis of schizophrenia is made only if prominent delusions or hallucinations, in addition to the other required symptoms of schizophrenia, are also present for at least 1 month (or less if successfully treated).

Specify if: First episode, currently in acute, partial, or full remission; Multiple episodes, currently in acute, partial or full remission; Continuous; Unspecified; With catatonia
Specify current severity.

Reprinted with permission from the Diagnostic and Statistical Manual of Mental Disorders, Fifth Edition *(Copyright 2013). American Psychiatric Association.*

gene expression in peripheral blood samples of patients admitted with acute psychosis and found that a specific combination of genes (CDK4, MCM7, and POLD 4) differentiated these patients from controls. This finding suggests that the combination could be a genetic biomarker for schizophrenia and may also clarify aspects of pathophysiology in schizophrenia. The authors conclude that the messenger ribonucleic acid (mRNA) expression changes that occur in CDK4 are potentially both trait and state biomarkers for schizophrenia. Research is ongoing to identify genetic influences in schizophrenia that will hone our understanding of the multivariate influences in the development of this disease and perhaps identify treatment implications.

In monozygotic twins, the rate of schizophrenia is four to five times greater than the rate for dizygotic (fraternal) twins and approximately 50 times that of the general population (Sadock et al., 2015). Identical twins reared apart are at the same risk for schizophrenia as those reared together. Genetic makeup alone cannot account for the development of this disease, however;

in about half of cases, only one of a pair of identical twins develops schizophrenia.

Biochemical Factors

The oldest and most thoroughly explored biological theory to explain schizophrenia attributes a pathogenic role to abnormal brain biochemistry. Notions of a "chemical disturbance" as an explanation for mental illness were suggested by some theorists as early as the mid-19th century.

The Dopamine Hypothesis

This theory suggests that schizophrenia or schizophrenia-like symptoms may be caused by an excess of dopamine-dependent neuronal activity in the brain (Fig. 24–1). This excess activity may be related to increased production or release of the substance at nerve terminals, increased receptor sensitivity, too many dopamine receptors, or a combination of these mechanisms (Sadock et al., 2015).

Pharmacological support for this hypothesis exists. Amphetamines, which increase levels of dopamine,

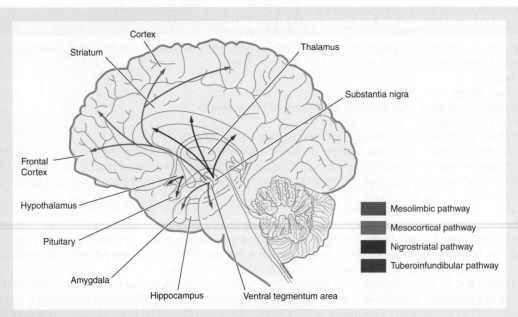

FIGURE 24–1 Neurobiology of schizophrenia.

NEUROTRANSMITTERS

A number of neurotransmitters have been implicated in the etiology of schizophrenia: dopamine, norepinephrine, serotonin, glutamate, and gamma-aminobutyric acid (GABA). The dopaminergic system has been most widely studied and closely linked to the symptoms associated with the disease.

AREAS OF THE BRAIN AFFECTED

Four major dopaminergic pathways (the pathways that transmit dopamine to different areas of the brain) have been identified:
- *Mesolimbic pathway:* Originates in the ventral tegmentum area (VTA) and projects to areas of the limbic system, including the nucleus accumbens, amygdala, and hippocampus. The mesolimbic pathway is associated with functions of memory, emotion, arousal, and pleasure. Excess activity in the mesolimbic tract has been implicated in the positive symptoms of schizophrenia (e.g., hallucinations, delusions). Dopamine blockade in this pathway is the target of antipsychotic medication to reduce hallucinations and delusions.
- *Mesocortical pathway:* Originates in the VTA and projects into the cortex. The mesocortical pathway is concerned with cognition, social behavior, planning, problem-solving, motivation, and reinforcement in learning. Negative symptoms of schizophrenia (e.g., flat affect, apathy, lack of motivation, and anhedonia) have been associated with diminished activity in the mesocortical tract.
- *Nigrostriatal pathway:* Originates in the substantia nigra and terminates in the striatum of the basal ganglia. This pathway is associated with the function of motor control. Degeneration in this pathway is associated with Parkinson's disease, and since typical antipsychotics may also block dopamine here, drug-induced Parkinson-like extrapyramidal side effects and tardive dyskinesia occur.
- *Tuberoinfundibular pathway:* Originates in the hypothalamus and projects to the pituitary gland. It is associated with endocrine function, digestion, metabolism, hunger, thirst, temperature control, and sexual arousal. Dopamine blockade in this pathway is associated with an increase in prolactin levels (hyperprolactinemia), which can result in galactorrhea (milk discharge from the nipples) in both men and women, erectile disorder, and anorgasmia.

ANTIPSYCHOTIC MEDICATIONS

Type	Receptor Affinity	Associated Side Effects
Conventional (typical) antipsychotics: Phenothiazines	Strong D_2 (dopamine)	Extrapyramidal symptoms (EPS), hyperprolactinemia, neuroleptic malignant syndrome
Haloperidol		
Provide relief of psychosis, improvement in positive symptoms, worsening of negative symptoms.	Varying degrees of affinity for: ACh (acetylcholine)	Anticholinergic effects
	α_1 (norepinephrine)	Tachycardia, tremors, insomnia, postural hypotension
	H_1 (histamine)	Weight gain, sedation
	Weak 5-HT (serotonin)	Low potential for ejaculatory difficulty
Novel (atypical) antipsychotics: Clozapine, olanzapine, quetiapine, aripiprazole, risperidone, iloperidone,	Strong 5-HT	Sexual dysfunction, GI disturbance, headache
	Low to moderate D_2	Low potential for EPS

ANTIPSYCHOTIC MEDICATIONS—cont'd

Type	Receptor Affinity	Associated Side Effects
ziprasidone, paliperidone, asenapine, lurasidone Provide relief of psychosis, improvement in positive symptoms, improvement in negative symptoms.	Varying degrees of affinity for: ACh α-adrenergic H_1	 Anticholinergic effects Tachycardia, tremors, insomnia, postural hypotension Weight gain, sedation

induce symptoms that mimic those of psychosis. The antipsychotics (e.g., chlorpromazine or haloperidol) lower brain levels of dopamine by blocking dopamine receptors, thus reducing psychotic symptoms, including those induced by amphetamines.

Postmortem brain studies of individuals who had schizophrenia have revealed a significant increase in the average number of dopamine receptors in approximately two-thirds of cases. This finding suggests that an increased number of dopamine receptors may not be the central or sole issue in all individuals with schizophrenia. Clients with positive symptoms such as delusions and hallucinations (referred to as *positive* symptoms because they are "added" to the clinical picture) respond with greater efficacy to dopamine-reducing drugs than do clients with negative symptoms (deficits such as apathy, poverty of ideas, and loss of drive). More information about positive and negative symptoms is listed in Box 24–3.

Thus, the current position on the dopamine hypothesis is that positive symptoms of schizophrenia may be related to increased numbers of dopamine receptors in the brain, as these symptoms are ameliorated by antipsychotic drugs that block dopamine receptors.

Other Biochemical Hypotheses

Various other biochemicals have been implicated in the predisposition to schizophrenia. Abnormalities in the neurotransmitters norepinephrine, serotonin, acetylcholine, and gamma-aminobutyric acid and in neuroregulators such as prostaglandins and endorphins have been suggested. Excess of serotonin has been hypothesized to cause both positive and negative symptoms of schizophrenia. The effectiveness of medications such as clozapine (a strong serotonin antagonist) lends support to this hypothesis (Sadock et al., 2015).

Recent research has implicated the neurotransmitter glutamate in the etiology of schizophrenia. The *N*-methyl-D-aspartate (NMDA) receptor is activated by the neurotransmitters glutamate and glycine. Psychopharmacological studies have shown that the drug class of glutamate antagonists (e.g., phencyclidine [PCP], ketamine) can produce schizophrenia-like symptoms in individuals who do not have the disorder (Hashimoto, 2006; Stahl, 2013). In one study,

participants experiencing ketamine-induced schizophrenia-like psychotic symptoms were treated with a drug trial of a glycine transporter-1 inhibitor (D'Souza et al., 2012). This medication was shown to reduce psychotic symptoms induced by the NMDA receptor antagonism of ketamine, so it is hoped that it may also benefit schizophrenia treatment. Despite evidence of a glutamate link to schizophrenia (Hu et al., 2014), further research is needed on the implications for treatment. Previous studies have focused on trying to reduce glutamate levels in patients who have advanced illness, but current research has identified that glutamate levels may be more important in the *transition* to psychosis. This theory is supported by the fact that first episodes of psychosis are often precipitated by stress, and glutamate increases under stress (Nauert, 2015). When glutamate levels are very high, the hippocampus becomes hypermetabolic and then begins to atrophy. Hippocampal atrophy has been identified as a significant finding in many individuals with schizophrenia. Future research may find that targeting interventions on glutamate is beneficial in high-risk individuals or those in early stages of illness to prevent onset or slow the progression of the disease (Nauert, 2015).

Current conventional antipsychotic medications largely target the dopamine receptors in the brain. Newer second-generation antipsychotics have strong affinity for serotonergic receptors. The glutamate model of schizophrenia suggests possibilities for new biomarkers signaling early illness and for new approaches to prevention and early treatment.

Physiological Factors

A number of physical factors have been identified in the medical literature. However, their specific mechanisms in the etiology of schizophrenia are unclear.

Viral Infection

Sadock and colleagues (2015) report that epidemiological data indicate a high incidence of schizophrenia after prenatal exposure to influenza. They stated:

> Other data supporting a viral hypothesis are an increased number of physical anomalies at birth, an increased rate of pregnancy and birth complications,

seasonality of birth consistent with viral infection, geographical clusters of adult cases, and seasonality of hospitalizations. (p. 305)

The effect of autoimmune antibodies in the brain is being studied within the field of psychoneuroimmunology, and evidence suggests that these antibodies may be responsible for the development of at least some cases of schizophrenia following infection from a neurotoxic virus (particularly prenatal exposure to toxoplasma gondii) (Matheson, Shepherd, & Carr, 2014). The role of cytokines in inflammation and the specific effects of these chemicals in the brain are still being explored through ongoing research.

Anatomical Abnormalities

With the use of neuroimaging technologies, structural brain abnormalities have been observed in individuals with schizophrenia. Ventricular enlargement is the most consistent finding; however, some reduction in gray matter is also reported. As previously discussed, reduction in the volume of the hippocampus observed in neuroimaging studies may signal risk for transition to a first psychotic episode (Harrisberger et al., 2016). Studies that focus on risk for a first psychotic episode are important, as early treatment is associated with better outcomes. Ultimately, it is hoped that these studies will also point to preventive strategies.

Magnetic resonance imaging has revealed reduced symmetry in lobes of the brain and reductions in size of structures within the limbic system in clients with schizophrenia. Considerable evidence from postmortem studies has shown abnormalities in the prefrontal cortex, and people who have had prefrontal lobotomies are reported to manifest with many symptoms common to schizophrenia (Sadock et al., 2015).

Diffusion tensor imaging studies have identified widespread white matter abnormalities in schizophrenia (Viher et al., 2016). These abnormalities in white matter microstructure appear to be primarily associated with negative symptoms and psychomotor behavior abnormalities.

Long-term studies of patients with schizophrenia have noted brain volume reduction, particularly in the temporal and preventricular areas (Veijola et al., 2014). It has been postulated that long-term antipsychotic medication use may contribute to this reduction, but the implications are unclear. Veijola and associates found that symptom severity, level of functional ability, and decline in cognitive abilities were not correlated with this reduction in brain volume.

Electrophysiology

Several studies have evaluated 40 Hz auditory steady-state response, a measure of electrical activity in the brain, and identified neural circuit dysfunctions in people with schizophrenia. A recent meta-analysis (Thunè, Recasens, & Uhlhaas, 2016) of these studies demonstrates robust evidence of such dysfunction in schizophrenia. The meaning of these circuit dysfunctions is not well understood but may indicate another biomarker for identifying risk or illness.

Physical Conditions

Several medical conditions are known to cause acute psychotic episodes, including but not limited to Huntington's disease, hypo- or hyperthyroidism, hypoglycemia, calcium imbalances, temporal lobe epilepsy, Wilson's disease, central nervous system (CNS) neoplasms, encephalitis, meningitis, neurosyphilis, and stroke (Mathews et al., 2013). See Table 24–2 for a more comprehensive list.

Psychological Factors

Early conceptualizations of schizophrenia focused on family relationship factors as major influences in the development of the illness, probably in light of the conspicuous absence of information related to a biological connection. These early theories implicated poor parent-child communication, particularly condemning the mother as schizophrenogenic (inducing schizophrenia in her child) related to a troublesome communication style known as *double-bind communication*. This theory no longer holds credibility. Researchers now focus their studies on schizophrenia as a brain disorder. Even though family communication patterns are no longer a credible explanation for the etiology of schizophrenia, the symptoms of the disease can contribute to significant disruption in communication and relationships among family members. For this reason, psychosocial factors should always be part of a comprehensive assessment. Further, evidence suggests that childhood trauma, and particularly multiple traumatizations, are associated (in combination with many other influences) with the development of schizophrenia (Álvarez et al., 2015; Matheson et al., 2014). Trauma-informed care should also be part of a comprehensive psychosocial assessment.

Environmental Influences

Sociocultural Factors

Many studies have attempted to link schizophrenia to social class. Epidemiological statistics have shown that more individuals from lower socioeconomic classes experience symptoms associated with schizophrenia than do those from higher socioeconomic groups (Puri & Treasaden, 2011). This occurrence may be explained by the conditions associated with living in poverty, such as congested housing accommodations, inadequate nutrition, absence of prenatal care, few resources for dealing with stressful situations, and feelings of hopelessness for escaping the cycle of poverty.

An alternative view is that of the *downward drift hypothesis,* which suggests that because of the characteristic symptoms of the disorder, individuals with schizophrenia have difficulty maintaining gainful employment and "drift down" to a lower socioeconomic level (or fail to rise out of a lower socioeconomic group). Proponents of this view consider poor social conditions to be a consequence rather than a cause of schizophrenia.

Stressful Life Events

Studies have been conducted to determine whether psychotic episodes may be precipitated by stressful life events. No scientific evidence indicates that stress causes schizophrenia. It is probable, however, that stress may contribute to the severity and course of the illness. It is known that extreme stress can precipitate psychotic episodes, so it may also precipitate symptoms in an individual who possesses a genetic vulnerability to schizophrenia. Stressful life events also may be associated with exacerbation of schizophrenic symptoms and increased rates of relapse.

Cannabis and Genetic Vulnerability

Studies of genetic vulnerability for schizophrenia have linked certain genes (COMT and ATK1) to increased risk for psychosis, particularly for adolescents with this genetic vulnerability who use cannabinoids (Radhakrishnan, Wilkinson, & D'Souza, 2014). Both cannabis and synthetic cannabinoids can induce schizophrenia-like symptoms. In individuals with a preexisting psychosis, cannabinoids can exacerbate symptoms. More important, the increased risk for psychotic disorders such as schizophrenia when combined with cannabis use suggests the influence of lifestyle factors in the expression of genes and points to the possibility of multiple factors playing a role in the causality of this illness.

Theoretical Integration and the Transactional Model

The etiology of schizophrenia remains unclear. No single theory or hypothesis has substantiated a clear-cut explanation for the disease. It seems the more research that is conducted, the more evidence is compiled to support the concept of multiple causation in the development of schizophrenia. In a systematic review of the literature on schizophrenia, Matheson and associates (2014) summarize that the most robust evidence suggests that schizophrenia is a widespread neural dysfunction accompanied by various psychological effects that respond moderately well to psychosocial and biomedical therapy:

> Patients have relatively poor cognitive functioning, and subtle, but diverse, structural brain alterations, altered electrophysiological functioning and sleep patterns, minor physical anomalies, neurological soft signs, and sensory alterations. There are markers of infection, inflammation or altered immunological parameters; and there is increased mortality from a range of causes. Risk for schizophrenia is increased with cannabis use, pregnancy and birth complications, prenatal exposure to *Toxoplasma gondii,* childhood central nervous system viral infections, childhood adversities, urbanicity, and immigration (first and second generation), particularly in certain ethnic groups. Developmental motor delays and lower intelligence quotient in childhood and adolescence are apparent. (p. 3387)

Despite the wealth of research and knowledge that we have about schizophrenia, much more is needed before we will fully understand this illness.

One way to conceptualize the pathway to acute illness is through exploring influencing factors and the individual's response to these stressors. The dynamics of schizophrenia using the transactional model of stress and adaptation are presented in Figure 24–2.

Other Schizophrenia Spectrum and Psychotic Disorders

The *DSM-5* (APA, 2013) identifies a spectrum of psychotic disorders organized to reflect a gradient of psychopathology from least to most severe. Degree of severity is determined by the level, number, and duration of psychotic signs and symptoms.

Several disorders may carry the additional specification of *With Catatonic Features,* the criteria for which are presented in Box 24–2. The disorders to which this specifier may be applied include brief psychotic disorder, schizophreniform disorder, schizophrenia, schizoaffective disorder, and substance-induced psychotic disorder. It may also be applied to neurodevelopmental disorder, major depressive disorder, and bipolar disorders I and II (APA, 2013).

The *DSM-5* initiates the spectrum of disorders with Schizotypal Personality Disorder. For purposes of this textbook, this disorder is presented in Chapter 32, Personality Disorders.

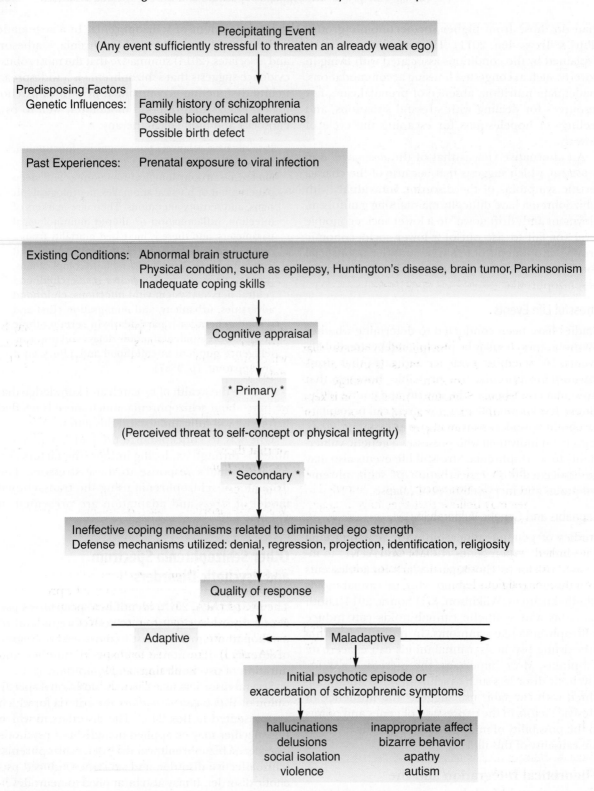

FIGURE 24–2 The dynamics of schizophrenia using the transactional model of stress and adaptation.

Delusional Disorder

Delusional disorder is characterized by the presence of delusions experienced for at least 1 month (APA, 2013). If present at all, hallucinations are not prominent, and behavior is not bizarre. The *DSM-5* states

that a specifier may be added to denote if the delusions are considered *bizarre* (i.e., if the thought is "clearly implausible, not understandable, and not derived from ordinary life experiences" [p. 91]). Subtypes of delusional disorder include the following.

BOX 24–2 **Diagnostic Criteria for Catatonia Specifier**

The clinical picture is dominated by three (or more) of the following symptoms:

1. Stupor (i.e., no psychomotor activity; not actively related to environment)
2. Catalepsy (i.e., passive induction of a posture held against gravity)
3. Waxy flexibility (i.e., slight, even resistance to positioning by examiner)
4. Mutism (i.e., no, or very little, verbal response [exclude if known aphasia])
5. Negativism (i.e., opposition or no response to instructions or external stimuli)
6. Posturing (i.e., spontaneous and active maintenance of a posture against gravity)
7. Mannerism (i.e., odd, circumstantial caricature of normal actions)
8. Stereotypy (i.e., repetitive, abnormally frequent, non-goal-directed movements)
9. Agitation, not influenced by external stimuli
10. Grimacing
11. Echolalia (i.e., mimicking another's speech)
12. Echopraxia (i.e., mimicking another's movements)

Reprinted with permission from the Diagnostic and Statistical Manual of Mental Disorders, Fifth Edition *(Copyright 2013). American Psychiatric Association.*

Erotomanic Type

With this type of delusion, the individual believes that someone, usually of a higher status, is in love with him or her. Famous persons are often the subjects of erotomanic delusions. Sometimes the delusion is kept secret, but some individuals may follow, contact, or otherwise try to pursue the object of their delusion.

Grandiose Type

Individuals with grandiose delusions have irrational ideas regarding their own worth, talent, knowledge, or power. They may believe that they have a special relationship with a famous person or even assume the identity of a famous person (believing that the actual person is an imposter). Grandiose delusions of a religious nature may lead to assumption of the identity of a deity or religious leader.

Jealous Type

The content of jealous delusions centers on the idea that the person's sexual partner is unfaithful. The idea is irrational and without cause, but the individual with the delusion searches for evidence to justify the belief. The sexual partner is confronted (and sometimes physically attacked) regarding the imagined infidelity. The imagined lover of the sexual partner may also be the object of the attack. Attempts to restrict the autonomy of the sexual partner in an effort to stop the imagined infidelity are common.

Persecutory Type

In persecutory delusions, the most common type, individuals believe they are being persecuted or malevolently treated in some way. Frequent themes include being plotted against, cheated or defrauded, followed and spied on, poisoned, or drugged. The individual may obsess about and exaggerate a slight rebuff (either real or imagined) until it becomes the focus of a delusional system. Repeated complaints may be directed at legal authorities, lack of satisfaction from which may result in violence toward the object of the delusion.

Somatic Type

Individuals with somatic delusions have fixed, false beliefs that they have some type of medical condition or that there has been an alteration in a body organ or its function.

Mixed Type

When the disorder is *mixed,* delusions are prominent, but no single theme is predominant.

Brief Psychotic Disorder

This disorder is identified by the sudden onset of psychotic symptoms that may or may not be preceded by a severe psychosocial stressor. These symptoms last at least a day but less than a month, and there is an eventual full return to the premorbid level of functioning (APA, 2013). The individual experiences emotional turmoil or overwhelming perplexity or confusion. Evidence of impaired reality may include incoherent speech, delusions, hallucinations, bizarre behavior, and disorientation. Individuals with preexisting personality disorders (most commonly, histrionic, narcissistic, paranoid, schizotypal, and borderline personality disorders) appear to be susceptible to this disorder (Sadock et al., 2015). Catatonic features may also be associated with this disorder (see Box 24–2).

Substance/Medication-Induced Psychotic Disorder

The prominent hallucinations and delusions associated with this disorder are directly attributable to substance intoxication or withdrawal or exposure to a medication or toxin. This diagnosis is made when the symptoms are more excessive and more severe than those usually associated with intoxication or withdrawal syndrome (APA, 2013). The medical history, physical examination, or laboratory findings provide evidence that the appearance of the symptoms occurred in association with substance intoxication or withdrawal or exposure to a medication or toxin. Substances believed to induce psychotic disorders are presented in Table 24–1. Catatonic features may also be associated with this disorder (see Box 24–2).

Psychotic Disorder Due to Another Medical Condition

The essential features of this disorder are prominent hallucinations and delusions that can be directly attributed to another medical condition (APA, 2013). The diagnosis is not made if the symptoms occur during the course of delirium. A number of medical conditions that can cause psychotic symptoms are presented in Table 24–2.

Catatonic Disorder Due to Another Medical Condition

Catatonic disorder is identified by the symptoms described in Box 24–2. This diagnosis is made when symptomatology evidenced from medical history, physical examination, or laboratory findings is directly attributable to the physiological consequences of another medical condition (APA, 2013). Types of medical conditions associated with **catatonia** include metabolic disorders (e.g., hepatic encephalopathy, diabetic ketoacidosis, hypo- and hyperthyroidism, hypo- and hyperadrenalism, hypercalcemia, and vitamin B_{12} deficiency) and neurological conditions (e.g., epilepsy, tumors, cerebrovascular disease, head

TABLE 24–1	Substances That May Cause Psychotic Disorders
Drugs of abuse	Alcohol Amphetamines and related substances Cannabis Cocaine Hallucinogens Inhalants Opioids Phencyclidine and related substances Sedatives, hypnotics, and anxiolytics
Medications	Anesthetics and analgesics Anticholinergic agents Anticonvulsants Antidepressant medication Antihistamines Antihypertensive agents Cardiovascular medications Antimicrobial medications Antineoplastic medications Antiparkinsonian agents Corticosteroids Disulfiram Gastrointestinal medications Muscle relaxants Nonsteroidal anti-inflammatory agents
Toxins	Anticholinesterase Organophosphate insecticides Nerve gases Carbon dioxide Carbon monoxide Volatile substances (e.g., fuel, paint, gasoline, toluene)

SOURCES: Black, D.W., & Andreasen, N.C. (2014). *Introductory textbook of psychiatry* (6th ed.). Washington, DC: American Psychiatric Publishing; Freudenreich, O. (2010). Differential diagnosis of psychotic symptoms: Medical "mimics." *Psychiatric Times, 27*(12), 52-61.

TABLE 24–2	General Medical Conditions That May Cause Psychotic Symptoms

Acute intermittent porphyria
Brain abscesses
Cerebrovascular disease
CNS infections
CNS trauma
Cushing's syndrome
Deafness
Encephalitis
Fluid or electrolyte imbalances
Hepatic disease
Herpes encephalitis
Huntington's disease
Hypoadrenocorticism
Hypo- or hyperparathyroidism
Hypo- or hyperthyroidism
Meningitis
Metabolic conditions (e.g., hypoxia; hypercarbia; hypoglycemia)
Migraine headache
Neoplasms
Neurosyphilis
Normal pressure hydrocephalus
Renal disease
Systemic lupus erythematosus
Temporal lobe epilepsy
Vitamin deficiency (e.g., B_{12})
Wilson's disease

SOURCES: Black, D.W., & Andreasen, N.C. (2014). *Introductory textbook of psychiatry* (6th ed.). Washington, DC: American Psychiatric Publishing; Freudenreich, O. (2010). Differential diagnosis of psychotic symptoms: Medical "mimics." *Psychiatric Times, 27*(12), 52-61. Sadock, B.J., Sadock, V.A., & Ruiz, P. (2015). *Synopsis of psychiatry: Behavioral sciences/clinical psychiatry* (11th ed.). Philadelphia: Lippincott Williams & Wilkins.

trauma, and encephalitis) (APA, 2013; Mathews et al., 2013).

Schizophreniform Disorder

The essential features of this disorder are identical to those of schizophrenia except that the duration, including prodromal, active, and residual phases, is at least 1 month but less than 6 months (APA, 2013). If the diagnosis is made while the individual is still symptomatic but has been so for less than 6 months, it is qualified as "provisional." The diagnosis is changed to schizophrenia if the clinical picture persists beyond 6 months. Schizophreniform disorder often has a good prognosis if the individual's affect is not blunted or flat, if there is a rapid onset of psychotic symptoms from the time the unusual behavior is noticed, or if premorbid social and occupational functioning was satisfactory (APA, 2013). Catatonic features may also be associated with this disorder (see Box 24–2).

Schizoaffective Disorder

This disorder is manifested by signs and symptoms of schizophrenia along with a strong element of symptomatology associated with the mood disorders (depression or mania). The client may appear depressed, with psychomotor retardation and suicidal ideation, or symptoms may include euphoria, grandiosity, and hyperactivity. The decisive factor in the diagnosis of schizoaffective disorder is the presence of hallucinations and/or delusions that occur for at least 2 weeks in the absence of a major mood episode (APA, 2013). However, prominent mood disorder symptoms must be evident for a majority of the time. The prognosis for schizoaffective disorder is generally better than that for other schizophrenic disorders but worse than that for mood disorders alone (Black & Andreasen, 2014). Catatonic features may also be associated with this disorder (see Box 24–2).

Application of the Nursing Process

Schizophrenia—Background Assessment Data

The diagnostic criteria for schizophrenia were presented earlier in this chapter. As previously stated, symptoms may present in phases, with schizophrenia representing the active phase of the disorder. Symptoms associated with the active phase are discussed in this section.

In the first step of the nursing process, the nurse gathers a database from which nursing diagnoses are derived and a plan of care is formulated. This step of the nursing process is extremely important because problem identification, objectives of care, and outcome criteria cannot be accurately determined without an accurate assessment.

Assessment of the client with schizophrenia is a complex process based on information gathered from a number of sources. Clients in an acute episode of their illness are seldom able to make significant contributions to their history. Data may be obtained from family members, if possible; from old medical records, if available; or from other individuals who have been in a position to report on the progression of the client's behavior.

The nurse must be familiar with behaviors common to the disorder to obtain an adequate assessment of the client with schizophrenia. Symptoms of schizophrenia are commonly described as positive or negative. Positive symptoms are those present in a person with schizophrenia that would not be present in a person without the illness, sometimes described as features that are "added." In contrast, negative symptoms are those that reflect a decrease in normal functions (functions that have been "taken away" by the illness). Most but not all clients exhibit a mixture of both types of symptoms.

Positive symptoms are associated with normal brain structures on computed tomography scan and respond relatively well to treatment. Sadock and associates (2015) identify that positive symptoms tend to become less severe over time, whereas the negative or "deficit" symptoms are socially debilitating and may increase in severity. Atypical antipsychotics have been advanced as more effective in treating negative symptoms, but researchers continue to search for medications that will specifically treat the several cognitive deficits that are most problematic for patients with schizophrenia. These deficits include memory, attention, language, and executive functions, and they can dramatically impact an individual's overall functional ability (Fioravanti, Bianchi, & Cinti, 2012).

The positive and negative symptoms associated with schizophrenia are described next. It is important to note that not all patients with schizophrenia experience all of these symptoms. Bora (2015) notes that in individuals who develop cognitive deficits, the age of onset is variable, and MacCabe and associates (2012) identify that a subgroup of individuals with schizophrenia have no cognitive impairment even in adulthood. Many factors contribute to functional impairment and decline beyond the symptoms themselves, including comorbid metabolic conditions, chronic substance use, stress, frequency and intensity of episodes, residual symptoms, and social defeat (Bora, 2015). A summary of positive and negative symptoms is presented in Box 24–3.

BOX 24–3 Positive and Negative Symptoms of Schizophrenia

POSITIVE SYMPTOMS

Delusions (Fixed, False Beliefs)

Persecutory—belief that one is going to be harmed by other(s)

Referential—belief that cues in the environment are specifically referring to them

Grandiose—belief that they have exceptional greatness

Somatic—beliefs that center on one's body functioning

Hallucinations (sensory perceptions without external stimuli)

Auditory (most common in schizophrenia)

Visual

Tactile

Olfactory

Gustatory

   (Note: Hallucinations may be a normal part of religious experience in cultural contexts)

Disorganized Thinking (Manifested in Speech)

Loose association

Tangentiality

Circumstantiality

Incoherence (includes word salad)

Neologisms

Clang associations

Echolalia

Grossly Disorganized or Abnormal Motor Behavior (Including Catatonia)

Hyperactivity

Hypervigilance

Hostility

Agitation

Childlike silliness

Catatonia (ranging from rigid or bizarre posture and decreased responsivity to complete lack of verbal or behavioral response to the environment)

Catatonic excitement (excessive and purposeless motor activity)

Stereotyped, repetitive movements

Unusual mannerisms or postures

NEGATIVE SYMPTOMS

Lack of Emotional Expression

Blunted affect

Lack of movement in head and hands that add expression in communication

Lack of intonation in speech

Decreased or Lack of Motivation to Complete Purposeful Activities (Avolition)

Neglect of activities of daily living

Decreased Verbal Communication (Alogia)

Decreased Interest in Social Interaction and Relationship (Asociality)

Withdrawal

Poor rapport

Diminished Ability for Abstract Thinking

Concrete interpretation of events and communication from others

Positive symptoms refer to symptoms that are present ("added") in people with schizophrenia and not typically present in people without the disease.
   Negative symptoms are referred to as deficits or impairments (things "taken away" by the illness) in individuals with schizophrenia.
SOURCES: American Psychiatric Association (APA). (2013). Diagnostic and statistical manual of mental disorders (5th ed.) Washington, DC: APA. Kay, S.R., Fiszbein, A., & Opler, L.A. (1987). The positive and negative syndrome scale (PANSS) for schizophrenia. Schizophrenia Bulletin,13(2), 261-276.

Positive Symptoms

Disturbances in Thought Content

Delusions Delusions are false personal beliefs inconsistent with the person's intelligence or cultural background. The individual continues to have the belief despite obvious proof that it is false or irrational.

Delusions are subdivided according to their content. Some of the more common ones are listed here.

■ **Delusion of persecution:** The individual feels threatened and believes that others intend harm or persecution toward him or her in some way (e.g., "The FBI has bugged my room and intends to kill me"; "I can't take a shower in this bathroom; the nurses have put a camera in there so that they can watch everything I do").

- **Delusion of grandeur:** The individual has an exaggerated feeling of importance, power, knowledge, or identity (e.g., "I am Jesus Christ").
- **Delusion of reference:** Events within the environment are referred by the psychotic person to himself or herself (e.g., "Someone is trying to get a message to me through the articles in this magazine [or newspaper or TV program]; I must break the code so that I can receive the message"). Delusions of reference are fixed false beliefs and are adhered to in spite of evidence to the contrary. *Ideas* of reference are less rigid than delusions of reference. For example, an individual with ideas of reference may think that other people in the room who are giggling must be laughing about him, but with additional information can acknowledge that there could be other explanations for their behavior.
- **Delusion of control or influence:** The individual believes certain objects or persons have control over his or her behavior (e.g., "The dentist put a filling in my tooth; I now receive transmissions through the filling that control what I think and do").
- **Somatic delusion:** The individual has a false idea about the functioning of his or her body (e.g., "I'm 70 years old, and I will be the oldest person ever to give birth. The doctor says I'm not pregnant, but I know I am").
- **Nihilistic delusion:** The individual has a false idea that the self, a part of the self, others, or the world is nonexistent or has been destroyed (e.g., "The world no longer exists"; "I have no heart").

Paranoia Individuals with **paranoia** have extreme suspiciousness of others and of their actions or perceived intentions (e.g., "I won't eat this food. I know it has been poisoned").

Magical Thinking With **magical thinking,** the person believes that his or her thoughts or behaviors have control over specific situations or people (e.g., the mother who believed if she scolded her son in any way he would be taken away from her). Magical thinking is common in children (e.g., "It's raining; the sky is sad"; "It snowed last night because I wished very, very hard that it would").

Disturbances in Thought Processes Manifested in Speech

Loose Associations Thinking is characterized by speech in which ideas shift from one unrelated subject to another. Typically, the individual with **loose associations** is unaware that the topics are unconnected. When the condition is severe, speech may be incoherent (e.g., "We wanted to take the bus, but the airport took all the traffic. Driving is the ticket when you want to get somewhere. No one needs a ticket to heaven. We have it all in our pockets").

Neologisms **Neologisms** are newly invented words that are meaningless to others but have symbolic meaning to the individual (e.g., "She wanted to give me a ride in her new *uniphorum*").

Clang Associations Choice of words is governed by sounds, often taking the form of rhyming, which forms a **clang association.** For instance, "It is very cold. I am cold and bold. The gold has been sold."

Word Salad A **word salad** is a group of words that appear to be put together randomly, without any logical connection (e.g., "Most forward action grows life double plays circle uniform").

Circumstantiality With **circumstantiality,** the individual delays in reaching the point of a communication because of unnecessary and tedious details. The point or goal is usually met but only with numerous interruptions by the interviewer to keep the person on track.

Tangentiality **Tangentiality** refers to a veering away from the topic of discussion and demonstrates difficulty in maintaining focus and attention.

Perseveration The individual who exhibits **perseveration** persistently repeats the same word or idea in response to different questions. It is the manifestation of a thought-processing disturbance in which the person gets stuck on a particular thought.

Echolalia **Echolalia** refers to repeating words or phrases spoken by another. In toddlers this is a normal phase in development, but in children with autism, echolalia may persist beyond the toddler years. In adulthood, echolalia is a significant neurological symptom of thought disturbance that occurs in schizophrenia, strokes, and other neurological disorders.

Disturbances in Perception

Hallucinations **Hallucinations,** or false sensory perceptions not associated with real external stimuli, may involve any of the five senses. Types of hallucinations include the following:

- **Auditory:** Auditory hallucinations are false perceptions of sound. Most commonly, these are voices, but the individual may report clicks, rushing noises, music, and other noises. Command hallucinations are "voices" that issue commands to the individual. They are potentially dangerous when the commands are for violence to self or others. Auditory hallucinations are the most common type in schizophrenia.
- **Visual:** These are false visual perceptions that may consist of formed images, such as those of people, or of unformed images, such as flashes of light. Visual hallucinations occur 27 percent of the time in individuals with schizophrenia (and 15 percent

in affective psychosis). They typically co-occur with auditory hallucinations and are associated with poorer outcomes (Waters et al., 2014).

■ **Tactile:** Tactile hallucinations are false perceptions of the sense of touch, often of something on or under the skin. One specific tactile hallucination is formication, the sensation that something is crawling on or under the skin.

■ **Gustatory:** This is a false perception of taste. Most commonly, gustatory hallucinations are described as unpleasant tastes.

■ **Olfactory:** Olfactory hallucinations are false perceptions of the sense of smell.

Illusions **Illusions** are misperceptions or misinterpretations of real external stimuli. These may occur during the prodromal phase and persist in the residual phase as well as during the active phase.

Echopraxia The client who exhibits **echopraxia** imitates movements made by others. The mechanisms underlying echopraxia in schizophrenia are not well understood, but current evidence suggests that it may involve a disturbance in mirror neuron activity in the presence of social cognition impairments and self-monitoring deficits, culminating in imitative psychomotor behavior (Urvakhsh et al., 2014).

Negative Symptoms

Disturbances in Affect

Affect describes the visual manifestations associated with an individual's feeling state or emotional tone.

Inappropriate Affect Affect is inappropriate when the individual's emotional tone is incongruent with the circumstances (e.g., a young woman who laughs when told of the death of her mother).

Bland or Flat Affect Affect is described as bland when the emotional tone is very weak. The individual with flat affect appears to be void of emotional tone (or overt expression of feelings).

Apathy

The client with schizophrenia often demonstrates an indifference to or disinterest in the environment. The bland or flat affect is a manifestation of the emotional apathy.

Avolition

Impaired volition has to do with the inability to initiate goal-directed activity. In the individual with schizophrenia, this may take the form of inadequate interest, lack of motivation, neglect of activities of daily living including personal hygiene and appearance, or inability to choose a logical course of action in a given situation. Impairment in social functioning may be reflected in social isolation, emotional detachment, and lack of regard for social convention.

Lack of Interest or Skills in Interpersonal Interaction

Some clients with acute schizophrenia cling to others and intrude on the personal space of others, exhibiting behaviors that are not socially and culturally acceptable. Others may exhibit ambivalence in social relationships. Still others may withdraw from relationships altogether (asociality).

Lack of Insight

Some individuals lack awareness of having any illness or disorder even when symptoms appear obvious to others. The term for this is **anosognosia.** The *DSM-5* identifies this symptom as the "most common predictor of nonadherence to treatment, and it predicts higher relapse rates, increased number of involuntary treatments, poorer psychosocial functioning, aggression, and poorer course of illness" (APA, 2013, p. 101).

Anergia

Anergia is a deficiency of energy. The individual with schizophrenia may lack sufficient energy to carry out activities of daily living or to interact with others.

Anhedonia

Anhedonia is the inability to experience pleasure. This is a particularly distressing symptom that compels some clients to attempt suicide.

Lack of Abstract Thinking Ability

Concrete thinking, or literal interpretations of the environment, represents a regression to an earlier level of cognitive development. Abstract thinking becomes impaired in some individuals with schizophrenia. For example, the client with schizophrenia would have great difficulty describing the abstract meaning of sayings such as "I'm climbing the walls" or "It's raining cats and dogs."

Associated Features

Waxy Flexibility

Waxy flexibility describes a condition in which the client with schizophrenia allows body parts to be placed in bizarre or uncomfortable positions. This symptom is associated with catatonia. Once placed in position, the arm, leg, or head remains in that position for long periods, regardless of how uncomfortable it is for the client. For example, the nurse may position the client's arm in an outward position to take a blood pressure measurement. When the cuff is removed, the client maintains the arm in the position in which it was placed to take the reading.

Posturing

This symptom is manifested by the voluntary assumption of inappropriate or bizarre postures.

Pacing and Rocking

Pacing back and forth and body rocking (a slow, rhythmic, backward-and-forward swaying of the trunk from the hips, usually while sitting) are common psychomotor behaviors of the client with schizophrenia.

Regression

Regression is the retreat to an earlier level of development. This primary defense mechanism of schizophrenia may be a dysfunctional attempt to reduce anxiety. It provides the basis for many of the behaviors associated with schizophrenia.

Eye Movement Abnormalities

Eye movement abnormalities may manifest in several ways including difficulty maintaining focus on a stationary object and difficulty with smooth pursuit of a moving object. Research (Benson et al., 2012) has found that simple eye movement tests can distinguish the abnormalities common in schizophrenia with exceptional accuracy.

Diagnosis and Outcome Identification

Using information collected during the assessment, the nurse completes the client database, from which the selection of appropriate nursing diagnoses is determined. Table 24–3 presents a list of client behaviors and the NANDA nursing diagnoses that correspond to those behaviors, which may be used in planning care for clients with psychotic disorders.

Outcome Criteria

The following criteria may be used for measurement of outcomes in the care of the client with schizophrenia.

The client:

■ Demonstrates an ability to relate satisfactorily with others

---

TABLE 24–3 Assigning Nursing Diagnoses to Behaviors Commonly Associated With Psychotic Disorders

BEHAVIORS	NURSING DIAGNOSES
Impaired communication (inappropriate responses), disordered thought sequencing, rapid mood swings, poor concentration, disorientation, stops talking in midsentence, tilts head to side as if to be listening	Disturbed sensory perception*
Delusional thinking; inability to concentrate; impaired volition; inability to problem-solve, abstract, or conceptualize; extreme suspiciousness of others; inaccurate interpretation of the environment	Disturbed thought processes*
Withdrawal; sad, dull affect; need-fear dilemma; preoccupation with own thoughts; expression of feelings of rejection or of aloneness imposed by others; uncommunicative; seeks to be alone	Social isolation
Risk factors: Aggressive body language (e.g., clenching fists and jaw, pacing, threatening stance); verbal aggression; catatonic excitement; command hallucinations; rage reactions; history of violence; overt and aggressive acts; goal-directed destruction of objects in the environment; self-destructive behavior; active, aggressive suicidal acts	Risk for violence: Self-directed or other-directed
Loose association of ideas, neologisms, word salad, clang associations, echolalia, verbalizations that reflect concrete thinking, poor eye contact, difficulty expressing thoughts verbally, inappropriate verbalization	Impaired verbal communication
Difficulty carrying out tasks associated with hygiene, dressing, grooming, eating, and toileting	Self-care deficit
Neglectful care of client in regard to basic human needs or illness treatment, extreme denial or prolonged overconcern regarding client's illness, depression, hostility and aggression	Disabled family coping
Inability to take responsibility for meeting basic health practices, history of lack of health-seeking behavior, lack of expressed interest in improving health behaviors, demonstrated lack of knowledge regarding basic health practices, anosognosia (lack of insight about illness)	Ineffective health maintenance
Unsafe, unclean, disorderly home environment; household members express difficulty in maintaining their home in a safe and comfortable condition	Impaired home maintenance

Adapted from Herdman, T.H., & Kamitsuru, S. (Eds.). (2014). *NANDA-I nursing diagnoses: Definitions and classification, 2015–2017.* Chichester, UK: Wiley Blackwell.
*These diagnoses have been resigned from the NANDA-I list of approved diagnoses. They are used in this instance because they are most compatible with the identified behaviors.

- Recognizes distortions of reality
- Has not harmed self or others
- Perceives self realistically
- Demonstrates the ability to perceive the environment correctly
- Maintains anxiety at a manageable level
- Relinquishes the need for delusions and hallucinations
- Demonstrates the ability to trust others
- Uses appropriate verbal communication in interactions with others
- Performs self-care activities independently

Planning and Implementation

The following section presents a group of selected nursing diagnoses, with short- and long-term goals and nursing interventions for each. In general, nursing interventions should be geared toward establishing trust, since suspiciousness is a common symptom in this disorder.

> Using a passive rather than a directive communication approach, which offers the client the opportunity to make his or her decisions about activities, treatment goals, and other aspects of care, is in the interest of establishing trust and incorporating a patient-centered approach.

In addition, nurses must be aware of their own attitudes in order to avoid perpetuating stigmatization of this client, since this concern has often been responsible for individuals avoiding treatment from health-care professionals. One way to reduce stigma is to become familiar with real people who suffer from this disorder rather than relying on fictitious representations (and sometimes, misrepresentations) of this population in popular media. (See the "Real People, Real Stories" introduction to Dr. Fred Frese).

Real People, Real Stories: Dr. Fred Frese

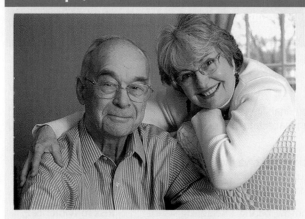

People with schizophrenia continue to be disenfranchised, misunderstood, and stigmatized. Even within health care, evidence has shown that some settings have been very hostile to people with severe mental illnesses. One way to begin combating stigmatization of people with mental illness is to get to know them personally. Dr. Fred Frese is a licensed psychologist and an internationally renowned speaker, writer, and advocate in the field of mental illness.

Karyn: Could you share a little bit about your history with schizophrenia?

Dr. Frese: I was 25 when I had my first episode. I was in the Marines and—I know I had seen the movie *The Manchurian Candidate* previously—and I began to think that the Vietnamese were using the same strategies from the movie to control us. When I let my commanding officer know my theories, I was hospitalized involuntarily, and for the next 10 years I was in and out of hospitals—mostly involuntarily—taking various medications, living many different places, and not employed.

Karyn: Were you getting any treatments or intervention that you thought were helpful to your recovery?

Dr. Frese: Well, at that time it was thought that schizophrenia was not an illness from which one could recover. Even recently, I've heard some folks who have a family member with schizophrenia say, "There's no way that anyone with this illness can get better." But that's starting to change, and now that the government, through SAMHSA [Substance Abuse and Mental Health Services Administration] is backing the recovery model approach, I think health care will improve. I remember being told that my brain was going to progressively deteriorate and that I would never be able to function on my own. All in all, I probably spent about a year of my life in hospitalizations. Once the laws changed and I knew you had to be of imminent harm to yourself or others in order to be hospitalized involuntarily, I talked some of the health professionals out of admitting me. During the last attempt to hospitalize me, I actually escaped and ran away, even though I was in pretty bad shape.

Karyn: So since you were knowledgeable about the laws, you could essentially be your own self-advocate and argue your case, so to speak?

Dr. Frese: Yes, and by that time, I was in grad school and had secured a job at what is now the Department of Mental Health and Addiction Services. I remember I was living in the hallway of some university housing, and one of the students, who saw me day after day just hanging around and not really doing anything, suggested that I might be eligible for a government job because of my military background. When I applied, the receptionist saw my history of mental health commitments and said I would never get the job, but I did. The last time I went to the hospital, I went voluntarily because I knew I needed more medication, but

Real People, Real Stories: Dr. Fred Frese—cont'd

they thought I needed to be hospitalized and I didn't; so I ran away.

Karyn: Sounds like you were managing a lot of stuff—grad school, working—and, at the same time, episodically struggling with symptoms of illness. You were working in the field of mental health, too. Was the work environment supportive?

Dr. Frese: Not always. It seemed like even among my coworkers, when something strange happened, they thought it was something wrong with me.

Karyn: What do you mean by "something strange"?

Dr. Frese: Like one time when they perceived I was spending too much time interacting with patients, they assumed I was "going off again," and next thing I knew, they called a "blue alert" and wanted to hospitalize me. But that time, the medical director just told me to take some time off. I never did find out why they called that blue alert.

Karyn: So you haven't been hospitalized for a very long time, and you are internationally renowned for all of your work and advocacy in the field of mental health. What do you think has contributed most to your recovery?

Dr. Frese: No, I haven't been hospitalized since I got married. I think that has been central in my recovery: having a person who you trust to give you feedback and let me know when I need more medication.

Karyn: What role do medications play in recovery?

Dr. Frese: It's very individual. We need more research to identify who, among people with schizophrenia, will benefit most by continuous medication versus episodic, reduced doses, or no medication. Genetic research is hopeful, but

we're not there yet. It's hard to advise any individual what to do without knowing their individual circumstances, and even knowing, it can be very hard.

Karyn: What do you think is most important for future nurses to know about what they should do or say when they encounter someone with schizophrenia in a health-care setting, such as ER, for example?

Dr. Frese: Even though Freud's theories about psychoanalysis and insight-oriented therapy have been shown in research to be not only not helpful in the treatment of people with schizophrenia but potentially harmful, these ideas continue to influence the thinking of health-care professionals. I would tell nurses to wean themselves away from psychoanalytic concepts in treating people with schizophrenia. There continue to be assumptions that something bad must have happened in this patient's childhood, and the family is probably to blame. It's not a good way to forge relationships and may prejudge or isolate the people that can provide invaluable support.

So I would say to future nurses, don't make assumptions about me because you see a diagnosis or the kind of medication I'm on, and don't try to blame anyone for my symptoms. Treat me with civility and respect, don't respond to me with shock and disbelief, bullying, or laughing at me. Listening to the patient is the best way to establish and maintain a relationship. Even if the patient is saying something that doesn't make any sense to you, the best response is, "That's very interesting; tell me more."

To learn more about Dr. Frese, go to www.fredfrese.com.

Some institutions use a case management model to coordinate care (see Chapter 9, The Nursing Process in Psychiatric-Mental Health Nursing, for more detailed explanation). In case management models, the plan of care may take the form of a critical pathway. In general, team approaches to the care of this client have been identified as essential to positive outcomes and recovery.

 Nurses need to collaborate effectively with other team members (including social workers, case managers, psychiatrists, chaplains, and counselors) to identify and respond to the complex care needs of this client.

Disturbed Sensory Perception: Auditory/Visual

Disturbed sensory perception has been resigned as a nursing diagnosis by NANDA International (NANDA-I), but it is retained in this text because of its appropriateness in describing specific behaviors. The diagnosis may be defined as sensory perceptions that are inconsistent with external stimuli and may include auditory, visual, tactile, olfactory, or gustatory perceptions. The following nursing interventions speak specifically to

auditory hallucinations, the most common type occurring in schizophrenia. Table 24–4 presents this nursing diagnosis in care plan format.

Client Goals

Outcome criteria include short- and long-term goals. Time lines are individually determined.

Short-term goal

■ Client will discuss content of hallucinations with nurse or therapist within 1 week.

Long-term goal

■ Client will be able to define and test reality, reducing or eliminating the occurrence of hallucinations.

This goal may not be realistic for the individual with severe and persistent illness who has experienced auditory hallucinations for many years. A more realistic goal may be:

■ Client will verbalize understanding that the voices are a result of his or her illness and demonstrate ways to interrupt the hallucination.

Table 24–4 | CARE PLAN FOR THE CLIENT WITH SCHIZOPHRENIA

NURSING DIAGNOSIS: DISTURBED SENSORY PERCEPTION: AUDITORY/VISUAL

RELATED TO: Panic anxiety, extreme loneliness, and withdrawal into the self

EVIDENCED BY: Inappropriate responses, disordered thought sequencing, rapid mood swings, poor concentration, disorientation

OUTCOME CRITERIA	NURSING INTERVENTIONS	RATIONALE
Short-Term Goal • Client discusses content of hallucinations with nurse or therapist within 1 week. **Long-Term Goals** • Client is able to define and test reality, reducing or eliminating the occurrence of hallucinations. *Note:* This goal may not be realistic for the individual with severe and persistent illness who has experienced auditory hallucinations for many years. A more realistic goal may be: • Client verbalizes understanding that the voices are a result of his or her illness and demonstrates ways to interrupt the hallucination.	1. Observe client for signs of hallucinations (listening pose, laughing or talking to self, stopping in midsentence). Ask, "Are you hearing the voices again?" 2. Avoid touching client without warning him or her that you are about to do so. 3. An attitude of acceptance encourages client to share the content of the hallucination with you. Ask, "What do you hear the voices saying to you?" 4. Do not reinforce the hallucination. Use "the voices" instead of words such as "they" that imply validation. Let client know that you do not share the perception. Say, "Even though I realize the voices are real to you, I do not hear any voices speaking." 5. Help client understand the connection between increased anxiety and the presence of hallucinations. 6. Try to distract client from the hallucination. 7. For some clients, auditory hallucinations persist after the acute psychotic episode has subsided. Listening to the radio or watching television helps distract some clients from attention to the voices. Others have benefited from an intervention called *voice dismissal*. With this technique, client is taught to say loudly, "Go away!" or "Leave me alone!" in a conscious effort to dismiss the auditory perception.	1. Early intervention may prevent aggressive response to command hallucinations. 2. Client may perceive touch as threatening and may respond in an aggressive manner. 3. This question is important to prevent possible injury to the client or others from command hallucinations. 4. It is important for the nurse to be honest, and client must accept the perception as unreal before hallucinations can be eliminated. 5. If client can learn to interrupt escalating anxiety, hallucinations may be prevented. 6. Involvement in interpersonal activities and explanation of the actual situation will help bring client back to reality. 7. These activities assist client to exert some conscious control over the hallucination.

Table 24–4 | CARE PLAN FOR THE CLIENT WITH SCHIZOPHRENIA–cont'd

NURSING DIAGNOSIS: IMPAIRED VERBAL COMMUNICATION

RELATED TO: Panic anxiety, regression, withdrawal, disordered, unrealistic thinking

EVIDENCED BY: Loose association of ideas, neologisms, word salad, clang association, echolalia, verbalizations that reflect concrete thinking, poor eye contact

OUTCOME CRITERIA	NURSING INTERVENTIONS	RATIONALE
Short-Term Goal • Client demonstrates the ability to remain on one topic, using appropriate, intermittent eye contact for 5 minutes with the nurse or therapist. Long-Term Goal • By time of discharge from treatment, client demonstrates ability to carry on a verbal communication in a socially acceptable manner with health-care providers and peers.	1. Attempt to decode incomprehensible communication patterns. Seek validation and clarification by stating, "Is it that you mean . . . ?" or "I don't understand what you mean by that. Would you please explain it to me?"	1. These techniques reveal how client is being perceived by others, while the responsibility for not understanding is accepted by the nurse.
	2. Maintain staff assignments as consistently as possible.	2. Consistency facilitates trust and understanding between client and nurse.
	3. The technique of verbalizing the implied is used with client who is mute (unable or unwilling to speak). Example: "That must have been a very difficult time for you when your mother left. You must have felt very alone."	3. This approach conveys empathy and may encourage client to disclose painful issues.
	4. Anticipate and fulfill client's needs until functional communication pattern returns.	4. Client safety and comfort are nursing priorities.
	5. Orient client to reality as required. Call client by name. Validate those aspects of communication that help differentiate between what is real and not real.	5. These techniques may facilitate restoration of functional communication patterns in client.
	6. Explanations must be provided at client's level of comprehension. Example: "Pick up the spoon, scoop some mashed potatoes into it, and put it in your mouth."	6. Because concrete thinking prevails, abstract phrases and clichés must be avoided, as they are likely to be misinterpreted.

NURSING DIAGNOSIS: SELF-CARE DEFICIT

RELATED TO: Withdrawal, regression, panic anxiety, perceptual or cognitive impairment, inability to trust

EVIDENCED BY: Difficulty carrying out tasks associated with hygiene, dressing, grooming, eating, toileting

OUTCOME CRITERIA	NURSING INTERVENTIONS	RATIONALE
Short-Term Goal • Client verbalizes a desire to perform activities of daily living (ADLs) by end of 1 week.	1. Provide assistance with self-care needs as required. Some clients who are severely withdrawn may require total care.	1. Client safety and comfort are nursing priorities.

Continued

Table 24–4 | CARE PLAN FOR THE CLIENT WITH SCHIZOPHRENIA–cont'd

OUTCOME CRITERIA	NURSING INTERVENTIONS	RATIONALE
Long-Term Goal • Client is able to perform ADLs in an independent manner and demonstrates a willingness to do so by time of discharge from treatment.	2. Encourage client to perform as many activities as possible independently. Provide positive reinforcement for independent accomplishments.	2. Independent accomplishment and positive reinforcement enhance self-esteem and promote repetition of desirable behaviors.
	3. Use concrete communication to show client what is expected. Provide step-by-step instructions for assistance in performing ADLs. Example: "Take your pajamas off and put them in the drawer. Take your shirt and pants from the closet and put them on. Comb your hair and brush your teeth."	3. Because concrete thinking prevails, explanations must be provided at client's concrete level of comprehension.
	4. Creative approaches may need to be taken with client who is not eating, such as allowing client to open own canned or packaged foods; family-style serving may also be an option.	4. These techniques may be helpful with client who is paranoid and may be suspicious that he or she is being poisoned with food or medication.
	5. If toileting needs are not being met, establish a structured schedule for client.	5. A structured schedule helps client establish a pattern so that he or she can develop a habit of toileting independently.

Interventions

■ Observe the client for signs of hallucinations (listening pose, laughing or talking to self, stopping in midsentence). Ask, "Are you hearing other voices?" "Are you able to distinguish those voices from my voice?" Early intervention may prevent aggressive responses to command hallucinations (such as voices telling the client to hurt or kill himself or herself).

■ Avoid touching the client, or ask for permission before doing so. The client may perceive touch as threatening and respond in an aggressive or defensive manner.

■ An attitude of acceptance will encourage the client to share the content of the hallucination with you. Ask, "What do you hear the voices saying to you?" This information is important in order to assess for risk of injury to the client or others from command hallucinations. Ask, "Do these voices seem familiar to you, or do they seem to be unfamiliar?" This question may shed some light on who the individual is associating with as the source of the voices.

CLINICAL PEARL

Do not reinforce the hallucination. Use "the voices" instead of words such as "they" that imply validation. Let the client know that you do not share the perception. For example, say, "Even though I realize that the voices are real to you, I do not hear any voices speaking." This statement conveys honesty and respect for the client's experience as real, and it provides a foundation for exploration of management and coping strategies.

■ Assess the client's level of anxiety and help him or her understand that increased anxiety may trigger hallucinations. If the client can learn to interrupt escalating anxiety, these episodes may be minimized or prevented.

■ Try to distract the client from the hallucination. Involvement in interpersonal activities and explanation of the actual situation will help the client focus on reality.

■ For some clients, auditory hallucinations persist after the acute psychotic episode has subsided. Listening to the radio or watching television helps distract some clients from the voices. Others have benefited from an intervention called *voice dismissal*. With this technique, the client is taught to say loudly, "Go away!" or "Leave me alone!" thereby exerting some conscious control over the behavior.

■ Assess for suicide risk. Some individuals have taken their own lives to escape from pervasive, troubling, or frightening hallucinations.

Disturbed Thought Processes

Disturbed thought processes has been resigned as a nursing diagnosis by NANDA-I, but it is retained in this text because of its appropriateness in describing specific behaviors. In this instance, it is evidenced by behaviors that indicate the presence of delusional thinking, suspiciousness, and inaccurate interpretation of the environment. The diagnosis is defined as a disruption in cognitive operations and activities.

Client Goals

Outcome criteria include short- and long-term goals. Time lines are individually determined.

Short-term goal

■ By the end of 2 weeks, client will recognize and verbalize that false ideas occur at times of increased anxiety.

Long-term goal

Depending on chronicity of the disease process, choose the most realistic long-term goal for the client:

■ By time of discharge from treatment, client's verbalizations will reflect reality-based thinking with no evidence of delusional ideation.

■ By time of discharge from treatment, client will be able to differentiate between delusional thinking and reality.

Interventions

■ Convey acceptance of the client's need for the false belief, but indicate that you do not share the belief. The client must understand that you do not view the idea as real.

■ Do not argue or deny the belief. Arguing with the client or denying the belief serves no useful purpose, because delusional ideas are not eliminated by this approach, and the development of a trusting relationship may be impeded.

CLINICAL PEARL

Use *reasonable doubt* as a therapeutic technique. For example, when a client says, "The FBI is wiretapping directly into my brain," the nurse may respond, "I understand that you believe this is true, but I personally find it hard to accept."

■ Reinforce and focus on reality. Although initially encouraging the client to describe his or her delusional thoughts may be helpful to understand the

client's experience and to establish trust, discourage long ruminations about the irrational thinking. Talk about real events and real people. See Box 24–4 for a list of interventions that may be helpful when working with a client who is highly suspicious.

Risk for Violence: Self-Directed or Other-Directed

Risk for self- or other-directed violence is defined by NANDA-I as "vulnerable to behaviors in which an individual demonstrates that he or she can be physically, emotionally, and/or sexually harmful either to self or to others" (Herdman & Kamitsuru, 2014, pp. 410–411).

Client Goals

Outcome criteria include short- and long-term goals. Time lines are individually determined.

Short-term goals

■ Within [a specified time], client will be able to recognize signs of increasing anxiety and agitation

---

BOX 24–4 Interventions When Working With Suspicious Clients

Clients who are prone to suspicious ideation are vulnerable to misinterpreting information and social cues in their environment, which can be a barrier to communication and relationship building. The following are some interventions to promote positive communication and establishment of trusting relationships.

• To promote the development of trust, use the same staff as much as possible; be honest and keep all promises.

• Avoid physical contact. Ask the client's permission before using touch to perform a procedure, such as taking blood pressure. Suspicious clients often perceive touch as threatening and may respond in an aggressive or defensive manner.

• Avoid laughing, whispering, or talking quietly where the client can see you but cannot hear what is being said.

• Extremely suspicious clients may believe they are being poisoned and refuse to eat food from an individually prepared tray. It may be necessary to provide canned food with a can opener or serve food family style.

• They may believe they are being poisoned with their medication and attempt to discard the tablets or capsules. Mouth checks may be necessary following medication administration to verify whether the client is actually swallowing the pills.

• Competitive activities may be threatening to suspicious clients. Activities that encourage a one-to-one relationship with the nurse or therapist are best.

• Maintain an assertive, matter-of-fact, yet genuine approach with suspicious clients. Approaches that are overly directive or cheerful may increase the patient's suspiciousness.

and report to staff (or other care provider) for assistance with intervention.

■ Client will not harm self or others.

Long-term goal

■ Client will not harm self or others.

Interventions

■ Maintain a low level of stimuli in the client's environment (low lighting, few people, simple decor, low noise level). Anxiety level rises in a stimulating environment. A suspicious, agitated client may perceive individuals as threatening.

■ Observe the client's behavior frequently while carrying out routine activities to avoid creating suspicion. Close observation is necessary so that intervention can occur if required to ensure the client's (and others') safety.

■ Assess for presence of suicidal ideation and/or command hallucinations that may be instructing the client to harm self or others, and remove all dangerous objects from the client's environment so that he or she may not use them to harm self or others.

> **CLINICAL PEARL**
>
> Intervene at the first sign of increased anxiety, agitation, or verbal or behavioral aggression. Offer empathetic response to the client's feelings: "You seem anxious [or frustrated, or angry] about this situation. How can I help?" Validation of the client's feelings conveys a caring attitude, and offering assistance reinforces trust.

■ It is important to maintain a calm attitude toward the client. As the client's anxiety increases, offer some alternatives: participating in physical activity (e.g., punching bag, exercise), talking about the situation, taking antianxiety medication. Offering alternatives gives the client a feeling of some control over the situation.

■ Have sufficient staff available to indicate a show of strength to client if it becomes necessary. This shows the client evidence of control over the situation and provides some physical security for staff.

■ If the client is not calmed by "talking down" or by medication and is posing an imminent threat to the safety of self or others, use of restraint may be necessary. The avenue of the least restrictive alternative must be selected when planning interventions for a violent client. Restraints should be used only as a last resort, after all other interventions have been unsuccessful, and only if the client is clearly at risk of harm to self or others.

■ If restraint is deemed necessary, ensure that sufficient staff is available to assist. Follow protocol established by the institution. As agitation decreases, assess the client's readiness for restraint removal or reduction. Remove one restraint at a time while assessing the client's response. This minimizes the risk of injury to the client and staff.

Impaired Verbal Communication

Impaired verbal communication is defined by NANDA-I as "decreased, delayed, or absent ability to receive, process, transmit, and/or use a system of symbols" (Herdman & Kamitsuru, 2014, p. 261). This care plan is also presented in Table 24–4.

Client Goals

Outcome criteria include short- and long-term goals. Time lines are individually determined.

Short-term goal

■ Client will demonstrate ability to remain on one topic, using appropriate, intermittent eye contact, for 5 minutes with the nurse or therapist.

Long-term goal

■ By time of discharge from treatment, client will demonstrate ability to carry on a verbal communication in a socially acceptable manner with healthcare providers and peers.

Interventions

■ Facilitate trust and understanding by maintaining staff assignments as consistently as possible. In a nonthreatening manner, explain to the client how his or her behavior and verbalizations are viewed by and may alienate others.

> **CLINICAL PEARL**
>
> Attempt to decode incomprehensible communication patterns. Seek validation and clarification by stating, "Is it that you mean . . . ?" or "I don't understand what you mean by that. Would you please explain it to me?" These techniques reveal to the client how he or she is being perceived by others and demonstrates active listening and interest in understanding what the client is trying to communicate.

■ Anticipate and fulfill the client's needs until functional communication has been established.

■ Orient the client to reality as required. Call the client by name. Validate those aspects of communication that help differentiate between what is real and not real. These techniques may facilitate restoration of functional communication patterns in the client.

CLINICAL PEARL

If the client is unable or unwilling to speak (mutism), using the technique of *verbalizing the implied* is therapeutic. For example, "That must have been very difficult for you when your mother left. You must have felt very alone." This approach conveys empathy, facilitates trust, and eventually may encourage the client to discuss painful issues.

■ Because concrete thinking may be a symptom, abstract phrases, clichés, and joking must be avoided, as they are likely to be misinterpreted. Explanations must be provided at the client's level of comprehension.

CLINICAL PEARL

Speak plainly and use concrete language to minimize misinterpretation by the client. For example, "Pick up the spoon, scoop some mashed potatoes into it, and put it in your mouth."

Concept Care Mapping

The concept map care plan (see Chapter 9) is a diagrammatic teaching and learning strategy that allows visualization of interrelationships between medical diagnoses, nursing diagnoses, assessment data, and treatments. An example of a concept map care plan for a client with schizophrenia is presented in Figure 24–3.

Client/Family Education

The role of client teacher is important in the psychiatric area, as it is in all areas of nursing. A list of topics for client/family education relevant to schizophrenia is presented in Box 24–5.

Evaluation

In the final step of the nursing process, a reassessment is conducted to determine if the nursing actions have been successful in achieving the objectives of care. Evaluation of the nursing actions for the client with exacerbation of schizophrenic psychosis may be facilitated by gathering information utilizing the following types of questions:

■ Has the client established trust with at least one staff member?
■ Is the anxiety level maintained at a manageable level?
■ Is delusional thinking still prevalent?
■ Is hallucinogenic activity evident? Does the client share content of hallucinations, particularly if commands are heard?
■ Is the client able to interrupt escalating anxiety with adaptive coping mechanisms?

■ Is the client easily agitated?
■ Is the client able to interact with others appropriately?
■ Does the client voluntarily attend therapy activities?
■ Is verbal communication comprehensible?
■ Is the client adhering to prescribed medications? Does the client verbalize the importance of taking medication regularly and on a long-term basis? Does he or she verbalize understanding of possible side effects and when to seek assistance from the physician?
■ Does the client spend time with others rather than isolating him or herself?
■ Is the client able to carry out all activities of daily living independently?
■ Is the client able to verbalize resources from which he or she may seek assistance outside the hospital?
■ Does the family have information regarding support groups in which they may participate and from which they may seek assistance in dealing with their family member who is ill?
■ If the client lives alone, does he or she have a source for assistance with home maintenance and health management?

Quality and Safety Education for Nurses (QSEN)

The Institute of Medicine (now the National Academy of Medicine), in its report *Health Professions Education: A Bridge to Quality* (Institute of Medicine [IOM], 2003), challenged faculties of medicine, nursing, and other health professions to ensure that their graduates have achieved a core set of competencies in order to meet the needs of the 21st-century health-care system. These competencies include *providing patient-centered care, working in interdisciplinary teams, employing evidence-based practice, applying quality improvement, maintaining safety,* and *utilizing informatics.* A QSEN teaching strategy is included in Box 24–6. The use of this type of activity is intended to arm the instructor and the student with guidelines for attaining the knowledge, skills, and attitudes necessary for achievement of quality and safety competencies in nursing.

Treatment Modalities for Schizophrenia and Other Psychotic Disorders

Psychological Treatments
Individual Psychotherapy

Individual recovery-oriented psychotherapy and cognitive therapies are evidence-based interventions in the treatment of the client with schizophrenia, but these should be adjuncts to a multifaceted team approach.

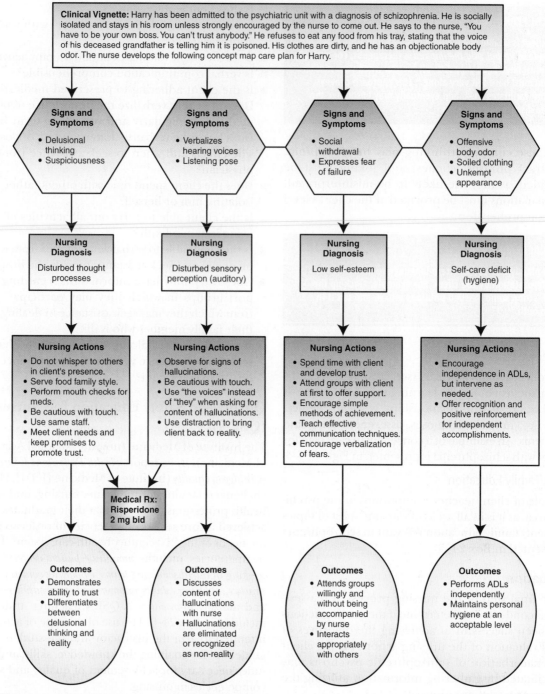

Clinical Vignette: Harry has been admitted to the psychiatric unit with a diagnosis of schizophrenia. He is socially isolated and stays in his room unless strongly encouraged by the nurse to come out. He says to the nurse, "You have to be your own boss. You can't trust anybody." He refuses to eat any food from his tray, stating that the voice of his deceased grandfather is telling him it is poisoned. His clothes are dirty, and he has an objectionable body odor. The nurse develops the following concept map care plan for Harry.

Signs and Symptoms
- Delusional thinking
- Suspiciousness

Signs and Symptoms
- Verbalizes hearing voices
- Listening pose

Signs and Symptoms
- Social withdrawal
- Expresses fear of failure

Signs and Symptoms
- Offensive body odor
- Soiled clothing
- Unkempt appearance

Nursing Diagnosis
Disturbed thought processes

Nursing Diagnosis
Disturbed sensory perception (auditory)

Nursing Diagnosis
Low self-esteem

Nursing Diagnosis
Self-care deficit (hygiene)

Nursing Actions
- Do not whisper to others in client's presence.
- Serve food family style.
- Perform mouth checks for meds.
- Be cautious with touch.
- Use same staff.
- Meet client needs and keep promises to promote trust.

Nursing Actions
- Observe for signs of hallucinations.
- Be cautious with touch.
- Use "the voices" instead of "they" when asking for content of hallucinations.
- Use distraction to bring client back to reality.

Nursing Actions
- Spend time with client and develop trust.
- Attend groups with client at first to offer support.
- Encourage simple methods of achievement.
- Teach effective communication techniques.
- Encourage verbalization of fears.

Nursing Actions
- Encourage independence in ADLs, but intervene as needed.
- Offer recognition and positive reinforcement for independent accomplishments.

Medical Rx:
Risperidone
2 mg bid

Outcomes
- Demonstrates ability to trust
- Differentiates between delusional thinking and reality

Outcomes
- Discusses content of hallucinations with nurse
- Hallucinations are eliminated or recognized as non-reality

Outcomes
- Attends groups willingly and without being accompanied by nurse
- Interacts appropriately with others

Outcomes
- Performs ADLs independently
- Maintains personal hygiene at an acceptable level

FIGURE 24–3 Concept map care plan for client with schizophrenia.

The primary focus in all cases must reflect efforts to decrease anxiety and increase trust.

Establishing a relationship is often particularly difficult because the individual with schizophrenia is desperately lonely yet defends against closeness and trust. He or she is likely to respond to attempts at closeness with suspiciousness, anxiety, aggression, or regression. Successful intervention may be achieved with honesty, simple directness, and a manner that respects the client's privacy and human dignity. Exaggerated warmth and professions of friendship are likely to be met with confusion and suspicion.

Once a therapeutic interpersonal relationship has been established, reality orientation is maintained through exploration of the client's behavior within relationships. Education is provided to help the client identify sources of real or perceived danger and ways of reacting appropriately. Methods for improving interpersonal communication, emotional expression, and frustration tolerance are attempted.

BOX 24–5 Topics for Client/Family Education Related to Schizophrenia

NATURE OF THE ILLNESS
1. What to expect as the illness progresses
2. Symptoms associated with the illness
3. Ways for family to respond to behaviors associated with the illness

MANAGEMENT OF THE ILLNESS
1. Connection of exacerbation of symptoms to times of stress
2. Appropriate medication management
3. Side effects of medications
4. Importance of not stopping medications
5. When to contact health-care provider
6. Relaxation techniques
7. Social skills training
8. Daily living skills training

SUPPORT SERVICES
1. Financial assistance
2. Legal assistance
3. Caregiver support groups
4. Respite care
5. Home health care
6. Residential treatment options

Group Therapy

Group therapy for individuals with schizophrenia has been shown to be effective, particularly with outpatients and when combined with drug treatment. Sadock and associates (2015) state:

> Group therapy for persons with schizophrenia generally focuses on real-life plans, problems, and relationships. Some investigators doubt that dynamic interpretation and insight therapy are valuable for typical patients with schizophrenia. But group therapy is effective in reducing social isolation, increasing the sense of cohesiveness, and improving reality testing for patients with schizophrenia. (p. 322)

Group therapy in inpatient settings is less productive. Inpatient treatment usually occurs when symptomatology and social disorganization are at their most intense. At this time, the least possible stimuli is most beneficial for the client. Because group therapy can be intensive and highly stimulating, it may be counterproductive early in treatment.

Group therapy for schizophrenia has been most useful over the long-term course of the illness. The social interaction, sense of cohesiveness, identification, and reality testing achieved within the group

BOX 24–6 QSEN TEACHING STRATEGY

Assignment: Using Evidence to Address Clinical Problems
Intervention With a Combative Client

Competency Domain: Evidence-Based Practice

Learning Objectives: Student will:
- Differentiate clinical opinion from research and evidence summaries.
- Explain the role of evidence in determining the best clinical practice for intervening with combative clients.
- Identify gaps between what is observed in the treatment setting and what has been identified as best practice.
- Discriminate between valid and invalid reasons for modifying evidence-based clinical practice based on clinical expertise or other reasons.
- Participate effectively in appropriate data collection and other research activities.
- Acknowledge own limitations in knowledge and clinical expertise before determining when to deviate from evidence-based best practices.

Strategy Overview:
1. Investigate the research related to intervening with a combative client.
2. Identify best practices described in the literature. How were these best practices determined?
3. Compare and contrast staff intervention with best practices described in the literature.
4. Investigate staff perceptions related to intervening with a combative client. How have they developed these perceptions?
5. Do staff members view any problems associated with their practice versus best practice described in the literature? If so, how would they like to see the problem addressed?
6. Describe ethical issues associated with intervening with a combative client.
7. What is your personal perception regarding the best evidence available to date related to intervening with a combative client? Are there situations that you can think of when you might deviate from the best practice model?
8. What questions do you have about intervening with a combative client that are not being addressed by current researchers?

Adapted from teaching strategy submitted by Pamela M. Ironside, Associate Professor, Indiana University School of Nursing, Indianapolis, IN. © 2009 QSEN; http://qsen.org. With permission.

setting have proven to be highly therapeutic processes for these clients. Groups that offer a supportive environment appear to be more helpful to clients with schizophrenia than those that follow a more confrontational approach.

Behavior Therapy

Behavior modification has a history of qualified success in reducing the frequency of bizarre, disturbing, and deviant behaviors and increasing appropriate behaviors. Features that have led to the most positive results include the following:

- Clearly defining goals and how they will be measured
- Attaching positive, negative, and aversive reinforcements to adaptive and maladaptive behavior
- Using simple, concrete instructions and prompts to elicit the desired behavior

Behavior therapy can be a powerful treatment tool for helping clients change undesirable behaviors. In the treatment setting, the health-care provider can use praise and other positive reinforcements to help the client with schizophrenia reduce the frequency of maladaptive or deviant behaviors. A limitation of this type of therapy is the inability of some individuals with schizophrenia to generalize what they have learned from the treatment setting to the community setting.

Social Treatments

Social Skills Training

Social skills training is used to help clients manage struggles with interpersonal relationships and communication, which are often complicated by clients' inability to accurately perceive responses in others. Mueser, Bond, and Drake (2002) describe this training as follows:

> The basic premise of social skills training is that complex interpersonal skills involve the smooth integration of a combination of simpler behaviors, including *nonverbal behaviors* (e.g., facial expression, eye contact); *paralinguistic features* (e.g., voice loudness and affect); *verbal content* (i.e., the appropriateness of what is said); and *interactive balance* (e.g., response latency, amount of time talking). These specific skills can be systematically taught, and, through the process of *shaping* (i.e., rewarding successive approximations toward the target behavior), complex behavioral repertoires can be acquired.

Social dysfunction is a hallmark of schizophrenia. Impairment in interpersonal relations is included as part of the defining diagnostic criteria for the condition in the *DSM-5* (APA, 2013). Considerable attention is now being given to enhancement of social skills in these clients.

The educational procedure in social skills training focuses on role-play. A series of brief scenarios are selected. These should be typical of situations clients experience in their daily lives and graduated in terms of level of difficulty. The health-care provider may serve as a role model for some behaviors. For example, "See how I sort of nod my head up and down and look at your face while you talk." This demonstration is followed by the client's role-playing. Immediate feedback is provided regarding the client's presentation. Only by countless repetitions does the response gradually become smooth and effortless.

Progress is geared toward the client's needs and limitations. The focus is on small units of behavior, and the training proceeds very gradually. Highly threatening issues are avoided, and emphasis is placed on functional skills that are relevant to activities of daily living. Milieu therapy, which focuses on the client's interaction within a social environment, may provide opportunities for social skills training.

Family Therapy

Schizophrenia is an illness that can puzzle, disrupt, and sometimes destroy families. Even when families appear to cope well, there is a notable impact on the mental and physical health of relatives when a family member has this illness.

The importance of the expanded role of family in the aftercare of those with schizophrenia has been recognized, thereby stimulating interest in family intervention programs designed to support the family system, prevent or delay relapse, and help to maintain the client in the community. These psychoeducational programs treat the family as a resource rather than a stressor, with the focus on concrete problem-solving and specific behaviors for coping with stress. These programs recognize the biological basis for schizophrenia and the impact that stress has on the client's ability to function. By providing the family with information about the illness and suggestions for effective coping, psychoeducational programs reduce the likelihood of the client's relapse and the possible emergence of mental illness in previously nonaffected relatives.

Mueser and associates (2002) stated that although models of family intervention with schizophrenia differ in their characteristics and methods, effective treatment programs share a number of common features:

- All programs are long term (usually 9 months to 2 years or more).
- They all provide the client and family with information about the illness and its management.
- They focus on improving adherence to prescribed medications.

■ They strive to decrease stress in the family and improve family functioning.

Asen (2002) suggested the following interventions with families of individuals with schizophrenia:

■ Forming a close alliance with the caregivers
■ Lowering the emotional climate within the family by reducing stress and burden on relatives
■ Increasing the ability of relatives to anticipate and solve problems
■ Reducing the expressions of anger and guilt by family members
■ Maintaining reasonable expectations for how the ill family member should perform
■ Encouraging relatives to set appropriate limits while maintaining some degree of separateness
■ Promoting desirable changes in the relatives' behaviors and belief systems

Family therapy typically consists of a brief program of family education about schizophrenia and a more extended program of family contact designed to reduce overt manifestations of conflict and improve patterns of family communication and problem-solving. The response to this type of therapy has been very dramatic. Studies have clearly revealed that a more positive outcome in the treatment of the client with schizophrenia can be achieved by including the family system in the program of care.

Assertive Community Treatment

Assertive community treatment (ACT) is an evidence-based program of case management that takes a team approach in providing comprehensive, community-based psychiatric treatment, rehabilitation, and support to persons with serious and persistent mental illness such as schizophrenia. Some states use other terms for this type of treatment, such as mobile treatment teams and community support programs. Assertive programs of treatment are individually tailored for each client, intended to be proactive, and include teaching basic living skills, helping clients work with community agencies, and assisting clients to develop a social support network. Vocational expectations are emphasized, and supported work settings (i.e., sheltered workshops) are an important part of the treatment program. Other services include substance abuse treatment, psychoeducational programs, family support and education, mobile crisis intervention, and attention to health-care needs.

Responsibilities are shared by multiple team members, including psychiatrists, nurses, social workers, vocational rehabilitation therapists, and substance abuse counselors. Services are provided in the person's home; within the neighborhood; in local restaurants, parks, or stores; or wherever assistance by the client is required. These services are available to the client 24 hours a day, 365 days a year, and ACT is considered a long-term intervention strategy. One recent study looked at the impact of a Housing First intervention (an intervention that prioritizes rapid re-housing for homeless individuals with schizophrenia) and found that when this type of intervention was combined with ACT, medication adherence improved from below 50 percent to 78 percent. Additionally, these combined interventions improved clients' integration in community, increased residential stability, and decreased criminal convictions (Rezansoff et al., 2016).

ACT has been shown to reduce the number of hospitalizations and decrease costs of care for these clients. Although it has been called "paternalistic" and "coercive" by its critics, ACT has provided much-needed services and increased quality of life for many clients who are unable to manage in a less-structured environment. One limitation is that treatment programs of this kind are time and labor intensive.

Recovery Model

Research provides support for recovery as an objective within reach for individuals with schizophrenia (Lysaker, Roe, & Buck, 2010). Lysaker and associates (2010) state:

> Recovery from schizophrenia, in the sense of a state in which persons experience no difficulties associated with the illness, can occur but the modal outcome seems to be one in which difficulties linked to symptoms, social function, and work appear periodically but can be successfully confronted. (p. 40)

Conceptual models of recovery from mental illness are presented in Chapter 21, The Recovery Model. The recovery model has been used primarily in caring for individuals with serious mental illness, such as schizophrenia and bipolar disorder. However, concepts of the model are amenable to use with all individuals experiencing emotional conditions that require assistance and desiring to take control and manage their lives more independently.

Weiden (2010) identifies two types of recovery with schizophrenia: functional and process. Functional recovery focuses on the individual's level of functioning in such areas as relationships, work, independent living, and other activities. He or she may or may not be experiencing active symptoms of schizophrenia.

Weiden (2010) suggests that recovery can also be considered a process. With process recovery, there is no defined end point. Recovery continues throughout the individual's life and involves collaboration between client and clinician. The individual identifies goals based on personal values or what he or she defines as giving meaning and purpose to life. The clinician and client work together to develop a treatment plan in alignment with the goals set forth by the client. In the process recovery model, the individual may still be experiencing symptoms. Weiden (2010) states:

> Patients do not have to be in remission, nor does remission automatically have to be a desired (or likely) goal when embarking on a recovery-oriented treatment plan. As long as the patient (and family) understands that a process recovery treatment plan is not to be confused with a promise of "cure" or even "remission," then one does not overpromise.

The concept of recovery in schizophrenia remains controversial among clinicians, and many challenges lie ahead for continued study. Recovery models have similarities with ACT in that they both necessarily engage the support of multiple resources, but recovery models also highlight the dimension of active engagement and empowerment of the client in decision-making. Some argue that this approach is difficult to implement with clients who lack insight about their illness or the need for treatment. Further, there is a lack of consistency in what constitutes "recovery," and many concepts exist.

 Still, the potential and hope is that as these models become better studied and more clearly defined, they will provide a treatment approach that is comprehensive, protective, and supportive of patient-centered care.

RAISE (Recovery After an Initial Schizophrenic Episode)

The RAISE approach to treatment for schizophrenia is based on a large National Institute of Mental Health (NIMH) initiative that began in 2008, and research findings published in 2015 have demonstrated several benefits of this approach. Insel (2015) describes the RAISE approach as

> coordinated specialty care for first episode psychosis. With coordinated specialty care the young person experiencing first episode psychosis works with a team of specialists to create a personal treatment plan, combining recovery-oriented psychotherapy, low-dose medication management, family education and support, case management, and work or education support. Coordinated specialty care emphasizes shared decision-making, including family members when possible.

The RAISE approach incorporates many elements from other treatment approaches, including community treatment, recovery model approaches, family approaches, and comprehensive care models. It adds the dimension of early intervention at the first episode of psychosis. The research findings after 5 years of studying this approach are promising for improving care to this population when intervention

begins at the earliest onset of psychotic symptoms. Positive outcomes have included greater adherence to treatment programs; greater improvement in symptoms, interpersonal relationships, and quality of life; more involvement in employment or educational pursuits; and less frequent hospitalizations than are seen for clients involved in more traditional treatment approaches (Insel, 2015).

The hope for this approach to treatment is that through early and comprehensive intervention, the long-term debilitating consequences of schizophrenia can be averted or minimized.

Psychopharmacological Treatment

Chlorpromazine (Thorazine) was first introduced in the United States in 1952. At that time, it was used in conjunction with barbiturates in surgical anesthesia. With increased use, the drug's psychic properties were recognized, and by 1954 it was marketed as an antipsychotic medication in the United States. The manufacture and sale of other antipsychotic drugs followed in rapid succession.

Antipsychotic medications are also called *neuroleptics,* historically referred to as major tranquilizers. They are effective in the treatment of acute and chronic manifestations of schizophrenia and in maintenance therapy to prevent exacerbation of schizophrenic symptoms. Without drug treatment, an estimated 72 percent of individuals who have experienced a psychotic episode relapse within a year. This relapse rate can be reduced to about 23 percent with continuous medication administration (Dixon, Lehman, & Levine, 2010).

The prognosis of schizophrenia has often been reported in a paradigm of thirds. One-third of individuals achieve significant and lasting improvement. They may never experience another episode of psychosis following the initial occurrence. One-third may achieve some improvement with intermittent relapses and residual disability. Their occupational level may have decreased because of their illness, or they may be socially isolated. Finally, one-third experience severe and permanent incapacity. They often do not respond to medication and remain severely ill for much of their lives. Men have poorer outcomes than women do; women respond better to treatment with antipsychotic medications.

As mentioned earlier, the efficacy of antipsychotic medications is enhanced by adjunct psychosocial therapy. Because the psychotic manifestations of the illness subside with use of the drugs, clients on medication are generally more cooperative with the psychosocial therapies. However, it takes several weeks for the antipsychotics to effectively treat positive symptoms, which often leads to discontinuation of the medication. Clients and families need to be educated about the importance of waiting, often for several weeks, to determine if the drug will be effective.

These medications are classified as either *typical* (first-generation, conventional antipsychotics) or *atypical* (the newer, novel antipsychotics). Examples of commonly used antipsychotic agents are presented in Table 24–5. A description of these medications follows. More detailed information is available in Chapter 4, Psychopharmacology.

Indications

Antipsychotic medications are used in the treatment of schizophrenia and other psychotic disorders. Selected agents are used in the treatment of bipolar mania (olanzapine, aripiprazole, chlorpromazine, quetiapine, risperidone, asenapine, ziprasidone, cariprazine).

Action

Typical antipsychotics work by blocking postsynaptic dopamine receptors in the basal ganglia, hypothalamus, limbic system, brainstem, and medulla. They also demonstrate varying affinity for cholinergic, alpha$_1$-adrenergic, and histaminic receptors. Antipsychotic effects may also be related to inhibition of dopamine-mediated transmission of neural impulses at the synapses.

Atypical antipsychotics are weaker dopamine receptor antagonists than conventional antipsychotics but more potent antagonists of the serotonin (5-hydroxytryptamine) type 2A (5HT$_{2A}$) receptors. They also exhibit antagonism for cholinergic, histaminic, and adrenergic receptors. A detailed discussion of contraindications, precautions, side effects, and drug interactions associated with antipsychotic medications is available in Chapter 4.

Side Effects

The effects of these medications are related to blockage of receptors for which they exhibit various degrees of affinity. Blockage of the dopamine receptors is thought to be responsible for controlling positive symptoms of schizophrenia. Dopamine blockage also results in **extrapyramidal symptoms** (EPS) and prolactin elevation (galactorrhea; **gynecomastia**). (A list of medications commonly used to treat EPS is included in Table 24–6). Cholinergic blockade causes anticholinergic side effects (dry mouth, blurred vision, constipation, urinary retention, tachycardia). Blockage of the alpha$_1$-adrenergic receptors produces dizziness, orthostatic hypotension, tremors, and reflex tachycardia. Histamine blockade is associated with weight gain and sedation.

The plan of care should include monitoring for the side effects from antipsychotic medications and

TABLE 24–5 **Antipsychotic Agents**			
CATEGORIES	GENERIC (TRADE NAME)	PREGNANCY CATEGORIES/ HALF-LIFE (hr)	DAILY DOSAGE RANGE (mg)
Typical antipsychotic agents (first generation; conventional)	Chlorpromazine	C/ 24	40–400
	Fluphenazine	C/ HCl: 18 hr Decanoate: 6.8–9.6 days	2.5–10
	Haloperidol (Haldol)	C/ ~18 (oral); ~3 wk (IM decanoate)	1–100
	Loxapine	C/ 8	20–250
	Perphenazine	C/ 9–12	12–64
	Pimozide (Orap)	C/ ~55	1–10
	Prochlorperazine	C/ 3–5 (oral); 6.9 (IV)	15–150
	Thioridazine	C/ 24	150–800
	Thiothixene (Navane)	C/ 34	6–30
	Trifluoperazine	C/ 18	4–40
Atypical antipsychotic agents (second generation; novel)	Aripiprazole (Abilify)	C/ 75–146	10–30
	Asenapine (Saphris)	C/ 24	10–20
	Brexpiprazole (Rexulti)	NA/ 19–91	2–4
	Cariprazine (Vraylar)	NA/ 48–96	1.5–6
	Clozapine (Clozaril)	B/ 8 (single dose); 12 (at steady state)	300–900
	Iloperidone (Fanapt)	C/ 18–33	12–24
	Lurasidone (Latuda)	B/ 18	40–80
	Olanzapine (Zyprexa)	C/ 21–54	5–20
	Paliperidone (Invega)	C/ 23	6–12
	Quetiapine (Seroquel)	C/ ~6	300–400
	Risperidone (Risperdal)	C/ 3–20	4–8
	Ziprasidone (Geodon)	C/ ~7 (oral); 2–5 (IM)	40–160

TABLE 24–6 Antiparkinsonian Agents Used to Treat Extrapyramidal Side Effects of Antipsychotic Drugs

Indication	Used to treat parkinsonism of various causes and drug-induced extrapyramidal reactions.
Action	Restores the natural balance of acetylcholine and dopamine in the CNS. The imbalance is a deficiency in dopamine that results in excessive cholinergic activity.
Contraindications/ precautions	Antiparkinsonian agents are contraindicated in individuals with hypersensitivity. Anticholinergics should be avoided by individuals with angle-closure glaucoma; pyloric, duodenal, or bladder neck obstructions; prostatic hypertrophy; or myasthenia gravis. 　　Caution should be used in administering these drugs to clients with hepatic, renal, or cardiac insufficiency; elderly and debilitated clients; those with a tendency toward urinary retention; or those exposed to high environmental temperatures.
Common side effects	Anticholinergic effects (dry mouth, blurred vision, constipation, paralytic ileus, urinary retention, tachycardia, elevated temperature, decreased sweating), nausea/GI upset, sedation, dizziness, orthostatic hypotension, exacerbation of psychoses.

CHEMICAL CLASS	GENERIC (TRADE NAME)	PREGNANCY CATEGORIES/ HALF-LIFE (hr)	DAILY DOSAGE RANGE (mg)
Anticholinergics	Benztropine (Cogentin) Biperiden (Akineton) Trihexyphenidyl	C/ UKN C/ 18.4–24.3 C/ 5.6–10.2	1–8 2–6 1–15
Antihistamines	Diphenhydramine (Benadryl)	C/ 4–15	25–200
Dopaminergic agonists	Amantadine	C/ 10–25	200–300

educating the client/family about safety precautions when taking antipsychotic medication. (A list of side effects and relevant nursing interventions is included in Chapter 4).

Client and Family Education Related to Antipsychotics

The client should:

■ Use caution when driving or operating dangerous machinery. Drowsiness and dizziness can occur.

■ Not discontinue the drug abruptly after long-term use. To do so might produce withdrawal symptoms, such as nausea, vomiting, dizziness, gastritis, headache, tachycardia, insomnia, and tremulousness.

■ Use sunblock lotion and wear protective clothing when spending time outdoors. Skin is more susceptible to sunburn, which can occur in as little as 30 minutes.

■ Report weekly (if receiving clozapine therapy) to have blood levels drawn and to obtain a weekly supply of the drug.

■ Report the occurrence of any of the following symptoms to the physician immediately: sore throat, fever, malaise, unusual bleeding, easy bruising, persistent nausea and vomiting, severe headache, rapid heart rate, difficulty urinating, muscle twitching, tremors, dark-colored urine, excessive urination, excessive thirst, excessive hunger, weakness, pale stools, yellow skin or eyes, muscular incoordination, or skin rash.

■ Rise slowly from a sitting or lying position to prevent a sudden drop in blood pressure.

■ Take frequent sips of water, chew sugarless gum, or suck on hard candy if dry mouth is a problem. Good oral care (frequent brushing and flossing) is very important.

■ Consult the physician regarding smoking while on antipsychotic therapy. Smoking increases the metabolism of antipsychotics, requiring an adjustment in dosage to achieve a therapeutic effect.

■ Dress warmly in cold weather and avoid extended exposure to very high or low temperatures. Body temperature is harder to maintain with this medication.

■ Avoid drinking alcohol while on antipsychotic therapy. These drugs potentiate each other's effects.

■ Avoid taking other medications (including over-the-counter products) without the physician's approval. Many medications contain substances that interact with antipsychotics in a way that may be harmful.

■ Be aware of possible risks of taking antipsychotics during pregnancy. Safe use during pregnancy has not been established. Antipsychotics are thought to readily cross the placental barrier; if so, a fetus could experience adverse effects of the drug. Inform the physician immediately if pregnancy occurs, is suspected, or is planned.

■ Be aware of side effects of antipsychotic drugs. Refer to written materials furnished by health-care providers for safe self-administration.

- Continue to take the medication, even if feeling well and as though it is not needed. Symptoms may return if medication is discontinued.
- Carry a card or other identification at all times describing medications being taken.

Smoking Cessation

Smoking cigarettes has long been identified as a particular health risk for clients with schizophrenia, since the prevalence is three times that of the general population; it is estimated that as many as 88 percent of those with schizophrenia and 70 percent of those with bipolar disorder are smokers (Kranjac, 2016). Besides the obvious health risks of chronic lung diseases and cancers, smoking decreases the effectiveness of some psychotropic medications. Varenicline (Chantix), a nicotine agonist used as a smoking deterrent, was once thought to increase symptoms and even suicide risk in those with severe mental illness. However, a recent meta-analysis (Wu et al., 2016) concluded that varenicline is effective for assisting with smoking cessation in this population and that "there was no clear evidence of neuropsychiatric or other adverse events compared with placebo" (p. 1554). In any scenario, assessing the client's motivation to stop smoking and exploring viable treatment options, including psychological interventions, is an important component of treatment.

CASE STUDY AND SAMPLE CARE PLAN

NURSING HISTORY AND ASSESSMENT

Frank is 22 years old. He joined the Marines just out of high school at age 18 for a 3-year enlistment. His final year was spent in Afghanistan. When his enlistment was up, he returned to his hometown and married a young woman with whom he had been a high school classmate. Frank has always been quiet, somewhat withdrawn, and had very few friends. He was the only child of a single mom who never married, and he does not know his father. His mother was killed in an automobile accident the spring before he enlisted in the Marines.

During the past year, he has become increasingly isolated and withdrawn. He is without regular employment but finds work as a day laborer when he can. His wife, Suzanne, works as a secretary and is the primary wage earner. Lately, Frank has become very suspicious of Suzanne and sometimes follows her to work. He also drops in on her at work and accuses her of having affairs with some of the men in the office.

Last evening when Suzanne got home from work, Frank was hiding in the closet. She didn't know he was home. When she started to undress, he jumped out of the closet holding a large kitchen knife and threatened to kill her "for being unfaithful." Suzanne managed to flee their home and ran to the neighbor's house and called the police.

Frank told the police that he received a message over the radio from his Marine commanding officer telling him that he couldn't allow his wife to continue to commit adultery, and the only way he could stop it was to kill her. The police took Frank to the emergency department of the VA Hospital, where he was admitted to the psychiatric unit. Suzanne is helping with the admission history.

Suzanne tells the nurse that she has never been unfaithful to Frank and she doesn't know why he believes that she has. Frank tells the nurse that he has been "taking orders from my commanding officer through my car radio ever since I got back from Afghanistan." He survived a helicopter crash in Afghanistan in which all were killed except Frank and one other man. Frank says, "I have to follow my CO's orders. God saved me to annihilate the impure."

Following an evaluation, the psychiatrist diagnoses Frank with schizophrenia. He orders olanzapine 10 mg PO to be given daily and olanzapine 10 mg IM q6h prn for agitation.

NURSING DIAGNOSES AND OUTCOME IDENTIFICATION

From the assessment data, the nurse develops the following nursing diagnoses for Frank:

1. **Risk for self-directed or other-directed violence** related to unresolved grief over loss of mother; survivor's guilt associated with helicopter crash; command hallucinations; and history of violence.
   a. **Short-term goals:**
      - Frank will seek out staff when anxiety and agitation start to increase.
      - Frank will not harm self or others.
   b. **Long-term goal:** Frank will not harm self or others.
2. **Disturbed sensory perception: Auditory** related to increased anxiety and agitation, withdrawal into self, and stress of sufficient intensity to threaten an already weak ego
   a. **Short-term goals:**
      - Frank will discuss the content of the hallucinations with the nurse.
      - Frank will maintain anxiety at a manageable level.
   b. **Long-term goal:** Frank will be able to define and test reality, reducing or eliminating the occurrence of hallucinations.

PLANNING AND IMPLEMENTATION

RISK FOR SELF-DIRECTED OR OTHER-DIRECTED VIOLENCE
1. Keep the stimuli as low as possible in Frank's environment.
2. Monitor Frank's behavior frequently, but in a manner of carrying out routine activities so as not to create suspiciousness on his part.
3. Watch for the following signs (considered the prodrome to aggressive behavior): increased motor activity, pounding,

Continued

CASE STUDY AND SAMPLE CARE PLAN—cont'd

slamming, tense posture, defiant affect, clenched teeth and fists, arguing, demanding, and challenging or threatening staff.

4. If client should become aggressive, maintain a calm attitude. Try talking. Offer medication. Provide physical activities.

5. If these interventions fail, indicate a show of strength with a team of staff members.

6. Utilize restraints only as a last resort and if Frank is clearly at risk of harm to himself or others.

7. Help Frank recognize unresolved grief and fixation in denial or anger stage of grief process.

8. Encourage him to talk about the loss of his mother and fellow Marines in Afghanistan.

9. Encourage him to talk about guilt feelings associated with survival when others died.

10. Make a short-term contract with Frank that he will seek out staff if considering harming himself or others. When this contract expires, make another, and so on.

DISTURBED SENSORY PERCEPTION: AUDITORY

1. Monitor Frank's behavior for signs that he is hearing voices: listening pose, talking and laughing to self, stopping in midsentence.

2. If these behaviors are observed, ask Frank, "Are you hearing the voices again?"

3. Encourage Frank to share the content of the hallucinations. This information is important for early intervention in case the content contains commands to harm himself or others.

4. Say to Frank, "I understand that the voice is real to you, but I do not hear any voices speaking." It is important for him to learn the difference between what is real and what is not real.

5. Try to help Frank recognize that the voices often appear at times when he becomes anxious about something and his agitation increases.

6. Help him to recognize this increasing anxiety, and teach him methods to keep it from escalating.

7. Use distracting activities to bring him back to reality. Involvement with real people and real situations will help to distract him from the hallucination.

8. Teach him to use *voice dismissal*. When he hears the CO's (or others') voice, he should shout, "Go away!" or "Leave me alone!" These commands may help to diminish the sounds and give him a feeling of control over the situation.

EVALUATION

The outcome criteria identified for Frank have been met. When feeling especially anxious or becoming agitated, he seeks out staff for comfort and for assistance in maintaining his anxiety at a manageable level. He establishes short-term contracts with staff not to harm himself. He is experiencing fewer auditory hallucinations and has learned to use voice dismissal to interrupt the behavior. He is beginning to recognize his position in the grief process and is working toward resolution at his own pace.

Summary and Key Points

■ Of all mental illnesses, schizophrenia undoubtedly results in the greatest amount of personal, emotional, and social costs. It presents an enormous threat to life and happiness, yet it remains an enigma to the medical community.

■ For many years, there was little agreement as to a definition of the concept of schizophrenia. The *DSM-5* (APA, 2013) identifies specific criteria for diagnosis of the disorder.

■ The initial symptoms of schizophrenia most often occur in early adulthood. Development of the disorder can be viewed in four phases: (1) premorbid, (2) prodromal, (3) active psychotic (schizophrenia), and (4) residual.

■ The cause of schizophrenia remains unclear. Research continues, and most contemporary psychiatrists view schizophrenia as a brain disorder with little if any emphasis on psychosocial influences.

■ Schizophrenia most likely results from a combination of influences including genetics, biochemical dysfunction, and physiological and environmental factors.

■ A spectrum of schizophrenic and other psychotic disorders has been identified. These include (on a gradient of psychopathology from least to most severe) schizotypal personality disorder, delusional disorder, brief psychotic disorder, substance-induced psychotic disorder, psychotic disorder associated with another medical condition, catatonic disorder associated with another medical condition, schizophreniform disorder, schizoaffective disorder, and schizophrenia.

■ Nursing care of the client with schizophrenia is accomplished using the six steps of the nursing process.

■ Nursing assessment is based on knowledge of symptomatology related to thought content and form, perception, affect, sense of self, volition, interpersonal functioning and relationship to the external world, and psychomotor behavior.

■ These behaviors are categorized as *positive* (an excess or distortion of normal functions) or *negative* (a diminution or loss of normal functions).

■ Antipsychotic medications remain the mainstay of treatment for psychotic disorders. Atypical antipsychotics have become the first line of therapy and treat both positive and negative symptoms of schizophrenia. They have a more favorable side-effect profile than the conventional (typical) antipsychotics.

■ Individuals with schizophrenia require long-term integrated treatment with pharmacological and other interventions. Some of these include individual psychotherapy, group therapy, behavior therapy, social skills training, milieu therapy, family therapy, and assertive community treatment. For the majority of clients, the most effective treatment appears to be a combination of psychotropic medication and psychosocial therapy.

■ Some clinicians are choosing a course of therapy based on a model of recovery, similar to that which has been used for many years with addiction. The basic premise of a recovery model is empowerment of the consumer. The recovery model is designed to allow consumers primary control over decisions about their own care and to enable persons with mental health problems to live a meaningful life in a community of their choice while striving to achieve their full potential.

■ Families generally require support and education about psychotic illnesses. The focus is on coping with the diagnosis, understanding the illness and its course, teaching about medication, and learning ways to manage symptoms.

■ The most current, evidence-based approach to treatment, RAISE, demonstrates that early intervention at the first episode of psychosis can significantly improve outcomes.

■ There is a risk for suicide (around 10 percent) among patients with schizophrenia, so suicide risk assessment should always be considered an essential evaluation component.

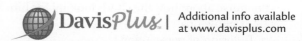

DavisPlus | Additional info available at www.davisplus.com

Review Questions
Self-Examination/Learning Exercise

Select the answer that is most appropriate for each of the following questions.

1. Josh, age 21, has been diagnosed with schizophrenia. He has been socially isolated and hearing voices telling him to kill his parents. He has been admitted to the psychiatric unit from the emergency department. The *initial* nursing intervention for Josh is to:
   a. Give him an injection of Thorazine.
   b. Ensure a safe environment for him and others.
   c. Place him in restraints.
   d. Order him a nutritious diet.

2. The primary goal in working with an actively psychotic, suspicious client would be to:
   a. Promote interaction with others.
   b. Decrease his anxiety and increase trust.
   c. Improve his relationship with his parents.
   d. Encourage participation in therapy activities.

3. The nurse is caring for a client with schizophrenia. Orders from the physician include 100 mg chlorpromazine IM STAT and then 50 mg PO bid; 2 mg benztropine PO bid prn. Why is chlorpromazine ordered?
   a. To reduce extrapyramidal symptoms
   b. To prevent neuroleptic malignant syndrome
   c. To decrease psychotic symptoms
   d. To induce sleep

Continued

Review Questions—cont'd
Self-Examination/Learning Exercise

4. The nurse is caring for a client with schizophrenia. Orders from the physician include 100 mg chlorpromazine IM STAT and then 50 mg PO bid; 2 mg benztropine PO bid prn. Because benztropine was ordered on a prn basis, which of the following assessments by the nurse would convey a need for this medication?
   a. The client's level of agitation increases.
   b. The client complains of a sore throat.
   c. The client's skin has a yellowish cast.
   d. The client develops muscle spasms.

5. Brandon, a client on the psychiatric unit, has been diagnosed with schizophrenia. He begins to tell the nurse about how the CIA is looking for him and will kill him if they find him. The most appropriate response by the nurse is:
   a. "That's ridiculous, Brandon. No one is going to hurt you."
   b. "The CIA isn't interested in people like you, Brandon."
   c. "Why do you think the CIA wants to kill you?"
   d. "I know you believe that, Brandon, but it's really hard for me to believe."

6. Brandon, a client on the psychiatric unit, has been diagnosed with schizophrenia. He begins to tell the nurse about how the CIA is looking for him and will kill him if they find him. Brandon's belief is an example of a:
   a. Delusion of persecution.
   b. Delusion of reference.
   c. Delusion of control or influence.
   d. Delusion of grandeur.

7. The nurse is interviewing a client on the psychiatric unit. The client tilts his head to the side, stops talking in midsentence, and listens intently. The nurse recognizes from these signs that the client is likely experiencing:
   a. Somatic delusions.
   b. Catatonic stupor.
   c. Auditory hallucinations.
   d. Pseudoparkinsonism.

8. The nurse is interviewing a client on the psychiatric unit. The client tilts his head to the side, stops talking in midsentence, and listens intently. The nurse recognizes these behaviors as a symptom of the client's illness. The most appropriate nursing intervention for this symptom is to:
   a. Ask the client to describe his physical symptoms.
   b. Ask the client to describe what he is hearing.
   c. Administer a dose of benztropine.
   d. Call the physician for additional orders.

9. When a client suddenly becomes aggressive and violent on the unit, which of the following approaches would be best for the nurse to use *first*?
   a. Provide large motor activities to relieve the client's pent-up tension.
   b. Administer a dose of prn chlorpromazine to keep the client calm.
   c. Call for sufficient help to control the situation safely.
   d. Convey to the client that his behavior is unacceptable and will not be permitted.

10. The primary focus of family therapy for clients with schizophrenia and their families is:
    a. To discuss concrete problem-solving and adaptive behaviors for coping with stress.
    b. To introduce the family to others with the same problem.
    c. To keep the client and family in touch with the health-care system.
    d. To promote family interaction and increase understanding of the illness.

Review Questions—cont'd
Self-Examination/Learning Exercise

11. A client recently admitted to the hospital reports to the nurse, "I don't understand why I was brought here. I was simply hanging out in my apartment and the police said I had to come with them." This is an example of what symptom of schizophrenia?
    a. Delusions of reference
    b. Loose association
    c. Anosognosia
    d. Auditory hallucinations

12. Recent research on the RAISE approach to treatment of schizophrenia incorporates which of the following elements as important to improving outcomes? (Select all that apply.)
    a. Early intervention at the first episode of psychosis
    b. Support for employment and/or educational pursuits
    c. Rapid high-dose loading with antipsychotic medication
    d. Court-ordered sanctions for treatment
    e. Recovery-focused psychotherapy

IMPLICATIONS OF RESEARCH FOR EVIDENCE-BASED PRACTICE

Castillo, E.G., Rosati, J., Williams, C., Pessin, N., & Lindy, D.C. (2015). Metabolic syndrome screening and assertive community treatment: A quality improvement study. *Journal of the American Psychiatric Nurses Association, 21*(4), 233-243.

DESCRIPTION OF THE STUDY: As part of a quality improvement study, the authors sought to improve physical health screening for metabolic syndrome in clients with severe mental illness (SMI) who were being treated in an assertive community treatment (ACT) program. An underlying assumption was that physical illnesses were not routinely being tracked and typically were not treated until after a medical event occurred. This was identified as a significant quality-of-care issue, since studies have shown that people with SMI generally have a 25-year shorter life span than the general population. One of the largest contributors (greater than suicide or injury) is metabolic syndrome and cardiometabolic sequelae such as hypertension, diabetes, and dyslipidemia. A large sample of clients ($N = 199$) agreed to participate in the study and were evaluated on five parameters that are diagnostic for metabolic syndrome: waist circumference, blood pressure, fasting blood glucose, triglycerides, and high-density lipoprotein cholesterol. ACT staff also provided additional support services to encourage adherence with laboratory test completion such as reminders, assistance with overcoming transportation barriers, and even accompanying clients to appointments when requested.

RESULTS OF THE STUDY: Although some of the identified barriers to adherence necessitated time-consuming support from staff, 141 clients completed all five parameters of screening. Fifty-three percent of the clients met criteria for

metabolic syndrome, and of those who did not meet criteria, only nine participants had *no* risk factors. As a result, the authors identified new preclinical or clinical diagnoses of hypertension for 68 percent of the clients, of diabetes for 15 percent of the clients, and of dyslipidemia for 53 percent of the clients. The authors concluded that the results justify routine screening for metabolic syndrome among those with SMI.

IMPLICATIONS FOR NURSING PRACTICE:

The Institute of Medicine (IOM, 2003) identifies quality improvement as a core competency needed by nurses to improve safe, effective nursing care. This study is an example of health-care professionals identifying a potential quality-of-care issue, studying the issue, and identifying outcomes needed to improve care based on the results of their study. Nurses, as they review current literature and think critically about the practice settings where they work, can take a leadership role in quality improvement studies such as this one. This particular study highlighted the fact that significant health-care risks for the SMI population can be missed unless screening for these risks is done routinely. The complex needs of the SMI client with regard to managing mental illness symptoms has, at times, taken precedence to the exclusion of attention to other health risks. Nurses need to be thoughtful about providing quality, holistic care to clients with SMI because some of these health risks contribute to a significantly shorter life span when they are not addressed.

TEST YOUR CRITICAL THINKING SKILLS

Sara, a 23-year-old single woman, has just been admitted to the psychiatric unit by her parents. They explain that over the past few months she has become increasingly withdrawn. She stays in her room alone but lately has been heard talking and laughing to herself.

Sara left home for the first time at age 18 to attend college. She performed well during her first semester, but when she returned after Christmas, she began to accuse her roommate of stealing her possessions. She started writing to her parents that her roommate wanted to kill her and that her roommate was turning everyone against her. She said she feared for her life. She started missing classes and stayed in her bed most of the time. Sometimes she locked herself in her closet. Her parents took her home, and she was hospitalized and diagnosed with schizophrenia. She has since been maintained on antipsychotic medication while taking a few classes at the local community college.

Sara tells the admitting nurse that she quit taking her medication 4 weeks ago because the pharmacist who fills the prescriptions is plotting to have her killed. She believes he is trying to poison her. She says she got this information from a television message. As Sara speaks, the nurse notices that she sometimes stops in mid-sentence and listens; sometimes she cocks her head to the side and moves her lips as though she is talking.

Answer the following questions related to Sara:

1. From the assessment data, what would be the most immediate nursing concern in working with Sara?
2. What is the nursing diagnosis related to this concern?
3. What interventions must be accomplished before the nurse can be successful in working with Sara?

💬 Communication Exercises

1. Hal, a patient on the psychiatric unit, has a diagnosis of schizophrenia. He lives in a halfway house, where last evening he began yelling that "aliens were on the way to take over our bodies! The message is coming through loud and clear!" The residence supervisor became frightened and called 911. As Hal was being admitted to the psychiatric unit he tells the nurse, "I'm special! I get messages from a higher being! We are in for big trouble!"
   - How would the nurse respond appropriately to this statement by Hal?
2. The nurse notices that Hal is sitting off by himself in a corner of the dayroom. He appears to be talking to himself and tilts his head to the side as if listening to something.
   - How would the nurse intervene with Hal in this situation?

3. Hal says to the nurse, "We must choose to take a ride. All alone we slip and slide. Now it's time to take a bride."
   - How would the nurse respond appropriately to this statement by Hal?

MOVIE CONNECTIONS

I Never Promised You a Rose Garden (schizophrenia) • *A Beautiful Mind* (schizophrenia) • *The Fisher King* (schizophrenia) • *Bennie & Joon* (schizophrenia) • *Out of Darkness* (schizophrenia) • *Conspiracy Theory* (paranoia) • *The Fan* (delusional disorder) • *The Soloist* (schizophrenia) • *Of Two Minds* (schizophrenia)

References

Álvarez, M.J., Masramon, H., Peña, C., Pont, M., Gourdier, C., Roura-Poch, P., & Arrufat, F. (2015). Cumulative effects of childhood traumas: Polytraumatization, dissociation, and schizophrenia. *Community Mental Health Journal, 51*(1), 54-62. doi:10.1007/s10597-014-9755-2

American Psychiatric Association (APA). (2013). *Diagnostic and statistical manual of mental disorders* (5th ed.) Washington, DC: APA.

Asen, E. (2002). Outcome research in family therapy: Family intervention for psychosis. *Advances in Psychiatric Treatment, 8,* 230-238. doi:10.1192/apt.8.3.230

Benson, P.J., Beedie, S.A., Shephard, E., Giegling, I., Rujescu, G., St. Clair, D. (2012). Simple viewing tests can detect eye movement abnormalities that distinguish schizophrenia cases from controls with exceptional accuracy. *Biological Psychiatry (72)* 9, 716-724.

Black, D.W., & Andreasen, N.C. (2014). *Introductory textbook of psychiatry* (6th ed.). Washington, DC: American Psychiatric Publishing.

Bora, E. (2015). Neurodevelopmental origin of cognitive impairment in schizophrenia. *Psychological Medicine, 45*(1), 1-9. doi:10.1017/S0033291714001263

Castillo, E.G., Rosati, J., Williams, C., Pessin, N., & Lindy, D.C. (2015). Metabolic syndrome screening and assertive community treatment: A quality improvement study. *Journal of the American Psychiatric Nurses Association, 21*(4), 233-243. doi:10.1177/1078390315598607

Clark, S.R., Baune, B.T., Schubert, K.O., Lavoie, S., Smesny, S., Rice, S.M., & Amminger, G.P. (2016). Prediction of transition from ultra-high risk to first-episode psychosis using a probabilistic model combining history, clinical assessment and fatty-acid biomarkers. *Translational Psychiatry, 6*(9), e897. doi:10.1038/tp.2016.170

Dixon, L.B., Lehman, A.F., & Levine, J. (2010). Conventional antipsychotic medications for schizophrenia. Retrieved from www.mental-health-matters.com

D'Souza, D.C., Singh, N., Elander, J., Carbuto, M., Pittman, B., Udo de Haes, J., . . . Schipper, J. (2012). Glycine transporter inhibitor attenuates the psychotomimetic effects of ketamine in healthy males: Preliminary evidence. *Neuropsychopharmacology 37*(4), 1036-1046. doi:10.1038/npp.2011.295

Fioravanti, M., Bianchi, V., & Cinti, M.E. (2012). Cognitive deficits in schizophrenia: An updated meta-analysis of the scientific evidence. *BMJ Psychiatry 12*(64), 1-20. doi:10.1186/1471-244X-12-64

Fohrman, D.A., & Stein, M.T. (2006). Psychosis: Six steps rule out medical causes in kids. *Journal of Family Practice Online, 5*(2). Retrieved from www.jfponline.com/pages.asp?aid=3887

Freudenreich, O. (2010). Differential diagnosis of psychotic symptoms: Medical "mimics." *Psychiatric Times, 27*(12), 52-61.

Harrisberger, F., Smieskova1, R., Vogler, C., Egli, T., Schmidt, A., Lenz, C, . . . Borgwardt, S. (2016). Impact of polygenic schizophrenia-related risk and hippocampal volumes on the onset of psychosis. *Translational Psychiatry, 6*, e868. doi:10.1038/tp.2016.143

Hashimoto, K. (2006). Glycine transporter inhibitors as therapeutic agents for schizophrenia. *Recent Patents on CNS Drug Discovery, 1*(1), 43-53. doi:https://doi.org/10.2174/157488906775245336

Herdman, T.H., & Kamitsuru, S. (Eds.). (2014). *NANDA-I nursing diagnoses: Definitions and classification, 2015–2017*. Chichester, UK: Wiley Blackwell.

Hu, W., MacDonald, M.L., Elswick, D.E., & Sweet, R.A. (2014). The glutamate hypothesis of schizophrenia: Evidence from human brain tissue studies. *Annals of the New York Academy of Sciences, 1338*(1), 38-57 [Abstract]. doi:.10.1111/nyas.12547

Insel, T. (2015). Director's blog: New hope for treating psychosis. Retrieved from www.nimh.nih.gov/about/director/2015/new-hope-for-treating-psychosis.shtml

Institute of Medicine. (2003). *Health professions education: A bridge to quality*. Washington, DC: National Academies Press.

Kay, S.R., Fiszbein, A., & Opler, L.A. (1987). The positive and negative syndrome scale (PANSS) for schizophrenia. *Schizophrenia Bulletin,13*(2), 261-276. doi:10.1093/schbul/13.2.261

Kranjac, D. (2016). Pharmacotherapy for smoking cessation in adults with neuropsychiatric illness. Retrieved from www.psychiatryadvisor.com/addiction/smoking-cessation-in-adults-with-neuropsychiatric-illness/article/518385

Lysaker, P.H., Roe, D., & Buck, K.D. (2010). Recovery and wellness amidst schizophrenia: Definitions, evidence, and the implications for clinical practice. *Journal of the American sychiatric Nurses Association, 16*(1), 36-42. doi:10.1177/1078390309353943

MacCabe, J.H., Wicks, S., Löfving, S., David, A.S., Berndtsson, Å., Gustafsson, . . . & Dalman, C. (2013). Decline in cognitive performance between ages 13 and 18 years and the risk for psychosis in adulthood: A Swedish longitudinal cohort study in males. *JAMA Psychiatry 70*(3), 261-270. doi:10.1001/2013.jamapsychiatry.43

Matheson, S.L., Shepherd, A.M., & Carr, V.J. (2014). How much do we know about schizophrenia and how well do we know it? Evidence from the Schizophrenia Library. *Psychological Medicine—London, 44*(6), 3387-3405. doi:10.1017/S0033291714000166

Mathews, M., Tesar, G.E., Fattal, O., & Muzina, D.J. (2013). Schizophrenia and acute psychosis. Retrieved from www.clevelandclinicmeded.com/medicalpubs/diseasemanagement/psychiatry-psychology/schizophrenia-acute-psychosis

Mueser, K.T., Bond, G.R., & Drake, R.E. (2002). Community-based treatment of schizophrenia and other severe mental disorders: Treatment outcomes. *Medscape Psychiatry & Mental Health eJournal*. Retrieved from www.medscape.com/viewarticle/430529

Nauert, R. (2015). Excess neurotransmitter in brain may trigger schizophrenia. *Psych Central*. Retrieved from http://psychcentral.com/news/2013/04/19/excess-neurotransmitter-in-brain-may-trigger-schizophrenia/53880.html

Okazaki, S, Boku, S, Otsuka, I, Mouri, K., Aoyama, S., Shiroiwa, K., . . . Hishimoto, A. (2016). The cell cycle-related genes as biomarkers for schizophrenia. *Progress Neuropsychopharmacology and Biological Psychiatry, 70*(suppl. 9), 85-91. doi:10.1016/j.pnpbp.2016.05.005

Puri, B.K., & Treasaden, I.H. (2011). *Textbook of psychiatry* (3rd ed.). Philadelphia: Churchill Livingstone Elsevier.

Radhakrishnan, R., Wilkinson, S. T., & D'Souza, D.C. (2014). Gone to pot—A review of the association between cannabis and psychosis. *Frontiers in Psychiatry 5*(54). doi:10.3389/fpsyt.2014.00054

Rezansoff, S., Moniruzzaman, A., Fazel, S., McCandless, L., Procyshyn, R., & Somers, J.M. (2016). Housing First improves adherence to antipsychotic medication among formerly homeless adults with schizophrenia: Results of a randomized controlled trial. *Schizophrenia Bulletin*. doi:10.1093/schbul/sbw136

Sadock, B.J., Sadock, V.A., & Ruiz, P. (2015). *Synopsis of psychiatry: Behavioral sciences/clinical psychiatry* (11th ed.). Philadelphia: Lippincott Williams & Wilkins.

Savill, M., Banks, C., Khanom, H., & Priebe, S. (2015). Do negative symptoms of schizophrenia change overtime? A meta-analysis of longitudinal data. *Psychological Medicine), 45*, 1613–1627. doi:10.1017/S0033291714002712

Stahl, S.M. (2013). *Stahl's essential psychopharmacology: Neuroscientific basis and practical applications* (4th ed.). New York: Cambridge University Press.

Thunè, H., Recasens, M., & Uhlhaas, P.J. (2016). The 40-Hz auditory steady-state response in patients with schizophrenia: A meta-analysis. *JAMA Psychiatry*. Retrieved from http://jamanetwork.com/journals/jamapsychiatry/article-abstract/2566207

Urvakhsh, M.M., Thirthalli, J., Aneelraj, D., Jadhav, P., Gangadhar, B.N., & Keshavan, M.S. (2014). Mirror neuron dysfunction in schizophrenia and its functional implications: A systematic review. *Schizophrenia Research, 160*(1-3), 9-19. doi:http://dx.doi.org/10.1016/j.schres.2014.10.040

Veijola, J., Guo, J.Y., Moilanen, J.S., Jaaskelainen, E., Miettunen, J., Kyllonen, M., . . . Murray, G. (2014). Longitudinal changes in total brain volume in schizophrenia: Relation to symptom severity, cognition and antipsychotic medication. *PLoS ONE, 9*(7), e101689. doi:10.1371/journal.pone.0101689

Viher, P.V., Stegmayer, K., Giezendanner, S., Federspiel, A., Bohlhalter, S., Vanbellingen, T., . . . Walthera, S. (2016). Cerebral white matter structure is associated with DSM-5 schizophrenia symptom dimensions. *Neuroimage: Clinical, 12*(suppl. 7), 93-99. doi:http://dx.doi.org/10.1016/j.nicl.2016.06.013

Waters, F., Collerton, D., Ffytche, D.H., Jardri, R., Pins, D., Dudley, R., . . . Laroi, F. (2014). Visual hallucinations in the psychosis spectrum and comparative information from neurodegenerative disorders and eye disease. *Schizophrenia Bulletin, 40*(suppl. 4), 233-245. doi:10.1093/schbul/sbu036

Weiden, P.J. (2010). Is recovery attainable in schizophrenia? *Medscape Psychiatry & Mental Health*. Retrieved from www.medscape.com/viewarticle/729750

Wu, Q., Gilbody, S., Peckham, E., Brabyn, S., & Parrott, S. (2016). Varenicline for smoking cessation and reduction in people with severe mental illnesses: Systematic review and meta-analysis. *Addiction, 111*(9):1554-67. doi:10.1111/add.13415. Epub 2016 Jun 9.

25

Depressive Disorders

CORE CONCEPTS

Depression

Mood

KEY TERMS

cognitive therapy

dysthymia

melancholia

postpartum depression

premenstrual dysphoric disorder

psychomotor retardation

OBJECTIVES

After reading this chapter, the student will be able to:

1. Recount historical perspectives of depression.
2. Discuss epidemiological statistics related to depression.
3. Describe various types of depressive disorders.
4. Identify predisposing factors in the development of depression.
5. Discuss implications of depression related to developmental stage.
6. Identify symptomatology associated with depression and use this information in client assessment.
7. Formulate nursing diagnoses and goals of care for clients with depression.
8. Identify topics for client and family teaching relevant to depression.
9. Describe appropriate nursing interventions for behaviors associated with depression.
10. Describe relevant criteria for evaluating nursing care of clients with depression.
11. Discuss various modalities relevant to treatment of depression.

HOMEWORK ASSIGNMENT

Please read the chapter and answer the following questions:

1. Alterations in which of the neurotransmitters are most closely associated with depression?
2. Depression in adolescence is very hard to differentiate from the normal stormy behavior associated with adolescence. What is the best clue for determining a problem with depression in adolescence?
3. Behaviors of depression often change with the diurnal variation in the level of neurotransmitters. Describe the difference in this phenomenon between moderate and severe depression.
4. All antidepressants carry a black-box warning. What is it?

Depression is likely the oldest and still one of the most frequently diagnosed psychiatric illnesses. Symptoms of depression have been described almost as far back as there is evidence of written documentation.

An occasional bout with the "blues," a feeling of sadness or downheartedness, is common among healthy people and considered a normal response to life's everyday disappointments. These episodes are short-lived as the individual adapts to the loss, change, or failure (real or perceived) that has been experienced. Pathological depression occurs when adaptation is ineffective and the symptoms are significant enough to impair functioning.

CORE CONCEPT

Mood

Mood is a pervasive and sustained emotion that may have a profound influence on a person's perception of the world. Examples of mood include depression, joy, elation, anger, and anxiety. Affect is described as the external, observable emotional reaction associated with an experience. A flat affect describes the state of a person who lacks emotional expression and is often seen in severely depressed clients.

This chapter focuses on the different manifestations of depressive illness and implications for nursing intervention. A historical perspective and epidemiological statistics related to depression are presented. Predisposing factors that have been implicated in the etiology of depression provide a framework for studying the dynamics of the disorder. Similarities and differences between depressive disorders and grief are discussed.

Depressive illnesses specific to individuals at various developmental stages are reviewed. An explanation of the symptomatology is presented as background knowledge for assessing the client with depression. Nursing care is described in the context of the six steps of the nursing process. Various medical treatment modalities are explored.

CORE CONCEPT

Depression

An alteration in mood expressed by feelings of sadness, despair, and pessimism. There is a loss of interest in usual activities, and somatic symptoms may be evident. Changes in appetite, sleep patterns, and cognition are common.

Historical Perspective

Many ancient cultures (e.g., Babylonian, Egyptian, Hebrew) have believed in the supernatural or divine origin of mood disorders. The Old Testament states in the Book of Samuel that King Saul's depression was inflicted by an "evil spirit" sent from God to "torment" him.

A clearly nondivine point of view regarding depression was held by the Greek medical community from the fifth century BC through the third century AD. This perspective represented the thinking of Hippocrates, Celsus, and Galen, among others. They strongly rejected the idea of divine origin and considered the brain the seat of all emotional states. Hippocrates believed that **melancholia** was caused by the effect of excess black bile, a heavily toxic substance produced in the spleen or intestine, on the brain. Melancholia is a severe form of depressive disorder in which symptoms are exaggerated and interest or pleasure in virtually all activities is lost.

During the Renaissance, several new theories evolved. Depression was viewed by some as being the result of obstructed air circulation, excessive brooding, or situations beyond the client's control. Depression was reflected in major literary works of the time, including Shakespeare's *King Lear*, *Macbeth*, and *Hamlet*.

Contemporary thinking has been substantially shaped by the works of Sigmund Freud, Emil Kraepelin, and Adolf Meyer. Having evolved from these early 20th-century models, current thinking about mood disorders generally encompasses the intrapsychic, behavioral, and biological perspectives. These perspectives support the notion of multiple causation in the development of mood disorders.

Epidemiology

Major depressive disorder (MDD) is one of the leading causes of disability in the United States. In addition to the disability posed by the disorder itself, recent research links depression to an increased risk for coronary artery disease (another leading cause of death), especially in women younger than age 65 (Jiang et al., 2016). In 2014, 6.6 percent of individuals ages 18 and older (15.6 million persons) had at least one major depressive episode in the past year (Substance Abuse and Mental Health Services Administration [SAMHSA], 2015). The lifetime prevalence of depression is about 17 percent, which makes it the most prevalent psychiatric disorder (Sadock, Sadock, & Ruiz, 2015). Further, there is evidence that the incidence of depression is increasing among American teens and young adults, particularly adolescent girls.

From 2005 to 2014, the incidence rose from 4.5 to 5.7 percent among teenage boys and from 13.1 to 17.3 percent for teenage girls (Mojtabai, Olfson, & Han, 2016). The reasons for these increases are unclear, but the overall preponderance has led to the consideration of depression by some researchers as "the common cold of psychiatric disorders" and this generation as an "age of melancholia."

Age and Gender

Research indicates that the incidence of depressive disorder is higher in women than it is in men by almost two to one. Sadock and associates (2015) report that this finding is "an almost universal observation, independent of country or culture" (p. 349). The gender difference is less pronounced between ages 44 and 65, but after age 65, women are again more likely than men to be depressed. This occurrence may be related to gender differences in social roles and economic and social opportunities and the shifts that occur with age. The construction of gender stereotypes, or *gender socialization*, promotes typical female characteristics, such as helplessness, passivity, and emotionality, that are associated with depression. In contrast, some studies have suggested that "masculine" characteristics are associated with higher self-esteem and less depression.

Social Class

Some studies have indicated an inverse relationship between social class and report of depressive symptoms. However, there has yet to be a definitive causal structure in the relationship between socioeconomic status and mental illness. A National Center for Health Statistics report identified that for the 45 to 64 age group, depression was five times more prevalent among those below the poverty level (National Center for Health Statistics [NCHS], 2012). One study identified a greater increase in depression with age when compared to more affluent individuals (Green & Benzeval, 2009). Nauert (2010) reports on research that revealed current treatments were less effective for working-class individuals than for middle-class counterparts, regardless of whether they received therapy or medication. This finding may be influential in higher levels of depression among lower socioeconomic class members. Whether these findings are related to lack of access to resources and early treatment, difficulty managing multiple stressors associated with socioeconomic well-being, or a combination of many factors requires further research.

Race and Culture

Studies have shown no consistent relationship between race and affective disorder. One problem encountered in reviewing racial comparisons involves the socioeconomic class of the race being investigated. Sample populations of nonwhite clients are often predominantly lower socioeconomic class populations that are compared with white populations from middle and upper social classes.

Other studies suggest a second problematic factor in the study of racial comparisons. Clinicians tend to underdiagnose mood disorders and overdiagnose schizophrenia in clients who have racial or cultural backgrounds different from their own (Sadock et al., 2015). This misdiagnosis may result from language barriers between clients and physicians who are unfamiliar with cultural aspects of nonwhite clients' language and behavior.

Marital Status

A number of studies have suggested that marriage has a positive effect on psychological well-being compared to those who are single or do not have a close relationship with another person. Other studies have suggested that marital status alone is not a valid indicator of risk for depression (Lapate et al., 2014; LaPierre, 2004). Some of those studies have identified age as an important variable in risk for depression among married and single individuals. Lapate and associates (2014) report that marital stress was associated with increased risk for depression, suggesting that social stress may also be an important variable to consider.

Seasonality

Studies exploring whether seasonality is a cause of depression have yielded varying results. The *Diagnostic and Statistical Manual of Mental Disorders, Fifth Edition (DSM-5)* (APA, 2013) uses the term *seasonal pattern* to describe and specify any depressive disorder that occurs at "characteristic times of the year" (p. 187). The authors note that episodes are most common in fall or winter, but some clients have recurrent summer episodes. Authors of one large study report that prevalence rates of depression with seasonal patterns have varied from 1 percent to 12 percent, but in their study of 5,549 patients from primary care settings, there was no evidence of seasonal patterns for major depressive disorder (Winthorst et al., 2011). In another study, Cobb and associates (2014) found that a small but significant peak in depression symptoms occurred in winter months, but over 20 years of following those clients, the winter seasonal pattern was not stable. Seasonal affective disorder (SAD) continues to be popularly referred to as a separate condition, although the *DSM-5* does not list it as a distinct diagnosis. Reported benefits of light therapy may support a seasonal cause for depression during winter months when there is often less exposure to natural sunlight, but more research is needed to determine a causal relationship.

Types of Depressive Disorders

Major Depressive Disorder

MDD is characterized by depressed mood or loss of interest or pleasure in usual activities, impaired social and occupational functioning that has existed for at least 2 weeks, no history of manic behavior, and symptoms that cannot be attributed to use of substances or a general medical condition. Additionally, the diagnosis of MDD is specified according to whether it is a *single episode* (the individual's first encounter with a major depressive episode) or *recurrent* (the individual has a history of previous major depressive episodes).

The diagnosis will also identify the degree of severity of symptoms (mild, moderate, or severe) and whether there is evidence of psychotic, catatonic, or melancholic features. The presence of anxiety and severity of suicide risk may also be noted. MDD is differentiated from schizoaffective disorder, a condition in which the individual expresses symptoms of a mood disorder as well as symptoms of schizophrenia. Read Josh's story on his experience with depression and an eventual diagnosis of schizoaffective disorder in the "Real People, Real Stories" feature. The *DSM-5* (APA, 2013) diagnostic criteria for major depressive episode are presented in Box 25–1.

Real People, Real Stories: Josh's Experience With Depression and Schizoaffective Disorder

(This individual preferred to remain anonymous, so his name has been changed.)

Consider reflecting on factors that may contribute to Josh's perceptions about his illness and his perceptions about the contributions of health-care providers in his recovery process.

Karyn: Tell me about the time when you first became aware that you had a mood disorder [Josh had told me he had depression. I was unaware when we began the interview that his actual diagnosis was schizoaffective disorder.]

Josh: I was in senior high school and was doing well. I was in advanced placement (AP) courses, and suddenly I got an F in AP English. Nothing like that had ever happened before. I started becoming more withdrawn. I was smoking pot with my friends, and I wonder now if that had an impact. I graduated high school, then attended college for two years until the symptoms really surfaced. I was cut from the soccer team, so there were some disappointments, but I became very withdrawn and depressed. I had suicide ideas and a plan. I had to take a break from school, and I just wasn't doing anything; I was just very withdrawn. Four years later I was diagnosed with schizoaffective disorder.

Karyn: What did you think about that diagnosis?

Josh: I thought it was wrong. I did have some difficulty tracking objects with my eyes, and I still do when I don't get enough sleep. I guess now that I think of it, there was a time in college when I thought my roommates were talking about me, and then I started thinking people in the next room were talking about me. I would read into things a lot. Sometimes I thought I saw something out of the corner of my eye, and sometimes I heard voices.

Karyn: It seems like that would be difficult, maybe even frightening, to have these symptoms and get this diagnosis. What was that like for you?

Josh: Yeah, it was, but I was glad to get a diagnosis because then I knew what I had to deal with. At the same time, though, I thought it was too quickly made and they were too quick to prescribe pills. If I had it to do over, I would have just trusted the doctors, but I rebelled against the drugs several times—sometimes because I was having side

effects like tardive dyskinesia; one time because I was convinced the meds were holding me back and even hurting me; and one time because I just gave up, since I didn't have any of the things I wanted, like marriage, a college degree, or a career. Sometimes I thought, "I can just be smarter than this, and I'll get over it." But I was very disorganized and incoherent. Each time I didn't take the pills, I became withdrawn, depressed, and hearing voices, and eventually I just couldn't find anything else to blame it on. I tried to hide the fact that I had stopped taking the pills, but it always became evident eventually. I stay on the medications now because I know I have to.

Karyn: You've come so far since then!

Josh: (smiles) Yeah, it took me eight years to finish my college degree, but now I have a good job in information technology at a large hospital system, and I live on my own. I was engaged, and although it didn't work out, I'm dating again and hopeful about pursuing a committed relationship.

Karyn: What do you think has been most important in supporting your recovery?

Josh: My parents supported me through all of it. They were my only support, and I didn't want other people to know my "stuff." I was able to stay with my parents until I got back on my feet, and that was really important. The last time I stopped taking my meds, I'd have to consult court records to remember everything that happened, but I know there were trespassing charges. I had run-ins with the police. I also had run-ins with my parents, who eventually called in a crisis team, and I was hospitalized against my will. I was in the hospital for around 30 days, and I saw people who were homeless and had no one supporting them, and they were really doing poorly. Knowing I had someplace to live really helped me. Also, I had a job and some successes at work, so that gave me focus. My job is largely mathematical and doesn't require a lot of social skills challenges. That was helpful for me because, while some people may be self-taught with social skills, I've always struggled with that. My job allows me to develop great insights, be quirky, and not have to try to figure people out.

Continued

Real People, Real Stories: Josh's Experience With Depression and Schizoaffective Disorder—cont'd

Karyn: What are your thoughts about the impact of the health-care providers with whom you've interacted?

Josh: I work in a hospital, so I have a great appreciation for their hard work. I saw an NP who gave me good advice and was very supportive. She asked some probing questions and confronted me at times, and that was challenging, but she was just doing her job and I was trying to hide from my illness. She told me the medications might end up being less effective if I didn't take them or stay on them early in my illness, so that may have encouraged me to keep taking them.

I had good community health services—a case worker, a psychiatrist, and a behavioral health specialist that I found to be particularly supportive because we talked about spiritual things, and that made it okay to explore other issues.

In the hospital, the nurses mostly worked at the station, and that was probably better for their safety, but still I could talk to them and they made it seem like it was okay that I was there. That was important because I wasn't sure what was happening to me, and they just talked about normal, everyday stuff. They seemed more like warm people than cold or clinical. I go to NAMI [National Alliance on Mental Illness] meetings now because I want to share the message with people who have a mental illness (and with their family members) that the professionals could see things I was unable to see at the time I was symptomatic, so it's important to trust the process. I also want families to know that having ongoing support from family members was a lifeline for me even when we were having run-ins and they were facilitating hospitalization against my will.

BOX 25–1 Diagnostic Criteria for Major Depressive Disorder

A. Five (or more) of the following symptoms have been present during the same 2-week period and represent a change from previous functioning; at least one of the symptoms is either (1) depressed mood or (2) loss of interest or pleasure. *Note:* Do not include symptoms that are clearly due to another medical condition.

1. Depressed mood most of the day, nearly every day, as indicated by either subjective report (e.g., feels sad, empty, or hopeless) or observation made by others (e.g., appears tearful). *Note:* In children and adolescents, can be irritable mood

2. Markedly diminished interest or pleasure in all, or almost all, activities most of the day, nearly every day (as indicated by either subjective account or observation)

3. Significant weight loss when not dieting or weight gain (e.g., a change of more than 5% of body weight in a month), or decrease or increase in appetite nearly every day. *Note:* In children, consider failure to make expected weight gain

4. Insomnia or hypersomnia nearly every day

5. Psychomotor agitation or retardation nearly every day (observable by others, not merely subjective feelings of restlessness or being slowed down)

6. Fatigue or loss of energy nearly every day

7. Feelings of worthlessness or excessive or inappropriate guilt (which may be delusional) nearly every day (not merely self-reproach or guilt about being sick)

8. Diminished ability to think or concentrate, or indecisiveness, nearly every day (either by subjective account or as observed by others)

9. Recurrent thoughts of death (not just fear of dying), recurrent suicidal ideation without a specific plan, or a suicide attempt or a specific plan for committing suicide

B. The symptoms cause clinically significant distress or impairment in social, occupation, or other important areas of functioning.

C. The episode is not attributable to the physiological effects of a substance or another medical condition.

Note: Criteria A–C represent a major depressive episode.

Note: Responses to a significant loss (e.g., bereavement, financial ruin, losses from a natural disaster, a serious medical illness or disability) may include the feelings of intense sadness, rumination about the loss, insomnia, poor appetite, and weight loss noted in Criterion A, which may resemble a depressive episode. Although such symptoms may be understandable or considered appropriate to the loss, the presence of a major depressive episode in addition to the normal response to a significant loss should also be carefully considered. This decision inevitably requires the exercise of clinical judgment based on the individual's history and the cultural norms for the expression of distress in the context of loss.

D. The occurrence of the major depressive episode is not better explained by schizoaffective disorder, schizophrenia, schizophreniform disorder, delusional disorder, or other specified and unspecified schizophrenia spectrum and other psychotic disorders.

E. There has never been a manic episode or a hypomanic episode.

Specify:

With anxious distress

With mixed features

With melancholic features

With atypical features

With mood-congruent psychotic features

With mood-incongruent psychotic features

With catatonia

With peripartum onset

With seasonal pattern

Persistent Depressive Disorder (Dysthymia)

Characteristics of **dysthymia** are similar to, if somewhat milder than, those ascribed to MDD. Individuals with this mood disturbance describe their mood as sad or "down in the dumps." There is no evidence of psychotic symptoms. The essential feature is a chronically depressed mood (or possibly an irritable mood in children or adolescents) for most of the day, more days than not, for at least 2 years (1 year for children and adolescents). The diagnosis is identified as *early onset* (occurring before age 21 years) or *late onset* (occurring at age 21 years or older). The *DSM-5* diagnostic criteria for persistent depressive disorder (dysthymia) are presented in Box 25–2.

Premenstrual Dysphoric Disorder

The essential features of **premenstrual dysphoric disorder** (PMDD) include markedly depressed mood, excessive anxiety, mood swings, and decreased interest in activities during the week prior to menses, improving shortly after the onset of menstruation, and becoming minimal or absent in the week postmenses (APA, 2013).

The *DSM-5* diagnostic criteria for PMDD are presented in Box 25–3.

Substance/Medication-Induced Depressive Disorder

The symptoms associated with a substance/medication-induced depressive disorder are considered the direct result of physiological effects of a substance (e.g., a drug of abuse, a medication, or toxin exposure). This disorder causes clinically significant distress or impairment in social, occupational, or other important areas of functioning. The depressed mood is associated with *intoxication* or *withdrawal* from substances such as alcohol, amphetamines, cocaine, hallucinogens, opioids, phencyclidine-like substances, sedatives, hypnotics, or anxiolytics. The symptoms meet the full criteria for a relevant depressive disorder (APA, 2013).

A number of medications have been known to evoke mood symptoms. Classifications include anesthetics, analgesics, anticholinergics, anticonvulsants, antihypertensives, antiparkinsonian agents, antiulcer agents, cardiac medications, oral contraceptives,

---

BOX 25–2 Diagnostic Criteria for Persistent Depressive Disorder (Dysthymia)

A. Depressed mood for most of the day, for more days than not, as indicated by either subjective account or observation by others, for at least 2 years. *Note:* In children and adolescents, mood can be irritable and duration must be at least 1 year.

B. Presence, while depressed, of two (or more) of the following:
1. Poor appetite or overeating
2. Insomnia or hypersomnia
3. Low energy or fatigue
4. Low self-esteem
5. Poor concentration or difficulty making decisions
6. Feelings of hopelessness

C. During the 2-year period (1 year for children or adolescents) of the disturbance, the individual has never been without the symptoms in Criteria A and B for more than 2 months at a time.

D. Criteria for a major depressive disorder may be continuously present for 2 years.

E. There has never been a manic episode or a hypomanic episode, and criteria have never been met for cyclothymic disorder.

F. The disturbance is not better explained by a persistent schizoaffective disorder, schizophrenia, delusional disorder, or other specified or unspecified schizophrenia spectrum and other psychotic disorder.

G. The symptoms are not attributable to the physiological effects of a substance (e.g., a drug of abuse, a medication) or another medical condition (e.g., hypothyroidism).

H. The symptoms cause clinically significant distress or impairment in social, occupational, or other important areas of functioning.

Specify if:

With anxious distress
With mixed features
With melancholic features
With atypical features
With mood-congruent psychotic features
With mood-incongruent psychotic features
With peripartum onset

Specify if:

With pure dysthymic syndrome
With persistent major depressive episode
With intermittent major depressive episodes, with current episode
With intermittent major depressive episodes, without current episode

Specify if:

In partial remission
In full remission

Specify if:

Early onset (onset before age 21 years)
Late onset (onset at age 21 years or older)

Specify if:

Mild
Moderate
Severe

Reprinted with permission from the Diagnostic and Statistical Manual of Mental Disorders, Fifth Edition *(Copyright 2013). American Psychiatric Association.*

BOX 25-3 Diagnostic Criteria for Premenstrual Dysphoric Disorder

A. In the majority of menstrual cycles, at least five symptoms must be present in the final week before the onset of menses, start to *improve* within a few days after the onset of menses, and become *minimal* or absent in the week postmenses.

B. One (or more) of the following symptoms must be present:
   1. Marked affective lability (e.g., mood swings; feeling suddenly sad or tearful or increased sensitivity to rejection)
   2. Marked irritability or anger or increased interpersonal conflicts
   3. Marked depressed mood, feelings of hopelessness, or self-deprecating thoughts
   4. Marked anxiety, tension, feelings of being keyed up or on edge

C. One (or more) of the following symptoms must additionally be present, to reach a total of *five* symptoms when combined with symptoms from Criterion B above.
   1. Decreased interest in usual activities (e.g., work, school, friends, hobbies)
   2. Subjective difficulty in concentration
   3. Lethargy, easy fatigability, or marked lack of energy
   4. Marked change in appetite; overeating; or specific food cravings
   5. Hypersomnia or insomnia

6. A sense of being overwhelmed or out of control
7. Physical symptoms, such as breast tenderness or swelling, joint or muscle pain, a sensation of "bloating," weight gain

Note: The symptoms in Criteria A–C must have been met for most menstrual cycles that occurred in the preceding year.

D. The symptoms are associated with clinically significant distress or interferences with work, school, usual social activities, or relationships with others (e.g., avoidance of social activities, decreased productivity, and efficiency at work, school, or home).

E. The disturbance is not merely an exacerbation of the symptoms of another disorder, such as major depressive disorder, panic disorder, persistent depressive disorder (dysthymia), or a personality disorder (although it may co-occur with any of these disorders).

F. Criteria A should be confirmed by prospective daily ratings during at least two symptomatic cycles. (*Note:* The diagnosis may be made provisionally prior to this confirmation).

G. The symptoms are not attributable to the physiological effects of a substance (e.g., a drug of abuse, a medication, or other treatment) or another medical condition (e.g., hyperthyroidism).

Reprinted with permission from the Diagnostic and Statistical Manual of Mental Disorders, Fifth Edition *(Copyright 2013). American Psychiatric Association.*

---

psychotropic medications, muscle relaxants, steroids, and sulfonamides. Some specific examples are included in the discussion of predisposing factors to depressive disorders.

Depressive Disorder Due to Another Medical Condition

This disorder is characterized by symptoms associated with a major depressive episode that are the direct physiological consequence of another medical condition (APA, 2013). The depression causes clinically significant distress or impairment in social, occupational, or other important areas of functioning. Types of physiological influences are included in the discussion on predisposing factors to depression.

Predisposing Factors

The etiology of depression is unclear. No single theory or hypothesis has been postulated that substantiates a clear-cut explanation for the disease. Evidence continues to mount in support of multiple causations, recognizing the combined effects of genetic, biochemical, and psychosocial influences on an individual's susceptibility to depression. A number of theoretical postulates are presented here.

Biological Theories

Genetics

Affective illness has been the subject of considerable research on the relevance of hereditary factors. A genetic link has been suggested in numerous studies; however, a definitive mode of genetic transmission has yet to be demonstrated.

Twin Studies

Twin studies suggest a strong genetic factor in the etiology of affective illness, including depressive disorders. Heritability is estimated at 40 to 50 percent (Lohoff, 2010). Twin studies looking specifically at the major depressive disorders–recurrent unipolar (MDD-RU) identify the risk for MDD-RU at 37 percent for twins "with a substantial component of unique individual environmental risk but little shared environmental risk" (Lohoff, 2010, p. 539). These findings suggest that while twin studies do identify genetic risk, they do not explain all depressions. Environmental risks not only are an important variable but are uniquely individual.

Family Studies

Most family studies have shown that major depression is more common among first-degree biological relatives of people with the disorder than among the general population (Black & Andreasen, 2014). The evidence to support an increased risk of depressive disorder in individuals with positive family history is quite compelling. It is unlikely that random environmental factors could cause the concentration of illness that is seen within families.

Adoption Studies

Support for heritability as an etiological influence in depression comes from studies of the adopted offspring of biological parents with depression. Some studies have found a threefold increase in depression among children of biological relatives with affective illness, but other studies have found no difference in the rate of mood disorders (Sadock et al., 2015). Conversely, adoption studies have also been used to examine the effects of being reared by an adoptive parent (particularly the maternal parent) with depression and the risks for depression in their nongenetically similar children. Interestingly, these studies have demonstrated an increased risk of depression (as well as oppositional defiant disorder and conduct disorder) in adopted children that cannot be explained by genetics (Natsuaki et al., 2014). Again, this finding suggests that environmental factors also play a role in the etiology of depressive illnesses.

Biochemical Influences

Biogenic Amines

It has been hypothesized that depressive illness may be related to a deficiency of the neurotransmitters norepinephrine, serotonin, and dopamine at functionally important receptor sites in the brain. Historically, the biogenic amine hypothesis of mood disorders grew out of the observation that reserpine, an antihypertensive that depletes the brain of amines such as norepinephrine, was associated with the development of a depressive syndrome. The catecholamine norepinephrine has been identified as a key component in the mobilization of the body to deal with stressful situations. Neurons that contain serotonin are critically involved in the regulation of many psychobiological functions, such as mood, anxiety, arousal, vigilance, irritability, thinking, cognition, appetite, aggression, sleep–wake cycles, eating, and intestinal motility. Tryptophan, the amino acid precursor of serotonin, has been shown to enhance the efficacy of antidepressant medications and on occasion to be effective as an antidepressant itself. The level of dopamine in the mesolimbic system of the brain is thought to exert a strong influence over human mood and behavior. A diminished supply of these biogenic amines inhibits the transmission of impulses from one neuronal fiber to another, causing a failure of the cells to fire or become charged (see Figure 25–1).

More recently, the biogenic amine hypothesis has been expanded to include another neurotransmitter, acetylcholine. Because cholinergic agents have profound effects on mood, electroencephalograms, sleep, and neuroendocrine function, it has been suggested that the problem in depression and mania may be an imbalance between the biogenic amines and acetylcholine. Cholinergic transmission is thought to be excessive in depression and inadequate in mania (Sadock et al., 2015). The precise role that any neurotransmitters play in the etiology of depression is unknown because these chemicals cannot be measured in the brain. It has been theorized that since selective serotonin reuptake inhibitors (SSRIs) are drugs that elevate serotonin levels, low serotonin levels in the brain must be responsible for depression. However, SSRIs also seem to be beneficial in the treatment of anxiety, leading to the hypothesis that low serotonin levels are responsible for anxiety. Further, too *much* serotonin has also been implicated in anxiety states and in schizophrenia. All of this seemingly contradictory information has led many current researchers to believe that neurotransmitters such as serotonin might be better explained as modulators of intense emotional states rather than associated with any one particular emotion (Sadock et al., 2015). As the body of research grows, increased knowledge regarding the biogenic amines undoubtedly will contribute to a greater capacity for understanding and treating affective illness.

Neuroendocrine Disturbances

Neuroendocrine disturbances may play a role in the pathogenesis or persistence of depressive illness. This notion has arisen in view of the marked disturbances in mood observed with the administration of certain hormones or in the presence of spontaneously occurring endocrine disease.

Hypothalamic-Pituitary-Adrenocortical Axis

In clients who are depressed, the normal system of hormonal inhibition fails, resulting in a hypersecretion of cortisol. This elevated serum cortisol is the basis for the dexamethasone suppression test that is sometimes used to determine if an individual has somatically treatable depression.

Hypothalamic-Pituitary-Thyroid Axis

Thyrotropin-releasing factor (TRF) from the hypothalamus stimulates the release of thyroid-stimulating hormone (TSH) from the anterior pituitary gland. In turn, TSH stimulates the thyroid gland. Diminished TSH response to administered TRF is observed in approximately 25 percent of depressed persons and appears to be associated with increased risk for relapse despite treatment with antidepressants (Sadock et al.,

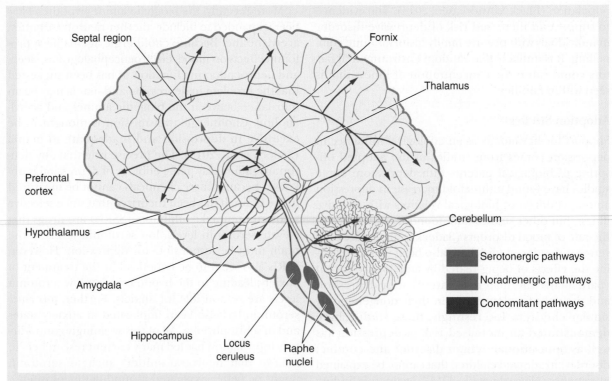

FIGURE 25–1 Neurobiology of depression.

NEUROTRANSMITTERS

Although other neurotransmitters have also been implicated in the pathophysiology of depression, disturbances in serotonin and norepinephrine have been the most extensively scrutinized.

Cell bodies of origin for the serotonin pathways lie within the raphe nuclei located in the brainstem. Those for norepinephrine originate in the locus ceruleus. Projections for both neurotransmitters extend throughout the forebrain, prefrontal cortex, cerebellum, and limbic system.

AREAS OF THE BRAIN AFFECTED

Areas of the brain affected by depression and the symptoms that they mediate include the following:
• Hippocampus: Memory impairments, feelings of worthlessness, hopelessness, and guilt
• Amygdala: Anhedonia, anxiety, reduced motivation
• Hypothalamus: Increased or decreased sleep and appetite; decreased energy and libido
• Other limbic structures: Emotional alterations
• Frontal cortex: Depressed mood; problems concentrating
• Cerebellum: Psychomotor retardation/agitation

MEDICATIONS AND THEIR EFFECTS ON THE BRAIN

All medications that increase serotonin, norepinephrine, or both can improve the emotional and vegetative symptoms of depression. Medications that produce these effects include those that block the presynaptic reuptake of the neurotransmitters or block receptors at nerve endings (tricyclics; SSRIs; SNRIs) and those that inhibit monoamine oxidase, an enzyme that is involved in the metabolism of the monoamines serotonin, norepinephrine, and dopamine (MAOIs).

Side effects of these medications relate to their specific neurotransmitter receptor–blocking action. Tricyclic (e.g., imipramine, amitriptyline) and tetracyclics (e.g. mirtazapine, maprotiline) block reuptake and/or receptors for serotonin, norepinephrine, acetylcholine, and histamine. SSRIs are selective serotonin reuptake inhibitors. Others, such as bupropion, venlafaxine, and duloxetine, block serotonin and norepinephrine reuptake, and also are weak inhibitors of dopamine.

Blockade of norepinephrine reuptake results in side effects of tremors, cardiac arrhythmias, sexual dysfunction, and hypertension. Blockade of serotonin reuptake results in side effects of gastrointestinal disturbances, increased agitation, and sexual dysfunction. Blockade of dopamine reuptake results in side effects of psychomotor activation. Blockade of acetylcholine reuptake results in dry mouth, blurred vision, constipation, and urinary retention. Blockade of histamine reuptake results in sedation, weight gain, and hypotension.

2015). About 4.6 percent of the U.S. population suffers from hypothyroidism (more women than men), and depression is a common symptom (in addition to a host of other symptoms) (National Institutes of Health [NIH], 2016a). Laboratory testing to evaluate TSH is relevant to distinguish between depressive disorders and thyroid disorders, since in thyroid disorders the symptoms of depression are treated with hormone replacement rather than antidepressants.

Physiological Influences

Depressive symptoms that occur as a consequence of a non-mood disorder or as an adverse effect of certain medications are called *secondary* depression. Secondary depression may be related to medication side effects, neurological disorders, electrolyte or hormonal disturbances, nutritional deficiencies, and other physiological or psychological conditions.

Medication Side Effects

A number of drugs, either alone or in combination with other medications, can produce a depressive syndrome. Most common are those that have a direct effect on the central nervous system, such as anxiolytics, antipsychotics, sedative-hypnotics (including barbiturates and opioids), and anticonvulsant mood stabilizers. Many drugs used to treat general medical conditions have also been associated with inducing depression (Vann, 2015), and several are listed here:

■ Antibacterial agents, antifungal agents, and antiviral agents
■ Antimalarials (including mefloquine)
■ Antihypertensives and statins (including beta blockers and calcium blockers)
■ Antineoplastics (including vincristine and zidovudine)
■ Dermatologics (including isotretinoin and finasteride)
■ Hormones (including contraceptives)
■ Nonnucleoside reverse transcriptase inhibitors (HIV medications)
■ Respiratory agents (leukotriene inhibitors)
■ Steroids
■ Smoking cessation agents (varenicline)
■ Vigabatrin (anticonvulsant)

Neurological Disorders

An individual who has suffered a cardiovascular accident (CVA) may experience despondency unrelated to the severity of the CVA. These are true mood disorders, and antidepressant drug therapy may be indicated. Brain tumors, particularly in the area of the temporal lobe, often cause symptoms of depression. Agitated depression may be part of the clinical picture associated with Alzheimer's disease, Parkinson's disease, and Huntington's disease. Agitation and restlessness may also represent underlying depression in the individual with multiple sclerosis.

Electrolyte Disturbances

Excessive levels of sodium bicarbonate or calcium can produce symptoms of depression, as can deficits in magnesium and sodium. Potassium is also implicated in the syndrome of depression. Symptoms have been observed with excesses of potassium in the body as well as in instances of potassium depletion.

Hormonal Disturbances

Depression is associated with dysfunction of the adrenal cortex and is commonly observed in both Addison's disease and Cushing's syndrome. Other endocrine conditions that may result in symptoms of depression include hypoparathyroidism, hyperparathyroidism, hypothyroidism, and hyperthyroidism.

An imbalance of the hormones estrogen and progesterone has been implicated in the predisposition to PMDD, although the exact etiology is unknown. The interaction of these hormonal changes has an impact on serotonin levels, which may contribute to the depression associated with this disorder. It is also noted that individuals with PMDD often have underlying depression and anxiety, so it is possible that hormone changes are exacerbating an already existing condition (Thielen, 2015).

Nutritional Deficiencies

Deficiencies in proteins, carbohydrates, vitamin B_1 (thiamine), vitamin B_2 (riboflavin), vitamin B_6 (pyridoxine), B_9 (folate), vitamin B_{12}, iron, zinc, calcium, chromium, iodine, lithium, selenium, potassium, and omega-3 fatty acids have all been associated with symptoms of depression (Sathyanarayana Rao et al., 2008; Schimelpfening, 2012). A recent large study also found that vitamin D deficiency was linked to depressive symptoms (Shin et al., 2016). It is not a surprise that individuals with anorexia nervosa, who have significant nutritional deficiencies, commonly have comorbid depression.

Other Physiological Conditions

Other conditions that have been associated with secondary depression include collagen disorders, such as systemic lupus erythematosus (SLE) and polyarteritis nodosa; cardiovascular disease, such as cardiomyopathy, congestive heart failure, and myocardial infarction; infections, such as encephalitis, hepatitis, mononucleosis, pneumonia, and syphilis; and metabolic disorders, such as diabetes mellitus and porphyria.

Psychosocial Theories

Psychoanalytical Theory

Freud (1957) presented his classic paper "Mourning and Melancholia" in 1917. He defined the distinguishing features of melancholia as:

a profoundly painful dejection, cessation of interest in the outside world, loss of the capacity to love, inhibition of all activity, and a lowering of the self-regarding feelings to a degree that finds utterances in self-reproaches and self-revilings, and culminates in a delusional expectation of punishment.

He observed that melancholia occurs after the loss of a loved object, either actually by death or emotionally by rejection, or the loss of some other abstraction of value to the individual. Freud indicated that in melancholia, the depressed patient's rage is internally directed because of identification with the lost object (Sadock et al., 2015).

Freud believed that the individual predisposed to melancholia experienced ambivalence in love relationships. He postulated, therefore, that once the loss is incorporated into the self (ego), the hostile part of the ambivalence that had been felt for the lost object is then turned inward against the ego.

Learning Theory

The model of "learned helplessness" arises out of Seligman's (1973) experiments with dogs. The animals were exposed to electrical stimulation from which they could not escape. Later, when they were given the opportunity to avoid the traumatic experience, they reacted with helplessness and made no attempt to escape. A similar state of helplessness exists in humans who have experienced numerous failures (either real or perceived). The individual abandons any further attempt to succeed. Seligman theorized that learned helplessness predisposes individuals to depression by imposing a feeling of lack of control over their life situations. They become depressed because they feel helpless; they have learned that whatever they do is futile. Learned helplessness can be especially damaging very early in life, because the sense of mastery over one's environment is an important foundation for future emotional development.

Object Loss Theory

The theory of object loss suggests that depressive illness occurs as a result of having been abandoned by or otherwise separated from a significant other during the first 6 months of life. Because the mother represents the child's main source of security during this period, she is considered the "object." This absence of attachment, which may be either physical or emotional, leads to feelings of helplessness and despair that contribute to lifelong patterns of depression in response to loss.

The concept of "anaclitic depression" was introduced in 1946 by psychiatrist René Spitz to refer to children who became depressed after being separated from their mothers for an extended period of time during the first year of life. The condition, as described by Spitz, included symptoms such as excessive crying, anorexia, withdrawal, **psychomotor retardation,** stupor, and a generalized impairment in the normal process of growth and development. Some researchers suggest that loss in adult life afflicts people much more severely in the form of depression if the individuals have suffered early childhood loss.

Cognitive Theory

Beck and colleagues (1979) proposed a theory suggesting that the primary disturbance in depression is cognitive rather than affective. The underlying cause of the depression is cognitive distortions that result in negative, defeated attitudes. Beck and colleagues identified three cognitive distortions that they believe serve as the basis for depression:

1. Negative expectations of the environment
2. Negative expectations of the self
3. Negative expectations of the future

These cognitive distortions arise out of a defect in cognitive development, and the individual feels inadequate, worthless, and rejected by others. Outlook for the future is one of pessimism and hopelessness.

Cognitive theorists believe that depression is the product of negative thinking. This is in contrast to the other theorists, who suggest that negative thinking occurs when an individual is depressed. **Cognitive therapy** focuses on helping the individual alter mood by changing the way he or she thinks. The individual is taught to control negative thought distortions that lead to pessimism, lethargy, procrastination, indecisiveness, and low self-esteem (see Chapter 19, Cognitive Therapy).

The Transactional Model

No single theory or hypothesis exists to substantiate a clear-cut explanation for depressive disorder. Evidence continues to mount in support of multiple causation. The transactional model recognizes the combined effects of genetic, biochemical, and psychosocial influences on an individual's susceptibility to depression. The dynamics of depression using the transactional model of stress and adaptation are presented in Figure 25–2.

Developmental Implications

Childhood

Only in recent years has a consensus developed among investigators identifying major depressive disorder as an entity in children and adolescents that can be identified using criteria similar to those used for adults. It is not uncommon, however, for the symptoms of

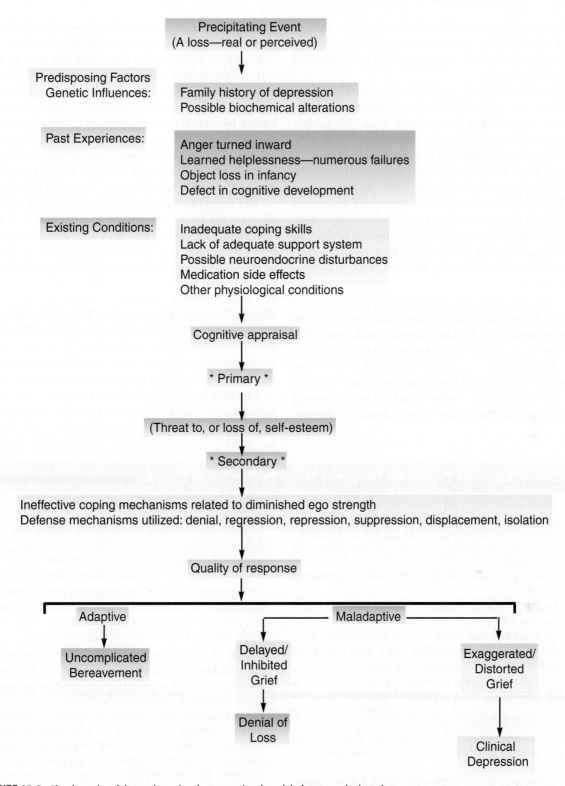

FIGURE 25–2 The dynamics of depression using the transactional model of stress and adaptation.

depression to be manifested differently in childhood, and the picture changes with age (Anxiety and Depression Association of America, 2016; Sadock et al., 2015):

■ **Up to age 3:** Signs may include feeding problems, tantrums, lack of playfulness and emotional expressiveness, failure to thrive, or delays in speech and gross motor development.

■ **Ages 3 to 5:** Common symptoms may include accident proneness, phobias, aggressiveness, and excessive self-reproach for minor infractions.

Mood-congruent auditory hallucinations are not uncommon. The incidence of depression among preschool children is estimated to be between 0.3 and 0.9 percent.

■ **Ages 6 to 8:** There may be vague physical complaints and aggressive behavior. Children in this age group may cling to parents and avoid new people and challenges. They may lag behind their classmates in social skills and academic competence.

■ **Ages 9 to 12:** Common symptoms include morbid thoughts, excessive worrying, and poor self-esteem. These children may reason that they are depressed because they have disappointed their parents in some way. There may be lack of interest in playing with friends. The incidence of depression among school-aged children is estimated to be around 2 to 3 percent.

Other symptoms of childhood depression may include hyperactivity, delinquency, school problems, psychosomatic complaints, sleeping and eating disturbances, social isolation, delusional thinking, and suicidal thoughts or actions. The APA (2013) has included a new diagnostic category in the Depressive Disorders chapter of the *DSM-5*. This childhood disorder is called *disruptive mood dysregulation disorder*.

The diagnostic criteria for disruptive mood dysregulation disorder are presented in Box 25–4.

Children may become depressed for various reasons. In many depressed children, there is a genetic predisposition toward the condition, which is then precipitated by a stressful situation. Common precipitating factors include physical or emotional detachment by the primary caregiver, parental separation or divorce, death of a loved one (person or pet), a move, academic failure, or physical illness. In any event, the common denominator is loss.

The focus of therapy with depressed children is to alleviate the child's symptoms and strengthen his or her coping and adaptive skills, with the hope of possibly preventing future psychological problems. Some studies have shown that untreated childhood depression may lead to subsequent problems in adolescence and adult life. Most children are treated on an outpatient basis. Hospitalization of the depressed child usually occurs only if he or she is actively suicidal, when the home environment precludes adherence to a treatment regimen, or if the child needs to be separated from the home because of psychosocial deprivation.

Parental and family therapy are commonly used to help the younger depressed child. Recovery is

---

BOX 25–4 Diagnostic Criteria for Disruptive Mood Dysregulation Disorder

A. Severe recurrent temper outbursts manifested verbally (e.g., verbal rages) and/or behaviorally (e.g., physical aggression toward people or property) that are grossly out of proportion in intensity or duration to the situation or provocation.

B. The temper outbursts are inconsistent with developmental level.

C. The temper outbursts occur, on average, three or more times per week.

D. The mood between temper outbursts is persistently irritable or angry most of the day, nearly every day, and is observable by others (e.g., parents, teachers, peers).

E. Criteria A–D have been present for 12 or more months. Throughout that time, the individual has not had a period lasting 3 or more consecutive months without all of the symptoms of Criteria A–D.

F. Criteria A and D are present in at least two of three settings (i.e., at home, at school, with peers) and are severe in at least one of these.

G. The diagnosis should not be made for the first time before age 6 or after age 18 years.

H. By history or observation, the age at onset of Criteria A–E is before 10 years.

I. There has never been a distinct period lasting more than 1 day during which the full symptom criteria, except duration,

for a manic or hypomanic episode have been met. *Note:* Developmentally appropriate mood elevation, such as occurs in the context of a highly positive event or its anticipation, should not be considered as a symptom of mania or hypomania.

J. The behaviors do not occur exclusively during an episode of major depressive disorder and are not better explained by another mental disorder (e.g., autism spectrum disorder, posttraumatic stress disorder, separation anxiety disorder, persistent depressive disorder [dysthymia]).

Note: This diagnosis cannot coexist with oppositional defiant disorder, intermittent explosive disorder, or bipolar disorder, though it can coexist with others, including major depressive disorder, attention-deficit/hyperactivity disorder, conduct disorder, and substance use disorders. Individuals whose symptoms meet criteria for both disruptive mood dysregulation disorder and oppositional defiant disorder should only be given the diagnosis of disruptive mood dysregulation disorder. If an individual has ever experienced a manic or hypomanic episode, the diagnosis of disruptive mood dysregulation disorder should not be assigned.

K. The symptoms are not attributable to the physiological effects of a substance or to another medical or neurological condition.

---

facilitated by emotional support and guidance to family members. Children older than age 8 usually participate in family therapy. In some situations, individual treatment may be appropriate for older children. Medications such as antidepressants can be important in the treatment of children, especially for the more serious and recurrent forms of depression. The SSRIs have been used with success, particularly in combination with psychosocial therapies. However, because there has been some concern that the use of antidepressant medications may cause suicidal behavior in young people, the U.S. Food and Drug Administration (FDA) has applied a black-box warning (described in the next section) to all antidepressant medications. The National Institute of Mental Health (2016) stated:

> In some cases, children, teenagers, and young adults under 25 may experience an increase in suicidal thoughts or behavior when taking antidepressants, especially in the first few weeks after starting or when the dose is changed. This warning from the U.S. Food and Drug Administration (FDA) also says that patients of all ages taking antidepressants should be watched closely, especially during the first few weeks of treatment.

Adolescence

Depression may be even harder to recognize in an adolescent than in a younger child. Feelings of sadness, loneliness, anxiety, and hopelessness associated with depression may be perceived as the normal emotional stresses of growing up. Therefore, many young people whose symptoms are attributed to the "normal adjustments" of adolescence do not get the help they need. Depression is a major cause of suicide among teens, and suicide is the second-leading cause of death in the 15- to 24-year-old age group (NCHS, 2015).

Common symptoms of depression in the adolescent are inappropriately expressed anger, aggressiveness, running away, delinquency, social withdrawal, sexual acting out, substance abuse, restlessness, and apathy. Loss of self-esteem, sleeping and eating disturbances, and psychosomatic complaints are also common.

What, then, differentiates mood disorder from the typical stormy behavior of adolescence? A visible manifestation of *behavioral change that lasts for several weeks* is the best clue for a mood disorder. Examples include the normally outgoing and extroverted adolescent who has become withdrawn and isolates herself, the good student who previously received consistently high marks but is now failing and skipping classes, and the usually self-confident teenager who is now inappropriately irritable and defensive with others.

Adolescents become depressed for all the same reasons discussed under childhood depression. In adolescence, however, depression is a common manifestation of the stress and independence conflicts associated with the normal maturation process. Depression may also be the response to death of a parent, other relative, or friend or to a breakup with a boyfriend or girlfriend. This perception of abandonment by parents or the closest peer relationship is thought to be the most frequent immediate precipitant to adolescent suicide.

Treatment of the depressed adolescent is often conducted on an outpatient basis. Hospitalization may be required in cases of severe depression or threat of imminent suicide, when a family situation is such that treatment cannot be carried out in the home, when the physical condition precludes self-care of biological needs, or when the adolescent has indicated possible harm to self or others in the family.

In addition to supportive psychosocial intervention, antidepressant therapy may be part of the treatment of adolescent mood disorders. However, as mentioned previously, the FDA has issued a public health advisory warning the public about the increased risk of suicidal thoughts and behavior in children and adolescents being treated with antidepressant medications. The black-box warning label on all antidepressant medications describes this risk and emphasizes the need for close monitoring of clients started on these medications. The advisory language does not prohibit the use of antidepressants in children and adolescents. Rather, it warns of the increased risk of suicidal ideation and encourages prescribers to balance this risk with clinical need.

Fluoxetine (Prozac) has been approved by the FDA to treat depression in children aged 8 and older, and escitalopram (Lexapro) was approved in 2009 for treatment of MDD in adolescents aged 12 and older. The other SSRI medications, such as sertraline, citalopram, and paroxetine, and the serotonin-norepinephrine reuptake inhibitor (SNRI) antidepressants duloxetine, venlafaxine, and desvenlafaxine have not been approved for treatment of depression in children or adolescents, although they have been prescribed to children by physicians in "off-label use"—a use other than the FDA-approved use. In June 2003, the FDA recommended that paroxetine not be used in children and adolescents for the treatment of MDD. The FDA analysis of antidepressant medications, as reported by the Mayo Clinic (2016a), identified that 4 percent of those taking antidepressants had an increase in suicidal thoughts and that none of the children in the study actually took his or her own life. Nonetheless, the potential risk is considered significant enough to carefully evaluate risks versus benefits before prescribing antidepressants to children and adolescents.

Senescence

Depression is the most common psychiatric disorder of the elderly, who make up 14.5 percent of the general population of the United States (Administration on Aging, 2016). This is not surprising considering the disproportionate value our society places on youth, vigor, and uninterrupted productivity. These societal attitudes continually nurture the feelings of low self-esteem, helplessness, and hopelessness that become more pervasive and intensive with advanced age. Further, the aging individual's adaptive coping strategies may be seriously challenged by major stressors, such as financial problems, physical illness, changes in bodily functioning, and an increasing awareness of approaching death. The problem is often intensified by the numerous losses individuals experience during this period in life, such as spouse, friends, children, home, and independence. A phenomenon called *bereavement overload* occurs when individuals experience so many losses in their lives that they are not able to resolve one grief response before another begins. Bereavement overload predisposes elderly individuals to depressive illness. The elderly population is growing, and it is estimated that by 2030, one in five Americans will be over the age of 65 (CDC, 2013). Evidence-based treatments for depression will continue to be a focal point of care for this population.

Although they make up only about 14.5 percent of the population, the elderly account for a proportionately larger percentage of suicides in the United States. In the 65 to 84 age group, the prevalence of suicide is 16.6 percent; the rate of suicide in those 85 years of age and older jumps to 19.3 percent (American Foundation for Suicide Prevention, 2016). The highest number of these cases is among white men at almost four times the national rate.

Some symptoms of depression in the elderly are similar to those in younger adults. However, depressive syndromes are often confused by other illnesses associated with the aging process. Symptoms of depression are often misdiagnosed as neurocognitive disorder (NCD) when in fact the memory loss, confused thinking, or apathy symptomatic of NCD actually may be the result of depression. This condition is often referred to as *pseudodementia*. The early awakening and reduced appetite typical of depression are common among many older people who are not depressed. Compounding this situation is that many medical conditions, such as endocrinological, neurological, nutritional, and metabolic disorders, often present with classic symptoms of depression. Many medications commonly used by the elderly, such as antihypertensives, corticosteroids, and analgesics, can also produce a depressant effect.

Depression accompanies many illnesses that are common among older people, such as Parkinson's disease, cancer, arthritis, and the early stages of Alzheimer's disease. Treating depression in these situations can reduce unnecessary suffering and help afflicted individuals cope with their medical problems.

The most effective treatment of depression in the elderly individual is thought to be a combination of psychosocial and biological approaches. Antidepressant medications are administered with consideration for age-related physiological changes in absorption, distribution, elimination, and brain receptor sensitivity. Because of these changes, plasma concentrations of these medications can reach very high levels despite moderate oral doses. Anticholinergic side effects associated with tricyclic antidepressants can be problematic for the elderly, and SSRIs have been associated with inducing significant hyponatremia in this population, so careful evaluation and monitoring is essential.

Electroconvulsive therapy (ECT) is an important alternative for treatment of major depression in the elderly, especially considering the problematic side effects of antidepressants in this population. The response to ECT appears to be slower with advancing age, and the therapeutic effects are of limited duration. Research has identified ECT as generally safe for the acute treatment of late-life depression (Van der Wurff et al., 2003). It may be considered the treatment of choice for the elderly individual who is an acute suicidal risk or is unable to tolerate antidepressant medications. Confusion, a side effect of ECT that typically last a few minutes to several hours, is generally more pronounced in the elderly (Mayo Clinic, 2016b).

Other therapeutic approaches include interpersonal, behavioral, cognitive, group, and family psychotherapies. Appropriate treatment of the depressed elderly individual can bring relief from suffering and offer a new lease on life with a feeling of renewed productivity.

Postpartum Depression

The severity of depression in the postpartum period varies from a feeling of the blues, to moderate depression, to severe depression with psychotic features. About 50 percent of these episodes actually begin prior to delivery (APA, 2013), and the onset of symptoms during pregnancy, including the "baby blues," increases risk for major depression in the postpartum period. Major depression with psychotic features occurs in about 1 or 2 out of 1,000 postpartum women.

Symptoms of the baby blues include worry, sadness, and fatigue after having a baby. These symptoms affect about 80 percent of mothers and usually subside on their own within a week or two (NIH, 2016b).

Symptoms of moderate **postpartum depression** have been described as depressed mood varying from day to day, with more bad days than good, worsening toward evening and associated with fatigue, irritability, loss of appetite, sleep disturbances, and loss of libido. In addition, the new mother expresses a great deal of concern about her inability to care for her baby. These symptoms begin somewhat later than those attributable to the baby blues and take from a few weeks to several months to abate.

Postpartum depression with psychotic features is characterized by depressed mood, agitation, indecision, lack of concentration, guilt, and an abnormal attitude toward bodily functions. The symptoms can be severe and incapacitating. There may be lack of interest in or rejection of the baby or a morbid fear that the baby may be harmed, accompanied by delusions and hallucinations. Risks of suicide and infanticide should not be overlooked. There is a 30 to 50 percent likelihood of postpartum psychosis recurring with subsequent pregnancies (APA, 2013).

The etiology of postpartum depression remains unclear. Baby blues may be associated with hormonal changes, tryptophan metabolism, or alterations in membrane transport during the early postpartum period. Besides being exposed to these same somatic changes, the woman who experiences moderate to severe symptoms probably possesses a vulnerability to depression related to heredity, upbringing, early life experiences, personality, or social circumstances. A history of depression appears to be a risk factor for postpartum depression (Sword et al., 2012). The etiology of postpartum depression may very likely be a combination of hormonal, metabolic, and psychosocial influences.

Treatment of postpartum depression varies with the severity of the illness. Psychotic depression may be treated with antidepressant medication along with supportive psychotherapy, group therapy, and possibly family therapy. Moderate depression may be relieved with supportive psychotherapy and continuing assistance with home management until the symptoms subside. Baby blues usually needs no treatment beyond a word of reassurance from the physician or nurse that these feelings are common and will soon pass. Extra support and comfort from significant others also is important.

Application of the Nursing Process

Background Assessment Data

Symptomatology of depression can be viewed on a continuum from transient symptoms to severe depression according to severity of the illness. All individuals become depressed from time to time in response to life's disappointments, and these symptoms tend to be transient. Severe depression, however, is marked by significant distress that interferes with social, occupational, cognitive, and emotional functioning.

The individual who is severely depressed may also demonstrate a loss of contact with reality. This level is associated with a complete lack of pleasure in all activities, and ruminations about suicide are common. MDD is an example of severe depression. A continuum of depression is presented in Figure 25–3.

A number of assessment rating scales are available for measuring severity of depressive symptoms. Some are meant to be clinician administered, whereas others may be self-administered. Examples of self-rating scales include the Zung Self-Rating Depression Scale and the Beck Depression Inventory. One of the most widely used clinician-administered scales is the Hamilton Depression Rating Scale (HDRS). It has been reviewed and revised over the years and exists today in several versions. The original version (see Box 25–5) contains 17 items and is designed to measure mood, guilty feelings, suicidal ideation, sleep disturbances, anxiety levels, and weight loss.

Symptoms of depression can be described as alterations in four spheres of human functioning: (1) affective, (2) behavioral, (3) cognitive, and (4) physiological. Alterations within these spheres differ according to degree of severity of symptomatology.

Transient Depression

Symptoms at this level of the continuum are not necessarily dysfunctional; in fact, they may be considered part of the broad range of typical human emotional

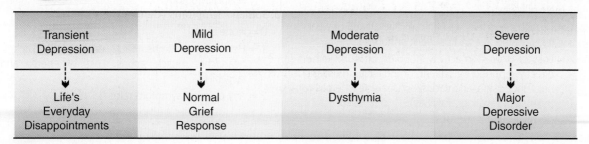

FIGURE 25–3   A continuum of depression.

BOX 25–5 Hamilton Depression Rating Scale (HDRS)

Instructions: For each item, circle the number to select the one "cue" that best characterizes the patient.

1. Depressed Mood (sadness, hopeless, helpless, worthless)

0 = Absent

1 = These feeling states indicated only on questioning

2 = These feeling states spontaneously reported verbally

3 = Communicates feeling states nonverbally, i.e., through facial expression, posture, voice, tendency to weep

4 = Patient reports virtually only these feeling states in spontaneous verbal and nonverbal communication

2. Feelings of Guilt

0 = Absent

1 = Self-reproach; feels he/she has let people down

2 = Ideas of guilt or rumination over past errors or sinful deeds

3 = Present illness is a punishment. Delusions of guilt

4 = Hears accusatory or denunciatory voices and/or experiences threatening visual hallucinations

3. Suicide

0 = Absent

1 = Feels life is not worth living

2 = Wishes he/she were dead or any thoughts of possible death to self

3 = Suicidal ideas or gesture

4 = Attempts at suicide (any serious attempt rates 4)

4. Insomnia: Early in the Night

0 = No difficulty falling asleep

1 = Complains of occasional difficulty falling asleep, i.e., more than 1/2 hour

2 = Complains of nightly difficulty falling asleep

5. Insomnia: Middle of the Night

0 = No difficulty

1 = Complains of being restless and disturbed during the night

2 = Waking during the night—any getting out of bed rates 2 (except for purposes of voiding)

6. Insomnia: Early Hours of the Morning

0 = No difficulty

1 = Waking in early hours of the morning, but goes back to sleep

2 = Unable to fall asleep again if he/she gets out of bed

7. Work and Activities

0 = No difficulty

1 = Thoughts and feelings of incapacity, fatigue, or weakness related to activities, work, or hobbies

2 = Loss of interest in activity, hobbies, or work—either directly reported by patient, or indirectly in listlessness, indecision, and vacillation (feels he/she has to push self to work or activities)

3 = Decrease in actual time spent in activities or decrease in productivity. Rate 3 if patient does not spend at least 3 hours a day in activities (job or hobbies), excluding routine chores

4 = Stopped working because of present illness. Rate 4 if patient engages in no activities except routine chose, or if does not perform routine chores unassisted

8. Psychomotor Retardation (slowness of thought and speech, impaired ability to concentrate, decreased motor activity)

0 = Normal speech and thought

1 = Slight retardation during the interview

2 = Obvious retardation during the interview

3 = Interview difficult

4 = Complete stupor

9. Agitation

0 = None

1 = Fidgetiness

2 = Playing with hands, hair, etc.

3 = Moving about, can't sit still

4 = Hand wringing, nail biting, hair pulling, biting of lips

10. Anxiety (Psychic)

0 = No difficulty

1 = Subjective tension and irritability

2 = Worrying about minor matters

3 = Apprehensive attitude apparent in face or speech

4 = Fears expressed without questioning

11. Anxiety (Somatic): Physiological concomitants of anxiety (e.g., dry mouth, indigestion, diarrhea, cramps, belching, palpitations, headache, tremor, hyperventilation, sighing, urinary frequency, sweating, flushing)

0 = Absent

1 = Mild

2 = Moderate

3 = Severe

4 = Incapacitating

12. Somatic Symptoms (Gastrointestinal)

0 = None

1 = Loss of appetite, but eating without encouragement. Heavy feelings in abdomen

2 = Difficulty eating without urging from others. Requests or requires medication for constipation or gastrointestinal symptoms

13. Somatic Symptoms (General)

0 = None

1 = Heaviness in limbs, back, or head. Backaches, headache, muscle aches. Loss of energy and fatigability

2 = Any clear-cut symptom rates 2

BOX 25–5 Hamilton Depression Rating Scale (HDRS)—cont'd

14. **Genital Symptoms** (e.g., loss of libido, impaired sexual performance, menstrual disturbances)
    0 = Absent
    1 = Mild
    2 = Severe
15. **Hypochondriasis**
    0 = Not present
    1 = Self-absorption (bodily)
    2 = Preoccupation with health
    3 = Frequent complaints, requests for help, etc.
    4 = Hypochondriacal delusions
16. **Loss of Weight** (Rate *either* A *or* B)
    A. **According to subjective patient history:**
       0 = No weight loss
       1 = Probably weight loss associated with present illness
       2 = Definite weight loss associated with present illness

B. **According to objective weekly measurements:**
    0 = Less than 1 lb weight loss in week
    1 = Greater than 1 lb weight loss in week
    2 = Greater than 2 lb weight loss in week
17. **Insight**
    0 = Acknowledges being depressed and ill
    1 = Acknowledges illness but attributes cause to bad food, climate, overwork, virus, need for rest, etc.
    2 = Denies being ill at all

SCORING:
    0–6 = No evidence of depressive illness
    7–17 = Mild depression
    18–24 = Moderate depression
    >24 = Severe depression

TOTAL SCORE_____

SOURCE: *Hamilton, M. (1960). A rating scale for depression.* Journal of Neurology, Neurosurgery, & Psychiatry, 23, *56-62. The HDRS is in the public domain.*

responses that accompany everyday disappointments in life. Transient depression subsides quickly, and the individual is able to refocus on other goals and achievements. Alterations include the following:

■ **Affective:** Sadness, dejection, feeling downhearted, having the blues
■ **Behavioral:** Some crying possible
■ **Cognitive:** Some difficulty getting mind off of one's disappointment
■ **Physiological:** Feeling tired and listless

Mild Depression

Symptoms at the mild level of depression are like those associated with uncomplicated grieving. Alterations at the mild level include the following:

■ **Affective:** Denial of feelings, anger, anxiety, guilt, helplessness, hopelessness, sadness, despondency
■ **Behavioral:** Tearfulness, regression, restlessness, agitation, withdrawal
■ **Cognitive:** Preoccupation with the loss, self-blame, ambivalence, blaming others
■ **Physiological:** Anorexia or overeating, insomnia or hypersomnia, headache, backache, chest pain, or other symptoms associated with the loss of a significant other

Moderate Depression

Dysthymia (also called persistent depressive disorder) is an example of moderate depression and represents a more problematic disturbance, which, according to the *DSM-5*, is characterized by symptoms that are enduring for at least 2 years (APA, 2013). Symptoms associated with this disorder include the following:

■ **Affective:** Feelings of sadness, dejection, helplessness, powerlessness, hopelessness; gloomy and pessimistic outlook; low self-esteem; difficulty experiencing pleasure in activities
■ **Behavioral:** Sluggish physical movements (i.e., psychomotor retardation); slumped posture; slowed speech; limited verbalizations, possibly consisting of ruminations about life's failures or regrets; social isolation with a focus on the self; increased use of substances possible; self-destructive behavior possible; decreased interest in personal hygiene and grooming
■ **Cognitive:** Slowed thinking processes; difficulty concentrating and directing attention; obsessive and repetitive thoughts, generally portraying pessimism and negativism; verbalizations and behavior reflecting suicidal ideation
■ **Physiological:** Anorexia or overeating; insomnia or hypersomnia; sleep disturbances; amenorrhea; decreased libido; headaches; backaches; chest pain; abdominal pain; low energy level; fatigue and listlessness; feeling best early in the morning and continually worse as the day progresses (possibly related to the diurnal variation in the level of neurotransmitters that affect mood and level of activity)

Severe Depression

Severe depression (also called major depressive disorder) is characterized by an intensification of the symptoms described for moderate depression (see Box 25–2). Symptoms at the severe level of depression include the following:

- **Affective:** Feelings of total despair, hopelessness, and worthlessness; flat (unchanging) affect, appearing devoid of emotional tone; prevalent feelings of nothingness and emptiness; apathy; loneliness; sadness; inability to feel pleasure.
- **Behavioral:** Psychomotor retardation so severe that physical movement may literally come to a standstill, or psychomotor behavior manifested by rapid, agitated, purposeless movements; slumped posture; sitting in a curled-up position; walking slowly and rigidly; virtually nonexistent communication (when verbalizations do occur, they may reflect delusional thinking); no personal hygiene and grooming; social isolation is common, with virtually no inclination toward interaction with others
- **Cognitive:** Prevalent delusional thinking, with delusions of persecution and somatic delusions being most common; confusion, indecisiveness, and an inability to concentrate; hallucinations reflecting misinterpretations of the environment; excessive self-deprecation, self-blame, and thoughts of suicide

NOTE: Because of the low energy level and slow thought processes, the individual may be unable to follow through on suicidal ideas. However, the desire is strong at this level.

- **Physiological:** A general slowdown of the entire body, reflected in sluggish digestion, constipation, and urinary retention; amenorrhea; impotence; diminished libido; anorexia; weight loss or weight gain associated with appetite changes; changes in sleep patterns, including difficulty falling asleep and awakening very early in the morning; feeling worse early in the morning and somewhat better as the day progresses (as with moderate depression, this may reflect the diurnal variation in the level of neurotransmitters that affect mood and activity)

Diagnosis and Outcome Identification

Using information collected during the assessment, the nurse completes the client database from which the selection of appropriate nursing diagnoses is determined. Table 25–1 presents a list of client behaviors and the NANDA-I nursing diagnoses that correspond to those behaviors, which may be used in planning care for the depressed client.

TABLE 25–1 Assigning Nursing Diagnoses to Behaviors Commonly Associated With Depression

BEHAVIORS	NURSING DIAGNOSES
Depressed mood; feelings of hopelessness and worthlessness; anger turned inward in the self; misinterpretations of reality; suicidal ideation, plan, and available means	Risk for suicide
Depression, preoccupation with thoughts of loss, self-blame, grief avoidance, inappropriate expression of anger, decreased functioning in life roles	Complicated grieving
Expressions of helplessness, uselessness, guilt, and shame; hypersensitivity to slight or criticism; negative, pessimistic outlook; lack of eye contact; self-negating verbalizations	Low self-esteem
Apathy, verbal expressions of having no control, dependence on others to fulfill needs	Powerlessness
Expresses anger toward God, expresses lack of meaning in life, sudden changes in spiritual practices, refuses interactions with significant others or with spiritual leaders	Spiritual distress
Withdrawn, uncommunicative, seeks to be alone, dysfunctional interaction with others, discomfort in social situations	Social isolation/Impaired social interaction
Inappropriate thinking, confusion, difficulty concentrating, impaired problem-solving ability, inaccurate interpretation of environment, memory deficit	Disturbed thought processes*
Weight loss, poor muscle tone, pale conjunctiva and mucous membranes, poor skin turgor, weakness	Imbalanced nutrition: Less than body requirements
Difficulty falling asleep, difficulty staying asleep, lack of energy, difficulty concentrating, verbal reports of not feeling well rested	Insomnia
Uncombed hair, disheveled clothing, offensive body odor	Self-care deficit (hygiene, grooming)

*This diagnosis has been resigned from the NANDA-I list of approved diagnoses. It is used in this instance because it is most compatible with the identified behaviors.

Outcome Criteria

The following criteria may be used for measurement of outcomes in the care of the depressed client.

The client:

- Has experienced no physical harm to self
- Discusses feelings with staff and family members
- Expresses hopefulness
- Sets realistic goals for self
- Is no longer afraid to attempt new activities
- Is able to identify aspects of self-control over life situation
- Expresses personal satisfaction and support from spiritual practices
- Interacts willingly and appropriately with others
- Is able to maintain reality orientation
- Is able to concentrate, reason, solve problems, and make decisions
- Eats a well-balanced diet with snacks, to prevent weight loss and maintain nutritional status
- Sleeps 6 to 8 hours per night and reports feeling well rested
- Bathes, washes and combs hair, and dresses in clean clothing without assistance

Planning and Implementation

The following section presents a group of selected nursing diagnoses, with short- and long-term goals and nursing interventions for each.

Some institutions use a case management model to coordinate care (see Chapter 9, The Nursing Process in Psychiatric-Mental Health Nursing, for more detailed explanation). In case management models, the plan of care may take the form of a critical pathway.

Risk for Suicide

Risk for suicide is defined as "vulnerable to self-inflicted, life-threatening injury" (Herdman & Kamitsuru, 2014, p. 417). For additional information on interventions for this diagnosis see Chapter 17, Suicide Prevention.

Client Goals

Outcome criteria include short- and long-term goals. Time lines are individually determined.

Short-term goals

- Client will seek out staff when feeling urge to harm self.
- Client will not harm self.

Long-term goal

- Client will not harm self.

Interventions

- Create a safe environment for the client. Remove all potentially harmful objects from client's access (sharp objects, straps, belts, ties, glass items, alcohol).

Supervise closely during meals and medication administration. Perform room searches as deemed necessary.

> **CLINICAL PEARL**
>
> Ask the client directly, "Have you thought about killing yourself?" or "Have you thought about harming yourself in any way?" "If so, what do you plan to do? Do you have the means to carry out this plan?" "How strong are your intentions to die?" The risk of suicide is greatly increased if the client has developed a plan, has strong intentions, and especially if means exist for the client to execute the plan.

- Assess frequently for the presence and lethality risk of suicidal ideation. The intensity of suicide ideation can change over the course of hours or days, so it is important to assess subjective and objective data to evaluate current risk. Discussion of suicidal feelings with a trusted individual provides some relief to the client.
- Convey an attitude of unconditional acceptance of the client as a worthwhile individual. (See Chapter 17 for more detailed information about relevant assessment and intervention strategies.)
- Encourage the client to actively participate in establishing a safety plan. (See Chapter 17 for guidelines on establishing safety plans). Suicidal clients are often very ambivalent about their feelings. Discussion of strategies for maintaining safety with a trusted individual may provide assistance before the client experiences a crisis situation.

> **CLINICAL PEARL** Be direct. Talk openly and matter-of-factly about suicide. Listen actively and encourage expression of feelings, including anger. Accept the client's feelings in a nonjudgmental manner.

- Maintain close observation of the client. Depending on level of suicide precaution, provide one-to-one contact, constant visual observation, or checks at least every 15 minutes conducted at irregular intervals. Place the client in a room close to the nurse's station; do not assign to a private room. Accompany the client to off-ward activities if attendance is indicated and, if necessary, to the bathroom. Close observation is necessary to ensure that the client does not harm self in any way. Being alert for suicidal and escape attempts facilitates being able to prevent or interrupt harmful behavior.
- Maintain special care in administration of medications. This prevents saving up to overdose or discarding and not taking.
- Make rounds at frequent, *irregular* intervals (especially at night, toward early morning, at change of shift, or other predictably busy times for staff). This prevents staff surveillance from becoming

predictable. Awareness of client's location is important, especially when staff is busy, unavailable, or less observable.

■ Encourage verbalizations of honest feelings. Through exploration and discussion, help the client identify symbols of hope in his or her life.

■ Encourage the client to express angry feelings within appropriate limits. Provide a safe method of hostility release. Help the client identify the true source of anger and work on adaptive coping skills for use outside the treatment setting. Depression and suicidal behaviors may be viewed as anger turned inward on the self. If this anger can be verbalized in a nonthreatening environment, the client may be able to eventually resolve these feelings.

■ Identify community resources that the client may use as a support system and from whom he or she may request help if feeling suicidal once discharged from the hospital. Having a concrete plan for seeking assistance during a crisis may discourage or prevent self-destructive behaviors.

■ Orient the client to reality, as required. Point out sensory misperceptions or misinterpretations of the environment. Take care not to belittle the client's fears or indicate disapproval of verbal expressions.

■ Most importantly, spend time with client. This provides a feeling of safety and security while also conveying the message, "I want to spend time with you because I think you are a worthwhile person."

Complicated Grieving

Complicated grieving is defined as "a disorder that occurs after the death of a significant other [or any other loss of significance to the individual], in which the experience of distress accompanying bereavement fails to follow normative expectations and manifests in functional impairment" (Herdman & Kamitsuru, p. 339). Table 25–2 presents this nursing diagnosis in care plan format.

Client Goals

Outcome criteria include short- and long-term goals. Time lines are individually determined.

Short-term goals

■ Client will express anger about the loss.
■ Client will identify coping strategies and rational thought patterns in response to loss.

Table 25–2 | CARE PLAN FOR THE DEPRESSED CLIENT

NURSING DIAGNOSIS: COMPLICATED GRIEVING

RELATED TO: Real or perceived loss, bereavement overload

EVIDENCED BY: Denial of loss, inappropriate expression of anger, idealization of or obsession with lost object, inability to carry out activities of daily living

OUTCOME CRITERIA	NURSING INTERVENTIONS	RATIONALE
Short-Term Goals: • Client expresses anger about the loss. • Client verbalizes behaviors associated with normal grieving. Long-Term Goal: • Client is able to recognize his or her own position in the grief process while progressing at own pace toward resolution.	1. Determine the stage of grief in which client is fixed. Identify behaviors associated with this stage. 2. Develop a trusting relationship with client. Show empathy, concern, and unconditional positive regard. Be honest and keep all promises. 3. Convey an accepting attitude, and enable client to express feelings openly. 4. Encourage client to express anger. Do not become defensive if the initial expression of anger is displaced on the nurse or therapist. Help client explore angry feelings so that they may be directed toward the actual intended person or situation.	1. Accurate baseline assessment data are necessary to effectively plan care for the grieving client. 2. Trust is the basis for a therapeutic relationship. 3. An accepting attitude conveys to client that you believe he or she is a worthwhile person. Trust is enhanced. 4. Verbalization of feelings in a nonthreatening environment may help client come to terms with unresolved issues.

Table 25–2 | CARE PLAN FOR THE DEPRESSED CLIENT–cont'd

OUTCOME CRITERIA	NURSING INTERVENTIONS	RATIONALE
	5. Help client to discharge pent-up anger through participation in large motor activities (e.g., brisk walks, jogging, physical exercises, volleyball, punching bag, exercise bike).	5. Physical exercise provides a safe and effective method for discharging pent-up tension.
	6. Teach the normal stages of grief and behaviors associated with each stage. Help client to understand that feelings such as guilt and anger toward the lost concept are appropriate and acceptable during the grief process and should be expressed rather than held inside.	6. Knowledge of acceptability of the feelings associated with normal grieving may help to relieve some of the guilt that these responses generate.
	7. Encourage client to review the relationship with the lost concept. With support and sensitivity, point out the reality of the situation in areas where misrepresentations are expressed.	7. Client must give up an idealized perception and be able to accept both positive and negative aspects about the lost concept before the grief process is complete.
	8. Communicate to client that crying is acceptable. Use of touch may also be therapeutic.	8. Some cultures believe it is important to remain stoic and refrain from crying openly. Individuals from certain cultures are uncomfortable with touch. It is important to be aware of cultural influences before employing these interventions.
	9. Encourage client to reach out for spiritual support during this time in whatever form is desirable to him or her. Assess spiritual needs of client, and assist as necessary in the fulfillment of those needs.	9. Client may find comfort in religious rituals with which he or she is familiar.

Long-term goal

■ Client will be able to recognize his or her own position in the grief process while progressing at own pace toward resolution.

Interventions

■ Determine the stage of grief in which the client is fixed. Identify behaviors associated with this stage. It is important to obtain accurate baseline assessment data to effectively plan care for the grieving client.

■ Develop a trusting relationship with the client. Show empathy, concern, and unconditional positive regard. Be honest and keep all promises. Convey an accepting attitude, and encourage the client to express feelings openly.

■ Encourage the client to express anger. Do not become defensive if the initial expression of anger is displaced on the nurse or therapist. Help the client explore angry feelings so that the feelings may be directed toward the actual intended person or situation.

■ Help the client to discharge pent-up anger through participation in large motor activities (e.g., brisk walks, jogging, physical exercises, volleyball, punching bag, exercise bike). Physical exercise provides a safe and effective method for discharging pent-up tension.

■ Teach the stages of grief and behaviors associated with each stage. Help the client understand that feelings such as guilt and anger toward the lost concept/entity are appropriate and acceptable during the grief process and should be expressed rather than held inside. Knowledge of acceptability of the feelings associated with grieving may help relieve some of the guilt that these responses generate.

■ Encourage the client to review the relationship with the lost concept/entity. With support and sensitivity, point out the reality of the situation in areas where misrepresentations are expressed. The client must give up an idealized perception and be able to accept both positive and negative aspects about the lost concept/entity before the grief process is complete.

■ Communicate to the client that crying is acceptable. This can be accomplished by verbal reassurance and, in some cases, with caring touch. Use of touch must also consider cultural influences and trauma history before including this as part of the intervention.

■ Assist the client in problem-solving as he or she attempts to determine methods for more adaptive coping with the experienced loss. Provide positive feedback for strategies identified and decisions made.

■ Encourage the client to reach out for spiritual support during this time in whatever form is desirable to him or her. Assess spiritual needs of the client and assist as necessary in the fulfillment of those needs. (See Chapter 6, Cultural and Spiritual Concepts Relevant to Psychiatric-Mental Health Nursing, for more information about spiritual assessment and interventions.)

■ Encourage the client to attend a support group of individuals who are experiencing life situations similar to his or her own. Help the client to locate a group of this type.

Low Self-Esteem/Self-Care Deficit

Low self-esteem is defined as "negative self-evaluating/feelings about self or self-capabilities [either long-standing or in response to a current situation]" (Herdman & Kamitsuru, pp. 271–274). *Self-care deficit* is defined as "impaired ability to perform or complete [activities of daily living (ADLs)] for self" (Herdman & Kamitsuru, 2014, pp. 242–245).

Client Goals

Short-term goals

■ Client will verbalize attributes he or she likes about self.
■ Client will participate in activities of daily living (ADLs) with assistance from health-care provider.

Long-term goals

■ By time of discharge from treatment, the client will exhibit increased feelings of self-worth as

evidenced by verbal expression of positive aspects of self, past accomplishments, and future prospects.

■ By time of discharge from treatment, the client will exhibit increased feelings of self-worth by setting realistic goals and trying to reach them, thereby demonstrating a decrease in fear of failure.

■ By time of discharge from treatment, the client will satisfactorily accomplish ADLs independently.

Interventions

■ Be accepting of the client, and spend time with him or her even though pessimism and negativism may seem objectionable. Focus on strengths and accomplishments and minimize failures.

■ Promote attendance in therapy groups that offer the client simple methods of accomplishment. Encourage the client to be as independent as possible.

■ Encourage the client to recognize areas of change and provide assistance toward this effort.

■ Teach assertiveness techniques: the ability to recognize the differences among passive, assertive, and aggressive behaviors and the importance of respecting the human rights of others while protecting one's own basic human rights. Self-esteem is enhanced by the ability to interact with others in an assertive manner.

■ Teach effective communication techniques, such as the use of "I" messages.

■ Emphasize ways to avoid making judgmental statements.

■ Encourage independence in the performance of ADLs, but intervene when client is unable to perform.

> **CLINICAL PEARL**
>
> **Offer recognition and positive reinforcement for independent accomplishments. (Example: "Mrs. J., I see you have put on a clean dress and combed your hair.")**

■ Show the client how to perform activities with which he or she is having difficulty. When a client is depressed, he or she may require simple, concrete demonstrations of activities that would be performed without difficulty under normal conditions.

■ Keep strict records of food and fluid intake. Offer nutritious snacks and fluids between meals. The client may be unable to tolerate large amounts of food at mealtimes and may therefore require additional nourishment at other times during the day to receive adequate nutrition.

■ Before bedtime, provide nursing measures that promote sleep, such as back rub; warm bath; warm, nonstimulating drinks; soft music; and relaxation exercises.

Powerlessness

Powerlessness is defined as "the lived experience of lack of control over a situation, including a perception that one's actions do not significantly affect an outcome" (Herdman & Kamitsuru, 2014, p. 343).

Client Goals

Short-term goal

■ Client will participate in decision-making regarding own care within 5 days.

Long-term goal

■ Client will be able to effectively problem-solve ways to take control of his or her life situation by time of discharge from treatment, thereby decreasing feelings of powerlessness.

Interventions

■ Encourage the client to take as much responsibility as possible for his or her own self-care practices. In the most acute stage of severe depression, clients may have extreme difficulty making decisions. At this point, it may be more helpful to use *active communication* to help the client accomplish even basic ADLs. For example, "It's time to eat lunch," rather than, "Would you like to eat lunch now?" Ongoing assessment is important so that the client can be encouraged to make choices as soon as possible. Providing the client with choices whenever possible will increase feelings of control. For example,
  ▪ Include the client in setting the goals of care he or she wishes to achieve.
  ▪ Allow the client to establish own schedule for self-care activities.
  ▪ Provide the client with privacy as need is determined.
  ▪ Provide positive feedback for decisions made. Respect the client's right to make those decisions independently, and refrain from attempting to influence him or her toward those that may seem more logical.

■ Help the client set realistic goals. Unrealistic goals set the client up for failure and reinforce feelings of powerlessness.

■ Help the client identify areas of his or her life situation that can be controlled. The client's emotional condition interferes with his or her ability to solve problems. Assistance is required to perceive the benefits and consequences of available alternatives accurately.

■ Discuss with the client areas of life that are not within his or her ability to control. Encourage verbalization of feelings related to this inability in an effort to deal with unresolved issues and accept what cannot be changed.

Concept Care Mapping

The concept map care plan is an approach to planning and organizing nursing care (see Chapter 9) that allows visualization of interrelationships between medical diagnoses, nursing diagnoses, assessment data, and treatments. An example of a concept map care plan for a client with depression is presented in Figure 25–4.

Client and Family Education

The role of client teacher is important in the psychiatric area, as it is in all areas of nursing. A list of topics for client and family education relevant to depression is presented in Box 25–6.

Evaluation of Care for the Depressed Client

In the final step of the nursing process, a reassessment is conducted to determine if the nursing actions have been successful in achieving the objectives of care. Evaluation of the nursing actions for the depressed client may be facilitated by gathering information using the following types of questions:

■ Has self-harm to the individual been avoided?

■ Have suicidal ideations subsided?

■ Does the individual know where to seek assistance outside the hospital when suicidal thoughts occur?

■ Has the client discussed the recent loss with staff and family members?

■ Is he or she able to verbalize feelings and behaviors associated with each stage of the grieving process and recognize own position in the process?

■ Has obsession with and idealization of the lost object subsided?

■ Is anger toward the lost object expressed appropriately?

■ Does the client set realistic goals for self?

■ Is he or she able to verbalize positive aspects about self, past accomplishments, and future prospects, including a desire to live?

■ Can the client identify areas of life situation over which he or she has control?

■ Is the client able to participate in usual religious practices and feel satisfaction and support from them?

■ Is the client seeking out interaction with others in an appropriate manner?

■ Does the client maintain reality orientation with no evidence of delusional thinking?

■ Is he or she able to concentrate and make decisions concerning own self-care?

■ Is the client selecting and consuming foods sufficiently high in nutrients and calories to maintain weight and nutritional status?

■ Does the client sleep without difficulty and wake feeling rested?

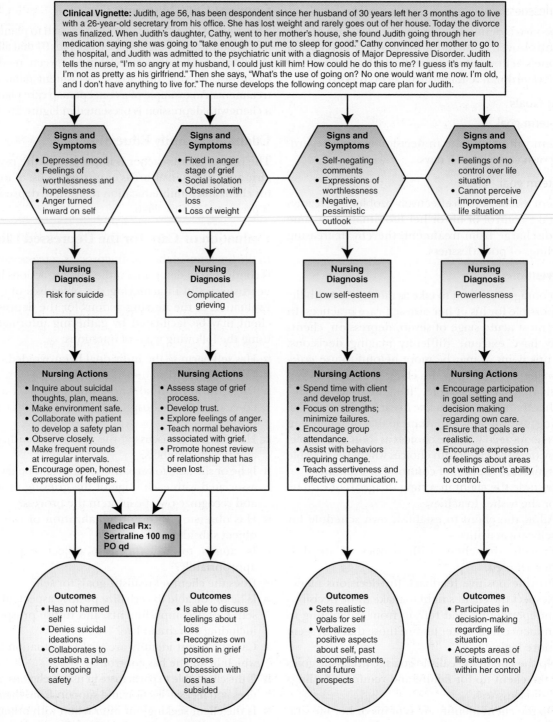

FIGURE 25–4 Concept map care plan for a client with depression.

■ Does the client show pride in appearance by attending to personal hygiene and grooming?
■ Have somatic complaints subsided?

Quality and Safety Education for Nurses (QSEN)

Health Professions Education: A Bridge to Quality (Institute of Medicine, 2003) challenged faculties of medicine,

nursing, and other health professions to ensure that their graduates have achieved a core set of competencies in order to meet the needs of the 21st-century healthcare system. These competencies include *providing patient-centered care, working in interdisciplinary teams, maintaining safety, employing evidence-based practice, applying quality improvement,* and *utilizing informatics.* A QSEN teaching strategy is included in Box 25–7. This type of activity is

BOX 25–6 Topics for Client and Family Education Related to Depression

NATURE OF THE ILLNESS
1. Stages of grief and symptoms associated with each stage
2. What is depression?
3. Why do people get depressed?
4. What are the symptoms of depression?

MANAGEMENT OF THE ILLNESS
1. Medication management
   a. Nuisance side effects
   b. Side effects to report to physician
   c. Importance of taking regularly
   d. Length of time to take effect
   e. Diet (related to MAO Inhibitors)
2. Assertiveness techniques
3. Stress-management techniques
4. Ways to increase self-esteem
5. Electroconvulsive therapy

SUPPORT SERVICES
1. Suicide hotline
2. Support groups
3. Legal and/or financial assistance

intended to arm the instructor and student with guidelines for attaining the knowledge, skills, and attitudes necessary for achievement of quality and safety competencies in nursing.

Treatment Modalities for Depression

Individual Psychotherapy

Research has documented both the importance of close and satisfactory attachments in the prevention of depression and the role of disrupted attachments in the development of depression. With this concept in mind, interpersonal psychotherapy focuses on the client's current interpersonal relations. Interpersonal psychotherapy with the depressed person proceeds through three phases and interventions.

Phase I

During the first phase, the client is assessed to determine the extent of the illness. Complete information is given to the individual regarding the nature of depression, symptom pattern, frequency, clinical course, and alternative treatments. If the level of depression is severe, interpersonal psychotherapy has been shown

BOX 25–7 QSEN TEACHING STRATEGY

Assignment: Staff Workarounds
Placing a Client on Suicide Precautions

Competency Domains: Evidence-Based Practice; Patient-Centered Care; Quality Improvement; Safety; Teamwork and Collaboration

Learning Objectives: Student will:
• Demonstrate skills in identifying gaps between practice on the unit and what has been identified as best practice.
• Demonstrate skills at finding professional practice standards and research literature related to placing a client on suicide precautions.
• Demonstrate skills in accounting for patient preferences within the boundaries of safe and therapeutic practice.
• Demonstrate attitudes and behaviors that show that they value teamwork and want to contribute to maintaining standards of safe and effective care.

Strategy Overview: This assignment is meant to familiarize the student with standardized nursing policies, procedures, standards of care, and other evidence-based nursing practice guidelines and to encourage students to observe actual nursing practice on the units to note compliance with, deviations from, or "workarounds" for those policies, procedures, standards, and guidelines by registered nurses (RNs) when implementing nursing procedures. The following aspects of the assignment can guide students in preparation for clinical conference discussion, in writing a paper, or in putting together a poster presentation.

1. Identify a need to place a client on suicide precautions.
2. Find the current written nursing policy or procedure in place for your institution or unit, and answer these questions:
   a. How easy or difficult was it to find the policy/procedure?
   b. Did the RNs know where to find the written policy/procedure?
   c. How was the policy/procedure originally disseminated to the staff?
   d. Is the policy/procedure evidence based?
      (Review the current practice standards from professional organizations and/or oversight and accreditation groups [e.g., The Joint Commission, CDC] and/or the research literature.)

continued

BOX 25–7 QSEN TEACHING STRATEGY—cont'd

3. Observe RNs on the unit putting a client on suicide precautions and describe:
   a. What steps the RN took.
   b. In what ways the RN deviated from the written policy/procedure.
   c. What prompted the RN to make the deviations she or he made.
   d. As many details as you can recollect.
4. Discuss why RNs may or may not follow the institution's written policies and procedures. Reflect on the opportunities and challenges of evidence-based practice and the implementation into actual bedside nursing practice.
5. Discuss what the proper response should be when you, as an RN, discover unsafe practice that deviates from standards, policies, or procedures.

Adapted from teaching strategy submitted by Lisa Day, Assistant Clinical Professor, UCSF, School of Nursing, San Francisco, CA. © 2009 QSEN; http://qsen.org. With permission.

more effective if conducted in combination with antidepressant medication. The client is encouraged to continue working and participating in regular activities during therapy. A mutually agreeable therapeutic contract is negotiated.

Phase II

Treatment at this phase focuses on helping the client resolve complicated grief reactions. This may include resolving the ambivalence with a lost relationship and assistance with establishing new relationships. Other areas of treatment focus may include interpersonal disputes between the client and a significant other, difficult role transitions at various developmental life cycles, and correction of interpersonal deficits that may interfere with the client's ability to initiate or sustain interpersonal relationships.

Phase III

During the final phase of interpersonal psychotherapy, the therapeutic alliance is terminated. With emphasis on reassurance, clarification of emotional states, improvement of interpersonal communication, testing of perceptions, and performance in interpersonal settings, interpersonal psychotherapy has been successful in helping depressed persons recover enhanced social functioning.

Group Therapy

Group therapy forms an important dimension of multimodal treatment for the depressed client. Once an acute phase of the illness has passed, groups can provide an atmosphere in which individuals may discuss issues in their lives that cause, maintain, or arise from having a serious affective disorder. The element of peer support provides a feeling of security, as troublesome or embarrassing issues are discussed and resolved. Some groups have other specific purposes, such as helping to monitor medication-related issues or serving as an avenue for promoting education related to the affective disorder and its treatment. Therapy

groups help members gain a sense of perspective on their condition and encourage them to link up with others who have common problems. A sense of hope is conveyed when the individual is able to see that he or she is not alone or unique in experiencing affective illness.

Self-help groups offer another avenue of support for the depressed client. These groups are usually peer led and are not meant to substitute for or compete with professional therapy. Rather, they offer supplementary support that frequently enhances compliance with the medical regimen. Examples of self-help groups are the Depression and Bipolar Support Alliance (DBSA), Depressives Anonymous, Recovery International, and GriefShare (grief recovery support groups). Although self-help groups are not psychotherapy groups, they do provide important adjunctive support experiences, which often have therapeutic benefit for participants.

Family Therapy

The ultimate objectives in working with families of clients with mood disorders are to resolve the symptoms and initiate or restore adaptive family functioning. Similar to group therapy, the most effective approach appears to be a combination of psychotherapeutic and pharmacotherapeutic treatments. Sadock and associates (2015) stated:

> Family therapy is indicated if the disorder jeopardizes the patient's marriage or family functioning or if the mood disorder is promoted or maintained by the family situation. Family therapy examines the role of the mood-disordered member in the overall psychological well-being of the whole family; it also examines the role of the entire family in the maintenance of the patient's symptoms. (p. 373)

Cognitive Therapy

In cognitive therapy, the individual is taught to control thought distortions that are a factor in the development and maintenance of mood disorders. In the cognitive model, depression is characterized by a triad of negative distortions related to expectations of the environment, self, and future. The environment and activities within it are viewed as unsatisfying, the self is unrealistically devalued, and the future is perceived as hopeless.

The general goals in cognitive therapy are to obtain symptom relief as quickly as possible, assist the client in identifying dysfunctional patterns of thinking and behaving, and guide the client to evidence and logic that effectively tests the validity of the dysfunctional thinking (see Chapter 19, Cognitive Therapy). Therapy focuses on changing "automatic thoughts" that occur spontaneously and contribute to the distorted affect. Following are examples of automatic thoughts that may be common cognitive distortions in depression:

■ **Personalizing:** "I'm the only one who failed."
■ **All or nothing:** "I'm a complete failure."
■ **Mind reading:** "He thinks I'm foolish."
■ **Discounting positives:** "The other questions were so easy. Any dummy could have gotten them right."

The client is asked to describe evidence that both supports and disputes the automatic thought. The logic underlying the inferences is then reviewed with the client. Another technique involves evaluating what would most likely happen if the client's automatic thoughts were true. Implications of the consequences are then discussed.

Clients should not become discouraged if one technique seems not to be working. No single technique works with all clients. He or she should be reassured that any of a number of techniques may be used, and both therapist and client may explore these possibilities.

Cognitive therapy has offered encouraging results in the treatment of depression. In fact, the results of several studies with depressed clients show that in some cases cognitive therapy may be equally as or even more effective than antidepressant medication (Amick et al., 2015; Page & Hooke, 2012; Siddique et al., 2012).

Electroconvulsive Therapy

ECT is the induction of a grand mal (generalized) seizure through the application of electrical current to the brain. ECT is effective with clients who are acutely suicidal and in the treatment of severe depression, particularly in those clients who are also experiencing psychotic symptoms and those with psychomotor retardation and neurovegetative changes, such as disturbances in sleep, appetite, and energy. It is often considered for treatment only after a trial of therapy with antidepressant medication has proved ineffective (see Chapter 20, Electroconvulsive Therapy, for a detailed discussion of ECT).

Transcranial Magnetic Stimulation

Transcranial magnetic stimulation (TMS) is a procedure that is used to treat depression by stimulating nerve cells in the brain. TMS involves the use of very short pulses of magnetic energy to stimulate nerve cells at localized areas in the cerebral cortex, similar to the electrical activity observed with ECT. However, unlike with ECT, the electrical waves generated by TMS do not result in generalized seizure activity (George, Taylor, & Short, 2013). The waves are passed through a coil placed on the scalp to areas of the brain involved in mood regulation. It is noninvasive and considered generally safe. A typical course of treatment is 40-minute sessions, three to five times a week for 4 to 6 weeks (Raposelli, 2015). Some clinicians believe that TMS holds a great deal of promise in the treatment of depression, whereas others remain skeptical. In a study at King's College in London, researchers compared the efficacy of TMS with ECT in the treatment of severe depression (Eranti et al., 2007). They concluded that ECT is substantially more effective for the short-term treatment of depression and indicated the need for further intense clinical evaluation of TMS. In one study (Connolly et al., 2012), identified that 24.7 percent of patients receiving TMS were in remission at 6 weeks. Effectiveness ratings for ECT have varied from 17 to 70 percent. Although the effectiveness ratings may seem small or highly variable, both treatments provide an option for clients who are otherwise treatment-resistant. Magnezi and associates (2016) compared ECT to TMS and found that although ECT was more effective than TMS and additionally relieved anxiety symptoms, ECT had a much higher incidence (60%) of adverse effects, mostly related to memory loss. From the client's perspective, TMS was still deemed preferable to ECT (if it was covered by insurance), which may be related to the stigma associated with ECT.

George and associates (2013) stated:

> Since FDA approval, TMS has been generally safe and well tolerated with a low incidence of treatment discontinuation, and the therapeutic effects once obtained appear at least as durable as other antidepressant treatments. TMS also shows promise in several other psychiatric disorders, particularly treating acute and chronic pain. (p. 17)

More recently, researchers compared TMS to pharmacotherapy and found both effective but identified TMS as more cost effective (Raposelli, 2015). Currently, not all insurance companies cover this treatment, so from the client's standpoint, it may be a more expensive alternative. Raposelli reports that up to 40 percent of clients with MDD do not respond to pharmacotherapy, so again, alternatives such as ECT and TMS may offer hope of recovery for treatment-resistant conditions.

Vagal Nerve Stimulation and Deep Brain Stimulation

When studied in the treatment of epilepsy, vagal nerve stimulation (VNS) was found to improve the client's mood. This treatment involves implanting an electronic device in the skin to stimulate the vagus nerve. The mechanism of action is not known, but preliminary studies have shown that many clients with chronic recurrent depression improved when treated with VNS (Sadock et al., 2015). Trials are ongoing to determine its effectiveness.

Another new approach is deep brain stimulation (DBS), a form of psychosurgery. In this procedure, as in VNS, an electrode is implanted with the intent of stimulating brain function. Unlike VNS, however, DBS involves a deep implant that requires craniotomy. DBS has been well studied to determine its safety and effectiveness for other conditions, and controlled trials are ongoing. Currently, DBS is reserved for clients with severe, incapacitating depression or obsessive-compulsive disorder who have not responded to any more conservative treatments (Sadock et al., 2015).

Light Therapy

The prevalence of depression with a seasonal pattern is reported to be up to 10 percent but varies on the basis of geographic location (Kurlansik & Ibay, 2013). The *DSM*-5 identifies this disorder as Major Depressive Disorder, Recurrent, With Seasonal Pattern. It has commonly been known as seasonal affective disorder (SAD).

Theories suggest that SAD is related to the presence of the hormone melatonin (Cotterell, 2010), which is produced by the pineal gland. Melatonin plays a role in the regulation of biological rhythms for sleep and activation. It is produced during the cycle of darkness and shuts off in the light of day. During the months of longer darkness hours, there is increased production of melatonin, which seems to trigger the symptoms of SAD in susceptible people. Other research has pointed to seasonal serotonin transporter fluctuations associated with variation in exposure to daylight (McMahon et al., 2016).

Light therapy, or exposure to light, has been shown an effective treatment for SAD. The light therapy is administered by a 10,000-lux light box, which contains white fluorescent light tubes covered with a plastic screen that blocks ultraviolet rays. The individual sits in front of the box with eyes open (although one should not look directly into the light). Therapy usually begins with 10- to 15-minute sessions and gradually progresses to 30 to 45 minutes. The mechanism of action is believed to be related to retinal stimulation, which triggers a reduction of melatonin and an increase in serotonin in the brain (Rodriguez, 2015). A recent study demonstrated benefits of bright light therapy in nonseasonal affective disorders as well (Lam et al., 2015). Some people notice improvement rapidly, within a few days, whereas others may take several weeks to feel better. Side effects appear to be dosage related and include headache, eyestrain, nausea, irritability, photophobia (eye sensitivity to light), or insomnia agitation, but these are usually mild and short-lived (Kurlansik & Ibay, 2013). Light therapy and antidepressants have shown comparable efficacy in studies of SAD treatment. One study compared the efficacy of light therapy for SAD to daily treatment with 20 mg of fluoxetine (Lam et al., 2015). The authors concluded, "Light treatment showed earlier response onset and lower rate of some adverse events relative to fluoxetine, but there were no other significant differences in outcome between light therapy and antidepressant medication" (p. 805). Although improvement is often noted within 2 weeks, most clients relapse in the short term. Treatment should therefore be continued until an expected time of spontaneous remission, such as the change in season to spring or summer (Kurlansik & Ibay, 2013).

Psychopharmacology

Antidepressant medication is generally considered first-line treatment for severe clinical depression and is used in the treatment of other depressive disorders. These include tricyclic, tetracyclic, monoamine oxidase inhibitors (MAOIs), SSRIs, SNRIs, and SSRI/SNRI combination drugs. Examples of commonly used antidepressant medications are presented in Table 25–3. A detailed description of these medications can be found in Chapter 4, Psychopharmacology. In addition to the side effects and safety issues addressed in Chapter 4, it is important to highlight that antidepressant medication can be lethal in overdose, so depressed, suicidal patients must be observed closely and suicide risk assessed frequently in the use of this treatment modality.

> **CLINICAL PEARL** All antidepressants carry an FDA black-box warning for increased risk of suicidality in children and adolescents.

> **CLINICAL PEARL** As antidepressant drugs take effect and mood begins to lift, the individual may have increased energy with which to implement a suicide plan. Suicide potential often increases as level of depression decreases. The nurse should be particularly alert to sudden lifts in mood.

TABLE 25-3 Medications Used in the Treatment of Depression

CHEMICAL CLASS	GENERIC (TRADE) NAME*	PREGNANCY CATEGORIES/ HALF-LIFE (hr)	DAILY ADULT DOSAGE RANGE (mg)†	THERAPEUTIC PLASMA RANGES
Tricyclics	Amitriptyline	D/ 31–46	50–300	110–250 (including metabolite)
	Amoxapine	C/ 8	50–300	200–500
	Clomipramine (Anafranil)	C/ 19–37	25–250	80–100
	Desipramine (Norpramin)	C/ 12–24	25–300	125–300
	Doxepin	C/ 8–24	25–300	100–200 (including metabolite)
	Imipramine (Tofranil)	D/ 11–25	30–300	200–350 (including metabolite)
	Nortriptyline (Aventyl; Pamelor)	D/ 18–44	30–100	50–150
	Protriptyline (Vivactil)	C/ 67–89	15–60	100–200
	Trimipramine (Surmontil)	C/ 7–30	50–300	180 (including metabolite)
Selective Serotonin Reuptake Inhibitors (SSRIs)	Citalopram (Celexa)	C/ ~35	20–40	Not well established
	Escitalopram (Lexapro)	C/ 27–32	10–20	Not well established
	Fluoxetine (Prozac; Sarafem)	C/ 1–16 days (including metabolite)	20–80	Not well established
	Fluvoxamine (Luvox)	C/ 13.6–15.6	50–300	Not well established
	Paroxetine (Paxil)	D/ 21 (CR: 15–20)	10–50 (CR: 12.5–75)	Not well established
	Sertraline (Zoloft)	C/ 26–104 (including metabolite)	25–200	Not well established
	Vilazodone (Viibryd) (also acts as a partial serotonergic agonist)	C/ 25	40	Not well established
	Vortioxetine (Trintellix)	C/ 66	5–20	Not well established
Monoamine Oxidase Inhibitors	Isocarboxazid (Marplan)	C/ Not established	20–60	Not well established
	Phenelzine (Nardil)	C/ 2–3	45–90	Not well established
	Tranylcypromine (Parnate)	C/ 2.4–2.8	30–60	Not well established
	Selegiline Transdermal System (Emsam)	C/ 18–25 (including metabolites)	6/24-hr– 12/24-hr patch	Not well established
Atypical Antidepressants	Bupropion (Wellbutrin, Zyban)		200–450	Not well established
	Forfivo XL		450	
	Maprotiline	B/ 21–25	25–225	200–300 (including metabolite)
	Mirtazapine (Remeron)	C/ 20–40	15–45	Not well established
	Nefazodone‡ (Serzone)	C/ 2–4	200–600	Not well established
	Trazodone	C/ 4–9	150–600	800–1,600
Serotonin- Norepinephrine Reuptake Inhibitors (SNRIs)	Desvenlafaxine (Pristiq)	C/ 11	50–400	Not well established
	Duloxetine (Cymbalta)	C/ 8–17	40–60	Not well established
	Venlafaxine (Effexor)	C/ 5–11 (including metabolite)	75–375	Not well established

Continued

TABLE 25–3 **Medications Used in the Treatment of Depression–cont'd**				
CHEMICAL CLASS	GENERIC (TRADE) NAME*	PREGNANCY CATEGORIES/ HALF-LIFE (hr)	DAILY ADULT DOSAGE RANGE (mg)†	THERAPEUTIC PLASMA RANGES
Psychotherapeutic Combinations	Olanzapine and fluoxetine (Symbyax)	C/ (see individual drugs)	6/25–12/50	Not well established
	Chlordiazepoxide and fluoxetine (Limbitrol)	D/ (see individual drugs)	20/50– 40/100	Not well established
	Perphenazine and amitriptyline (Etrafon)	C–D/ (see individual drugs)	6/30–16/200	Not well established

*Drugs without trade names are available in generic form only.
†Dosage requires slow titration; onset of therapeutic response may be 1 to 4 weeks.
‡Bristol-Myers Squibb voluntarily removed its brand of nefazodone (Serzone) from the market in 2004. The generic equivalent is currently available through various other manufacturers.

Client and Family Education Related to Antidepressants

The client should:

- Continue to take the medication even though symptoms have not subsided. The therapeutic effect may not be seen for as long as 4 weeks. If after this length of time no improvement is noted, the physician may prescribe a different medication.
- Use caution when driving or operating dangerous machinery. Drowsiness and dizziness can occur. If these side effects become persistent or interfere with ADLs, the client should report them to the physician. Dosage adjustment may be necessary.
- Not discontinue use of the drug abruptly. To do so might produce withdrawal symptoms, such as nausea, vertigo, insomnia, headache, malaise, nightmares, and return of symptoms for which the medication was prescribed.
- Use sunblock lotion and wear protective clothing when spending time outdoors. The skin may be sensitive to sunburn.
- Report occurrence of any of the following symptoms to the physician immediately: sore throat, fever, malaise, yellowish skin, unusual bleeding, easy bruising, persistent nausea/vomiting, severe headache, rapid heart rate, difficulty urinating, anorexia/weight loss, seizure activity, stiff or sore neck, and chest pain.
- Rise slowly from a sitting or lying position to prevent a sudden drop in blood pressure.
- Take frequent sips of water, chew sugarless gum, or suck on hard candy if dry mouth is a problem. Good oral care (frequent brushing and flossing) is very important.
- Not consume the following foods or medications while taking MAOIs: aged cheese, wine (especially Chianti), beer, chocolate, colas, coffee, tea, sour cream, smoked and processed meats, beef or chicken liver, canned figs, soy sauce, overripe and fermented foods, pickled herring, raisins, caviar, yogurt, yeast products, broad beans, cold remedies, diet pills. To do so could cause a life-threatening hypertensive crisis.
- Avoid smoking while receiving tricyclic therapy. Smoking increases the metabolism of tricyclics, requiring an adjustment in dosage to achieve the therapeutic effect.
- Avoid drinking alcohol while taking antidepressant therapy. These drugs potentiate the effects of each other.
- Avoid use of other medications (including over-the-counter medications) without physician's approval while receiving antidepressant therapy. Many medications contain substances that could precipitate a life-threatening hypertensive crisis in combination with antidepressant medication.
- Notify physician immediately if inappropriate or prolonged penile erections occur while taking trazodone. If the erection persists longer than 1 hour, seek emergency department treatment. This condition is rare but has occurred in some men who have taken trazodone. If measures are not instituted immediately, impotence can result.
- Not "double up" on medication if a dose of bupropion (Wellbutrin) is missed unless advised to do so by the physician. Taking bupropion in divided doses will decrease the risk of seizures and other adverse effects.
- Follow the correct procedure for applying the selegiline transdermal patch:
  - Apply to dry, intact skin on upper torso, upper thigh, or outer surface of upper arm.
  - Apply approximately same time each day to new spot on skin after removing and discarding old patch.
  - Wash hands thoroughly after applying the patch.

- Avoid exposing application site to direct heat (e.g., heating pads, electric blankets, heat lamps, hot tub, or prolonged direct sunlight).
    - If patch falls off, apply new patch to a new site and resume previous schedule.
- Be aware of possible risks of taking antidepressants during pregnancy. Safe use during pregnancy and lactation has not been fully established. These drugs are believed to readily cross the placental barrier; if so, the fetus could experience adverse effects of the drug. Inform the physician immediately if pregnancy occurs, is suspected, or is planned.
- Be aware of the side effects of antidepressants. Refer to written materials furnished by health-care providers for safe self-administration.
- Carry a card or other identification at all times describing the medications being taken.

Pharmacogenomics

Recent genetic studies have demonstrated that variations in genes can predict whether a person will respond to SSRIs (Lee, 2015). This is important because, as Lee notes, between 30 and 50 percent of people do not respond to the first antidepressant they have been prescribed. It is no wonder that patients and family members often express frustration as medicines and doses are changed in an effort to find the right antidepressant and dose that will be effective for the individual. Genotyping has also demonstrated benefits in identifying which individuals may be more prone to certain side effects. One study cited by Lee demonstrated that Asian populations with a specific genotype were at increased risk for sexual dysfunction side effects associated with SSRIs. This could be useful information because sexual dysfunction is a primary reason that many people choose to stop taking these medications. Currently, this area of study is in its infancy, and further study is needed to identify benefits of routine testing, cost effectiveness, and their ability to provide timely results so that therapy can be initiated promptly.

CASE STUDY AND SAMPLE CARE PLAN

NURSING HISTORY AND ASSESSMENT

Sam is a 45-year-old white male admitted to the psychiatric unit of a general medical center by his family physician, Dr. Jones, who reported that Sam had become increasingly despondent over the past month. His wife reported that he had made statements such as, "Life is not worth living," and "I think I could just take all those pills Dr. Jones prescribed at one time; then it would all be over." Sam says he loves his wife and children and does not want to hurt them but feels they no longer need him. He states, "They would probably be better off without me." His wife appears to be very concerned about his condition, although in his despondency, he seems oblivious to her feelings. His mother (a widow) lives in a neighboring state, and he sees her infrequently. His father was an alcoholic and physically abused Sam and his siblings. He admits that he is somewhat bitter toward his mother for allowing him and his siblings to "suffer from the physical and emotional brutality of their father." His siblings and their families live in distant states, and he sees them rarely, during holiday gatherings.

Sam earned a college degree while working full time at night to pay his way. He is employed in the administration department of a large corporation. Over the past 12 years, Sam has watched while a number of his peers were promoted to management positions. Sam has been considered for several of these positions but has never been selected. Last month, a management position became available for which Sam felt he was qualified. He applied for this position, believing he had a good chance of being promoted. However, his wife reports that when the announcement was made that the position had been given to a younger man who had been with the company only 5 years, Sam initially expressed anger and then seemed to accept the decision. But over the past few weeks, he has become increasingly withdrawn. He speaks to very few people at the office and is falling behind in his work. At home, he eats very little, talks to family members only when they ask a direct question, withdraws to his bedroom very early in the evening, and does not come out until time to leave for work the next morning. Today, he refused to get out of bed or to go to work, and he told his wife he has nothing to live for. His wife convinced him to talk to their family doctor, who admitted him to the hospital after hearing Sam acknowledge that he desires to end his life. The referring psychiatrist diagnosed Sam with Major Depressive Disorder.

NURSING DIAGNOSES AND OUTCOME IDENTIFICATION

From the assessment data, the nurse develops the following nursing diagnoses for Sam:

1. **Risk for suicide** related to depressed mood and expressions of having nothing to live for.
    a. **Short-Term Goals:**
        - Sam will discuss suicide ideation and intentions with staff.
        - Sam will collaborate with the nurse to identify a plan for maintaining safety.

Continued

CASE STUDY AND SAMPLE CARE PLAN—cont'd

b. **Long-Term Goal:**
- Sam will not harm himself during his hospitalization.

2. **Complicated grieving** related to unresolved losses (job promotion and unsatisfactory parent-child relationships) evidenced by expressed anger over loss of a job opportunity and desire to end his life.
   a. **Short-Term Goal:**
   - Sam will discuss anger toward boss and parents within 1 week.
   b. **Long-Term Goal:**
   - Sam will verbalize his position in the grief process and begin movement in the progression toward resolution by time of discharge from treatment.

PLANNING AND IMPLEMENTATION

RISK FOR SUICIDE

The following nursing interventions have been identified for Sam's care:

1. Develop a trusting relationship with Sam that facilitates open, nonjudgmental discussion of suicide ideation and related thoughts and feelings.
2. Ask Sam directly, "Have you thought about killing yourself? If so, what do you plan to do? Do you have the means to carry out this plan?"
3. Create a safe environment. Remove all potentially harmful objects from immediate access (sharp objects, straps, belts, ties, glass items).
4. Assess suicide risk each shift and identify any changes in level of hopelessness. Encourage verbalizations of honest feelings. Through exploration and discussion, help Sam to identify symbols of hope in his life (participating in activities he finds satisfying outside of his job).
5. Allow Sam to express angry feelings within appropriate limits. Encourage use of the exercise room and other activities for releasing energy appropriately. Help him identify the true source of his anger, and work on adaptive coping skills for use outside the hospital (e.g., jogging, exercise club available to employees of his company).
6. Identify community resources that he may use as a support system and from whom he may request help if feeling suicidal (e.g., suicidal or crisis hotline; psychiatrist or social worker at community mental health center; hospital HELP line).
7. Introduce Sam to support and education groups for adult children of alcoholics (ACoA).
8. Spend time with Sam. This will help him to feel safe and secure while conveying the message that he is a worthwhile person.

COMPLICATED GRIEVING

The following nursing interventions have been identified for Sam:

1. Discuss with Sam the stages in the grief process and encourage him to explore his feelings so that he may come to realize the connection between grief and his anger.

2. Develop a trusting relationship with Sam. Show empathy and caring. Be honest and keep all promises.
3. Convey an accepting attitude—one in which Sam is not afraid to express his feelings openly.
4. Allow him to verbalize feelings of anger. The initial expression of anger may be displaced on to the health-care provider. Do not become defensive if this should occur. Have Sam write letters *(not to be mailed)* to his boss and to his parents stating his true feelings toward them. Discuss these feelings with him, then destroy the letters.
5. Assist Sam to discharge pent-up anger through participation in large motor activities (brisk walks, jogging, physical exercises, volleyball, punching bag, exercise bike, or other equipment).
6. Help Sam to understand that feelings such as guilt and anger toward his boss and parents are appropriate and acceptable during the grieving process. Help him also to understand that he must work through these feelings and move past this stage in order to eventually feel better. Knowledge of acceptability of the feelings associated with normal grieving may help to relieve some of the guilt that these responses generate. Knowing why he is experiencing these feelings may also help to resolve them.
7. Encourage Sam to review the relationship with his parents. Educate Sam about common roles and behaviors of members in an alcoholic family. Encourage Sam to identify his roles and behaviors within his family of origin. Assist Sam in problem-solving as he attempts to determine methods for more adaptive coping. Suggest alternatives to automatic negative thinking (e.g., thought-stopping techniques). Provide positive feedback for strategies identified and decisions made.
8. Encourage Sam to reach out for spiritual support during this time in whatever form is desirable to him. Assess spiritual needs (see Chapter 6, Cultural and Spiritual Concepts Relevant to Psychiatric-Mental Health Nursing), and assist as necessary in the fulfillment of those needs. Sam may find comfort in religious rituals with which he is familiar.

EVALUATION

The outcome criteria identified for Sam have been met. He sought out staff when feelings of suicide surfaced and has identified a safety plan for which he reports willingness to engage. He has not harmed himself in any way. He verbalizes no further thought of suicide and expresses hope for the future. He is able to verbalize names of resources outside the hospital from whom he may request help if thoughts of suicide return. Sam is able to verbalize normal stages of the grief process and behaviors associated with each stage. He is able to identify his own position in the grief process and express honest feelings related to the loss of his job promotion and satisfactory parent-child relationships. He expresses willingness to continue exploring behaviors and coping mechanisms through a local ACoA meeting.

Summary and Key Points

- Depression is one of the oldest recognized psychiatric illnesses that is still prevalent today. It is so common, in fact, that it has been referred to as the "common cold of psychiatric disorders."
- The cause of depressive disorders is not entirely known. A number of factors, including genetics, biochemical influences, and psychosocial experiences likely enter into the development of the disorder.
- Secondary depression occurs in response to other physiological disorders.
- Symptoms of depression occur along a continuum according to the degree of severity from transient to severe.

- The disorder occurs in all developmental levels, including childhood, adolescence, senescence, and during the puerperium.
- Treatment of depression includes individual therapy, group and family therapy, cognitive therapy, electroconvulsive therapy, light therapy, transcranial magnetic stimulation, and psychopharmacology.
- Nursing care of the depressed client is provided using the six steps of the nursing process.

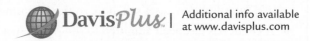

Davis*Plus* | Additional info available at www.davisplus.com

Review Questions
Self-Examination/Learning Exercise

Select the answer that is most appropriate for each of the following questions.

1. Margaret, age 68, is a widow of 6 months. Since her husband died, her sister reports that Margaret has become socially withdrawn, has lost weight, and does little more each day than visit the cemetery where her husband is buried. She told her sister today that she "doesn't have anything more to live for." She has been hospitalized with major depressive disorder. The *priority* nursing diagnosis for Margaret would be:
   a. Imbalanced nutrition: less than body requirements.
   b. Complicated grieving.
   c. Risk for suicide.
   d. Social isolation.

2. The physician orders sertraline (Zoloft) 50 mg PO bid for Margaret, a 68-year-old woman with major depressive disorder. After 3 days of taking the medication, Margaret says to the nurse, "I don't think this medicine is doing any good. I don't feel a bit better." What is the most appropriate response by the nurse?
   a. "Cheer up, Margaret. You have so much to be happy about."
   b. "Sometimes it takes a few weeks for the medicine to bring about an improvement in symptoms."
   c. "I'll report that to the physician, Margaret. Maybe he will order something different."
   d. "Try not to dwell on your symptoms, Margaret. Why don't you join the others down in the dayroom?"

3. The goal of cognitive therapy with depressed clients is to:
   a. Identify and change dysfunctional patterns of thinking.
   b. Resolve the symptoms and initiate or restore adaptive family functioning.
   c. Alter the neurotransmitters that are creating the depressed mood.
   d. Provide feedback from peers who are having similar experiences.

4. Education for the client who is taking MAOIs should include which of the following?
   a. Fluid and sodium replacement when appropriate, frequent drug blood levels, signs and symptoms of toxicity
   b. Lifetime of continuous use, possible tardive dyskinesia, advantages of an injection every 2 to 4 weeks
   c. Short-term use, possible tolerance to beneficial effects, careful tapering of the drug at end of treatment
   d. Tyramine-restricted diet, prohibitive concurrent use of over-the-counter medications without physician notification

Continued

Review Questions—cont'd
Self-Examination/Learning Exercise

5. A client expresses interest in alternative treatments for depression with seasonal variations and asks the nurse about light therapy. Which of the following are evidence-based teaching points that the nurse may share with the client? (Select all that apply.)
   a. Light therapy has demonstrated effectiveness that is comparable to antidepressants.
   b. Light therapy should be used regularly until the season changes.
   c. Light therapy should be used only when ECT has proven to be ineffective.
   d. Side effects such as headache, nausea, or agitation, when they occur, are usually mild and transient.
   e. Light therapy causes sedation, so the best time to use it is before bedtime.

6. A client has just been admitted to the psychiatric unit with a diagnosis of major depressive disorder. Which of the following behavioral manifestations might the nurse expect to assess? (Select all that apply.)
   a. Slumped posture
   b. Delusional thinking
   c. Feelings of despair
   d. Feels best early in the morning and worse as the day progresses
   e. Anorexia

7. A client with depression asks the nurse, "Why would they be checking my thyroid function when I clearly have depression and I'm not overweight?" Which of these is an accurate response?
   a. An underactive thyroid gland can manifest as depression.
   b. Depression has been proven to be a hormonal illness.
   c. Thyroid hormone replacement is a first-line treatment for most clients with depression.
   d. All of the above.

8. A client whose husband died 6 months ago is diagnosed with major depressive disorder. She says to the nurse, "I start feeling angry that Harold died and left me all alone; he should have stopped smoking years ago! But then I start feeling guilty for feeling that way." What is an appropriate response by the nurse?
   a. "Yes, he should have stopped smoking. Then he probably wouldn't have gotten lung cancer."
   b. "I can understand how you must feel."
   c. "Those feelings are a normal part of the grief response."
   d. "Just think about the good times that you had while he was alive."

9. An acutely depressed client isolates herself in her room and just sits and stares into space. Which of these is the best example of an active communication approach with this client?
   a. "Do you like exercise?"
   b. "Come with me. I will go with you to group therapy."
   c. "Would you like to go to group therapy, stay in bed, or come out to the day lounge for some activities?"
   d. "Why do you stay in your room all the time?"

10. Sally is admitted to the hospital with major depressive disorder and repeatedly makes negative statements about herself. Which of the following interventions are identified as those that will promote positive self-esteem in the patient? (Select all that apply.)
    a. Teach assertive communication skills.
    b. Make observations to Sally when she completes a goal or task.
    c. Instruct Sally that you will not talk with her unless she stops talking negatively about herself.
    d. Offer to spend time with Sally using a nonjudgmental, accepting approach.

IMPLICATIONS OF RESEARCH FOR EVIDENCE-BASED PRACTICE

Pessagno, R.A., & Hunker, D. (2012). Using short-term group psychotherapy as an evidence-based intervention for first-time mothers at risk for postpartum depression. *Perspectives in Psychiatric Care, 49*(3), 202-209. doi:10.1111/j.1744-6163.2012.00350.x

DESCRIPTION OF THE STUDY: The purpose of this study was to determine if an 8-week, short-term psychotherapy group decreased the risk of developing postpartum depression (PPD) among first-time mothers at risk for PPD. The sample consisted of 16 women between the ages of 20 and 38 (mean 28.5 yr). All were Caucasian, and the majority were Catholic. Thirteen were married, two were partnered, and one participant was single. Two psychotherapy groups with eight women in each group met once a week for 8 weeks beginning one month after discharge from the hospital. Each session lasted 90 minutes, and both groups were led by the same advanced practice psychiatric nurse practitioner. All participants completed the Edinburgh Postnatal Depression Scale (EPDS) within 3 days of giving birth, and all scored 11 or higher, which was targeted as a high risk for PPD score by the participant hospital (a community hospital in New Jersey). The psychotherapy groups followed an unstructured format, with an interpersonal-focused theoretical model. The authors stated, "This focus was structured to provide optimal opportunity in developing skills relative to their new maternal roles as new mothers, coping with depression and stress, honing communication skills with their husbands and partners, and sharing their individual, weekly experiences."

The EPDS was administered to all participants at the end of the 8 sessions.

RESULTS OF THE STUDY: The mean preintervention score on the EPDS for group 1 was 16.13, and for group 2, the mean score was 15.5, placing participants from both groups at high risk for PPD. Following the intervention, the mean score for group 1 participants was 6.38 and for group 2 was 6.63. The EPDS was administered at 6 months postintervention to determine the long-term effects. At that time, both groups demonstrated a significant decrease in scores on the EPDS, indicating a continued effect of the group intervention for participants. The authors stated, "This is suggestive that group psychotherapy can have long-term effects to reduce risk for PPD for first-time mothers."

IMPLICATIONS FOR NURSING PRACTICE: The results of this study indicate that, particularly in those states that mandate screening for PPD, implementing nonpharmacologic interventions such as short-term group psychotherapy provides a choice for women who decide against the use of medication. The authors stated, "In today's mental health services market, significant focus is placed on the importance of medication management skills of the psychiatric APN, yet the intervention in this project supports the need for continued education and training of advanced practice psychiatric nursing as psychotherapists with group psychotherapy skills."

IMPLICATIONS OF RESEARCH FOR EVIDENCE-BASED PRACTICE

Schomerus, G., Matschinger, H., & Angermeyer, M.C. (2014). Causal beliefs of the public and social acceptance of persons with mental illness: A comparative analysis of schizophrenia, depression, and alcohol dependence. *Psychological Medicine 44*(2), 303-314. doi:10.1017/S003321971300072X

DESCRIPTION OF THE STUDY: The aim of the study was to identify whether biological explanations for mental illness (including schizophrenia, depression, and alcohol dependence) improved people's perceptions about and tolerance of people with these conditions. This study was conducted in Germany with a large sample ($N = 3,642$). The researchers used path models to compare different variables such as beliefs that these illnesses are caused by biogenetic factors, current stress, and/or childhood adversity. Then, on the basis of those beliefs, the researchers identified the participants' attitudes and social acceptance of patients with a mental illness.

RESULTS OF THE STUDY: Biogenetic beliefs as a cause for mental illness were associated with lower acceptance

of people with schizophrenia and depression but higher acceptance of individuals with alcohol dependence. Lower social acceptance was related to the perceptions of differentness and dangerous that were believed to be "etched in stone" if the illness is genetic in origin (an oversimplification of the influence of genetic factors). Current stress as a cause for mental illness was associated with higher acceptance of people with schizophrenia, while belief in childhood adversity as a cause was associated with lower acceptance of people with depression.

IMPLICATIONS FOR NURSING PRACTICE: Stigmatization (a devaluing attitude about peoples' ability to function in society because of an illness or disability) has been identified as a major barrier to recovery for people with mental illnesses. This study provides evidence that we need to be thoughtful as we educate patients and families. In reality, and based on current evidence, mental illnesses are probably caused by many factors, including genetic vulnerability, current stress, and past trauma. Often, mental illnesses are explained strictly as biogenetic diseases of the brain, and this explanation

Continued

IMPLICATIONS OF RESEARCH FOR EVIDENCE-BASED PRACTICE—cont'd

sometimes is misrepresented as completely known when, in fact, much of our current knowledge about causality in mental illness is theoretical. The researchers conclude that we may not be helping our clients or combating stigma when we try to oversimplify causality explanations.

When interpreting findings from a study such as this one, it is important to consider what variables might influence the findings. For example, might cultural beliefs about mental illness and biogenetics in Germany differ from those in other parts of the world? These questions become the foundation for additional research. Interestingly, the researchers cite a study by Hansell and associates in 2011* that reviewed Web sites in the United States and found that

information provided by universities and government agencies more often provided a balanced view of potential causative factors where nongovernment agencies and pharmaceutical Web sites tended to overemphasize biological causes. Nurses need to be cautious about the reliability of their sources for information to maintain the public trust in the information that is shared. The bottom line is that, as nurses, we need to ensure that we are providing balanced information, based on current evidence, when we provide patient education. This is critical to providing accurate information to clients and families and, as the study suggests, may help in the battle against stigmatization of people with mental illness.

*Hansell, J., Bailin, A.P., Franke, K.A., Kraft, J.M., Wu, H.Y., . . . Kazi, N.F. (2011). Conceptually sound thinking about depression: An Internet survey and its implications. Professional Psychology: Research and Practice, 42(5): 382-390. doi:10.1037/a0025608.

TEST YOUR CRITICAL THINKING SKILLS

Carol is a 17-year-old high school senior. She will graduate in 1 month and has plans to attend the state university a few hours from her home. Carol has always made good grades in school, has participated in many activities, and is a pep squad cheerleader. She had been dating the star quarterback, Alan, since last summer, and they had spoken a number of times about going to the senior prom together. About a month before the prom, Alan broke up with Carol and began dating Salima, whom he subsequently took to the prom. Since that time, Carol has become despondent. She does not go out with her friends, she dropped out of the pep squad, her grades have fallen, and she has lost 10 pounds. She attends classes most of the time, but evenings and weekends she spends in her room alone listening to her music, crying, and sleeping. Her parents have become very concerned and contacted the family physician, who has had Carol admitted to the psychiatric unit of the local hospital. The admitting psychiatrist has made the diagnosis of Major Depressive Disorder. Carol tells the nurse, "Sometimes I drive around and try to find Alan and Salima. I don't know why he broke up with me. I hate myself! I just want to die!"

Answer the following questions related to Carol:

1. What is the primary nursing diagnosis that is identified for Carol?
2. To determine the seriousness of this problem, what are important nursing assessments that must be made?
3. What medication might the physician order for Carol?
4. What concern has the FDA identified that is associated with this medication?

💬 Communication Exercises

1. Carrie, age 75, is a patient on the psychiatric unit with a diagnosis of Major Depressive Disorder. She says to the nurse, "I never knew my life would end up like this. I've lost my husband, all my friends, and my home."
   • How would the nurse respond appropriately to this statement by Carrie?
2. "I have spent my whole life taking care of others. Now someone else has to take care of me. I feel so useless."
   • How would the nurse respond appropriately to this statement by Carrie?
3. "I don't know why anyone would want to bother taking care of me. I really have nothing left to live for."
   • How would the nurse respond appropriately to this statement by Carrie?

MOVIE CONNECTIONS

Prozac Nation (depression) • *The Butcher Boy* (depression) • *Night, Mother* (depression) • *The Prince of Tides* (depression/suicide)

References

Administration on Aging. (2016). Aging statistics. Retrieved from www.aoa.acl.gov/aging_statistics/index.aspx

American Foundation for Suicide Prevention. (2016). Suicide statistics. Retrieved from https://afsp.org/about-suicide/suicide-statistics

American Psychiatric Association. (2013). *Diagnostic and statistical manual of mental disorders* (5th ed.). Washington, DC: American Psychiatric Publishing.

Amick, H.R., Gartlehner, G., Gaynes, B.N., Forneris, C., Asher, G.N., Morgan, L.C., . . . Lohr, K.N. (2015). Comparative benefits and harms of second generation antidepressants and cognitive behavioral therapies in initial treatment of major depressive disorder: Systematic review and meta-analysis. *British Medical Journal, 351,* h6019. doi:http://dx.doi.org/10.1136/bmj.h6019

Anxiety and Depression Association of America. (2016). Anxiety and depression in children. Retrieved from https://www.adaa.org/living-with-anxiety/children/anxiety-and-depression

Black, D.W., & Andreasen, N.C. (2014). *Introductory textbook of psychiatry* (6th ed.). Washington, DC: American Psychiatric Publishing.

Centers for Disease Control and Prevention (CDC). (2013). *The state of aging and health in America 2013.* Atlanta, GA: CDC.

Cobb, B.S., Coryell, W.H., Cavanough, J., Keller, M., Solomon, D., Endicott, J., . . . Fiedorowicz, J.G. (2014). Seasonal variation of depressive symptoms in unipolar major depressive disorder. *Comprehensive Psychiatry 55*(8), 1891-1899. doi:10.1016/j.comppsych.2014.07.021

Connolly, K.R., Helmer, A., Christancho, M.A., Christancho, P., & O'Reardon, J.P. (2012). Effectiveness of transcranial magnetic stimulation in clinical practice post FDA approval in the United States: Results observed with the first 100 consecutive cases at an academic medical center. *Journal of Clinical Psychiatry, 73*(4), 567-573. doi:10.4088/JCP.11m07413

Cotterell, D. (2010). Pathogenesis and management of seasonal affective disorder. *Progress in Neurology and Psychiatry 14*(5), 18-25. doi:10.1002/pnp.173

Eranti, S., Mogg, A., Pluck, G., Landau, S., Purvis, R., Brown, R.G., . . . McLoughlin, D.M. (2007). A randomized, controlled trial with 6-month follow-up of repetitive transcranial magnetic stimulation and electroconvulsive therapy for severe depression. *American Journal of Psychiatry, 164*(1), 73-81. doi:10.1176/ajp.2007.164.1.73

George, M.S., Taylor, J.J., & Short, E.B. (2013). The expanding evidence base for rTMS treatment of depression. *Current Opinion in Psychiatry, 26*(1), 13-18. doi:10.1097/YCO.0b013e32835ab46d

Green, M.J., & Benzeval, M. (2009). Social class differences in anxiety and depression across the life course: Evidence from three cohorts in the west of Scotland. *Journal of Epidemiology and Community Mental Health, 63*(Suppl. 2), 19. doi:10.1136/jech.2009.096701s

Herdman, T.H., & Kamitsuru, S. (Eds.). (2014). *NANDA-I nursing diagnoses: Definitions and classification, 2015–2017.* Chichester, UK: Wiley Blackwell.

Institute of Medicine. (2003). *Health professions education: A bridge to quality.* Washington, DC: National Academies Press.

Jiang, X., Asmaro, R., O'Sullivan, D.O., Budnik, E., & Schnatz, P.F. (2016). Depression may be one of the strongest risk factors for coronary artery disease in women aged <65 years: A 10-year prospective longitudinal study. Abstract S-17. Presented at NAMS 2016 Annual Meeting; October 5–8, 2016; Orlando, FL.

Kurlansik, S.L., & Ibay, A.D. (2013). Seasonal affective disorder. *Indian Journal of Clinical Practice. 24*(7), 607-610.

Lam, R.W., Levitt, A.J., Levitan, R.D., Michelak, E., Morehouse, R., Rammasubbu, R., . . . Tam, E.M. (2015). Efficacy of bright light treatment, fluoxetine, and the combination in patients with non-seasonal major depressive disorder: A randomized clinical trial. *JAMA Psychiatry, 73*(1), 56-63. doi:10.1001/jamapsychiatry.2015.2235

Lapate, R.C., Van Reekum, C.M., Schaefer, S.M., Greischar, L.L., Norris, C.J., Bachhuber, D., . . . Davidson, R.J. (2014). Prolonged marital stress is associated with short-lived responses to positive stimuli. *Psychophysiology 51*(6), 499-509. doi:10.1111/psyp.12203

LaPierre, T.A. (2004). An investigation of the role of age and life stage in the moderation and mediation of the effect of marital status on depression. Paper presented at the annual meeting of the American Sociological Association, Hilton San Francisco & Renaissance Parc 55 Hotel, San Francisco, August 14, 2004. Retrieved from www.allacademic.com/meta/p109917_index.html

Lee, K.C. (2015). Using pharmacogenomics to aid antidepressant prescribing. *Psychiatry Advisor.* Retrieved from www.psychiatryadvisor.com/mood-disorders/using-pharmacogenomics-to-aid-antidepressant-prescribing/article/394244/2

Lohoff, F.W. (2010). Overview of the genetics of major depressive disorder. *Current Psychiatry Reports, 12*(6), 539-546. doi:10.1007/s11920-010-0150-6

Magnezi, R., Aminov, E., Shmuel, D., Dreifuss, M., & Dannon, P. (2016). Comparison between neurostimulation techniques repetitive transcranial magnetic stimulation vs electroconvulsive therapy for the treatment of resistant depression: Patient preference and cost-effectiveness. *Patient Preference and Adherence, 10,*1481-1487. doi:10.2147/PPA.S105654

Mayo Clinic. (2016a). Antidepressants for children and teens. Retrieved from www.mayoclinic.org/diseases-conditions/teen-depression/in-depth/antidepressants/art-20047502

Mayo Clinic. (2016b). Electroconvulsive therapy. Retrieved from www.mayoclinic.org/tests-procedures/electroconvulsive-therapy/basics/risks/prc-20014161

McMahon, B., Andersen, S.B., Madsen, M.K., Hjordt, L.V., Hageman, I., Dam, H., . . . Knudsen, G.M. (2016). Seasonal difference in brain serotonin transporter binding predicts symptom severity in patients with seasonal affective disorder. *Brain, 139*(Pt 5), 1605-1614. doi:10.1093/brain/aww043

Mojtabai, R., Olfson, M., & Han, B. (2016). National trends in the prevalence and treatment of depression in adolescents and young adults. *Pediatrics, 138*(6), 9. doi:10.1542/peds.2016-1878

National Center for Health Statistics. (2012). *Health, United States, 2011: With special feature on socioeconomic status and health.* Hyattsville, MD: U.S. Department of Health and Human Services.

National Center for Health Statistics. (2015). Faststats. Retrieved from www.cdc.gov/nchs/fastats/depression.htm

National Institutes of Health. (2016a). Hypothyroidism. Retrieved from https://www.niddk.nih.gov/health-information/health-topics/endocrine/hypothyroidism/Pages/fact-sheet.aspx

National Institutes of Health. (2016b). Postpartum depression facts. Retrieved from https://www.nimh.nih.gov/health/publications/postpartum-depression-facts/index.shtml

National Institute of Mental Health. (2016). Depression. Retrieved from https://www.nimh.nih.gov/health/topics/depression/index.shtml

Natsuaki, M.N., Shaw, D.S., Neiderhiser, J.M, Ganiban, J., Gordon, H.T., Reiss, D., & Leve, L.D. (2014). Raised by depressed parents: Is it an environmental risk? *Clinical Child and Family Psychology Review, 17*(4), 357-367 doi:10.1007/s10567-014-0169-z.

Nauert, R. (2010). Social class influences depression treatment. *Psych Central.* Retrieved from http://psychcentral.com/news/2010/11/08/social-class-influences-depression-treatment/20632.html

Page, A.C., & Hooke, G.R. (2012). Effectiveness of cognitive-behavioral therapy modified for inpatients with depression. *International Scholarly Research Notices, 2012*(4). doi:http://dx.doi.org/10.5402/2012/461265

Pessagno, R.A., & Hunker, D. (2012). Using short-term group psychotherapy as an evidence-based intervention for first-time mothers at risk for postpartum depression. *Perspectives in Psychiatric Care, 49*(3), 202-209. doi:10.1111/j.1744-6163.2012.00350.x

Raposelli, D. (2015). Is TMS cost effective? *Psychiatric Times.* Retrieved from www.psychiatrictimes.com/major-depressive-disorder/tms-cost-effective

Rodriguez, T. (2015). Using bright light therapy beyond seasonal affective disorder. *Psychiatry Advisor.* Retrieved from www.psychiatryadvisor.com/mood-disorders/depression-mood-winter-season-light-sad-antidepressant/article/457643

Sadock, B.J., Sadock, V.A., & Ruiz, P. (2015). *Synopsis of psychiatry: Behavioral sciences/clinical psychiatry* (11th ed.). Philadelphia: Lippincott Williams & Wilkins.

Sathyanarayana Rao, T.S., Asha, M.R., Ramsh, B.M., & Jagannatha Rao, K.S. (2008). Understanding nutrition, depression, and mental illness. *Indian Journal of Psychiatry, 50*(2), 77-82. doi:10.4103/0019-5545.42391

Schimelpfening, N. (2012). A good vitamin supplement could be just what the doctor ordered. Retrieved from http://depression.about.com/cs/diet/a/vitamin.htm

Schomerus, G., Matschinger, H., & Angermeyer, M.C. (2014). Causal beliefs of the public and social acceptance of persons with mental illness: A comparative analysis of schizophrenia, depression, and alcohol dependence. *Psychological Medicine 44*(2), 303-314. doi:10.1017/S003321971300072X

Shin, Y.C., Jung, C.H., Kim, H.J., Kim, E.J., &, Lim, S.W. (2016). The associations among vitamin D deficiency, C-reactive protein, and depressive symptoms. *Journal of Psychosomatic Research, 90*, 98-104. doi:http://dx.doi.org/10.1016/j.jpsychores.2016.10.001

Siddique, J., Chung, J.Y., Brown, C.H., & Miranda, J. (2012). Comparative effectiveness of medication versus cognitive-behavioral therapy in a randomized controlled trial of low-income young minority women with depression. *Journal of Consulting and Clinical Psychology, 80*(6), 995-1006. doi:10.1037/a0030452

Substance Abuse and Mental Health Services Administration, Center for Behavioral Health Statistics and Quality. (2015). Results from the 2014 National Survey on Drug Use and Health: Mental health detailed tables [Table 1.45A]. Retrieved from www.samhsa.gov/data/sites/default/files/NSDUH-MHDetTabs2014/NSDUH-MHDet-Tabs2014.htm#tab1-45a

Sword, W., Clark, A.M., Hegadoren, K., Brooks, S., & Kingston, D. (2012). The complexity of postpartum mental health and illness: A critical realist study. *Nursing Inquiry, 19*(1), 51-62. doi:10.1111/j.1440-1800.2011.00560.x

Thielen, J. (2015). Premenstrual syndrome. *Mayo Clinic.* Retrieved from www.mayoclinic.org/diseases-conditions/premenstrual-syndrome/expert-answers/pmdd/faq-20058315

Van der Wurff, F.B., Stek, M.L., Hoogendijk, W.J.G., & Beekman, A.T.F. (2003). Electroconvulsive therapy for the depressed elderly [review content assessed as up-to-date: January 21, 2007]. *Cochrane Database of Systematic Reviews 2003,* Issue 2, Art. no.: CD003593, doi:10.1002/14651858.CD003593

Vann, M.R. (2015). Prescription drugs that cause depression. Retrieved from www.everydayhealth.com/depression/prescription-drugs-that-cause-depression.aspx

Winthorst, W., Post, W., Meesters, Y., Penninx, B., & Nolen, W.A. (2011). Seasonality in depressive and anxiety symptoms among primary care patients and in patients with depressive and anxiety disorders; results from the Netherlands Study of Depression and Anxiety. *BMC Psychiatry.* 11(1), 1-18. doi:10.1186/1471-244X-11-198

Classical References

Beck, A.T., Rush, A.J., Shaw, B.F., & Emery, G. (1979). *Cognitive theory of depression.* New York: Guilford Press.

Freud, S. (1957). *Mourning and melancholia,* vol. 14 (standard ed.). London: Hogarth Press. (Original work published 1917.)

Seligman, M.E.P. (1973). Fall into helplessness. *Psychology Today, 7,* 43-48.

Bipolar and Related Disorders

26

CORE CONCEPTS

Mania

KEY TERMS

bipolar disorder	delirious mania	hypomania
cyclothymic disorder	flight of ideas	

OBJECTIVES
After reading this chapter, the student will be able to:

1. Recount historical perspectives of bipolar disorder.
2. Discuss epidemiological statistics related to bipolar disorder.
3. Describe various types of bipolar disorders.
4. Identify predisposing factors in the development of bipolar disorder.
5. Discuss implications of bipolar disorder related to developmental stage.
6. Identify symptomatology associated with bipolar disorder and use this information in client assessment.

7. Formulate nursing diagnoses and goals of care for clients experiencing a manic episode.
8. Identify topics for client and family teaching relevant to bipolar disorder.
9. Describe appropriate nursing interventions for clients experiencing a manic episode.
10. Describe relevant criteria for evaluating nursing care of clients experiencing a manic episode.
11. Discuss various modalities relevant to treatment of bipolar disorder.

HOMEWORK ASSIGNMENT
Please read the chapter and answer the following questions:

1. What is the most common medication that has been known to trigger manic episodes?
2. What is the speech pattern of a person experiencing a manic episode?
3. What is the difference between cyclothymic disorder and bipolar disorder?
4. Why should a person on lithium therapy have blood levels drawn regularly?

Mood was defined in Chapter 25, Depressive Disorders, as a pervasive and sustained emotion that may have a profound influence on a person's perception of the world. Examples of mood include depression, joy, elation, anger, and anxiety. *Affect* is described as the external, observable emotional reaction associated with an experience.

The previous chapter focused on the consequences of complicated grieving as it is manifested by depressive disorders. This chapter addresses mood disorders as they are manifested by cycles of mania and depression—called **bipolar disorder.** A historical perspective and epidemiological statistics related to bipolar disorder are presented. Predisposing factors that have been implicated in the etiology of bipolar disorder provide a framework for studying the dynamics of the disorder.

The implications of bipolar disorder relevant to children and adolescents are discussed. An explanation of the symptomatology is presented as background knowledge for assessing the client with bipolar disorder. Nursing care is described in the context of the six steps of the nursing process. Various medical treatment modalities are explored.

CORE CONCEPT

Mania

An alteration in mood that may be expressed by feelings of elation, inflated self-esteem, grandiosity, hyperactivity, agitation, racing thoughts, and accelerated speech. Mania can occur as part of the psychiatric disorder bipolar disorder, as part of some other medical conditions, or in response to some substances.

Historical Perspective

Documentation of the symptoms associated with bipolar disorder dates back to about the second century in ancient Greece. Aretaeus of Cappadocia, a Greek physician, is credited with associating these extremes of mood as part of the same illness. He described patients who could at times laugh and play all night and day but at other times appeared "torpid, dull, and sorrowful" (Burton, 2012). His view that these mood swings were part of the same illness did not gain acceptance until much later.

In early writings, mania was categorized with all forms of "severe madness." In 1025, the Persian physician Avicenna wrote *The Canon of Medicine* in which he described mania as "bestial madness characterized by rapid onset and remission, with agitation and irritability."

The modern concept of manic-depressive illness began to emerge in the 19th century. In 1854, Jules Baillarger presented information to the French Imperial Academy of Medicine in which he used the term *dual-form insanity* to describe the illness. In the same year, Jean-Pierre Falret described the same disorder, one with alternating periods of depression and manic excitation, with the term *circular insanity* (Burton, 2012). Falret also noted that this disorder appeared to have genetic underpinnings, a belief that is adhered to today (Krans & Cherney, 2016).

Contemporary thinking about bipolar disorder has been shaped by the works of Emil Kraepelin, who first coined the term *manic-depressive* in 1913. He added that this disorder was characterized by acute episodes followed by relatively symptom-free periods. In 1980, the American Psychiatric Association adopted the term *bipolar disorder* as the diagnostic category for manic-depressive illness in the third edition of the *Diagnostic and Statistical Manual of Mental Disorders.* This term identified a period of mood elevation and excitation as a defining characteristic of the disorder that distinguishes it from other mood or psychotic disorders. In addition, it replaced the term *mania* because descriptions of people as "maniacs" were considered stigmatizing (Krans & Cherney, 2016).

Epidemiology

Bipolar disorder affects approximately 5.7 million American adults, or about 2.6 percent of the U.S. population aged 18 and older in a given year. Of these cases, 82.9 percent are considered severe (National Institute of Mental Health [NIMH], 2015). In terms of gender, the incidence of bipolar disorder is roughly equal, with a ratio of women to men of about 1.2 to 1. The average age of onset for bipolar disorder is 25 years, and following the first manic episode, the disorder tends to be recurrent. Unlike depressive disorders, bipolar disorder appears to occur more frequently among the higher socioeconomic classes (Sadock, Sadock, & Ruiz, 2015). Bipolar disorder is the sixth-leading cause of disability in the middle-age group, but for those who respond to lithium treatment (about 33% of those treated with lithium), bipolar disorder is completely treatable, with no further episodes. Unfortunately, many individuals go for years without an accurate diagnosis or treatment, and for some the consequences can be devastating.

Types of Bipolar Disorders

A bipolar disorder is characterized by mood swings from profound depression to extreme euphoria (mania), with intervening periods of normalcy. Delusions or hallucinations may or may not be part of the clinical picture, and onset of symptoms may reflect a seasonal pattern.

During a manic episode, the mood is elevated, expansive, or irritable. The disturbance is sufficiently severe to cause marked impairment in occupational functioning or in usual social activities or relationships with others, or to require hospitalization to prevent harm to self or others. Motor activity is excessive and frenzied. Psychotic features may be present. The *Diagnostic and Statistical Manual of Mental Disorders, Fifth Edition (DSM-5)* (APA, 2013) diagnostic criteria for a manic episode are presented in Box 26–1.

BOX 26–1 Diagnostic Criteria for Manic Episode

A. A distinct period of abnormally and persistently elevated, expansive, or irritable mood, and abnormally and persistently increased goal-directed activity or energy, lasting at least 1 week and present most of the day, nearly every day (or any duration if hospitalization is necessary).

B. During the period of mood disturbance and increased energy or activity, three (or more) of the following symptoms (four if the mood is only irritable) are present to a significant degree, and represent a noticeable change from usual behavior:
   1. Inflated self-esteem or grandiosity.
   2. Decreased need for sleep (e.g., feels rested after only 3 hours of sleep).
   3. More talkative than usual or pressure to keep talking.
   4. Flight of ideas or subjective experience that thoughts are racing.
   5. Distractibility (i.e., attention too easily drawn to unimportant or irrelevant external stimuli), as reported or observed.
   6. Increase in goal-directed activity (either socially, at work or school, or sexually) or psychomotor agitation (i.e., purposeless non-goal-directed activity).
   7. Excessive involvement in activities that have a high potential for painful consequences (e.g., engaging in unrestrained buying sprees, sexual indiscretions, or foolish business investments).

C. The mood disturbance is sufficiently severe to cause marked impairment in social or occupational functioning or to necessitate hospitalization to prevent harm to self or others, or there are psychotic features.

D. The episode is not attributable to the physiological effects of a substance (e.g., a drug of abuse, a medication, or other treatment) or to another medical condition. *Note:* A full manic episode that emerges during antidepressant treatment (e.g., medication, electroconvulsive therapy) but persists at a fully syndromal level beyond the physiological effect of that treatment is sufficient evidence for a manic episode and, therefore, a bipolar I diagnosis.

Reprinted with permission from the Diagnostic and Statistical Manual of Mental Disorders, Fifth Edition *(Copyright 2013). American Psychiatric Association.*

A somewhat milder degree of this clinical symptom picture is called **hypomania.** Hypomania is not severe enough to cause marked impairment in social or occupational functioning or to require hospitalization, and it does not include psychotic features. The *DSM-5* diagnostic criteria for a hypomanic episode are presented in Box 26–2.

The diagnostic picture for depression associated with bipolar disorder is similar to that described for major depressive disorder, with one major distinction: the client must have a history of one or more manic episodes. When the presentation includes symptoms associated with both depression and mania, the diagnosis is further specified as *with mixed features.*

Bipolar I Disorder

Bipolar I disorder is the diagnosis given to an individual who is experiencing a manic episode or has a history of one or more manic episodes. The client may also have experienced episodes of depression. This diagnosis is further specified by the current or most recent behavioral episode experienced. For example, the specifier might be *single manic episode* (to describe individuals having a first episode of mania) or *current* (or most recent) *episode manic, hypomanic, mixed,* or *depressed* (to describe individuals who have had recurrent mood episodes). Psychotic or catatonic features may also be noted.

Bipolar II Disorder

The bipolar II disorder diagnostic category is characterized by recurrent bouts of major depression with episodic occurrence of hypomania. The individual who is assigned this diagnosis may present with symptoms (or history) of depression or hypomania. The client has never experienced a full manic episode, and the symptoms are "not severe enough to cause marked impairment in social or occupational functioning or to necessitate hospitalization" (APA, 2013, p. 133). The diagnosis may specify whether the current or most recent episode is hypomanic, depressed, or with mixed features. If the current syndrome is a major depressive episode, psychotic or catatonic features may be noted.

Cyclothymic Disorder

The essential feature of **cyclothymic disorder** is a chronic mood disturbance of at least 2 years' duration, involving numerous periods of elevated mood that do not meet the criteria for a hypomanic episode and numerous periods of depressed mood of insufficient severity or duration to meet the criteria for major depressive episode. The individual is never without the symptoms for more than 2 months. The *DSM-5* criteria for cyclothymic disorder are presented in Box 26–3.

Substance/Medication-Induced Bipolar Disorder

The disturbance of mood associated with this disorder is considered to be the direct result of physiological effects of a substance (e.g., ingestion of or withdrawal from a drug of abuse or a medication). The mood disturbance may involve elevated, expansive, or irritable mood with inflated self-esteem, decreased need for

---

BOX 26–2 Diagnostic Criteria for Hypomanic Episode

A. A distinct period of abnormally and persistently elevated, expansive, or irritable mood and abnormally and persistently increased activity or energy, lasting at least 4 consecutive days and present most of the day, nearly every day.

B. During the period of mood disturbance and increased energy and activity, three (or more) of the following symptoms (four if the mood is only irritable) have persisted, represent a noticeable change from usual behavior, and have been present to a significant degree:

1. Inflated self-esteem or grandiosity.
2. Decreased need for sleep (e.g., feels rested after only 3 hours of sleep).
3. More talkative than usual or pressure to keep talking.
4. Flight of ideas or subjective experience that thoughts are racing.
5. Distractibility (i.e., attention too easily drawn to unimportant or irrelevant external stimuli), as reported or observed.
6. Increase in goal-directed activity (either socially, at work or school, or sexually) or psychomotor agitation.
7. Excessive involvement in pleasurable activities that have a high potential for painful consequences (e.g., engaging in unrestrained buying sprees, sexual indiscretions, or foolish business investments).

C. The episode is associated with an unequivocal change in functioning that is uncharacteristic of the individual when not symptomatic.

D. The disturbance in mood and the change in functioning are observable by others.

E. The episode is not severe enough to cause marked impairment in social or occupational functioning or to necessitate hospitalization. If there are psychotic features, the episode is, by definition, manic.

F. The episode is not attributable to the physiological effects of a substance (e.g., a drug of abuse, a medication, or other treatment).

NOTE: A full hypomanic episode that emerges during antidepressant treatment (medication, electroconvulsive therapy) but persists at a fully syndromal level beyond the physiological effect of that treatment is sufficient evidence for a hypomanic episode diagnosis. However, caution is indicated so that one or two symptoms (particularly increased irritability, edginess or agitation following antidepressant use) are not taken as sufficient for diagnosis of a hypomanic episode, nor necessarily indicative of a bipolar diathesis.

Reprinted with permission from the Diagnostic and Statistical Manual of Mental Disorders, Fifth Edition (Copyright 2013). American Psychiatric Association.

BOX 26–3 Diagnostic Criteria for Cyclothymic Disorder

A. For at least 2 years (at least 1 year in children and adolescents) there have been numerous periods with hypomanic symptoms that do not meet criteria for hypomanic episode and numerous periods with depressive symptoms that do not meet the criteria for a major depressive episode.

B. During the above 2-year period (1 year in children and adolescents), the hypomanic and depressive periods have been present for at least half the time and the individual has not been without the symptoms for more than 2 months at a time.

C. Criteria for a major depressive, manic, or hypomanic episode have never been met.

D. The symptoms in Criterion A are not better explained by schizoaffective disorder, schizophrenia, schizophreniform disorder, delusional disorder, or other specified or unspecified schizophrenia spectrum and other psychotic disorder.

E. The symptoms are not attributable to the physiological effects of a substance (e.g., a drug of abuse, a medication) or another medical condition (e.g., hyperthyroidism).

F. The symptoms cause clinically significant distress or impairment in social, occupational, or other important areas of functioning.

Specify if:

With anxious distress

Reprinted with permission from the Diagnostic and Statistical Manual of Mental Disorders, Fifth Edition (Copyright 2013). American Psychiatric Association.

---

sleep, and distractibility. The disorder causes clinically significant distress or impairment in social, occupational, or other important areas of functioning.

Mood disturbances are associated with *intoxication* from substances such as alcohol, amphetamines, cocaine, hallucinogens, inhalants, opioids, phencyclidine,

sedatives, hypnotics, and anxiolytics. Symptoms can also occur during *withdrawal* from substances such as alcohol, amphetamines, cocaine, sedatives, hypnotics, and anxiolytics.

A number of medications have been known to evoke mood symptoms. Classifications include anesthetics, analgesics, anticholinergics, anticonvulsants, antihypertensives, antiparkinsonian agents, antiulcer agents, cardiac medications, oral contraceptives, psychotropic medications, muscle relaxants, steroids, and sulfonamides. Some specific examples are included in the discussion of predisposing factors associated with bipolar disorders.

Bipolar Disorder Due to Another Medical Condition

This disorder is characterized by an abnormally and persistently elevated, expansive, or irritable mood and excessive activity or energy judged to be the direct physiological consequence of another medical condition (APA, 2013). The mood disturbance causes clinically significant distress or impairment in social, occupational, or other important areas of functioning. Types of physiological influences are included in the discussion of predisposing factors associated with bipolar disorders.

Predisposing Factors

The exact etiology of bipolar disorder has yet to be determined. Scientific evidence supports a chemical imbalance in the brain, although the cause of the imbalance remains unclear. Theories that consider a combination of hereditary factors and environmental triggers (stressful life events) appear to hold the most credibility.

Biological Theories
Genetics

Research suggests that bipolar disorder strongly reflects an underlying genetic vulnerability. Evidence from family, twin, and adoption studies exists to support this observation. A large study that looked at genetic variations associated with five major mental illnesses found that schizophrenia and bipolar disorders had about 15 percent of genetic variations in common (NIMH, 2013).

Twin Studies

Twin studies have indicated a concordance rate for bipolar disorder among monozygotic twins at 60 to 80 percent, compared to 10 to 20 percent in dizygotic twins. Because monozygotic twins have identical genes and dizygotic twins share only approximately half their genes, this is strong evidence that genes play a major role in the etiology. However, since identical twins do not always both develop the illness, other factors must also be involved. It is likely that many different genes as well as environmental factors are involved, although researchers do not yet know how these factors interact to cause bipolar disorder (NIMH, 2012).

Family Studies

In general, family studies have shown that if one parent has a mood disorder, the risk that a child will have a mood disorder is between 10 and 25 percent (Sadock et al., 2015). Sadock and associates report that "a family history of bipolar disorder conveys a greater risk for mood disorders in general and, specifically, a much greater risk for bipolar disorder" (p. 352). If both parents have the disorder, the risk is two to three times greater. This has also been the case in studies of children born to parents with bipolar disorder who were adopted at birth and reared by adoptive parents without evidence of the disorder.

Other Genetic Studies

Soreff and McInnes (2012) state:

Studies from the first series of genome-wide association studies have given combined support for two particular genes, *ANK3* (ankyrin G) and *CACNA1C* (alpha 1C subunit of the L-type voltage-gated calcium channel) in a sample of 4,387 cases and 6,209 controls.

The *ANK3* protein, located on the first part of the axon, is involved in making the determination of whether a neuron will fire. Studies have shown that lithium carbonate, the most common medication used to prevent manic episodes, reduces expression of *ANK3* (Leussis et al., 2013). The *CACNA1C* protein regulates the influx and outflow of calcium from the cells and is the site of action of the calcium channel blockers sometimes used in the treatment of bipolar disorder.

Recent research looking specifically at factors associated with lithium's effectiveness identified "a number of candidate genes related to neurotransmitters, intracellular signaling, neuroprotection, circadian rhythms, and other pathogenic mechanisms of bipolar disorder [that] were found to be associated with lithium's prophylactic response" (Rybakowski, 2014, p. 353). Evidence from another recent study identified that common gene sets demonstrated altered expression in patients with schizophrenia, bipolar disorder, and depression (Darby, Yolken, & Sabunciyan, 2016). Specifically, ribosomal genes were overexpressed, and those involved with neuronal connections such as gamma-aminobutyric acid (GABA) signaling were underexpressed. The researchers suggest that this finding may lead the way to RNA processing and protein synthesis as targets for therapeutic intervention. Ongoing genetic research will continue to shed light on the genetic influences in the development of bipolar disorder and the genetic factors that influence treatment response.

Biochemical Influences
Biogenic Amines

Early studies have associated symptoms of mania with a functional excess of norepinephrine and dopamine.

The neurotransmitter serotonin is believed to remain low in both depression and mania, but the exact mechanisms and biochemical influences are complex and not yet completely understood. For example, even though low serotonin is thought to play a role in both depression and manic states, selective serotonin reuptake inhibitors (SSRIs) sometimes trigger manic episodes and rapid cycling of mood swings in clients with bipolar disorders. Likely, multiple factors influence serotonin's role in this illness. Acetylcholine is another neurotransmitter believed to be related to symptoms in bipolar disorder. Medications that have an effect on cholinergic transmission, particularly cholinergic agonists, can reduce symptoms in mania (Sadock et al., 2015). Excessive levels of glutamate, an excitatory neurotransmitter, have been associated with bipolar disorder. Many of the mood stabilizers used to treat bipolar disorder inhibit the actions of glutamate. The primary support for neurotransmitter hypotheses is the effects that neuroleptic drugs have on the levels of these biogenic amines and the resulting reduction in symptoms of the disorder.

Although several neurotransmitters have been implicated in influencing symptoms, the cause of bipolar disorder remains unknown.

Physiological Influences

Neuroanatomical Factors

Neuroanatomical changes have been correlated with dysfunction in the prefrontal cortex, basal ganglia, temporal and frontal lobes of the forebrain, and parts of the limbic system including the amygdala, thalamus, and striatum. The different symptoms in bipolar disorder may be correlated to those specific areas of dysfunction (Semeniken & Dudás, 2012). Sadock and associates (2015) report that widely replicated positive emission tomography (PET) demonstrates decreased anterior brain function on the left side in depression and greater right-side reductions in brain activity in mania. Although causality of bipolar disorder cannot yet be defined as solely a neuroanatomical disorder, it is clear that mood disorders, including bipolar disorder, involve pathology in the brain.

Medication Side Effects

Certain medications used to treat somatic illnesses have been known to trigger a manic response. The most common of these are the steroids frequently used to treat chronic illnesses such as multiple sclerosis and systemic lupus erythematosus. Some clients whose first episode of mania occurred during steroid therapy have reported spontaneous recurrence of manic symptoms years later. Amphetamines, antidepressants, and high doses of anticonvulsants and narcotics also have the potential for initiating a manic episode.

Psychosocial Theories

Interest in psychosocial theories has declined in recent years with the focus of research on genetic and biochemical predisposing factors. Consequently, conditions such as schizophrenia and bipolar disorder are more often viewed as diseases of the brain with biological etiologies. However, several studies have confirmed a link between childhood trauma (emotional, physical, and sexual abuse) and the development of bipolar disorder (Aas et al., 2016; Etain et al., 2013; Janiri et al., 2015; Watson et al., 2013). Aas and associates (2016) identify that childhood trauma interacts with genes along several different pathways, which influences not only an increased risk for bipolar disorder but also earlier onset, more severe symptoms, substance use, and suicide risk. As research continues, the interaction of genetics and psychosocial stressors becomes more apparent. More research is needed to translate these connections into practical applications for treatment or prevention.

The Transactional Model of Stress and Adaptation

Bipolar disorder clearly results from an interaction between genetic, biological, and psychosocial determinants. The transactional model takes into consideration these etiological influences as well as those associated with past experiences, existing conditions, and the individual's perception of the event. Figure 26–1 depicts the dynamics of bipolar mania using the transactional model of stress and adaptation.

Developmental Implications

Childhood and Adolescence

The lifetime prevalence of adolescent bipolar disorders is estimated to be about 1 percent. In younger children, the incidence is very rare, but children and adolescents are often difficult to diagnose (Sadock et al., 2015). In the past decade, diagnosis of bipolar I disorder in youth has rapidly increased, which prompted researchers to look more closely at factors contributing to this trend. A connection is thought to exist between attention-deficit/hyperactivity disorder (ADHD) and the development of bipolar disorder in youth, but research has not supported this theory (Hassan et al., 2011; Sadock et al., 2015).

Studies also found that youth given this diagnosis more often manifested with a host of atypical symptoms, including nondiscrete mood episodes, chronic irritability, and temper tantrums. The *DSM-5* incorporated a new diagnosis, *disruptive mood dysregulation disorder,* that more aptly describes this symptom profile. Since then, a longitudinal study of children with

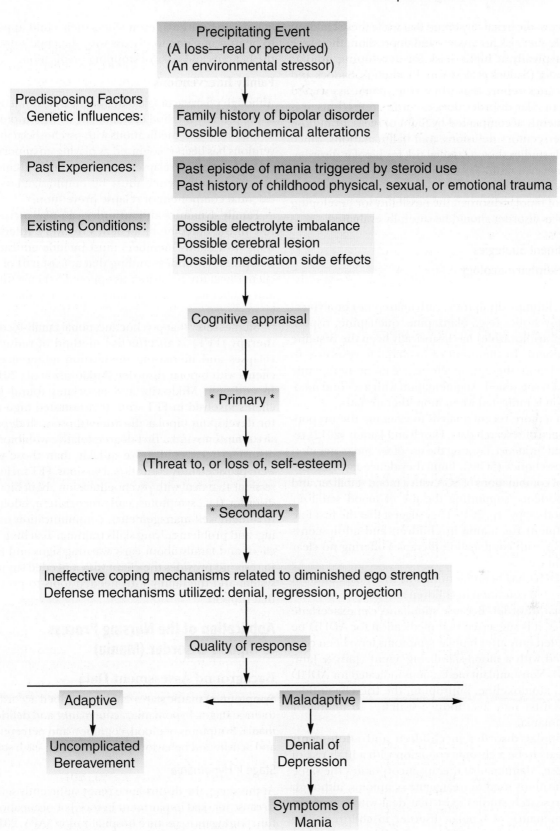

FIGURE 26–1 The dynamics of bipolar mania using the transactional model of stress and adaptation.

nonepisodic irritability found that while these children had higher risk for anxiety and depression, they were not typically at higher risk for developing bipolar disorder (Sadock et al., 2015). In addition, Sadock and associates report that when true mania associated with bipolar disorder does occur in adolescents, it is frequently accompanied by flight of ideas, grandiose or persecutory delusions, and hallucinations. Since family studies show a familial risk for bipolar disorder, whenever a child is exhibiting mood-related symptoms (including depression) and there is a family history of bipolar disorder, the possibility for developing bipolar disorder should be carefully evaluated.

Treatment Strategies

Psychopharmacology

Monotherapy with the traditional mood stabilizers (e.g., lithium, divalproex, carbamazepine) or atypical antipsychotics (e.g., olanzapine, quetiapine, risperidone, aripiprazole) has historically been the first-line treatment. In the event of inadequate response to initial monotherapy, an alternative monotherapeutic agent is suggested. Augmentation with a second medication is indicated when monotherapy fails.

In a more recent analysis to examine the preponderance of research data, Hazell and Jairam (2012) reported "evidence favoring the use of second-generation antipsychotics (SGAs), limited evidence favoring the use of combinations of SGA with a mood stabilizer, and no evidence supporting the use of mood stabilizer monotherapy" (p. 264). They suggest that the first-line treatment for mania in children and adolescents is SGA, with combination therapies offering no clear advantage.

ADHD has been identified as the most common comorbid condition in children and adolescents with bipolar disorder. Because stimulants can exacerbate mania, it is suggested that medication for ADHD be initiated only after bipolar symptoms have been controlled with a mood-stabilizing agent (Jain & Jain, 2014). Nonstimulant medications indicated for ADHD (e.g., atomoxetine, bupropion, the tricyclic antidepressants) may also induce switches to mania or hypomania.

Bipolar disorder in children and adolescents appears to be a chronic condition with a high risk of relapse. Maintenance therapy incorporates the same medications used to treat acute symptoms, although few research studies exist that deal with long-term maintenance of bipolar disorder in children. The American Academy of Child and Adolescent Psychiatry (AACAP) instructs parents to consider bipolar disorder a chronic illness much like diabetes and epilepsy (2010). As such, many people will require long-term or lifelong medication treatment. The AACAP encourages parents, even when their child appears to be in remission, to discuss with the child's doctor the benefits and risks of stopping medication.

Family Interventions

Although pharmacological treatment is acknowledged as the primary method of stabilizing acute symptoms, a combination of medications with psychosocial interventions has been recognized as playing an important role in preventing relapses and improving adjustment. Treatment adherence must be emphasized as an essential component of relapse prevention.

Family dynamics and attitudes can play a crucial role in the outcome of a client's recovery. Interventions with family members must include education that promotes understanding that at least part of the client's negative behaviors, as opposed to being willful and deliberate, are attributable to an illness that must be managed.

Studies show that psychoeducational family-focused therapy (FFT) is an effective method of reducing relapses and increasing medication adherence in clients with bipolar disorder (Miklowitz et al., 2013). In addition, Miklowitz and associates found that clients involved in FFT who demonstrated high risk for developing bipolar disorder (those with depressive symptoms and a first-degree relative with bipolar disorder) recovered more quickly than those who were provided only educational sessions. FFT includes sessions that deal with psychoeducation about bipolar disorder (i.e., symptoms, early recognition, etiology, treatment, self-management), communication training, and problem-solving skills training. Teaching the client and family about early warning signs and how to respond provides the client with a needed support system and the family with needed tools to provide that support.

Application of the Nursing Process to Bipolar Disorder (Mania)

Background Assessment Data

Symptoms of manic states can be described according to three stages: hypomania, acute mania, and **delirious mania.** Symptoms of mood, cognition and perception, and activity and behavior are presented for each stage.

Stage I: Hypomania

At this stage, the disturbance is not sufficiently severe to cause marked impairment in social or occupational functioning or to require hospitalization (APA, 2013).

Mood

The mood of a hypomanic person is cheerful and expansive. An underlying irritability surfaces rapidly when the person's wishes and desires go unfulfilled, however. The nature of the hypomanic person is volatile and fluctuating (see Box 26–2).

Cognition and Perception

Perceptions of the self are exalted—the individual has ideas of great worth and ability. Thinking is flighty, with a rapid flow of ideas. Perception of the environment is heightened, but the individual is so easily distracted by irrelevant stimuli that goal-directed activities are difficult.

Activity and Behavior

Hypomanic individuals exhibit increased motor activity. They are perceived as being extroverted and sociable and thus attract numerous acquaintances. However, they lack the depth of personality and warmth to formulate close friendships. They talk and laugh a great deal, usually very loudly and often inappropriately. Increased libido is common. Some individuals experience anorexia and weight loss. The exalted self-perception leads some hypomanic individuals to engage in inappropriate behaviors, such as phoning the President of the United States or running up debt on a credit card without having the resources to pay.

Stage II: Acute Mania

Symptoms of acute mania may progress in intensification from those experienced in hypomania, or they may be manifested directly. Most individuals experience marked impairment in functioning and require hospitalization (see Box 26–1).

Mood

Acute mania is characterized by euphoria and elation. The person appears to be on a continuous "high." However, the mood is always subject to frequent variation, easily changing to irritability and anger or even to sadness and crying.

Cognition and Perception

Cognition and perception become fragmented and often psychotic in acute mania. Accelerated thinking proceeds to racing thoughts; overconnection of ideas; and rapid, abrupt movement from one thought to another (**flight of ideas**) and may be manifested by a continuous flow of accelerated, pressured speech (loquaciousness) to the point that conversing with this individual may be extremely difficult. When flight of ideas is severe, speech may be disorganized and incoherent. Distractibility becomes all-pervasive. Attention can be diverted by even the smallest of stimuli. Hallucinations and delusions (usually paranoid and grandiose) are common.

Activity and Behavior

Psychomotor activity is excessive. Sexual interest is increased. There is poor impulse control and low frustration tolerance. The individual who is normally discreet may become socially and sexually uninhibited. Excessive spending is common. In acute mania, the individual typically has little insight into his or her behavior and communication. This lack of insight manifests at times as unreliable reporting of events and denial of problems when confronted by friends or family, which may be interpreted as lying. Energy seems inexhaustible, and the need for sleep is diminished. An individual experiencing acute mania may go for many days without sleep and still not feel tired. Hygiene and grooming may be neglected. Dress may be disorganized, flamboyant, or bizarre, and the use of excessive makeup or jewelry is common.

Stage III: Delirious Mania

Delirious mania is a grave form of the disorder characterized by severe clouding of consciousness and an intensification of the symptoms associated with acute mania. This condition has become relatively rare since the availability of antipsychotic medication.

Mood

The mood of the delirious person is very labile. He or she may exhibit feelings of despair, quickly converting to unrestrained merriment and ecstasy or becoming irritable or totally indifferent to the environment. Panic-level anxiety may be evident.

Cognition and Perception

Cognition and perception are characterized by a clouding of consciousness, with accompanying confusion, disorientation, and sometimes stupor. Other common manifestations include religiosity, delusions of grandeur or persecution, and auditory or visual hallucinations. The individual is extremely distractible and incoherent.

Activity and Behavior

Psychomotor activity is frenzied and characterized by agitated, purposeless movements. The safety of these individuals is at stake unless this activity is curtailed. Exhaustion, injury to self or others, and eventually death could occur without intervention.

Diagnosis and Outcome Identification

Using information collected during the assessment, the nurse completes the client database, from which the selection of appropriate nursing diagnoses is determined. Table 26–1 presents a list of client behaviors and the NANDA International nursing diagnoses that correspond to those behaviors, which may be used in planning care for the client experiencing a manic episode.

Outcome Criteria

The following criteria may be used for measuring outcomes in the care of the client experiencing a manic episode.

TABLE 26–1 Assigning Nursing Diagnoses to Behaviors Commonly Exhibited by Individuals Experiencing a Manic Episode

BEHAVIORS	NURSING DIAGNOSES
Extreme hyperactivity; increased agitation and lack of control over purposeless and potentially injurious movements	Risk for injury
Manic excitement, delusional thinking, hallucinations, impulsivity	Risk for violence: Self-directed or other-directed
Loss of weight, amenorrhea, refusal or inability to sit still long enough to eat	Imbalanced nutrition: Less than body requirements
Delusions of grandeur and persecution; inaccurate interpretation of the environment	Disturbed thought processes*
Auditory and visual hallucinations; disorientation	Disturbed sensory-perception*
Inability to develop satisfying relationships, manipulation of others for own desires, use of unsuccessful social interaction behaviors	Impaired social interaction
Difficulty falling asleep, sleeping only short periods	Insomnia

*These diagnoses have been resigned from the NANDA-I list of approved diagnoses. They are used in this instance because they are most compatible with the identified behaviors.

The client:

■ Exhibits no evidence of physical injury
■ Has not harmed self or others
■ Is no longer exhibiting signs of physical agitation
■ Eats a well-balanced diet with snacks to prevent weight loss and maintain nutritional status
■ Verbalizes an accurate interpretation of the environment
■ Verbalizes that hallucinatory activity has ceased and demonstrates no outward behavior indicating hallucinations
■ Accepts responsibility for own behaviors
■ Does not manipulate others for gratification of own needs
■ Interacts appropriately with others
■ Is able to fall asleep within 30 minutes of retiring
■ Is able to sleep 6 to 8 hours per night without medication

Planning and Implementation

The following section presents a group of selected nursing diagnoses, with short- and long-term goals and nursing interventions for each. Some institutions use a case management model to coordinate care (see Chapter 9, The Nursing Process in Psychiatric-Mental Health Nursing, for a more detailed explanation). In case management models, the plan of care may take the form of a critical pathway.

Risk for Violence: Self-Directed or Other-Directed

Risk for self- or other-directed violence is defined as "vulnerable to behaviors in which an individual demonstrates that he or she can be physically, emotionally, and/or sexually harmful to [self or to others]" (Herdman & Kamitsuru, 2014, pp. 410–411).

Client Goals

Outcome criteria include short- and long-term goals. Time lines are individually determined.

Short-term goals

■ Within [a specified time], client will recognize signs of increasing anxiety and agitation and report to staff (or other care provider) for assistance with intervention.
■ Client will not harm self or others.

Long-term goal

■ Client will not harm self or others.

Interventions

■ Maintain a low level of stimuli in the client's environment (low lighting, few people, simple decor, low noise level). Anxiety level rises in a stimulating environment. A suspicious, agitated client may perceive individuals as threatening.
■ Assess for concurrent substance use issues. There is a high incidence of comorbid substance use disorders in clients with bipolar disorder. Substance use issues can increase the client's risk for harm to self or others. In addition, the use of mood-altering chemicals beyond what is prescribed can make the evaluation of pharmacotherapy more difficult. (See Chapter 23, Substance-Related and Addictive Disorders, for more information on substance use disorders and relevant nursing interventions.)

- Observe the client's behavior frequently. Do this while carrying out routine activities so as to avoid creating suspiciousness in the individual. Close observation is necessary so that intervention can occur if required to ensure client (and others') safety.
- Remove all dangerous objects from the client's environment so the client may not use them to harm self or others in an agitated, confused state.
- Intervene at the first sign of increased anxiety, agitation, or verbal or behavioral aggression. Offer empathetic response to client's feelings: "You seem anxious (or frustrated, or angry) about this situation. How can I help?" Validation of the client's feelings conveys a caring attitude and offering assistance reinforces trust. Since the client may be highly distractible, providing a distraction can aid in diffusing anxiety and agitation as well.
- It is important to maintain a calm attitude toward the client. As the client's anxiety increases, offer some alternatives: participating in a physical activity (e.g., punching bag, physical exercise), talking about the situation, taking antianxiety medication. Offering alternatives to the client gives him or her a feeling of some control over the situation.
- Have sufficient staff available to indicate a show of strength to the client if it becomes necessary. This

shows the client evidence of control over the situation and provides some physical security for staff.
- If the client is not calmed by "talking down" or by medication, use of mechanical restraints may be necessary.

> **CLINICAL PEARL** The avenue of the "least restrictive alternative" must be selected when planning interventions for a violent client. Restraints should be used only as a last resort, after all other interventions have been unsuccessful and the client is clearly at risk of harm to self or others.

- If restraint is deemed necessary, ensure that sufficient staff is available to assist. Follow protocol established by the institution.
- As agitation decreases, assess the client's readiness for restraint removal or reduction. Remove one restraint at a time while assessing the client's response. This minimizes the risk of injury to client and staff.

Impaired Social Interaction

Impaired social interaction is defined as "insufficient or excessive quantity or ineffective quality of social exchange" (Herdman & Kamitsuru, 2014, p. 301). Table 26–2 presents this nursing diagnosis in care plan format.

Table 26–2 | CARE PLAN FOR THE CLIENT EXPERIENCING A MANIC EPISODE

NURSING DIAGNOSIS: IMPAIRED SOCIAL INTERACTION

RELATED TO: Delusional thought processes (grandeur and/or persecution); underdeveloped ego and low self-esteem

EVIDENCED BY: Inability to develop satisfying relationships and manipulation of others for own desires

OUTCOME CRITERIA	NURSING INTERVENTIONS	RATIONALE
Short-Term Goal: • Client verbalizes which of his or her interaction behaviors are appropriate and which are inappropriate within 1 week. **Long-Term Goal:** • Client demonstrates use of appropriate interaction skills as evidenced by lack of, or marked decrease in, manipulation of others to fulfill own desires.	1. Recognize the purpose manipulative behaviors serve for client: to reduce feelings of insecurity by increasing feelings of power and control. 2. Set limits on manipulative behaviors. Explain to client what is expected and what the consequences are if limits are violated. Terms of the limitations must be agreed on by all staff who will be working with client. 3. Do not argue, bargain, or try to reason with client. Merely state the limits and expectations. Confront client as soon as possible when interactions with others	1. Understanding the motivation behind the manipulation may facilitate acceptance of the individual and his or her behavior. 2. Client is unable to establish own limits, so this must be done for him or her. Unless administration of consequences for violation of limits is consistent, manipulative behavior will not be eliminated. 3. Because the client may be vulnerable to impulsive, reckless, or pleasure seeking behavior without considering consequences, he or she should receive immediate feedback when behavior is unacceptable. Consistency in enforcing

Continued

Table 26–2 | CARE PLAN FOR THE CLIENT EXPERIENCING A MANIC EPISODE—cont'd

OUTCOME CRITERIA	NURSING INTERVENTIONS	RATIONALE
	are manipulative or exploitative. Follow through with established consequences for unacceptable behavior.	the consequences is essential if positive outcomes are to be achieved. Inconsistency creates confusion and encourages testing of limits.
	4. Provide positive reinforcement for nonmanipulative behaviors. Explore feelings and help client seek more appropriate ways of dealing with them.	4. Positive reinforcement enhances self-esteem and promotes repetition of desirable behaviors.
	5. Help client recognize that he or she must accept the consequences of own behaviors and refrain from attributing them to others.	5. Client must accept responsibility for own behaviors before adaptive change can occur.
	6. Help client identify positive aspects about self, recognize accomplishments, and feel good about them.	6. As self-esteem is increased, client will feel less need to manipulate others for own gratification.

Client Goals

Outcome criteria include short- and long-term goals. Time lines are individually determined.

Short-term goal

■ Client will verbalize which of his or her interaction behaviors are appropriate and which are inappropriate within 1 week.

Long-term goal

■ Client will demonstrate use of appropriate interaction skills as evidenced by lack of, or marked decrease in, manipulation of others to fulfill own desires.

Interventions

■ Recognize the purpose these behaviors serve for the client: to reduce feelings of insecurity by increasing feelings of power and control. Understanding the motivation behind the manipulation may help to facilitate acceptance of the individual and his or her behavior.

■ Set limits on manipulative behaviors. Explain to the client what is expected and what the consequences are if the limits are violated. Terms of the limitations must be agreed on by all staff who will be working with the client. The client is unable to establish own limits, so this must be done for him or her. Unless administration of consequences for violation of limits is consistent, manipulative behavior will not be

eliminated. Comorbid borderline personality disorder has been identified as a risk in patients with bipolar disorder. (See Chapter 32, Personality Disorders, for more information on borderline personality disorder features and nursing interventions.)

■ Do not argue, bargain, or try to reason with the client. Merely state the limits and expectations. Individuals with mania can be very charming in their efforts to fulfill their own desires. Confront the client as soon as possible when interactions with others are manipulative or exploitative. Follow through with established consequences for unacceptable behavior. Because of the strong id influence on the client's behavior, he or she should receive immediate feedback when behavior is unacceptable. Consistency in enforcing the consequences is essential if positive outcomes are to be achieved. Inconsistency creates confusion and encourages testing of limits.

■ Provide positive reinforcement for nonmanipulative behaviors. Explore feelings and help the client seek more appropriate ways of dealing with them.

■ Help the client recognize that he or she must accept the consequences of behaviors and refrain from attributing them to others. The client must accept responsibility for own behaviors before adaptive change can occur.

■ Help the client identify positive aspects about self, recognize accomplishments, and feel good about them. As self-esteem increases, the client will feel less need to manipulate others for own gratification.

Imbalanced Nutrition: Less Than Body Requirements/Insomnia

Imbalanced nutrition: Less than body requirements is defined as "intake of nutrients insufficient to meet metabolic needs" (Herdman & Kamitsuru, 2014, p. 161). *Insomnia* is defined as "a disruption in amount and quality of sleep that impairs functioning" (p. 209).

Client Goals

Outcome criteria include short- and long-term goals. Time lines are individually determined.

Short-term goals

- Client will consume sufficient finger foods and between-meal snacks to meet recommended daily allowances of nutrients.
- Within 3 days, with the aid of a sleeping medication, client will sleep 4 to 6 hours without awakening.

Long-term goals

- Client will exhibit no signs or symptoms of malnutrition.
- By time of discharge from treatment, client will be able to acquire 6 to 8 hours of uninterrupted sleep without medication.

Interventions

- In collaboration with the dietitian, determine the number of calories required to provide adequate nutrition for maintenance or realistic (according to body structure and height) weight gain. Determine client's likes and dislikes, and provide favorite foods if possible. The client is more likely to eat foods that he or she particularly enjoys.
- Provide the client with high-protein, high-calorie, nutritious finger foods and drinks that can be consumed "on the run." Because of the hyperactive state, the client has difficulty sitting still long enough to eat a meal. He or she is more likely to consume food and drinks that can be carried around and eaten with little effort. Have juice and snacks available on the unit at all times. Regular nutritious intake is required to compensate for increased caloric requirements of hyperactivity.
- Maintain an accurate record of intake, output, and calorie count. Weigh the client daily. Administer vitamin and mineral supplements as ordered by the physician. Monitor laboratory values, and report significant changes to the physician. It is important to carefully monitor data that provide an objective assessment of the client's nutritional status.
- Assess the client's activity level. He or she may ignore or be unaware of feelings of fatigue. Observe for signs such as increasing restlessness; fine tremors; slurred speech; and puffy, dark circles under eyes. The client could collapse from exhaustion if hyperactivity is uninterrupted and rest is not achieved.
- Monitor sleep patterns. Provide a structured schedule of activities that includes established times for naps or rest. Accurate baseline data are important in planning care to help the client with this problem. A structured schedule, including time for short naps, will help the hyperactive client achieve much-needed rest.
- Client should avoid intake of caffeinated drinks, such as tea, coffee, and colas. Caffeine is a central nervous system (CNS) stimulant and may interfere with the client's achievement of rest and sleep.
- Before bedtime, provide nursing measures that promote sleep, such as back rub; warm bath; warm, nonstimulating drinks; soft music; and relaxation exercises.
- Administer sedative medications as ordered to help client achieve sleep until normal sleep pattern is restored.

Concept Care Mapping

The concept map care plan (see Chapter 9) is a diagrammatic teaching and learning strategy that allows visualization of interrelationships between medical diagnoses, nursing diagnoses, assessment data, and treatments. An example of a concept map care plan for a client experiencing a manic episode is presented in Figure 26–2.

Client and Family Education

The role of client-teacher is important in the psychiatric area, as it is in all areas of nursing. A list of topics for client and family education relevant to bipolar disorder is presented in Box 26–4.

Evaluation of Care for the Client Experiencing a Manic Episode

In the final step of the nursing process, a reassessment is conducted to determine if the nursing actions have been successful in achieving the objectives of care. Evaluation of the nursing actions for the client experiencing a manic episode may be facilitated by gathering information using the following types of questions.

- Has the individual avoided personal injury?
- Has violence to client or others been prevented?
- Has agitation subsided?
- Have nutritional status and weight been stabilized? Is the client able to select foods to maintain adequate nutrition?
- Have delusions and hallucinations ceased? Is the client able to interpret the environment correctly?

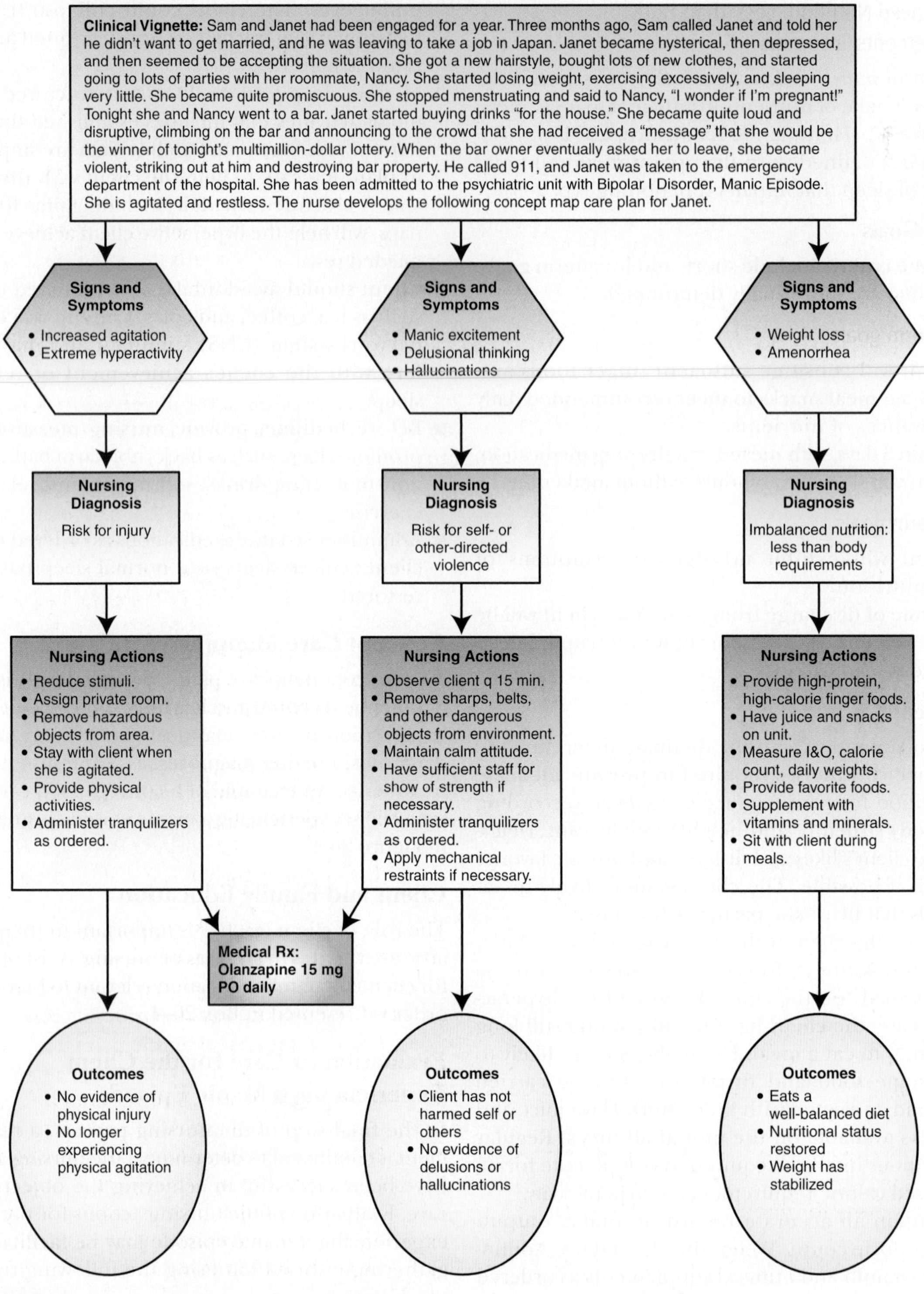

Clinical Vignette: Sam and Janet had been engaged for a year. Three months ago, Sam called Janet and told her he didn't want to get married, and he was leaving to take a job in Japan. Janet became hysterical, then depressed, and then seemed to be accepting the situation. She got a new hairstyle, bought lots of new clothes, and started going to lots of parties with her roommate, Nancy. She started losing weight, exercising excessively, and sleeping very little. She became quite promiscuous. She stopped menstruating and said to Nancy, "I wonder if I'm pregnant!" Tonight she and Nancy went to a bar. Janet started buying drinks "for the house." She became quite loud and disruptive, climbing on the bar and announcing to the crowd that she had received a "message" that she would be the winner of tonight's multimillion-dollar lottery. When the bar owner eventually asked her to leave, she became violent, striking out at him and destroying bar property. He called 911, and Janet was taken to the emergency department of the hospital. She has been admitted to the psychiatric unit with Bipolar I Disorder, Manic Episode. She is agitated and restless. The nurse develops the following concept map care plan for Janet.

Signs and Symptoms
- Increased agitation
- Extreme hyperactivity

Signs and Symptoms
- Manic excitement
- Delusional thinking
- Hallucinations

Signs and Symptoms
- Weight loss
- Amenorrhea

Nursing Diagnosis

Risk for injury

Nursing Diagnosis

Risk for self- or other-directed violence

Nursing Diagnosis

Imbalanced nutrition: less than body requirements

Nursing Actions
- Reduce stimuli.
- Assign private room.
- Remove hazardous objects from area.
- Stay with client when she is agitated.
- Provide physical activities.
- Administer tranquilizers as ordered.

Nursing Actions
- Observe client q 15 min.
- Remove sharps, belts, and other dangerous objects from environment.
- Maintain calm attitude.
- Have sufficient staff for show of strength if necessary.
- Administer tranquilizers as ordered.
- Apply mechanical restraints if necessary.

Nursing Actions
- Provide high-protein, high-calorie finger foods.
- Have juice and snacks on unit.
- Measure I&O, calorie count, daily weights.
- Provide favorite foods.
- Supplement with vitamins and minerals.
- Sit with client during meals.

Medical Rx:
Olanzapine 15 mg PO daily

Outcomes
- No evidence of physical injury
- No longer experiencing physical agitation

Outcomes
- Client has not harmed self or others
- No evidence of delusions or hallucinations

Outcomes
- Eats a well-balanced diet
- Nutritional status restored
- Weight has stabilized

FIGURE 26–2 Concept map care plan for a client with bipolar mania.

■ Is the client able to make decisions about own self-care? Has hygiene and grooming improved?

■ Is behavior socially acceptable? Is client able to interact with others in a satisfactory manner? Has the client stopped manipulating others to fulfill own desires?

■ Is the client able to sleep 6 to 8 hours per night and awaken feeling rested?

■ Does the client understand the importance of maintenance medication therapy? Does he or she understand that symptoms may return if medication is discontinued?

BOX 26–4 Topics for Client and Family Education Related to Bipolar Disorder

NATURE OF THE ILLNESS
1. Causes of bipolar disorder
2. Cyclic nature of the illness
3. Symptoms of depression
4. Symptoms of mania

MANAGEMENT OF THE ILLNESS
1. Medication management
   a. Lithium
   b. Others
      1) Carbamazepine
      2) Valproic acid
      3) Clonazepam
      4) Verapamil
      5) Lamotrigine
      6) Gabapentin
      7) Topiramate
      8) Oxcarbazepine
      9) Olanzapine
      10) Risperidone
      11) Chlorpromazine
      12) Aripiprazole
      13) Quetiapine
      14) Ziprasidone
      15) Asenapine
   c. Side effects
   d. Symptoms of lithium toxicity
   e. Importance of regular blood tests
   f. Adverse effects
   g. Importance of not stopping medication, even when feeling well
2. Assertive techniques
3. Anger management

SUPPORT SERVICES
1. Crisis hotline
2. Support groups
3. Individual psychotherapy
4. Legal and/or financial assistance

■ Can the client taking lithium verbalize early signs of lithium toxicity? Does he or she understand the necessity for monthly blood level checks?

Treatment Modalities for Bipolar Disorder (Mania)

Individual Psychotherapy

In a review of the evidence on psychotherapy for clients with bipolar disorder, Swartz and Swanson (2014) conclude that bipolar-specific psychotherapies in conjunction with medication treatment have better outcomes than medication alone. Evidence supports the benefits of psychoeducation, cognitive-behavioral therapy (CBT), FFT, interpersonal and social rhythm therapy (IPSRT), and integrated care management (Strakowski, 2016).

IPSRT is a type of therapy specifically designed for bipolar patients. Developed by Frank (2005), IPSRT focuses on helping clients regulate social rhythms or daily activities such as the sleep–wake cycle and exercise routines that may otherwise disrupt underlying biological rhythms and contribute to mood disturbances. In combination with this strategy, IPSRT also engages principles of interpersonal therapy to help clients address relationship problems.

Group Therapy

Once an acute phase of the illness has passed, groups can provide an atmosphere in which individuals may discuss issues in their lives that cause, maintain, or arise from having a serious affective disorder. Both group psychoeducation and group CBT have demonstrated benefits for this population (Swartz & Swanson, 2014). The element of peer support may provide a feeling of security, as troublesome or embarrassing issues are discussed and resolved. Some groups have other specific purposes, such as helping to monitor medication-related issues or serving as an avenue for promoting education related to the affective disorder and its treatment.

Support groups help members gain a sense of perspective on their condition and tangibly encourage them to connect with others who have common problems. A sense of hope is conveyed when the individual is able to see that he or she is not alone or unique in experiencing affective illness.

Self-help groups offer another avenue of support for the individual with bipolar disorder. These groups are usually peer led and are not meant to substitute for or compete with professional therapy. They offer supplementary support that frequently enhances compliance with the medical regimen. Examples of self-help groups are the Depression and Bipolar Support Alliance (DBSA) and the Child and Adolescent Bipolar Foundation, which put individuals in touch with their local support groups. Although self-help groups are not psychotherapy groups, they do provide important adjunctive support experiences that often have therapeutic benefit for participants.

Family Therapy

The ultimate objectives in working with families of clients with mood disorders are to resolve the symptoms and initiate or restore adaptive family functioning. Some studies with bipolar disorder have shown that behavioral family treatment combined with medication substantially reduces relapse rate compared with medication therapy alone.

Sadock and associates (2015) state:

> Family therapy is indicated if the disorder jeopardizes the patient's marriage or family functioning or if the mood disorder is promoted or maintained by the family situation. Family therapy examines the role of the mood-disordered member in the overall psychological well-being of the whole family; it also examines the role of the entire family in the maintenance of the patient's symptoms. (p. 373)

Family functioning and marital relationships are often disrupted in clients with bipolar disorder, especially when symptoms are contributing to disloyalty in the marriage and to financial problems related to the client's excessive spending behaviors. Whether intervention occurs in the form of family education, support, formal therapy, or a combination of these approaches, it is clear that families need to be involved in treatment whenever possible.

Cognitive Therapy

In cognitive therapy, the individual is taught to control thought distortions that are considered a factor in the development and maintenance of mood disorders. In the cognitive model, depression is characterized by a triad of negative distortions related to expectations of the environment, self, and future. The environment and activities within it are viewed as unsatisfying, the self is unrealistically devalued, and the future is perceived as hopeless. In the same model, mania is characterized by exaggeratedly positive cognitions and perceptions. The individual perceives the self as highly valued and powerful. Life is experienced with overstated self-assurance, and the future is viewed with unrealistic optimism.

The general goals in cognitive therapy are to obtain symptom relief as quickly as possible, assist the client in identifying dysfunctional patterns of thinking and behaving, and guide the client to evidence and logic that effectively tests the validity of the dysfunctional thinking (see Chapter 19, Cognitive Therapy). Therapy focuses on changing "automatic thoughts" that occur spontaneously and contribute to the distorted affect. Examples of automatic thoughts in bipolar mania include the following:

- **Personalizing:** "I'm the only reason my husband is a successful businessman."
- **All or nothing:** "Everything I do is great."
- **Mind reading:** "She thinks I'm wonderful."
- **Discounting negatives:** "None of those mistakes are really important."

The client is asked to describe evidence that both supports and disputes the automatic thought. The logic underlying the inferences is then reviewed with the client. Another technique involves evaluating what would most likely happen if the client's automatic thoughts were true. Implications of the consequences are then discussed.

Clients should not become discouraged if one technique does not seem to be working. No single technique works with all clients. He or she should be reassured that any of a number of techniques may be used, and both therapist and client may explore these possibilities.

The Recovery Model

Research provides support for recovery as an obtainable objective for individuals with bipolar disorder. Conceptual models of recovery from mental illness are presented in Chapter 21, The Recovery Model. The recovery model has been used primarily in caring for individuals with serious mental illness, such as schizophrenia and bipolar disorder. However, concepts of the model can be used with all individuals experiencing emotional conditions that require assistance and who have a desire to take control and manage their lives more independently.

In bipolar disorder, recovery is a continuous process. The individual identifies goals based on personal values or what he or she defines as giving meaning and purpose to life. The clinician and client work together to develop a treatment plan that is in alignment with the goals set forth by the client. In the recovery process, the individual may still be experiencing symptoms. Weiden (2010) states:

> Patients do not have to be in remission, nor does remission automatically have to be a desired (or likely) goal when embarking on a recovery-oriented treatment plan. As long as the patient (and family) understands that a process recovery treatment plan is not to be confused with a promise of "cure" or even "remission," then one does not overpromise.

In the process of recovery, the client and clinician work on strategies to help the individual with bipolar disorder take control of and manage his or her illness. Some of these strategies include the following (Carolla, 2013; National Alliance on Mental Illness [NAMI], 2008):

- Exhibiting self-awareness
- Becoming an expert on the disorder
- Taking medications regularly
- Recognizing earliest symptoms
- Identifying and reducing sources of stress
- Knowing when to seek help
- Developing a personal support system
- Managing lifestyle factors such as sleep time and exercise
- Developing a plan for emergencies

During the process of recovery, individuals actively work on the strategies they have identified to keep themselves well. The clinician serves as a support person to help the individual take the necessary steps to achieve the goals he or she has previously set forth.

Although there is no cure for bipolar disorder, there are effective treatments and interventions. Recovery is possible when the client is empowered and actively engaged in a multifaceted illness management approach.

Electroconvulsive Therapy

Episodes of acute mania are occasionally treated with electroconvulsive therapy (ECT), particularly when the client does not tolerate or fails to respond to lithium or other drug treatment or when life is threatened by dangerous behavior or exhaustion. See Chapter 20, Electroconvulsive Therapy, for a detailed discussion of ECT.

Psychopharmacology With Mood-Stabilizing Agents

For many years, the drug of choice for treatment and management of bipolar mania was lithium carbonate. However, in recent years a number of investigators and clinicians in practice have achieved satisfactory results with other medications, including anticonvulsant drugs that have a mood-stabilizing effect, either alone or in combination with lithium. (See Chapter 4, Psychopharmacology, for a detailed discussion of indications, actions, contraindications, and other safety issues related to mood-stabilizing agents.)

Both lithium and mood stabilizers demonstrate effectiveness in managing bipolar depression. Three products are currently approved by the U.S. Food and Drug Administration (FDA) for that purpose: the combination of olanzapine and fluoxetine, quetiapine, and lurasidone (Strakowski, 2016). Antidepressants have shown little evidence of effectiveness in treating bipolar depression as an adjunct to mood stabilizers. Additionally, Strakowski identifies that antidepressants carry as high as a 40 percent risk of potentially triggering a switch from depression to mania in individuals with bipolar disorder.

Clients who respond to lithium can be virtually symptom free over the long term. About 33 percent of people treated with lithium respond positively (Rybakowski, 2014), so having other pharmacological treatments available is important in the treatment of this illness. Since bipolar disorder is a chronic, episodic illness, most people will remain on medication throughout their lives. See Table 26–3 for a list of commonly used medications in the treatment of bipolar disorder. Lithium, like other medications, has side effects. Most notably, its therapeutic range (0.6–1.2 mEq/L) can have toxic side effects and is potentially fatal when exceeded.

Client and Family Education for Lithium
The client should:

■ Take medication on a regular basis, even when feeling well. Discontinuation can result in return of symptoms.

■ Not drive or operate dangerous machinery until lithium levels are stabilized. Drowsiness and dizziness can occur.

■ Not skimp on dietary sodium intake. He or she should eat a variety of healthy foods and avoid "junk" foods. The client should drink six to eight large glasses of water each day and avoid excessive use of beverages containing caffeine (coffee, tea, colas), which promote increased urine output.

■ Notify the physician if vomiting or diarrhea occurs. These symptoms can result in sodium loss and an increased risk of lithium toxicity.

■ Carry a card or other identification noting that he or she is taking lithium.

■ Be aware of appropriate diet should weight gain become a problem. Include adequate sodium and other nutrients while decreasing number of calories.

■ Be aware of risks of becoming pregnant while receiving lithium therapy. Use information furnished by health-care providers regarding methods of contraception. Notify the physician as soon as possible if pregnancy is suspected or planned.

■ Be aware of side effects and symptoms associated with toxicity. Notify the physician if any of the following symptoms occur: persistent nausea and vomiting, severe diarrhea, ataxia, blurred vision, tinnitus, excessive urine output, increasing tremors, or mental confusion.

■ Refer to written materials furnished by health-care providers while receiving self-administered maintenance therapy. Keep appointments for outpatient follow-up; have serum lithium level checked every 1 to 2 months or as advised by physician.

Client and Family Education for Anticonvulsant Mood Stabilizers
The client should:

■ Refrain from discontinuing the drug abruptly. Physician will administer orders for tapering the drug when therapy is to be discontinued.

■ Report the following symptoms to the physician immediately: skin rash, unusual bleeding, spontaneous bruising, sore throat, fever, malaise, dark urine, and yellow skin or eyes.

■ Not drive or operate dangerous machinery until reaction to the medication has been established.

TABLE 26-3 Mood Stabilizing Agents

CLASSIFICATION: GENERIC (TRADE)	PREGNANCY CATEGORY/ HALF-LIFE/ INDICATIONS	MECHANISM OF ACTION	CONTRAINDICATIONS/ PRECAUTIONS	DAILY ADULT DOSAGE RANGE/ THERAPEUTIC PLASMA RANGE
ANTIMANIC				
Lithium carbonate (Eskalith, Lithobid)	D/ 24 hr/ ■ Prevention and treatment of manic episodes of bipolar disorder *Unlabeled uses:* ■ Neutropenia ■ Cluster headaches (prophylaxis) ■ Alcohol dependence ■ Bulimia ■ Postpartum affective psychosis ■ Corticosteroid-induced psychosis	Not fully understood but may modulate the effects of various neurotransmitters (e.g., norepinephrine, serotonin, dopamine, glutamate, and GABA) that are thought to play a role in the symptomatology of bipolar disorder (may take 1–3 weeks for symptoms to subside)	Hypersensitivity Cardiac or renal disease, dehydration, sodium depletion, brain damage, pregnancy and lactation Caution with thyroid disorders, diabetes, urinary retention, history of seizures, and the elderly	Acute mania: 1,800–2,400 mg Maintenance: 900–1,200 mg/ Acute mania: 1.0–1.5 mEq/L Maintenance: 0.6–1.2 mEq/L
ANTICONVULSANTS				
Carbamazepine (Tegretol)	D/ 25–65 hr (initial): 12–17 hr (repeated doses)/ ■ Epilepsy ■ Trigeminal neuralgia *Unlabeled uses:* ■ Bipolar disorder ■ Resistant schizophrenia ■ Management of alcohol withdrawal ■ Restless legs syndrome ■ Postherpetic neuralgia	Action in the treatment of bipolar disorder is unclear	Hypersensitivity With MAOIs, lactation Caution with elderly; liver, renal, cardiac disease; pregnancy	200–1,600 mg/ 4–12 mcg/mL
Clonazepam (Klonopin)	C/ 18–60 hr/ ■ Petit mal, akinetic, and myoclonic seizures ■ Panic disorder *Unlabeled uses:* ■ Acute manic episodes ■ Uncontrolled leg movements during sleep ■ Neuralgias	Action in the treatment of bipolar disorder is unclear	Hypersensitivity, glaucoma, liver disease, lactation Caution in elderly; liver, renal disease; pregnancy	0.5–20 mg/ 0.02–0.08 mcg/mL
Valproic acid (Depakene; Depakote)	D/ 5–20 hr/ ■ Epilepsy ■ Manic episodes ■ Migraine prophylaxis ■ Adjunct therapy in schizophrenia	Action in the treatment of bipolar disorder is unclear	Hypersensitivity, liver disease Caution in elderly; renal, cardiac diseases; pregnancy and lactation	5 mg/kg–60 mg/kg/ 50–150 mcg/mL
Lamotrigine (Lamictal)	C/ ~33 hr/ ■ Epilepsy *Unlabeled use:* ■ Bipolar disorder	Action in the treatment of bipolar disorder is unclear	Hypersensitivity Caution in renal and hepatic insufficiency, pregnancy, lactation, and children <16 years old	100–200 mg/ Not established

Drug	Half-life / Uses	Action / Mechanism	Contraindications / Precautions	Dosage (Adult / Child)
Gabapentin (Neurontin)	C/ 5–7 hr/ ■ Epilepsy ■ Postherpetic neuralgia *Unlabeled uses:* ■ Bipolar disorder ■ Migraine prophylaxis ■ Neuropathic pain ■ Tremors associated with multiple sclerosis	Action in the treatment of bipolar disorder is unclear	Hypersensitivity and children <3 years Caution in renal insufficiency, pregnancy, lactation, children, and the elderly	900–1,800 mg/ Not established
Topiramate (Topamax)	C/ 21 hr/ ■ Epilepsy ■ Migraine prophylaxis *Unlabeled uses:* ■ Bipolar disorder ■ Cluster headaches ■ Bulimia ■ Binge eating disorder ■ Weight loss in obesity	Action in the treatment of bipolar disorder is unclear	Hypersensitivity Caution in renal and hepatic impairment, pregnancy, lactation, children, and the elderly	50–400 mg/ Not established
Oxcarbazepine (Trileptal)	C/ 2–9 hr/ ■ Epilepsy *Unlabeled uses:* ■ Bipolar disorder ■ Diabetic neuropathy ■ Neuralgia	Action in the treatment of bipolar disorder is unclear	Hypersensitivity Caution in renal and hepatic impairment, pregnancy, lactation, children, and the elderly	600–2,400 mg/ Not established
ANTIPSYCHOTICS ALL ANTIPSYCHOTICS:				
Olanzapine (Zyprexa)	C/ 21–54 hr/ ■ Schizophrenia ■ Acute manic episodes ■ Management of bipolar disorder ■ Agitation associated with schizophrenia or mania *Unlabeled uses:* ■ Obsessive-compulsive disorder	Efficacy in schizophrenia is achieved through a combination of dopamine and serotonin type 2 (5HT₂) antagonism. Mechanism of action in the treatment of mania is unknown. Action may be mediated via effects on dopamine and serotonin (5HT2a) receptor antagonism	Hypersensitivity, children, lactation Caution with hepatic or cardiovascular disease, history of seizures, coma or other CNS depression, prostatic hypertrophy, narrow-angle glaucoma, diabetes or risk factors for diabetes, pregnancy, elderly and debilitated patients, history of suicide attempts	10–20 mg/ Not established
Olanzapine and fluoxetine (Symbyax)	C/ (see individual drugs)/ ■ Treatment of depressive episodes associated with bipolar disorder			6/25–12/50 mg/ Not established
Aripiprazole (Abilify)	C/ 50–80 hr/ ■ Bipolar mania ■ Schizophrenia			10–30 mg/ Not established

Continued

TABLE 26–3 Mood Stabilizing Agents—cont'd

CLASSIFICATION: GENERIC (TRADE)	PREGNANCY CATEGORY/ HALF-LIFE/ INDICATIONS	MECHANISM OF ACTION	CONTRAINDICATIONS/ PRECAUTIONS	DAILY ADULT DOSAGE RANGE/ THERAPEUTIC PLASMA RANGE
Lurasidone (Latuda)	B/ 18 hr/ ■ Depressive episodes in bipolar I disorder ■ Schizophrenia			20–120 mg/ Not established
Chlorpromazine	C/ 24 hr/ ■ Bipolar mania ■ Schizophrenia ■ Emesis, hiccoughs ■ Acute intermittent porphyria ■ Preoperative apprehension *Unlabeled uses:* ■ Migraine headaches			75–400 mg/ Not established
Quetiapine (Seroquel)	C/ 6 hr/ ■ Schizophrenia ■ Acute manic episodes			100–800 mg/ Not established
Risperidone (Risperdal)	C/ 3–20 hr/ ■ Bipolar mania ■ Schizophrenia *Unlabeled uses:* ■ Severe behavioral problems in children ■ Behavioral problems associated with autism ■ Obsessive-compulsive disorder			1–6 mg/ Not established
Ziprasidone (Geodon)	C/ 7 hr (oral)/ ■ Bipolar mania ■ Schizophrenia ■ Acute agitation in schizophrenia			40–160 mg/ Not established
Asenapine (Saphris)	C/ 24 hr/ ■ Schizophrenia ■ Bipolar mania			10–20 mg/ Not established

- Avoid consuming alcoholic beverages and non-prescription medications without approval from physician.
- Carry a card at all times identifying the name of medications being taken.

> **CLINICAL PEARL** The FDA requires that all antiepileptic (anticonvulsant) drugs carry a warning label indicating that use of the drugs increases risk for suicidal thoughts and behaviors. Patients being treated with these medications should be monitored for the emergence or worsening of depression, suicidal thoughts or behavior, or any unusual changes in mood or behavior.

Client and Family Education for Calcium Channel Blocker

The client should:

- Take medication with meals if gastrointestinal upset occurs.
- Use caution when driving or when operating dangerous machinery. Dizziness, drowsiness, and blurred vision can occur.
- Refrain from discontinuing the drug abruptly. To do so may precipitate cardiovascular problems. Physician will administer orders for tapering the drug when therapy is to be discontinued.
- Report occurrence of any of the following symptoms to physician immediately: irregular heartbeat, shortness of breath, swelling of the hands and feet, pronounced dizziness, chest pain, profound mood swings, severe and persistent headache.
- Rise slowly from a sitting or lying position to prevent a sudden drop in blood pressure.
- Avoid taking other medications (including over-the-counter medications) without physician's approval.
- Carry a card at all times describing medications being taken.

Client and Family Education for Antipsychotics

The client should:

- Use caution when driving or operating dangerous machinery. Drowsiness and dizziness can occur.
- Refrain from discontinuing the drug abruptly after long-term use. To do so might produce withdrawal symptoms, such as nausea, vomiting, dizziness, gastritis, headache, tachycardia, insomnia, and tremulousness. Physician will administer orders for tapering the drug when therapy is to be discontinued.

- Use sunblock lotion and wear protective clothing when spending time outdoors. Skin is more susceptible to sunburn, which can occur in as little as 30 minutes.
- Report the occurrence of any of the following symptoms to the physician immediately: sore throat, fever, malaise, unusual bleeding, easy bruising, persistent nausea and vomiting, severe headache, rapid heart rate, difficulty urinating, muscle twitching, tremors, dark-colored urine, excessive urination, excessive thirst, excessive hunger, weakness, pale stools, yellow skin or eyes, muscular incoordination, or skin rash.
- Rise slowly from a sitting or lying position to prevent a sudden drop in blood pressure.
- Take frequent sips of water, chew sugarless gum, or suck on hard candy, if dry mouth is a problem. Good oral care (frequent brushing, flossing) is very important.
- Consult the physician regarding smoking while on antipsychotic therapy. Smoking increases the metabolism of these drugs, requiring an adjustment in dosage to achieve a therapeutic effect.
- Dress warmly in cold weather, and avoid extended exposure to very high or low temperatures. Body temperature is harder to maintain with this medication.
- Avoid drinking alcohol while on antipsychotic therapy. These drugs potentiate each other's effects.
- Avoid taking other medications (including over-the-counter products) without the physician's approval. Many medications contain substances that interact with antipsychotic medications in a way that may be harmful.
- Be aware of possible risks of taking antipsychotics during pregnancy. Safe use during pregnancy has not been established. Antipsychotics are thought to readily cross the placental barrier; if so, a fetus could experience adverse effects of the drug. Inform the physician immediately if pregnancy occurs, is suspected, or is planned.
- Be aware of side effects of antipsychotic medications. Refer to written materials furnished by health-care providers for safe self-administration.
- Continue to take the medication even if feeling well. Symptoms may return if medication is discontinued.
- Carry a card or other identification at all times describing medications being taken.

CASE STUDY AND SAMPLE CARE PLAN

NURSING HISTORY AND ASSESSMENT

Candace, age 32, recently moved to New York City from Omaha, Nebraska, where she had been working as a television reporter. She felt that Omaha had become "too boring" and wanted to experience the big city life. Candace has a history of bipolar I disorder and has been maintained on lithium since she was 23 years old. Since she arrived in New York City, she has run out of her medication and has not found a doctor to have her prescription renewed. She has been staying in an inexpensive apartment and living on savings. She has been seeking employment in her chosen line of work, but it has been 2 months now, and she has been unable to find a job. She is becoming anxious as her savings have depleted. She has lost weight and has trouble sleeping.

Today, after two failed interviews, Candace went to a bar and began drinking. She ordered several rounds of drinks for everyone in the bar and told the bartender to "put it on my tab." The bartender called the police when Candace refused to pay her tab and became loud and belligerent. He said she began shouting that she knew the mayor, and he was going to help her find a job, and if they didn't leave her alone, she would tell the mayor how they were treating her. She took out her cell phone and said she was calling the mayor. When others in the room began laughing at her, she began cursing and saying that they "would be sorry one day that they laughed at her." When the police arrived, Candace was resistant and had to be physically restrained. The police took Candace to the emergency department of the community hospital, where she was admitted with a diagnosis of Bipolar I Disorder, current episode manic. The psychiatrist ordered olanzapine 10 mg IM STAT, olanzapine 10 mg PO qd, lithium carbonate 600 mg PO bid, and vitamin supplement daily. He ordered lithium level to be drawn prior to first dose of lithium.

NURSING DIAGNOSES AND OUTCOME IDENTIFICATION

From the assessment data, the admitting nurse develops the following nursing diagnoses for Candace:

1. **Risk for self- or other-directed violence** related to manic hyperactivity, delusional thinking, impulsivity
   a. Short-Term Goal:
      ■ Agitation and hyperactivity will be maintained at manageable level with the administration of tranquilizing medication.
   b. **Long-Term Goal:**
      ■ Candace will not harm self or others during hospitalization.
2. **Imbalanced nutrition: Less than body requirements** related to lack of appetite and excessive physical agitation, evidenced by loss of weight.
   a. **Short-Term Goal:**
      ■ Candace will consume sufficient finger foods and between-meal snacks to meet recommended daily allowances of nutrients.
   b. **Long-Term Goal:**
      ■ Candace will begin to regain weight and exhibit no signs or symptoms of malnutrition.

PLANNING AND IMPLEMENTATION

RISK FOR SELF- OR OTHER-DIRECTED VIOLENCE
The following nursing interventions have been identified for Candace:

1. Place Candace in a private room near the nurse's station. Observe her behavior frequently.
2. Remove all dangerous objects from her environment.
3. Plan some physical activities for Candace (e.g., treadmill, punching bag) and regular rest periods during the day.
4. Administer tranquilizing medication as ordered by physician.
5. Monitor lithium levels three times during first week of therapy. Monitor for signs and symptoms of toxicity (e.g., ataxia, blurred vision, severe diarrhea, persistent nausea and vomiting, tinnitus).
6. Ensure that sufficient staff is available to intervene should Candace become agitated and aggressive.

IMBALANCED NUTRITION: LESS THAN BODY REQUIREMENTS
The following nursing interventions have been identified for Candace:

1. Consult dietitian to determine appropriate diet for Candace to restore nutrition and gain weight. Ensure that her diet includes foods that she particularly likes.
2. Ensure that Candace has access to finger foods and between-meal snacks if she cannot or will not sit still to eat off a meal tray.
3. Maintain an accurate record of intake, output, and calorie count.
4. Obtain daily weights.
5. Administer vitamin supplement, as ordered by physician.
6. Sit with Candace during mealtime.

EVALUATION

The outcome criteria identified for Candace have been met. She has not harmed herself or others in any way. She is able to verbalize names of resources outside the hospital from whom she may request help if needed. With help from the social worker, she has applied for unemployment assistance and will begin receiving help within 2 weeks. She has gained 3 pounds in the hospital and verbalizes understanding of the importance of maintaining good nutrition. She is taking her medication regularly, and has a follow-up appointment with the psychiatric nurse practitioner, who will see Candace biweekly and ensure that she is compliant with medication and laboratory requirements. Candace verbalizes understanding of the importance of taking her medication on a continuous basis. She has a hopeful but realistic attitude about finding work in New York City and states that she will give herself a deadline after which she plans to return to her home in Omaha where she will be near family and friends.

Summary and Key Points

■ Bipolar disorder is manifested by mood swings from profound depression to extreme elation and euphoria.

■ Genetic influences have been strongly implicated in the development of bipolar disorder. Various physiological factors, such as biochemical and electrolyte alterations, as well as cerebral structural changes, have been implicated. Side effects of certain medications may also induce symptoms of mania. No single theory can explain the etiology of bipolar disorder, and it is likely that the illness is caused by a combination of factors.

■ Symptoms of mania may be observed on a continuum of three phases, each identified by the degree of severity: phase I, hypomania; phase II, acute mania; and phase III, delirious mania.

■ The symptoms of bipolar disorder may occur in children and adolescents as well as in adults.

■ Treatment of bipolar disorder includes individual therapy, group and family therapy, cognitive therapy, ECT, and psychopharmacology. For the majority of clients, the most effective treatment appears to be a combination of psychotropic medication and psychosocial therapy.

■ Some clinicians choose a course of therapy based on a model of recovery similar to that used for many years to treat addiction. The basic premise of a recovery model is empowerment of the consumer; it is designed to allow consumers primary control over decisions about their own care and to enable a person with a mental health problem to live a meaningful life in a community of choice while striving to achieve his or her full potential.

■ For many years, the pharmacological treatment of choice for bipolar mania was lithium carbonate. A number of other medications are now being used with satisfactory results, including anticonvulsants and antipsychotics.

■ There is a narrow margin between the therapeutic and toxic levels of lithium. Serum lithium levels must be monitored regularly while on maintenance therapy.

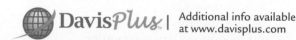

DavisPlus | Additional info available at www.davisplus.com

Review Questions
Self-Examination/Learning Exercise

Select the answer that is most appropriate for each of the following questions.

1. Margaret, a 68-year-old widow, is brought to the emergency department by her sister-in-law. Margaret has a history of bipolar disorder and has been maintained on medication for many years. Her sister-in-law reports that Margaret quit taking her medication a few months ago, thinking she no longer needed it. Margaret is agitated, pacing, demanding, and speaking very loudly. Her sister-in-law reports that Margaret eats very little, is losing weight, and almost never sleeps. "I'm afraid she's going to just collapse!" Margaret is admitted to the psychiatric unit. What is the *priority* nursing diagnosis for Margaret?
   a. Imbalanced nutrition: Less than body requirements related to not eating
   b. Risk for injury related to hyperactivity
   c. Disturbed sleep pattern related to agitation
   d. Ineffective coping related to denial of depression

2. Margaret, age 68, is diagnosed with bipolar I disorder, current episode manic. She is extremely hyperactive and has lost weight. One way to promote adequate nutritional intake for Margaret is to:
   a. Sit with her during meals to ensure that she eats everything on her tray.
   b. Have her sister-in-law bring all her food from home because she knows Margaret's likes and dislikes.
   c. Provide high-calorie, nutritious finger foods and snacks that Margaret can eat "on the run."
   d. Tell Margaret that she will be on room restriction until she starts gaining weight.

3. The physician orders lithium carbonate 600 mg tid for a newly diagnosed client with bipolar I disorder. There is a narrow margin between the therapeutic and toxic levels of lithium. Therapeutic range for *acute* mania is:
   a. 1.0 to 1.5 mEq/L.
   b. 10 to 15 mEq/L.
   c. 0.5 to 1.0 mEq/L.
   d. 5 to 10 mEq/L.

Continued

Review Questions—cont'd
Self-Examination/Learning Exercise

4. Although historically lithium has been the medication of choice for mania, several others have been used with good results. Which of the following are used in the treatment of bipolar disorder? (Select all that apply.)
   a. Olanzapine (Zyprexa)
   b. Oxycodone (OxyContin)
   c. Carbamazepine (Tegretol)
   d. Gabapentin (Neurontin)
   e. Tranylcypromine (Parnate)

5. Margaret, a 68-year-old widow experiencing a manic episode, is admitted to the psychiatric unit after being brought to the emergency department by her sister-in-law. Margaret yells, "My sister-in-law is just jealous of me! She's trying to make it look like I'm insane!" This behavior is an example of:
   a. A delusion of grandeur.
   b. A delusion of persecution.
   c. A delusion of reference.
   d. A delusion of control or influence.

6. What is the most common comorbid condition in children with bipolar disorder?
   a. Schizophrenia
   b. Substance disorders
   c. Oppositional defiant disorder
   d. Attention-deficit/hyperactivity disorder

7. A nurse is educating a client about his lithium therapy and explaining signs and symptoms of lithium toxicity. Which of the following would she instruct the client to be on the alert for?
   a. Fever, sore throat, malaise
   b. Tinnitus, severe diarrhea, ataxia
   c. Occipital headache, palpitations, chest pain
   d. Skin rash, marked rise in blood pressure, bradycardia

8. A client experiencing a manic episode enters the milieu area dressed in a provocative and physically revealing outfit. Which of the following is the most appropriate intervention by the nurse?
   a. Tell the client she cannot wear this outfit while she is in the hospital.
   b. Do nothing, and allow her to learn from the responses of her peers.
   c. Quietly walk with her back to her room and help her change into something more appropriate.
   d. Explain to her that if she wears this outfit, she must remain in her room.

9. The nurse is prioritizing nursing diagnoses in the plan of care for a client experiencing a manic episode. Number the diagnoses in order of the appropriate priority.
   _____ Disturbed sleep pattern evidenced by sleeping only 4 to 5 hours per night
   _____ Risk for injury related to manic hyperactivity
   _____ Impaired social interaction evidenced by manipulation of others
   _____ Imbalanced nutrition: Less than body requirements evidenced by loss of weight and poor skin turgor

10. A child with bipolar disorder also has attention-deficit/hyperactivity disorder (ADHD). How would these comorbid conditions most likely be treated?
    a. No medication would be given for either condition.
    b. Medication would be given for both conditions simultaneously.
    c. The bipolar condition would be stabilized before ADHD medication would be given.
    d. The ADHD would be treated before consideration of the bipolar disorder.

IMPLICATIONS OF RESEARCH FOR EVIDENCE-BASED PRACTICE

Morriss, R., Lobban, F., Riste, L., Davies, L., Holland, F., Long, R., . . . Jones, S. (2016). Clinical effectiveness and acceptability of structured group psychoeducation versus optimised unstructured peer support for patients with remitted bipolar disorder (PARADES): A pragmatic, multi-centre, observer-blind, randomised controlled superiority trial. *The Lancet Psychiatry, 3*(11), 1029-1038. doi:10.1016/S2215-0366(16)30302-9

DESCRIPTION OF THE STUDY: This study sought evidence for efficacy of group psychoeducation versus peer support for patients with bipolar disorder in remission. The participants ($N = 304$) were randomly assigned to one of the two intervention strategies, and efficacy was measured by time from randomization to the next bipolar episode.

RESULTS OF THE STUDY: The researchers found that there was no significant difference in effectiveness between the two interventions. However, in the subset of participants with fewer than eight previous bipolar episodes, psychoeducation did improve outcomes.

IMPLICATIONS FOR NURSING PRACTICE: Both peer support and group psychoeducation demonstrated good outcomes, but as the researchers note, findings suggest that early intervention with group psychoeducation may have important benefits for clients with bipolar disorder. Nurses play an important role both in providing psychoeducation and referring clients for group treatment. Assessing the client's history of bipolar episodes and providing psychoeducation early in the illness process may improve outcomes. Nurses can also play an active role in conducting and participating in similar research to identify which interventions demonstrate the best evidence of positive outcomes. This forms the foundation for evidence-based practice.

TEST YOUR CRITICAL THINKING SKILLS

Alice, age 29, had been working in the typing pool of a large corporation for 6 years. Her immediate supervisor recently retired, and Alice was promoted to supervisor, in charge of 20 people in the department. Alice was flattered by the promotion but anxious about the additional responsibility of the position. Shortly after the promotion, she overheard two of her former coworkers saying, "Why in the world did they choose her? She's not the best one for the job. I know *I* certainly won't be able to respect her as a boss!" Hearing these comments added to Alice's anxiety and self-doubt.

Shortly after Alice began her new duties, her friends and coworkers noticed a change. She had a great deal of energy and worked long hours on her job. She began to speak very loudly and rapidly. Her roommate noticed that Alice slept very little yet seldom appeared tired. Every night she would go out to bars and dances. Sometimes she brought men she had just met home to the apartment, something she had never done before. She bought lots of clothes and makeup and had her hair restyled in a more youthful look. She failed to pay her share of the rent and bills but came home with a brand new convertible. She lost her temper and screamed at her roommate, "Mind your own business!" when asked to pay her share.

She became irritable at work, and several of her subordinates reported her behavior to the corporate manager. When the manager confronted Alice about her behavior, she lost control, shouting, cursing, and striking out at anyone and anything that happened to be within her reach. The security officers restrained her and took her to the emergency department of the hospital, where she was admitted to the psychiatric unit. She had no previous history of psychiatric illness.

The psychiatrist assigned a diagnosis of Bipolar I Disorder and wrote orders for olanzapine (Zyprexa) 10 mg IM STAT, olanzapine 15 mg PO daily, and lithium carbonate 600 mg tid.

Answer the following questions related to Alice:
1. What are the most important considerations for the nurse who is taking care of Alice?
2. Why was Alice given the diagnosis of Bipolar I Disorder?
3. The doctor should order a lithium level drawn after 4 to 6 days. For what symptoms should the nurse be on alert?
4. Why did the physician order olanzapine in addition to the lithium carbonate?

Communication Exercise

1. Bob, a newly admitted client diagnosed with bipolar disorder, states to the nurse, "I was looking at the sky, blue is the color of my eyes, too. I went to Florida on a plane."
   • How might the nurse respond to this client's statement?
2. John, who is in a manic phase of bipolar disorder, is jumping from chair to chair in the patient lounge during visiting hours, loudly proclaiming to the visitors that he is a famous gymnast. He begins doing somersaults, nearly tripping a visitor.
   • How might the nurse respond to the client at this point?

MOVIE CONNECTIONS

Lust for Life (bipolar disorder) • *Call Me Anna* (bipolar disorder) • *Blue Sky* (bipolar disorder) • *A Woman Under the Influence* (bipolar disorder)

References

Aas, M., Henry, C., Andreassen, O.A. Bellivier, F., Melle, I., & Etain, B. (2016). The role of childhood trauma in bipolar disorders. *International Journal of Bipolar Disorders, 4*(2), 1-10. doi:10.1186/s40345-015-0042-0

American Academy of Child and Adolescent Psychiatry. (2010). Parents medication guide for bipolar disorder in children and adolescents. Retrieved from www.parentsmedguide.org

American Psychiatric Association. (2013). *Diagnostic and statistical manual of mental disorders* (5th ed.). Washington, DC: American Psychiatric Publishing.

Burton, N. (2012). A short history of bipolar disorder. Retrieved from https://www.psychologytoday.com/blog/hide-and-seek/201206/short-history-bipolar-disorder

Carolla, B. (2013). Putting people in the bipolar driver's seat. Retrieved from www.nami.org/About-NAMI/NAMI-News/Putting-People-in-the-Bipolar-Driver's-Seat

Darby, M.M., Yolken, R.H., & Sabunciyan, S. (2016). Consistently altered expression of gene sets in postmortem brains of individuals with major psychiatric disorders. *Translational Psychiatry, 6*(9), e890. doi:10.1038/tp.2016.173

Etain, B., Aas, M., Andreassen, O.A., Lorentzen, S., Dieset, I., Gard, S., . . . Henry, C. (2013). Childhood trauma is associated with severe clinical characteristics of bipolar disorders. *Journal of Clinical Psychiatry, 74*(10), 991-998.

Frank E. (2005). *Treating bipolar disorder: A clinician's guide to interpersonal and social rhythm therapy.* New York: Guilford Press.

Hassan, A., Agha, S.S., Langley, K., & Thapar, A. (2011). Prevalence of bipolar disorder in children and adolescents with attention-deficit hyperactivity disorder. *British Journal of Psychiatry, 198*(3), 195-198. doi:10.1192/bjp.bp.110.078741

Hazell, P., & Jairam, R. (2012). Acute treatment of mania in children and adolescents. *Current Opinion in Psychiatry, 25*(4), 264-270. doi:10.1097/YCO.0b013e328353d467

Herdman, T.H., & Kamitsuru, S. (Eds.). (2014). *NANDA-I nursing diagnoses: Definitions and classification, 2015–2017.* Chichester, UK: Wiley Blackwell.

Jain, R., & Jain, S. (2014). Facing the diagnostic challenge of comorbid bipolar disorder and ADHD. Retrieved from www.psychiatryadvisor.com/adhd/facing-the-diagnostic-challenge-of-comorbid-bipolar-disorder-and-adhd/article/370068

Janiri, D., Sani, G., Danese, E., Simonetti, A., Ambrosi, E., Angeletti, G., . . . Girardi, P. (2015). Childhood traumatic experiences of patients with bipolar disorder type I and type II. *Journal of Affective Disorders, 175*(8), 92-97. doi:http://dx.doi.org/10.1016/j.jad.2014.12.055

Krans, B., & Cherney, K. (2016). The history of bipolar disorder. Retrieved from www.healthline.com/health/bipolar-disorder/history-bipolar#1

Leussis, M.P., Berry-Scott, E.M., Saito, M., Jhuang, H., Haan, G., Alkan, O., . . . Petryshen, T.L. (2013). The ANK3 bipolar disorder gene regulates psychiatric-related behaviors that are modulated by lithium and stress. *Biological Psychiatry, 73*(7), 683-696. doi:10.1016/j.biopsych.2012.10.016

Miklowitz, D.J., Schneck, C.D., Singh, M.K., Taylor, D.O., George, E.L., Cosgrove, V., . . . Chang, K.D. (2013). Early intervention for symptomatic youth at risk for bipolar disorder: A randomized trial of family-focused therapy. *Journal of the American Academy of Child and Adolescent Psychiatry, 52*(2), 121-131. doi:http://dx.doi.org/10.1016/j.jaac.2012.10.007

Morriss, R., Lobban, F., Riste, L., Davies, L., Holland, F., Long, R., . . . Jones, S. (2016). Clinical effectiveness and acceptability of structured group psychoeducation versus optimised unstructured peer support for patients with remitted bipolar disorder (PARADES): A pragmatic, multicentre, observer-blind, randomised controlled superiority trial. *The Lancet Psychiatry, 3*(11), 1029-1038. doi:10.1016/S2215-0366(16)30302-9

National Alliance on Mental Illness. (2008). Understanding bipolar disorder and recovery. Retrieved from www.nami.org

National Institute of Mental Health. (2012). Bipolar disorder in adults. Retrieved from www.nimh.nih.gov/health/publications/bipolar-disorder-in-adults/bipolar_disorder_adults_cl508_144295.pdf

National Institute of Mental Health. (2013). New data reveal the extent of genetic overlap between major mental disorders: Schizophrenia, bipolar disorder share the most common genetic variation [press release]. Retrieved from www.nimh.nih.gov/news/science-news/2013/new-data-reveal-extent-of-genetic-overlap-between-major-mental-disorders.shtml

National Institute of Mental Health. (2015). Bipolar disorder among adults. Retrieved from www.nimh.nih.gov/health/statistics/prevalence/bipolar-disorder-among-adults.shtml

Rybakowski, J. (2014). Factors associated with lithium efficacy in bipolar disorder *Harvard Review of Psychiatry, 22*(6), 353-357. doi:10.1097/HRP.0000000000000006

Sadock, B.J., Sadock, V.A., & Ruiz, P. (2015). *Synopsis of psychiatry: Behavioral sciences/clinical psychiatry* (11th ed.). Philadelphia: Lippincott Williams & Wilkins.

Semeniken, K.R., & Dudás, B. (2012). Bipolar disorder: Diagnosis, neuroanatomical and biochemical background. In M. Juruena (Ed.), *Clinical, research and treatment approaches to affective disorders.* Rijeka, Croatia: InTech.

Soreff, S., & McInnes, L.A. (2012). Bipolar affective disorder. *E-medicine: Psychiatry.* Retrieved from http://emedicine.medscape.com/article/286342-overview

Strakowski, S. (2016). A guide to treating unipolar and bipolar depression. Retrieved from www.medscape.com/viewarticle/871539#vp_6

Swartz, H., & Swanson, J. (2014). Psychotherapy for bipolar disorder in adults: A review of the evidence. *American Psychiatric Publishing, 12*(3), 251-266. doi:10.1176/appi.focus.12.3.251

Watson, S., Gallagher, P., Dougall, D., Porter, R., Moncrieff, J., Ferrier, I.N., & Young, A.H. (2013). Childhood trauma in bipolar disorder. *Australian and New Zealand Journal of Psychiatry. 48*(6), 564-70. doi:10.1177/0004867413516681

Weiden, P.J. (2010). Is recovery attainable in schizophrenia? *Medscape Psychiatry & Mental Health.* Retrieved from www.medscape.com/viewarticle/729750

Anxiety, Obsessive-Compulsive, and Related Disorders

27

CORE CONCEPTS

Anxiety

Compulsions

Obsessions

Panic

Phobia

KEY TERMS

agoraphobia

flooding

generalized anxiety disorder

habit-reversal therapy

hoarding disorder

implosion therapy

obsessive-compulsive disorder

panic disorder

social anxiety disorder

specific phobia

systematic desensitization

OBJECTIVES

After reading this chapter, the student will be able to:

1. Differentiate among stress, anxiety, and fear.
2. Discuss historical aspects and epidemiological statistics related to anxiety, obsessive-compulsive, and related disorders.
3. Differentiate between normal anxiety and psychoneurotic anxiety.
4. Describe types of anxiety, obsessive-compulsive, and related disorders, and identify symptomatology associated with each. Use this information in client assessment.
5. Identify predisposing factors in the development of anxiety, obsessive-compulsive, and related disorders.

6. Formulate nursing diagnoses and outcome criteria for clients with anxiety, obsessive-compulsive, and related disorders.
7. Describe appropriate nursing interventions for behaviors associated with anxiety, obsessive-compulsive, and related disorders.
8. Identify topics for client and family teaching relevant to anxiety, obsessive-compulsive, and related disorders.
9. Evaluate nursing care of clients with anxiety, obsessive-compulsive, and related disorders.
10. Discuss various modalities relevant to treatment of anxiety, obsessive-compulsive, and related disorders.

HOMEWORK ASSIGNMENT

Please read the chapter and answer the following questions:

1. What are the symptoms of a person with agoraphobia?
2. What neurotransmitter has been implicated in the development of obsessive-compulsive disorder?

3. What are some predisposing factors that have been associated with hair-pulling disorder?
4. What is the primary nursing intervention for a person in panic anxiety?

Singer, actor, and producer Barbra Streisand relates her experience of dealing with an anxiety disorder following a performance in which she forgot the lyrics to a song:

> I couldn't come out of it . . . it was shocking to me to forget the words. So I didn't have any sense of humor about it. Some performers do really well when they forget the words. They forget the words all the time but they somehow have humor about it. I remember I didn't have a sense of humor about it. I was quite shocked. I didn't sing and charge people for 27 years because of that night. . . . I was like "God, I don't know. What if I forget the words again?" (ABC News, 2005)

Barbra Streisand, who was diagnosed with social anxiety disorder, has a story similar to that of many others who experience anxiety disorders. The interference with occupational, social, and other areas of functioning can be profound. Streisand has sought therapy and medication and has since returned to performing on stage. Her story highlights not only the impact that anxiety disorders can have on one's functioning but also that treatment can be successful and improve one's quality of life.

CORE CONCEPT

Anxiety

A feeling of discomfort, apprehension, or dread related to anticipation of danger, the source of which is often nonspecific or unknown. Anxiety is considered a disorder (or pathological) when fears and anxieties are excessive (in a cultural context) and there are associated behavioral disturbances such as interference with social and occupational functioning (American Psychiatric Association [APA], 2013).

Individuals face anxiety on a daily basis. Anxiety, which provides the motivation for achievement, is a necessary force for survival. The term *anxiety* is often used interchangeably with the word *stress;* however, they are not the same. Stress, or more properly, a *stressor,* is an external pressure that is brought to bear on the individual. Anxiety is the subjective emotional response to that stressor. (See Chapter 2, Mental Health and Mental Illness: Historical and Theoretical Concepts, for an overview of anxiety as a psychological response to stress.)

Anxiety may be distinguished from *fear* in that anxiety is an emotional process, whereas fear is a cognitive one. Fear involves the intellectual appraisal of a threatening stimulus; anxiety involves the emotional response to that appraisal.

This chapter focuses on disorders that are characterized by exaggerated and often disabling anxiety reactions. Historical aspects and epidemiological statistics are presented. Predisposing factors that have been implicated in the etiology of the disorders provide a framework for studying the dynamics of phobias, obsessive-compulsive disorders, generalized anxiety disorder, panic disorder, and other anxiety disorders. Various theories of causation are presented, although it is most likely that a combination of factors contribute to the etiology of these disorders. The neurobiology of anxiety disorders is presented in Figure 27–1.

An explanation of the symptomatology is presented as background knowledge for assessing the client with an anxiety or obsessive-compulsive disorder. Nursing care is described in the context of the nursing process. Various treatment modalities are explored.

Historical Aspects

Individuals have experienced anxiety throughout the ages. Yet anxiety, like fear, was not clearly defined or isolated as a separate entity by psychiatrists or psychologists until the 19th and 20th centuries. In fact, what we now know as anxiety was once solely identified by its physiological symptoms, focusing largely on the cardiovascular system. Clinicians used a myriad of diagnostic terms in attempting to identify these symptoms. For example, cardiac neurosis, DaCosta's syndrome, irritable heart, nervous tachycardia, neurocirculatory asthenia, soldier's heart, vasomotor neurosis, and vasoregulatory asthenia are just a few of the names under which anxiety has been concealed over the years (Sadock, Sadock, & Ruiz, 2015).

Freud first introduced the term *anxiety neurosis* in 1895. Freud wrote, "I call this syndrome 'anxiety neurosis' because all its components can be grouped round the chief symptom of anxiety" (Freud, 1959). This notion attempted to negate the previous concept of the problem as strictly physical, although it was some time before physicians of internal medicine were ready to accept psychological implications for the symptoms. In fact, it was not until the years during World War II that the psychological dimensions of various functional heart conditions were recognized.

For many years, anxiety disorders were viewed as purely psychological or purely biological in nature. Researchers now focus on the interrelatedness of mind and body, and anxiety disorders provide an excellent example of this complex relationship. It is likely that various factors, including genetic, developmental, environmental, and psychological, play a role in the etiology of anxiety disorders.

Epidemiological Statistics

Anxiety disorders are the most common of all psychiatric illnesses and result in considerable functional

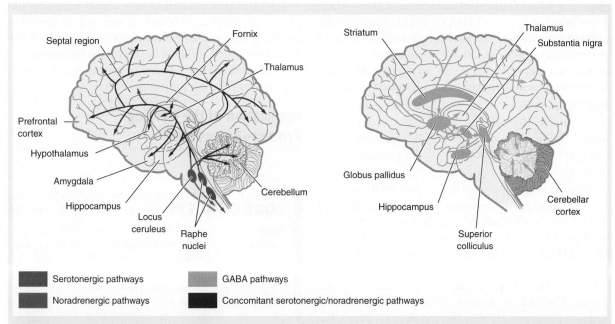

Serotonergic pathways   GABA pathways

Noradrenergic pathways   Concomitant serotonergic/noradrenergic pathways

FIGURE 27–1 Neurobiology of anxiety disorders.

NEUROTRANSMITTERS

Although other neurotransmitters have also been implicated in the pathophysiology of anxiety disorders, disturbances in serotonin, norepinephrine, and gamma-aminobutyric acid (GABA) appear to be most significant.

Cell bodies of origin for the serotonin pathways lie within the raphe nuclei located in the brainstem. Serotonin is thought to be decreased in anxiety disorders (based on the efficacy of SSRIs in the treatment of anxiety disorders), but some studies suggest that serotonin may have a modulating effect in response to intense emotions in general. Cell bodies for norepinephrine originate in the locus ceruleus. Norepinephrine is thought to be increased in anxiety disorders. GABA is the major inhibitory neurotransmitter in the brain, involved in the reduction and slowing of cellular activity. It is synthesized from glutamic acid, with vitamin B_6 as a cofactor. It is found in almost every region of the brain. GABA is thought to be decreased in anxiety disorders (allowing for increased cellular excitability).

AREAS OF THE BRAIN AFFECTED

Areas of the brain affected by anxiety disorders and the symptoms that they mediate include the following:
• Amygdala: Fear; particularly important in panic and phobic disorders
• Hippocampus: Associated with memory related to fear responses
• Locus ceruleus: Arousal
• Brainstem: Respiratory activation; heart rate
• Hypothalamus: Activation of stress response
• Frontal cortex: Cognitive interpretations
• Thalamus: Integration of sensory stimuli
• Basal ganglia: Tremor

Anxiolytic Agents	Action	Side Effects
Benzodiazepines	Increases the affinity of the GABA$_A$ receptor for GABA	Sedation, dizziness, weakness, ataxia, decreased motor performance, dependence, withdrawal
SSRIs SNRIs	SSRIs: Block reuptake of serotonin into the presynaptic nerve terminal, increasing synaptic concentration of serotonin	SSRIs: Nausea, diarrhea, headache, insomnia, somnolence, sexual dysfunction
	SNRIs: Inhibit reuptake of neuronal serotonin and norepinephrine; mild reuptake of dopamine	SNRIs: Headache, dry mouth, nausea, somnolence, dizziness, insomnia, asthenia, constipation, diarrhea
Noradrenergic Agents (e.g., propranolol, clonidine)	Propranolol: Blocks beta adrenergic receptor activity	Propranolol: Bradycardia, hypotension, weakness, fatigue, impotence, gastrointestinal upset, bronchospasm
	Clonidine: Stimulates alpha-adrenergic receptors	Clonidine: Dry mouth, sedation, fatigue, hypotension
Barbiturates	CNS depression. Also produces effects in the hepatic and cardiovascular systems	Somnolence, agitation, confusion, ataxia, dizziness, bradycardia, hypotension, constipation
Buspirone	Partial agonist of 5-HT$_{1A}$ receptor	Dizziness, drowsiness, dry mouth, headache, nervousness, nausea, insomnia

impairment and distress (Anxiety and Depression Association of America [ADAA], 2016). Statistics vary widely, but most agree that anxiety disorders are more common in women than in men by at least two to one. Prevalence rates (ADAA, 2016) for anxiety disorders within the general population are identified as follows:

Specific phobias	8.7 percent
Social anxiety disorder	6.8 percent
Posttraumatic stress disorder	3.5 percent
Generalized anxiety disorder	3.1 percent
Panic disorder	2.7 percent
Obsessive-compulsive disorder	1 percent

The prevalence for any anxiety disorder is estimated at 18.1 percent for adults and 25.2 percent for children aged 13 to 18 years of age (National Institute of Mental Health [NIMH], 2015). Common comorbidities include another anxiety disorder, depression, and substance abuse. Vulnerability to comorbidities include parental psychiatric history, childhood trauma, and negative life events (Hofmeijer-Sevink et al., 2012), but regardless of the contributing factors, comorbidities are associated with poorer outcomes, higher healthcare utilization, and greater impairment in functioning. Studies of familial patterns suggest that a familial predisposition to anxiety disorders probably exists.

How Much Is Too Much?

Anxiety is usually considered a normal reaction to a realistic danger or threat to biological integrity or self-concept. Normal anxiety dissipates when the danger or threat is no longer present.

It is difficult to draw a precise line between normal and abnormal anxiety. Normality is determined by societal standards; what is considered normal in Chicago, Illinois, may not be so in Cairo, Egypt. There may even be regional differences within a country or cultural differences within a region. So what criteria can be used to determine if an individual's anxious response is normal? Anxiety can be considered abnormal or pathological if

1. It is out of proportion to the situation that is creating it.

EXAMPLE

Mrs. K. witnessed a serious automobile accident 4 weeks ago when she was out driving in her car, and since that time, she refuses to drive even to the grocery store a few miles from her house. When he is available, her husband must take her wherever she needs to go.

2. The anxiety interferes with social, occupational, or other important areas of functioning.

EXAMPLE

Because of the anxiety associated with driving her car, Mrs. K. has been forced to quit her job in a downtown bank for lack of transportation.

It is clear that when anxiety becomes excessive and persistent, humans respond in a variety of ways that are likely a complex interaction of genetic vulnerability, biochemical influences, and environmental factors. Various manifestations of pathological anxiety are discussed in the following section.

Application of the Nursing Process—Assessment

CORE CONCEPT

Panic

A sudden, overwhelming feeling of terror or impending doom. This most severe form of emotional anxiety is usually accompanied by behavioral, cognitive, and physiological signs and symptoms considered extremely intense and frightening.

Panic Disorder
Background Assessment Data

Panic disorder is characterized by recurrent *panic attacks,* the onset of which is unpredictable and manifested by intense apprehension, fear, or terror, often associated with feelings of impending doom (clients often fear they are dying) and accompanied by intense physical discomfort. The physical sensations can be so intense that the individual believes he or she is having a heart attack or other critical illness. The symptoms come on suddenly and unexpectedly; that is, they do not occur immediately before or on exposure to a situation that usually causes anxiety (as in specific phobia). They are not triggered by situations in which the person is the focus of others' attention (as in social anxiety disorder). The role of organic factors in the etiology has been ruled out.

The *Diagnostic and Statistical Manual of Mental Disorders, Fifth Edition (DSM-5)* (APA, 2013) states that at least four of the following symptoms must be present to identify the presence of a panic attack.

- Palpitations, pounding heart, or accelerated heart rate
- Sweating
- Trembling or shaking
- Sensations of shortness of breath or smothering
- Feelings of choking
- Chest pain or discomfort
- Nausea or abdominal distress
- Feeling dizzy, unsteady, lightheaded, or faint
- Chills or heat sensations

- Paresthesias (numbness or tingling sensations)
- Derealization (feelings of unreality) or depersonalization (feelings of being detached from oneself)
- Fear of losing control or going crazy
- Fear of dying

The attacks usually last minutes or, more rarely, hours. The individual often experiences varying degrees of nervousness and apprehension between attacks. Symptoms of depression are common.

The average age of onset of panic disorder is the late 20s. Frequency and severity of the panic attacks vary widely. Some individuals may have attacks of moderate severity weekly; others may have less severe or limited-symptom attacks several times a week. Still others may experience panic attacks separated by weeks or months. The disorder may last for a few weeks or months or for a number of years. Sometimes the individual experiences periods of remission and exacerbation. Limited-symptom attacks ("fearful spells" that do not meet criteria for panic attacks) may be a risk factor for later panic attacks and panic disorder. Genetic vulnerability, tendency toward negative emotions, history of childhood physical and sexual abuse, and smoking have also been identified as risk factors (APA, 2013).

Generalized Anxiety Disorder
Background Assessment Data

Generalized anxiety disorder (GAD) is characterized by persistent, unrealistic, and excessive anxiety and worry that have occurred more days than not for at least 6 months and cannot be attributed to specific organic factors, such as caffeine intoxication or hyperthyroidism. The anxiety and worry are associated with muscle tension, restlessness, or feeling keyed up or on edge (APA, 2013). These symptoms are like those often associated with anxiety in the general population, but unlike the typical experience of anxiety, the symptoms in generalized anxiety disorder are intense enough to cause clinically significant impairment in social, occupational, or other important areas of functioning. The individual often avoids activities or events that may result in negative outcomes or spends considerable time and effort preparing for such activities. Anxiety and worry often result in procrastination in behavior or decision-making, and the individual repeatedly seeks reassurance from others.

The disorder may begin in childhood or adolescence, but onset is not uncommon after age 20. Depressive symptoms are common, and numerous somatic complaints may also be a part of the clinical picture. GAD tends to be chronic, with frequent stress-related exacerbations and fluctuations in the course of the illness.

Theories of Etiology Related to Panic and Generalized Anxiety Disorders

Psychodynamic Theory

The psychodynamic view focuses on the inability of the ego to intervene when conflict occurs between the id and the superego, producing anxiety. For various reasons (unsatisfactory parent-child relationship; conditional love or provisional gratification), ego development is delayed. When developmental defects in ego functions compromise the capacity to modulate anxiety, the individual resorts to unconscious mechanisms to resolve the conflict. Use of defense mechanisms rather than coping and management skills results in maladaptive responses to anxiety.

Cognitive Theory

The main thesis of the cognitive view is that faulty, distorted, or counterproductive thinking patterns accompany or precede maladaptive behaviors and emotional disorders (Sadock et al., 2015). A disturbance in this central mechanism of cognition results in a consequent disturbance in feeling and behavior. Because of distorted thinking, anxiety is maintained by erroneous or dysfunctional appraisal of a situation. There is a loss of ability to reason regarding the problem, whether it is physical or interpersonal. The individual feels vulnerable in a given situation, and the distorted thinking results in an irrational appraisal, fostering a negative outcome.

Biological Aspects

Research investigations into the psychobiological correlation of panic and generalized anxiety disorders have implicated a number of possibilities.

Genetics Genetic studies have identified variations on specific genes that may be associated with anxiety disorders (including panic disorder and obsessive-compulsive disorder), and some studies suggest that genetic variations may affect the sensitivity of emotional processing centers in the brain (Ressler & Smoller, 2016). Twin studies identify a 30 to 40 percent risk of heritability. But as Ressler and Smoller point out, genetic findings are indicative of risk rather than determinants of illness, and many current genetic studies are ironically teaching us more about the impact of environmental factors in interaction with genes rather than genetic influences alone.

Neuroanatomical Structural brain imaging studies in clients with panic disorder have implicated pathological involvement in the temporal lobes, particularly the hippocampus and the amygdala (Sadock et al., 2015). Dysfunctions in the limbic system (often referred to as "the emotional brain") and the frontal cerebral cortex have also been noted in clients with anxiety disorders.

Biochemical Abnormal elevations of blood lactate have been noted in clients with panic disorder. Likewise, infusion of sodium lactate into clients with anxiety produced symptoms of panic disorder. Studies have suggested that people with panic disorders may be more sensitive to hypercapnia (which increases lactate levels), and carbon dioxide (CO_2) challenge tests have supported this sensitivity (Amaral et al., 2013). Additionally, studies of various medications and treatments such as cognitive-behavioral therapy have demonstrated decreased sensitivity to CO_2 inhalation after treatment, suggesting a relationship between lactate levels and anxiety reduction.

Neurochemical Stronger evidence exists for the involvement of the neurotransmitter norepinephrine in the etiology of panic disorder. Norepinephrine is known to mediate arousal and causes hyperarousal and anxiety. This fact has been demonstrated by a notable increase in anxiety following the administration of drugs that increase the synaptic availability of norepinephrine, such as yohimbine. The neurotransmitters serotonin and gamma aminobutyric acid (GABA) are thought to be decreased in anxiety disorders. These hypotheses are related to the efficacy of benzodiazepines, which enhance the activity of GABA, and the efficacy of selective serotonin reuptake inhibitors (SSRIs), which enhance the activity of serotonin. Similarly, deep-breathing exercises have been shown to elevate thalamic GABA levels through stimulation of vagal nerve pathways with a subsequent reduction in heart rate and improvement in emotional regulation and stress responses (Gerbard & Brown, 2016). Studies of serotonin's function in anxiety disorders have had mixed results (Sadock et al., 2015).

CORE CONCEPT

Phobia

A persistent, intensely felt, and irrational fear of a specific object, activity, or situation that results in a compelling desire to avoid the feared stimulus (Venes, 2014). Responses typically include intense anxiety or panic attacks.

Phobias

Two of the more common phobia disorders include **agoraphobia** and social anxiety disorder (social phobia). Agoraphobia has a 12-month prevalence rate of 0.8 percent, and approximately 40 percent of those cases are considered severe (NIMH, 2015). Social anxiety disorder has a 12-month prevalence rate of 7 percent (APA, 2013).

Agoraphobia

Background Assessment Data

The literal Greek translation of the word *agoraphobia* is "fear of the marketplace." This term defines the fear that some clients have of being in open shops and markets, although it may be more related to fears of being vulnerable and in a less secure environment (Black & Andreasen, 2014). The individual experiences fear of being in places or situations from which escape might be difficult or in which help might not be available in the event that panic symptoms should occur. It is possible that the individual may have experienced the symptom(s) in the past and is preoccupied with fears of their recurrence. The *DSM-5* diagnostic criteria for agoraphobia are presented in Box 27–1.

Onset of symptoms most commonly occurs in the 20s and 30s and persists for many years. It is diagnosed more commonly in women than in men. Impairment can be severe. In extreme cases, the individual is unable to leave his or her home without being accompanied by a friend or relative. If this is not possible, the person may become totally confined to his or her home.

Social Anxiety Disorder (Social Phobia)

Background Assessment Data

Social anxiety disorder is an excessive fear of situations in which a person might do something embarrassing or be evaluated negatively by others. The individual has extreme concerns about being exposed to possible scrutiny by others and fears social or performance situations in which embarrassment may occur (APA, 2013). In some instances, the fear may be quite defined, such as the fear of speaking or eating in a public place, fear of using a public restroom, or fear of writing in the presence of others. In other cases, the social phobia may involve general social situations, such as saying things or answering questions in a manner that would provoke laughter on the part of others. Exposure to the phobic situation usually results in feelings of panic anxiety, with sweating, tachycardia, and dyspnea.

Onset of symptoms of this disorder often begins in late childhood or early adolescence and runs a chronic, sometimes lifelong, course. It appears to be more common in women than in men (Puri & Treasaden, 2011). Impairment interferes with social or occupational functioning and causes marked distress. The *DSM-5* diagnostic criteria for social anxiety disorder are presented in Box 27–2.

Specific Phobia

Background Assessment Data

Specific phobia is identified by fear of specific objects or situations that could conceivably cause harm (e.g., snakes, heights), but the person's reaction to them is excessive, unreasonable, and inappropriate.

BOX 27–1 **Diagnostic Criteria for Agoraphobia**

A. Marked fear or anxiety about two (or more) of the following five situations:
1. Using public transportation (e.g., automobiles, buses, trains, ships, planes)
2. Being in open spaces (e.g., parking lots, marketplaces, bridges)
3. Being in enclosed places (e.g., shops, theaters, cinemas)
4. Standing in line or being in a crowd
5. Being outside of the home alone

B. The individual fears these situations because of thoughts that escape might be difficult or help might not be available in the event of panic-like symptoms or other incapacitating or embarrassing symptoms (e.g., fear of falling in the elderly, fear of incontinence).

C. The agoraphobic situations almost always provoke fear or anxiety.

D. The agoraphobic situations are actively avoided, require the presence of a companion, or are endured with intense fear or anxiety.

E. The fear or anxiety is out of proportion to the actual danger posed by the agoraphobic situations and to the sociocultural context.

F. The fear, anxiety, or avoidance is persistent, typically lasting 6 months or more.

G. The fear, anxiety, or avoidance causes clinically significant distress or impairment in social, occupational, or other important areas of functioning.

H. If another medical condition (e.g., inflammatory bowel disease, Parkinson's disease) is present, the fear, anxiety, or avoidance is clearly excessive.

I. The fear, anxiety, or avoidance is not better explained by the symptoms of another mental disorder—for example, the symptoms are not confined to specific phobia, situational type; do not involve only social situations (as in social anxiety disorder); and are not related exclusively to obsessions (as in obsessive-compulsive disorder), perceived defects or flaws in physical appearance (as in body dysmorphic disorder), reminders of traumatic events (as in posttraumatic stress disorder), or fear of separation (as in separation anxiety disorder).

Reprinted with permission from the Diagnostic and Statistical Manual of Mental Disorders, Fifth Edition *(Copyright 2013). American Psychiatric Association.*

BOX 27–2 **Diagnostic Criteria for Social Anxiety Disorder (Social Phobia)**

A. Marked fear or anxiety about one or more social situations in which the individual is exposed to possible scrutiny by others. Examples include social interactions (e.g., having a conversation, meeting unfamiliar people), being observed (e.g., eating or drinking), and performing in front of others (e.g., giving a speech). *Note:* In children, the anxiety must occur in peer settings and not just during interactions with adults.

B. The individual fears that he or she will act in a way or show anxiety symptoms that will be negatively evaluated (i.e., will be humiliating or embarrassing; will lead to rejection or offend others).

C. The social situations almost always provoke fear or anxiety. *Note*: In children, the fear or anxiety may be expressed by crying, tantrums, freezing, clinging, shrinking, or failing to speak in social situations.

D. The social situations are avoided or endured with intense fear or anxiety.

E. The fear or anxiety is out of proportion to the actual threat posed by the social situation and to the sociocultural context.

F. The fear, anxiety, or avoidance is persistent, typically lasting 6 months or more.

G. The fear, anxiety, or avoidance causes clinically significant distress or impairment in social, occupation, or other important areas of functioning.

H. The fear, anxiety, or avoidance is not attributable to the physiological effects of a substance (e.g., a drug of abuse, a medication) or another medical condition.

I. The fear, anxiety, or avoidance is not better explained by the symptoms of another mental disorder, such as panic disorder, body dysmorphic disorder, or autism spectrum disorder.

J. If another medical condition (e.g., Parkinson's disease, obesity, disfigurement from burns or injury) is present, the fear, anxiety, or avoidance is clearly unrelated or is excessive.

Specify if:
Performance only: If the fear is restricted to speaking or performing in public

Reprinted with permission from the Diagnostic and Statistical Manual of Mental Disorders, Fifth Edition *(Copyright 2013). American Psychiatric Association.*

Specific phobias are often identified when other anxiety disorders have become a focus of clinical attention. Treatment is generally aimed at the primary diagnosis because it usually produces the greatest distress and interferes with functioning more so than does a specific phobia. A diagnosis of specific phobia is made only when the irrational fear restricts the individual's activities and interferes with his or her daily living.

The phobic person may be no more (or less) anxious than anyone else until exposed to the phobic object or situation. Exposure to the phobic stimulus produces overwhelming symptoms of panic, including palpitations, sweating, dizziness, and difficulty breathing. In fact, these symptoms may occur in response to the individual's merely *thinking* about the phobic stimulus. Invariably, the person recognizes that his or her fear is excessive or unreasonable but is powerless to change, even though the individual may occasionally endure the phobic stimulus when experiencing intense anxiety.

Phobias may begin at almost any age. Those that begin in childhood often disappear without treatment, but those that begin or persist into adulthood usually require assistance with therapy. The disorder is diagnosed more often in women than in men.

Even though the disorder is relatively common among the general population, people seldom seek treatment unless the phobia interferes with ability to function. Obviously, the individual who has a fear of snakes but who lives on the 23rd floor of an urban, high-rise apartment building is not likely to be bothered by the phobia unless he or she decides to move to an area where snakes are prevalent. On the other hand, a fear of elevators may very well interfere with this individual's daily functioning.

Specific phobias are classified according to the phobic stimulus. A list of some of the identified phobias appears in Table 27–1. This list is by no means all-inclusive. People can become phobic about almost any object or situation, and anyone with a little knowledge of Greek or Latin can produce a phobia classification, thereby making possibilities for the list almost infinite.

Theories of Etiology Related to Phobias

The cause of phobias is unknown. However, various theories exist that may offer insight into the etiology.

Psychoanalytic Theory

Freud's classic theory associated phobias with a symbolic displacement of anxiety rooted in castration anxiety. Modern-day psychoanalysts accept this concept of phobic development but believe that castration anxiety is not the sole source of phobias. They believe that other unconscious fears may also be expressed in a symbolic manner as phobias. For example, a female child who was sexually abused by an adult male family friend when he was taking her for a ride in his boat grew up with an intense, irrational fear of all water vessels. Psychoanalytic theory postulates that fear of the man was repressed and displaced onto boats. Boats became an unconscious symbol for the feared person, but one that the young girl viewed as safer because her fear of boats prevented her from having to confront the real fear.

TABLE 27–1 **Classifications of Specific Phobias**	
CLASSIFICATION	**FEAR**
Acrophobia	Height
Ailurophobia	Cats
Algophobia	Pain
Anthophobia	Flowers
Anthropophobia	People
Aquaphobia	Water
Arachnophobia	Spiders
Astraphobia	Lightning
Belonephobia	Needles
Brontophobia	Thunder
Claustrophobia	Closed spaces
Cynophobia	Dogs
Dementophobia	Insanity
Equinophobia	Horses
Gamophobia	Marriage
Herpetophobia	Lizards, reptiles
Homophobia	Homosexuality
Murophobia	Mice
Mysophobia	Dirt, germs, contamination
Numerophobia	Numbers
Nyctophobia	Darkness
Ochophobia	Riding in a car
Ophidiophobia	Snakes
Pyrophobia	Fire
Scoleciphobia	Worms
Siderodromophobia	Railroads or train travel
Taphophobia	Being buried alive
Thanatophobia	Death
Trichophobia	Hair
Triskaidekaphobia	The number 13
Xenophobia	Strangers
Zoophobia	Animals

Learning Theory

Classic conditioning in the case of phobias may be explained as follows: a stressful stimulus produces an "unconditioned" response of fear. When the stressful stimulus is repeatedly paired with a harmless object, eventually the harmless object alone produces a "conditioned" response: fear. The fear becomes a phobia when the individual consciously avoids the harmless object to escape fear.

Some learning theorists hold that fears are conditioned responses and thus are learned by imposing rewards for certain behaviors. In the instance of phobias, when the individual avoids the phobic object, he or she escapes fear, which is indeed a powerful reward.

Phobias also may be acquired by direct learning or imitation (modeling; e.g., a mother who exhibits fear toward an object will provide a model for the child, who may also develop a phobia of the same object).

Cognitive Theory

Cognitive theorists espouse that anxiety is the product of faulty cognitions or anxiety-inducing self-instructions. Two types of faulty thinking have been investigated: negative self-statements and irrational beliefs. Cognitive theorists believe that some individuals engage in negative and irrational thinking that produces anxiety reactions. The individual begins to seek out avoidance behaviors to prevent the anxiety reactions, and phobias result.

Somewhat related to the cognitive theory is the involvement of locus of control. Johnson and Sarason (1978) suggested that individuals with internal locus of control and those with external locus of control might respond differently to life change. These researchers proposed that locus of control orientation may be an important variable in the development of phobias. Individuals with an external control orientation experiencing anxiety attacks in a stressful period are likely to mislabel the anxiety and attribute it to external sources (e.g., crowded areas) or to a disease (e.g., heart attack). They may perceive the experienced anxiety as outside of their control. Figure 27–2 depicts a graphic model of the relationship between locus of control and the development of phobias.

Biological Aspects

Neuroanatomical Specific areas in the prefrontal cortex and the amygdala play a role in storing and recalling information about threatening or potentially deadly events. Similar future events can trigger those memories, after which the amygdala triggers release of fight-or-flight hormones and the individual experiences heightened stress and fear as though the original threat was happening again (Nordqvist, 2016). Other researchers (Dias & Ressler, 2014) have found

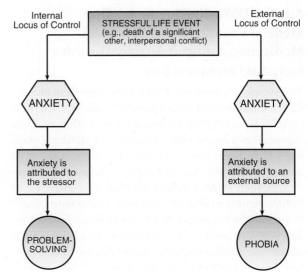

FIGURE 27–2 Locus of control as a variable in the etiology of phobias.

that parental traumatic exposure creates gene "memories" that are passed down to subsequent generations via parental gametes which are then expressed as phobias in their offspring.

Temperament Children experience fears as a part of normal development. Most infants are afraid of loud noises. Common fears of toddlers and preschoolers include strangers, animals, darkness, and fears of being separated from parents or attachment figures. During the school-age years, there is fear of death and anxiety about school achievement. Fears of social rejection and sexual anxieties are common among adolescents.

Innate fears represent a part of the overall characteristics or tendencies one is born with that influence how he or she responds to specific situations. Innate fears usually do not reach phobic intensity but may have the capacity for such development if reinforced by events in later life. For example, a 4-year-old girl is afraid of dogs. By age 5, however, she has overcome her fear and plays with her own dog and the neighbors' dogs without fear. Then, when she is 19, she is bitten by a stray dog and develops a phobia of dogs.

Life Experiences

Certain early experiences may set the stage for phobic reactions later in life. Some researchers believe that phobias, particularly specific phobias, are symbolic of original anxiety-producing objects or situations that have been repressed. For example,

- A child who is punished by being locked in a closet develops a phobia of elevators or other closed places.
- A child who falls down a flight of stairs develops a phobia of high places.
- A young woman who survived a plane crash during childhood in which both her parents were killed has a phobia of airplanes.

Anxiety Disorder Due to Another Medical Condition and Substance/Medication-Induced Anxiety Disorder
Background Assessment Data

The symptoms associated with these disorders are the direct physiological consequence of another medical condition, substance intoxication or withdrawal, or exposure to a medication. A number of medical conditions have been associated with the development of anxiety symptoms. Some of these include cardiac conditions, such as myocardial infarction, congestive heart failure, and mitral valve prolapse; endocrine conditions, such as hypoglycemia, hypo- or hyperthyroidism, and pheochromocytoma; respiratory conditions, such as chronic obstructive pulmonary disease and hyperventilation; and neurological conditions, such as complex partial seizures, neoplasms, and encephalitis.

Nursing care of clients with this disorder must take into consideration the underlying cause of the anxiety. Holistic nursing care is essential to ensure that the client's physiological and psychosocial needs are met. Nursing actions appropriate for the specific medical condition must be considered.

The diagnosis of substance-induced anxiety disorder is made only if the anxiety symptoms are in excess of those usually associated with the intoxication or withdrawal syndrome and warrant independent clinical attention. Evidence of intoxication or withdrawal must be available from history, physical examination, or laboratory findings to substantiate the diagnosis. Substance-induced anxiety disorder may be associated with use of the following substances: alcohol, amphetamines, cocaine, hallucinogen, sedatives, hypnotics, anxiolytics, caffeine, cannabis, or other substances (APA, 2013). Nursing care of the client with substance-induced anxiety disorder must take into consideration the nature of the substance and the context in which the symptoms occur; that is, intoxication or withdrawal.

CORE CONCEPT
Obsessions
Intrusive thoughts that are recurrent and stressful. Although they are recognized by the individual as irrational they continue to be repetitive and cannot be ignored.

CORE CONCEPT
Compulsions
Repetitive ritualistic behaviors or mental acts an individual feels driven to perform which are intended to reduce the anxiety associated with obsessive thoughts (APA, 2013).

Obsessive-Compulsive Disorder
Background Assessment Data

The manifestations of **obsessive-compulsive disorder** (OCD) include the presence of obsessions, compulsions, or both, the severity of which is significant enough to cause distress or impairment in social, occupational, or other important areas of functioning (APA, 2013). The individual recognizes that the behavior is excessive or unreasonable, but because of the feeling of relief from discomfort that it promotes, is compelled to continue the act. Common compulsions include hand washing, ordering, checking, praying, counting, and repeating words silently (APA, 2013).

The disorder is equally common among men and women. It may begin in childhood but more often begins in adolescence or early adulthood. The course is usually chronic and may be complicated by depression or substance abuse. OCD is identified more frequently in single people than in married people, but this finding probably reflects the difficulty that individuals with this disorder have with maintaining interpersonal relationships (Sadock et al., 2015). The *DSM-5* diagnostic criteria for OCD are presented in Box 27–3.

Body Dysmorphic Disorder
Background Assessment Data

Body dysmorphic disorder is characterized by the exaggerated belief that the body is deformed or defective in some specific way. The most common complaints involve imagined or slight flaws of the face or head, such as wrinkles or scars, the shape of the nose, excessive facial hair, and facial asymmetry (Puri & Treasaden, 2011). Other complaints may have to do with some aspect of the ears, eyes, mouth, lips, or teeth. Some clients may present with complaints involving other parts of the body, and in some instances a true defect is present. The significance of the defect is unrealistically exaggerated, however, and the person's concern is grossly excessive. These beliefs are differentiated from delusions in that individuals with body dysmorphic disorder are aware that their beliefs are exaggerated. In some cases, though, people with body dysmorphic disorder also develop psychotic disorders.

People with body dysmorphic disorder often have other comorbid mental disorders. One study found that 90 percent of people with body dysmorphic disorder had major depressive disorder, about 70 percent had an anxiety disorder (often OCD), and 30 percent had experienced a psychotic disorder (Sadock et al., 2015). Social and occupational impairment may occur because of the excessive anxiety experienced by the individual in relation to the imagined defect. The person's medical history may reflect numerous visits

---

BOX 27–3 Diagnostic Criteria for Obsessive-Compulsive Disorder

A. Presence of obsessions, compulsions, or both:

Obsessions are defined by (1) and (2)

1. Recurrent and persistent thoughts, urges, or images that are experienced, at some time during the disturbance, as intrusive and unwanted, and that in most individuals cause marked anxiety or distress.
2. The individual attempts to ignore or suppress such thoughts, urges, or images, or to neutralize them with some other thought or action (i.e., by performing a compulsion).

Compulsions are defined by (1) and (2):

1. Repetitive behaviors (e.g., hand washing, ordering, checking) or mental acts (e.g., praying, counting, repeating words silently) that the person feels driven to perform in response to an obsession or according to rules that must be applied rigidly.
2. The behaviors or mental acts are aimed at preventing or reducing anxiety or distress, or preventing some dreaded event or situation; however, these behaviors or mental acts either are not connected in a realistic way with what they are designed to neutralize or prevent, or are clearly excessive. *Note:* Young children may not be able to articulate the aims of these behaviors or mental acts.

B. The obsessions or compulsions are time-consuming (e.g., take more than 1 hour a day) or cause clinically significant distress or impairment in social, occupational, or other important areas of functioning.

C. The obsessive-compulsive symptoms are not attributable to the direct physiological effects of a substance (e.g., a drug of abuse, a medication) or another medical condition.

D. The disturbance is not better explained by the symptoms of another mental disorder (e.g., excessive worries, as in generalized anxiety disorder; preoccupation with appearance, as in body dysmorphic disorder; difficulty discarding or parting with possessions, as in hoarding disorder; hair pulling, as in trichotillomania [hair-pulling disorder]; skin picking, as in excoriation [skin-picking] disorder; stereotypies, as in stereotypic movement disorder; ritualized eating behavior, as in eating disorders; preoccupation with substances or gambling, as in substance-related and addictive disorders; preoccupation with having an illness, as in illness anxiety disorder; sexual urges or fantasies, as in paraphilic disorders; impulses, as in disruptive, impulse-control, and conduct disorders; guilty ruminations, as in major depressive disorder; thought insertion or delusional preoccupations, as in schizophrenia spectrum and other psychotic disorders; or repetitive patterns of behavior, as in autism spectrum disorder).

Specify if:

With good or fair insight

With poor insight

With absent insight/delusional beliefs

Specify if:

Tic-related

Reprinted with permission from the Diagnostic and Statistical Manual of Mental Disorders, Fifth Edition *(Copyright 2013). American Psychiatric Association.*

---

to plastic surgeons and dermatologists in an unrelenting drive to correct the imagined defect. He or she may undergo unnecessary surgical procedures toward this effort.

The *DSM-5* diagnostic criteria for body dysmorphic disorder are presented in Box 27–4.

Trichotillomania (Hair-Pulling Disorder)
Background Assessment Data

The *DSM-5* defines this disorder as the recurrent pulling out of one's hair that results in hair loss (APA, 2013). The impulse is preceded by an increasing sense of tension and results in a sense of release or gratification from pulling out the hair. The most common sites for hair pulling are the scalp, eyebrows, and eyelashes, but it may occur in any area of the body on which hair grows. The areas of hair loss are often found on the opposite side of the body from the dominant hand. Pain is seldom reported to accompany the hair pulling, although tingling and pruritus in the area are not uncommon.

Comorbid psychiatric disorders are common with hair-pulling disorder. The most frequent comorbidities include major depressive disorder, GAD, OCD, other impulse control disorders, and substance use disorder (Kaplan, 2012).

The disorder usually begins in childhood and is seven times more prevalent in children (between the ages of 4 and 17) than adults (Yasgur, 2015). It may be accompanied by nail biting, head banging, scratching, biting, or other acts of self-mutilation. This phenomenon occurs more often in women than in men. Studies indicate that it affects about 4 percent of the population (Yasgur, 2015).

Hoarding Disorder
Background Assessment Data

The *DSM-5* defines the essential feature of **hoarding disorder** as "persistent difficulties discarding or parting with possessions, regardless of their actual value" (APA, 2013, p. 248). Additionally, the diagnosis may be specified as *with excessive acquisition*, which identifies

BOX 27–4 Diagnostic Criteria for Body Dysmorphic Disorder

A. Preoccupation with one or more perceived defects or flaws in physical appearance that are not observable or appear slight to others.

B. At some point during the course of the disorder, the individual has performed repetitive behaviors (e.g., mirror checking, excessive grooming, skin picking, reassurance seeking) or mental acts (e.g., comparing his or her appearance with that of others) in response to the appearance concerns.

C. The preoccupation causes clinically significant distress or impairment in social, occupational, or other important areas of functioning.

D. The appearance preoccupation is not better explained by concerns with body fat or weight in an individual whose symptoms meet diagnostic criteria for an eating disorder.

Specify if:

With muscle dysmorphia

Specify if:

With good or fair insight
With poor insight
With absent insight/delusional beliefs

---

the excessive need for continual acquiring of items (either by buying them or by other means). In previous editions of the *DSM*, hoarding was considered a symptom of OCD. However, in the *DSM-5*, it has been reclassified as a diagnosable disorder.

Individuals with hoarding disorder collect items until virtually all surfaces within the home are covered. There may be only narrow pathways winding through stacks of clutter. Some individuals also hoard food and animals, keeping dozens or hundreds of pets, often in unsanitary conditions (Mayo Clinic, 2014a).

Hoarding disorder affects an estimated 700,000 to 1.4 million Americans, but few receive adequate treatment (Symonds & Janney, 2013). More men than women are diagnosed with the disorder, and it is almost three times more prevalent in older adults (aged 55–94) than in younger adults (aged 34–44) (APA, 2013). The symptoms, regardless of when they begin, appear to become more severe with each decade of life. Associated symptoms include perfectionism, indecisiveness, anxiety, depression, distractibility, and difficulty planning and organizing tasks (APA, 2013; Symonds & Janney, 2013). In addition to OCD, hoarding is associated with high comorbidity for dependent, avoidant, schizotypal, and paranoid personality disorders (Sadock et al., 2015). Research has shown that hoarding disorder runs in families and there may be a genetic vulnerability.

Treatment of hoarding disorder has been met with mixed results. It is often difficult to convince individuals with the disorder that they are actually ill. Change is slow, and the relapse rate is high; when possessions or animals are taken away, they are often quickly replaced to provide emotional comfort (Mayo Clinic, 2014a). Psychoeducation about the disorder is almost always the initial intervention, and treatment is most commonly a combination of cognitive-behavioral therapy and psychopharmacology with SSRIs. Families and friends may misinterpret hoarding behavior as laziness or uncleanliness. Psychoeducation that includes the client's identified support system assists the client in a recovery plan. Some experts have identified unresolved grief issues as associated with hoarding behavior, which may provide another avenue for psychological intervention.

Theories of Etiology in Obsessive-Compulsive and Related Disorders

Psychoanalytic Theory

Psychoanalytic theorists propose that individuals with OCD have underdeveloped egos (for any of a variety of reasons: unsatisfactory parent-child relationship, conditional love, or provisional gratification). The psychoanalytical concept views clients with OCD as having regressed to earlier developmental stages of the infantile superego—the harsh, exacting, punitive characteristics that now reappear as part of the psychopathology. Regression and use of defense mechanisms (isolation, undoing, displacement, reaction formation) produces the clinical symptoms of obsessions and compulsions (Sadock et al., 2015).

Learning Theory

Learning theorists explain obsessive-compulsive behavior as a conditioned response to a traumatic event. The traumatic event produces anxiety and discomfort, and the individual learns to prevent the anxiety and discomfort by avoiding the situation with which they are associated. This type of learning is called *passive avoidance* (staying away from the source). When passive avoidance is not possible, the individual learns to engage in behaviors that provide relief from the anxiety and discomfort associated with the traumatic situation. This type of learning is called *active avoidance* and describes the behavior pattern of the individual with OCD (Sadock et al., 2015).

According to this classic conditioning interpretation, a traumatic event should mark the beginning of the obsessive-compulsive behaviors. However, in a significant number of cases, the onset of the behavior is gradual, and the clients relate the onset of their problems to life stress in general rather than to one or more traumatic events.

Psychosocial Influences

The onset of trichotillomania can be related to stressful situations in more than a quarter of cases. Additional factors that have been implicated include disturbances in mother-child relationship, fear of abandonment, and recent object loss. Trichotillomania has at times been connected to childhood trauma, but Woods (as cited by Kaplan, 2012) indicates that only 5 percent of patients have comorbid trichotillomania and post-traumatic stress disorder (PTSD).

Biological Aspects

Genetics Trichotillomania demonstrates a 38 percent heritability in monozygotic twins and no concordance in dizygotic twins. Researchers identify that multiple genes are likely involved in biological vulnerability (Kaplan, 2012). Structural abnormalities in various areas of the brain and alterations in the serotonin and endogenous opioid systems have also been noted.

Genetics also may play a role in the development of hoarding disorder. Family and twin studies indicate that approximately 50 percent of individuals who hoard report having a relative who also hoards (APA, 2013).

Neuroanatomy Recent findings suggest that neurobiological disturbances may play a role in the pathogenesis and maintenance of OCD. Abnormalities in various regions of the brain have been implicated in the neurobiology of OCD. Neuroimaging and neurocognitive assessment have identified an impairment in motor inhibition responses (the ability to stop an action once initiated) in patients with OCD and trichotillomania (Kaplan, 2012). In individuals with hoarding disorder, neuroimaging studies have indicated less activity in the cingulate cortex, the area of the brain that connects the emotional part of the brain with the parts that control higher-level thinking (Saxena, 2013). Yasgur (2015) reports that "animal models and brain imaging studies of patients with trichotillomania suggest abnormalities in neural regions involved in cognition (frontal cortex), affect regulation (amygdala-hippocampal formation), and habit learning (putamen). One study suggests that TTM may be associated with altered reward processing within the central nervous system."

Physiology Electrophysiological studies, sleep electroencephalogram studies, and neuroendocrine studies have suggested that there are commonalities between depressive disorders and OCD (Sadock et al., 2015). Neuroendocrine commonalities were suggested in studies in which about one-third of OCD clients show nonsuppression on the dexamethasone-suppression test and decreased growth hormone secretion with clonidine infusions.

Biochemical Factors A number of studies have implicated the neurotransmitter serotonin as influential in the etiology of obsessive-compulsive behaviors. Drugs that have been used successfully in alleviating the symptoms of OCD are clomipramine and the SSRIs, all of which are believed to block the neuronal reuptake of serotonin, thereby potentiating serotoninergic activity in the central nervous system (see Figure 27–1). The serotonergic system may also be a factor in the etiology of body dysmorphic disorder. This can be reflected in a high incidence of comorbidity with major mood disorder and anxiety disorder and the positive responsiveness of the condition to the serotonin-specific drugs.

Transactional Model of Stress and Adaptation

Anxiety, obsessive-compulsive, and related disorders are most likely caused by multiple factors. In Figure 27–3, a graphic depiction of this theory of multiple causation is presented in the transactional model of stress and adaptation.

Assessment Scales

A number of assessment rating scales are available for measuring severity of anxiety symptoms. Some are meant to be clinician administered, whereas others may be self-administered. Examples of self-rating scales include the Beck Anxiety Inventory and the Zung Self-Rated Anxiety Scale. One of the most widely used clinician-administered scales is the Hamilton Anxiety Rating Scale (HAM-A), which is used in both clinical and research settings. The scale consists of 14 items and measures both psychic and somatic anxiety symptoms (psychological distress and physical complaints associated with anxiety). A copy of the HAM-A is presented in Box 27–5.

Diagnosis and Outcome Identification

Nursing diagnoses are formulated from the data gathered during the assessment phase and with background knowledge regarding predisposing factors to the disorder. Table 27–2 presents a list of client behaviors and the NANDA International (NANDA-I) nursing diagnoses that correspond to those behaviors, which may be used in planning care for clients with anxiety, obsessive-compulsive, and related disorders.

Outcome Criteria

The following criteria may be used for measurement of outcomes in the care of the client with anxiety disorders.

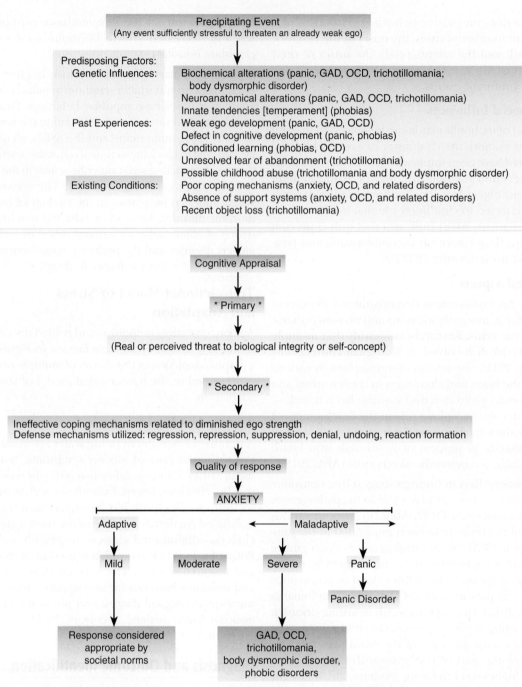

FIGURE 27–3 The dynamics of anxiety, obsessive-compulsive, and related disorders using the transactional model of stress and adaptation.

The client:

■ Is able to recognize signs of escalating anxiety and intervene before reaching panic level (*panic and generalized anxiety disorders*)

■ Is able to maintain anxiety at manageable level and make independent decisions about life situations (*panic and generalized anxiety disorders*)

■ Functions adaptively in the presence of the phobic object or situation without experiencing panic anxiety (*phobic disorder*)

■ Verbalizes a future plan of action for responding in the presence of the phobic object or situation without developing panic anxiety (*phobic disorder*)

■ Is able to maintain anxiety at a manageable level without resorting to the use of ritualistic behavior (*OCD*)

■ Demonstrates more adaptive coping strategies for dealing with anxiety than ritualistic behaviors (*OCD*)

■ Verbalizes a realistic perception of his or her appearance and expresses feelings that reflect a positive body image (*body dysmorphic disorder*)

BOX 27–5 Hamilton Anxiety Rating Scale (HAM-A)

Below are descriptions of symptoms commonly associated with anxiety. Assign the client the rating between 0 and 4 (for each of the 14 items) that best describes the extent to which he/she has these symptoms.

| 0 = Not present | 1 = Mild | 2 = Moderate | 3 = Severe | 4 = Very severe |

Rating

1. Anxious mood

_____

Worries, anticipation of the worst, fearful anticipation, irritability

2. Tension

_____

Feelings of tension, fatigability, startle response, moved to tears easily, trembling, feelings of restlessness, inability to relax

3. Fears

_____

Of dark, of strangers, of being left alone, of animals, of traffic, of crowds

4. Insomnia

_____

Difficulty in falling asleep, broken sleep, unsatisfying sleep and fatigue on waking, dreams, nightmares, night terrors

5. Intellectual

_____

Difficulty in concentration, poor memory

6. Depressed mood

_____

Loss of interest, lack of pleasure in hobbies, depression, early waking, diurnal swing

7. Somatic (muscular)

_____

Pains and aches, twitching, stiffness, myoclonic jerks, grinding of teeth, unsteady voice, increased muscular tone

Rating

8. Somatic (sensory)

_____

Tinnitus, blurred vision, hot/cold flushes, feelings of weakness, tingling sensation

9. Cardiovascular symptoms

_____

Tachycardia, palpitations, pain in chest, throbbing of vessels, feeling faint

10. Respiratory symptoms

_____

Pressure or constriction in chest, choking feelings, sighing, dyspnea

11. Gastrointestinal symptoms

_____

Difficulty swallowing, flatulence, abdominal pain and fullness, burning sensations, nausea/vomiting, borborygmi, diarrhea, constipation, weight loss

12. Genitourinary symptoms

_____

Urinary frequency, urinary urgency, amenorrhea, menorrhagia, loss of libido, premature ejaculation, impotence

13. Autonomic symptoms

_____

Dry mouth, flushing, pallor, tendency to sweat, giddiness, tension headache,

14. Behavior at interview

_____

Fidgeting, restlessness or pacing, tremor of hands, furrowed brow, strained face, sighing or rapid respiration, facial pallor, swallowing, clearing throat

Client's Total Score _____

SCORING:

14–17 = Mild anxiety

18–24 = Moderate anxiety

25–30 = Severe anxiety

SOURCE: Hamilton, M. (1959). The assessment of anxiety states by rating. British Journal of Medical Psychology, 32(1), 50-55. The HAM-A is in the public domain.

TABLE 27–2 Assigning Nursing Diagnoses to Behaviors Commonly Associated With Anxiety, Obsessive-Compulsive, and Related Disorders

BEHAVIORS	NURSING DIAGNOSES
Palpitations, trembling, sweating, chest pain, shortness of breath, fear of going crazy, fear of dying *(panic disorder);* excessive worry, difficulty concentrating, sleep disturbance *(generalized anxiety disorder)*	Anxiety (severe/panic)
Verbal expressions of having no control over life situation; nonparticipation in decision-making related to own care or life situation; expressions of doubt regarding role performance *(panic and generalized anxiety disorders)*	Powerlessness

Continued

TABLE 27–2 Assigning Nursing Diagnoses to Behaviors Commonly Associated With Anxiety, Obsessive-Compulsive, and Related Disorders–cont'd	
BEHAVIORS	**NURSING DIAGNOSES**
Behavior directed toward avoidance of a feared object or situation *(phobic disorder)*	Fear
Stays at home alone, afraid to venture out alone *(agoraphobia)*	Social isolation
Ritualistic behavior; obsessive thoughts, inability to meet basic needs; severe level of anxiety *(OCD)*	Ineffective coping
Inability to fulfill usual patterns of responsibility because of need to perform rituals *(OCD)*	Ineffective role performance
Preoccupation with imagined defect; verbalizations that are out of proportion to any actual physical abnormality that may exist; numerous visits to plastic surgeons or dermatologists seeking relief *(body dysmorphic disorder)*	Disturbed body image
Repetitive and impulsive pulling out of one's hair *(trichotillomania)*	Ineffective impulse control

■ Verbalizes and demonstrates more adaptive strategies for coping with stressful situations *(trichotillomania)*

Planning and Implementation

Care Plan for the Client With Anxiety, OCD, and Related Disorders

The following section presents a group of selected nursing diagnoses, with short- and long-term goals and nursing interventions for each.

Some institutions use a case management model to coordinate care (see Chapter 9, The Nursing Process in Psychiatric-Mental Health Nursing, for more detailed explanation). In case management models, the plan of care may take the form of a critical pathway.

Anxiety (Panic)

Anxiety is defined as a "vague uneasy feeling of discomfort or dread accompanied by an autonomic response (the source often nonspecific or unknown to the individual); a feeling of apprehension caused by anticipation of danger. It is an alerting signal that warns of impending danger and enables the individual to take measures to deal with threat" (Herdman & Kamitsuru, 2014, p. 323). Table 27–3 presents this nursing diagnosis in care plan format.

Table 27–3 | CARE PLAN FOR THE CLIENT WITH ANXIETY, OBSESSIVE-COMPULSIVE, AND RELATED DISORDERS		
NURSING DIAGNOSIS: PANIC ANXIETY		
RELATED TO: Real or perceived threat to biological integrity or self-concept		
EVIDENCED BY: Any or all of the physical symptoms identified by the DSM-5		
OUTCOME CRITERIA	**NURSING INTERVENTIONS**	**RATIONALE**
Short-Term Goal: • The client verbalizes ways to intervene in escalating anxiety within 1 week.	1. Stay with client and offer reassurance of safety and security. Do not leave client in panic anxiety alone.	1. Client may fear for his or her life. Presence of a trusted individual provides a feeling of security and assurance of personal safety.
Long-Term Goal: • By time of discharge from treatment, the client is able to recognize symptoms of onset of	2. Maintain a calm, nonthreatening, matter-of-fact approach.	2. Anxiety is contagious and may be transferred from staff to client or vice versa. Client develops a feeling of security in the presence of a calm staff person.

Table 27–3 | CARE PLAN FOR THE CLIENT WITH ANXIETY, OBSESSIVE-COMPULSIVE, AND RELATED DISORDERS—cont'd

OUTCOME CRITERIA	NURSING INTERVENTIONS	RATIONALE
anxiety and intervene before reaching panic level.	3. Use simple words and brief messages, spoken calmly and clearly, to explain hospital experiences.	3. In an intensely anxious situation, client is unable to comprehend anything but the most elemental communication.
	4. Hyperventilation may occur during periods of extreme anxiety. Hyperventilation causes the amount of carbon dioxide in the blood to decrease, possibly resulting in lightheadedness, rapid heart rate, shortness of breath, numbness or tingling in the hands or feet, and syncope. If hyperventilation occurs, assist client to breathe into a small paper bag held over the mouth and nose. Six to 12 natural breaths should be taken, alternating with short periods of diaphragmatic breathing.	4. Hyperventilation may result in injury to client, and client safety is a nursing priority. The technique here should not be used with clients who have coronary or respiratory disorders, such as coronary artery disease, asthma, or chronic obstructive pulmonary disease.
	5. Keep immediate surroundings low in stimuli (dim lighting, few people, simple decor).	5. A stimulating environment may increase level of anxiety.
	6. Administer tranquilizing medication, as ordered by physician. Assess for effectiveness and for side effects.	6. Antianxiety medication provides relief from the immobilizing effects of anxiety.
	7. When level of anxiety has been reduced, explore possible reasons for occurrence.	7. Recognition of precipitating factor(s) is the first step in teaching client to interrupt escalation of anxiety.
	8. Teach signs and symptoms of escalating anxiety, and ways to interrupt its progression (relaxation techniques, such as deep-breathing exercises and meditation, or physical exercise, such as brisk walks and jogging).	8. Relaxation techniques result in a physiological response opposite that of the anxiety response. Physical activities discharge excess energy in a healthful manner.

Client Goals

Outcome criteria include short- and long-term goals. Time lines are individually determined.

Short-term goal

■ The client will verbalize ways to intervene in escalating anxiety within 1 week.

Long-term goal

■ By time of discharge from treatment, the client will be able to recognize symptoms of onset of anxiety and intervene before reaching panic stage.

Interventions

■ Do not leave a client who is experiencing panic anxiety alone. Stay with him or her and offer reassurance of safety and security. At this level of anxiety, clients often express a fear of dying or of "going crazy." They need the presence of and assurance of their safety from a trusted individual.

■ Maintain a calm, nonthreatening, matter-of-fact approach. Anxiety is contagious and can be transferred from staff to client or vice versa. The presence of a calm person provides a feeling of security to an anxious client.

■ Use simple words and brief messages, spoken calmly and clearly, to explain hospital experiences to the client. In an intensely anxious situation, the client is unable to comprehend anything but the most elementary communication.

■ Hyperventilation may occur during periods of extreme anxiety. Hyperventilation causes the amount of CO_2 in the blood to decrease, possibly resulting in lightheadedness, rapid heart rate, shortness of breath, numbness or tingling in the hands or feet, and syncope. If hyperventilation occurs, assist the client to breathe into a small paper bag held over the mouth and nose. Six to 12 natural breaths should be taken, alternating with short periods of diaphragmatic breathing. This technique should not be used with clients who have coronary or respiratory disorders, such as coronary artery disease, asthma, or chronic obstructive pulmonary disease.

■ Keep the immediate surroundings low in stimuli (dim lighting, few people, simple decor). A stimulating environment may increase the level of anxiety.

■ Administer antianxiety medications as ordered by the physician. Assess the medication for effectiveness and for adverse side effects.

■ When the level of anxiety has been reduced, explore with the client possible reasons for its occurrence. If the client is going to learn to interrupt escalating anxiety, he or she must first learn to recognize the factors that precipitate its onset.

■ Teach the client the signs and symptoms of escalating anxiety. Discuss ways to interrupt its progression, such as relaxation techniques, deep-breathing exercises, physical exercises, brisk walks, jogging, and meditation. The client will determine which method is most appropriate for him or her. Relaxation techniques result in a physiological response opposite that of the anxiety response, and physical activities discharge excess energy in a healthful manner.

Fear

Fear is defined as the "response to perceived threat that is consciously recognized as a danger" (Herdman & Kamitsuru, 2014, p. 336).

Client Goals

Outcome criteria include short- and long-term goals. Time lines are individually determined.

Short-term goal

■ Client will discuss the phobic object or situation with the health-care provider within (time specified).

Long-term goal

■ By time of discharge from treatment, client will be able to function in the presence of the phobic object or situation without experiencing panic anxiety.

Interventions

■ Explore the client's perception of threat to physical integrity or threat to self-concept. Reassure the client of his or her safety and security. It is important to understand the client's perception of the phobic object or situation in order to assist with the desensitization process.

■ Discuss the reality of the situation with the client in order to recognize aspects that can be changed and those that cannot. The client must accept the reality of the situation (aspects that cannot change) before the work of reducing the fear can progress. For example, a man who has a fear of flying and whose employment position requires long-distance air travel must accept that he needs to conquer the fear of flying if he is going to stay in this particular job.

■ Include the client in making decisions related to the selection of alternative coping strategies. For example, the client may choose to either avoid the phobic stimulus or attempt to eliminate the fear associated with it. Encouraging the client to make choices promotes feelings of empowerment and serves to increase feelings of self-worth.

■ If the client elects to work on elimination of the fear, the techniques of systematic desensitization or implosion therapy may be employed. (See the explanation of these techniques under "Treatment Modalities" at the end of this chapter.) Systematic desensitization is a plan of behavior modification designed to expose the individual gradually to the situation or object (either in reality or through fantasizing) until the fear is no longer experienced. With implosion therapy the individual is "flooded" with stimuli related to the phobic situation or object (rather than in gradual steps) until anxiety associated with the object or situation is no longer experienced. Fear is decreased as the physical and psychological sensations diminish in response to repeated exposure to the phobic stimulus under nonthreatening conditions.

■ Encourage the client to explore underlying feelings that may be contributing to irrational fears and to face them rather than suppress them. Exploring underlying feelings may help the client confront unresolved conflicts and develop more adaptive coping abilities.

Ineffective Coping

Ineffective coping is defined as the "inability to form a valid appraisal of the stressors, inadequate choices of practiced responses, and/or inability to use available resources" (Herdman & Kamitsuru, 2014, p. 326).

Client Goals

Outcome criteria include short- and long-term goals. Time lines are individually determined.

Short-term goal

■ Within 1 week, the client will decrease participation in ritualistic behavior by half.

Long-term goal

■ By the time of discharge from treatment, the client will demonstrate the ability to cope effectively without resorting to obsessive-compulsive behaviors or increased dependency.

Interventions

■ Work with the client to determine the types of situations that increase anxiety and result in ritualistic behaviors. If the client is going to learn to interrupt escalating anxiety, he or she must first learn to recognize the factors that precipitate its onset.

■ Initially meet the client's dependency needs as required. To suddenly and completely eliminate all avenues for dependency would create intense anxiety on the part of the client. Encourage independence and give positive reinforcement for independent behaviors. Positive reinforcement enhances self-esteem and may encourage repetition of the desired behaviors.

■ In the beginning of treatment, allow plenty of time for rituals. Do not be judgmental or verbalize disapproval of the behavior. To deny the client this activity may precipitate panic level of anxiety. Also, low levels of anxiety provide a better foundation for exploring thoughts, feelings, and associated behaviors, and mild anxiety is most beneficial for teaching and learning.

■ Support the client's efforts to explore the meaning and purpose of the behavior. He or she is most likely unaware of the relationship between emotional problems and compulsive behaviors. Knowledge and recognition of this fact is important before change can occur.

■ Provide a structured schedule of activities for the client, including adequate time for the completion of rituals. The anxious individual needs a great deal of structure in his or her life. Assistance is needed with decision-making, and structure provides a sense of security and comfort to deal with activities of daily living.

■ Gradually begin to limit the amount of time allotted for ritualistic behavior as the client becomes more involved in other activities. Anxiety is minimized when the client is able to replace ritualistic behaviors with more adaptive ones. Give positive reinforcement for nonritualistic behaviors.

■ Help the client learn ways to interrupt obsessive thoughts and ritualistic behavior with techniques such as thought-stopping (see Chapter 19, Cognitive Therapy) and relaxation techniques, including physical exercise or other constructive activity with which the client feels comfortable. Knowledge and practice of coping techniques that are more adaptive will help the client change and let go of maladaptive responses to anxiety.

Disturbed Body Image

Disturbed body image is defined as the "confusion in mental picture of one's physical self" (Herdman & Kamitsuru, 2014, p. 275).

Client Goals

Outcome criteria include short- and long-term goals. Time lines are individually determined.

Short-term goal

■ Client will verbalize understanding that changes in bodily structure or function are exaggerated out of proportion to the change that actually exists. (Time frame for this goal must be determined according to individual client's situation.)

Long-term goal

■ Client will verbalize perception of own body that is realistic to actual structure or function by time of discharge from treatment.

Interventions

■ Assess the client's perception of his or her body image. Keep in mind that this image is real to the client even though he or she may recognize it as an exaggeration. Assessment information is necessary in developing an accurate plan of care. Denial of the client's feelings impedes the development of a trusting, therapeutic relationship.

■ Help the client to see that his or her body image is distorted or out of proportion in relation to the significance of an actual physical anomaly. Recognition that a misperception exists is necessary before the client can accept reality and reduce the significance of the imagined defect.

■ Encourage verbalization of fears and anxieties associated with identified stressful life situations. Discuss alternative adaptive coping strategies. Verbalization of feelings with a trusted individual may help the client come to terms with unresolved issues. Knowledge of alternative coping strategies may help the client respond to stress more adaptively in the future.

■ Involve the client in activities that reinforce a positive sense of self not based on appearance. When the client is able to develop self-satisfaction based on accomplishments and unconditional acceptance, significance of the imagined defect or minor physical anomaly will diminish.

- Make referrals to support groups of individuals with similar histories (e.g., Adult Children of Alcoholics [ACOA], Victims of Incest, Survivors of Suicide [SOS], Adults Abused as Children).

Ineffective Impulse Control

Ineffective impulse control is defined as "a pattern of performing rapid, unplanned reactions to internal or external stimuli without regard for the negative consequences of these reactions to the impulsive individual or to others" (Herdman & Kamitsuru, 2014, p. 256).

Client Goals

Outcome criteria include short- and long-term goals. Time lines are individually determined.

Short-term goal

- Client will verbalize adaptive ways to cope with stress by means other than pulling out own hair (time dimension to be individually determined).

Long-term goal

- Client will be able to demonstrate adaptive coping strategies in response to stress and a discontinuation of pulling out own hair (time dimension to be individually determined).

Interventions

- Support the client in his or her effort to stop hair pulling. Help the client understand that it is possible to discontinue the behavior. The client realizes that the behavior is maladaptive but feels helpless to stop. Support from the nurse builds trust.
- Ensure that a nonjudgmental attitude is conveyed and criticism of the behavior is avoided. An attitude of acceptance promotes feelings of dignity and self-worth.
- Assist the client with **habit reversal training** (HRT), which has been shown to be an effective tool in treatment of hair-pulling disorder. HRT involves three components:
  - **Awareness training:** Help the client become aware of times when the hair pulling most often occurs (e.g., the client learns to recognize urges, thoughts, or sensations that precede the behavior; the therapist points out to the client each time the behavior occurs). Awareness helps the client identify situations in which the behavior occurs or is most likely to occur and gives the client a feeling of increased self-control.
  - **Competing response training:** In this step, the client learns to substitute another response to the

urge to pull his or her hair. For example, when a client experiences a hair-pulling urge, suggest that the individual ball up his or her hands into fists, tightening arm muscles, and "locking" his or her arms so as to make hair pulling impossible at that moment. Substituting an incompatible behavior may help to extinguish the undesirable behavior.
  - **Social support:** Encourage family members to participate in the therapy process and offer positive feedback for attempts at habit reversal. Positive feedback enhances self-esteem and increases the client's desire to continue with the therapy. It also provides cues for family members to use in their attempts to help the client in treatment.
- Once the client has become aware of hair-pulling times, suggest that the client hold something (a ball, paperweight, or other item) in his or her hand at times when hair pulling is anticipated. Occupying the hands can help to prevent behaviors from occurring without the client's awareness.
- Practice stress management techniques: deep breathing, meditation, stretching, physical exercise, listening to soft music. Hair pulling is thought to occur at times of increased anxiety.
- Offer support and encouragement when setbacks occur. Help the client to understand the importance of not quitting when it seems that change is not happening as quickly as he or she would like. Although some people see a decrease in the behavior within a few days, most take several months to notice the greatest change.

Concept Care Mapping

The concept map care plan (see Chapter 9) is a diagrammatic teaching and learning strategy that allows visualization of interrelationships between medical diagnoses, nursing diagnoses, assessment data, and treatments. An example of a concept map care plan for the client with an anxiety disorder is presented in Figure 27–4.

Client and Family Education

The role of client teacher is important in the psychiatric area, as it is in all areas of nursing. A list of topics for client and family education relevant to anxiety disorders is presented in Box 27–6.

Evaluation

In the final step of the nursing process, a reassessment is conducted in order to determine if the nursing actions have been successful in achieving the objectives

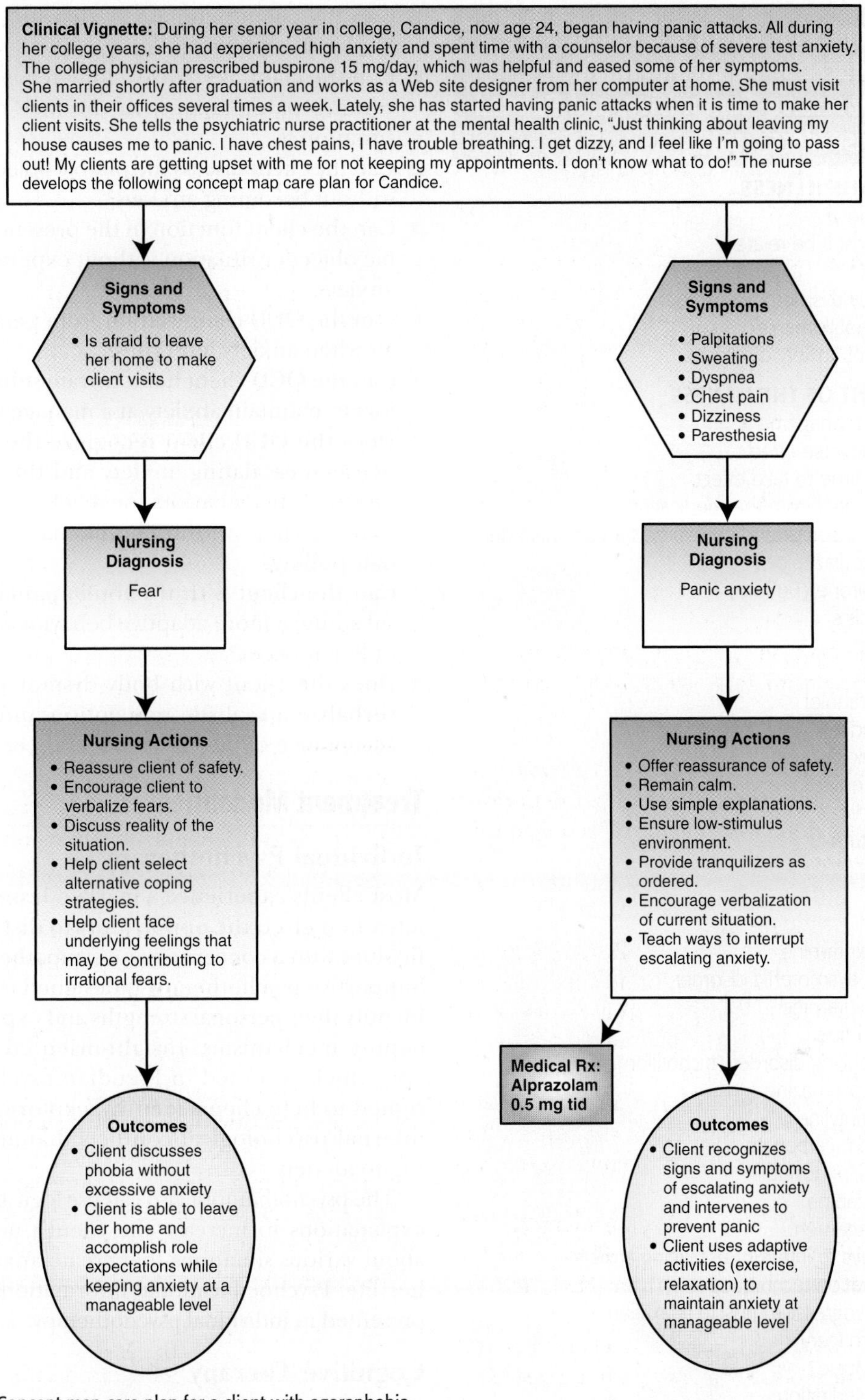

Clinical Vignette: During her senior year in college, Candice, now age 24, began having panic attacks. All during her college years, she had experienced high anxiety and spent time with a counselor because of severe test anxiety. The college physician prescribed buspirone 15 mg/day, which was helpful and eased some of her symptoms. She married shortly after graduation and works as a Web site designer from her computer at home. She must visit clients in their offices several times a week. Lately, she has started having panic attacks when it is time to make her client visits. She tells the psychiatric nurse practitioner at the mental health clinic, "Just thinking about leaving my house causes me to panic. I have chest pains, I have trouble breathing. I get dizzy, and I feel like I'm going to pass out! My clients are getting upset with me for not keeping my appointments. I don't know what to do!" The nurse develops the following concept map care plan for Candice.

Signs and Symptoms

- Is afraid to leave her home to make client visits

Signs and Symptoms

- Palpitations
- Sweating
- Dyspnea
- Chest pain
- Dizziness
- Paresthesia

Nursing Diagnosis

Fear

Nursing Diagnosis

Panic anxiety

Nursing Actions

- Reassure client of safety.
- Encourage client to verbalize fears.
- Discuss reality of the situation.
- Help client select alternative coping strategies.
- Help client face underlying feelings that may be contributing to irrational fears.

Nursing Actions

- Offer reassurance of safety.
- Remain calm.
- Use simple explanations.
- Ensure low-stimulus environment.
- Provide tranquilizers as ordered.
- Encourage verbalization of current situation.
- Teach ways to interrupt escalating anxiety.

Medical Rx: Alprazolam 0.5 mg tid

Outcomes

- Client discusses phobia without excessive anxiety
- Client is able to leave her home and accomplish role expectations while keeping anxiety at a manageable level

Outcomes

- Client recognizes signs and symptoms of escalating anxiety and intervenes to prevent panic
- Client uses adaptive activities (exercise, relaxation) to maintain anxiety at manageable level

FIGURE 27–4   Concept map care plan for a client with agoraphobia.

of care. Evaluation of the nursing actions for the client with an anxiety, OCD, or related disorder may be facilitated by gathering information utilizing the following types of questions:

■ Can the client recognize signs and symptoms of escalating anxiety?

■ Can the client use learned skills to interrupt the escalating anxiety before it reaches the panic level?
■ Can the client demonstrate the activities (e.g., relaxation techniques, physical exercise) most appropriate for him or her that can be used to maintain anxiety at a manageable level?

BOX 27–6 **Topics for Client and Family Education Related to Anxiety, Obsessive-Compulsive, and Related Disorders**

NATURE OF THE ILLNESS
1. What is anxiety?
2. To what might it be related?
3. What is OCD?
4. What is body dysmorphic disorder?
5. What is trichotillomania?
6. Symptoms of anxiety disorders.

MANAGEMENT OF THE ILLNESS
1. Medication management:
   • Possible adverse effects
   • Length of time to take effect
   • What to expect from the medication
   a. For panic disorder and generalized anxiety disorder
      (1) Benzodiazepines
      (2) Buspirone (BuSpar)
      (3) Tricyclics
      (4) SSRIs
      (5) SNRIs
      (6) Propranolol
      (7) Clonidine
   b. For phobic disorders
      (1) Benzodiazepines
      (2) Tricyclics
      (3) Propranolol
      (4) SSRIs
   c. For OCD
      (1) SSRIs
      (2) Clomipramine
   d. For body dysmorphic disorder
      (1) Clomipramine
      (2) Fluoxetine
   e. For hair-pulling disorder (trichotillomania)
      (1) Chlorpromazine
      (2) Amitriptyline
      (3) Lithium carbonate
      (4) SSRIs/pimozide
      (5) Olanzapine
2. Stress management
   a. Teach ways to interrupt escalating anxiety
      (1) Relaxation techniques
         (a) Progressive muscle relaxation
         (b) Imagery
         (c) Music
         (d) Meditation
         (e) Yoga
         (f) Physical exercise

SUPPORT SERVICES
1. Crisis hotline
2. Support groups
3. Individual psychotherapy

■ Can the client maintain anxiety at a manageable level without medication?
■ Can the client verbalize a long-term plan for preventing panic anxiety in the face of a stressful situation?
■ Can the client discuss the phobic object or situation without becoming anxious?
■ Can the client function in the presence of the phobic object or situation without experiencing panic anxiety?
■ Can the OCD client refrain from performing rituals when anxiety level rises?
■ Can the OCD client demonstrate substitute behaviors to maintain anxiety at a manageable level?
■ Does the OCD client recognize the relationship between escalating anxiety and the dependence on ritualistic behaviors for relief?
■ Can the client with trichotillomania refrain from hair pulling?
■ Can the client with trichotillomania successfully substitute a more adaptive behavior when urges to pull hair occur?
■ Does the client with body dysmorphic disorder verbalize a realistic perception and satisfactory acceptance of personal appearance?

Treatment Modalities

Individual Psychotherapy

Most clients experience a marked lessening of anxiety when given the opportunity to discuss their difficulties with a concerned and sympathetic therapist. Supportive psychotherapy is designed to help clients identify their personal strengths and explore adaptive coping mechanisms. Insight-oriented psychotherapy, which is rooted in Freudian psychology is designed to help clients identify, explore, and resolve internal psychological conflicts that are contributing to anxiety.

The psychotherapist also can use logical and rational explanations to increase the client's understanding about various situations that create anxiety in his or her life. Psychoeducational information may also be presented in individual psychotherapy.

Cognitive Therapy

The cognitive model relates to how individuals respond in stressful situations to their subjective cognitive appraisal of the event. Anxiety is experienced when the cognitive appraisal is one of danger with which the individual perceives that he or she is unable to cope. Impaired cognition can contribute to anxiety and related disorders when the individual's appraisals are chronically negative. Automatic negative appraisals provoke self-doubts, negative evaluations, and negative predictions. Anxiety is maintained by this dysfunctional appraisal of a situation.

Cognitive therapy strives to assist the individual to reduce anxiety responses by altering cognitive distortions. Anxiety is described as being the result of exaggerated, *automatic* thinking.

Cognitive therapy for anxiety is brief and time-limited, usually lasting from 5 to 20 sessions. Brief therapy discourages the client's dependency on the therapist, which is prevalent in anxiety disorders, and encourages the client's self-sufficiency.

A sound therapeutic relationship is a necessary condition for effective cognitive therapy. For the therapeutic process to occur, the client must be able to talk openly about fears and feelings. A major part of treatment consists of encouraging the client to face frightening situations to be able to view them realistically, and talking about them is one way of achieving this goal. Treatment is a collaborative effort between client and therapist.

Rather than offering suggestions and explanations, the therapist uses questions to encourage the client to correct his or her anxiety-producing thoughts. The client is encouraged to become aware of the thoughts, examine them for cognitive distortions, substitute more balanced thoughts, and eventually develop new patterns of thinking.

Cognitive therapy is very structured and orderly, which is important for the client with an anxiety or related disorder who is often confused and lacks self-assurance. The focus is on solving current problems. Together, the client and therapist work to identify and correct maladaptive thoughts and behaviors that maintain a problem and block its solution.

Cognitive therapy is based on education. The premise is that one develops anxiety because he or she has learned inappropriate ways of thinking about and responding to life experiences. The belief is that, with practice, individuals can learn more effective ways of responding to these experiences through cognitive reframing. Homework assignments, a central feature of cognitive therapy, provide an experimental, problem-solving approach to overcoming long-held anxieties. Through fulfillment of these personal "experiments," the effectiveness of specific strategies and techniques is determined.

Behavior Therapy

Behavior modification has been used to treat trichotillomania. Various techniques have been tried, including covert desensitization and HRT. These may include a system of positive and negative reinforcements in an effort to modify the hair-pulling behaviors. With HRT, in an attempt to extinguish the unwanted behavior, the individual learns to become more aware of the hair pulling, identify times of occurrence, and substitute a more adaptive coping strategy. (See interventions listed under the nursing diagnosis "Ineffective Impulse Control.")

Other forms of behavior therapy include **systematic desensitization** and **implosion therapy,** or **flooding.** They are commonly used to treat clients with phobic disorders and modify the stereotyped behavior of clients with OCD. They have also been shown to be effective in a variety of other anxiety-producing situations.

Systematic Desensitization

In systematic desensitization, the client is gradually exposed to the phobic stimulus in either a real or imagined situation. The concept was introduced by Joseph Wolpe in 1958 and is based on behavioral conditioning principles. Emphasis is placed on reciprocal inhibition or counterconditioning.

Reciprocal inhibition is described as the restriction of anxiety prior to the effort of reducing avoidance behavior. The rationale behind this concept is that because relaxation is antagonistic to anxiety, individuals cannot be anxious and relaxed at the same time.

Systematic desensitization with reciprocal inhibition involves two main elements:

1. Training in relaxation techniques
2. Progressive exposure to a hierarchy of fear stimuli while in the relaxed state

The individual is instructed in the art of relaxation using techniques most effective for him or her (e.g., progressive relaxation, mental imagery, tense and relax, meditation). When the individual has mastered the relaxation technique, exposure to the phobic stimulus is initiated. He or she is asked to present a hierarchal arrangement of situations pertaining to the phobic stimulus in order from most disturbing to least disturbing. While in a state of maximum relaxation, the client may be asked to imagine the phobic stimulus. Initial exposure is focused on a concept of the phobic stimulus that produces the least amount of fear or anxiety. In subsequent sessions, the individual is gradually exposed to stimuli that are more fearful. Sessions may be executed in fantasy, in real-life (in vivo) situations, or sometimes in a combination of both. Following is a case study describing systematic desensitization.

Implosion Therapy (Flooding)

Implosion therapy, or flooding, is a therapeutic process in which the client must imagine, for a prolonged period of time, situations or participate in real-life situations that he or she finds extremely frightening. Relaxation training is not a part of this technique. Plenty of time must be allowed for these sessions because brief periods may be ineffective or even harmful.

CASE STUDY: SYSTEMATIC DESENSITIZATION

Carlos was afraid to ride on elevators. He had been known to climb 24 flights of stairs in an office building to avoid riding the elevator. Carlos's own insurance office had plans for moving the company to a high-rise building soon, with offices on the 32nd floor. Carlos sought assistance from a therapist for help to treat this fear. He was taught to achieve a sense of calmness and well-being by using a combination of mental imagery and progressive relaxation techniques. In the relaxed state, Carlos was initially instructed to imagine the entry level of his office building, with a clear image of the bank of elevators. In subsequent sessions, and always in the relaxed state, Carlos progressed to images of walking onto an elevator, having the elevator door close after he had entered, riding the elevator to the 32nd floor, and emerging from the elevator once the doors were opened. The progression included being accompanied in the activities by the therapist and eventually accomplishing them alone.

Therapy for Carlos also included in vivo sessions in which he was exposed to the phobic stimulus in real-life situations (always after achieving a state of relaxation). This technique, combining imagined and in vivo procedures, proved successful for Carlos, and his employment in the high-rise complex was no longer in jeopardy because of his fear of elevators.

A session is terminated when the client responds with considerably less anxiety than at the beginning of the session.

In implosion therapy, the therapist "floods" the client with information concerning situations that trigger anxiety in him or her. The therapist describes anxiety-provoking situations in vivid detail and is guided by the client's response; the more anxiety provoked, the more expedient is the therapeutic endeavor. The same theme is continued as long as it arouses anxiety. The therapy is continued until a topic no longer elicits inappropriate anxiety on the part of the client. Sadock and associates (2015) state:

> Many patients refuse flooding because of the psychological discomfort involved. It is also contraindicated when intense anxiety would be hazardous to a patient (e.g., those with heart disease or fragile psychological adaptation). The technique works best with specific phobias. (p. 879)

Psychopharmacology

Antianxiety Agents

Antianxiety drugs are also called *anxiolytics* and historically were referred to as *minor tranquilizers*. Antianxiety agents are used in the treatment of anxiety disorders, anxiety symptoms, acute alcohol withdrawal, skeletal muscle spasms, convulsive disorders, status epilepticus, and preoperative sedation. Their use and efficacy for periods greater than 4 months have not been evaluated. Benzodiazepines have been the traditional medication treatment for acute anxiety states and are an important adjunct in treatment because a reduction in anxiety is essential for learning and adaptation. Because these medications are addictive, they are used typically as a short-term intervention. Buspirone and other SSRIs have demonstrated efficacy in treating anxiety disorders as well and are not addictive. (See Chapter 4, Psychopharmacology, for a detailed description of contraindications, precautions, and other safety issues related to this class of drugs.)

Examples of commonly used antianxiety agents are presented in Table 27–4.

Medications for Specific Disorders

For Panic and Generalized Anxiety Disorders

Anxiolytics The benzodiazepines have been used with success in the acute treatment of generalized anxiety disorder. They can be prescribed on an as-needed basis when the client is feeling particularly anxious. Alprazolam, lorazepam, and clonazepam have been particularly effective in the treatment of panic disorder. The major risks with benzodiazepine therapy are physical dependence and tolerance, which may encourage abuse. Because withdrawal symptoms can be life threatening, clients must be warned against abrupt discontinuation of the drug and should be tapered off the medication at the end of therapy. Because of this addiction potential, the benzodiazepines have been surpassed as first-line choice of treatment by the SSRIs, the serotonin and norepinephrine reuptake inhibitors (SNRIs), and buspirone.

The antianxiety agent buspirone is effective in about 60 to 80 percent of clients with generalized anxiety disorder (Sadock et al., 2015). One disadvantage of buspirone is its 10- to 14-day delay in alleviating symptoms. However, the benefit of lack of physical dependence and tolerance with buspirone may make it the drug of choice in the treatment of generalized anxiety disorder.

Antidepressants Several antidepressants are effective as major antianxiety agents. The tricyclics clomipramine and imipramine have been used with success in clients experiencing panic disorder. However, since the advent of SSRIs, the tricyclics are less widely used because of their tendency to produce severe side effects at the high doses required to relieve symptoms of panic disorder.

TABLE 27–4 Antianxiety Agents

CHEMICAL CLASS	GENERIC (TRADE) NAME	CONTROLLED CATEGORIES	PREGNANCY CATEGORIES/ HALF-LIFE (hr)	DAILY ADULT DOSAGE RANGE (mg)	COMMON SIDE EFFECTS OF ANTIANXIETY AGENTS
Antihistamines	Hydroxyzine (Vistaril)		C/ 3	100–400	■ Drowsiness, confusion, lethargy.
Benzodiazepines	Alprazolam (Xanax, Niravam)	CIV	D/ 6.3–26.9	0.75–4	■ Tolerance; physical and psychological dependence (does not apply to buspirone). Client should be tapered off long-term use.
	Chlordiazepoxide (Librium)	CIV	D/ 5–30	15–100	
	Clonazepam (Klonopin)	CIV	D/ 18–50	1.5–20	
	Clorazepate (Tranxene)	CIV	D/ 40–50	15–60	■ Potentiates the effects of other CNS depressants. Client should not take alcohol or other CNS depressants with the medication.
	Diazepam (Valium, Diastat)	CIV	D/ 20–80	4–40	
	Lorazepam (Ativan)	CIV	D/ 10–20	2–6	
	Oxazepam (Serax)	CIV	D/ 5–20	30–120	■ May aggravate symptoms of depression.
	Midazolam (Versed)*	CIV	D/ 2–6 Adults	5 mg	■ Orthostatic hypotension. Client should rise slowly from lying or sitting position.
Carbamate derivative	Meprobamate (Miltown, Equanil)	CIV	D/ 6–17	400–1,600	■ Paradoxical excitement. If symptoms opposite of desired effect occur, notify physician immediately.
Azaspirodecanedione	Buspirone		B/ 14	15–60	■ Dry mouth. ■ Nausea and vomiting. May be taken with food or milk. ■ Blood dyscrasias. Symptoms of sore throat, fever, malaise, easy bruising, or unusual bleeding should be reported to the physician immediately. ■ Delayed onset (with buspirone). Lag time of 10–14 days for anxiety symptoms to diminish with buspirone. Buspirone is not recommended for prn administration.

*Primarily used for preoperative sedation, antianxiety, and conscious sedation.
NOTE: Antidepressants (which are also used in the treatment of anxiety disorders) are listed in Chapter 25, Depressive Disorders.

The SSRIs have been effective in the treatment of panic disorder. Paroxetine, fluoxetine, and sertraline have been approved by the U.S. Food and Drug Administration (FDA) for this purpose. Venlafaxine, an SNRI, is also FDA approved for treatment of panic disorder. Clients with panic disorder appear to be sensitive to treatment with antidepressants, so doses are lower initially and titrated slowly.

SSRIs and SNRIs are first-line treatments for generalized anxiety disorder (Mayo Clinic, 2014b). The FDA has approved paroxetine (Paxil), escitalopram (Lexapro), duloxetine (Cymbalta), and extended-release venlafaxine (Effexor XR) in the treatment of generalized anxiety disorder. Atypical antidepressants such as nefazodone (Serzone) and mirtazapine (Remeron), while not FDA-approved for anxiety disorder treatment, have also been identified as beneficial (Bhatt, 2016).

Antihypertensive Agents Several studies have called attention to the effectiveness of beta blockers (e.g., propranolol) and alpha$_2$-receptor agonists (e.g., clonidine) in the amelioration of anxiety symptoms (Bhatt, 2016). Propranolol has potent effects on the somatic manifestations of anxiety (e.g., palpitations, tremors), with less dramatic effects on the psychic component of anxiety. It appears to be most effective in the treatment of acute situational anxiety (e.g., performance anxiety; test anxiety), but it is not the first-line drug of choice in the treatment of panic disorder and generalized anxiety disorder. Propranolol also demonstrated effectiveness in reducing hyperarousal states for up to 1 week after patients with PTSD had a flashback (Bhatt, 2016).

Clonidine is effective in blocking the acute anxiety effects in conditions such as opioid and nicotine withdrawal. However, it has had limited usefulness in the long-term treatment of panic and generalized anxiety disorders, particularly because of the development of tolerance to its antianxiety effects.

Anticonvulsants Pregabalin (Lyrica), which is a GABA derivative, may have benefits in treating anxiety disorders, but it is a schedule V controlled substance and therefore may pose a risk for dependence or drug diversion (Bhatt, 2016).

For Phobic Disorders

Anxiolytics The benzodiazepines have been successful in the treatment of social anxiety disorder (social phobia). Controlled studies have shown the efficacy of alprazolam and clonazepam in reducing symptoms of social anxiety. Both are well tolerated and have a rapid onset of action. However, because of their potential for abuse and dependence, they are not considered first-line choice of treatment.

Antidepressants The tricyclic imipramine and the monoamine oxidase inhibitor (MAOI) phenelzine have been effective in diminishing symptoms of agoraphobia and social anxiety disorder. In recent years, the SSRIs have become the first-line treatment of choice for social anxiety disorder, and paroxetine and sertraline have been approved for this purpose. Additional clinical trials have indicated efficacy with other antidepressants, including nefazodone, venlafaxine, and bupropion. Specific phobias generally are not treated with medication unless panic attacks accompany the phobia.

Antihypertensive Agents The beta blockers propranolol and atenolol have been tried with success in clients experiencing anticipatory performance anxiety or "stage fright." This type of phobic response produces symptoms such as sweaty palms, racing pulse, trembling hands, dry mouth, labored breathing, nausea, and memory loss. The beta blockers appear to be quite effective in reducing these symptoms in some individuals.

For Obsessive-Compulsive Disorder

Antidepressants The SSRIs fluoxetine (Prozac), paroxetine (Paxil), sertraline (Zoloft), and fluvoxamine (Luvox) have been approved by the FDA for the treatment of OCD. Doses in excess of what is effective for treating depression may be required for OCD. Common side effects include sleep disturbances, headache, and restlessness. These effects are often transient and are less troublesome than those of the tricyclics.

The tricyclic antidepressant clomipramine (Anafranil) was the first drug approved by the FDA in the treatment of OCD. Clomipramine is more selective for serotonin reuptake than any of the other tricyclics. Its efficacy in the treatment of OCD is well established, although the adverse effects, such as those associated with all the tricyclics, may make it less desirable than the SSRIs.

For Body Dysmorphic Disorder

Antidepressants The most positive results of pharmacological therapy with body dysmorphic disorder have been with clomipramine (Anafranil) and fluoxetine (Prozac). These medications have been shown to reduce symptoms in more than 50 percent of clients with the disorder (Sadock et al., 2015).

For Trichotillomania (Hair-Pulling Disorder)

No medications have demonstrated consistent benefits for clients with trichotillomania, but SSRIs have yielded moderate results for some clients with this condition (Elston & Ellis, 2016).

CASE STUDY AND SAMPLE CARE PLAN

NURSING HISTORY AND ASSESSMENT

Stephanie is a 34-year-old mother of a 7-year-old girl named April. Stephanie's husband, Chris, brought her to the emergency department when she began complaining of chest pain and shortness of breath. Diagnostic testing ruled out cardiac problems, and Stephanie was referred for psychiatric evaluation. Chris was present at the admission interview. He explained to the nurse that Stephanie has become increasingly "nervous and high-strung" over the past few years. Four years ago, April, then 3 years old, was attending nursery school 2 days a week. April came down with a very severe case of influenza that developed into pneumonia. She was hospitalized, and her prognosis was questionable for a short while, although she eventually made a complete recovery. Since that time, however, Stephanie has been extremely anxious about her family's health. She is fastidious about housekeeping and scrubs her floors three times a week. She launders the bedclothes daily and uses bleach on all the countertops and door handles several times a day. She washes the woodwork twice a week. She washes her hands incessantly, and they are red and noticeably chapped. Chris explained that Stephanie becomes very upset if she is not able to perform all of her cleaning chores according to her self-assigned schedule. This afternoon, April came home from school with a note from the teacher saying that a child in April's class had been diagnosed with a case of meningitis. Chris told the nurse, "Stephanie just lost it. She got all upset and started crying and had trouble breathing. Then she got those pains in her chest. That's when I brought her to the hospital." Stephanie is admitted to the psychiatric unit with a diagnosis of Obsessive-Compulsive Disorder. The physician orders alprazolam 0.5 mg tid and paroxetine 20 mg every morning.

The night nurse finds her up at 2 a.m. scrubbing the shower with a hand towel. She refuses to sleep in the bed, stating that it must certainly be contaminated. When the day nurse makes morning rounds, she finds Stephanie in the bathroom washing her hands.

NURSING DIAGNOSES AND OUTCOME IDENTIFICATION

From the assessment data, the nurse develops the following nursing diagnoses for Stephanie:

1. **Panic anxiety** related to perceived threat to biological integrity evidenced by chest pain and shortness of breath.
   a. **Short-Term Goal:** Client will be able to relax with effects of medication.
   b. **Long-Term Goal:** Client will be able to maintain anxiety at manageable level.
2. **Ineffective coping** related to panic anxiety and weak ego strength evidenced by compulsive cleaning and washing hands.
   a. **Short-Term Goal:** Client will reduce amount of time performing rituals within 3 days.
   b. **Long-Term Goal:** Client will demonstrate ability to cope effectively without resorting to ritualistic behavior.

PLANNING AND IMPLEMENTATION

PANIC ANXIETY

The following nursing interventions have been identified for Stephanie:

1. Stay with Stephanie and reassure her that she is safe and that she is not going to die.
2. Maintain a calm, nonthreatening manner.
3. Speak very clearly and calmly, and use simple words and messages.
4. Keep the lights low, the noise level down as much as possible, and as few people in her environment as is necessary.
5. Administer the alprazolam and paroxetine as ordered by the physician. Monitor for effectiveness and side effects.
6. After several days, when the anxiety has subsided, discuss with Stephane the causes that precipitated this attack.
7. Teach her the signs that indicate her anxiety level is rising.
8. Teach strategies that she may employ to interrupt the escalation of the anxiety. She may choose which is best for her: relaxation exercises, physical exercise, meditation.

INEFFECTIVE COPING

The following nursing interventions have been identified for Stephanie:

1. Initially, allow Stephanie all the time she needs to wash her hands, straighten up her room, change her own sheets, and so on. To deny her these rituals would result in panic anxiety.
2. Initiate discussions with Stephanie about her behavior. She ultimately must come to understand that these rituals are her way of keeping her anxiety under control.
3. Within a couple of days, begin to limit the amount of time Stephanie may spend on her rituals. Assign her to groups and activities that take up her time and distract her from her obsessions.
4. Explore with Stephanie the types of situations that cause her anxiety to rise. Help her to correlate these times of increased anxiety to initiation of the ritualistic behavior.
5. Help her with problem-solving and with making decisions about more adaptive ways to respond to situations that cause her anxiety to rise.
6. Explore her fears surrounding the health of her daughter. Help her to recognize which fears are legitimate and which are irrational.
7. Discuss possible activities in which she may participate that may distract from obsessions about contamination. Make suggestions, and encourage her to follow through. Examples may include enrollment in classes at the local community college, volunteer work at the local hospital, or part-time employment.
8. Explain to her that she will likely be discharged from the hospital with a prescription for paroxetine. Teach her about the medication, how it should be taken, possible side effects, and what to report to the physician.
9. Suggest that she may benefit from attendance in an anxiety disorder support group. If she is interested, help locate one that would be convenient and appropriate for her.

Continued

CASE STUDY AND SAMPLE CARE PLAN—cont'd

EVALUATION

The outcome criteria for Stephanie have been met. She has remained calm during her hospital stay with the use of the medication. The use of ritualistic behavior in the hospital setting diminished rapidly. She has discussed situations that she knows cause her anxiety to rise. She has learned relaxation exercises and practices them daily. She plans to start jogging and has the phone number for an anxiety support group that she plans to call. She says that she hopes the support group will help her maintain rationality about her daughter's health. She knows about paroxetine and plans to take it every morning.

Summary and Key Points

- Anxiety is a necessary force for survival and has been experienced by humanity throughout the ages.
- Anxiety was first described as a physiological disorder and identified by its physical symptoms, particularly the cardiac symptoms. The psychological implications for the symptoms were not recognized until the early 1900s.
- Anxiety is considered a normal reaction to a realistic danger or threat to biological integrity or self-concept.
- Normality of the anxiety experienced in response to a stressor is defined by societal and cultural standards.
- Anxiety disorders are more common in women than in men by at least two to one.
- Studies of familial patterns suggest that a familial predisposition to anxiety disorders probably exists.
- The *DSM-5* identifies several broad categories of anxiety and related disorders. They include panic and generalized anxiety disorders, phobic disorders, and OCD and related disorders, such as body dysmorphic disorder and trichotillomania. Anxiety disorders may also be the result of other medical conditions and intoxication or withdrawal from substances.
- Panic disorder is characterized by recurrent panic attacks, the onset of which are unpredictable and manifested by intense apprehension, fear, and physical discomfort.
- Generalized anxiety disorder is characterized by chronic, unrealistic, and excessive anxiety and worry.
- Social anxiety disorder is an excessive fear of situations in which a person might do something embarrassing or be evaluated negatively by others.
- Specific phobia is a marked, persistent, and excessive or unreasonable fear when in the presence of or when anticipating an encounter with a specific object or situation.
- Agoraphobia is a fear of being in places or situations from which escape might be difficult or in which help might not be available in the event that the person becomes anxious.
- OCD involves recurrent obsessions or compulsions that are severe enough to interfere with social and occupational functioning.
- Body dysmorphic disorder is an exaggerated belief that the body is deformed or defective in some specific way.
- Trichotillomania (also known as hair-pulling disorder) is a disorder of impulse characterized by the recurrent pulling out of one's own hair that results in noticeable hair loss.
- Hoarding disorder is defined by the persistent difficulty in discarding or parting with possessions, regardless of their actual value.
- A number of elements, including psychosocial factors, biological influences, and learning experiences, most likely contribute to the development of these disorders.
- Treatment of anxiety and related disorders includes individual psychotherapy, cognitive therapy, behavior therapy (including implosion therapy, systematic desensitization, and HRT), and psychopharmacology.
- Nurses can help clients with anxiety and related disorders gain insight and increase self-awareness in relation to their illness.
- Intervention focuses on assisting clients to learn techniques with which they may interrupt the escalation of anxiety before it reaches unmanageable proportions and to replace maladaptive behavior patterns with new, more adaptive, coping skills.

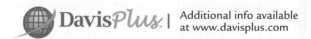 **DavisPlus** | Additional info available at www.davisplus.com

Review Questions
Self-Examination/Learning Exercise

Select the answer that is most appropriate for each of the following questions.

1. Ms. T. has been diagnosed with agoraphobia. Which behavior would be most characteristic of this disorder?
   a. Ms. T. experiences panic anxiety when she encounters snakes.
   b. Ms. T. refuses to fly in an airplane.
   c. Ms. T. will not eat in a public place.
   d. Ms. T. stays in her home for fear of being in a place from which she cannot escape.

2. Which of the following is the most appropriate therapy for a client with agoraphobia?
   a. 10 mg Valium qid
   b. Group therapy with other agoraphobics
   c. Facing the fear in gradual step progression
   d. Hypnosis

3. With implosion therapy, a client with phobic anxiety would be:
   a. Taught relaxation exercises.
   b. Subjected to graded intensities of the fear.
   c. Instructed to stop the therapeutic session as soon as anxiety is experienced.
   d. Presented with massive exposure to a variety of stimuli associated with the phobic object or situation.

4. A client with OCD spends many hours each day washing her hands. The most likely reason she washes her hands so much is that it:
   a. Relieves her anxiety.
   b. Reduces the probability of infection.
   c. Gives her a feeling of control over her life.
   d. Increases her self-concept.

5. The *initial* care plan for a client with OCD who washes her hands obsessively would include which of the following nursing interventions?
   a. Keep the client's bathroom locked so she cannot wash her hands all the time.
   b. Structure the client's schedule so that she has plenty of time for washing her hands.
   c. Place the client in isolation until she promises to stop washing her hands so much.
   d. Explain the client's behavior to her, since she is probably unaware that it is maladaptive.

6. A client with OCD says to the nurse, "I've been here 4 days now, and I'm feeling better. I feel comfortable on this unit, and I'm not ill-at-ease with the staff or other patients anymore." In light of this change, which nursing intervention is most appropriate?
   a. Give attention to the ritualistic behaviors each time they occur, and point out their inappropriateness.
   b. Ignore the ritualistic behaviors, and they will be eliminated for lack of reinforcement.
   c. Set limits on the amount of time the client may engage in the ritualistic behavior.
   d. Continue to allow the client all the time she wants to carry out the ritualistic behavior.

7. Annie has trichotillomania. She is receiving treatment at the mental health clinic with habit-reversal therapy. Which of the following elements would be included in this therapy? (Select all that apply.)
   a. Awareness training
   b. Competing response training
   c. Social support
   d. Hypnotherapy
   e. Aversive therapy

Continued

Review Questions—cont'd
Self-Examination/Learning Exercise

8. Joselyn is a new patient at the mental health clinic. She has been diagnosed with body dysmorphic disorder. Which of the following medications is the psychiatric nurse practitioner most likely to prescribe for Joselyn?
   a. Alprazolam (Xanax)
   b. Diazepam (Valium)
   c. Fluoxetine (Prozac)
   d. Olanzapine (Zyprexa)

9. A client who is experiencing a panic attack has just arrived at the emergency department. Which is the *priority* nursing intervention for this client?
   a. Stay with the client and reassure of safety.
   b. Administer a dose of diazepam.
   c. Leave the client alone in a quiet room so that she can calm down.
   d. Encourage the client to talk about what triggered the attack.

10. Jareth has a diagnosis of generalized anxiety disorder. His physician has prescribed buspirone 15 mg daily. Jareth says to the nurse, "Why do I have to take this every day? My friend's doctor ordered Xanax for him, and he only takes it when he is feeling anxious." Which of the following would be an appropriate response by the nurse?
    a. "Xanax is not effective for generalized anxiety disorder."
    b. "Buspirone must be taken daily in order to be effective."
    c. "I will ask the doctor if he will change your dose of buspirone to prn so that you don't have to take it every day."
    d. "Your friend really should be taking the Xanax every day."

IMPLICATIONS OF RESEARCH FOR EVIDENCE-BASED PRACTICE

Uebelacker, L.A., Weisberg, R., Millman, M., Yen, S., & Keller, M. (2013). Prospective study of risk factors for suicidal behavior in individuals with anxiety disorders. *Psychological Medicine, 43,* 1465-1474. doi:10.1017/50033291712002504

DESCRIPTION OF THE STUDY: Recognizing that there is an increased risk of suicide among people with anxiety disorders, the researchers initiated a prospective study of 676 individuals with a diagnosed anxiety disorder to identify associated factors that might predict an increased incidence of suicide attempts in this population. They studied the sample population for 12 years in an attempt to identify whether specific types of anxiety disorders, comorbid psychiatric disorders, physical health, or social/occupational functioning were associated with future risk of suicide attempts in people with anxiety disorders.

RESULTS OF THE STUDY: As the researchers hypothesized, comorbid posttraumatic stress disorder, major depressive disorder (MDD), intermittent depressive disorder (IDD), epilepsy, pain, and poor social/occupational functioning all predicted a shorter time to a suicide attempt. MDD and IDD were independent predictors of time to a suicide attempt even when they controlled for a past history of suicide attempts. No specific type of anxiety disorder predicted a shorter time to suicide attempts. The researchers conclude that the most powerful predictors of future suicide attempts in this sample of people with anxiety disorders was previous history of suicide attempts and comorbid mood disorders.

IMPLICATIONS FOR NURSING PRACTICE: Suicide is a major health problem in the United States, and the increase in incidence has prompted researchers to explore variables that are most associated with suicide risk. The findings in this study highlight the importance of assessing for symptoms of depression and suicidal ideation in individuals with anxiety disorders. (See Chapter 17, Suicide Prevention, for a more thorough discussion of current assessment tools and interventions associated with risks for suicide.) Current research on the topic of suicide is rapidly expanding the evidence base related to this health concern, so nurses in any practice setting need to remain informed of the latest research to improve safety and quality care for this population.

TEST YOUR CRITICAL THINKING SKILLS

Sarah, age 25, was taken to the emergency department by her friends. They were at a dinner party when Sarah suddenly clasped her chest and started having difficulty breathing. She complained of nausea and was perspiring profusely. She had calmed down some by the time they reached the hospital. She denied any pain, and electrocardiogram and laboratory results were unremarkable.

Sarah told the admitting nurse that she had a history of these "attacks." She began having them in her sophomore year of college. She knew her parents had expectations that she should follow in their footsteps and become an attorney. They also expected her to earn grades that would promote acceptance by a top Ivy League university. Sarah experienced her first attack when she made a B in English during her third semester of college. Since that time, she has experienced these symptoms sporadically, often in conjunction with her perception of the need to excel. She graduated with top honors from Harvard.

Last week, Sarah was promoted within her law firm. She was assigned her first solo case of representing a couple whose baby had died at birth and who were suing the physician for malpractice. She has experienced these panic symptoms daily for the past week, stating, "I feel like I'm going crazy!"

Sarah is transferred to the psychiatric unit. The psychiatrist diagnoses panic disorder.

Answer the following questions related to Sarah:

1. What would be the priority nursing diagnosis for Sarah?
2. What is the priority nursing intervention with Sarah?
3. What medical treatment might you expect the physician to prescribe?

Communication Exercises

1. John, who was just admitted to the psychiatric unit with panic disorder, approaches the nurse with complaints of numbness in his fingers and shortness of breath.
   - What would be some appropriate responses by the nurse?
2. After attending a group that discussed irrational thinking patterns, John asks the nurse, "How does this cognitive behavior therapy work?"
   - What would be some appropriate responses to John's question?

🎬 MOVIE CONNECTIONS

As Good As It Gets (OCD) • *The Aviator* (OCD) • *What About Bob?* (phobias) • *Copycat* (agoraphobia) • *Analyze This* (panic disorder) • *Vertigo* (specific phobia)

References

ABC News. (2005). Barbra Streisand looks back on twenty-five years. Retrieved from http://abcnews.go.com/Primetime/Entertainment/story?id=1147020&page=1

Amaral, J.M., Spadaro, P.T., Pereira, V.M., Oliveira e Silva, A.C., & Nardi, A.E. (2013). The carbon dioxide challenge test in panic disorder: A systematic review of preclinical and clinical research. *Revista Brasileira de Psiquiatria, 35*(3), 318-331. doi:http://dx.doi.org/10.1590/1516-4446-2012-1045

American Psychiatric Association. (2013). *Diagnostic and statistical manual of mental disorders* (5th ed.). Washington, DC: American Psychiatric Publishing.

Anxiety and Depression Association of America. (2016). Facts and statistics. Retrieved from https://www.adaa.org/about-adaa/press-room/facts-statistics

Bhatt, N. (2016). Anxiety disorders. Retrieved from http://emedicine.medscape.com/article/286227-overview#a2

Black, D.W., & Andreasen, N.C. (2014). *Introductory textbook of psychiatry* (6th ed.). Washington, DC: American Psychiatric Publishing.

Dias, B.G., & Ressler, K.J. (2014). Parental olfactory experience influences behavior and neural structure in subsequent generations. *Nature Neuroscience 17,* 86-96. doi:10.1038/nn.3594

Elston, D.M., & Ellis, C.R. (2016). Trichotillomania. Retrieved from http://emedicine.medscape.com/article/1071854-overview#a3

Gerbard, P.L. & Brown, R.P. (2016). Neurobiology and neurophysiology of breath practices in psychiatric care. *Psychiatric Times.* Retrieved from www.psychiatrictimes.com/special-reports/neurobiology-and-neurophysiology-breath-practices-psychiatric-care

Herdman, T.H., & Kamitsuru, S. (Eds.). (2014). *NANDA-I nursing diagnoses: Definitions and classification, 2015–2017.* Chichester, UK: Wiley Blackwell.

Hofmeijer-Sevink, M.K., Batelaan, N.M., van Megen, H.J., Penninx, B.W., Cath, D.C., van den Hout, M.A., & van Balkom, A.J. (2012). Clinical relevance of comorbidity in anxiety disorders: A report from the Netherlands Study of Depression and Anxiety (NESDA). *Journal of Affective Disorders, 137*(1-3), 106-112. doi:http://dx.doi.org/10.1016/j.jad.2011.12.008

Kaplan, K. (2012). Update on trichotillomania. *Psychiatric Times.* Retrieved from www.psychiatrictimes.com/apa2012/update-trichotillomania

Mayo Clinic. (2014a). Hoarding. Retrieved from www.mayoclinic.com/health/hoarding/DS00966

Mayo Clinic. (2014b). Generalized anxiety disorder. Retrieved from www.mayoclinic.org/diseases-conditions/generalized-anxiety-disorder/basics/treatment/con-20024562

National Institute of Mental Health (NIMH). (2015). Health topics. Retrieved from www.nimh.nih.gov/index.shtml

Nordqvist, C. (2016). Phobias: Causes, symptoms, and diagnosis. Retrieved from www.medicalnewstoday.com/articles/249347.php

Puri, B.K., & Treasaden, I.H. (2011). *Textbook of psychiatry* (3rd ed.). Philadelphia: Churchill Livingstone Elsevier.

Ressler, K., & Smoller, J. (2016). The genetics of anxiety disorders. Retrieved from https://www.adaa.org/resources-professionals/podcasts/genetics-anxiety-disorders

Sadock, B.J., Sadock, V.A., & Ruiz, P. (2015). *Synopsis of psychiatry: Behavioral sciences/clinical psychiatry* (11th ed.). Philadelphia: Lippincott Williams & Wilkins.

Saxena, S. (2013). Medicines for the treatment of hoarding. *International OCD Foundation.* Retrieved from www.ocfoundation.org/hoarding/medication.aspx

Symonds, A., & Janney, R. (2013). Shining a light on hoarding disorder. *Nursing 2013, 43*(10), 22-28. doi:10.1097/01.NURSE.0000434310.68016.18

Uebelacker, L.A., Weisberg, R., Millman, M., Yen, S., & Keller, M. (2013). Prospective study of risk factors for suicidal behavior in individuals with anxiety disorders. *Psychological Medicine, 43,* 1465-1474. doi:10.1017/50033291712002504

Venes, D. (Ed.). (2014). *Taber's medical dictionary* (22nd ed.). Philadelphia: F.A. Davis.

Yasgur, B. S. (2015). Managing trichotillomania: A coordinated approach to compulsive hair pulling. *Psychiatry Advisor.* Retrieved from www.psychiatryadvisor.com/obsessive-compulsive-disorders/managing-trichotillomania-compulsive-hair-pulling/article/432260/?

Classical References

Freud, S. (1959). On the grounds for detaching a particular syndrome from neurasthenia under the description "anxiety neurosis." In *The standard edition of the complete psychological works of Sigmund Freud* (Vol. 3). London: Hogarth Press.

Hamilton, M. (1959). The assessment of anxiety states by rating. *British Journal of Medical Psychology, 32*(1), 50-55. doi:10.1111/j.2044-8341.1959.tb00467.x

Johnson, J.H., & Sarason, I.B. (1978). Life stress, depression and anxiety: Internal-external control as moderator variable. *Journal of Psychosomatic Research, 22*(3), 205-208. doi:http://dx.doi.org/10.1016/0022-3999(78)90025-9

Trauma- and Stressor-Related Disorders

28

CORE CONCEPTS

Stress
Trauma

KEY TERMS

acute stress disorder   adjustment disorder   posttraumatic stress disorder

OBJECTIVES
After reading this chapter, the student will be able to:

1. Discuss historical aspects and epidemiological statistics related to trauma- and stressor-related disorders.
2. Describe various types of trauma- and stressor-related disorders and identify symptomatology associated with each; use this information in client assessment.
3. Identify predisposing factors in the development of trauma- and stressor-related disorders.

4. Formulate nursing diagnoses and goals of care for clients with trauma- and stressor-related disorders.
5. Describe appropriate nursing interventions for behaviors associated with trauma- and stressor-related disorders.
6. Evaluate the nursing care of clients with trauma- and stressor-related disorders.
7. Discuss various modalities relevant to treatment of trauma- and stressor-related disorders.

HOMEWORK ASSIGNMENT
Please read the chapter and answer the following questions:

1. What two variables are considered to be the best predictors of posttraumatic stress disorder (PTSD) according to the psychosocial theory?
2. What is associated with the onset of an adjustment disorder?

3. What are the elements that determine one's response (and subsequent adjustment) to a stressful situation?
4. What agents are considered first-line psychopharmacological treatment for PTSD?

In 2011, a massive earthquake and tsunami claimed the lives of thousands and destroyed communities in eastern Japan. Yuri Sato, a public health nurse charged with helping survivors, shares her courageous experience (Frances, 2015):

> As public health nurses, our immediate task was to treat the injured and sick; collect and dispense medicines; and respond to the desperate conditions of the townspeople. We launched and managed an aid station and

a welfare evacuation site for those in need of urgent nursing care; established countermeasures against infectious disorders; and arranged for emergency food supplies and sanitation. . . .With the entire town disaster-stricken, I was overcome with a sense of doubt and anxiety. Questions continually spun around in my mind: "What is mental health care when all of us have suffered so greatly?" But with everyone in mourning, we were single-mindedly focused on not losing any more lives to suicide or accident. . . . People continued to be unable to accept the deaths of family members, relatives and friends—and the fact that so many were still missing. I often heard "I should have died," "Why did I survive?" or "I want my time to come soon." I also felt this way, but had too much work to do to linger on my own losses and feelings about them.

Traumas such as these test the very fiber of our human spirit and emotional well-being. Anyone hearing Ms. Sato's recollections would agree that the events were (and are) painfully traumatic. For some, the stress associated with trauma continues to cause enduring, significant distress and interference with their ability to function. This leads to conditions called trauma and stressor-related disorders.

The *Diagnostic and Statistical Manual of Mental Disorders, Fourth Edition, Text Revision (DSM-IV-TR)* (American Psychiatric Association [APA], 2000) classified **posttraumatic stress disorder** (PTSD) and **acute stress disorder** with anxiety disorders. **Adjustment disorder** carried its own classification and was identified as "a psychological response to an identifiable stressor or stressors" (APA, 2000, p. 679). In the *DSM-5* (APA, 2013), these disorders have been combined into a single chapter, Trauma- and Stressor-Related Disorders. This reclassification "reflects increased recognition of trauma as a precipitant, emphasizing common etiology over common phenomenology" (Friedman et al., 2011, p. 737).

This chapter focuses on disorders that occur following exposure to an identifiable stressor or an extreme traumatic event. Epidemiological statistics are presented, and predisposing factors associated with the etiology of these disorders are discussed. An explanation of the symptomatology is presented as background knowledge for assessing clients with trauma- and stressor-related disorders. Nursing care is described in the context of the nursing process. Various treatment modalities are explored.

Historical and Epidemiological Data

The concept of a posttrauma response has been referred to as *shell shock, battle fatigue, accident neurosis,* and *posttraumatic neurosis.* Reports of symptoms and syndromes with PTSD-like features have existed in writing throughout the centuries. In the early part of the 20th century, traumatic neurosis was viewed as the ego's inability to master the degree of disorganization brought about by a traumatic experience. Very little was written about posttraumatic neurosis between 1950 and 1970. This absence was followed in the 1970s and 1980s with expansive research and writing on the subject. Many of the papers written during this time were about Vietnam veterans. Clearly, the renewed interest in PTSD was linked to the psychological casualties of the Vietnam War.

The diagnostic category of PTSD did not appear until the third edition of the *DSM* in 1980, after a need was indicated by increasing numbers of problems with Vietnam veterans and victims of multiple disasters. The *DSM-IV-TR* (2000) described the trauma that precedes PTSD as an event that is outside the range of usual human experience, such as rape, war, physical attack, torture, or natural or manmade disaster.

About 60 percent of men and 50 percent of women are exposed to a traumatic event in their lifetimes (Department of Veterans Affairs, 2016). Women are more likely to experience sexual assault and childhood sexual abuse, whereas men are more likely to experience accidents, physical assaults, combat, or proximity to death or injury. Although the prevalence of trauma exposure is high, less than 10 percent of trauma victims develop PTSD. The disorder appears to be more common in women than in men.

Historically, as previously stated, individuals who experienced stress reactions that followed exposure to an extreme traumatic event were given the diagnosis of PTSD. Accordingly, stress reactions from "normal" daily events (e.g., divorce, failure, rejection) were characterized as adjustment disorders (Friedman, 1996).

A number of studies have indicated that adjustment disorders are probably quite common. Sadock, Sadock, and Ruiz, (2015) report:

> Adjustment disorders are one of the most common psychiatric diagnoses for disorders of patients hospitalized for medical and surgical problems. In one study, 5 percent of people admitted to a hospital over a 3-year period were classified as having an adjustment disorder. Up to 50 percent of people with specific medical problems or stressors have been diagnosed with adjustment disorders. (p. 446)

Adjustment disorders are more common in women, unmarried persons, and adolescents (Black & Andreasen, 2014). It can occur at any age, from childhood to senescence.

Application of the Nursing Process—Trauma-Related Disorders

CORE CONCEPT

Trauma

An extremely distressing experience that causes severe emotional shock and may have long-lasting psychological effects.

Posttraumatic Stress Disorder and Acute Stress Disorder

Background Assessment Data

Puri and Treasaden (2011) describe PTSD as "a reaction to an extreme trauma, which is likely to cause pervasive distress to almost anyone, such as natural or man-made disasters, combat, serious accidents, witnessing the violent death of others, being the victim of torture, terrorism, rape, or other crimes" (p. 197). These symptoms are not related to common experiences such as uncomplicated bereavement, marital conflict, or chronic illness but are associated with events that would be markedly distressing to almost anyone. The individual may experience the trauma alone or in the presence of others.

Characteristic symptoms include reexperiencing the traumatic event, a sustained high level of anxiety or arousal, or a general numbing of responsiveness. Intrusive recollections or nightmares of the event are common. Some individuals may be unable to remember certain aspects of the trauma.

Symptoms of depression are common with this disorder and may be severe enough to warrant a diagnosis of a depressive disorder in addition to PTSD. In the case of a life-threatening trauma shared with others, survivors often describe painful guilt feelings about surviving when others lost their lives. They may also express trauma and guilt feelings about the things they had to do to survive. Substance abuse, anger and aggressive behavior, and relationship problems are common. The full symptom picture must be present for more than 1 month and cause significant interference with social, occupational, and other areas of functioning. The disorder can occur at any age. Symptoms may begin within the first 3 months after the trauma, or there may be a delay of several months or even years. The *DSM-5* diagnostic criteria for PTSD are presented in Box 28–1.

The *DSM-5* describes a disorder similar to PTSD called *acute stress disorder (ASD)*. There are similarities between the two disorders in terms of precipitating traumatic events and symptomatology, but in ASD the symptoms are time-limited, lasting up to 1 month following the trauma. By definition, if the symptoms last longer than 1 month, the diagnosis would be PTSD. The *DSM-5* diagnostic criteria for ASD are presented in Box 28–2.

BOX 28–1 Diagnostic Criteria for Posttraumatic Stress Disorder

Note: The following criteria apply to adults, adolescents, and children older than 6 years.

A. Exposure to actual or threatened death, serious injury, or sexual violence, in one (or more) of the following ways:
   1. Directly experiencing the traumatic event(s).
   2. Witnessing, in person, the event(s) as it occurred to others.
   3. Learning that the traumatic event(s) occurred to a close family member or close friend. In cases of actual or threatened death of a family member or friend, the event(s) must have been violent or accidental.
   4. Experiencing repeated or extreme exposure to aversive details of the traumatic event(s) (e.g., first responders collecting human remains; police officers repeatedly exposed to details of child abuse). *Note:* Criterion A4 does not apply to exposure through electronic media, television, movies, or pictures, unless this exposure is work-related.
B. Presence of one (or more) of the following intrusion symptoms associated with the traumatic event(s), beginning after the traumatic event(s) occurred:
   1. Recurrent, involuntary, and intrusive distressing memories of the traumatic event(s) *Note*: In children older than 6 years, repetitive play may occur in which themes or aspects of the traumatic event(s) are expressed.
   2. Recurrent distressing dreams in which the content and/or affect of the dream is related to the traumatic event(s). *Note*: In children, there may be frightening dreams without recognizable content.
   3. Dissociative reactions (e.g., flashbacks) in which the individual feels or acts as if the traumatic event(s) were recurring. (Such reactions may occur on a continuum, with the most extreme expression being a complete loss of awareness of present surroundings.) *Note*: In children, trauma-specific reenactment may occur in play.
   4. Intense or prolonged psychological distress at exposure to internal or external cues that symbolize or resemble an aspect of the traumatic event(s).
   5. Marked physiological reactions to internal or external cues that symbolize or resemble an aspect of the traumatic event(s).
C. Persistent avoidance of stimuli associated with the traumatic event(s) beginning after the traumatic event(s) occurred, as evidenced by one or both of the following:
   1. Avoidance of or efforts to avoid distressing memories, thoughts, or feelings about or closely associated with the traumatic event(s).
   2. Avoidance of or efforts to avoid external reminders (people, places, conversations, activities, objects, situations) that arouse distressing memories, thoughts, or feelings about or closely associated with the traumatic event(s).
D. Negative alterations in cognitions and mood associated with the traumatic event(s), beginning or worsening after the traumatic event(s) occurred, as evidenced by two or more of the following:
   1. Inability to remember an important aspect of the traumatic event(s) (typically due to dissociative amnesia and not to other factors such as head injury, alcohol, or drugs).
   2. Persistent and exaggerated negative beliefs or expectations about oneself, others, or the world (e.g., "I am bad," "No one can be trusted," "The world is completely dangerous," "My whole nervous system is permanently ruined").
   3. Persistent, distorted cognitions about the cause or consequences of the traumatic event(s) that lead the individual to blame himself/herself or others.

Continued

BOX 28–1 Diagnostic Criteria for Posttraumatic Stress Disorder—cont'd

4. Persistent negative emotional state (e.g., fear, horror, anger, guilt, or shame).
5. Markedly diminished interest or participation in significant activities.
6. Feelings of detachment or estrangement from others.
7. Persistent inability to experience positive emotions (e.g., inability to experience happiness, satisfaction, or loving feelings).

E. Marked alterations in arousal and reactivity associated with the traumatic event(s), beginning or worsening after the traumatic event(s) occurred, as evidenced by two or more of the following:
1. Irritable behavior and angry outbursts (with little or no provocation) typically expressed as verbal or physical aggression toward people or objects.
2. Reckless or self-destructive behavior.
3. Hypervigilance.
4. Exaggerated startle response.

5. Problems with concentration.
6. Sleep disturbance (e.g., difficulty falling or staying asleep or restless sleep).

F. Duration of the disturbance (Criteria B, C, D, and E) is more than 1 month.

G. The disturbance causes clinically significant distress or impairment in social, occupation, or other important areas of functioning.

H. The disturbance is not attributable to the physiological effects of a substance (e.g., medication, alcohol) or another medical condition.

Specify whether:

With dissociative symptoms (depersonalization or derealization)

With delayed expression (full diagnostic criteria not met until at least 6 months after the event)

Reprinted with permission from the Diagnostic and Statistical Manual of Mental Disorders, Fifth Edition *(Copyright 2013). American Psychiatric Association.*

BOX 28–2 Diagnostic Criteria for Acute Stress Disorder

A. Exposure to actual or threatened death, serious injury, or sexual violation, in one (or more) of the following ways:
1. Directly experiencing the traumatic event(s).
2. Witnessing, in person, the event(s) as it occurred to others.
3. Learning that the event(s) occurred to a close family member or close friend. *Note:* In cases of actual or threatened death of a family member or friend, the event(s) must have been violent or accidental.
4. Experiencing repeated or extreme exposure to aversive details of the traumatic event(s) (e.g., first responders collecting human remains, police officers repeatedly exposed to details of child abuse). *Note*: This does not apply to exposure through electronic media, television, movies, or pictures, unless this exposure is work related.

B. Presence of nine (or more) of the following symptoms from any of the five categories of intrusion, negative mood, dissociation, avoidance, and arousal, beginning or worsening after the traumatic event(s) occurred:

INTRUSION SYMPTOMS

1. Recurrent, involuntary, and intrusive distressing memories of the traumatic event(s). *Note*: In children, repetitive play may occur in which themes or aspects of the traumatic event(s) are expressed.
2. Recurrent distressing dreams in which the content and/or affect of the dream are related to the event(s). *Note*: In children, there may be frightening dreams without recognizable content.
3. Dissociative reactions (e.g., flashbacks) in which the individual feels or acts as if the traumatic event(s) were recurring. (Such reactions may occur on a continuum,

with the most extreme expression being a complete loss of awareness of present surroundings.) *Note*: In children, trauma-specific reenactment may occur in play.
4. Intense or prolonged psychological distress or marked physiological reactions in response to internal or external cues that symbolize or resemble an aspect of the traumatic event(s).

NEGATIVE MOOD

5. Persistent inability to experience positive emotions (e.g., inability to experience happiness, satisfaction, or loving feelings).

DISSOCIATIVE SYMPTOMS

6. An altered sense of the reality of one's surroundings or oneself (e.g., seeing oneself from another's perspective, being in a daze, time slowing).
7. Inability to remember an important aspect of the traumatic event(s) (typically due to dissociative amnesia and not to other factors such as head injury, alcohol, or drugs).

AVOIDANCE SYMPTOMS

8. Efforts to avoid distressing memories, thoughts, or feelings about or closely associated with the traumatic event(s).
9. Efforts to avoid external reminders (people, places, conversations, activities, objects, situations) that arouse distressing memories, thoughts, or feelings about or closely associated with the traumatic event(s).

AROUSAL SYMPTOMS

10. Sleep disturbance (e.g., difficulty falling or staying asleep, or restless sleep).

BOX 28-2 Diagnostic Criteria for Acute Stress Disorder—cont'd

11. Irritable behavior and angry outbursts (with little or no provocation), typically expressed as verbal or physical aggression toward people or objects.
12. Hypervigilance.
13. Problems with concentration.
14. Exaggerated startle response.
C. Duration of the disturbance (symptoms in Criteria B) is 3 days to 1 month after trauma exposure. *Note:* Symptoms typically begin immediately after the trauma, but persistence for at least 3 days and up to a month is needed to meet disorder criteria.
D. The disturbance causes clinically significant distress or impairment in social, occupational, or other important areas of functioning.
E. The disturbance is not attributable to the direct physiological effects of a substance (e.g., medication or alcohol) or another medical condition (e.g., mild traumatic brain injury), and is not better explained by brief psychotic disorder.

Reprinted with permission from the Diagnostic and Statistical Manual of Mental Disorders, Fifth Edition *(Copyright 2013). American Psychiatric Association.*

Predisposing Factors to Trauma-Related Disorders

Psychosocial Theory

The widely accepted psychosocial model seeks to explain why certain persons exposed to massive trauma develop trauma-related disorders and others do not. Variables include characteristics that relate to (1) the traumatic experience, (2) the individual, and (3) the recovery environment.

The Traumatic Experience

Specific characteristics of the trauma have been identified as crucial in the determination of an individual's long-term response to stress:

■ Severity and duration of the stressor
■ Extent of anticipatory preparation for the event
■ Exposure to death
■ Numbers affected by life threat
■ Amount of control over recurrence
■ Location where the trauma was experienced (e.g., familiar surroundings, at home, in a foreign country)

The Individual

Variables that are considered important in determining an individual's response to trauma include the following:

■ Degree of ego-strength
■ Effectiveness of coping resources
■ Presence of preexisting psychopathology
■ Outcomes of previous experiences with stress and trauma
■ Behavioral tendencies (temperament)
■ Current psychosocial developmental stage
■ Demographic factors (e.g., age, socioeconomic status, education)

The Recovery Environment

The quality of the environment in which the individual attempts to work through the traumatic experience is correlated with the outcome. Environmental variables include the following:

■ Availability of social supports
■ The cohesiveness and protectiveness of family and friends
■ The attitudes of society regarding the experience
■ Cultural and subcultural influences

In research with Vietnam veterans, the best predictors of PTSD were the severity of the stressor and the degree of psychosocial isolation in the recovery environment.

Learning Theory

Learning theorists view negative reinforcement as behavior that leads to a reduction in an aversive experience, thereby reinforcing and resulting in repetition of the behavior. Avoidance behaviors and psychic numbing in response to a trauma are mediated by negative reinforcement (behaviors that decrease the emotional pain of the trauma). Behavioral disturbances, such as anger, aggression, and drug and alcohol abuse, are the behavioral patterns that are reinforced by their capacity to reduce objectionable feelings.

Cognitive Theory

These models take into consideration the cognitive appraisal of an event and focus on assumptions that an individual makes about the world. Epstein (1991) outlines three fundamental beliefs that most people construct within a personal theory of reality:

1. The world is benevolent and a source of joy.
2. The world is meaningful and controllable.
3. The self is worthy (e.g., lovable, good, and competent).

As life situations occur, some disequilibrium is expected until accommodation for the changed circumstance has been made and it becomes assimilated into one's personal theory of reality. An individual is vulnerable to trauma-related disorders when the fundamental beliefs are invalidated by a trauma that cannot be comprehended and a sense of helplessness and hopelessness prevail. One's appraisal of the environment can be drastically altered.

Biological Aspects

Exposure to trauma has been associated with hyperarousal of the sympathetic nervous system, excessive amygdala activity, and decreased hippocampus volume, all of which are neurobiological reactions to heightened stress. Dysfunctions in the hypothalamic-pituitary-adrenal (HPA) axis, either from chronic stress or exposure to an extreme stressor, have been linked to many psychiatric illnesses including PTSD, depression, Alzheimer's disease, and substance abuse and to medical conditions such as inflammatory disorders and cardiovascular disease (Valentino & Van Bockstaele, 2015). In addition, neuroendocrine abnormalities, including serotonin, glutamate, thyroid, and endogenous opioids (among others), have been associated with stress responses and PTSD. Valentino and Van Bockstaele (2015) identify that the activation of endogenous opioids both reduces stress and mimics the stress response depending on which opioid receptors are activated. Studies have shown that opioids administered shortly after exposure to a trauma reduced the incidence of PTSD, suggesting a protective effect. Chronic activation, however, may sensitize neurons in a way that increases vulnerability to stress-induced relapse. Lanius (2013) discusses the effects of repeated activation of opioid receptors, including the effect of increasing one's addiction potential to other drugs or even to the learned experience of relief when traumatic stress is reexperienced. He identifies that opiate antagonists such as naltrexone have demonstrated effectiveness in treatment.

Other biological systems have also been implicated in the symptomatology of PTSD. Norepinephrine, dopamine, and benzodiazepine receptors are other neurotransmitters believed to be dysregulated in individuals with PTSD. Whether these factors are suggestive of vulnerability to PTSD or whether these changes result from the brain's efforts to process trauma remains unclear. As with other disorders, it is likely that a complex dynamic of biological, social, and psychological factors is involved.

Trauma-Informed Care

Experts highlight the importance of trauma-informed care as essential to improving the quality of care for clients both in and outside of behavioral health care settings (Hopper, Bassuk, & Olivet, 2010; Substance Abuse and Mental Health Services Administration [SAMHSA], 2015). The National Center for

Trauma-Informed Care (SAMHSA, 2015) calls national attention to this critical approach. Trauma-informed care generally describes a philosophical approach that values awareness and understanding of trauma when assessing, planning, and implementing care. SAMHSA advances the following principles in defining this approach. Trauma-informed care

- *Realizes* the widespread impact of trauma and various paths for recovery.
- *Recognizes* the signs and symptoms of trauma in clients, families, staff, and all those involved with the system.
- *Responds* by fully integrating knowledge about trauma in policies, procedures, and practices.
- Seeks to actively resist *retraumatization*.

Hopper and associates (2010) discuss applying this approach with the homeless population (a significant problem for people with severe mental illness). The authors describe the many traumatic experiences that culminate in homelessness and the often co-occurring illnesses such as depression, substance abuse, and severe mental illness. To ignore the significance of trauma or to provide uninformed care leaves this population vulnerable to revictimization and "further complicates their service needs" (p. 81). Childhood trauma, including physical, emotional, and sexual abuse, is also often identified as significant in the development of behavioral problems, eating disorders, some personality disorders, depression, and substance abuse. Health-care providers, if they do not fully understand the impact of previous trauma on the client's current health concerns, may unwittingly retraumatize clients. Even interventions such as seclusion and restraint, which are designed to protect the client's safety when they are at imminent risk of harm to themselves or others, may be retraumatizing to a client with a history of trauma.

Inherent in this definition is the importance of health-care providers being aware of the impact of trauma on themselves, as it may impact their effectiveness in providing care to clients.

 Interventions that are considered trauma-informed highlight the importance of respect for the client, collaboration and connection, providing information about the connections between trauma and other health concerns, instilling hope, and empowering the trauma survivor to guide and direct his or her recovery plan (the essence of patient-centered care).

Diagnosis and Outcome Identification

Nursing diagnoses are formulated from the data gathered during the assessment phase and with background knowledge regarding predisposing factors to the disorder. Following are some common nursing diagnoses for clients with trauma-related disorders:

■ Posttrauma syndrome related to distressing events outside the range of usual human experience, evidenced by flashbacks, intrusive recollections, nightmares, psychological numbness related to the event, dissociation, or amnesia
■ Complicated grieving related to loss of self as perceived before the trauma or other actual or perceived losses incurred during or after the event, evidenced by irritability and explosiveness, self-destructiveness, substance abuse, verbalization of survival guilt, or guilt about behavior required for survival

The following criteria may be used for measurement of outcomes in the care of the client with a trauma-related disorder.

The client:

■ Can acknowledge the traumatic event and the impact it has had on his or her life
■ Is experiencing fewer flashbacks, intrusive recollections, and nightmares than he or she was on admission (or at the beginning of therapy)
■ Can demonstrate adaptive coping strategies (e.g., relaxation techniques, mental imagery, music, art)

■ Can concentrate and has made realistic goals for the future
■ Includes significant others in the recovery process and willingly accepts their support
■ Verbalizes no ideas or intent of self-harm
■ Has worked through feelings of survivor's guilt
■ Gets enough sleep to avoid risk of injury
■ Verbalizes community resources from which he or she may seek assistance in times of stress
■ Attends support group of individuals who have recovered or are recovering from similar traumatic experiences
■ Verbalizes desire to put the trauma in the past and progress with his or her life

Planning and Implementation

The following section presents a group of selected nursing diagnoses, with short- and long-term goals and nursing interventions for each.

Posttrauma Syndrome

Posttrauma syndrome is defined as "a sustained maladaptive response to a traumatic, overwhelming event" (Herdman & Kamitsuru, 2014, p. 315). Table 28–1 presents this nursing diagnosis in care plan format.

Table 28–1 | CARE PLAN FOR THE CLIENT WITH A TRAUMA-RELATED DISORDER

NURSING DIAGNOSIS: POSTTRAUMA SYNDROME

RELATED TO: Distressing event considered to be outside the range of usual human experience

EVIDENCED BY: Flashbacks, intrusive recollections, nightmares, psychological numbness related to the event, dissociation, or amnesia

OUTCOME CRITERIA	NURSING INTERVENTIONS	RATIONALE
Short-Term Goals: • Client will begin a healthy grief resolution, initiating the process of psychological healing (within time frame specific to individual). • Client will demonstrate ability to deal with emotional reactions in an individually appropriate manner. Long-Term Goal: • Client will integrate the traumatic experience into his or her persona, renew significant relationships, and establish meaningful goals for the future.	1. a. Assign the same staff as often as possible. b. Use a nonthreatening, matter-of-fact, but friendly approach. c. Respect client's wishes regarding interaction with individuals of opposite sex at this time (especially important if the trauma was rape). d. Be consistent; keep all promises; convey acceptance; spend time with client. 2. Stay with client during periods of flashbacks and nightmares. Offer reassurance of safety and security and that these symptoms are not uncommon following a trauma	1. A posttrauma client may be suspicious of others in his or her environment. All of these interventions serve to facilitate a trusting relationship. 2. Presence of a trusted individual may calm fears for personal safety and reassure client that he or she is not "going crazy."

Continued

Table 28–1 | CARE PLAN FOR THE CLIENT WITH A TRAUMA-RELATED DISORDER–cont'd

OUTCOME CRITERIA	NURSING INTERVENTIONS	RATIONALE
	of the magnitude he or she has experienced.	
	3. Obtain accurate history from significant others about the trauma and client's specific response.	3. Various types of traumas elicit different responses in clients (e.g., human-engendered traumas often generate a greater degree of humiliation and guilt in victims than trauma associated with natural disasters).
	4. Encourage client to talk about the trauma at his or her own pace. Provide a nonthreatening, private environment, and include a significant other if client wishes. Acknowledge and validate client's feelings as they are expressed.	4. This debriefing process is the first step in the progression toward resolution.
	5. Discuss coping strategies used in response to the trauma, as well as those used during stressful situations in the past. Determine those that have been most helpful, and discuss alternative strategies for the future. Include available support systems, including religious and cultural influences. Identify maladaptive coping strategies (e.g., substance use, psychosomatic responses) and practice more adaptive coping strategies for possible future posttrauma responses.	5. Resolution of the posttrauma response is largely dependent on the effectiveness of the coping strategies employed.
	6. Assist client to try to comprehend the trauma if possible. Discuss feelings of vulnerability and the individual's "place" in the world following the trauma.	6. Posttrauma response is largely a function of the shattering of basic beliefs the victim holds about self and world. Assimilation of the event into one's persona requires that some degree of meaning associated with the event be incorporated into the basic beliefs, which will affect how the individual eventually comes to reappraise self and world (Epstein, 1991).

Client Goals

Outcome criteria include short- and long-term goals. Time lines are individually determined.

Short-term goals

■ The client will begin a healthy grief resolution, initiating the process of psychological healing (within time frame specific to individual).

■ The client will demonstrate ability to deal with emotional reactions in an individually appropriate manner.

Long-term goal

■ The client will integrate the traumatic experience into his or her persona, renew significant relationships, and establish meaningful goals for the future.

Interventions

■ A posttrauma client may be suspicious of others in his or her environment. Establishing a trusting relationship with this individual is essential before care can be given. To promote trust, assign the same staff as often as possible. Use a nonthreatening, matter-of-fact but friendly approach. Ask for permission before using touch as an intervention. Respect the client's wishes regarding interaction with individuals of opposite gender at this time (especially important if the trauma was rape). Be consistent and keep all promises, and convey an attitude of unconditional acceptance.

■ Stay with the client during periods of flashbacks and nightmares. Offer reassurance of safety and security and that these symptoms are not uncommon following a trauma of the magnitude he or she has experienced. The presence of a trusted individual may help to calm fears for personal safety and reassure the anxious client that he or she is not "going crazy."

■ Obtain an accurate history from significant others about the trauma and the client's specific response. Various types of traumas elicit different responses in clients. For example, human-engendered traumas often generate a greater degree of humiliation and guilt in victims than does trauma associated with natural disasters.

■ Encourage the client to talk about the trauma *at his or her own pace*. Provide a nonthreatening, private environment, and include a significant other if the client wishes. Acknowledge and validate the client's feelings as they are expressed. This debriefing process is the first step in the progression toward resolution.

■ Discuss coping strategies used in response to the trauma, as well as those used during stressful situations in the past. Determine those that have been most helpful and discuss alternative strategies for the future. Clients who have suffered multiple or sustained traumas may find longer-term PTSD-focused therapy to be beneficial. Include available support systems, including religious and cultural influences. Identify maladaptive coping strategies, such as substance use or psychosomatic responses, and practice more adaptive coping strategies for possible future posttrauma responses. Resolution of the posttrauma response is largely dependent on the effectiveness of the coping strategies employed.

■ Assist the individual to comprehend the trauma if possible. Discuss feelings of vulnerability and the individual's "place" in the world following the trauma. Posttrauma response is largely a function of the shattering of basic beliefs the survivor holds about self and world. Assimilation of the event into one's persona requires that some degree of meaning associated with the event be incorporated into the basic beliefs, which will affect how the individual eventually comes to reappraise self and world (Epstein, 1991).

Complicated Grieving

Complicated grieving is defined as "a disorder that occurs after the death of a significant other [or any other loss of significance to the individual], in which the experience of distress accompanying bereavement fails to follow normative expectations and manifests in functional impairment" (Herdman & Kamitsuru, 2014, p. 339).

Client Goals

Outcome criteria include short- and long-term goals. Time lines are individually determined.

Short-term goal

■ Client will verbalize feelings (guilt, anger, self-blame, hopelessness) associated with the trauma.

Long-term goal

■ Client will demonstrate progress in dealing with stages of grief and will verbalize a sense of optimism and hope for the future.

Interventions

■ Acknowledge feelings of guilt or self-blame the client may express. Guilt at having survived a trauma in which others died is common. The client needs to discuss these feelings and recognize that he or she is not responsible for what happened but must take responsibility for his or own recovery.

■ Assess stage of grief in which the client is fixed. Discuss normalcy of feelings and behaviors related to stages of grief. Knowledge of grief stage is necessary for accurate intervention. Guilt may be generated if client believes it is unacceptable to have these feelings. Knowing they are normal can provide a sense of relief.

■ Assess impact of the trauma on the client's ability to resume regular activities of daily living. Consider employment, marital relationship, and sleep patterns. Following a trauma, individuals are at high risk for physical injury because of disruption in ability to concentrate and problem-solve and lack of sufficient sleep. Isolation and avoidance behaviors may interfere with interpersonal relatedness.

■ Assess for self-destructive ideas and behavior. The trauma may result in feelings of hopelessness and worthlessness, leading to high risk for suicide.

■ Assess for maladaptive coping strategies such as substance abuse. These behaviors interfere with and delay the recovery process.

■ Identify available community resources from which the individual may seek assistance if problems with complicated grieving persist. Support groups for victims of various types of trauma exist within most communities. The presence of support systems in the recovery environment has been identified as a major predictor in the successful recovery from trauma.

Concept Care Mapping

The concept map care plan (see Chapter 9, The Nursing Process in Psychiatric-Mental Health Nursing) is a diagrammatic teaching and learning strategy that allows visualization of interrelationships between medical diagnoses, nursing diagnoses, assessment data, and treatments. An example of a concept map care plan for a client with a trauma-related disorder is presented in Figure 28–1.

Evaluation

Reassessment is conducted to determine if the nursing actions have been successful in achieving the objectives of care. Evaluation of the nursing actions for the client with a trauma-related disorder may be facilitated by gathering information using the following types of questions:

■ Can the client discuss the traumatic event without experiencing panic anxiety?

■ Does the client voluntarily discuss the traumatic event?

■ Can the client discuss changes that have occurred in his or her life because of the traumatic event?

■ Does the client have flashbacks?

■ Can the client sleep without medication?

■ Does the client have nightmares?

■ Has the client learned new, adaptive coping strategies for assistance with recovery?

■ Can the client demonstrate successful use of these new coping strategies in times of stress?

■ Can the client verbalize stages of grief and the normal behaviors associated with each?

■ Can the client recognize his or her own position in the grieving process?

■ Is guilt being alleviated?

■ Has the client maintained or regained satisfactory relationships with significant others?

■ Can the client look to the future with optimism?

■ Does the client attend a regular support group for victims of similar traumatic experiences?

■ Does the client have a plan of action for dealing with symptoms if they recur?

Application of the Nursing Process— Stressor-Related Disorders

Adjustment Disorders—Background Assessment Data

> ## CORE CONCEPT
> **Stress**
> Perceptions, emotions, anxieties, interpersonal, social, or economic events that are considered threatening to one's physical health, personal safety or well-being (Venes, 2014).

An adjustment disorder is characterized by a maladaptive reaction to an identifiable stressor or stressors that results in the development of clinically significant emotional or behavioral symptoms (APA, 2013). The response occurs within 3 months after onset of the stressor and persists for no longer than 6 months after the stressor or its consequences have ended.

The individual shows impairment in social and occupational functioning or exhibits symptoms that are in excess of an expected reaction to the stressor. The symptoms are expected to remit soon after the stressor is relieved or, if the stressor persists, when a new level of adaptation is achieved.

The stressor itself can be almost anything, but an individual's response to a particular stressor cannot be predicted. If an individual is highly predisposed or vulnerable to maladaptive response, a severe form of the disorder may follow what most people would consider only a mild or moderate stressor. Conversely, a less vulnerable individual may develop only a mild form of the disorder in response to what others might consider a severe stressor.

A number of clinical presentations are associated with adjustment disorders. The following categories, identified by the *DSM-5* (APA, 2013), are distinguished by the predominant features of the maladaptive response.

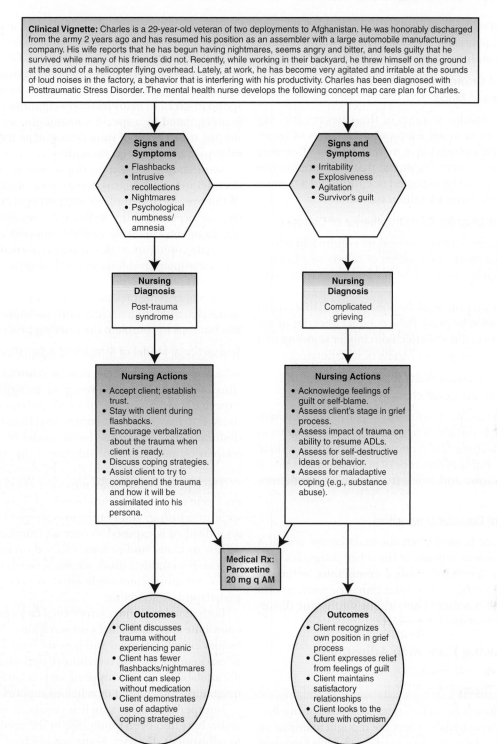

Clinical Vignette: Charles is a 29-year-old veteran of two deployments to Afghanistan. He was honorably discharged from the army 2 years ago and has resumed his position as an assembler with a large automobile manufacturing company. His wife reports that he has begun having nightmares, seems angry and bitter, and feels guilty that he survived while many of his friends did not. Recently, while working in their backyard, he threw himself on the ground at the sound of a helicopter flying overhead. Lately, at work, he has become very agitated and irritable at the sounds of loud noises in the factory, a behavior that is interfering with his productivity. Charles has been diagnosed with Posttraumatic Stress Disorder. The mental health nurse develops the following concept map care plan for Charles.

Signs and Symptoms
- Flashbacks
- Intrusive recollections
- Nightmares
- Psychological numbness/amnesia

Signs and Symptoms
- Irritability
- Explosiveness
- Agitation
- Survivor's guilt

Nursing Diagnosis
Post-trauma syndrome

Nursing Diagnosis
Complicated grieving

Nursing Actions
- Accept client; establish trust.
- Stay with client during flashbacks.
- Encourage verbalization about the trauma when client is ready.
- Discuss coping strategies.
- Assist client to try to comprehend the trauma and how it will be assimilated into his persona.

Nursing Actions
- Acknowledge feelings of guilt or self-blame.
- Assess client's stage in grief process.
- Assess impact of trauma on ability to resume ADLs.
- Assess for self-destructive ideas or behavior.
- Assess for maladaptive coping (e.g., substance abuse).

Medical Rx: Paroxetine 20 mg q AM

Outcomes
- Client discusses trauma without experiencing panic
- Client has fewer flashbacks/nightmares
- Client can sleep without medication
- Client demonstrates use of adaptive coping strategies

Outcomes
- Client recognizes own position in grief process
- Client expresses relief from feelings of guilt
- Client maintains satisfactory relationships
- Client looks to the future with optimism

FIGURE 28–1 Concept map care plan for a client with posttraumatic stress disorder.

Adjustment Disorder With Depressed Mood

This category is the most commonly diagnosed adjustment disorder. The clinical presentation is one of predominant mood disturbance, although less pronounced than that of major depressive disorder. The symptoms, such as depressed mood, tearfulness, and feelings of hopelessness, exceed what is an expected or normative response to an identified stressor.

Adjustment Disorder With Anxiety

This category denotes a maladaptive response to a stressor in which the predominant manifestation is anxiety.

For example, the symptoms may reveal nervousness, worry, and jitteriness. The clinician must differentiate this diagnosis from those of anxiety disorders.

Adjustment Disorder With Mixed Anxiety and Depressed Mood

The predominant features of this category include disturbances in mood (depression, feelings of hopelessness and sadness) and manifestations of anxiety (nervousness, worry, jitteriness) that are more intense than what would be expected or considered a normative response to an identified stressor.

Adjustment Disorder With Disturbance of Conduct

This category is characterized by conduct in which there is violation of the rights of others or of major age-appropriate societal norms and rules. Examples include truancy, vandalism, reckless driving, fighting, and defaulting on legal responsibilities. Differential diagnosis must be made from conduct disorder or antisocial personality disorder, both longer standing and pervasive responses to a variety of situations.

Adjustment Disorder With Mixed Disturbance of Emotions and Conduct

The predominant features of this category include emotional disturbances (e.g., anxiety or depression) as well as disturbances of conduct in which there is violation of the rights of others or of major age-appropriate societal norms and rules (e.g., truancy, vandalism, fighting).

Adjustment Disorder Unspecified

This subtype is used when the maladaptive reaction is not consistent with any of the other categories. The individual may have physical complaints, withdraw from relationships, or exhibit impaired work or academic performance, but without significant disturbance in emotions or conduct.

Predisposing Factors to Adjustment Disorders

Biological Theory

Chronic disorders, such as neurocognitive or intellectual developmental disorders, are thought to impair an individual's ability to adapt to stress, causing increased vulnerability to adjustment disorder. Genetic factors also may influence individual risks for maladaptive response to stress (Sadock et al., 2015).

Psychosocial Theories

Some proponents of psychoanalytic theory view adjustment disorder as a maladaptive response to stress caused by early childhood trauma, increased dependency, and retarded ego development. Freud (1964) theorized that traumatic childhood experiences created points of fixation to which the individual would be likely to regress during times of stress. Other psychoanalysts put considerable weight on birth characteristics that contribute to the manner in which individuals respond to stress. In many instances, adjustment disorder is precipitated by a specific meaningful stressor connecting with a point of vulnerability in an individual of otherwise adequate ego strength.

Some studies relate a predisposition to adjustment disorder to factors such as developmental stage, timing of the stressor, and available support systems. When a stressor occurs and the individual does not have the developmental maturity, available support systems, or adequate coping strategies to adapt, normal functioning is disrupted, resulting in psychological or somatic symptoms. The disorder also may be related to a dysfunctional grieving process. The individual may remain in the denial or anger stage, with inadequate defense mechanisms to complete the grieving process.

Transactional Model of Stress and Adaptation

Why are some individuals able to confront stressful situations adaptively and even gain strength from the experience, while others not only fail to cope adaptively but may even encounter psychopathological dysfunction? The transactional model of stress and adaptation takes into consideration the interaction between the individual and the environment.

The type of stressor that one experiences may influence one's adaptation. Sudden shock stressors occur without warning, and continuous stressors are those an individual is exposed to over an extended period. Although many studies have focused on individuals' responses to sudden shock stressors, continuous stressors were more commonly cited as precipitants to maladaptive functioning.

Both situational and interpersonal factors most likely contribute to an individual's stress response. Situational factors include personal and general economic conditions; occupational and recreational opportunities; and the availability of social supports such as family, friends, neighbors, and cultural or religious support groups.

Interpersonal factors such as constitutional vulnerability have also been implicated in the predisposition to adjustment disorder. Some studies have indicated that a child with a difficult temperament (defined as one who cries loudly and often; adapts to changes slowly; and has irregular patterns of hunger, sleep, and elimination) is at greater risk of developing a behavior disorder. Other intrapersonal factors that might influence one's ability to adjust to a painful life change include social skills, coping strategies, the presence of psychiatric illness, degree of flexibility, and level of intelligence.

Diagnosis and Outcome Identification

Nursing diagnoses are formulated from the data gathered during the assessment phase and with background knowledge regarding predisposing factors to the disorder. Nursing diagnoses that may be used for the client with an adjustment disorder include the following:

- Complicated grieving related to real or perceived loss of any concept of value to the individual, evidenced by interference with life functioning, developmental regression, or somatic complaints
- Risk-prone health behavior related to change in health status requiring modification in lifestyle (e.g., chronic illness, physical disability), evidenced by inability to problem-solve or set realistic goals for the future (appropriate diagnosis for the person with adjustment disorder if the precipitating stressor was a change in health status)
- Anxiety (moderate to severe) related to situational and/or maturational crisis evidenced by restlessness, increased helplessness, and diminished productivity

Outcome Criteria

The following criteria may be used for measurement of outcomes in the care of the client with an adjustment disorder.

The client:

- Verbalizes acceptable behaviors associated with each stage of the grief process
- Demonstrates a reinvestment in the environment
- Accomplishes activities of daily living independently
- Demonstrates ability for adequate occupational and social functioning
- Verbalizes awareness of change in health status and the effect it will have on lifestyle
- Solves problems and sets realistic goals for the future
- Demonstrates ability to cope effectively with change in lifestyle

Planning and Implementation

The following section presents a group of selected nursing diagnoses, with short- and long-term goals and nursing interventions for each.

Complicated Grieving

Complicated grieving is defined as "a disorder that occurs after the death of a significant other [or any other loss of significance to the individual], in which the experience of distress accompanying bereavement fails to follow normative expectations and manifests in functional impairment" (Herdman & Kamitsuru, 2014, p. 339).

Client Goals

Outcome criteria include short- and long-term goals. Time lines are individually determined.

Short-term goal

- By end of 1 week, client will express anger toward lost entity.

Long-term goal

- The client will be able to verbalize behaviors associated with the normal stages of grief and identify own position in grief process, while progressing at own pace toward resolution.

Interventions

- Determine the stage of grief in which client is fixed. Identify behaviors associated with this stage. Accurate baseline assessment data are necessary to plan effective care for the grieving client.
- Develop a trusting relationship with the client. Show empathy and caring. Be honest and keep all promises. Trust is the basis for a therapeutic relationship.
- Convey an accepting attitude so the client is not afraid to express feelings openly. An accepting attitude conveys that you believe he or she is a worthwhile person. Trust is enhanced.
- Allow the client to express anger. Do not become defensive if the initial expression of anger is displaced on the nurse or therapist. Help the client explore angry feelings so that they may be directed toward the intended object or person. Verbalization of feelings in a nonthreatening environment may help the client come to terms with unresolved issues.
- Assist the client to discharge pent-up anger through participation in large motor activities (e.g., brisk walks, jogging, physical exercises, volleyball, punching bag, exercise bike). Physical exercise provides a safe and effective method for discharging pent-up tension.
- Explain to the client the normal stages of grief and the behaviors associated with each stage. Help the client to understand that feelings such as guilt and anger toward the lost entity/concept are natural and acceptable during the grief process. Knowledge of the acceptability of the feelings associated with normal grieving may help to relieve some of the guilt that these responses generate.
- Encourage the client to review his or her perception of the loss or change. With support and sensitivity, point out the reality of the situation in areas where misrepresentations are expressed. The client must give up an idealized perception and be able to accept both positive and negative aspects about the painful life change before the grief process is complete.

■ Communicate to the client that crying is acceptable. The use of touch is therapeutic and appropriate with most clients. Knowledge of cultural influences specific to the client is important before employing this technique. Touch is considered inappropriate in some cultures.

■ Help the client solve problems as he or she attempts to determine methods for more adaptive coping with the stressor. Provide positive feedback for strategies identified and decisions made. Positive reinforcement enhances self-esteem and encourages repetition of desirable behaviors.

■ Encourage the client to reach out for spiritual support during this time in whatever form is desirable. Assess client's spiritual needs and assist as necessary in the fulfillment of those needs. For some individuals, spiritual support can enhance successful adaptation to painful life experiences.

Risk-Prone Health Behavior

Risk-prone health behavior is defined as "impaired ability to modify lifestyle/behaviors in a manner that improves health status" (Herdman & Kamitsuru, 2014, p. 145).

Client Goals

Outcome criteria include short- and long-term goals. Time lines are individually determined.

Short-term goals

■ The client and primary nurse will discuss the kinds of lifestyle changes that will occur because of the change in health status.

■ With the help of the primary nurse, the client will formulate a plan of action for incorporating those changes into his or her lifestyle.

■ The client will demonstrate movement toward independence, considering the change in health status.

Long-term goal

■ The client will demonstrate competence to function independently to his or her optimal ability, considering the change in health status, by the time of discharge from treatment.

Interventions

■ Encourage the client to talk about his or her lifestyle prior to the change in health status. Discuss coping mechanisms that were used at stressful times in the past. It is important to identify the client's strengths so that they may be used to facilitate adaptation to the change or loss that has occurred.

■ Encourage the client to discuss the change or loss and particularly to express anger associated with it. Anger is a normal stage in the grieving process and, if not released in an appropriate manner, may be turned inward on the self, leading to pathological depression.

■ Encourage the client to express fears associated with lifestyle alterations imposed by the chronic illness, physical disability, or other change in health status. Change often creates a feeling of disequilibrium, and the individual may respond with fears that are irrational or unfounded. The client may benefit from feedback that corrects misperceptions about how life will be with the change in health status.

■ Provide assistance with activities of daily living as required, but encourage independence to the limit that the client's ability allows. Give positive feedback for activities accomplished independently. Independent accomplishments and positive feedback enhance self-esteem and encourage repetition of desired behaviors. Successes also provide hope that adaptive functioning is possible and decrease feelings of powerlessness.

■ Help the client with decision-making regarding incorporation of the change or loss into his or her lifestyle. Identify problems the change or loss is likely to create. Discuss alternative solutions, weighing potential benefits and consequences of each alternative. Support the client's decision in the selection of an alternative. The great amount of anxiety that usually accompanies a major lifestyle change often interferes with an individual's ability to solve problems and to make appropriate decisions. The client may need assistance with this process to progress toward successful adaptation.

■ Use role-play to practice stressful situations that might occur in relation to the health status change. Role-playing decreases anxiety and provides a feeling of security by developing a plan of action for responding in an appropriate manner when a stressful situation occurs.

■ Ensure that the client and family are fully knowledgeable regarding the physiology of the change in health status and understand the necessity of such knowledge for optimal wellness. Encourage them to ask questions, and provide printed material with additional explanation. Knowing what to expect regarding the change or loss decreases anxiety and enhances the capacity for wellness.

■ Ensure that the client can identify resources within the community from which he or she may seek assistance in adapting to the change in health status. Examples include self-help or support groups and public health nurse, counselor, or social worker. Encourage the client to keep follow-up appointments with his or her physician and to call the physician's office prior to the follow-up date if problems or concerns arise. Support services provide a feeling of security that one is not alone and a means to prevent decompensation when stress becomes intolerable.

Concept Care Mapping

Individuals with adjustment disorders may have several physical and mental health issues that impact effective intervention. The concept map care plan (see Chapter 9) is a diagrammatic teaching and learning strategy that allows visualization of interrelationships between medical diagnoses, nursing diagnoses, assessment data, and treatments. An example of a concept map care plan for a client with an adjustment disorder is presented in Figure 28–2.

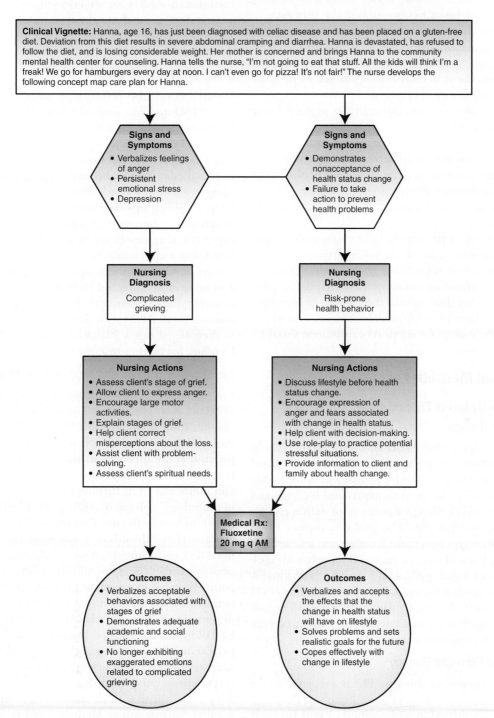

Clinical Vignette: Hanna, age 16, has just been diagnosed with celiac disease and has been placed on a gluten-free diet. Deviation from this diet results in severe abdominal cramping and diarrhea. Hanna is devastated, has refused to follow the diet, and is losing considerable weight. Her mother is concerned and brings Hanna to the community mental health center for counseling. Hanna tells the nurse, "I'm not going to eat that stuff. All the kids will think I'm a freak! We go for hamburgers every day at noon. I can't even go for pizza! It's not fair!" The nurse develops the following concept map care plan for Hanna.

Signs and Symptoms
- Verbalizes feelings of anger
- Persistent emotional stress
- Depression

Signs and Symptoms
- Demonstrates nonacceptance of health status change
- Failure to take action to prevent health problems

Nursing Diagnosis
Complicated grieving

Nursing Diagnosis
Risk-prone health behavior

Nursing Actions
- Assess client's stage of grief.
- Allow client to express anger.
- Encourage large motor activities.
- Explain stages of grief.
- Help client correct misperceptions about the loss.
- Assist client with problem-solving.
- Assess client's spiritual needs.

Nursing Actions
- Discuss lifestyle before health status change.
- Encourage expression of anger and fears associated with change in health status.
- Help client with decision-making.
- Use role-play to practice potential stressful situations.
- Provide information to client and family about health change.

Medical Rx:
Fluoxetine 20 mg q AM

Outcomes
- Verbalizes acceptable behaviors associated with stages of grief
- Demonstrates adequate academic and social functioning
- No longer exhibiting exaggerated emotions related to complicated grieving

Outcomes
- Verbalizes and accepts the effects that the change in health status will have on lifestyle
- Solves problems and sets realistic goals for the future
- Copes effectively with change in lifestyle

FIGURE 28–2 Concept map care plan for a client with an adjustment disorder.

Evaluation

Reassessment is conducted to determine if the nursing actions have been successful in achieving the objectives of care. Evaluation of the nursing actions for the client with an adjustment disorder may be facilitated by gathering information using the following types of questions:

- Does the client verbalize understanding of the grief process and his or her position in the process?
- Does the client recognize his or her adaptive and maladaptive behaviors associated with the grief response?
- Does the client demonstrate evidence of progression along the grief response?
- Can the client accomplish activities of daily living independently?
- Does the client demonstrate the ability to perform occupational and social activities adequately?
- Does the client discuss the change in health status and modification of lifestyle it will affect?
- Does the client demonstrate acceptance of the modification?
- Can the client participate in decision-making and problem-solving for his or her future?
- Does the client set realistic goals for the future?
- Does the client demonstrate new adaptive coping strategies for dealing with the change in lifestyle?
- Can the client verbalize available resources to whom he or she may go for support or assistance should it be necessary?

Treatment Modalities

Trauma-Related Disorders
Cognitive Therapy

Cognitive therapy for PTSD and ASD strives to help the individual recognize and modify trauma-related thoughts and beliefs. The individual learns to modify the relationships between thoughts and feelings and to identify and challenge inaccurate or extreme automatic negative thoughts. The goal is to replace these negative thoughts with more accurate and less distressing thoughts and to cope more effectively with feelings such as anger, guilt, and fear. The individual is assisted to modify the appraisal of self and the world as it has been affected by the trauma and to regain hope and optimism about safety, trust, power and control, esteem, and intimacy.

Prolonged Exposure Therapy

Prolonged exposure therapy (PE) is a type of behavioral therapy similar to implosion therapy or flooding. It can be conducted in an imagined or real (in vivo) situation. In the imagined situation, the individual is exposed to repeated and prolonged mental recounting of the traumatic experience. In vivo exposure involves systematic confrontation, within safe limits, of trauma-related situations that are feared and avoided. This intense emotional processing of the traumatic event serves to neutralize the memories so that they no longer result in anxious arousal or escape and avoidance behaviors. PE has four main parts: (1) education about the treatment, (2) breathing retraining for relaxation, (3) imagined exposure through repeated discussion about the trauma with a therapist, and (4) exposure to real-world situations related to the trauma.

Group and Family Therapy

Group therapy has been strongly advocated for clients with PTSD and has proved especially effective with military veterans (Sadock et al., 2015). The importance of being able to share their experiences with empathetic fellow veterans, to talk about problems in social adaptation, and to discuss options for managing aggression toward others has been emphasized. Some PTSD groups are informal and leaderless, such as self-help or support groups, and some are led by experienced group therapists who may have had some first-hand experience with trauma. Some groups involve family members, recognizing that they may also be severely affected by symptoms of PTSD. For example, family members of military veterans sometimes develop PTSD symptoms as a result of exposure to their loved one's PTSD (see Chapter 38, Military Families, for further discussion of this topic).

Eye Movement Desensitization and Reprocessing

Eye movement desensitization and reprocessing (EMDR) is a type of psychotherapy that was developed in 1989 by psychologist Francine Shapiro. It "has evolved from a simple technique into an integrative psychotherapy approach with a theoretical model that emphasizes the brain's information processing system and memories of disturbing experiences as the basis of pathology" (Shapiro, 2007, p. 3). EMDR has been shown to be an effective therapy for PTSD and other trauma-related disorders. It has been used with other disorders, including depression, adjustment disorder, phobias, addictions, generalized anxiety disorder, and panic disorder. However, at present, EMDR has been empirically validated only for trauma-related disorders such as PTSD and ASD (Aetna Healthcare, 2013). EMDR is contraindicated in clients who have neurological impairments (e.g., seizure disorders), clients who are suicidal or experiencing psychosis, those with severe dissociative disorders or unstable substance abuse, and those with detached retina or glaucoma (Center for Integrative Medicine, 2013).

The exact biological mechanisms by which EMDR achieves its therapeutic effects are unknown. Some studies have indicated that eye movements cause a decrease in imagery vividness and distress and an increase in memory access. The process involves rapid eye movements while processing painful emotions. The EMDR International Association (2016) stresses that "processing" does not mean "talking about it" but rather "setting up a learning state that will allow experiences that are causing problems to be 'digested' and stored appropriately in your brain." While concentrating on a particular emotion or physical sensation surrounding the traumatic event, the client is asked to focus his or her eye movements on the therapist's fingers as the therapist moves them from left to right and back again. Although some individuals report rapid results with this therapy, research has indicated that between 5 and 12 sessions are required to achieve lasting treatment effects. The treatment encompasses an eight-phase process.

Phase 1: History and Treatment Planning The therapist takes a thorough history and develops a treatment plan. The problem for which the client is seeking treatment and current symptoms are discussed. However, the client is not required to discuss the traumatic event in detail unless he or she chooses to do so. Instead, emphasis is placed on the emotions and physical sensations surrounding the traumatic event.

Phase 2: Preparation The therapist teaches the client certain self-care techniques (e.g., relaxation techniques) for dealing with emotional disturbances that may arise during or between sessions. Self-care is an important component of EMDR. The client must develop a sense of trust in the therapist during this phase.

Phase 3: Assessment The therapist asks the client to identify a specific scene or picture from the event identified in phase 1 that best represents the memory. The client is then directed to express a negative self-belief associated with the memory (e.g., "I am bad" or "I'm in danger"). The next step is to identify a self-statement that he or she would *rather* believe (e.g., "I am good" or "I'm safe now"). When the self-statements have been identified, the client is asked to rate the validity of each of the statements on the Validity of Cognition (VOC) scale from 1 (completely false) to 7 (completely true). The client is also asked to rank the disturbing emotions on the 0 to 10 Subjective Units of Disturbance (SUD) scale (with 0 meaning not disturbing at all and 10 meaning the worst feeling he or she has ever had).

Phase 4: Densensitization The client gives attention to the negative beliefs and disturbing emotions associated with the traumatic event while focusing his or her vision on the back-and-forth motion of the therapist's finger. All personal feelings and physical reactions experienced during this time are noted. Following each

set of rapid eye movements, the therapist reassesses the level of disturbance associated with the feelings, images, and beliefs. This desensitization process continues until the distress level (as measured by the SUD scale) is reduced to 0 or 1.

Phase 5: Installation The client gives attention to the positive belief that he or she has identified to replace the negative belief associated with the trauma. This is accomplished while simultaneously visually tracking the therapist's finger. Following each set of rapid eye movements, the client is asked to rate the positive belief on the VOC scale. The goal is to strengthen the positive belief or self-statement until it is accepted as completely true (a score of 7 on the VOC scale).

Phase 6: Body Scan When positive cognition has been strengthened, the therapist asks the client to concentrate on any lingering physical sensations. While focusing on the traumatic event, the client is asked to identify any areas of the body where residual tension is experienced. Because positive self-beliefs must be on a physical as well as an intellectual level, phase 6 is not complete until the client is able to think about or discuss the traumatic event (or the feelings associated with it) without experiencing bodily tension.

Phase 7: Closure Closure ensures that the client leaves each session feeling better than he or she felt at the beginning. If the processing that took place during the session is not complete, the therapist will direct the client through a variety of self-calming relaxation techniques to help him or her regain emotional equilibrium. The client is briefed about what to expect between sessions. Until processing of the trauma is complete, disturbing images, thoughts, and emotions may arise between therapy sessions. The therapist instructs the client to record these experiences in a journal so that they may be used as targets for processing in future therapy sessions.

Phase 8: Reevaluation Reevaluation begins each new therapy session. The therapist assesses whether the positive changes have been maintained, determines if previous target areas need reprocessing, and identifies any new target areas that need attention.

Clients often feel relief quite rapidly with EMDR. However, to achieve lasting results, it is important that each of the eight phases be completed. Treatment is not complete until "EMDR therapy has focused on the past memories that are contributing to the problem, the present situations that are disturbing, and what skills the client may need for the future" (EMDR Network, 2013).

Psychopharmacology

Antidepressants The selective serotonin reuptake inhibitors (SSRIs) are now considered first-line treatment of choice for PTSD because of their efficacy, tolerability, and safety ratings (Sadock et al., 2015). Paroxetine and sertraline have been approved by the FDA for this purpose. The tricyclic antidepressants amitriptyline and imipramine have been supported by several well-controlled studies. MAO inhibitors (e.g., phenelzine) and trazodone have also been effective in the treatment of PTSD.

Anxiolytics Alprazolam has been prescribed for PTSD clients for its antidepressant and antipanic effects. Other benzodiazepines have also been used despite the absence of controlled studies demonstrating their efficacy in PTSD. Their addictive properties make them less desirable than some of the other medications in the treatment of posttrauma clients.

Buspirone, which has serotonergic properties similar to the SSRIs, may also be useful. Further controlled trials with this drug are needed to validate its efficacy in treating PTSD.

Antihypertensives The beta blocker propranolol and alpha$_2$-receptor agonist clonidine have been successful in alleviating some of the symptoms associated with PTSD. In clinical trials, marked reductions in nightmares, intrusive recollections, hypervigilance, insomnia, startle responses, and angry outbursts were reported with the use of these drugs.

Other Medications Carbamazepine, valproic acid, and lithium carbonate have been reported to alleviate symptoms of intrusive recollections, flashbacks, nightmares, impulsivity, irritability, and violent behavior in PTSD clients. Sadock and associates (2015) report that little positive evidence exists concerning the use of antipsychotics in PTSD. They suggest that these drugs "should be reserved for the short-term control of severe aggression and agitation" (p. 621).

Ketamine, an anesthetic agent which has demonstrated benefits in treatment of depression and obsessive-compulsive disorder, was found in clinical trials (Feder et al., 2014) to benefit some patients with PTSD. It is a modulator of glutaminergic activity at *N*-methyl-D-aspartate receptors and serotonergic activity at $5HT_1$ receptors that is believed to disrupt the fear associated with trauma. Currently, ketamine is not FDA approved for this use but is prescribed as an off-label use. It is administered intravenously at subanesthetic doses and usually involves a series of treatments. Jeffreys (2016) cautions that its effects are short term and there is potential for addiction.

The endocannabinoid system may be another avenue for treatment, since decreased levels of endogenous cannabinoids have been found in PTSD patients (Jeffreys, 2016). Although direct stimulation of this pathway has demonstrated negative effects on PTSD, indirect stimulation of this pathway might provide some additional treatment options.

Prazosin, an alpha$_1$ antagonist, has demonstrated benefit in reducing nightmares and enhancing normal dreaming patterns in clients with PTSD (Gore, 2015), and recent research has identified benefits for daytime PTSD symptoms as well (Jeffreys, 2016). Low-dose glucocorticoids are being studied for possible benefit in decreasing recall of traumatic memories, but more research is needed (Gore, 2015).

Adjustment Disorders

Various treatments are used for clients with adjustment disorders. The primary focus of intervention is to maximize the potential for adaptation.

Individual Psychotherapy

Individual psychotherapy is the most common treatment for adjustment disorder. Individual psychotherapy allows the client to examine the stressor that is causing the problem, possibly assign personal meaning to the stressor, and confront unresolved issues that may be exacerbating this crisis. Treatment works to remove these blocks to adaptation so that normal developmental progression can resume. Techniques are used to clarify links between the current stressor and past experiences and assist with the development of more adaptive coping strategies.

Family Therapy

The focus of treatment is shifted from the individual to the system of relationships in which the individual is involved. The maladaptive response of the identified client is viewed as symptomatic of a dysfunctional family system. All family members are included in the therapy, and treatment serves to improve the functioning within the family network. Emphasis is placed on communication, family rules, and interaction patterns among the family members.

Behavior Therapy

The goal of behavior therapy is to replace ineffective response patterns with more adaptive ones. The situations that promote ineffective responses are identified, and carefully designed reinforcement schedules along with role modeling and coaching are used to alter the maladaptive response patterns. This type of treatment is very effective when implemented in an inpatient setting where the client's behavior and its consequences may be more readily controlled.

Self-Help Groups

Group experiences, with or without a professional facilitator, provide an arena in which members may consider and compare their responses to individuals with similar life experiences. Members benefit from learning that they are not alone in their painful experiences. Hope is derived from knowing that others have survived and even grown from similar traumas. Members of the group exchange advice, share coping strategies, and provide support and encouragement for each other.

Crisis Intervention

In crisis intervention, the therapist or other intervener becomes part of the individual's life situation. Because of increased anxiety, the individual with adjustment disorder is unable to problem-solve, so he or she requires guidance and support from another to help mobilize the resources needed to resolve the crisis. Crisis intervention is short term and relies heavily on orderly problem-solving techniques and structured activities that are focused on change. The ultimate goal of crisis intervention in the treatment of adjustment disorder is to resolve the immediate crisis, restore adaptive functioning, and promote personal growth.

Psychopharmacology

Adjustment disorder is not commonly treated with medications because (1) their effect may be temporary and only mask the real problem, interfering with the possibility of finding a more permanent solution; and (2) psychoactive drugs carry the potential for physiological and psychological dependence.

When the client with adjustment disorder has symptoms of anxiety or depression, the physician may prescribe antianxiety or antidepressant medication. These medications are considered only adjuncts to psychotherapy and should not be given as primary therapy. They are given to alleviate symptoms so that the individual may more effectively cope while attempting to adapt to the stressful situation.

CASE STUDY AND SAMPLE CARE PLAN

NURSING HISTORY AND ASSESSMENT

Marissa, age 22, was born in a small town in Oklahoma. She lived there her whole life, even living at home while she attended a nearby college to earn a baccalaureate degree in education. She is an only child, and her parents were in their 40s when she was born. She was engaged throughout her college years to her high school sweetheart, Dave, who graduated 6 months ago from the state university with a degree in aeronautical engineering.

Upon his graduation, he accepted a position with NASA at Kennedy Space Center in Florida. Marissa and Dave were married 5 months ago and moved to a small apartment in Cape Canaveral, where Dave began his work with NASA. The plan was for Marissa to seek employment upon their arrival, but she has been unable to move ahead with those plans. She stays in the apartment most days, talking on the phone to her parents and crying about how much she misses them and her home in Oklahoma. She has met very few people and has no desire to do so. She sleeps a lot and has lost weight. She has been having severe headaches. Her husband has become very concerned about her and made an appointment for her with a private physician. Following a complete and unremarkable physical examination, the physician referred Marissa to the mental health clinic, where she was admitted to the day treatment center with a diagnosis of Adjustment Disorder with Depressed Mood.

NURSING DIAGNOSES AND OUTCOME IDENTIFICATION

From the assessment data, the nurse develops the following nursing diagnoses for Marissa:

1. **Complicated grieving** related to feelings of loss associated with leaving her parents and her lifetime home.
   a. **Short-Term Goal:** Within 1 week, Marissa will express anger about the loss associated with her move.

   b. **Long-Term Goal:** Marissa will be able to verbalize behaviors associated with the normal stages of grief and identify her own position in the grief process, while progressing at her own pace toward resolution.

2. **Relocation stress syndrome** related to move away from parents and familiar environment in which she had spent her whole life.
   a. **Short-Term Goal:** Within 1 week, Marissa will verbalize at least one positive aspect regarding relocation to her new environment.

   b. **Long-Term Goal:** Within 1 month, Marissa will demonstrate positive adaptation to her new environment as evidenced by involvement in activities, expression of satisfaction with new acquaintances, and elimination of previously evident physical and psychological symptoms associated with the relocation.

PLANNING AND IMPLEMENTATION

COMPLICATED GRIEVING

The following nursing interventions have been identified for Marissa:

1. Determine the stage of grief in which Marissa is fixed. Identify behaviors associated with this stage.
2. Develop a trusting relationship with Marissa. Show empathy and caring. Be honest and keep all promises.
3. Convey an accepting attitude so that Marissa is not afraid to express her feelings openly.
4. Allow Marissa to express her anger. Do not become defensive if the initial expression of anger is displaced on nurse or therapist. Help Marissa explore angry feelings so that they may be directed toward the intended object or situation.
5. Help Marissa discharge pent-up anger through participation in large motor activities (e.g., brisk walks, jogging, physical exercises, or activity of her choice).

Continued

CASE STUDY AND SAMPLE CARE PLAN—cont'd

6. Explain to Marissa the normal stages of grief and the behaviors associated with each stage. Help her to understand that these feelings are normal and acceptable during a grief process.
7. Encourage Marissa to review her personal perception of the move. With support and sensitivity, point out the reality of the situation in areas where misrepresentations are expressed.
8. Help Marissa solve problems as she attempts to determine methods for more adaptive coping with the life change. Provide positive feedback for strategies identified and decisions made.
9. Encourage Marissa to reach out for spiritual support during this time in whatever form is desirable to her. Assess her spiritual needs and assist as necessary in the fulfillment of those needs.

RELOCATION STRESS SYNDROME
The following nursing interventions have been identified for Marissa:
1. Encourage Marissa to discuss feelings (concerns, fears, anger) regarding this relocation.
2. Encourage Marissa to discuss how the change will affect her life. Ensure that Marissa is involved in decision-making and problem-solving regarding the move.
3. Help Marissa identify positive aspects about the move.

4. Help Marissa identify resources within the new community from which assistance with various types of services may be obtained.
5. Identify groups within the community that specialize in helping individuals adapt to relocation. Examples include Newcomers' Club, Welcome Wagon International, and school and church organizations.
6. Refer Marissa to a support group (e.g., Depression and Bipolar Support Alliance [DBSA]).

EVALUATION
The outcome criteria for Marissa have been met. She is no longer having headaches and has regained some of her weight. She has joined a chapter of DBSA and has made some new acquaintances. She has applied to become a substitute teacher in the local school district, and she and Dave have joined the local Methodist church, where they have started to socialize with several couples their age. They have also adopted Molly, a 2-year-old mutt from the local shelter, who showers Marissa with love and keeps her company when no one else is around. They take daily walks together. Marissa still talks to her parents on the phone daily but no longer has feelings of despair about living so far away from them. Her parents provide encouragement and give her positive feedback for achieving a satisfactory adaptation to her new environment. They are planning a visit to see Marissa and Dave in the near future.

Summary and Key Points

- PTSD is the development of characteristic symptoms following exposure to an extreme traumatic stressor involving a personal threat to physical integrity or to the integrity of others. Symptoms may begin within the first 3 months after the trauma, or there may be a delay of several months or even years.
- The symptoms are associated with events that would be markedly distressing to almost anyone and include reexperiencing the trauma, a sustained high level of anxiety or arousal, or a general numbing of responsiveness.
- A disorder that is similar in terms of precipitating traumatic events and symptomatology to PTSD is ASD. In ASD, the symptoms are time limited, lasting up to 1 month following the trauma. If the symptoms last longer than 1 month, the diagnosis would be PTSD.
- Predisposing factors to trauma-related disorders include psychosocial, learning, cognitive, and biological influences.
- Adjustment disorders are relatively common. Some studies indicate they are the most commonly ascribed psychiatric diagnoses.
- Clinical symptoms associated with adjustment disorders include inability to function socially or occupationally in response to an identifiable stressor.

- Adjustment disorder is distinguished by the predominant features of the maladaptive response. These include depression, anxiety, mixed anxiety and depression, disturbance of conduct, and mixed disturbance of emotions and conduct.
- Of the two types of stressors discussed (i.e., sudden shock and continuous), more individuals respond with maladaptive behaviors to long-term continuous stressors.
- Treatment modalities for PTSD include cognitive therapy, prolonged exposure therapy, group and family therapy, eye movement desensitization and reprocessing, and psychopharmacology.
- Treatment modalities for adjustment disorders include individual psychotherapy, family therapy, behavior therapy, self-help groups, crisis intervention, and medications to treat anxiety or depression.
- Nursing care of individuals with trauma- and stressor-related disorders is accomplished using the steps of the nursing process.

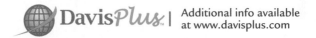 **DavisPlus** | Additional info available at www.davisplus.com

Review Questions
Self-Examination/Learning Exercise

Select the answer that is most appropriate for each of the following questions.

1. John, a veteran of the war in Iraq, is diagnosed with PTSD. He says to the nurse, "I can't figure out why God took my buddy instead of me." From this statement, the nurse assesses which of the following in John?
   a. Repressed anger
   b. Survivor's guilt
   c. Intrusive thoughts
   d. Spiritual distress

2. John, a veteran of the war in Iraq, is diagnosed with PTSD. He experiences a nightmare during his first night in the hospital. He explains to the nurse that he was dreaming about gunfire all around and people being killed. The nurse's most appropriate *initial* intervention is to:
   a. Administer alprazolam as ordered prn for anxiety.
   b. Call the physician and report the incident.
   c. Stay with John and reassure him of his safety.
   d. Have John listen to a tape of relaxation exercises.

3. John, a veteran of the war in Iraq, is diagnosed with PTSD. Which of the following therapy regimens would most appropriately be ordered for John?
   a. Paroxetine and group therapy
   b. Diazepam and implosion therapy
   c. Alprazolam and behavior therapy
   d. Carbamazepine and cognitive therapy

4. Which of the following may be influential in the predisposition to PTSD?
   a. Unsatisfactory parent-child relationship
   b. Excess of the neurotransmitter serotonin
   c. Distorted, negative cognitions
   d. Severity of the stressor and availability of support systems

5. Nina recently left her husband of 10 years. She was very dependent on him and is having difficulty adjusting to an independent lifestyle. She has been hospitalized with a diagnosis of adjustment disorder with depressed mood. What is the *priority* nursing diagnosis for Nina?
   a. Risk-prone health behavior related to loss of dependency
   b. Complicated grieving related to breakup of marriage
   c. Ineffective communication related to problems with dependency
   d. Social isolation related to depressed mood

6. Nina, who is depressed following the breakup of a very stormy marriage, says to the nurse, "I feel so bad. I thought I would feel better once I left, but I feel worse!" Which is the *best* response by the nurse?
   a. "Cheer up, Nina. You have a lot to be happy about."
   b. "You are grieving the loss of your marriage. It's natural for you to feel badly."
   c. "Try not to dwell on how you feel. If you don't think about it, you'll feel better."
   d. "You did the right thing, Nina. Knowing that should make you feel better."

7. Nina has been hospitalized with adjustment disorder with depressed mood following the breakup of her marriage. Which of the following is true regarding the diagnosis of adjustment disorder?
   a. Nina will require long-term psychotherapy to achieve relief.
   b. Nina likely inherited a genetic tendency for the disorder.
   c. Nina's symptoms will likely remit once she has accepted the change in her life.
   d. Nina probably would not have experienced adjustment disorder if she had a higher level of intelligence.

Continued

Review Questions—cont'd
Self-Examination/Learning Exercise

8. The physician orders sertraline (Zoloft) for a client who is hospitalized with adjustment disorder with depressed mood. This medication is intended to:
   a. Increase energy and elevate mood.
   b. Stimulate the central nervous system.
   c. Prevent psychotic symptoms.
   d. Produce a calming effect.

   Zoloft ↑ energy ↑ mood

9. An individual who is diagnosed with *adjustment disorder with disturbance of conduct* most likely:
   a. Violates the rights of others to feel better.
   b. Expresses symptoms that reveal a high level of anxiety.
   c. Exhibits severe social isolation and withdrawal.
   d. Is experiencing a complicated grieving process.

10. Emma, age 16, has recently been diagnosed with diabetes mellitus. She must watch her diet and take an oral hypoglycemic medication daily. She has become very depressed, and her mother reports that Emma refuses to change her diet and often skips her medication. Emma has been hospitalized for stabilization of her blood sugar. The psychiatric nurse practitioner has been called in as a consult. Which of the following nursing diagnoses by the psychiatric nurse would be a priority for Emma at this time?
    a. Anxiety related to hospitalization evidenced by noncompliance
    b. Low self-esteem related to feeling different from her peers evidenced by social isolation
    c. Risk for suicide related to new diagnosis of diabetes mellitus
    d. Risk-prone health behavior related to denial of seriousness of her illness evidenced by refusal to follow diet and take medication

11. Trauma-informed care is a philosophical approach that includes which of the following principles? (Select all that apply.)
    a. Nurses need to be aware of the potential for trauma in any client and provide care that minimizes the risk of revictimization or retraumatization.
    b. Medications need to be given before any other interventions are considered.
    c. Trauma-informed care highlights the importance of providing care that protects the physical, psychological, and emotional safety of the client.
    d. Trauma-informed care is based on the principle that traumas are not correlated with depression or increased risk for suicide.

TEST YOUR CRITICAL THINKING SKILLS

Alice, age 48, underwent a mastectomy of the right breast after her mammogram revealed a lump that proved malignant when biopsied. Since her surgery 6 weeks ago, Alice has refused to see any of her friends. She stays in her bedroom, speaks to her husband only when he speaks first, is having difficulty sleeping, and eats very little. She refuses to look at the mastectomy scar and has refused to see the Reach to Recovery representative who has tried several times to help fit her with a prosthesis. Her husband has become very worried about her and spoke to the family doctor, who recommended a psychiatrist. She has been admitted to the psychiatric unit with a diagnosis of adjustment disorder with depressed mood.
   Answer the following questions about Alice:

1. What would be the primary nursing diagnosis for Alice?
2. Describe a short-term goal and a long-term goal for Alice.
3. Discuss a priority nursing intervention in working with Alice.

References

Aetna Healthcare. (2013). Clinical policy bulletin: Eye movement desensitization and reprocessing (EMDR) therapy. Retrieved from www.aetna.com/cpb/medical/data/500_599/0583.html

American Psychiatric Association (APA). (2000). *Diagnostic and statistical manual of mental disorders, Fourth Edition, Text Revision (DSM-IV-TR)*. Washington, DC: American Psychiatric Publishing.

American Psychiatric Association (APA). (2013) *Diagnostic and statistical manual of mental disorders* (5th ed.). Washington, DC: American Psychiatric Publishing.

Black, D.W., & Andreasen, N.C. (2014). *Introductory textbook of psychiatry*. (6th ed.) Washington, DC: American Psychiatric Publishing.

Center for Integrative Medicine. (2013). Eye movement desensitization and reprocessing. Retrieved from www.upmc.com/Services/integrative-medicine/outpatient-services/Pages/eye-movement.aspx

Department of Veterans Affairs. (2016). How common is PTSD? Retrieved from www.ptsd.va.gov/public/PTSD-overview/basics/how-common-is-ptsd.asp

EMDR International Association. (2016). What is the actual EMDR session like? Retrieved from https://emdria.site-ym.com/?120

EMDR Network. (2013). A brief description of EMDR therapy: Eight phases of treatment. Retrieved from www.emdrnetwork.org/description.html

Epstein, S. (1991). Beliefs and symptoms in maladaptive resolutions of the traumatic neurosis. In D. Ozer, J.M. Healy, Jr., & A.J. Stewart (Eds.), *Perspectives on personality* (Vol. 3). London: Jessica Kingsley.

Feder, A., Parides, M.K., Murrough, J.W., Perez, A.M., Morgan, J.E., Saxena, S., . . . Charney, D.S. (2014). Efficacy of intravenous ketamine for treatment of chronic posttraumatic stress disorder: A randomized clinical trial. *JAMA Psychiatry, 71*(6), 681-688. doi:10.1001/jamapsychiatry.2014.62

Frances, A. (2015). "We should live"—Surviving after catastrophic death. *Psychiatric Times*. Retrieved from www.psychiatrictimes.com/major-depressive-disorder/we-should-live-surviving-after-catastrophic-death

Friedman, M.J. (1996). PTSD diagnosis and treatment for mental health clinicians. *Community Mental Health Journal, 32*(2), 173-189. doi:10.1007/BF02249755

Friedman, M.J., Resick, P.A., Bryant, R.A., Strain, J., Horowitz, M., & Spiegel, D. (2011). Classification of trauma and stressor-related disorders in DSM-5. *Depression and Anxiety, 28*(9), 737-749. doi:10.1002/da.20845

Gore, A. (2015). Posttraumatic stress disorder medication. Retrieved from http://emedicine.medscape.com/article/288154-medication#1

Herdman, T.H., & Kamitsuru, S. (Eds.). (2014). *NANDA-I nursing diagnoses: Definitions and classification, 2015–2017*. Chichester, UK: Wiley Blackwell.

Hopper, E. K., Bassuk, E.L., & Olivet, J. (2010). Shelter from the storm: Trauma-informed care in homelessness services settings. *The Open Health Services and Policy Journal, 3*(2), 80-100. doi:10.2174/1874924001003010080

Jeffreys, M. (2016). Clinician's guide to medications for PTSD. Retrieved from www.ptsd.va.gov/professional/treatment/overview/clinicians-guide-to-medications-for-ptsd.asp

Lanius, U. (2013). Neurobiology and treatment of traumatic dissociation. Retrieved from www.isst-d.org/downloads/AnnualConference/2013/Baltimore2013handout.pdf

Puri, B.K., & Treasaden, I.H. (2011). *Textbook of psychiatry*. Philadelphia: Churchill Livingstone Elsevier.

Sadock, B.J., Sadock, V.A., & Ruiz, P. (2015). *Synopsis of psychiatry: Behavioral sciences/clinical psychiatry* (11th ed.). Philadelphia: Lippincott Williams & Wilkins.

Shapiro, F. (2007). EMDR and case conceptualization from an adaptive information processing perspective. In F. Shapiro, F.W. Kaslow, & L. Maxfield (Eds.), *Handbook of EMDR and family therapy processes* (pp. 3-34). Hoboken, NJ: Wiley.

Substance Abuse and Mental Health Services Administration. (2015). Trauma informed care and alternatives to seclusion and restraint. Retrieved from https://www.samhsa.gov/nctic/trauma-interventions

Valentino, R.J., & Van Bockstaele, E. (2015). Endogenous opioids: The downside to opposing stress. *Neurobiology of Stress, 1*, 23-32. doi:http://dx.doi.org/10.1016/j.ynstr.2014.09.006

Venes, D. (Ed.). (2014). *Taber's medical dictionary* (22nd ed.). Philadelphia: F.A. Davis.

Classical References

Freud, S. (1964). New introductory lectures on psychoanalysis and other works. In *The standard edition of the complete psychological works of Sigmund Freud* (Vol. 22). London: Hogarth Press.

29 Somatic Symptom and Dissociative Disorders

CHAPTER OUTLINE

KEY TERMS

OBJECTIVES

After reading this chapter, the student will be able to:

1. Discuss historical aspects and epidemiological statistics related to somatic symptom and dissociative disorders.
2. Describe various types of somatic symptom and dissociative disorders and identify symptomatology associated with each; use this information in client assessment.
3. Identify predisposing factors in the development of somatic symptom and dissociative disorders.
4. Formulate nursing diagnoses and goals of care for clients with somatic symptom and dissociative disorders.
5. Describe appropriate nursing interventions for behaviors associated with somatic symptom and dissociative disorders.
6. Evaluate the nursing care of clients with somatic symptom and dissociative disorders.
7. Discuss modalities relevant to treatment of somatic symptom and dissociative disorders.

HOMEWORK ASSIGNMENT

Please read the chapter and answer the following questions:

1. Past experience with serious or life-threatening physical illness, either personal or that of a close family member, can predispose an individual to what somatic symptom disorder?
2. In an individual with dissociative identity disorder, what most commonly precipitates transition from one personality to another?
3. Conversion symptoms most commonly occur in an individual for what reason?
4. Somatic symptom and dissociative disorders are the physical and behavioral responses to what unconscious phenomenon?

Disorders with primarily somatic symptoms are characterized by physical symptoms suggesting medical disease but without demonstrable organic pathology. For this reason, most clients with a somatic symptom or related disorder are seen in primary care and hospital settings rather than in mental health-care settings. It is important to note that the inability of modern medicine to determine the existence of pathophysiology to explain a client's symptoms is not sufficient to diagnose him or her with a mental illness. Somatic symptom and related disorders are classified as mental disorders by the *Diagnostic and Statistical Manual of Mental Disorders, Fifth Edition (DSM-5)* when the excessive focus on somatic symptoms is beyond any medical explanation *and* it causes significant distress and impairment in one's functioning (APA, 2013).

The *DSM-5* identifies a specific disorder called *somatic symptom disorder* and several related disorders including *illness anxiety disorder, conversion disorder, factitious disorders, psychological factors affecting other medical conditions,* and others (APA, 2013). The common focus of these diagnoses is distress and impairment secondary to somatic symptoms, as described previously. The prevalence of somatic symptom disorder in primary care settings has been estimated to be as high as 11 percent and hypochondriasis (no longer a diagnostic category in the *DSM-5* but similar to illness anxiety disorder) from 4 to 6 percent (Yates, 2014). The prevalence of conversion disorders, based on studies of hospital psychiatric consults, is estimated to be as high as 15 percent. The wide variation of these estimates highlights the difficulties associated with consensus about diagnosing and reporting these conditions.

Dissociative disorders are defined by a disturbance of or alteration in the usually integrated functions of consciousness, memory, and identity (Black & Andreasen, 2014). Dissociative responses occur when anxiety becomes overwhelming and the personality becomes disorganized. Defense mechanisms that normally govern consciousness, identity, and memory break down, and behavior occurs with little or no participation on the part of the conscious personality. Types of dissociative disorders described by the *DSM-5* include *depersonalization derealization disorder, dissociative amnesia, dissociative identity disorder,* and others.

This chapter focuses on disorders characterized by severe repressed anxiety that manifests as physical symptoms, fear of illness, and dissociative behaviors. Historical and epidemiological statistics are presented. Predisposing factors that have been implicated in the etiology of these responses provide a framework for studying the dynamics of somatic symptom and dissociative disorders. An explanation of the symptomatology of these disorders is presented as background

knowledge for assessing the client, and nursing care is described in the context of the nursing process. Additional treatment modalities are explored.

Historical Aspects

Historically, somatic symptom disorders were identified as *hysterical neuroses.* The concept of hysteria is at least 4,000 years old and probably originated in Egypt. The name has been in use since the time of Hippocrates.

Over the years, symptoms of hysterical neuroses have been associated with witchcraft, demonology, and sorcery; dysfunction of the nervous system; and unexpressed emotion. They have also historically been viewed as primarily an affliction of women. Critics have argued that the depiction of women as prone to hysteria not only is sexist but has interfered with women receiving adequate medical evaluation for symptoms. Somatic symptom disorders are thought to occur in response to repressed severe anxiety. Freud observed that under hypnosis, clients with hysterical neurosis could recall past memories and emotional experiences that would relieve their symptoms. This observation led to his proposal that unexpressed emotion can be "converted" into physical symptoms.

CORE CONCEPT

Dissociation

An unconscious defense mechanism in which there is separation of identity, memory, and cognition from affect; the segregation of ideas and memories about oneself from their emotional and historical underpinnings (Sadock, Sadock, & Ruiz, 2015; Venes, 2014).

Freud (1962) viewed dissociation as a type of repression, an active defense mechanism used to remove threatening or unacceptable mental contents from conscious awareness. He also described the defense of ego-splitting in the management of incompatible mental contents. Although the study of dissociative processes dates back to the 19th century, scientists still know remarkably little about the phenomena. Questions remain unanswered: Are dissociative disorders psychopathological processes or ego-protective devices? Are dissociative processes under voluntary control, or are they a totally unconscious effort? In either case, they may serve to reduce a person's awareness and anxiety associated with events that are perceived as extremely stressful.

While symptoms such as dissociation are often an unconscious defense mechanism, some individuals consciously fabricate symptoms. The syndrome of fabricating symptoms for emotional gain was first described by Richard Asher in 1951 in an article in *The Lancet*. He described a pattern of behavior in which individuals fabricated or embellished their histories and signs and symptoms of illness. He termed this condition **Munchausen syndrome** after Baron Friedrich Hieronymus Freiherr von Munchhausen, a German cavalry officer and nobleman, who was known for his fabricated stories and fanciful exaggerations about himself (Asher, 1951). Currently the *DSM-5* describes these syndromes as **factitious disorders.** These include *factitious disorders imposed on self,* or when someone deceptively induces injury or illness in another person, *factitious disorder imposed on another.*

Epidemiological Statistics

The prevalence of somatic symptom disorder is estimated to be anywhere from 0.1 to 11.6 percent (Yates, 2014). Although historically this disorder has been thought to be more prevalent in women, Sadock and associates (2015) identify it as a disorder that affects men and women equally. The *DSM-5* (APA, 2013) suggests that the higher reported prevalence in women may be related to the fact that females tend to report somatic symptoms more often than males do.

Lifetime prevalence rates of conversion disorder vary widely. Statistics within the general population have ranged from 5 to 30 percent. The disorder occurs more frequently in women than in men and more frequently in adolescents and young adults than in other age groups. A higher prevalence exists in lower socioeconomic groups, rural populations, those with less education, and military personnel who have been exposed to combat situations (Black & Andreasen, 2014; Sadock et al., 2015).

The prevalence of illness anxiety disorder, closely associated with the now-deleted diagnosis of hypochondriasis, is especially difficult to establish because this disorder is new in the *DSM-5*. The best estimate is based on data about the prevalence of hypochondriasis, estimated at between 3 and 8 percent (APA, 2013). Some people who were previously diagnosed with hypochondriasis might better meet diagnostic criteria for somatic symptom disorder under this new classification. There are similarities in these two disorders, but in somatic symptom disorder, the primary symptom is significant somatic sensations, whereas in illness anxiety disorder, there are few to no somatic symptoms but anxiety or fear about having or acquiring an illness is a primary concern. More research is needed to better understand the epidemiological statistics for each of these disorders. Hypochondriasis was relabeled to illness anxiety disorder at least in part to eliminate myths and stigmas associated with the former diagnosis (Dimsdale, 2015). Illness anxiety disorder is equally

common among men and women, and onset most commonly occurs in early adulthood. Data on the prevalence of factitious disorder is limited, so the frequency of the disorder is unknown. Estimates based on samples of hospital patients identify that about 1 percent meet criteria for factitious disorder (APA, 2013). Factitious disorder imposed on another is most often perpetrated by mothers against infants but accounts for less than 0.04 percent of reported cases of child abuse in the United States (Sadock et al., 2015).

Dissociative syndromes, although often portrayed in fictional media, are statistically quite rare. However, when they do occur, they may present dramatic clinical pictures of severe disturbance in normal personality functioning. Dissociative amnesia occurs most frequently under conditions of war or during natural disasters. In recent years, the number of reported cases has increased, possibly attributable to increased awareness of the phenomenon and subsequent identification of cases that were previously undiagnosed. It appears to be equally common in men and women. Dissociative amnesia can occur at any age but is difficult to diagnose in children because it is easily confused with inattention or oppositional behavior.

Estimates of the prevalence of dissociative identity disorder (DID, previously called *multiple personality disorder*) also vary. The disorder occurs from five to nine times more frequently in women than in men (Sadock et al., 2015). Onset likely occurs in childhood, although manifestations of the disorder may not be recognized until late adolescence or early adulthood.

The prevalence of severe episodes of depersonalization-derealization disorder is unknown. Single brief episodes may occur in as many as half of all adults, particularly when under severe psychosocial stress; when sleep deprived; during travel to unfamiliar places; or when intoxicated with hallucinogens, marijuana, or alcohol (Black & Andreasen, 2014). Symptoms usually begin in adolescence or early adulthood. The disorder is chronic, with periods of remission and exacerbation. The incidence of depersonalization-derealization disorder is high under conditions of sustained traumatization, such as in military combat or prisoner-of-war camps. It has also been reported in many individuals who endure near-death experiences.

Application of the Nursing Process

Background Assessment Data: Types of Somatic Symptom Disorders
Somatic Symptom Disorder

Somatic symptom disorder is a syndrome of multiple somatic symptoms that cannot be explained medically and are associated with psychosocial distress and frequent visits to health-care professionals to seek assistance. Symptoms may be vague, dramatized, or exaggerated in presentation, and an excessive amount of time and energy is devoted to worry and concern about the symptoms. Individuals with somatic symptom disorder are so convinced that their symptoms are related to organic pathology that they adamantly reject and are often irritated by any implication that stress or psychosocial factors play a role in their conditions. The disorder is chronic, with symptoms beginning before age 30. Anxiety and depression are frequent comorbidities, and consequently, there is an increased risk for suicide attempts (Yates, 2014).

The disorder usually runs a fluctuating course, with periods of remission and exacerbation. Clients often receive medical care from several physicians, sometimes concurrently, leading to the possibility of dangerous treatment combinations. They have a tendency to seek relief through overmedicating with prescribed analgesics or antianxiety agents. Drug abuse and dependence are common complications of somatic symptom disorder. The *DSM-5* diagnostic criteria for somatic symptom disorder are presented in Box 29–1.

Illness Anxiety Disorder

Illness anxiety disorder is defined as an unrealistic or inaccurate interpretation of physical symptoms or sensations, leading to preoccupation about and fear of having a serious disease. The fear becomes disabling and persists despite appropriate reassurance that no organic pathology can be detected. Symptoms may be minimal or absent, but the individual is highly anxious about and suspicious of the presence of an undiagnosed, serious medical illness (APA, 2013).

Individuals with illness anxiety disorder are extremely conscious of bodily sensations and changes and may become convinced that a rapid heart rate indicates they have heart disease or that a small sore is skin cancer. They are profoundly preoccupied with their bodies and are totally aware of even the slightest change in feeling or sensation. The response to these small changes, however, is usually unrealistic and exaggerated.

Some individuals with illness anxiety disorder have a long history of "doctor shopping" and are convinced that they are not receiving the proper care. Others avoid seeking medical assistance because to do so would increase their anxiety to intolerable levels. Depression is common, and obsessive-compulsive traits frequently accompany the disorder. Preoccupation with the fear of serious disease may interfere with social or occupational functioning. Some individuals are able to function appropriately on the job, however, while limiting their physical complaints to non-work time.

Individuals with illness anxiety disorder are so apprehensive and fearful that they become alarmed at the slightest intimation of serious illness. Even reading about a disease or hearing that someone they know has been diagnosed with an illness precipitates alarm. Both somatic symptom disorder and illness anxiety disorder have similar features to what was previously called hypochondriasis, but the *DSM-5* identifies two separate disorders to distinguish between individuals who are primarily preoccupied with perceived

---

BOX 29–1 Diagnostic Criteria for Somatic Symptom Disorder

A. One or more somatic symptoms that are distressing or result in significant disruption in daily life.

B. Excessive thoughts, feelings, or behaviors related to the somatic symptoms or associated health concerns as manifested by at least one of the following:
   1. Disproportionate and persistent thoughts about the seriousness of one's symptoms.
   2. Persistently high level of anxiety about health or symptoms.
   3. Excessive time and energy devoted to these symptoms or health concerns.

C. Although any one symptom may not be continuously present, the state of being symptomatic is persistent (typically more than 6 months).

Specify if:

With predominant pain (the somatic symptoms predominantly involve pain)

Persistent (a persistent course is characterized by severe symptoms, marked impairment, and long duration [more than 6 months])

Specify current severity:

Mild (only one of the symptoms specified in Criterion B is fulfilled)

Moderate (two or more of the symptoms specified in Criterion B are fulfilled)

Severe (two or more of the symptoms specified in Criterion B are fulfilled, plus there are multiple somatic complaints [or one very severe somatic symptom])

physical symptoms (somatic symptom disorder) and those who are primarily focused on fear of illness in general (illness anxiety disorder).

The *DSM-5* diagnostic criteria for illness anxiety disorder are presented in Box 29–2.

Conversion Disorder (Functional Neurological Symptom Disorder)

Conversion disorder is a loss of or change in body function that cannot be explained by any known medical disorder or pathophysiological mechanism. There is likely a psychological component involved in the initiation, exacerbation, or perpetuation of the symptom, although it may or may not be identifiable.

Conversion symptoms affect voluntary motor or sensory functioning suggestive of neurological disease. Examples include paralysis, **aphonia** (inability to produce voice), seizures, coordination disturbance, difficulty swallowing, urinary retention, akinesia, blindness, deafness, double vision, **anosmia** (inability to perceive smell), loss of pain sensation, and hallucinations. Abnormal limb shaking with impaired or loss of consciousness that resembles epileptic seizures is another type of conversion disorder symptom, referred to as *psychogenic* or *nonepileptic seizures.* **Pseudocyesis** (false pregnancy) is a conversion symptom and may represent a strong desire to be pregnant.

The *DSM-5* clarifies that "although the diagnosis [of conversion disorder] requires that the symptom is not explained by neurological disease, it should not be made simply because results from investigations are normal or because the symptom is 'bizarre.' There must be clear evidence of incompatibility with neurological disease" (APA, 2013, p. 319). For example, if a client appears to be having a seizure but the EEG is normal, the eyes are closed and resist opening, and there is no urinary incontinence, conversion disorder may be diagnosed. Multiple causes likely play a role in etiology.

While not diagnostic of a conversion disorder, some clients display an apparent indifference to symptoms that seem very serious to others. This feature is coined *la belle indifference* (Sadock et al., 2015). Most symptoms of conversion disorder resolve within a few weeks. About 20 percent of individuals with the diagnosis have a relapse within 1 year. The *DSM-5* states the prognosis is better when the symptoms are of short duration, when the client accepts the diagnosis, when there is absence of comorbid physical disease, and when there are no identified maladaptive personality traits (APA, 2013). The *DSM-5* diagnostic criteria for conversion disorder are presented in Box 29–3.

Psychological Factors Affecting Other Medical Conditions

Psychological factors play a role in virtually all medical conditions. However, in this disorder, it is evident that psychological or behavioral factors are clearly implicated in the development, exacerbation, or delayed recovery from a medical condition.

The *DSM-5* diagnostic criteria for psychological factors affecting other medical conditions are presented in Box 29–4.

Factitious Disorder

Factitious disorders involve conscious, intentional feigning of physical or psychological symptoms (Black & Andreasen, 2014). Individuals with factitious disorder pretend to be ill in order to receive emotional care

---

BOX 29–2 **Diagnostic Criteria for Illness Anxiety Disorder**

A. Preoccupation with having or acquiring a serious illness.

B. Somatic symptoms are not present or, if present, are only mild in intensity. If another medical condition is present or there is a high risk for developing a medical condition (e.g., strong family history is present), the preoccupation is clearly excessive or disproportionate.

C. There is a high level of anxiety about health, and the individual is easily alarmed about personal health status.

D. The individual performs excessive health-related behaviors (e.g., repeatedly checks his or her body for signs of illness) or exhibits maladaptive avoidance (e.g., avoids doctors' appointments and hospitals).

E. Illness preoccupation has been present for at least 6 months, but the specific illness that is feared may change over that period of time.

F. The illness-related preoccupation is not better explained by another mental disorder, such as somatic symptom disorder, panic disorder, generalized anxiety disorder, body dysmorphic disorder, obsessive-compulsive disorder, or delusional disorder, somatic type.

Specify whether:

Care-seeking type: Medical care, including physician visits or undergoing tests and procedures, is frequently used.

Care-avoidant type: Medical care is rarely used.

Reprinted with permission from the Diagnostic and Statistical Manual of Mental Disorders, Fifth Edition *(Copyright 2013). American Psychiatric Association.*

BOX 29–3 **Diagnostic Criteria for Conversion Disorder (Functional Neurological Symptom Disorder)**

A. One or more symptoms of altered voluntary motor or sensory function.
B. Clinical findings provide evidence of incompatibility between the symptom and recognized neurological or medical conditions.
C. The symptom or deficit is not better explained by another medical or mental disorder.
D. The symptom or deficit causes clinically significant distress or impairment in social, occupational, or other important areas of functioning or warrants medical evaluation.

Specify symptom type:

With weakness or paralysis
With abnormal movement
With swallowing symptoms
With speech symptom
With attacks or seizures
With anesthesia or sensory loss
With special sensory symptom
With mixed symptoms

Specify if:

Acute episode
Persistent

Specify if:

With psychological stressor
Without psychological stressor

Reprinted with permission from the Diagnostic and Statistical Manual of Mental Disorders, Fifth Edition *(Copyright 2013). American Psychiatric Association.*

BOX 29–4 **Diagnostic Criteria for Psychological Factors Affecting Other Medical Conditions**

A. A medical symptom or condition (other than a mental disorder) is present.
B. Psychological or behavioral factors adversely affect the general medical condition in one of the following ways:
   1. The factors have influenced the course of the medical condition as shown by a close temporal association between the psychological factors and the development or exacerbation of, or delayed recovery from, the medical condition.
   2. The factors interfere with the treatment of the medical condition (e.g., poor adherence).
   3. The factors constitute additional well-established health risks for the individual.
   4. The factors influence the underlying pathophysiology, precipitating or exacerbating symptoms or necessitating medical attention.
C. The psychological and behavioral factors in Criterion B are not better explained by another mental disorder (e.g., panic disorder, major depressive disorder, posttraumatic stress disorder).

Specify current severity:

Mild: Increases medical risk
Moderate: Aggravates underlying medical condition
Severe: Results in medical hospitalization or emergency room visit
Extreme: Results in severe, life-threatening risk

Reprinted with permission from the Diagnostic and Statistical Manual of Mental Disorders, Fifth Edition *(Copyright 2013). American Psychiatric Association.*

---

and support commonly associated with the role of "patient." Even though the behaviors are deliberate and intentional, there may be an associated compulsive element that diminishes personal control. Individuals with this disorder characteristically become skilled at presenting their "symptoms" so well that they successfully gain admission to hospitals and treatment centers. To accomplish this, they may aggravate existing symptoms, induce new ones, or even inflict painful injuries on themselves (Sadock et al., 2015). The disorder has also been identified as *Munchausen syndrome*, and symptoms may be psychological, physical, or a combination of both.

The disorder may be imposed on oneself or on another person (previously called *factitious disorder by proxy*). In the latter case, physical symptoms are intentionally imposed on a person under the care of the perpetrator. Diagnosis of factitious disorder can be difficult, as individuals become very inventive in their quest to produce symptoms. "The most common case of factitious disorder by proxy involves a mother who deceives medical personnel into believing her child is ill" (Sadock et al., 2015, p. 492). This may be accomplished by lying about the child's medical history, manipulating data such as by contaminating laboratory samples, and inducing illness or injury in their child through use of substances or other physical assaults.

The *DSM-5* diagnostic criteria for factitious disorder are presented in Box 29–5.

Predisposing Factors Associated With Somatic Symptom and Related Disorders

Genetic

Studies have shown an increased incidence of somatic symptom disorder, conversion disorder, and illness anxiety disorder in first-degree relatives, implying a possible inheritable predisposition. In somatic symptom disorder, there is evidence of genetic overlap with some other mental disorders, including eating disorders (Soares & Grossman, 2012; Yates, 2014; Yutzy & Parish, 2008).

Biochemical

Studies have indicated that tryptophan catabolism may be abnormal in clients with somatic symptom disorders (Yate, 2014). Decreased levels of serotonin and endorphins may play a role in the sensation of pain.

Neuroanatomical

Brain dysfunction has been proposed by some researchers as a factor in factitious disorders (Sadock et al., 2015). The hypothesis is that impairment in information processing contributes to the aberrant behaviors associated with the disorder. Sadock and associates report that brain imaging studies have found hypometabolism in the dominant hemisphere, hypermetabolism in the nondominant hemisphere, and impaired hemispheric communication in conversion disorders (p. 474). Other reports of brain imaging studies have identified reduced volume of the amygdala as well as reduced connectivity between the amygdala and brain centers controlling executive and motor functions in one or more somatic symptom disorders (Yates, 2014).

Psychodynamic

Some psychodynamicists view illness anxiety disorder as an ego defense mechanism. Physical complaints are the expression of low self-esteem and feelings of worthlessness, because it is easier to feel something is

---

BOX 29–5 Diagnostic Criteria for Factitious Disorder

FACTITIOUS DISORDER IMPOSED ON SELF

A. Falsification of physical or psychological signs or symptoms, or induction of injury or disease, associated with identified deception.

B. The individual presents himself or herself to others as ill, impaired, or injured.

C. The deceptive behavior is evident even in the absence of obvious external rewards.

D. The behavior is not better explained by another mental disorder, such as delusional disorder or other psychotic disorder.

Specify:

Single episode

Recurrent episodes

FACTITIOUS DISORDER IMPOSED ON ANOTHER (PREVIOUSLY FACTITIOUS DISORDER BY PROXY)

A. Falsification of physical or psychological signs or symptoms, or induction of injury or disease in another, associated with identified deception.

B. The individual presents another individual (victim) to others as ill, impaired, or injured.

C. The deceptive behavior is evident even in the absence of obvious external rewards.

D. The behavior is not better explained by another mental disorder, such as delusional disorder or other psychotic disorder.

Note: The perpetrator, not the victim, receives this diagnosis.
Specify:

Single episode

Recurrent episodes

Reprinted with permission from the Diagnostic and Statistical Manual of Mental Disorders, Fifth Edition *(Copyright 2013). American Psychiatric Association.*

wrong with the body than to feel something is wrong with the self. Another psychodynamic view of illness anxiety disorder (as well as somatic symptom disorder, predominantly pain) is related to a defense against guilt. The individual views the self as "bad," based on real or imagined past misconduct, and considers physical suffering the deserved punishment required for atonement. This view has also been related to individuals with factitious disorders.

The psychodynamic theory of conversion disorder proposes that emotions associated with a traumatic event that the individual cannot express because of moral or ethical unacceptability are "converted" into physical symptoms. The unacceptable emotions are repressed and converted to a somatic symptom that is symbolic in some way of the original emotional trauma.

Some reports suggest that individuals with factitious disorders were victims of child abuse or neglect. Frequent childhood hospitalizations provided a reprieve from the traumatic home situation and a loving and caring environment that was absent in the child's family. This theory proposes that the individual with factitious disorder is attempting to recapture the only positive support he or she may have known by seeking out the environment in which it was received as a child. Regarding factitious disorder imposed on another, Sadock and associates (2015) have stated, "One apparent purpose of the behavior is for the caretaker to indirectly assume the sick role; another is to be relieved of the caretaking role by having the child hospitalized" (p. 492).

Family Dynamics

Some families have difficulty expressing emotions openly and resolving conflicts verbally. When this occurs, the child may become ill, and a shift in focus is made from the open conflict to the child's illness, leaving unresolved the underlying issues that the family cannot confront openly. Thus, **somatization** in the child brings some stability to the family as harmony replaces discord and the child's welfare becomes the common concern. The child in turn receives positive reinforcement for the illness. This shift in focus from family discord to concern for the child is sometimes called **tertiary gain.**

Learning Theory

Somatic complaints are often reinforced when the sick role relieves the individual from the need to deal with a stressful situation, whether it be within society or within the family. The sick person learns that he or she may avoid stressful obligations; may postpone unwelcome challenges; is excused from troublesome duties **(primary gain);** becomes the prominent focus of attention because of the illness **(secondary gain);** or relieves conflict within the family as concern is shifted to the ill person and away from the real issue **(tertiary gain).** These types of positive reinforcements virtually guarantee repetition of the response.

Past experience with serious or life-threatening physical illness, either personal or that of close family members, can predispose an individual to illness anxiety disorder. Once an individual has experienced a threat to biological integrity, he or she may develop a fear of recurrence. This generates an exaggerated response to minor physical changes, leading to excessive anxiety and health concerns.

Transactional Model of Stress and Adaptation

The etiology of somatic symptom disorders is most likely influenced by multiple factors. In Figure 29–1, a graphic depiction of this theory of multiple causation is presented in the transactional model of stress and adaptation.

Background Assessment Data: Types of Dissociative Disorders

Dissociative Amnesia

> # CORE CONCEPT
> **Amnesia**
> Partial or total, permanent or transient loss of memory. The term is often applied to episodes during which patients forget recent events (although they may conduct themselves appropriately) and after which no memory of the period persists. Such episodes may be caused by strokes, seizures, trauma, senility, alcoholism, or intoxication (Venes, 2014).

Dissociative amnesia is an inability to recall important personal information, usually of a traumatic or stressful nature, that is too extensive to be explained by ordinary forgetfulness and is not due to the direct effects of substance use or a neurological or other medical condition (APA, 2013). The *DSM-5* states that the most common types of dissociative amnesia are localized, selective, and generalized. Localized and selective amnesia are related to a specific stressful event. For example, the individual with **localized amnesia** is unable to recall all incidents associated with a stressful period. It may be broader than just a single event, such as the inability to remember months or years of child abuse (APA, 2013). In **selective amnesia,** the individual can recall only certain incidents associated with a stressful event for a specific period after the event. In **generalized amnesia,** the individual has amnesia for his or her identity and total life history.

The individual with amnesia usually appears alert and may give no indication to observers that anything is wrong, although some clients may present

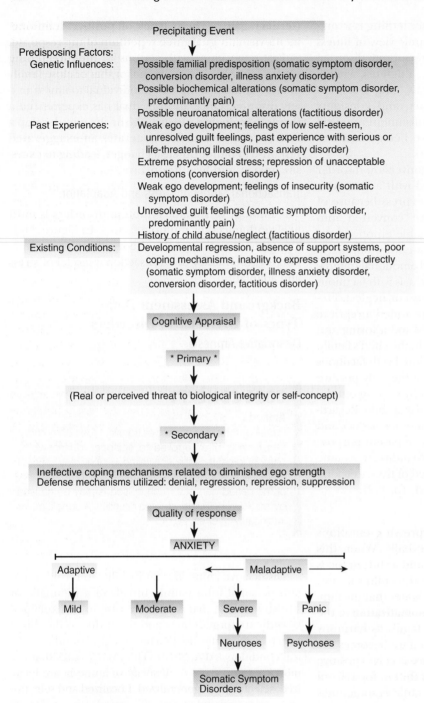

Precipitating Event

Predisposing Factors:
Genetic Influences: Possible familial predisposition (somatic symptom disorder, conversion disorder, illness anxiety disorder)
Possible biochemical alterations (somatic symptom disorder, predominantly pain)
Possible neuroanatomical alterations (factitious disorder)

Past Experiences: Weak ego development; feelings of low self-esteem, unresolved guilt feelings, past experience with serious or life-threatening illness (illness anxiety disorder)
Extreme psychosocial stress; repression of unacceptable emotions (conversion disorder)
Weak ego development; feelings of insecurity (somatic symptom disorder)
Unresolved guilt feelings (somatic symptom disorder, predominantly pain)
History of child abuse/neglect (factitious disorder)

Existing Conditions: Developmental regression, absence of support systems, poor coping mechanisms, inability to express emotions directly (somatic symptom disorder, illness anxiety disorder, conversion disorder, factitious disorder)

Cognitive Appraisal

* Primary *

(Real or perceived threat to biological integrity or self-concept)

* Secondary *

Ineffective coping mechanisms related to diminished ego strength
Defense mechanisms utilized: denial, regression, repression, suppression

Quality of response

ANXIETY

Adaptive   Maladaptive

Mild   Moderate   Severe   Panic

Neuroses   Psychoses

Somatic Symptom Disorders

FIGURE 29–1 The dynamics of somatic symptom disorders using the transactional model of stress and adaptation.

with alterations in consciousness, with conversion symptoms, or in trance states. Clients suffering from amnesia are often brought to general hospital emergency departments by police who have found them wandering confusedly around the streets.

Onset of an amnestic episode usually follows severe psychosocial stress. Termination is typically abrupt and followed by complete recovery. Recurrences are unusual. A specific subtype of dissociative amnesia is *with dissociative fugue.* Dissociative **fugue** is characterized by a sudden, unexpected travel away from customary places or by bewildered wandering, with the inability to recall some or all of one's past. An individual in a fugue state may not be able to recall personal identity and sometimes assumes a new identity (Black & Andreasen, 2014).

The *DSM-5* diagnostic criteria for dissociative amnesia are presented in Box 29–6.

BOX 29–6 **Diagnostic Criteria for Dissociative Amnesia**

A. An inability to recall important autobiographical information, usually of a traumatic or stressful nature, that is inconsistent with ordinary forgetting. *Note*: Dissociative amnesia most often consists of localized or selective amnesia for a specific event or events; or generalized amnesia for identity and life history.

B. The symptoms cause clinically significant distress or impairment in social, occupational, or other important areas of functioning.

C. The disturbance is not attributable to the physiological effects of a substance (e.g., alcohol or other drug of abuse, a medication) or a neurological or other medical condition (e.g., partial complex seizures, transient global amnesia, sequelae of a closed head injury/traumatic brain injury, other neurological condition).

D. The disturbance is not better explained by dissociative identity disorder, posttraumatic stress disorder, acute stress disorder, somatic symptom disorder, or major or mild neurocognitive disorder.

Specify if:

With dissociative fugue (apparently purposeful travel or bewildered wandering that is associated with amnesia for identity or for other important autobiographical information)

Reprinted with permission from the Diagnostic and Statistical Manual of Mental Disorders, Fifth Edition (Copyright 2013). American Psychiatric Association.

Dissociative Identity Disorder

Dissociative identity disorder (DID) was formerly called multiple personality disorder and is characterized by the existence of two or more personality states in a single individual. These different personality states are sometimes referred to as *alter identities* or just *alters*. Only one of the personalities is evident at any given moment, and one of them is dominant most of the time over the course of the disorder. Each personality is unique and composed of a complex set of memories, behavior patterns, and social relationships that surface at different times. Transition from one personality state to another may be sudden or gradual and is sometimes quite dramatic. Sadock and associates (2015) state, "Patients often describe a profound sense of concretized internal division or personified internal conflicts between parts of themselves . . . these parts may have proper names or be designated by their predominant affect or function, for example, 'the angry one' or 'the wife'" (p. 460).

DID has been a controversial disorder since it gained attention after the 1976 movie *Sybil*, which portrayed the presumed true story of a woman who reported having 16 different personalities. Diagnosis of this disorder increased significantly in the years following the movie, and in 1980 the APA formally recognized the disorder as a psychiatric illness (Haberman, 2014). Since then, critics have reported that both the patient "Sybil" and her psychiatrist acknowledged her case as fabrication. Dr. David Speigel, a psychiatrist who was involved in promoting the American Psychiatric Association's adoption of DID as the preferred term for this condition, is quoted in Haberman's review (2014) as saying "[the term] multiple personality carries with it the implication that they really have more than one personality. The problem is fragmentation of identity, not that you really are 12 people . . . that you have not more than one but less than one personality."

Although questions persist about whether this disorder has been overdiagnosed, there are certainly individuals who present with fragmented identity. Most have been victims of severe childhood physical and sexual abuse. It is not uncommon for clients with DID to also manifest with symptoms of other dissociative disorders such as amnesia, fugue states, depersonalization, and derealization (Sadock et al., 2015). Generally, there is amnesia for the events that took place when another personality was being manifested, and clients report "gaps" in autobiographical histories, "lost time" or "blackouts." They may "wake up" in unfamiliar situations with no idea where they are, how they got there, or the identities of the people around them. They may be accused of lying when they deny remembering or being responsible for events or actions.

Dissociative identity disorder is not always incapacitating. Some individuals with DID maintain responsible positions, complete graduate degrees, and are successful spouses and parents before diagnosis and while in treatment. Before they are diagnosed with DID, many individuals are misdiagnosed with depression, borderline and antisocial personality disorders, schizophrenia, epilepsy, or bipolar disorder. The *DSM-5* diagnostic criteria for DID are presented in Box 29–7.

Depersonalization-Derealization Disorder

Depersonalization-derealization disorder is characterized by a temporary change in the quality of self-awareness, which often takes the form of feelings of unreality, changes in body image, feelings of detachment from the environment, or a sense of observing oneself from outside the body. For example, a soldier in recalling an experience in combat describes observing himself from a distance and wondering what he would do if *he* were in that situation. **Depersonalization** (a disturbance in the perception of oneself) is differentiated from **derealization,** which describes an alteration in the perception of the external environment. Both of

BOX 29–7 Diagnostic Criteria for Dissociative Identity Disorder

A. Disruption of identity characterized by two or more distinct personality states, which may be described in some cultures as an experience of possession. The disruption in identity involves marked discontinuity in sense of self and sense of agency, accompanied by related alterations in affect, behavior, consciousness, memory, perception, cognition, and/or sensory-motor functioning. These signs and symptoms may be observed by others or reported by the individual.

B. Recurrent gaps in the recall of everyday events, important personal information, and/or traumatic events that are inconsistent with ordinary forgetting.

C. The symptoms cause clinically significant distress or impairment in social, occupational, or other important areas of functioning.

D. The disturbance is not a normal part of a broadly accepted cultural or religious practice. *Note*: In children, the symptoms are not better explained by imaginary playmates or other fantasy play.

E. The symptoms are not attributable to the physiological effects of a substance (e.g., blackouts or chaotic behavior during alcohol intoxication) or another medical condition (e.g., complex partial seizures).

Reprinted with permission from the Diagnostic and Statistical Manual of Mental Disorders, Fifth Edition *(Copyright 2013). American Psychiatric Association.*

these phenomena also occur in a variety of psychiatric illnesses such as schizophrenia, depression, anxiety states, and neurocognitive disorders. As previously stated, the symptoms of depersonalization and derealization are very common. It is estimated that approximately half of all adults have experienced transient episodes of these symptoms, identified as the third-most

commonly reported psychiatric symptoms after depression and anxiety (Sadock et al., 2015, p. 454). Diagnosis of the disorder is made only if the symptoms cause significant distress or impairment in functioning.

The *DSM-5* describes this disorder as persistent or recurrent episodes of depersonalization, derealization, or both (APA, 2013). There may be a mechanical or dreamlike feeling or a belief that the body's physical characteristics have changed. If derealization is present, objects in the environment are perceived as altered in size or shape. Other people in the environment may seem automated or mechanical.

These distorted perceptions are experienced as disturbing and often accompanied by anxiety, depression, fear of going insane, obsessive thoughts, somatic complaints, and an alteration in the subjective sense of time. The age of onset is typically late adolescence or early adulthood, and it is two to four times more common in women than in men (Sadock et al., 2015).

The *DSM-5* diagnostic criteria for depersonalization-derealization disorder are presented in Box 29–8.

Predisposing Factors Associated With Dissociative Disorders

Genetics

The overwhelming majority of adults with DID (85% to 97%) have a history of physical and sexual abuse. Although genetic factors are being studied, preliminary research does not show evidence of significant genetic contribution (Sadock et al., 2015, p. 458).

Neurobiological

Some clinicians have suggested a possible correlation between neurological alterations and dissociative disorders. Although available information is inadequate, dissociative amnesia may be related to neurophysiological

BOX 29–8 Diagnostic Criteria for Depersonalization-Derealization Disorder

A. The presence of persistent or recurrent depersonalization, derealization, or both:
1. **Depersonalization:** Experiences of unreality, detachment, or being an outside observer with respect to one's thoughts, feelings, sensations, body, or actions (e.g., perceptual alterations, distorted sense of time, unreal or absent self, emotional and/or physical numbing).
2. **Derealization:** Experiences of unreality or detachment with respect to surroundings (e.g., individuals or objects are experienced as unreal, dreamlike, foggy, lifeless, or visually distorted).
B. During the depersonalization or derealization experiences, reality testing remains intact.
C. The symptoms cause clinically significant distress or impairment in social, occupational, or other important areas of functioning.
D. The disturbance is not attributable to the physiological effects of a substance (e.g., a drug of abuse, medication) or another medical condition (e.g., seizures).
E. The disturbance is not better explained by another mental disorder, such as schizophrenia, panic disorder, major depressive disorder, acute stress disorder, posttraumatic stress disorder, or another dissociative disorder.

Reprinted with permission from the Diagnostic and Statistical Manual of Mental Disorders, Fifth Edition *(Copyright 2013). American Psychiatric Association.*

dysfunction. Areas of the brain that have been associated with memory include the hippocampus, amygdala, fornix, mammillary bodies, thalamus, and frontal cortex.

Depersonalization has been evidenced with migraines and with marijuana use, responds to selective serotonin reuptake inhibitors (SSRIs), and is seen in cases where L-tryptophan, a serotonin precursor, is depleted. These facts suggest some level of serotonergic involvement in this dissociative symptom (Sadock et al., 2015). Some studies have suggested a possible link between DID and certain neurological conditions, such as temporal lobe epilepsy and severe migraine headaches. Electroencephalographic abnormalities have been observed in some clients with DID.

Psychodynamic Theory

Freud (1962) believed that dissociative behaviors occurred when individuals repressed distressing mental contents from conscious awareness. He believed that the unconscious was a dynamic entity in which repressed mental contents were stored and unavailable to conscious recall. Current psychodynamic explanations of dissociation are based on Freud's concepts. The repression of mental contents is believed to protect the client from extreme emotional pain triggered by either disturbing external circumstances or anxiety-provoking internal urges and feelings. In the case of depersonalization and derealization, the pain and anxiety are expressed as feelings of unreality or detachment from the environment of the painful situation.

Psychological Trauma

A growing body of evidence points to the etiology of dissociative disorders as a response to traumatic experiences that overwhelm the individual's capacity to cope by any means other than dissociation. In DID, these experiences are most often physical, sexual, or psychological abuse by a parent or significant other in the child's life. The most widely accepted explanation for DID is that it begins as a survival strategy to help children cope with horrifying sexual, physical, or psychological abuse and evolves into a fragmented identity as the victim struggles to integrate conflicting aspects of personality into a cohesive whole. Dissociative amnesia is frequently related to acute and extreme trauma but may also develop in the clinical presentation of DID or in response to combat trauma during wartime.

Transactional Model of Stress and Adaptation

The etiology of dissociative disorders is likely influenced by multiple factors. In Figure 29–2, a graphic depiction of this theory of multiple causation is presented in the transactional model of stress and adaptation.

Diagnosis and Outcome Identification

Nursing diagnoses are formulated from the data gathered during the assessment phase and with background knowledge regarding predisposing factors to the disorder. Table 29–1 presents a list of client behaviors and the NANDA nursing diagnoses that correspond to those behaviors, which may be used in planning care for clients with somatic symptom and dissociative disorders.

Outcome Criteria

The following criteria may be used for measurement of outcomes in the care of the client with somatic symptom and dissociative disorders.

The client:

- Effectively uses adaptive coping strategies during stressful situations without resorting to physical symptoms (*somatic symptom disorder*)
- Interprets bodily sensations rationally, verbalizes understanding of the significance of the irrational fear, and has decreased the number and frequency of physical complaints (*illness anxiety disorder and somatic symptom disorder*)
- Is free of physical disability and is able to verbalize understanding of the possible correlation between the loss of or alteration in function and extreme emotional stress (*conversion disorder*)
- Can recall events associated with a traumatic or stressful situation (*dissociative amnesia*)
- Can verbalize the extreme anxiety that precipitated the dissociation (*depersonalization-derealization disorder*)
- Can demonstrate more adaptive coping strategies to avert dissociative behaviors in the face of severe anxiety (*depersonalization-derealization disorder*)
- Verbalizes understanding of the existence of multiple personality states and the purposes they serve (*dissociative identity disorder*)
- Is able to maintain a sense of reality during stressful situations (*depersonalization-derealization disorder*)

Planning and Implementation

The following section presents a group of selected nursing diagnoses, with short- and long-term goals and nursing interventions for each.

Ineffective Coping

Ineffective coping is defined as the "inability to form a valid appraisal of the stressors, inadequate choices of practiced responses, and/or inability to use available resources" (Herdman & Kamitsuru, 2014, p. 326). This nursing diagnosis may be relevant to any somatic symptom and related disorders as well as to clients with dissociative disorders.

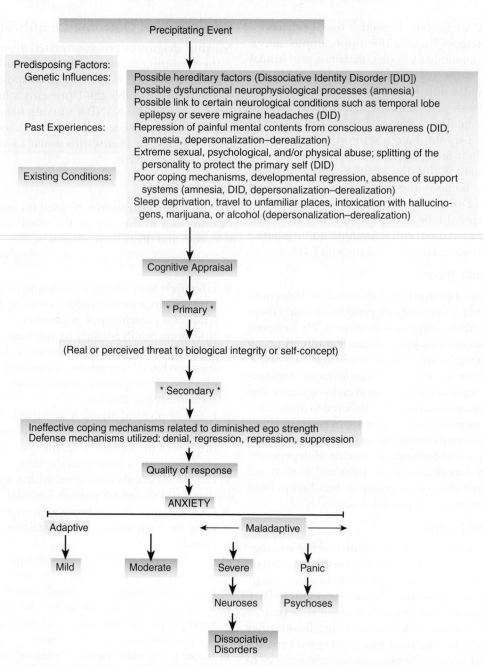

FIGURE 29–2 The dynamics of dissociative disorders using the transactional model of stress and adaptation.

Client Goals

Outcome criteria include short- and long-term goals. Time lines are individually determined.

Short-term goal

■ Within (specified time), client will verbalize understanding of correlation between physical symptoms and psychological problems.

Long-term goal

■ By time of discharge from treatment, client will demonstrate ability to cope with stress by means other than preoccupation with physical symptoms.

Interventions

■ Monitor the physician's ongoing assessments, laboratory reports, and other data to maintain assurance that the possibility of organic pathology is clearly ruled out. Review findings with the client. Accurate medical assessment is vital for the provision of adequate and appropriate care. Honest explanation may help the client understand the psychological implications.

■ Recognize and accept that the physical complaint is real to the client even though no organic etiology can be identified. Denial of the client's feelings is

TABLE 2–2 Assigning Nursing Diagnoses to Behaviors Commonly Associated With Somatic Symptom and Dissociative Disorders

BEHAVIORS	NURSING DIAGNOSES
Verbalization of numerous physical complaints in the absence of any pathophysiological evidence; focus on the self and physical symptoms *(somatic symptom disorder)*	Ineffective coping; chronic pain
History of "doctor shopping" for evidence of organic pathology to substantiate physical symptoms; statements such as, "I don't know why the doctor put me on the psychiatric unit. I have a physical problem" *(somatic symptom disorder)*	Deficient knowledge (psychological causes for physical symptoms)
Preoccupation with and unrealistic interpretation of bodily signs and sensations *(illness anxiety disorder)*	Fear (of having a serious disease)
Loss or alteration in physical functioning without evidence of organic pathology *(conversion disorder)* Alteration in the perception or experience of the self or the environment *(depersonalization-derealization disorder)*	Disturbed sensory perception*
Need for assistance to carry out self-care activities such as eating, dressing, maintaining hygiene, and toileting due to alteration in physical functioning *(conversion disorder)*	Self-care deficit
History of numerous exacerbations of physical illness; inappropriate or exaggerated behaviors; denial of emotional problems *(psychological factors affecting other medical conditions)*	Deficient knowledge (psychological factors affecting medical condition); Ineffective denial
Loss of memory *(dissociative amnesia)*	Impaired memory
Verbalizations of frustration over lack of control and dependence on others *(dissociative amnesia)*	Powerlessness
Unresolved grief; depression; self-blame associated with childhood abuse *(dissociative identity disorder [DID])*	Risk for suicide
Presence of more than one personality within the individual *(DID)*	Disturbed personality identity
Feigning of physical or psychological symptoms to gain attention *(factitious disorder)*	Ineffective coping

*This diagnosis has been resigned from the NANDA-I list of approved diagnoses. It is used in this instance because it is most compatible with the identified behaviors.

nontherapeutic and interferes with establishment of a trusting relationship.

■ Provide pain medication as prescribed by physician. Client comfort and safety are nursing priorities.

■ Identify gains that the physical symptoms are providing for the client: increased dependency, attention, and distraction from other problems. Identification of underlying motivation is important in assisting the client with problem resolution.

■ Initially, fulfill the client's most urgent dependency needs, but gradually withdraw attention to physical symptoms. Minimize time given in response to physical complaints. Anxiety and maladaptive behaviors will increase if dependency needs are ignored initially. Gradual withdrawal of positive reinforcement will discourage repetition of maladaptive behaviors.

■ Explain to the client that any new physical complaints will be referred to the physician and give no further attention to them. Follow up on the physician's assessment of the complaint. The possibility

of organic pathology must always be considered. Failure to do so could jeopardize client safety.

■ Encourage the client to verbalize fears and anxieties. Explain that attention will be withdrawn if rumination about physical complaints begins and follow through. Without consistency of limit setting, change will not occur.

■ Help the client recognize that physical symptoms often occur because of, or are exacerbated by, specific stressors. Discuss alternative coping strategies that client may use in response to stress (e.g., relaxation exercises, physical activities, assertiveness skills). The client may need help with problem-solving. Give positive reinforcement for adaptive coping strategies.

■ Have the client keep a diary of appearance, duration, and intensity of physical symptoms. A separate record of situations that the client finds especially stressful should also be kept. Comparison of these records may provide objective data from which to observe the relationship between physical symptoms and stress.

■ Help the client identify ways to achieve recognition from others without resorting to physical symptoms. Positive recognition from others enhances self-esteem and minimizes the need for attention through maladaptive behaviors.

■ Discuss how interpersonal relationships are affected by the client's narcissistic behavior. Explain how this behavior alienates others. The client may not realize how he or she is perceived by others.

■ Provide instruction in relaxation techniques and assertiveness skills. These approaches decrease anxiety and increase self-esteem, which facilitate adaptive responses to stressful situations.

Fear (of Having a Serious Disease)

Fear is defined as the "response to perceived threat that is consciously recognized as a danger" (Herdman & Kamitsuru, 2014, p. 336). This nursing diagnosis is particularly relevant to clients with illness anxiety disorder but may pertain also to clients with somatic symptom disorder and some dissociative disorders.

Client Goals

Outcome criteria include short- and long-term goals. Time lines are individually determined.

Short-term goal

■ Client will verbalize that fears associated with bodily sensations are irrational (within time limit deemed appropriate for specific individual).

Long-term goal

■ Client interprets bodily sensations correctly.

Interventions

■ Monitor the physician's ongoing assessments and laboratory reports. Organic pathology must be clearly ruled out.

■ Refer all new physical complaints to the physician. To ignore all physical complaints could place the client's safety in jeopardy.

■ Assess the function the client's illness is fulfilling for him or her (e.g., unfulfilled needs for dependency, nurturing, caring, attention, or control). This information may provide insight into reasons for maladaptive behavior and provide direction for planning client care.

■ Identify times during which the preoccupation with physical symptoms worsens. Determine the extent of correlation of physical complaints with times of increased anxiety. The client may be unaware of the psychosocial implications of the physical complaints. Knowledge of the relationship is the first step in the process for creating change.

■ Convey empathy. Let the client know that you understand how a specific symptom may conjure up fears of previous life-threatening illness. Unconditional acceptance and empathy promote a therapeutic nurse-client relationship.

■ Initially allow the client a limited amount of time (e.g., 10 minutes each hour) to discuss physical symptoms. Because preoccupation with physical symptoms has been his or her primary method of coping for so long, complete prohibition of this activity would likely raise the client's anxiety level significantly, further exacerbating the behavior.

■ Help the client determine what techniques may be most useful for him or her to implement when fear and anxiety are exacerbated (e.g., relaxation techniques, mental imagery, thought-stopping techniques, physical exercise). All of these techniques are effective in reducing anxiety and may assist the client in the transition from focusing on fear of physical illness to the discussion of honest feelings.

■ Gradually increase the limit on amount of time spent each hour in discussing physical symptoms. If the client violates the limits, withdraw attention. Lack of positive reinforcement may help to extinguish the maladaptive behavior.

■ Encourage the client to discuss feelings associated with fear of serious illness. Verbalization of feelings in a nonthreatening environment facilitates expression and resolution of disturbing emotional issues. When the client can express feelings directly, there is less need to express them through physical symptoms.

■ Role-play the client's plan for dealing with the fear the next time it assumes control and before anxiety becomes disabling. Anxiety and fears are minimized when the client has achieved a degree of comfort through practicing a plan for dealing with stressful situations in the future.

Disturbed Sensory Perception

Disturbed sensory perception, no longer identified as a NANDA-I diagnosis, is retained here and may be defined as an impaired or exaggerated sensory perception. This may include an exaggerated sensation of pain, impairment of function or mobility without medical basis, other somatic sensations, and distorted perception of the self (depersonalization) or distorted perception of the environment (derealization). The nursing diagnosis of disturbed sensory perception is relevant to clients with somatic symptom disorders, conversion disorder symptoms, and depersonalization derealization disorder. Table 29–2 presents this nursing diagnosis in care plan format.

Client Goals

Outcome criteria include short- and long-term goals. Time lines are individually determined.

Table 29–2 | CARE PLAN FOR THE CLIENT WITH CONVERSION DISORDER

NURSING DIAGNOSIS: DISTURBED SENSORY PERCEPTION

RELATED TO: Repressed severe anxiety

EVIDENCED BY: Loss or alteration in physical functioning, without evidence of organic pathology

OUTCOME CRITERIA	NURSING INTERVENTIONS	RATIONALE
Short-Term Goal • Client will verbalize understanding of emotional problems as a contributing factor to the alteration in physical functioning (within time limit appropriate for specific individual). **Long-Term Goal** • Client will demonstrate recovery of lost or altered function.	1. Monitor physician's ongoing assessments, laboratory reports, and other data to ensure that possibility of organic pathology is clearly ruled out.	1. Failure to do so may jeopardize client safety.
	2. Identify primary or secondary gains that the physical symptom may be providing for the client (e.g., increased dependency, attention, protection from experiencing a stressful event).	2. Primary and secondary gains are often etiological factors and may be used to assist in problem resolution.
	3. Do not focus on the disability, and encourage client to be as independent as possible. Intervene only when client requires assistance.	3. Positive reinforcement would encourage continual use of the maladaptive response for secondary gains, such as dependency.
	4. Maintain nonjudgmental attitude when providing assistance to the client. The physical symptom is not within the client's conscious control and is very real to him or her.	4. A judgmental attitude interferes with the nurse's ability to provide therapeutic care for the client.
	5. Do not reinforce the client's attempts to use the disability as a manipulative tool to avoid participation in therapeutic activities. Withdraw attention if client continues to focus on physical limitation.	5. Lack of reinforcement may help to extinguish the maladaptive response.
	6. Encourage the client to verbalize fears and anxieties. Help identify physical symptoms as a coping mechanism that is used in times of extreme stress.	6. Clients with conversion disorder are usually unaware of the psychological implications of their illness.
	7. Help client identify coping mechanisms that he or she could use when faced with stressful situations rather than retreating from reality with a physical disability.	7. Client needs assistance with problem-solving at this severe level of anxiety.
	8. Give positive reinforcement for identification or demonstration of alternative, more adaptive coping strategies.	8. Positive reinforcement enhances self-esteem and encourages repetition of desirable behaviors.

Short-term goal

■ The client will verbalize understanding of emotional problems as a contributing factor to the alteration in sensory perceptions (within time limit appropriate for specific individual).

Long-term goal

■ The client will demonstrate recovery of lost or altered function.

Interventions

■ Monitor the physician's ongoing assessments, laboratory reports, and other data to ensure that the possibility of organic pathology is clearly ruled out. Failure to do so may jeopardize the client's safety.

■ Identify primary or secondary gains that the physical symptom is providing for the client (e.g., increased dependency, attention, protection from experiencing a stressful event). These are considered to be etiological factors and may be used to assist in problem resolution.

■ Do not focus on the disability, and encourage the client to be as independent as possible. Intervene only when the client requires assistance. Positive reinforcement would encourage continued use of the maladaptive response for secondary gains, such as dependency.

■ Maintain a nonjudgmental attitude when providing assistance with self-care activities to the client. The physical symptom is not within the client's conscious control and is very real to him or her.

■ Do not reinforce the client's use of the disability as a manipulative tool to avoid participating in therapeutic activities. Withdraw attention if the client continues to focus on the physical limitation. Lack of reinforcement may help to extinguish the maladaptive response.

■ Encourage the client to verbalize fears and anxieties. Help identify physical symptoms as a coping mechanism that is used in times of extreme stress. Clients with conversion disorder are usually unaware of the psychological implications of their illness.

■ Help the client identify coping mechanisms that he or she could use when faced with stressful situations rather than retreating from reality with a physical disability. The client needs assistance with problem-solving at this severe level of anxiety.

■ Give positive reinforcement for identification or demonstration of alternative, more adaptive coping strategies.

■ Discuss ways the client may more adaptively respond to stress, and use role-play to practice using these new methods. Having practiced through role-play helps to prepare the client to face stressful situations by using these new behaviors when they occur in real life.

For clients experiencing depersonalization, also use the following interventions:

■ Provide support and encouragement during times of depersonalization. Clients manifesting these symptoms may express fear and anxiety. They do not understand the response and may express a fear of going insane. Support and encouragement from a trusted individual provide a feeling of security when fears and anxieties are manifested.

■ Explain the depersonalization behaviors and the purpose they usually serve for the client. This knowledge may help to minimize fears and anxieties associated with their occurrence. Help relate these behaviors to times of severe psychological stress that client has experienced. The client may be unaware that the occurrence of depersonalization behaviors is related to severe anxiety. Knowledge of this relationship is the first step in the process of behavioral change.

Deficient Knowledge (Psychological Factors Affecting Medical Condition)

Deficient knowledge is defined as "absence or deficiency of cognitive information related to a specific topic" (Herdman & Kamitsuru, 2014, p. 257). This nursing diagnosis may be relevant to clients with any somatic or related disorder as well as to clients with dissociative disorders.

Client Goals

■ Outcome criteria include short- and long-term goals. Time lines are individually determined.

Short-term goal

■ Client will cooperate with plan for teaching provided by primary nurse.

Long-term goal

■ By time of discharge from treatment, client will be able to verbalize psychological factors affecting his or her physical condition.

Interventions

■ Assess the client's level of knowledge regarding effects of psychological problems on the body. An adequate database is necessary for the development of an effective teaching plan.

■ Assess the client's level of anxiety and readiness to learn. Learning does not occur beyond the moderate level of anxiety.

■ Discuss physical examinations and laboratory tests that have been conducted. Explain the purpose and results of each. Fear of the unknown may contribute to an elevated level of anxiety. The client has the right to know about and accept or refuse any medical treatment.

■ Explore the client's feelings and fears as he or she demonstrates readiness. Go slowly. These feelings may have been suppressed or repressed for so long that their disclosure may be a very painful experience. Be supportive. Expression of feelings in the presence of a trusted individual and in a nonthreatening environment may encourage the individual to confront unresolved issues.

■ Have the client keep a diary of appearance, duration, and intensity of physical symptoms. A separate record of situations the client finds especially stressful should also be kept. Comparison of these records may provide objective data from which to observe the relationship between physical symptoms and stress.

■ Help the client identify needs that are being met through the sick role. Together, formulate more adaptive means for fulfilling these needs. Practice by role-playing. Repetition through practice serves to reduce discomfort in the actual situation.

■ Provide instruction in assertiveness techniques, especially the ability to recognize the differences among passive, assertive, and aggressive behaviors and the importance of respecting the rights of others while protecting one's own basic rights. These skills will preserve the client's self-esteem while also improving his or her ability to form satisfactory interpersonal relationships.

■ Discuss adaptive methods of stress management, such as relaxation techniques, physical exercise, meditation, and breathing exercises. Use of these adaptive techniques may decrease appearance of physical symptoms in response to stress.

Impaired Memory

Impaired memory is defined as an "inability to remember or recall bits of information or behavioral skills" (Herdman & Kamitsuru, 2014, p. 259). This nursing diagnosis is particularly relevant in clients with dissociative disorders such as dissociative amnesia.

Client Goals

Outcome criteria include short- and long-term goals. Time lines are individually determined.

Short-term goal

■ The client will verbalize understanding that the loss of memory is related to a stressful situation and begin discussing the stressful situation with nurse or therapist.

Long-term goal

■ The client will recover deficits in memory and develop more adaptive coping mechanisms to deal with stressful situations.

Interventions

■ Obtain as much information as possible about the client from family and significant others if possible. Consider likes, dislikes, important people, activities, music, and pets. A comprehensive baseline assessment is necessary for the development of an effective plan of care.

■ Do not confront the client with information he or she does not appear to remember. Individuals who are exposed to painful information from which the amnesia is providing protection may decompensate even further into a psychotic state.

■ Instead, expose the client to stimuli that represent pleasant experiences from the past, such as smells associated with enjoyable activities, beloved pets, and music the client enjoys. As memory begins to return, engage the client in activities that may provide additional stimulation. Recall often occurs during activities that simulate life experiences.

■ Listen empathically when the client discusses situations that have been especially stressful and explore the feelings associated with those times. Verbalization of feelings in a nonthreatening environment may help the client come to terms with unresolved issues that may be contributing to the dissociative process.

■ Identify specific conflicts that remain unresolved and help the client identify possible solutions. Provide instruction regarding more adaptive ways to respond to anxiety. Unless these underlying conflicts are resolved, any improvement in coping behaviors must be viewed as temporary.

■ Provide positive feedback for decisions made. Respect the client's right to make those decisions independently and refrain from attempting to influence him or her toward those that may seem more logical. Independent choice provides a feeling of control, decreases feelings of powerlessness, and increases self-esteem.

Disturbed Personal Identity

Disturbed personal identity is defined as the "inability to maintain an integrated and complete perception of self" (Herdman & Kamitsuru, 2014, p. 268). This nursing diagnosis is particularly relevant for the client with dissociative identity disorder.

Client Goals

Outcome criteria include short- and long-term goals. Time lines are individually determined.

Short-term goals

■ The client will verbalize understanding about the existence of multiple personality states within the self.

■ The client will be able to recognize stressful situations that precipitate transition from one personality to another.

Long-term goals

■ The client will verbalize understanding of the reasons for fragmented identity.

■ The client will enter into and cooperate with long-term therapy, with the ultimate goal of integration into one personality.

Interventions

■ The nurse must develop a trusting relationship with the client. Trust is the basis of a therapeutic relationship. Listen nonjudgmentally when the client transitions from one personality state to another. Help the client understand the existence of the subpersonalities and the need each serves in the personal identity of the individual. The client may initially be unaware of the dissociative response. Knowledge of the needs each personality fulfills is the first step in the integration process and the client's ability to face unresolved issues without dissociation.

■ Help the client identify stressful situations that precipitate transition from one personality to another. Carefully observe and record these transitions. Identification of stressors is required to assist the client in responding more adaptively and eliminate the need for transition to another personality.

■ Use nursing interventions necessary to deal with maladaptive behaviors associated with individual subpersonalities. For example, if one personality is suicidal, precautions must be taken to guard against the client's self-harm. If another personality has a tendency toward physical hostility, precautions must be taken to protect others.

> **CLINICAL PEARL It may be possible to seek assistance from one of the subpersonalities. For example, a strong-willed personality may help to control the behaviors of a suicidal personality.**

■ Help subpersonalities understand that their "being" will not be destroyed, but rather integrated into a unified identity within the individual. Because the subpersonalities function as separate entities, the idea of total elimination generates fear and defensiveness.

■ Provide support during disclosure of painful experiences and reassurance when the client becomes discouraged with lengthy treatment.

Concept Care Mapping

The concept map care plan (see Chapter 9, The Nursing Process in Psychiatric-Mental Health Nursing) is a diagrammatic teaching and learning strategy that allows visualization of interrelationships between medical diagnoses, nursing diagnoses, assessment data, and treatments. Examples of concept map care plans for clients with somatic symptom and dissociative disorders are presented in Figures 29–3 and 29–4.

Evaluation

Reassessment is conducted to determine if the nursing actions have been successful in achieving the objectives of care. Evaluation of the nursing actions for the client with a somatic symptom disorder may be facilitated by gathering information using the following types of questions:

■ Can the client recognize signs and symptoms of escalating anxiety?

■ Can the client intervene with adaptive coping strategies to interrupt the escalating anxiety before physical symptoms are exacerbated?

■ Can the client verbalize an understanding of the correlation between physical symptoms and times of escalating anxiety?

■ Does the client have a plan for dealing with increased stress to prevent exacerbation of physical symptoms?

■ Does the client demonstrate a decrease in ruminations about physical symptoms?

■ Have fears of serious illness diminished?

■ Does the client demonstrate full recovery from previous loss or alteration of physical functioning?

Evaluation of the nursing actions for the client with a dissociative disorder may be facilitated by gathering information using the following types of questions:

■ Has the client's memory been restored?

■ Can the client connect occurrence of psychological stress to loss of memory?

■ Does the client discuss fears and anxieties with members of the staff in an effort toward resolution?

■ Can the client discuss the presence of various personalities within the self?

■ Can he or she verbalize why these personalities exist?

■ Can the client verbalize situations that precipitate transition from one personality to another?

■ Can the client maintain a sense of reality during stressful situations?

■ Can the client verbalize a correlation between stressful situations and the onset of depersonalization behaviors?

■ Can the client demonstrate more adaptive coping strategies for dealing with stress without resorting to dissociation?

Treatment Modalities

Somatic Symptom Disorders
Individual Psychotherapy

The goal of psychotherapy is to help clients develop healthy and adaptive behaviors and encourage them to move beyond their somatization and become able to manage their lives more effectively. The focus is on

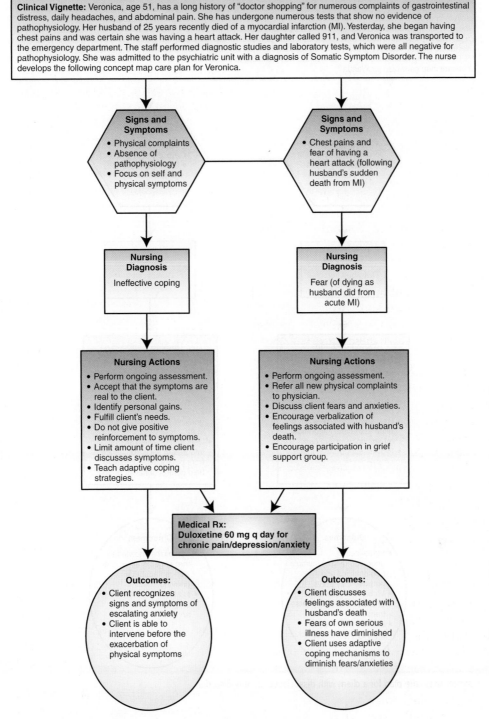

Clinical Vignette: Veronica, age 51, has a long history of "doctor shopping" for numerous complaints of gastrointestinal distress, daily headaches, and abdominal pain. She has undergone numerous tests that show no evidence of pathophysiology. Her husband of 25 years recently died of a myocardial infarction (MI). Yesterday, she began having chest pains and was certain she was having a heart attack. Her daughter called 911, and Veronica was transported to the emergency department. The staff performed diagnostic studies and laboratory tests, which were all negative for pathophysiology. She was admitted to the psychiatric unit with a diagnosis of Somatic Symptom Disorder. The nurse develops the following concept map care plan for Veronica.

Signs and Symptoms
- Physical complaints
- Absence of pathophysiology
- Focus on self and physical symptoms

Signs and Symptoms
- Chest pains and fear of having a heart attack (following husband's sudden death from MI)

Nursing Diagnosis

Ineffective coping

Nursing Diagnosis

Fear (of dying as husband did from acute MI)

Nursing Actions
- Perform ongoing assessment.
- Accept that the symptoms are real to the client.
- Identify personal gains.
- Fulfill client's needs.
- Do not give positive reinforcement to symptoms.
- Limit amount of time client discusses symptoms.
- Teach adaptive coping strategies.

Nursing Actions
- Perform ongoing assessment.
- Refer all new physical complaints to physician.
- Discuss client fears and anxieties.
- Encourage verbalization of feelings associated with husband's death.
- Encourage participation in grief support group.

Medical Rx:
Duloxetine 60 mg q day for chronic pain/depression/anxiety

Outcomes:
- Client recognizes signs and symptoms of escalating anxiety
- Client is able to intervene before the exacerbation of physical symptoms

Outcomes:
- Client discusses feelings associated with husband's death
- Fears of own serious illness have diminished
- Client uses adaptive coping mechanisms to diminish fears/anxieties

FIGURE 29–3   Concept map care plan for a client with somatic symptom disorder.

personal and social difficulties that the client experiences in daily life as well as the achievement of practical solutions for these difficulties.

Treatment is initiated with a complete physical examination to rule out organic pathology. Clients may be more amenable to psychotherapeutic treatment, particularly stress management, when it is conducted in a medical setting. Frequent, regular physical examinations are recommended to reassure clients that their concerns are being heard (Sadock et al., 2015; Yates, 2014) and may also provide an ongoing opportunity for education and stress management. The use of psychotherapy in the treatment of illness anxiety disorder is controversial (Sadock et al., 2015). Individual

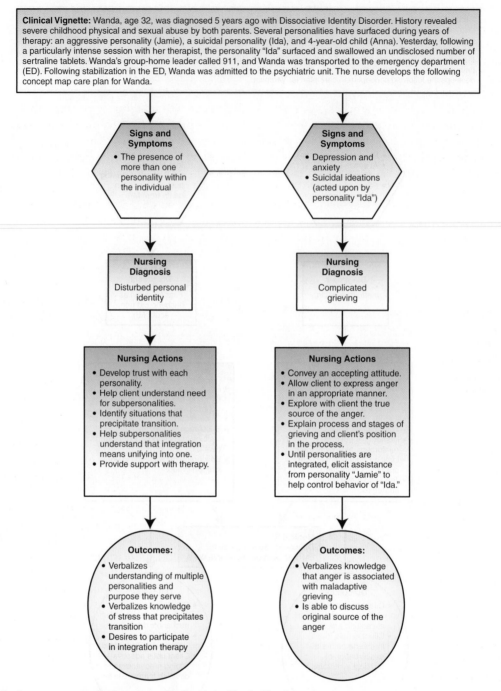

FIGURE 29-4 Concept map care plan for a client with dissociative identity disorder.

insight-oriented psychotherapy has not been proven effective (Yates, 2014).

Group Psychotherapy

Group therapy may be helpful for somatic symptom disorders because it provides a setting where clients can share their experiences of illness, learn to verbalize thoughts and feelings, and be confronted by group members and leaders when they reject responsibility for maladaptive behaviors. It is the treatment of choice for both somatic symptom disorder and illness anxiety disorder, in part because it provides the social support and anxiety reduction that these clients need.

Cognitive-Behavioral Therapy (CBT) and Psychoeducation

Yates (2014) reports that several studies support CBT as an effective strategy for reducing depressive symptoms in clients with somatic diseases. Psychoeducation has also been identified as beneficial and includes teaching the patient that the symptoms may be related to or exacerbated by stress and anxiety. This teaching should be done in the context of a trusting relationship between the health-care provider and the client because the client may resist the suggestion that physical symptoms could have a psychological foundation. Psychoeducation for family members and other support persons focuses on teaching these individuals to reward the client's autonomy, self-sufficiency, and independence while taking care not to reinforce passivity and dependence associated with the sick role. This process becomes more difficult when the client is very regressed and the sick role is well established. In conversion disorder, symptoms usually abate spontaneously, but behavior therapy may be beneficial.

Psychopharmacology

Based on studies of somatization disorder, medication treatment is not effective unless it used to treat underlying depression or anxiety (Sadock et al., 2015; Yates, 2014). When antidepressant therapy is warranted, SSRIs are generally preferred. Anxiety may be treated in the short term with antianxiety agents such as benzodiazepines, but long-term use should be avoided because of the potential for addiction.

In the treatment of conversion disorders, parenteral amobarbital or lorazepam may be helpful in revealing historical information related to trauma.

Dissociative Amnesia

Many cases of dissociative amnesia resolve spontaneously when the individual is removed from the stressful situation. For more refractory conditions, intravenous administration of amobarbital is useful in the retrieval of lost memories. Most clinicians recommend supportive psychotherapy to reinforce adjustment to the psychological impact of the retrieved memories and associated emotions.

In some instances, psychotherapy is used as the primary treatment. Techniques of persuasion and free or directed association are used to help the client remember. In other cases, hypnosis may be required to mobilize the memories. Hypnosis is sometimes facilitated by the use of pharmacological agents, such as sodium amobarbital. Supportive psychotherapy, group psychotherapy, and cognitive therapy may be employed once the memories have been obtained through hypnosis to help the client integrate the memories into his or her conscious state. Cognitive therapy has an added benefit of helping clients recall details about traumatic events when he or she begins to correct cognitive distortions about these traumas (Sadock et al., 2015).

Dissociative Identity Disorder

The goal of therapy for the client with DID is to optimize the client's function and potential. The achievement of **integration** (a blending of all the personalities into one) is usually considered desirable, but some clients choose not to pursue this lengthy therapeutic regimen. In these cases, resolution, or a smooth collaboration among the subpersonalities, may be all that is realistic.

Intensive long-term psychotherapy with the DID client is directed toward uncovering the underlying psychological conflicts, helping him or her gain insight into these conflicts, and striving to synthesize the various identities into one integrated personality. The therapist who engages in psychotherapy with this client must be skilled in various approaches, including insight-oriented psychotherapy, cognitive therapy, and especially trauma-informed and posttraumatic stress disorder (PTSD) treatment approaches. Clients are assisted to recall past traumas in detail. They must mentally reexperience the abuse that caused their illness. This process, called **abreaction,** or "remembering with feeling," is so painful that clients may actually cry, scream, and feel the pain that they felt at the time of the abuse.

During therapy, each personality is actively explored and encouraged to become aware of the others across previously amnestic barriers. Traumatic memories associated with the different personality manifestations, especially those related to childhood abuse, are examined. The course of treatment is often difficult and anxiety-provoking to client and therapist alike, especially when aggressive or suicidal personalities dominate. In these instances, brief periods of hospitalization may be necessary as an interim supportive measure.

When integration is achieved, the individual is able to integrate all the feelings, experiences, memories, skills, and talents that were previously in the command of the various personalities. He or she learns how to function effectively without the necessity for creating separate identities to cope with life. This is possible only after years of intense psychotherapy, and even then, recovery is often incomplete.

Depersonalization-Derealization Disorder

Information about the treatment of depersonalization-derealization disorder is sparse and inconclusive. Various psychiatric medications have been tried, both singly and in combination: antidepressants, mood stabilizers, anticonvulsants, and antipsychotics. Results have been sporadic at best. If other psychiatric disorders, such as schizophrenia, are evident, they too may be treated pharmacologically. For clients with evident intrapsychic conflict, analytically oriented insight psychotherapy may be useful. Some clients with depersonalization-derealization disorders have benefited from hypnotherapy or CBT.

CASE STUDY AND SAMPLE CARE PLAN

NURSING HISTORY AND ASSESSMENT

Jake is a 54-year-old client of the psychiatric outpatient department of the VA Medical Center. At age 42, Jake was diagnosed with colon cancer and underwent a colon resection. Since that time, he has had regular follow-up exams, with no recurrence of the cancer and no residual effects. He did not require follow-up chemotherapy or radiation therapy. For 10 years, Jake has had yearly physical and laboratory examinations. He regularly complains to his family physician of mild abdominal pain, sensations of "fullness," "bowel rumblings," and what he calls a "firm mass," which he says he can sometimes feel in his lower left quadrant. The physician has performed x-rays of the entire gastrointestinal (GI) tract, an esophagoscopy, gastroscopy, and colonoscopy. All results were negative for organic pathology. Rather than being relieved, Jake appears resentful and disappointed that the physician has not been able to reveal a pathological problem. Jake's job is in jeopardy because of excessive use of sick leave. The family physician has referred Jake for psychiatric evaluation. Jake was admitted as an outpatient with the diagnosis of Illness Anxiety Disorder. He has been assigned to Lisa, a psychiatric nurse practitioner.

In her assessment, Lisa learns that Jake has pretty much lived his adult life in isolation. He was never close to his parents, who worked and seldom had time for Jake or his sister. Jake told Lisa, "My parents really didn't care about me. They were too busy taking care of the farm. Dad wanted me to take over the farm, but I was never interested. I liked working on cars, and went to vocational school to learn how to be a mechanic. I thought they would be proud of me, but they never cared. I think they only had kids so they would have some help on the farm. When I left home, they really didn't care if they ever saw me again." He has never been married nor had a really serious relationship. "Women don't like me much. I spend most of my time alone. I guess I don't really like people, and they don't really like me."

NURSING DIAGNOSES AND OUTCOME IDENTIFICATION

From the assessment data, the nurse develops the following nursing diagnoses for Jake:

1. **Fear** (of cancer recurrence) related to history of colon cancer evidenced by numerous complaints of the GI tract and insistence that something is wrong despite objective tests that rule out pathophysiology.
   a. **Short-Term Goal:** Client will verbalize that fears associated with bodily sensations are irrational.
   b. **Long-Term Goal:** Client interprets bodily sensations correctly.
2. **Chronic low self-esteem** related to unfulfilled childhood needs for nurturing and caring evidenced by transformation of internalized anger into physical complaints and hostility toward others.
   a. **Short-Term Goal:** Within 2 weeks, client will verbalize aspects about self that he likes.

b. **Long-Term Goal:** By discharge from treatment, client will demonstrate acceptance of self as a person of worth, as evidenced by setting realistic goals, limiting physical complaints and hostility toward others, and verbalizing positive prospects for the future.

PLANNING AND IMPLEMENTATION

FEAR (OF CANCER RECURRENCE)
The following nursing interventions have been identified for Jake:

1. Monitor the physician's ongoing assessments and laboratory reports to ensure that pathology is clearly ruled out.
2. Refer any new physical complaints to the physician.
3. Assess what function these physical complaints are fulfilling for Jake. Is it a way for him to get attention that he cannot get in any other way?
4. Show empathy for his feelings. Let him know that you understand how GI symptoms may bring about fears of the colon cancer.
5. Encourage Jake to talk about his fears of cancer recurrence. What feelings did he have when it was first diagnosed? How did he deal with those feelings? What are his fears at this time?
6. Have Jake keep a diary of the appearance of the symptoms. In a separate diary, have Jake keep a record of situations that create stress for him. Compare these two records. Correlate whether symptoms appear at times of increased anxiety.
7. Help Jake determine techniques that may be useful for him to implement when fear and anxiety are exacerbated (e.g., relaxation techniques; mental imagery; thought-stopping techniques; physical exercise).
8. Offer positive feedback when Jake responds to stressful situations with coping strategies other than physical complaints.

CHRONIC LOW SELF-ESTEEM
The following nursing interventions have been identified for Jake:

1. Convey acceptance and unconditional positive regard, and remain nonjudgmental at all times.
2. Encourage Jake to participate in decision-making regarding his care and in life situations.
3. Help Jake to recognize and focus on strengths and accomplishments. Minimize attention given to past (real or perceived) failures.
4. Encourage Jake to talk about feelings related to his unsatisfactory relationship with his parents.
5. Discuss things in his life that Jake would like to change. Help him determine what *can* be changed and what changes are not realistic.
6. Encourage participation in group activities and in therapy groups that offer simple methods of achievement. Give recognition and positive feedback for actual accomplishments.

CASE STUDY AND SAMPLE CARE PLAN—cont'd

7. Teach assertiveness techniques and effective communication techniques.
8. Offer positive feedback for appropriate social interactions with others. Role-play with Jake situations that he finds particularly stressful. Help him to understand that ruminations about himself and his health may cause others to reject him socially.
9. Help Jake to set realistic goals for his future.

EVALUATION

Some of the outcome criteria for Jake have been met, and some are ongoing. He has come to realize that the fears about his "symptoms" are not rational. He understands that the physician has performed adequate diagnostic procedures to rule out illness. He still has fears of cancer occurrence and discusses these fears with the nurse practitioner on a weekly basis. He has kept his symptoms and stressful situations diaries and has correlated the appearance of some of the symptoms to times of increased anxiety. He has started running and tries to use this as a strategy to keep the anxiety from escalating out of proportion and bringing on new physical symptoms. He continues to discuss feelings associated with his childhood, and the nurse has helped him see that he has had numerous accomplishments in his life, even though they were not recognized by his parents or others. He has joined a support group for depressed persons and states that he "has made a few friends." He has made a long-term goal of joining a church with the hope of meeting new people. He is missing fewer workdays because of illness, and his job is no longer in jeopardy.

Summary and Key Points

- Somatic symptom and related disorders and dissociative disorders are associated with anxiety that occurs at the severe level. The anxiety is repressed and manifested in the form of symptoms and behaviors associated with these disorders.
- Somatic symptom and related disorders affect about 4 to 8 percent (although estimates range from 0.1% to 11.6%) of the general population. Types of somatic disorders include somatic symptom disorder, illness anxiety disorder, conversion disorder, psychological factors affecting other medical conditions, factitious disorder, and other specified or unspecified somatic symptom and related disorders.
- Somatic symptom disorder is manifested by physical symptoms that may be vague, dramatized, or exaggerated in presentation. No evidence of organic pathology can be identified.
- Illness anxiety disorder is an unrealistic preoccupation with fear of having a serious illness. This disorder may follow a personal experience or the experience of a close family member with serious or life-threatening illness.
- The individual with conversion disorder experiences a loss of or alteration in bodily functioning, unsubstantiated by medical or pathophysiological explanation. Psychological factors may be evident by the primary or secondary gains the individual achieves from experiencing the physiological manifestation.
- With the diagnosis of psychological factors affecting medical condition, psychological or behavioral factors have been implicated in the development, exacerbation, or delayed recovery from a medical condition.
- In factitious disorder, the individual falsifies physical or psychological signs or symptoms or induces injury on the self or another person in order to receive attention from medical personnel.
- A dissociative response has been described as a defense mechanism to protect the ego in the face of overwhelming anxiety.
- Dissociative responses result in an alteration in the normally integrative functions of identity, memory, or consciousness.
- Classification of dissociative disorders includes dissociative amnesia, DID, depersonalization-derealization disorder, and other specified or unspecified dissociative disorders.
- The individual with dissociative amnesia is unable to recall important personal information that is too extensive to be explained by ordinary forgetfulness.
- The prominent feature of DID is the existence of two or more personality states within a single individual. An individual may have many personality states, each of which allows him or her to endure painful stimuli that the identity is too fragmented to integrate as one whole personality.
- Depersonalization-derealization disorder is characterized by an alteration in the perception of oneself and/or the environment. Depersonalization is described as a feeling of unreality or detachment from one's body. Derealization is an experience of unreality or detachment with respect to one's surroundings.

■ Individuals with somatic symptom and dissociative disorders often receive initial health care in areas other than psychiatry.

■ Nurses can assist clients with these disorders by helping them understand the role of anxiety in symptom development and identify and establish new, more adaptive cognitive and behavior patterns. Nurses should provide trauma-informed care and be aware of resources for referral to specialists in trauma care and PTSD treatment.

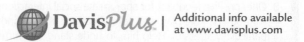 Additional info available at www.davisplus.com

Review Questions
Self-Examination/Learning Exercise

Select the answer that is most appropriate for each of the following questions.

1. Lorraine has been diagnosed with somatic symptom disorder. Which of the following symptom profiles would you expect when assessing Lorraine?
   a. Multiple somatic symptoms in several body systems
   b. Fear of having a serious disease
   c. Loss or alteration in sensorimotor functioning
   d. Belief that her body is deformed or defective in some way

2. Which of the following ego defense mechanisms describes the underlying psychodynamics of somatic symptom disorder?
   a. Denial of depression
   b. Repression of anxiety
   c. Suppression of grief
   d. Displacement of anger

3. Nursing care for a client with somatic symptom disorder would focus on helping her to:
   a. Eliminate the stress in her life.
   b. Discontinue her numerous physical complaints.
   c. Take her medication only as prescribed.
   d. Learn more adaptive coping strategies.

4. Lorraine, a client diagnosed with somatic symptom disorder, states, "My doctor thinks I should see a psychiatrist. I can't imagine why he would make such a suggestion." What is the most common basis for Lorraine's statement?
   a. She thinks her doctor wants to get rid of her as a client.
   b. She does not understand the correlation of symptoms and stress.
   c. She thinks psychiatrists are only for "crazy" people.
   d. She thinks her doctor has made an error in diagnosis.

5. Lorraine, a client diagnosed with somatic symptom disorder, tells the nurse about a pain in her side. She says she has not experienced it before. Which is the most appropriate response by the nurse?
   a. "I don't want to hear about another physical complaint. You know they are all in your head. It's time for group therapy now."
   b. "Let's sit down here together and you can tell me about this new pain you are experiencing. You'll just have to miss group therapy today."
   c. "I will report this pain to your physician. In the meantime, group therapy starts in 5 minutes."
   d. "I will call your physician and see if he will order a new pain medication for your side. The one you have now doesn't seem to provide relief. Why don't you get some rest for now?"

Review Questions—cont'd
Self-Examination/Learning Exercise

6. Ellen has a history of childhood physical and sexual abuse. She was diagnosed with dissociative identity disorder 6 years ago and has been admitted to the psychiatric unit following a suicide attempt. What is the primary nursing diagnosis for Ellen?
   a. Disturbed personal identity related to childhood abuse
   b. Disturbed sensory perception related to repressed anxiety
   c. Impaired memory related to disturbed thought processes
   d. Risk for suicide related to unresolved grief

7. In establishing trust with Ellen, a client with the diagnosis of dissociative identity disorder, the nurse must:
   a. Try to relate to Ellen as though she did not have multiple personalities.
   b. Listen nonjudgmentally and respond empathically when Ellen transitions to different personality states.
   c. Ignore behaviors that Ellen attributes to other subpersonalities.
   d. Explain to Ellen that he or she will work with her only if the primary personality is maintained.

8. What is the ultimate goal of therapy for a client with dissociative identity disorder?
   a. Integration of the personalities into one
   b. The ability to switch from one personality to another voluntarily
   c. The ability to select one personality as the dominant self
   d. Recognition that the various personalities exist

9. The ultimate goal of therapy for a client with dissociative identity disorder is most likely achieved through:
   a. Crisis intervention and directed association.
   b. Psychotherapy and hypnosis.
   c. Psychoanalysis and free association.
   d. Insight psychotherapy and dextroamphetamines.

10. Lucille has a diagnosis of illness anxiety disorder. Which of the following symptoms would be consistent with this diagnosis?
    a. Complains of a multitude of incapacitating physical symptoms
    b. Manifests with pseudoseizures or pseudocyesis
    c. Takes substances to induce vomiting in order to convince the nurse that she needs treatment
    d. Expresses persistent fears of having life-threatening disease
    e. All of the above

IMPLICATIONS OF RESEARCH FOR EVIDENCE-BASED PRACTICE

Brand, R., Classen, C., Lanius, R., Loewenstein, R., McNary, S., Pain, C., & Putnam, F. (2009). A naturalistic study of dissociative identity disorder and dissociative disorder not otherwise specified patients treated by community clinicians. *Psychological Trauma: Theory, Research, Practice, and Policy, 1*(2), 153-171. doi:http://dx.doi.org/10.1037/a0016210

DESCRIPTION OF THE STUDY: This study examined an international sample of clients ($N = 280$) receiving a similar five-phase treatment model for dissociative disorders by community clinicians. The researchers sought to identify whether the treatment was as effective as treatments for PTSD and conditions comorbid with dissociative disorders.

RESULTS OF THE STUDY: In the late stages of this 30-month treatment program, the effects of treatment were similar to those of treatment for chronic PTSD associated with childhood trauma and depression comorbid with borderline personality disorder. In addition, patients and therapists reported fewer incidents of self-injury, fewer hospitalizations, higher levels of adaptive functioning, less dissociation, and fewer PTSD symptoms. The researchers conclude that considering the

Continued

IMPLICATIONS OF RESEARCH FOR EVIDENCE-BASED PRACTICE—cont'd

prevalence, severity, chronicity and high costs of health care associated with dissociative disorders, extended treatment may be beneficial and justifies more research.

IMPLICATIONS FOR NURSING PRACTICE:

 Awareness of evidence-based research is identified as an essential QSEN (Quality and Safety Education for Nurses) competency (QSEN Institute, 2014). Studies such as this one not only inform

clinical practice for nurses in advanced practice roles but provide a foundation for registered nurses to educate patients about treatment options that have demonstrated efficacy. Patients can be educated that evidence supports the benefit of extended treatment for dissociative disorders. Sharing evidence-based information about treatment options may also encourage patients to follow through with a longer-term treatment program when there is evidence to support that it is effective.

TEST YOUR CRITICAL THINKING SKILLS

Tom was admitted to the psychiatric unit from the emergency department of a general hospital in the Midwest. The owner of a local bar called the police when Tom suddenly seemed to "lose control. He just went ballistic." The police reported that Tom did not know where he was or how he got there. He kept saying, "My name is John Brown, and I live in Philadelphia." When the police ran an identity check on Tom, they found that he was indeed John Brown from Philadelphia, and his wife had reported him missing a month ago. Mrs. Brown explained that about 12 months before his disappearance, her husband, who was a shop foreman at a large manufacturing plant, had been having considerable difficulty at work. He had been passed over for a promotion, and his supervisor was very critical of his work. Several of his staff had left the company for other jobs, and without enough help, Tom had been unable to meet shop deadlines. Work stress made him very difficult to live with at home. Previously an easygoing, extroverted individual, he became withdrawn and extremely critical of his wife and children. Immediately preceding his disappearance, he had had a violent argument with his 18-year-old son, who called Tom a "loser" and stormed out of the house to stay with some friends. It was the day after this argument that Tom disappeared. The psychiatrist assigns a diagnosis of Dissociative Amnesia, with dissociative fugue.

Answer the following questions related to Tom:

1. Describe the *priority* nursing intervention with Tom as he is admitted to the psychiatric unit.
2. What approach should be taken to help Tom with his problem?
3. What is the long-term goal of therapy for Tom?

🎬 MOVIE CONNECTIONS

Bandits (illness anxiety disorder) • *Hannah and Her Sisters* (illness anxiety disorder) • *Send Me No Flowers* (illness anxiety disorder) • *Dead Again* (amnesia) • *Mirage* (amnesia) • *Suddenly Last Summer* (amnesia) • *Sybil* (DID) • *The Three Faces of Eve* (DID) • *Identity* (DID)

References

American Psychiatric Association. (2013). *Diagnostic and statistical manual of mental disorders* (5th ed.). Washington, DC: American Psychiatric Publishing.

Black, D.W., & Andreasen, N.C. (2014). *Introductory textbook of psychiatry* (6th ed.). Washington, DC: American Psychiatric Publishing.

Brand, R., Classen, C., Lanius, R., Loewenstein, R., McNary, S., Pain, C., & Putnam, F. (2009). A naturalistic study of dissociative identity disorder and dissociative disorder not otherwise specified patients treated by community clinicians. *Psychological Trauma: Theory, Research, Practice, and Policy, 1*(2), 153-171. doi:http://dx.doi.org/10.1037/a0016210

Dimsdale, J. (2015). Illness anxiety disorder. *Merck Manual: Professional Version.* Retrieved from www.merckmanuals.com/professional/psychiatric-disorders/somatic-symptom-and-related-disorders/illness-anxiety-disorder

Haberman, C. (2014). Debate persists over diagnosing mental disorders, long after "Sybil." *New York Times.* Retrieved from www.nytimes.com/2014/11/24/us/debate-persists-over-diagnosing-mental-health-disorders-long-after-sybil.html?_r=0

Herdman, T.H., & Kamitsuru, S. (Eds.). (2014). *NANDA-I nursing diagnoses: Definitions and classification, 2015–2017.* Chichester, UK: Wiley Blackwell.

QSEN Institute. (2014). *Competencies.* Retrieved from http://qsen.org/competencies/

Sadock, B.J., Sadock, V.A., & Ruiz, P. (2015). *Synopsis of psychiatry: Behavioral sciences/clinical psychiatry* (11th ed.). Philadelphia: Lippincott Williams & Wilkins.

Soares, N., & Grossman, L. (2012, November 29). Conversion disorder. *Emedicine Pediatrics.* Retrieved from http://emedicine.medscape.com/article/917864-overview

Venes, D. (2014). *Taber's medical dictionary* (22nd ed.). Philadelphia: F.A. Davis.

Yates, W. (2014). Somatic symptom disorders. *Medscape.* Retrieved from http://emedicine.medscape.com/article/294908-overview

Yutzy, S.H., & Parish, B.S. (2008). Somatoform disorders. In R.E. Hales, S.C. Yudofsky, & G.O. Gabbard (Eds.), *Textbook of psychiatry* (5th ed., pp. 609-664). Washington, D.C.: American Psychiatric Publishing.

Classical References

Asher, R. (1951). Munchausen's syndrome. *The Lancet, 257*(6650), 339-341.

Freud, S. (1962). The neuro-psychoses of defense. In J. Strachey (Ed.), *Standard edition of the complete psychological works of Sigmund Freud,* vol. 3. London: Hogarth Press. (Original work published 1984.)

Issues Related to Human Sexuality and Gender Dysphoria

30

CORE CONCEPTS

Gender

Sexuality

KEY TERMS

anorgasmia

cisgender

delayed ejaculation

exhibitionistic disorder

fetishistic disorder

frotteuristic disorder

gay

homosexuality

lesbian

orgasm

pedophilic disorder

premature (early) ejaculation

sensate focus

sexual masochism disorder

sexual sadism disorder

transgender (trans)

transvestic disorder

voyeuristic disorder

OBJECTIVES

After reading this chapter, the student will be able to:

1. Describe developmental processes associated with human sexuality.
2. Discuss variations in sexual orientation.
3. Formulate nursing diagnoses and goals of care for clients with gender dysphoria.
4. Identify appropriate nursing interventions for clients with gender dysphoria.
5. Evaluate care of clients with gender dysphoria.
6. Discuss historical and epidemiological aspects of paraphilic disorders.
7. Identify various types of paraphilic disorders.
8. Discuss predisposing factors associated with the etiology of paraphilic disorders..
9. Describe the physiology of the human sexual response.
10. Conduct a sexual history.
11. Formulate nursing diagnoses, goals, and interventions for clients with sexual dysfunction disorders.
12. Identify topics for client/family education relevant to sexual dysfunction disorders.
13. Describe various treatment modalities for clients with sexual disorders.

HOMEWORK ASSIGNMENT

Please read the chapter and answer the following questions:

1. At about what age do children become aware of their own gender?
2. What types of psychosocial factors may predispose individuals to sexual desire disorders?
3. What medications have been implicated in the etiology of erectile disorder?
4. Which physiological mechanisms contribute to sexual dysfunctions?

Humans are sexual beings. Sexuality is a basic human need and an innate part of the total personality. It influences our thoughts, actions, and interactions and is involved in aspects of physical and mental health.

Society's attitude toward sexuality is changing. Clients are more open to seeking assistance in matters that pertain to sexuality. Although not all nurses need to be educated as sex therapists, they can readily integrate information on sexuality into the care they give by focusing on preventive, therapeutic, and educational interventions to assist individuals to attain, regain, or maintain sexual wellness.

This chapter focuses on disorders associated with sexual functioning and gender dysphoria. Primary consideration is given to the categories of paraphilic disorders and sexual dysfunctions as classified in the *Diagnostic and Statistical Manual of Mental Disorders, Fifth Edition (DSM-5)* (American Psychiatric Association [APA], 2013). An overview of human sexual development throughout the life span is presented to help nurses better understand typical versus atypical desires and behaviors. Historical and epidemiological information associated with sexual disorders is included. Predisposing factors that have been implicated in the etiology of sexual disorders and gender dysphoria provide a framework for studying the dynamics of these conditions. Various medical treatment modalities are explored, and variations in sexual orientation are discussed.

Symptomatology is presented as background knowledge for assessing clients with sexual disorders and gender dysphoria. A tool for acquiring a sexual history is provided. Nursing care is described in the context of the nursing process.

> ## CORE CONCEPT
>
> ### Sexuality
> Sexuality is the constitution and life of an individual relative to characteristics regarding intimacy. It reflects the totality of the person and does not relate exclusively to the sex organs or sexual behavior.

Development of Human Sexuality

Birth Through Age 12

Although the sexual identity of an infant is determined before birth by chromosomal factors and physical appearance of the genitals, postnatal factors can greatly influence the way developing children perceive themselves sexually. Masculinity and femininity as well as gender roles are, for the most part, culturally defined.

For example, differentiation of roles may be initiated at birth by painting a child's room pink or blue.

It is not uncommon for infants to touch and explore their genitals. In fact, research on infantile sexuality indicates that both male and female infants are capable of sexual arousal and **orgasm** (Berman & Berman, 2014).

By age 2 to 3 years, children know what gender they are. They know that they are like the parent of the same gender and different from the parent of the opposite gender and from other children of the opposite gender. They become acutely aware of anatomical gender differences during this time.

By age 4 or 5, children may engage in heterosexual play, such as "playing doctor." Through heterosexual play, children form a concept of relationships with a member of the opposite gender. It is not uncommon for children to act out in play behaviors they have seen in their parents or significant others, including touching, kissing, and arguing. Although these activities are a part of normal sexual development, they can sometimes signal issues such as sexual abuse. For example, if a child is engaging in play with other children that is nonconsensual, if there is a significant age discrepancy between the children involved, or if the language being used to describe the heterosexual play seems to be age-inappropriate, further assessment is warranted. Open, nonjudgmental communication such as, "Tell me more about where you learned this," encourages children to discuss issues about sexuality and provides a foundation for instruction.

Children increasingly gain experience with masturbation during childhood, although not all children masturbate during this period. Most children begin self-exploration and genital self-stimulation as soon as they are able to gain sufficient control over their physical movements (King & Regan, 2014).

Late childhood and preadolescence may be characterized by heterosexual or homosexual play. Generally, the activity involves no more than touching the other's genitals but may include a wide range of sexual behaviors (Masters, Johnson, & Kolodny, 1995). Girls at this age become interested in menstruation, and both genders are interested in learning about fertility, pregnancy, and birth. Interest in the opposite gender typically increases. Children of this age become self-conscious about their bodies and are concerned with physical attractiveness.

Children ages 10 to 12 are preoccupied with pubertal changes and the beginnings of romantic sexual attraction. Prepubescent boys may engage in group sexual activities such as genital exhibition or group masturbation. Homosexual sex play is not uncommon. Prepubescent girls may engage in some genital exhibition, but they are usually not as preoccupied with the genitalia as are boys of this age.

Adolescence

Adolescence represents an acceleration in terms of biological changes and psychosocial and sexual development. This time of turmoil is challenged by awakening endocrine forces and a new set of psychosocial tasks. These tasks include issues relating to sexuality, such as how to deal with new or more powerful sexual feelings, whether to participate in various types of sexual behavior, how to recognize love, how to prevent unwanted pregnancy, and how to define age-appropriate gender roles.

Biologically, puberty begins for the female adolescent with breast enlargement, widening of the hips, and growth of pubic and ancillary hair. Onset of menstruation is variable but usually occurs between the ages of 11 and 13 years. Some children may begin menstruating as early as age 8. Malnutrition is one factor that influences a delay in onset of menses. In the male adolescent, growth of pubic hair and enlargement of the testicles begin at 12 to 16 years of age. Penile growth and the ability to ejaculate usually occur between the ages of 13 to 17. There is a marked growth of the body between ages 11 and 17, accompanied by the growth of body and facial hair, increased muscle mass, and a deeper voice.

Sexuality is slower to develop in the female than in the male adolescent. The notion that women show steady increases in sexual responsiveness that peak in their middle 20s or early 30s while sexual maturity for men is usually reached in the late teens dates back to Alfred Kinsey's research in the 1950s. However, it is more accurate to say that each person's sexuality is a unique, complex interplay among many variables. Masturbation is a common sexual activity among male and female adolescents.

Many individuals have their first experience with sexual intercourse during the adolescent years. According to data collected between September 2014 and December 2015, 41 percent of high school students surveyed admitted to having had sexual intercourse, and 43 percent said they did not use a condom the last time they had intercourse (Kann et al., 2016). Although the general trend has been toward safer sex practices in this age group, these statistics reflect an ongoing need for education about health risks and preventive measures. The American culture has ambivalent feelings about adolescent sexuality. Psychosexual development is desired, but most parents want to avoid anything that may encourage teenage sex. The rise in number of cases of sexually transmitted infections (STIs), some of which are life threatening, also contributes to fears associated with unprotected sexual activity in all age groups.

In June 2006, the U.S. Food and Drug Administration (FDA) licensed Gardasil, the first vaccine developed to prevent cervical cancer and other diseases caused by certain strains of human papillomavirus (HPV). A second vaccine, Cervarix, was approved by the FDA in October 2009. If administered prior to exposure to HPV, these vaccines can protect women from ultimately developing cervical cancer caused by these specific strains. The Centers for Disease Control and Prevention (CDC) (2012) recommends routine administration of the vaccine to all girls aged 11 or 12 years with three doses of either vaccine. The vaccine is also recommended for girls and women aged 13 through 26 who have not already received the vaccine or have not completed all booster shots. In October 2011, the CDC's Advisory Committee on Immunization Practices (ACIP) recommended routine use of the quadrivalent vaccine, Gardasil, in males aged 11 or 12 years (CDC, 2011b). The ACIP also recommended vaccination for males aged 13 through 21 years who have not been vaccinated previously or who have not completed the 3-dose series; males aged 22 through 26 years may also be vaccinated. In 2015, a 9-valent HPV vaccine became available and was recommended by the ACIP as one of three HPV vaccines that may be used. This most current vaccine is identified as protective against 14 percent more HPV cancers for women and 5 percent more for men (Petrosky et al., 2015).

Some state legislatures have proposed making administration of the HPV vaccine mandatory for girls aged 9 to 12 years. However, some parents believe these types of laws circumvent their rights and may send the message that these young women are protected and thereby promote promiscuity. One recent study regarding this issue indicates that this concern is unfounded. Evidence has supported that HPV vaccination in the recommended age group was not associated with increased sexual activity–related outcomes or increase in unsafe sexual practices (Bednarczyk et al., 2012; Jena, Goldman, & Seabury, 2015). Currently, the controversy is ongoing, with supporters of a mandate saying that states have a rare opportunity to fight a cancer that kills 3700 American women every year, and to be effective, it must be given before a woman has been infected with the virus. But opponents say states—and parents—should be trying to prevent premarital sex instead of requiring a vaccination with the assumption that it is going to happen.

Adulthood

This period of the life cycle begins at approximately 20 years of age and continues to age 65. Sexuality associated with older adults is discussed more thoroughly in Chapter 34, The Aging Individual.

Marital Sex

Choosing a partner is one of the major tasks in the early years of this life stage. Current cultural perspective reflects that marriage has survived as a mainstream institution. The United States has marriage rates of approximately 70 percent, although for the last decade, approximately 50 percent of marriages have ended in divorce (CDC, 2015). Changing attitudes about sex, living arrangement options, and marriage as a lifelong institution may be just a few of the factors contributing to this trend. Still, intimacy in marriage is one of the most common forms of sexual expression for adults. The average American couple has sex about two or three times per week in their 20s, with the frequency gradually declining to about once weekly for those 45 years of age and over. Many adults continue to masturbate even though they are married and have ready access to heterosexual sex. This behavior is perfectly normal, although it often evokes feelings of guilt and may be kept secret.

Extramarital Sex

Studies present widely variable results for surveys of extramarital sex. Even the most carefully conducted surveys are based on the reliability of self-reporting, and these reports may be skewed by people's hesitancy to acknowledge a behavior they perceive as contrary to societal expectations. King and Regan (2014) report estimates that about one-third of married men and one-fourth of married women have engaged in extramarital sex during their marriages. Allen and Atkins, as cited by Hughes (2012), analyzed data on 16,090 individuals over almost two decades from 1991 to 2008 to identify trends over time and concluded that about 17.7 percent of ever-married individuals and about 10 percent more men than women reported having an extramarital affair. They calculated the probability of divorce following an extramarital affair at 50 percent, but as Hughes notes, the factors within a marriage that contribute to extramarital affairs and ultimately to divorce are complex and multifaceted and therefore cannot be reduced to a simple cause-and-effect relationship.

Sex and the Single Person

Attitudes about sexual intimacy among singles—never married, divorced, or widowed—vary among individuals. Some single people pursue relationships, casual or committed, that they believe will enrich their lives. Others cherish their independent, single status and have no desire for marriage or a sexual partner.

Many divorced men and women return to having an active sex life following separation from their spouses. More widowed men than widowed women return to an active sex life after the loss of their partners, perhaps in part because men may be more comfortable choosing women partners younger than themselves, and also because widows outnumber widowers by more than 4 to 1 (Administration on Aging, 2013).

The "Middle" Years—40 to 65

With the advent of the middle years, a decrease in hormone production initiates a number of changes in the sex organs as well as in the rest of the body. The average age of naturally occurring menopause for women in North America is 51 years, although changes can be noted from about 40 to 60 years of age (Kingsberg & Krychman, 2016). The decrease in the amount of estrogen results in loss of natural vaginal lubrication, possibly making intercourse painful. Other symptoms may include insomnia, hot flashes, headaches, heart palpitations, and depression. Hormonal supplements may alleviate some of these symptoms, although controversy still exists within the medical community regarding the safety of menopausal hormone therapy.

With the decrease of androgen production during these years, men also experience sexual changes. The amount of ejaculate may decrease, and ejaculation may be less forceful. The testes decrease in size, and erections may be less frequent and less rigid. By age 50, the refractory period increases, and men may require 8 to 24 hours after orgasm before another erection can be achieved.

Biological drives decrease and interest in sexual activity may decrease during these middle years. A man's declining interest in sexual activity may be influenced by needing longer stimulation to reach orgasm and decreased intensity of pleasure. Women, however, stabilize at the same level of sexual activity as at the previous stage in the life cycle and often have a greater capacity for orgasm in middle adulthood than in young adulthood (Sadock, Sadock, & Ruiz, 2015).

Variations in Sexual Orientation

Several labels have been used to describe variations in sexual orientation. One current acronym, LGBTQIA, attempts to describe the range of preferences (including lesbian, gay, bisexual, transgender, queer, intersex, and asexual). The term *lesbian* refers to women with a homosexual orientation; *gay* refers to males with homosexual orientation; *bisexual* refers to people who are oriented to both heterosexual and homosexual relationships; *transgender* refers to individuals who are inclined toward a gender different from their biologically assigned gender; *queer* is a term that has more recently been identified within the LGBTQIA community to describe people who are either uncertain about or uncomfortable with conventional, binary labels; *intersexual* relates to individuals who describe themselves as sexually ambiguous; and *asexual* refers to those who have no sexual orientation or preference. Together, those with minority orientations are often described as the "LGBTQIA community." The following discussion focuses on the most common of these orientations, homosexuality and bisexuality.

Homosexuality

Same-sex relationships exist in all known human cultures and all mammalian species for which it has been studied. The term **homosexuality** is derived from the Greek root *homo*, meaning "same," and refers to sexual preference for individuals of the same gender. The term **gay** is used to refer to men who prefer same-sex relationships. The term **lesbian** also has Greek roots and is used to identify females who prefer same-sex relationships. Most men in same-sex relationships prefer the term *gay* because it focuses less on the sexual aspects of the orientation. A heterosexual person may be commonly referred to as "straight."

To provide informed, supportive care to all patients, it is important to understand the evolution of medical information and societal perceptions regarding homosexuality. Beginning in the late 1800s, homosexuality was classified as a mental illness. This remained the case until 1973, when the APA finally removed the classification from the *DSM*, affirming that homosexuality was one expression of sexuality, not a mental disorder. Still, homosexuality remained classified as a mental disorder in the World Health Organization's *International Classification of Diseases* until 1992, when it was finally removed.

Despite the advances made within the medical and mental health communities, U.S. state legislation prohibiting sexual behavior that could not result in reproduction ("sodomy laws") was slower to change. In 2003, when these laws still remained in 13 states, the U.S. Supreme Court finally issued a broad-scoped decision that essentially invalidated all sodomy laws (King & Regan, 2014). Then, on June 26, 2015, the Supreme Court declared same-sex marriage legal in all 50 states. Justice Anthony Kennedy, who wrote the majority opinion, said of same-sex couples in the case: "They ask for equal dignity in the eyes of the law. The Constitution grants them that right" (Chappell, 2015).

Despite these recent changes, some experts believe that some Americans' attitudes toward homosexuals can still best be described as homophobic. *Homophobia* is a negative attitude toward or fear of homosexuality or nonheterosexuals. Homophobic behaviors include extreme prejudice against, abhorrence of, and discomfort around nonheterosexuals. The impact of these prejudices, beliefs, or behaviors can create a climate of fear or stress for members of the homosexual community and their families.

Health-care providers must ensure that those of all sexual orientations receive care with dignity, which is the right of every human being. In 2013, for the first time, the CDC collected health data based on sexual orientation in an effort to pursue a goal of the national initiative *Healthy People 2020* (Institute of Medicine, 2003) to improve the health, safety, and well-being of lesbian, gay, and bisexual (LGB) individuals (CDC, 2014). One of the research findings was a higher than average incidence of alcohol use (five or more drinks a day) in this population, suggesting that a good health assessment should include screening for substance abuse issues. Other studies have identified concerns about increased risks for suicide attempts and suicides among LGB individuals, especially in men (Mathy et al., 2011; Ploderl et al., 2013). Whether this risk is associated with sexual orientation itself or the stresses associated with being a stigmatized minority group, nurses play an important role in promoting the safety and well-being for this population by screening for depression and suicide ideation in each health-care encounter.

Relationship patterns are as varied among homosexuals as they are among heterosexuals. They may remain single or live with one partner for an extended period of time; they may divorce or remain married for a lifetime. As a nurse and health-care provider, what matters is understanding that variations in sexual orientation are commonplace, with no relationship whatsoever to mental illness. Unconditional acceptance of each individual is an essential component of compassionate, successful nursing.

Bisexuality

A bisexual person is not exclusively heterosexual or homosexual, but engages in sexual activity with members of both genders. Bisexuals are also sometimes referred to as *ambisexual*. According to the 2013 National Health Interview Survey (CDC, 2014) 0.4 percent men and 0.9 percent women identified themselves as bisexual.

A diversity of sexual preference exists among those who identify themselves as bisexual. Some individuals prefer men and women equally, whereas others have a preference for one gender but also accept sexual activity with the other gender. Some may alternate between homosexual and heterosexual activity for long periods; others may have both a male and a female lover at the same time. Whereas some individuals maintain their bisexual orientation throughout their lives, others may eventually become exclusively homosexual or heterosexual.

Gender Dysphoria

> ## CORE CONCEPT
> **Gender**
> The condition of being either male or female.

Gender identity is a person's sense of being male or female—that is, the awareness of one's masculinity or femininity. The term **cisgender** refers to a personal identity that is the same as the gender assigned at birth. **Transgender** describes a state in which an individual experiences incongruence between his or her biological/assigned gender and gender identity. Colloquially, this term is sometimes abbreviated to simply *trans*. Gender identity does not dictate to whom one is attracted: in other words, transgender individuals may or may not have same-sex couples relationships (Lowry & Vega, 2016). The *DSM-5* stipulates that a diagnosis of gender dysphoria, in addition to incongruence between assigned gender and expressed gender, requires that the client expresses significant distress in school, social, occupational, and performance functions for at least 6 months. It is not sufficient to make a diagnosis solely on a parent's or other people's discomfort with someone's gender identity. Changes in labeling and criteria for diagnosis reflect efforts within the psychiatric community to depathologize variances in gender. Stroumsa (2014) points out that there is increasing agreement among psychiatrists that transgender identity is not an "illness" to be "cured." However, when struggles with gender identity cause suffering, the individual may benefit from treatment. Although most cases of gender dysphoria begin in childhood, those who seek treatment may be of any age.

The *DSM-5* categorizes diagnosis of the condition in two groups: gender dysphoria in children and gender dysphoria in adolescents and adults. For purposes of this text, differentiation between the age groups is discussed, but the major focus is on gender dysphoria as it emerges in childhood. Nurses who work in areas of primary prevention with children can have the greatest effect in responding to the needs of this population.

There was a great deal of controversy in the psychiatric community about whether gender dysphoria should be included in the *DSM-5* (APA, 2013). The transgender community protested to the psychiatric work group that "different is not a disease." The work group attempted to address some of the concerns of the transgender community, taking into consideration the stigma associated with inclusion of the diagnosis but also the need for inclusion in terms of access to adequate treatment and care. If the diagnosis was not included, those who chose to seek medical-surgical and/or psychiatric treatment may have been denied third-party assistance. The term *gender dysphoria* was adopted to minimize the stigma connected to the previous label and emphasize the emotional component of the condition.

Course and Epidemiology

An estimated 1 in 30,000 men and 1 in 100,000 women identify as transgender (Sadock et al., 2015). In other words, most (approximately 75%) transgender individuals are biological males desiring reassignment to female gender (MTF), and the remaining 25 percent are females desiring to be male (FTM). Some transgender individuals choose to find ways of living with their cross-gender identity without surgically altering their bodies. Others have a strong desire to change their physical bodies to reflect their core gender identities. Transgender ideation and expression sometimes dissipates after early childhood; however, if it persists into adolescence, it appears to be an established identity.

Predisposing Factors
Biological Influences

The etiology of transgender identity is unknown. There is no significant evidence linking this condition to hormone or chromosome variations (Gooren, 2011). Some small postmortem studies of brain tissue have demonstrated that MTF transgender individuals (also referred to as *trans women*) had typically female patterns of sexual differentiation in both the stria terminalis and the hypothalamic uncinate nucleus, leading researchers to suggest that perhaps this is a sexual differentiation issue that affects the brain (Garcia-Falgueras & Swaab, 2008).

Family Dynamics

Gender roles are certainly culturally influenced as parents encourage masculine or feminine behaviors in their children. However, there is no clear evidence that psychological factors or family dynamics cause gender dysphoria (Gooren, 2011). Parents may present with anxiety over their child's gender-nonconforming behavior based on their attitudes and perceptions. Likewise, children may present with symptoms of anxiety and depression related to negative attitudes toward their gender-nonconforming behaviors. Interestingly, researchers have observed that many children who show gender-nonconforming behavior do not grow up to become transgender, and many people who identify themselves as transgender in adulthood were not identified as gender nonconforming in childhood (Sadock et al., 2015).

Application of the Nursing Process to Gender Dysphoria in Children

Background Assessment Data (Symptomatology)

Some children may resist wearing clothing or playing with toys that are typical for their assigned genders. This resistance is often part of normal childhood behavior. But when these behaviors persist into later childhood and adolescence, they may indicate a stable gender identity. Gender dysphoria is not diagnosed unless symptoms of distress emerge, such as marked distress associated with gender identity, concerns such as depression related to the desire to be the opposite gender, disgust with one's own genitals, or fear and anxiety related to others learning about their gender identity. These children may be subjected to teasing and rejection by their peers and disapproval from family members. This occurs early in childhood for boys but often does not occur before adolescence in girls, because masculine behavior in girls is more culturally accepted than feminine behavior in boys. Because of this rejection, interpersonal relationships are hampered. The *DSM-5* diagnostic criteria for gender dysphoria in children are presented in Box 30–1.

Diagnosis and Outcome Identification

Based on the data collected during the nursing assessment, possible nursing diagnoses for the child with gender dysphoria may include the following:

■ Impaired social interaction related to socially and culturally nonconforming behaviors
■ Low self-esteem related to rejection by peers and/or family members

The following criteria may be used for measurement of outcomes in the care of the child with gender dysphoria.

The client:

■ Demonstrates trust in a therapist
■ Demonstrates development of a close relationship with parents
■ Verbalizes positive self-esteem
■ Demonstrates evidence of social skills and assertive communication in relationship with family and peers
■ Verbalizes and demonstrates comfort with gender identity

Planning and Implementation

Table 30–1 provides a plan of care for the child with gender dysphoria. Nursing diagnoses are presented along with outcome criteria, appropriate nursing interventions, and rationales.

BOX 30–1 Diagnostic Criteria for Gender Dysphoria in Children

A. A marked incongruence between one's experienced/expressed gender and assigned gender, of at least 6 months' duration, as manifested by at least six of the following indicators (one of which must be Criterion A1):
   1. A strong desire to be of the other gender or an insistence that he or she is the other gender (or some alternative gender different from one's assigned gender).
   2. In boys (assigned gender), a strong preference for cross-dressing or simulating female attire; in girls (assigned gender), a strong preference for wearing only typical masculine clothing and a strong resistance to the wearing of typical feminine clothing.
   3. A strong preference for cross-gender roles in make-believe or fantasy play.
   4. A strong preference for the toys, games, or activities stereotypically used or engaged in by the other gender.
   5. A strong preference for playmates of the other gender.
   6. In boys (assigned gender), a strong rejection of typically masculine toys, games, and activities and a strong avoidance of rough-and-tumble play; or in girls (assigned gender), a strong rejection of typically feminine toys, games, and activities.
   7. A strong dislike of one's sexual anatomy.
   8. A strong desire for the primary and/or secondary sex characteristics that match one's experienced gender.
B. The condition is associated with clinically significant distress or impairment in social, occupational, or other important areas of functioning.

Specify if:
   With a disorder of sex development (e.g., a congenital adrenogenital disorder such as congenital adrenal hyperplasia or androgen insensitivity syndrome).

Reprinted with permission from the Diagnostic and Statistical Manual of Mental Disorders, Fifth Edition *(Copyright 2013). American Psychiatric Association.*

Evaluation

The final step of the nursing process is to determine whether nursing interventions have been effective in achieving the intended outcomes. This evaluation process requires that the nurse reassess the client's behaviors and determine if the changes at which the interventions had been directed have occurred. For the child with gender dysphoria, this evaluation may be accomplished by using the following types of questions:

■ Does the client perceive that a problem existed that required a change in behavior for resolution?
■ What is the client's response to any negative peer reaction?
■ Can the client verbalize positive statements about self?
■ Can the client discuss past accomplishments without dwelling on the perceived failures?

Table 30–1 | CARE PLAN FOR THE CHILD WITH GENDER DYSPHORIA

NURSING DIAGNOSIS: INEFFECTIVE COPING ASSOCIATED WITH GENDER IDENTITY

RELATED TO: Biological factors or parenting patterns that encourage culturally unacceptable behaviors for assigned gender

EVIDENCED BY: Wearing clothing of and engaging in activities associated with the opposite gender; verbalized discomfort and distress related to assigned gender

OUTCOME CRITERIA	NURSING INTERVENTIONS	RATIONALE
Short-Term Goals • Client will verbalize knowledge of behaviors that are appropriate and culturally acceptable for assigned gender. • Client will verbalize personal feelings and behavior about assigned gender. • Parents will demonstrate knowledge about gender-nonconforming behaviors and gender dysphoria. Long-Term Goal • Client will express personal satisfaction and feelings of being comfortable within self-concept and gender identity.	1. Spend time with client and show positive regard. 2. Be aware of personal feelings and attitudes toward client and his or her behavior. 3. Educate parents about issues children face when engaging in gender-nonconforming behaviors and describe current knowledge about gender dysphoria. 4. Allow client to describe his or her perception of the problem.	1. Trust and unconditional acceptance are essential to the establishment of a therapeutic nurse–client relationship. 2. Attitudes influence behavior. The nurse must not allow negative attitudes to interfere with the effectiveness of interventions. 3. Including parents in the care plan for children is an important aspect of providing care for minor children. Providing current education to parents offers opportunities to discuss their roles and to provide supportive care. 4. It is important to know how the client perceives the problem before attempting to intervene.

NURSING DIAGNOSIS: IMPAIRED SOCIAL INTERACTION

RELATED TO: Socially and culturally nonconforming behaviors

EVIDENCED BY: Ridicule from peers and self-imposed social isolation

OUTCOME CRITERIA	NURSING INTERVENTIONS	RATIONALE
Short-Term Goal • Client will verbalize possible reasons for ineffective interactions with others Long-Term Goal • Client will interact with others using behaviors that promote personal safety and self-esteem.	1. Once client feels comfortable with new behaviors in role-playing or one-to-one nurse–client interactions, new behaviors may be tried in group situations. If possible, remain with client during initial interactions with others. This intervention may include identification of safe and supportive peer groups. 2. Offer support if client is feeling hurt from peer ridicule. Matter-of-factly discuss behaviors that elicited the ridicule. Offer no personal reaction to the behavior.	1. The presence of a trusted individual provides security for client in a new situation and also provides the potential for feedback to client about his or her behavior. 2. Personal reaction from the nurse would be considered judgmental. Validation of client's feelings is important, yet it is also important that client understand why his or her behavior was the subject of ridicule and how to avoid it in the future.

Table 30-1 | CARE PLAN FOR THE CHILD WITH GENDER DYSPHORIA—cont'd

OUTCOME CRITERIA	NURSING INTERVENTIONS	RATIONALE
	3. The goal is to create a trusting, nonthreatening atmosphere for the client in an attempt to improve social interactions.	3. Long-term studies have not yet revealed the significance of therapy with these children for psychosexual relationship development in adolescence or adulthood. One variable that must be considered is the evidence of psychopathology within the families of these children.

NURSING DIAGNOSIS: LOW SELF-ESTEEM

RELATED TO: Rejection by peers

EVIDENCED BY: Lack of eye contact, negative self-evaluation, social withdrawal

OUTCOME CRITERIA	NURSING INTERVENTIONS	RATIONALE
Short-Term Goal • Client will verbalize positive statements about self, including past accomplishments and future prospects. **Long-Term Goal** • Client will verbalize and demonstrate behaviors that indicate self-satisfaction with gender identity, ability to interact with others, and a sense of self as a worthwhile person.	1. Encourage child to engage in activities in which he or she is likely to achieve success. 2. Help child to focus on aspects of his or her life for which positive feelings exist. Discourage rumination about situations that are perceived as failures or over which child has no control. Give positive feedback for these behaviors. 3. Help child identify behaviors or aspects of life he or she would like to change. If realistic, assist child in problem-solving ways to bring about the change. 4. Offer to be available for support to child when he or she is feeling rejected by peers.	1. Successful endeavors enhance self-esteem. 2. Rumination about perceived failures only further diminishes feelings of self-worth. Positive feedback increases self-esteem. 3. Having some control over his or her life may decrease feelings of powerlessness and increase feelings of self-worth and self-satisfaction. 4. Having an available support person who does not judge child's behavior and who provides unconditional acceptance assists child to progress toward acceptance of self as a worthwhile person.

■ Has the client shown progress toward accepting self as a worthwhile person regardless of others' responses to his or her behavior?

Treatment Issues

Determining whether a child is truly experiencing gender dysphoria should be done cautiously because gender-related behaviors vary widely in this age group. When this issue is identified as real gender dysphoria

(e.g., the child is manifesting significant distress, symptoms of clinical depression, or suicidal ideation), treatment should include evaluation and management of concurrent mental health problems, social support systems, and in later childhood, nonjudgmental exploration of the individual's desires with regard to sexual reassignment.

Some practitioners still engage in treatment models that attempt to "repair" or change the person's gender identity, but this approach is contrary to position statements by the American Psychiatric Association (Byne et al., 2012) and the practice guidelines established by the American Academy of Child and Adolescent Psychiatry (Adelson, 2012).

Another treatment model suggests that children who have differing gender identity are dysphoric only because of their image within the culture. In this view, children should be accepted as they see themselves—different from their assigned gender—and supported in their efforts to live as the gender in which they feel most comfortable. One option for treatment is pubertal delay for adolescents aged 12 to 16 years who have suffered with extreme lifelong gender dysphoria and who have supportive parents who encourage the child to pursue a desired change in gender (Adelson, 2012; Byne et al., 2012; Gibson & Catlin, 2010). A gonadotropin-releasing hormone agonist is administered to suppress changes associated with puberty. The treatment is reversible if the adolescent later decides not to pursue the gender change. When the medication is withdrawn, external sexual development proceeds, and the individual has avoided permanent surgical intervention. If he or she decides as an adult to advance to surgical intervention, pubertal delay may facilitate transition because secondary sex characteristics have not been clearly established. The type of treatment one chooses for gender dysphoria (if any) is a matter of personal choice. However, issues associated with mental health concerns, such as depression, anxiety, social isolation, anger, self-esteem, and parental conflict, must be addressed.

Children who demonstrate gender-nonconforming behaviors are often targets of bullying and violence. Nurses can play a key role in educating families and providing support to identify safe, supportive peer groups for these children (Nicholson & McGuiness, 2014).

Gender Dysphoria in Adolescents and Adults

An individual who identifies as transgender has anatomical characteristics of one gender but has the self-perception of being the opposite gender. Gender Dysphoria refers to a clinically significant mood disturbance related to transgender identity issues. Individuals with this disorder may not feel comfortable wearing the clothes of their assigned gender and often engage in cross-dressing. They may find their own genitals repugnant and may repeatedly seek treatment for hormonal and surgical gender reassignment. Depression and anxiety are common

mood disturbances in this population, often attributed by the individual to his or her inability to live in the desired gender role. (Refer to the previous section on gender dysphoria in children for predisposing factors to this condition.)

Treatment Issues

Intervention with adolescents and adults with gender dysphoria is multifaceted. Evidence suggests that the longer people live with gender dysphoria before seeking treatment, the greater the likelihood of suicide attempts and completions (Nicholson & McGuiness, 2014). With a 41 percent lifetime prevalence of suicide attempts among transgender individuals and 33 percent identifying that they postponed preventive care because of discrimination or disrespect from health-care providers (Stroumsa, 2014), we must improve our abilities to provide holistic, nonjudgmental care. Adolescents rarely have the desire or motivation to alter their cross-gender roles, and in the interest of patient-centered care, nurses must listen carefully to the desires and treatment preferences expressed by the client. Some adults seek therapy to learn how to cope with their sexual identities, whereas others directly and immediately request hormonal therapy and surgical sex reassignment. The transgender person may intensely desire to have the genitalia and physical appearance of the assigned gender changed to conform to his or her gender identity. This change requires a great deal more than surgical alteration of physical features. In most cases, the individual must undergo extensive psychological testing and counseling as well as live in the role of the desired gender for up to 2 years before surgery.

Hormonal treatment is initiated during this period. Male clients receive estrogen, which results in a redistribution of body fat in a more "feminine" pattern, enlargement of the breasts, softening of the skin, and reduction in body hair. Women receive testosterone, which also causes a redistribution of body fat, growth of facial and body hair, enlargement of the clitoris, and deepening of the voice. Menstruation ceases (amenorrhea) within a few months of the advent of testosterone treatment.

Surgical treatment for MTF transgender reassignment involves removal of the penis and testes and creation of an artificial vagina. Care is taken to preserve sensory nerves in the area so that the individual may continue to experience sexual stimulation.

Surgical treatment for FTM transgender reassignment is more complex. A mastectomy and sometimes a hysterectomy are performed. A penis and scrotum are constructed from tissues in the genital and abdominal area, the vaginal orifice is closed, and nerves are preserved to maintain sensation. A penile implant is used to attain erection.

Both men and women continue to receive maintenance hormone therapy following surgery. One study reported that after completion of gender reassignment, the satisfaction rate was 87 percent for MTF patients and 97 percent for FTM patients, and suicide rates decreased (Nicholson & McGuiness, 2014). Black and Andreasen (2014) state, "Many patients will continue to benefit from psychotherapy following surgery to assist them in adjusting to their new gender role" (p. 340).

Nursing care of the post-gender-reassignment surgical client is similar to that of most other postsurgical clients. Particular attention is given to maintaining comfort, preventing infection, preserving integrity of the surgical site, maintaining elimination, and meeting nutritional needs. Psychosocial needs may have to do with body image, fears and insecurities about relating to others, and being accepted in the new gender role. Meeting these needs can begin with nursing in a nonthreatening, nonjudgmental, healing atmosphere. For an example of communication that reflects a nonjudgmental, patient-centered approach, see "Real People, Real Stories: Erin."

Real People, Real Stories: Erin

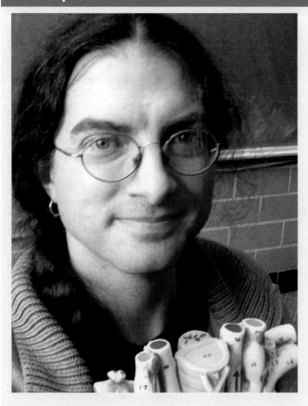

Introduction: Patient-centered care is identified as an important competency for nurses and health-care professionals by the Institute of Medicine's 2003 report. Listening to the patient and his or her identified needs is a key way to develop this competency. Erin's story may not represent the experience of everyone who is transgender, but is presented here as an example of a health-care provider listening and encouraging a client to clarify her needs.

Nurse: Tell me about your background with regard to gender identity.

Erin: I didn't fit in as a boy and knew that, maybe as early as age 6. The only thing I was familiar with was drag queens on television, and they weren't me. Not until college did I recognize this thing called "transgender." In high school, I tried to overcompensate by listening to loud macho music, heavy metal. I had cross-dressed in theater settings but not outside of that.

Nurse: Did you experience any difficulties in school or relationships that were related to your gender identity?

Erin: There was bullying and some violence but not gender-role related, more because I was performing male roles but not very well, and teenagers are morons.

Nurse: What was it like in college after you learned about transgender identity?

Erin: In college was where I found a name for my feelings. I knew that trying to behave as a male was acting, and I didn't want to do that. I started experimenting with going out as a woman on Halloween. I was terrified though. What if I saw someone I knew? How would I explain this costume? What if I got beat up? I had an okay time. I went to a place where I wouldn't be recognized, but I was on guard all night.

Nurse: Did you have any support systems there?

Erin: I sought out safe spaces, largely gay spaces where I could spend some time "out" and figure out who would be safe to "come out" to. The first time I came out to someone not gay or transgender was difficult, and so I laid some hints and groundwork, doing more stereotypical stuff like baking and cooking. When I did formally come out I was very worked up and agitated, but to them it was a nonissue.

Nurse: So your friends were more accepting than you thought they would be! How about your family relationships?

Erin: I was living full time as a woman and attending grad school before I came out to my parents. They are pretty progressive. Dad was a chaplain who worked with AIDS patients early on. I'm not aware of any major conflicts with

Continued

Dad; he might have wanted me to be more athletic but wasn't pushy, and I was an athlete in high school, running cross country and track. Again, I got very worked up, but if there was a negative reaction from them, I never saw it. I have one uncle who is a conservative Christian that I don't talk with much, but there's no overt conflict, just distance. I'm the oldest of three siblings, but my sisters don't live nearby. We're not very close and never have been. I'm closer to my mom than my sisters, and our relationship is okay. I've been enormously fortunate; I am the exception. Some people I know have been kicked out or even had their lives threatened by family members when they came out.

Nurse: What kinds of health care have you sought out related to your gender identity?

Erin: To make the transition more physical, I used "gray market" hormone therapies that I purchased online, in part for fear of expense because endocrinologists and psychologists were required to get the okay for hormone therapy from insurance, and the costs were prohibitive. I didn't have insurance. The hormones were effective but also shot down my libido. I took them for about three years.

Nurse: Have you ever been interested in or explored sexual reassignment surgery?

Erin: Sexual reassignment is not a priority for me, although it's not off the table. I'm ambivalent. I'm not sufficiently dysphoric that I feel like I need major surgeries or major expense.

Nurse: Have you ever sought counseling for mental health concerns?

Erin: I have had counseling on and off for stress and depression related to gender issues but not because I wanted counseling about gender identity. My counseling experiences were helpful in that I learned more effective life skills and coping skills. To find a counselor, I looked for a resource listed in a gay resources guide. With another counseling encounter, I was open during the intake assessment about my gender issues, and they assigned me to someone more familiar with transgender populations. So in general, I've had positive experiences with counseling.

Nurse: Are there any experiences you've had in seeking health care that were not positive?

Erin: I haven't encountered any health professionals who were overtly hostile. Sometimes they were unfamiliar with transgender populations or uncomfortable but not unwilling to work with me. Mostly I've encountered nonverbal signals of discomfort.

Nurse: What do you want or need most from health-care professionals when you seek them out?

Erin: I don't need for someone to know the latest things about reassignment surgery or hormone treatments; that stuff can be looked up. I need honesty about what someone knows or doesn't know and some reassurance that the person is engaged and interested in helping me. Asking about mood, social supports, and coping skills are important screening questions. If someone disrespects me, I would go somewhere else, but I don't ignore my health-care needs because of fear of disrespect or discrimination. I just don't care.

Nurse: That may be a testimony to your self-esteem.

Erin: I've been very fortunate with friends, family, and health-care workers with regard to their response to me, but since I am also somewhat "acting" in my performance as a female and I kind of live somewhere in between genders, some people might be uncomfortable or unfamiliar with that. But I think that that is probably a pretty common experience for transgender individuals.

Nurse: I have been concerned when I've read that there is a high incidence of depression and suicide attempts in transgender individuals. Have you ever struggled with depression or suicidal ideation?

Erin: I've been on antidepressants, and although I have had some decreased sex drive, it's a trade-off I'm willing to take. I have had periods where I didn't want to get out of bed or leave the house and periods in the past where I had suicide ideas but have never attempted. I realized that wasn't where I wanted to be, so I went back to therapy and got back on meds.

Nurse: That's so important! Depression can be a downward spiral, and getting some kind of help before it becomes too severe can be a lifesaving decision.

Sexual Disorders

Paraphilic Disorders

The term *paraphilia* is used to identify repetitive or preferred sexual fantasies or behaviors that involve (1) nonhuman objects, (2) suffering or humiliation of oneself or one's partner, or (3) nonconsenting persons (Black & Andreasen, 2014).

According to the *DSM-5*, a paraphilia is labeled a paraphilic *disorder* only when specific types of sexual fantasies or behaviors are recurrent over a period of at least 6 months and cause the individual clinically significant distress or impairment in social, occupational, or other important areas of functioning (APA, 2013). Many paraphilic behaviors are illegal sex acts, so an individual may come to the attention of legal authorities before he or she is introduced to psychiatric treatment for this disorder. The general prognosis for controlling or curing paraphilias is poor when associated with an early age of onset, high frequency of behaviors, lack of guilt about the act, and substance abuse (Sadock et al., 2015). Nonetheless, Fedoroff (2016) notes that, contrary to popular opinion, when individuals with paraphilic disorders *seek* treatment, outcomes are frequently positive.

Epidemiological Statistics

Relatively limited data exist on the prevalence or course of paraphilic disorders. Most available information has been obtained from studies of incarcerated sex offenders and from outpatient psychiatric services for individuals with paraphilic disorders outside the criminal justice system. Data suggest that most people with paraphilic disorders who seek outpatient treatment do so for pedophilic disorder (45%), exhibitionistic disorder (25%), or voyeuristic disorder (12%).

Most individuals with paraphilic disorders are men, and the behavior is generally established in adolescence (Black & Andreasen, 2014). The behavior peaks between ages 15 and 25 and gradually declines so that, by age 50, the occurrence of paraphilic acts is very low, except for those behaviors that occur in isolation or with a cooperative partner. It is not uncommon for individuals with paraphilias to exhibit multiple paraphilias (APA, 2013).

Types of Paraphilic Disorders

The following types of paraphilic disorders are identified by the *DSM-5:*

Exhibitionistic Disorder

Exhibitionistic disorder is characterized by recurrent and intense sexual arousal (manifested by fantasies, urges, or behaviors of at least 6 months' duration) from the exposure of one's genitals to an unsuspecting individual (APA, 2013). Masturbation may occur during the exhibitionism. In most cases of exhibitionism, the perpetrators are men and the victims are women. Evidence has demonstrated that victims identify several negative outcomes as a consequence of the occurrence, including "feelings of violation, changes in behavior, and even long-term psychological distress" (Clark et al., 2016).

The urges for genital exposure intensify when the exhibitionist has excessive free time or is under significant stress. Most people who engage in exhibitionism have rewarding sexual relationships with adult partners but concomitantly expose themselves to others.

Fetishistic Disorder

Fetishistic disorder involves recurrent and intense sexual arousal (manifested by fantasies, urges, or behaviors of at least 6 months' duration) from the use of either inanimate objects or specific nongenital body part(s) (APA, 2013). A common sexual focus is on objects intimately associated with the human body

(e.g., shoes, gloves, stockings). The fetish object is usually used during masturbation or incorporated into sexual activity with another person in order to produce sexual excitement.

Onset of a fetishistic disorder usually occurs during adolescence. The disorder is chronic, and the complication arises when the individual becomes progressively more intensely aroused by sexual behaviors that exclude a sexual partner. Requirement of the fetish object for sexual arousal may become so intense that to be without it results in impotence. The person with the fetish and his partner may become so distant that the partner eventually terminates the relationship.

Frotteuristic Disorder

Frotteuristic disorder is the recurrent and intense sexual arousal (manifested by urges, behaviors, or fantasies of at least 6 months' duration) involving touching or rubbing against a nonconsenting person (APA, 2013). Sexual excitement is derived from the actual touching or rubbing, not from the coercive nature of the act. Almost without exception, the gender of the frotteur is male.

The individual usually chooses to commit the act in crowded places, such as on buses or subways during rush hour. In this way, he can provide rationalization for his behavior should someone complain and can more easily escape arrest. The frotteur waits in a crowd until he identifies a victim, then he follows her and allows the rush of the crowd to push him against her. He fantasizes a relationship with his victim while rubbing his genitals against her thighs and buttocks or touching her genitalia or breasts with his hands. He often escapes detection because of the victim's initial shock and denial that such an act has been committed in this public place.

Pedophilic Disorder

The essential feature of **pedophilic disorder** is sexual arousal derived from prepubescent or early pubescent children equal to or greater than that derived from physically mature persons. *DSM-5* criteria specify that the behavior has lasted at least 6 months and is manifested by fantasies or sexual urges on which the individual has acted or which cause significant distress or impairment in social, occupational, or other important areas of functioning (APA, 2013). The age of the perpetrator with pedophilic disorder is at least 16 years, and he or she is at least 5 years older than the child victimized. This category of paraphilic disorder is the most common of sexual assaults.

Most child molestations involve genital fondling or oral sex. Vaginal or anal penetration of the child is most common in cases of incest. Sexual abuse of a child may include a wide range of behaviors, including speaking to the child in a sexual manner, indecent exposure and masturbation in the presence of the child, and inappropriate touching or acts of penetration (oral, vaginal, and anal) (King & Regan, 2014). Onset usually occurs during adolescence, and the disorder is often chronic.

Sexual Masochism Disorder

The identifying feature of **sexual masochism disorder** is recurrent and intense sexual arousal (manifested by urges, behaviors, or fantasies of at least 6 months' duration) from the act of being humiliated, beaten, bound, or otherwise made to suffer (APA, 2013). These masochistic activities may be fantasized (e.g., being raped) and may be performed alone (e.g., self-inflicted pain) or with a partner (e.g., being restrained, spanked, or beaten by the partner). Some masochistic activities, particularly those involving sexual arousal by oxygen deprivation, have resulted in death. The disorder is usually chronic and can progress to the point at which the individual cannot achieve sexual satisfaction without masochistic fantasies or activities.

Sexual Sadism Disorder

The *DSM-5* identifies the essential feature of **sexual sadism disorder** as recurrent and intense sexual arousal (manifested by urges, behaviors, or fantasies of at least 6 months' duration) from the physical or psychological suffering of another individual (APA, 2013). The sadistic activities may be fantasized or acted on with a consenting or nonconsenting partner. In all instances, sexual excitation occurs in response to the suffering of the victim. Examples of sadistic acts include restraint, beating, burning, rape, cutting, torture, and even killing.

The course of the disorder is usually chronic, with the severity of the sadistic acts often increasing over time. Activities with nonconsenting partners are usually terminated by legal apprehension.

Transvestic Disorder

Transvestic disorder involves recurrent and intense sexual arousal (as manifested by fantasies, urges, or behaviors of at least 6 months' duration) from dressing in the clothes of the opposite gender. The individual is commonly a heterosexual man who keeps a collection of women's clothing that he intermittently uses to dress in when alone. The sexual arousal may be produced by an accompanying fantasy of the individual as a woman with female genitalia or merely by the view of himself fully clothed as a woman without attention to the genitalia. As with other paraphilias, it is identified as a *disorder* only when these urges and behaviors cause marked distress to the individual or interfere with social, occupational, or other important areas of functioning.

Voyeuristic Disorder

Voyeuristic disorder is identified by recurrent and intense sexual arousal (manifested by urges, behaviors, or fantasies of at least 6 months' duration) involving the act of observing an unsuspecting individual who is naked, in the process of disrobing, or engaging in sexual activity (APA, 2013). Sexual excitement is achieved through the act of looking, and no contact with the person is attempted. Masturbation usually accompanies the "window peeping" but may occur later as the individual fantasizes about the voyeuristic act.

Onset of voyeuristic behavior commonly occurs during adolescence, but the minimum age for a diagnosis of voyeuristic disorder is 18 years (APA, 2013). Many individuals who engage in this behavior enjoy satisfying sexual relationships with an adult partner. Few apprehensions occur because most targets of voyeurism are unaware that they are being observed.

Predisposing Factors to and Theories of Etiology in Paraphilic Disorders

Biological Factors

Many studies have identified biologic abnormalities in individuals with paraphilias. Two common findings are that 74 percent have abnormal hormone levels and 24 percent have chromosomal abnormalities (Sadock et al., 2015). Temporal lobe diseases, such as psychomotor seizures or tumors, have been implicated in some individuals with paraphilic disorder. Abnormal levels of androgens also may contribute to inappropriate sexual arousal. The majority of studies have involved violent sex offenders, and the results cannot accurately be generalized.

Psychoanalytic Theory

The psychoanalytic approach defines an individual with paraphilic disorder as one who has failed the normal developmental process toward heterosexual adjustment (Sadock et al., 2015). This occurs when the individual fails to resolve the Oedipal crisis and either identifies with the parent of the opposite gender or selects an inappropriate object for libido cathexis.

Behavioral Theory

The behavioral model hypothesizes that whether or not an individual engages in paraphilic behavior depends on the type of reinforcement he or she receives following the behavior. The initial act may be committed for various reasons. Some examples include recalling memories of experiences from an individual's early life (especially the first shared sexual experience), modeling behavior of others who have carried out paraphilic acts, mimicking sexual behavior depicted in the media, and recalling past trauma such as one's own molestation (Sadock et al., 2015).

Once the initial act has been committed, the individual with paraphilic disorder consciously evaluates the behavior and decides whether to repeat it. A fear of punishment or perceived harm or injury to the victim, or a lack of pleasure derived from the experience, may extinguish the behavior. However, when negative consequences do not occur, when the act itself is highly pleasurable, or when the person with the paraphilic disorder immediately escapes and thereby avoids seeing any negative consequences experienced by the victim, the activity is more likely to be repeated.

Treatment Modalities for Paraphilic Disorders

Biological Treatment

Biological treatment of individuals with paraphilic disorders has focused on blocking or decreasing the level of circulating androgens. The most extensively used of the antiandrogenic medications are progestin derivatives that block testosterone synthesis or block androgen receptors. They do not influence the direction of sexual drive toward appropriate adult partners. Instead, they act to decrease libido by reducing serum testosterone levels to subnormal concentrations (Sadock et al., 2015). They are not meant to be the sole source of treatment and work best when given in conjunction with participation in individual or group psychotherapy.

Psychoanalytic Therapy

Psychoanalytic approaches have been tried in the treatment of paraphilic disorders. In this type of therapy, the therapist helps the client identify unresolved conflicts and traumas from early childhood. The therapy focuses on helping the individual resolve these early conflicts, thus relieving the anxiety that prevents him or her from forming appropriate sexual relationships. In turn, the individual has no further need for paraphilic fantasies.

Behavioral Therapy

Aversion therapy methods in the treatment of paraphilic disorders involve pairing noxious stimuli, such as electric shocks and bad odors, with the sexual impulse, which then diminishes. Behavioral therapy also includes skills training and cognitive restructuring in an effort to change the individual's maladaptive beliefs.

Other behavioral approaches to decreasing inappropriate sexual arousal have included *imaginal desensitization* and *satiation*. With imaginal desensitization, the client learns how to achieve a state of relaxation while recalling situations that triggered paraphilic behavior with the idea that relaxation will lead to less impulsivity in behavior. Satiation is a technique in which the postorgasmic individual repeatedly fantasizes deviant behaviors to the point of saturation with the deviant stimuli, consequently making the fantasies and behavior unexciting.

Role of the Nurse

Treatment of the person with a paraphilic disorder is often very frustrating for both the client and the therapist. Most individuals with paraphilic disorders deny that they have a problem and seek psychiatric care only after their inappropriate behavior comes to the attention of others. In secondary prevention, the focus is to diagnose and treat the problem as early as possible to minimize difficulties. One role of nurses may involve conducting a sexual history to identify the presence of paraphilic disorders. Developing skill in open, nonjudgmental communication when conducting a sexual history will help nurses assist clients to identify urges and behaviors that cause them distress. Individuals identified as suffering from paraphilic disorders should be referred to specialists who are accustomed to working with this population.

Nurses must also intervene to accomplish primary prevention. The focus of primary prevention in sexual disorders is to identify psychosocial stressors in childhood sexual development in an effort to prevent problems from developing. Again, developing skill in asking questions about sexual thoughts, concerns, and behaviors will enable nurses to provide interventions that encourage adaptive coping with stress and promote healthy sexual development.

Three major components of sexual development have been identified: (1) gender identity (one's sense of maleness or femaleness), (2) sexual responsiveness (arousal to appropriate stimuli), and (3) the ability to establish relationships with others. The questions that are asked in a sexual history collect information about the client's thoughts, feelings, and behaviors in each of these three domains, since distress in these areas may disrupt emotional, mental or behavioral health.

Nurses who work in pediatrics, psychiatry, public health, ambulatory clinics, schools, and any other facility requiring contact with children must be knowledgeable about human sexual development. Accurate assessment and early intervention by these nurses can substantially contribute to primary prevention of sexual disorders.

Sexual Dysfunctions

The Sexual Response Cycle

Because sexual dysfunctions occur as disturbances in any of the phases of the sexual response cycle, an understanding of anatomy and physiology is a prerequisite to considerations of pathology and treatment.

■ **Phase I—Desire:** During this phase, the desire to have sexual activity occurs in response to verbal, physical, or visual stimulation. Sexual fantasies can also bring about this desire.

■ **Phase II—Excitement:** This is the phase of sexual arousal and erotic pleasure. Physiological changes occur. The male responds with penile tumescence and erection. Female changes include vasocongestion in the pelvis, vaginal lubrication, and swelling of the external genitalia.

■ **Phase III—Orgasm:** Orgasm is identified as a peaking of sexual pleasure, with release of sexual tension and rhythmic contraction of the perineal muscles and reproductive organs. Orgasm in women is marked by simultaneous rhythmic contractions of the uterus, the lower third of the vagina, and the anal sphincter. In the man, a forceful emission of semen occurs in response to rhythmic spasms of the prostate, seminal vesicles, vas, and urethra.

■ **Phase IV—Resolution:** If orgasm has occurred, this phase is characterized by disgorgement of blood from the genitalia, creating a sense of general relaxation and well-being. If orgasm is not achieved, resolution may take several hours, producing pelvic discomfort and a feeling of irritability.

After orgasm, men experience a refractory period that may last from a few minutes to many hours, during which time they cannot be stimulated to further orgasm. Commonly, the length of the refractory period increases with age. Because women have no refractory period, they may be capable of multiple and successive orgasms (Sadock et al., 2015).

Historical and Epidemiological Aspects Related to Sexual Dysfunction

Treatments for sexual dysfunction have existed in most cultures throughout history. Meditation, aphrodisiacs, and tonics (primarily alcohol) are just a few of the remedies that have been promoted in the past. Concurrent with the cultural changes occurring during the sexual revolution of the 1960s and 1970s came an increase in scientific research into sexual physiology and sexual dysfunctions. Masters and Johnson (1966; 1970) pioneered this work with their studies on human sexual response and the treatment of sexual dysfunctions. Currently, treatment of sexual dysfunctions has found a place in medicine, with medications, surgeries, and psychological treatments as some of the available options.

Sexual dysfunction consists of an impairment or disturbance in any of the phases of the sexual response cycle. No one knows exactly how many people experience sexual dysfunctions. Knowledge exists only about those who seek some kind of treatment for the problem, and they may be few in number compared with those who have a dysfunction but suffer quietly and never seek therapy.

In 1970, Masters and Johnson reported that 50 percent of all American couples suffered from some type of sexual dysfunction. In 1984, Robins and fellow researchers estimated that 24 percent of the U.S. population would experience a sexual dysfunction at some time in their lives. A 1999 landmark survey (Laumann, Paik, & Rosen, 1999) identified the prevalence of sexual dysfunctions at 43 percent for women and 31 percent for men, highlighting that these dysfunctions are more common than previously thought. Data related to prevalence of sexual problems in the United States based on a more recent survey identified that the most prevalent sexual problems for men were premature ejaculation and erectile difficulties; for women the most prevalent sexual problems were lack of sexual interest and lubrication difficulties (Laumann et al., 2009). This survey included 1491 men and women aged 40 to 80, and a significant finding was that less than 25 percent of the individuals with a sexual problem sought help from a health-care provider.

Types of Sexual Dysfunction
Erectile Disorder

Erectile disorder is characterized by marked difficulty in obtaining or maintaining an erection during sexual activity or a decrease in erectile rigidity that interferes with sexual activity (APA, 2013). The problem persists for at least 6 months and causes the individual significant distress. *Primary erectile disorder* refers to cases in which the man has never been able to have intercourse; *secondary erectile disorder* refers to cases in which the man has difficulty getting or maintaining an erection but has been able to have vaginal or anal intercourse at least once.

Female Orgasmic Disorder

Female orgasmic disorder is defined by the *DSM-5* as a marked delay in or infrequency or absence of orgasm during sexual activity (APA, 2013). It may also be characterized by a reduced intensity of orgasmic sensation. The condition, which is sometimes referred to as **anorgasmia,** has lasted at least 6 months and causes the individual significant distress. Women who can achieve orgasm through noncoital clitoral stimulation but are not able to experience it during coitus in the absence of manual clitoral stimulation are not necessarily categorized as anorgasmic.

A woman is considered to have *primary orgasmic disorder* when she has never experienced orgasm by any kind of stimulation. *Secondary orgasmic disorder* exists if the woman has experienced at least one orgasm, regardless of the means of stimulation, but is no longer able to do so.

Delayed Ejaculation

Delayed ejaculation is characterized by marked delay in ejaculation or marked infrequency or absence of ejaculation during partnered sexual activity (APA, 2013). The condition has lasted for at least 6 months and causes the individual significant distress. With this disorder, the man is unable to ejaculate even though he has a firm erection and has had more than adequate stimulation. The severity of the problem may range from only occasional problems ejaculating *(secondary disorder)* to a history of never having experienced an orgasm *(primary disorder)*. In the most common version, the man cannot ejaculate during coitus but may be able to ejaculate as a result of other types of stimulation.

Premature (Early) Ejaculation

The *DSM-5* describes **premature (early) ejaculation** as persistent or recurrent ejaculation occurring within 1 minute of beginning partnered sexual activity and before the person wishes it to occur (APA, 2013). The condition has lasted at least 6 months and causes the individual significant distress. The diagnosis should take into account factors that affect the duration of the excitement phase, such as the person's age, the novelty of the sexual partner, and frequency of sexual activity (Sadock et al., 2015).

Premature (early) ejaculation is the most common sexual disorder for which men seek treatment. It is particularly common among young men who have a very high sex drive and have not yet learned to control ejaculation.

Female Sexual Interest/Arousal Disorder

This disorder is characterized by a reduced or absent interest or pleasure in sexual activity (APA, 2013). The individual typically does not initiate sexual activity and is commonly unreceptive to partner's attempts to initiate. There is an absence of sexual thoughts or fantasies and absent or reduced arousal in response to sexual or erotic cues. The condition has persisted for at least 6 months and causes the individual significant distress.

Male Hypoactive Sexual Desire Disorder

This disorder is defined by the *DSM-5* as a persistent or recurrent deficiency or absence of sexual fantasies and desire for sexual activity. In making the judgment of deficiency or absence, the clinician considers factors that affect sexual functioning, such as age and life circumstances (APA, 2013). The condition has persisted for at least 6 months and causes the individual significant distress.

An individual's absolute level of sexual desire may not be the problem; rather, the problem may be a discrepancy between the partners' levels of desire. Conflict may occur if one partner wants to have sexual relations more often than the other does. Care must be taken not to label one partner as pathological when the problem actually lies in the conflicting desire levels.

Genito-Pelvic Pain/Penetration Disorder

With this disorder, the individual experiences considerable difficulty with vaginal intercourse and attempts at penetration. Pain is felt in the vagina, around the vaginal entrance and clitoris, or deep in the pelvis. Fear and anxiety are associated with anticipation of pain or vaginal penetration. A tensing and tightening of the pelvic floor muscles occurs during attempted penetration (APA, 2013). The condition may be *lifelong* (present since the individual became sexually active) or *acquired* (began after a period of relatively normal sexual function). It has persisted for at least 6 months and causes the individual clinically significant distress.

Substance/Medication-Induced Sexual Dysfunction

With these disorders, the sexual dysfunction developed after substance intoxication or withdrawal or after exposure to a medication (APA, 2013). The dysfunction may involve pain, impaired desire, impaired arousal, or impaired orgasm. Some substances and medications that can interfere with sexual functioning include alcohol, amphetamines, cocaine, opioids, sedatives, hypnotics, anxiolytics, antidepressants, antipsychotics, and antihypertensives, among others.

Predisposing Factors to Sexual Dysfunction

Biological Factors

Sexual Desire Disorders Studies have correlated decreased levels of serum testosterone with hypoactive sexual desire disorder in men. Evidence also suggests a relationship between serum testosterone and increased female libido (Sadock et al., 2015). Diminished libido has been observed in both men and women with elevated levels of serum prolactin (Wisse, 2015). Various medications have been implicated in the etiology of hypoactive sexual desire disorder, including antihypertensives, antipsychotics, antidepressants, anxiolytics, and anticonvulsants. Alcohol and cocaine have also been associated with impaired desire, especially after chronic use. In 2015, the FDA approved the first drug for treatment of hypoactive sexual desire disorder in premenopausal women. This medication, flibanserin (Addyi), is a nonhormonal serotonin agonist and antagonist.

Sexual Arousal Disorders A decrease in estrogen levels when women are postpartum, postmenopausal, or receiving gonadotrophin-releasing hormone agonists may prohibit the vasocongestion and vaginal lubrication needed for painless intercourse. This may lead to decreased sexual desire (Basson, 2016; Kingsberg & Krychman, 2016). Various medications, particularly those with antihistaminic and anticholinergic properties, may also contribute to decreased ability for arousal in women.

Arteriosclerosis is a common cause of male erectile disorder as a result of arterial insufficiency (King & Regan, 2014). Various neurological disorders can contribute to erectile dysfunction as well. The most common neurologically based cause may be diabetes, which places men at high risk for neuropathy (Kim & Brosman, 2013). Other potential neurological causes include temporal lobe epilepsy and multiple sclerosis. Trauma (e.g., spinal cord injury, pelvic cancer surgery) can also result in erectile disorder. Several medications have been implicated in the etiology of this disorder, including antihypertensives, antipsychotics, antidepressants, and anxiolytics. Chronic use of alcohol has also been shown to be a contributing factor.

Orgasmic Disorders Some women report decreased ability to achieve orgasm following hysterectomy. Conversely, some report increased sexual activity and decreased sexual dysfunction following hysterectomy. Some medications (e.g., selective serotonin reuptake inhibitors [SSRIs]) may inhibit orgasm. Medical conditions such as depressive disorders, hypothyroidism, and diabetes mellitus may cause decreased sexual arousal and orgasm.

Biological factors associated with delayed male orgasm include surgery of the genitourinary tract (e.g., prostatectomy), neurological disorders (e.g., Parkinson's disease), and other diseases (e.g., diabetes mellitus). Medications that have been implicated include opioids, antihypertensives, antidepressants, and antipsychotics. Transient cases of the disorder may occur with excessive alcohol intake.

Although early ejaculation is commonly caused by psychological factors, general medical conditions or substance use may also be contributing influences. Physical factors are often involved in cases of secondary dysfunction. Examples include a local infection, such as prostatitis, or a degenerative neural disorder, such as multiple sclerosis.

Sexual Pain Disorders A number of organic factors can contribute to painful intercourse in women, including intact hymen, episiotomy scar, vaginal or urinary tract infection, ligament injuries, endometriosis, or ovarian cysts or tumors. Painful intercourse in men may also be caused by various organic factors. For example, infection caused by poor hygiene under the foreskin of an uncircumcised man can cause pain. Phimosis, a condition in which the foreskin cannot be pulled back, can also cause painful intercourse. An allergic reaction to various vaginal spermicides or irritation caused by vaginal infections may be a contributing factor. Finally, various prostate problems may cause pain on ejaculation.

Psychosocial Factors

Sexual Desire Disorders A variety of individual and relationship factors may contribute to hypoactive sexual desire disorder. Individual factors include fears associated with sex; history of sexual abuse and trauma; chronic stress, anxiety, depression; and aging-related concerns (e.g., changes in physical appearance). Among the relationship causes are interpersonal conflicts; current physical, verbal, or sexual abuse; extramarital affairs; and desire or practices that differ from those of one's partner. In general, the presence of sexual desire is influenced by sexual drives, self-esteem, accepting oneself as a sexual person, good stress management, and good relationship skills; disruption in any of these areas can contribute to lower desire (Sadock et al., 2015).

Sexual Arousal Disorders A number of psychological factors have been cited as possible impediments to female arousal. They include doubt, guilt, fear, anxiety, shame, conflict, embarrassment, tension, disgust, irritation, resentment, grief, hostility toward partner, and a puritanical or moralistic upbringing. Sexual abuse has been identified as a significant risk factor for desire and arousal disorders in women.

Problems with male sexual arousal may be related to chronic stress, anxiety, or depression. Developmental factors that hinder the ability to be intimate, that lead to a feeling of inadequacy or distrust, or that develop a sense of being unloving or unlovable may also result in impotence. Relationship factors that may affect erectile functioning include lack of attraction to one's partner, anger toward one's partner, or being in a relationship that is not characterized by trust. Regardless of the etiology of the erectile dysfunction, once it occurs the man may become increasingly anxious about his next sexual encounter. This anticipatory anxiety about achieving and maintaining an erection may then perpetuate the problem.

Orgasmic Disorders Numerous psychological factors are associated with inhibited female orgasm. They include fears of becoming pregnant or damage to the vagina, rejection by the sexual partner, hostility toward men, and feelings of guilt regarding sexual impulses (Sadock et al., 2015). Various developmental factors may also have relevance to orgasmic dysfunction. Examples include negative messages about sexuality from family; religion and culture; unwanted sexual experiences; or punishment for childhood sexual experimentation (Donahey, 2016).

Psychological factors are also associated with inhibited male orgasm (delayed ejaculation). In the primary disorder (in which the man has never experienced orgasm), the man often comes from a rigid, puritanical background. He perceives sex as sinful and the genitals as dirty, and he may have conscious or unconscious incest wishes and associated guilt (Sadock et al., 2015). In the case of secondary disorder (previously experienced orgasms that have now stopped), interpersonal difficulties are usually implicated. There may be some ambivalence about commitment, fear of pregnancy, or unexpressed hostility.

Premature ejaculation may be related to a lack of physical awareness on the part of a sexually inexperienced man. The ability to control ejaculation occurs as a gradual maturing process with a sexual partner in which foreplay becomes more give-and-take "pleasuring" rather than strictly goal-oriented. The man becomes aware of the sensations and learns to delay the point of ejaculatory inevitability. Relationship problems, negative cultural conditioning, anxiety over intimacy, and lack of comfort in the sexual relationship may also contribute to this disorder.

Sexual Pain Disorders Penetration disorders may occur in response to genito-pelvic pain experienced for various organic reasons stated in the "Biological Factors" section. Involuntary constriction within the vagina occurs in response to anticipatory pain, making intercourse difficult or impossible. The diagnosis does not apply if the etiology is determined to be due to another medical condition.

A variety of psychosocial factors have been identified in clients with sexual pain disorder. Clinicians report that frequently an individual with this disorder has been raised in a strict religious environment where sex was associated with sin (Sadock et al., 2015). Early traumatic sexual experiences (e.g., rape or incest) may also contribute to penetration disorder. Other etiological factors that may be important include painful childhood experiences with surgical, dental, or pelvic examination; phobias associated with pregnancy, STIs, or cancer; and catastrophizing or fear of pain (Bergeron, Rosen, & Corsini-Munt, 2016; King & Regan 2014; Sadock et al., 2015).

Application of the Nursing Process to Sexual Disorders

Assessment

Most assessment tools for taking a general nursing history contain some questions devoted to sexuality. Nurses may feel uncomfortable obtaining information about this subject. However, accurate data must be collected if problems are to be identified and resolutions attempted. Sexual health is an integral part of physical and emotional well-being. The nursing history is incomplete if items directed toward sexuality are not included.

Most nurses are not required to obtain a sexual history as in depth as the one presented in this chapter. However, for certain clients, a more extensive sexual history is required, including those who have medical or surgical conditions that may affect their sexuality; clients with infertility problems, STIs, or complaints of sexual inadequacy; clients who are pregnant or have gynecological problems; those seeking information on abortion or family planning; and individuals in premarital, marital, and psychiatric counseling.

The best approach for taking a sexual history is a nondirective one, meaning it is best to use the sexual history outline as a guideline but allow the interview to progress in a natural, less restrictive manner. The order of the questions should be adjusted according to the client's needs as identified during the interview. A nondirective approach allows time for the client to interject information related to feelings or concerns about his or her sexuality.

The language used should be understandable to the client. If he or she uses terminology that is unfamiliar, ask for clarification. Take level of education and cultural influences into consideration. Hispanic and Indian clients, for example, tend to be reluctant to talk about sexual matters and may feel more comfortable with a nurse of the same sex. In some cultures (such as Hispanic, Pakistani, and Arabic), discussing sexual matters with a male child requires the father rather than the mother to be present (Giger, 2017).

The nurse's attitude must convey warmth, openness, honesty, and objectivity. Personal feelings, attitudes, and values should be clarified and should not interfere with acceptance of the client. The nurse must remain nonjudgmental, which is conveyed by listening in an interested, matter-of-fact manner without overreacting to any information the client may present.

The content outline for a sexual history presented in Box 30–2 is not intended to be used as a rigid questionnaire but as a guideline from which the nurse may select appropriate topics for gathering information about the client's sexuality. The outline should be individualized according to client needs.

BOX 30-2 Sexual History Outline

The questions in this outline are a guide to identify issues that require further assessment and should not necessarily be followed in a rigid order. Rather, they provide a foundation for exploration of sexual health concerns in the context of a therapeutic nurse–client relationship.

The nurse initiates this assessment by

1. Acknowledging that he or she will be asking very personal questions about sexual health and activities.
2. Stating that the reason for asking these questions is to assist with any sexual health issues or concerns the patient may have.

PRESENT CONCERNS

Are there any specific concerns about sexuality or sexual health that you would like to discuss? If so, tell me more about these concerns.

GENERAL ASSESSMENT

Are you currently sexually active?

If no, have you ever been sexually active?

If yes, when was your last sexual encounter?

For Women

Contraceptive use? Presently? If so, for how long? If in the past, what were the dates?

Is there any possibility that you might now be pregnant?

Previous pregnancies? Any problems associated with pregnancies or childbirth?

When was your last menstrual period? Regular/irregular? Pain or heavy bleeding? Bleeding between periods?

SEXUAL HEALTH AND RISKS FOR SEXUALLY TRANSMITTED INFECTIONS (STIS)

Partners

How many sexual partners have you had within the last 12 months?

What are the gender(s) of your sexual partners within the last 12 months?

If you had only one partner, what was the length of the relationship?

If you had multiple partners, what was the history of encounters with past partners, drug use, condom use, safety considerations?

Practices

What kinds of sexual activities do you participate in? Genital? Anal? Oral?

Do you use any forms of protection against STIs? How often? What kinds?

Past History

Have you ever been diagnosed with an STI?

If so, how was it treated? Have you had any recurrent symptoms?

Have any current or past partners been diagnosed with an STI?

If so, were you tested for the same STIs?

Have you ever been tested for HIV?

Symptoms

Have you been aware of any painful urination, discharge, itching, swelling, pain, or skin changes on or around genitalia?

Do you have any other symptoms of concern, such as pain, rashes, or any other symptoms we haven't yet discussed?

HISTORY OF SEXUAL TRAUMA

Have any of your sexual encounters, past or present, been nonconsensual?

If so, please share whatever you feel comfortable telling me about this history.

Do you have any current concerns for your safety or well-being?

SEXUAL DYSFUNCTIONS

What medications are you currently taking, including over-the-counter and herbal remedies?

Are you aware of any changes in sexual function or desire since you began taking any of these medications?

What surgeries, medical treatments, or illnesses have you had?

Are you aware of any changes in sexual function or desire as a result of these?

How would you describe your level of satisfaction with your sexual responsiveness and sexual relationships?

Is sexual activity ever the source of pain, discomfort, or bleeding?

OTHER CONCERNS

Are there any other practices, urges, or concerns about sexuality or sexual health that you would like to discuss?

Adapted from Centers for Disease Control (CDC). (2011a). A guide to taking a sexual history [CDC Publication: 99-8445]. Retrieved from https://www.cdc. gov/std/treatment/sexualhistory.pdf

Diagnosis and Outcome Identification

Nursing diagnoses are formulated from data gathered during the assessment phase and with background knowledge regarding predisposing factors to the disorder. The following nursing diagnoses may be used for the client with sexual disorders:

■ Sexual dysfunction related to depression and conflict in relationship or certain biological or psychological contributing factors to the disorder, evidenced by loss of sexual desire or ability to perform.

■ Ineffective sexuality pattern related to conflicts with sexual orientation or variant preferences, evidenced by expressed dissatisfaction with sexual behaviors.

Outcome Criteria

The following criteria may be used for measurement of outcomes in the care of the client with sexual disorders.

The client:

- Correlates stressful situations that decrease sexual desire
- Communicates with partner about sexual situation without discomfort
- Verbalizes ways to enhance sexual desire
- Verbalizes resumption of sexual activity at level satisfactory to self and partner
- Correlates variant behaviors with times of stress
- Verbalizes fears about abnormality and inappropriateness of sexual behaviors
- Expresses desire to change variant sexual behavior
- Participates and cooperates with extended plan of behavior modification
- Expresses satisfaction with own sexuality pattern

Planning and Implementation

Table 30–3 provides a plan of care for the client with sexual disorders. Nursing diagnoses are presented, along with outcome criteria, appropriate nursing interventions, and rationales.

Concept Care Mapping

The concept map care plan is an innovative approach to planning and organizing nursing care (see Chapter 9, The Nursing Process in Psychiatric-Mental Health Nursing). It is a diagrammatic teaching and learning strategy that allows visualization of interrelationships between medical diagnoses, nursing diagnoses, assessment data, and treatments. An example of a concept map care plan for a client with a sexual disorder is presented in Figure 30–1.

Client and Family Education

The role of client teacher is important in the psychiatric area, as it is in all areas of nursing. A list of topics for client and family education relevant to sexual disorders is presented in Box 30–3.

Evaluation

Reassessment is necessary to determine whether selected interventions have been successful in helping the client overcome problems with sexual functioning.

Table 30–3 | CARE PLAN FOR THE CLIENT WITH A SEXUAL DISORDER

NURSING DIAGNOSIS: SEXUAL DYSFUNCTION

RELATED TO: Depression and conflict in relationship; biological or psychological contributing factors to the disorder

EVIDENCED BY: Loss of sexual desire or ability to perform

OUTCOME CRITERIA	NURSING INTERVENTIONS	RATIONALE
Short-Term Goals • Client will identify stressors that may contribute to loss of sexual function within 1 week. *OR* • Client will discuss pathophysiology of disease process that contributes to sexual dysfunction within 1 week. • *(For a client with permanent dysfunction due to disease process)* Client will verbalize willingness to seek professional assistance from a sex therapist to learn alternative ways of achieving sexual satisfaction with partner by [time is individually determined]. Long-Term Goal • Client will resume sexual activity at a level satisfactory to self and partner by [time is individually determined].	1. Assess client's sexual history and previous level of satisfaction in sexual relationship. 2. Assess client's perception of the problem. 3. Help client determine time dimension associated with onset of the problem, and discuss what was happening in life situation at that time. 4. Assess client's mood and level of energy. 5. Review medication regimen; observe for side effects.	1. Client history establishes a database from which to work and provides a foundation for goal setting. 2. Client's idea of what constitutes a problem may differ from that of the nurse. It is the client's perception on which the goals of care must be established. 3. Stress in all areas of life will affect sexual functioning. Client may be unaware of correlation between stress and sexual dysfunction. 4. Depression and fatigue decrease client's desire and enthusiasm for participation in sexual activity. 5. Many medications can affect sexual functioning. Evaluation of drug and individual response is important to ascertain whether drug is responsible for the problem.

Continued

Table 30–3 | CARE PLAN FOR THE CLIENT WITH A SEXUAL DISORDER—cont'd

OUTCOME CRITERIA	NURSING INTERVENTIONS	RATIONALE
	6. Encourage client to discuss the disease process that may be contributing to sexual dysfunction. Ensure that client is aware that alternative methods of achieving sexual satisfaction exist and can be learned through sex counseling if he or she and the partner desire to do so.	6. Client may be unaware of alternatives, leading to feelings of hopelessness about current situation. Education regarding various available options may increase feelings of self-worth and offer hope for the future.
	7. Provide information regarding sexuality and sexual functioning.	7. Increasing knowledge and correcting misconceptions can decrease feelings of powerlessness and anxiety and facilitate problem resolution.
	8. Refer for additional counseling or sex therapy if required.	8. Client and partner may need additional or more in-depth assistance if problems in sexual relationship are severe or remain unresolved.

NURSING DIAGNOSIS: INEFFECTIVE SEXUALITY PATTERN

RELATED TO: Conflicts with sexual orientation or variant preferences

EVIDENCED BY: Expressed dissatisfaction with sexual behaviors (e.g., voyeurism; transvestism)

OUTCOME CRITERIA	NURSING INTERVENTIONS	RATIONALE
Short-Term Goals • Client will verbalize aspects about sexuality that he or she would like to change. • Client and partner will communicate with each other ways in which each believes their sexual relationship could be improved. Long-Term Goals • Client will express satisfaction with own sexuality pattern. • Client and partner will express satisfaction with the sexual relationship.	1. Take sexual history, noting client's expression of areas of dissatisfaction with sexual pattern.	1. Knowledge of what client perceives as the problem is essential for providing the type of assistance he or she may need.
	2. Assess areas of stress in client's life, and examine relationship with sexual partner.	2. Variant sexual behaviors are often associated with added stress in client's life. The relationship with his or her partner may deteriorate as the individual eventually gains sexual satisfaction only from variant practices.
	3. Note cultural, social, ethnic, racial, and religious factors that may contribute to conflicts regarding variant sexual practices.	3. Client may be unaware of the influence these factors exert in creating feelings of discomfort, shame, and guilt regarding sexual attitudes and behavior.
	4. Be accepting and nonjudgmental.	4. Sexuality is a very personal and sensitive subject. Client is more likely to share this information if he or she does not fear being judged by the nurse.
	5. Assist therapist in a plan of behavior modification to help client who desires to decrease variant sexual behaviors.	5. Individuals with paraphilic disorders are treated by specialists who have experience in modifying variant sexual behaviors. Nurses can

Table 30–3 | CARE PLAN FOR THE CLIENT WITH A SEXUAL DISORDER–cont'd

OUTCOME CRITERIA	NURSING INTERVENTIONS	RATIONALE
		intervene by providing assistance with implementation of the plan for behavior modification.
	6. If altered sexuality patterns are related to illness or medical treatment, provide information to client and partner regarding correlation between the illness and the sexual alteration. Explain possible modifications in usual sexual pattern that client and partner may try in an effort to achieve a satisfying sexual experience despite the limitation.	6. Client and his or her partner may be unaware of alternative possibilities for achieving sexual satisfaction, or anxiety associated with the limitation may interfere with rational problem-solving.
	7. Teach client that sexuality is a normal human response and is not synonymous with any one sexual act; that it reflects the totality of the person and does not relate exclusively to sex organs or sexual behavior. Client must understand that *sexual* feelings are *human* feelings.	7. If client feels abnormal or unlike everyone else, self-concept is likely to be very low—even worthless. Helping client to understand that, even though the behavior is variant, the feelings and motivations are common, may help to increase feelings of self-worth and desire to change behavior.

Evaluation may be facilitated by gathering information using the following types of questions.

For the client with sexual dysfunction:

■ Has the client identified life situations that promote feelings of depression and decreased sexual desire?
■ Can he or she verbalize ways to deal with this stress?
■ Can the client satisfactorily communicate with sexual partner about the problem?
■ Have the client and sexual partner identified ways to enhance sexual desire and the achievement of sexual satisfaction for both?
■ Are the client and partner seeking assistance with relationship conflict?
■ Do both partners agree on what the major problem is? Do they have the motivation to attempt change?
■ Do the client and partner verbalize an increase in sexual satisfaction?

For the client with variant sexual behaviors:

■ Can the client correlate an increase in variant sexual behavior to times of severe stress?
■ Has the client been able to identify those stressful situations and verbalize alternative ways to deal with them?

■ Does the client express a desire to change variant sexual behavior and a willingness to cooperate with extended therapy to do so?
■ Does the client express an understanding about the normalcy of sexual feelings, aside from the inappropriateness of his or her behavior?
■ Are expressions of increased self-worth evident?

Treatment Modalities for Sexual Dysfunctions

Sexual Desire Disorders

Hypoactive Sexual Desire Disorder

Hypoactive sexual desire disorder has been treated in both men and women with the administration of testosterone. The masculinizing side effects make this approach unacceptable to women, and the evidence that it increases libido in men is inconclusive. In 2015, the FDA approved the first treatment specifically for sexual desire disorder in premenopausal women. The medication, flibanserin (Addyi), is a serotonin receptor agonist, but how it works to improve sexual desire is unknown (FDA, 2015). This drug has also been associated with severe hypotension and syncope and can be particularly serious in patients who drink alcohol during treatment. For these reasons, it carries a black

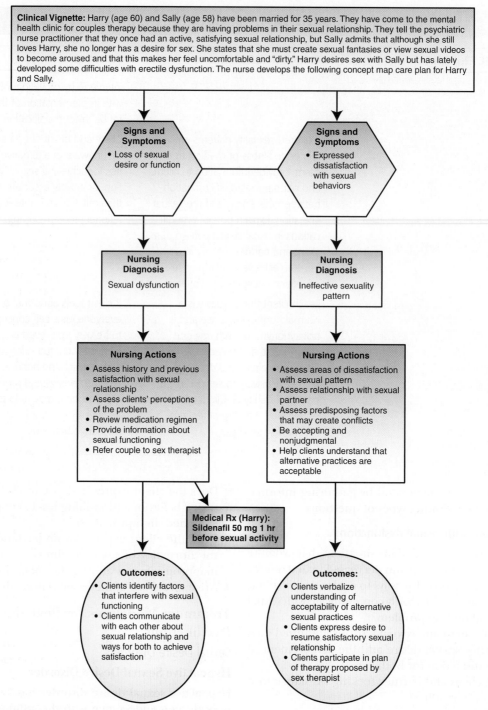

FIGURE 30–1 Concept map care plan for clients with sexual disorders.

box warning and may be prescribed only by practitioners who are certified to prescribe this medication. Basson (2016) identifies mental and relationship health as major factors determining sexual desire. Cognitive behavior therapy to identify and correct maladaptive thoughts and behaviors along with relationship therapy to improve communication and relationship skills have both been identified as effective psychological interventions.

If partner incompatibility is the suspected cause of hypoactive sexual desire disorder, the therapist may choose to shift from dealing with the sexual issue to helping a couple identify and deal with their incompatibility. Examples of incompatibility may include different preferences for type, amount, or frequency of sexual activities as well as conflicts around the emotional and physical expectations associated with sex.

Sexual Arousal Disorders

Female Sexual Interest/Arousal Disorder

The goal of treatment for female sexual interest/arousal disorder is to reduce the anxiety associated with sexual activity. Masters and Johnson (1970) reported successful results using their behaviorally oriented **sensate focus** exercises to treat this disorder. These exercises strive to reduce the goal-oriented demands of intercourse on both men and women, thus reducing performance pressures and anxiety associated with possible failure. The exercises include touching activities that initially exclude genital stimulation in order to increase comfort with physical intimacy and reduce anxiety associated with sexual performance.

The couple is instructed to take turns caressing each other's bodies. Initially, they are to avoid touching breasts and genitals and to focus on the sensations of being touched. The caressing progresses to include touching of the breasts and genitals, to touching each other simultaneously, and eventually to include intercourse. These non-goal-oriented exercises promote the sensual side of sexual interaction in a nonpressured, nonevaluative way (Masters et al., 1995).

Erectile Disorder

Sensate focus has also been used effectively for erectile disorder in men. Clinicians widely agree that even when significant organic factors have been identified, psychological factors may also be present and must be considered in treatment. The general public and the medical community agree that organic causes should be ruled out first, but nonetheless, biological factors influence a man's psychological state and psychosocial factors affect physiology (Levine, 2016). Not surprisingly, several studies support the benefits of combination medical and psychological therapy (Althof & Rosen, 2010). Group therapy, individual therapy, psychoeducation, and self-instruction manuals with telephone assistance from a therapist are some of the psychological interventions that have been used successfully in reducing the anxiety that may contribute to erectile difficulties. These studies demonstrated the added benefit of decreasing discontinuation rates and increasing sexual satisfaction compared to medical interventions alone.

Several medications have been approved by the FDA for the treatment of erectile disorder. They include avanafil (Stendra), sildenafil (Viagra), tadalafil (Cialis), and vardenafil (Levitra, Staxyn). These newer impotence agents block the action of phosphodiesterase-5 (PDE5), an enzyme that breaks down cyclic guanosine monophosphate, a compound required to produce an erection. This action only occurs, however, in the presence of nitric oxide, which is released during sexual arousal. PDE5 inhibitors do not result in sexual arousal. They work to achieve penile erection in the presence of sexual arousal. Adverse effects may include headache, facial flushing, indigestion, nasal congestion, dizziness, and visual changes (mild color tinges and blurred vision) (Vallerand, Sanoski, & Deglin, 2016).

In 2005, the FDA ordered that the manufacturers of these medications add a warning to their labels. This action was taken in response to 43 cases of sudden vision loss by individuals taking the drugs. It is not possible to ascertain whether the medications are responsible for nonarteritic ischemic optic neuropathy, a condition in which blood flow to the optic nerve is blocked. More recently, the FDA has issued an additional warning associated with PDE5, the risk of sudden hearing loss (Kim & Brosman, 2013). PDE5 inhibitors are contraindicated in concurrent use with nitrates. In 2016, the FDA identified an emerging trend in which many over-the-counter products, often marketed as dietary supplements for sexual enhancement or improved energy, were found to have sildenafil or sildenafil-like ingredients as well as controlled substances and other untested active ingredients. In the first 9 months of 2016, the FDA issued public notifications for more than 30 such products (a fraction of the number of products on the market) with warnings about potential dangers and drug interactions (FDA, 2017).

Yohimbine is a natural remedy used to treat erectile dysfunction and as such is not subject to FDA guidelines for medicines. Effectiveness does not necessarily equate with safety, so caution is advised when using such alternative medicines. Excessive doses can cause significant toxicity, and concomitant use with foods containing tyramine can lead to hypertensive crisis (Vallerand, Sanosky, & Deglin, 2016).

Althof and Rosen (2010) report that 90 percent of men with erectile dysfunction are being treated with PDE5 inhibitors, and the remaining 10 percent are treated with intraurethral suppositories; intra-cavernossal injections (both prostaglandin preparations); combination drugs that include papaverine phentolamine, and alprostadil vacuum tumescence therapy; and/or penile prosthesis surgery. Penile prostheses are usually reserved for erectile disorders that have not responded to other treatments. Two basic types are currently available: a bendable silicone implant and an inflatable device. The bendable variety requires a relatively simple surgical technique for insertion of silicone rods into the erectile areas of the penis. This results in a perpetual state of semierection for the client. The inflatable penile prosthesis produces an erection only when desired, and the appearance of the penis in both the flaccid and erect states is completely normal. Potential candidates for penile implantation should undergo careful psychological and physical screening. Although penile implants do not enable the client to recover the ability to ejaculate or to have an orgasm, men with prosthetic devices have generally reported satisfaction with their subsequent sexual functioning.

Orgasmic Disorders

Female Orgasmic Disorder

Many substances affect sexual function and the achievement of orgasm, so a thorough assessment for smoking, alcohol use, recreational drug use, and prescription medication is critical to effective treatment of female orgasmic disorder. Antidepressants, particularly SSRIs, can adversely affect orgasmic responsiveness, so treatment may include changes to the prescription drug regimen (Donahey, 2016).

Because anxiety may contribute to the lack of orgasmic ability in women, sensate focus is often advised to reduce anxiety, increase awareness of physical sensations, and transfer communication skills from the verbal to the nonverbal domain. Other therapeutic techniques include directed masturbation, vibrator use, bibliotherapy, communication skills training, visualization, and Kegel exercises (Donahey, 2016).

Treatment for secondary anorgasmia (in which the client has had orgasms in the past but is now unable to achieve them) focuses on the couple and their relationship. Therapy with both partners is essential to successful treatment of this disorder.

Delayed Ejaculation

Treatment for delayed ejaculation is very similar to that described for the anorgasmic woman. A combination of sensate focus and masturbatory training has been used with a high degree of success in the Masters and Johnson clinic. Treatment for male orgasmic disorder almost always includes the sexual partner.

Early Ejaculation

Masters and associates (1995) advocate what they suggest is a highly successful technique for the treatment of early ejaculation. Sensate focus is used with progression to genital stimulation. When the man reaches the point of imminent ejaculation, the woman is instructed to apply the "squeeze" technique: applying pressure at the base of the glans penis with her thumb and first two fingers. Pressure is held for about 4 seconds and then released. This technique is continued until the man is no longer on the verge of ejaculating. This technique is practiced during subsequent periods of sexual stimulation. Many other psychological therapies have been advanced as beneficial for treating early ejaculation, but the squeeze method is the only one with demonstrated evidence of effectiveness. However, even this treatment's effectiveness appears to be short term (Waldinger, 2016).

No medication has been approved by the FDA for the treatment of early ejaculation, but a number of studies have shown efficacy for this disorder with SSRIs (Benson et al., 2013). Some individuals may achieve positive results with single dosing prior to sexual relations, whereas others may require regular daily dosing to achieve an adequate blood level.

Genito-Pelvic Pain/Penetration Disorder

Treatment for painful intercourse begins with a thorough physical and gynecological examination. When organic pathology has been eliminated, the client's fears and anxieties underlying sexual functioning are investigated. Systematic desensitization has been used successfully to decrease fears and anxieties associated with painful intercourse.

Treatment of penetration disorder begins with education of the woman and her sexual partner regarding the anatomy and physiology of the disorder (i.e., what exactly is occurring during the vaginal reflex and possible etiologies). The involuntary nature of the disorder is stressed in an effort to alleviate the sexual partner's perception that this occurrence is an act of willful withholding by the woman.

Psychological treatment options with evidence of effectiveness include intensive exposure therapy, cognitive-behavioral therapy (CBT), and biofeedback (Bergeron et al., 2016). Bergeron and associates (2016) also report that in a 2.5-year follow-up study, CBT was equal over time to surgical interventions in alleviating pain during intercourse, according to client self-reports. In general, they recommended a multidisciplinary treatment approach for these disorders but note that, on the basis of the effectiveness of CBT, surgical interventions might be avoidable.

In systematic desensitization, the client is taught a series of tensing and relaxing exercises aimed at relaxation of pelvic musculature. This is followed by a procedure involving the systematic insertion of dilators of graduated sizes until the woman is able to accept the penis into the vagina without discomfort.

CASE STUDY AND SAMPLE CARE PLAN

NURSING HISTORY AND ASSESSMENT

Emma's obstetrician/gynecologist (OB/GYN) has referred her to the mental health clinic with a diagnosis of postpartum depression. Emma (age 30) tells Carol, the psychiatric nurse practitioner, that she and her husband Brett (age 32) have been married for 2 years and that she gave birth 4 months ago to their first child, a boy they named Jason. Jason has been a difficult baby, was diagnosed with colic, and is wakeful and cries much of the time. Emma is sleep deprived and continuously fatigued. Emma states, "I'm not depressed. I'm just exhausted! Brett is a computer analyst and is gone from home about 10 hours a day. When he gets home, we do what we can to put some dinner together and take care of Jason at the same time. By 9 o'clock, I'm ready to collapse, and Brett wants to go to bed and make love. I just don't have the energy. It's starting to cause a lot of friction in our marriage. Brett gets so angry when I refuse his advances. He also gets angry when I passively comply with his advances. To be honest, I'm just not interested in sex anymore. I certainly don't want to risk another pregnancy. But I also don't want to risk losing my husband. We used to have such a great sexual relationship, but that seems like a lifetime ago. I don't know what to do!"

NURSING DIAGNOSIS AND OUTCOME IDENTIFICATION

From the assessment data, the nurse develops the following nursing diagnosis for Emma: **Sexual dysfunction** related to extreme fatigue and depressed mood, evidenced by loss of sexual desire.

a. **Short-term goals:**
   ■ Client will identify ways to receive respite from child care.
   ■ Client will identify ways to devote time to regain satisfactory sexual relationship with husband.
b. **Long-term goal:**
   ■ Client will resume sexual activity at a level satisfactory to herself and her husband.

PLANNING AND IMPLEMENTATION

SEXUAL DYSFUNCTION
The following nursing interventions have been identified for Emma:

1. Take Emma's sexual history.
2. Determine the previous level of satisfaction in current sexual relationship.
3. Assess Emma's perception of the problem.
4. Suggest alternative strategies for resolution of the problem. (Because of Emma's fatigue and mild depression, she may not be able to adequately problem-solve the situation without assistance.)
   a. Respite from child care (e.g., babysitting service, Mom's Day Out program, sharing babysitting with other mothers or grandparents).
   b. Schedule regular "date nights" with husband.
   c. Schedule periodic weekends away with husband.
5. Provide information regarding sexuality and sexual functioning.
6. Discuss with Emma her fear of pregnancy. Provide information about various methods of contraception.
7. Make referral to sex therapist if Emma requests this service.

EVALUATION
The outcome criteria for Emma have been met. She was able to identify ways to receive respite from child care. She takes Jason to Mom's Day Out at her church every Friday morning. She now has an agreement with another new mother to trade one afternoon a week of babysitting duties. She inquired at the local community college in the department of early childhood education for names of students who would be interested in babysitting. Gina, a 19-year-old sophomore at the college, now babysits for Emma and Brett every Wednesday evening while they have a "date night." And one weekend a month, Brett's widowed mother stays with Jason while Emma and Brett have time away together. Emma's OB/GYN prescribed oral contraceptives, and Emma's fear of pregnancy has subsided. Her mood has lifted and she looks forward to her free time and time alone with her husband. She reports that her sexual desire has increased and that she and Brett now enjoy a satisfactory sexual relationship. She also states that she feels she is giving more quality care to Jason now that she has the periods of respite to which she looks forward every week.

Summary and Key Points

- Human sexuality influences all aspects of physical and mental health. Clients are becoming more open to discussing matters pertaining to sexuality, and it is therefore important for nurses to integrate information on sexuality into the care they give. This can be done by focusing on preventive, therapeutic, and educational interventions to assist individuals to attain, regain, or maintain sexual wellness.
- Variations in sexual orientation include lesbian, gay, bisexual, transgender, queer, intersexual (ambiguous), and asexual (LGBTQIA).
- Gender dysphoria occurs when one's transgender identity influences clinically significant distress in emotional, social, occupational, and performance functions.
- Individuals with gender dysphoria experience extreme discomfort in the assigned gender and desire to be, or insist that they are, the opposite gender.
- Paraphilic disorders are a group of behaviors involving sexual activity with nonhuman objects or with nonconsenting partners or that involve suffering to others.
- Types of paraphilic disorders include exhibitionistic, fetishistic, frotteuristic, pedophilic, sexual masochism, sexual sadism, transvestic, and voyeuristic disorders.
- Sexual dysfunctions are disturbances that occur in any of the phases of the normal human sexual response cycle.

- Types of sexual dysfunctions include sexual desire, sexual arousal, orgasmic, and sexual pain disorders.
- Biological treatment of paraphilic disorders involves decreasing the level of circulating androgens.
- Psychoanalytic treatment of paraphilic disorders focuses on helping the individual resolve early conflicts, thus relieving the anxiety that prevents him or her from forming appropriate sexual relationships.
- Psychological therapy for paraphilic disorders includes use of aversion therapy, behavior therapy, imaginal desensitization, and satiation.
- Nurses may best become involved in the treatment of paraphilic disorders at the primary level of prevention.
- Treatment of sexual dysfunction disorders involves a variety of techniques, including CBT, systematic desensitization, and sensate focus exercises.
- Several medications are available for the treatment of erectile disorder. These include sildenafil (Viagra), tadalafil (Cialis), avanafil (Stendra), and vardenafil (Levitra, Staxyn). Others include prostaglandin preparations and combination drugs that may include papaverine, phentolamine, and alprostadil.

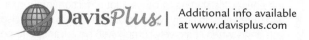

DavisPlus | Additional info available at www.davisplus.com

Review Questions
Self-Examination/Learning Exercise

Select the answer that is most appropriate for each of the following questions.

1. Anne, age 24, and her husband are seeking treatment at the sex therapy clinic. They have been married for 3 weeks and have never had sexual intercourse together. Pain and vaginal tightness prevent penile entry. Sexual history reveals Anne was raped when she was 15 years old. The physician would most likely assign which of the following diagnoses to Anne?
   a. Female orgasmic disorder
   b. Genito-pelvic pain/penetration disorder
   c. Female sexual interest/arousal disorder
   d. Sexual aversion disorder

Review Questions—cont'd
Self-Examination/Learning Exercise

2. Based on the scenario presented in question 1, which of the following would be the most appropriate *nursing* diagnosis for Anne?
   a. Pain related to vaginal constriction
   b. Ineffective sexuality patterns related to inability to have vaginal intercourse
   c. Sexual dysfunction related to history of sexual trauma
   d. Complicated grieving related to loss of self-esteem because of rape

3. A client comes to the mental health clinic with a complaint of lack of sexual desire. In the initial interview, what assessments would the nurse make? (Select all that apply.)
   a. Mood
   b. Level of energy
   c. Medications being taken
   d. Previous level of sexual activity

4. Which of the following medications may be prescribed for early ejaculation?
   a. Paroxetine
   b. Tadalafil
   c. Diazepam
   d. Imipramine

5. Carla watches her neighbor through his window each night as he undresses for bed. Later, she fantasizes about having sex with him. This is an example of which paraphilic disorder?
   a. Exhibitionistic disorder
   b. Voyeuristic disorder
   c. Frotteuristic disorder
   d. Pedophilic disorder

6. Frank drives his car up to a strange woman, stops, and asks her for directions. As she is explaining, he reveals his erect penis to her. This is an example of which paraphilic disorder?
   a. Sexual sadism disorder
   b. Sexual masochism disorder
   c. Frotteuristic disorder
   d. Exhibitionistic disorder

7. Tim, age 18, babysits for his 11-year-old neighbor, Jeff. Six months ago, Tim began fondling Jeff's genitals. They now engage in mutual masturbation each time they are together. This is an example of which paraphilic disorder?
   a. Fetishistic disorder
   b. Pedophilic disorder
   c. Exhibitionistic disorder
   d. Voyeuristic disorder

8. Fred rides a crowded subway every day. He stands beside a woman he finds very attractive. Just as the subway is about to stop, he places his hand on her breast and rubs his genitals against her buttock. As the door opens, he dashes out and away. Later, he fantasizes she is in love with him. This is an example of which paraphilia?
   a. Voyeuristic disorder
   b. Sexual sadism disorder
   c. Frotteuristic disorder
   d. Exhibitionistic disorder

Continued

Review Questions—cont'd
Self-Examination/Learning Exercise

9. A client with erectile disorder has a new prescription for sildenafil. The nurse who is providing education about this medication tells the client that which of the following are common side effects of this medication? (Select all that apply.)
   a. Headache
   b. Facial flushing
   c. Constipation
   d. Nasal congestion
   e. Indigestion

TEST YOUR CRITICAL THINKING SKILLS

Lindsey was hospitalized on the psychiatric unit with a depressive disorder. During her nursing assessment interview, she stated, "According to my husband, I can't do anything right—not even have sex." When asked to explain further, Lindsey said she and her husband had been married for 17 years. She said that in the beginning, they experienced a mutually satisfying sexual relationship and "made love" two or three times a week. Their daughter was born after they had been married 2 years, followed 2 years later by the birth of their son. They now have two teenagers (ages 15 and 13) who, by Lindsey's admission, require a great deal of her time and energy. She says, "I'm too tired for sex. And, besides, the kids might hear. I would be so embarrassed if they did. I walked in on my parents having sex once when I was a teenager, and I thought I would die! And my parents never mentioned it. It was just like it never happened! It was so awful! But sex is just so important to my husband, though, and we haven't had sex in months. We argue all the time about it. I'm afraid it's going to break us up."

Answer the following questions related to Lindsey.

1. Regarding her sexual relationship problem, what would be the nursing diagnosis for Lindsey?

2. What interventions for this problem might the nurse include in the treatment plan for Lindsey?
3. Regarding this problem, what would be a realistic goal for which Lindsey might strive?

Communication Exercises

Jamie is a 19-year-old male who came to the mental health clinic with complaints of worsening depression and feeling like he wants to die. He tells the nurse that he thinks he has gender issues, since he feels like a woman trapped in a man's body. What would be the appropriate response by the nurse at this point?

Jamie tells the nurse "I can't continue to live in this body, and I've been thinking of taking hormones to become more feminine." What would be an appropriate response by the nurse?

IMPLICATIONS OF RESEARCH FOR EVIDENCE-BASED PRACTICE

Mitchell, K., Jones, K.G., Wellings, K., Johnson, A.M., Graham, C.A., Datta, J., & Mercer, C. (2015). Estimating the prevalence of sexual function problems: The impact of morbidity criteria. *Journal of Sex Research, 53*(8), 955-967. doi:10.1080/00224499.2015.1089214

DESCRIPTION OF THE STUDY: This was a large, stratified probability survey ($N = 11,509$) designed to identify the prevalence of sexual dysfunctions using the *DSM-5* criteria. These diagnostic criteria were more stringent than those in the *DSM-IV-TR,* and the diagnosis of sexual dysfunctions historically has been criticized for medicalizing mild and transient sexual problems that are

"sufficiently common to be considered normal." The *DSM-5* added more stringent criteria, stating that symptoms must be present for at least 6 months and must occur at least 75 percent of the time.

RESULTS OF THE STUDY: The results of the study supported that the more stringent criteria did indeed identify clinically significant syndromes; 38.2 percent of men and 22 percent of women reported sexual dysfunctions, but only 4.2 and 3.6 percent respectively met DSM-V criteria. The study also found that depression and anxiety were contributing factors in sexual dysfunction, unemployment was a contributor for men, and nonvolitional sex was a

IMPLICATIONS OF RESEARCH FOR EVIDENCE-BASED PRACTICE—cont'd

contributing factor for women. Religiosity was not found to contribute to these dysfunctions, but the researchers report that this factor was difficult to firmly assess. Only about a third of those who met criteria for a clinically significant sexual dysfunction sought help. The researchers conclude that while historically the prevalence of sexual dysfunctions has been overstated, the numbers are still large (8.9 million in the United States and 1.8 million in the United Kingdom).

IMPLICATIONS FOR NURSING PRACTICE: This study broadens nurses' understanding of the prevalence of and contributing factors in sexual dysfunction. The finding that only a third of men and women reported their concerns to health-care providers supports the need for nurses to conduct a thorough sexual history and assessment. It also supports that asking relevant questions about the duration and frequency of a client's symptoms is helpful in prioritizing the clinical significance of the disorder.

 MOVIE CONNECTIONS

Mystic River (pedophilic disorder) • *Blue Velvet* (sexual masochism disorder) • *Looking for Mr. Goodbar* (sadism/masochism disorders) • *Normal* (transvestic disorder) • *TransAmerica* (gender dysphoria)

References

Adelson, S. (2012). Practice parameter on gay, lesbian, or bisexual sexual orientation, gender nonconformity, and gender discordance in children and adolescents. *Journal of the American Academy of Child and Adolescent Psychiatry, 51*(9), 957-974. doi:http://dx.doi.org/10.1016/j.jaac.2012.07.004

Administration on Aging. (2013). *A profile of older Americans: 2012.* Washington, DC: U.S. Department of Health and Human Services.

Allen, E.S., & Atkins, D.S. (2012). The association of divorce and extramarital sex in a representative U.S. sample. *Journal of Family Issues, 33*(11), 1477-1493. doi:10.1177/0192513X12439692

Althof, S.E., & Rosen, R.C. (2010). Combining medical and psychological interventions for the treatment of erectile dysfunction. In S. Levine, C. Risen, & S. Althof (Eds.), *Handbook of clinical sexuality for mental health professionals* (2nd ed., pp. 251-263). New York: Routledge.

American Psychiatric Association (APA). (2013). *Diagnostic and statistical manual of mental disorders* (5th ed.). Washington, DC: American Psychiatric Publishing.

Basson, R. (2016). Clinical challenges of sexual desire in younger women. In S. Levine, C. Risen, & S. Althof (Eds.), *Handbook of clinical sexuality for mental health professionals* (3rd ed., pp. 43-59). New York: Routledge.

Bednarczyk, R.A., Davis, R., Ault, K., Orenstein, W., & Omer, S.B. (2012). Sexual activity-related outcomes after human papillomavirus vaccination of 11- to 12-year-olds. *Pediatrics, 130*(5), 798-805.

Benson, A., Ost, L.B., Noble, M.J., & Lakin, M. (2013). Premature ejaculation. *MedscapeReference.* Retrieved from http://emedicine.medscape.com/article/435884-overview

Bergeron, S., Rosen, N.O., & Corsini-Munt, S. (2016). Painful sex. In S. Levine, C. Risen, & S. Althof (Eds.), *Handbook of clinical sexuality for mental health professionals* (3rd ed., pp. 71-85). New York: Routledge.

Berman, J., & Berman, L. (2014). *For women only: A revolutionary guide to overcoming sexual dysfunction and reclaiming your sex life* (2nd ed.). New York: Henry Holt. (Original work published 2005).

Black, D.W., & Andreasen, N.C. (2014). *Introductory textbook of psychiatry* (6th ed.). Washington, DC: American Psychiatric Publishing.

Byne, W., Bradley, S., Coleman, E., Eyler, A.E., Green, R., Menvielle, E., . . . Tompkins, D.A. (2012). Report of the APA task force on treatment of gender identity disorder. *American Journal of Psychiatry, 169*(8), 1-35.

Centers for Disease Control (CDC). (2011a). *A guide to taking a sexual history* [CDC Publication: 99-8445]. Retrieved from https://www.cdc.gov/std/treatment/sexualhistory.pdf

Centers for Disease Control and Prevention (CDC). (2011b). Recommendations on the use of quadrivalent human papillomavirus vaccine in males—Advisory Committee on Immunization Practices (ACIP), 2011. *Morbidity and Mortality Weekly Report, 60*(50), 1697-1728.

Centers for Disease Control and Prevention (CDC). (2012). Human papillomavirus—Associated cancers—United States, 2004–2008. *Morbidity and Mortality Weekly Report, 61*(15), 253-280.

Centers for Disease Control and Prevention (CDC). (2014). *Sexual orientation in the 2013 national health interview survey: A quality assessment.* Retrieved from https://www.cdc.gov/nchs/data/series/sr_02/sr02_169.pdf

Centers for Disease Control and Prevention (CDC). (2015). *National vital statistics system: National marriage and divorce rate trends. (United States 2000–2014).* Retrieved from http://www.cdc.gov/nchs/nvss/marriage_divorce_tables.htm

Chappell, W. (2015). Supreme court decrees same-sex marriage legal in all 50 states. *National Public Radio.* Retrieved from http://www.npr.org/sections/thetwo-way/2015/06/26/417717613/supreme-court-rules-all-states-must-allow-same-sex-marriages

Clark, S.K., Jeglic, E.L., Calkins, C., & Tatar, J.R. (2016). More than a nuisance: The prevalence and consequences of frotteurism and exhibitionism. *Sexual Abuse: A Journal of Research and Treatment, 28*(1) 3-19. doi:10.1177/1079063214525643

Donahey, K. (2016) Problems with orgasm. In S. Levine, C. Risen, & S. Althof (Eds.), *Handbook of clinical sexuality for mental health professionals* (3rd ed., pp. 60-70). New York: Routledge.

Fedoroff, J.P. (2016). Managing versus successfully treating paraphilic disorders: The paradigm is changing. In S. Levine, C. Risen, & S. Althof (Eds.), *Handbook of clinical sexuality for mental health professionals* (3rd ed., pp. 345-361). New York: Routledge.

Food and Drug Administration (FDA). (2015). *FDA approves first treatment for sexual desire disorder* [press release]. Retrieved from https://www.fda.gov/NewsEvents/Newsroom/PressAnnouncements/ucm458734.htm

Food and Drug Administration (FDA). (2017). *Tainted sexual enhancement products.* Retrieved from https://www.fda.gov/Drugs/ResourcesForYou/Consumers/BuyingUsing MedicineSafely/MedicationHealthFraud/ucm234539.htm

Garcia-Falgueras, A., & Swaab, D.F. (2008). A sex difference in the hypothalamic uncinate nucleus: Relationship to gender identity. *Brain, 131*(12), 3132-3146. doi:10.1093/brain/awn276

Gibson, B., & Catlin, A.J. (2010). Care of the child with the desire to change gender—Part I. *Pediatric Nursing, 36*(1), 53–59.

Giger, J.N. (2017). *Transcultural nursing: Assessment and intervention* (3rd ed.). St. Louis, MO: Mosby.

Gooren, L. (2011). Care of transsexual persons. *New England Journal of Medicine, 364*(13), 1251-1257.

Hughes, R. (2012). Does extramarital sex cause divorce? [blog post]. Retrieved from http://www.huffingtonpost.com/robert-hughes/does-extramarital-sex-cau_b_1567507.html

Institute of Medicine. (2003). *Health professions education: A bridge to quality.* Washington, DC: Institute of Medicine.

Jena, A.B., Goldman, D.P., & Seabury, S.A. (2015). Incidence of sexually transmitted infections after human papillomavirus vaccination among adolescent females. *JAMA Internal Medicine, 175*(4), 617-623. doi:10.1001/jamainternmed.2014.7886.

Kann, L., McManus, T., Harris, W.A., Shanklin, S.L., Flint, K.H., Hawkins, J., . . . Zaza, S. (2016). Youth risk behavior Surveillance—United States, 2015. *MMWR Surveillance Summary, 65*(No. SS-16), 1-174. doi:http://dx.doi.org/10.15585/mmwr.ss6506a1

Kim, E.D., & Brosman, S.A. (2013). *Erectile dysfunction.* Retrieved from http://emedicine.medscape.com/article/444220-overview.

King, B.M., & Regan, P. (2014). *Human sexuality today* (8th ed.). Upper Saddle River, NJ: Prentice Hall.

Kingsberg, S.A., & Krychman, M. (2016). Sexuality and menopause. In S. Levine, C. Risen, & S. Althof (Eds.), *Handbook of clinical sexuality for mental health professionals* (3rd ed., 86-94). New York: Routledge.

Laumann, E.O., Glasser, D.B., Neves, R.C.S., & Moreira, E.D. (2009). A population-based survey of sexual activity, sexual problems, and associated help-seeking behavior patterns in mature adults in the United States of America. *International Journal of Impotence Research, 21*(3), 171-178.

Laumann, E. O., Paik, A., & Rosen, R.C. (1999). Sexual dysfunction in the United States, prevalence and predictors. *JAMA, 281*(6), 537-544.

Levine, S.B. (2016). The mental health professional's treatment of erection problems. In S. Levine, C. Risen, & S. Althof (Eds.), *Handbook of clinical sexuality for mental health professionals* (3rd ed., 123-133). New York: Rutledge.

Lowry, F., & Vega, C.P. (2016). Health needs of transgender people poorly understood. *Medscape.* Retrieved from http://www.medscape.org/viewarticle/865405

Mathy, R.M., Cochran, S.D., Olsen, J., & Mays, V.M. (2011). The association between relationship markers of sexual orientation and suicide: Denmark, 1990–2001. *Social Psychiatry and Psychiatric Epidemiology, 46*(2), 111-117.

Mitchell, K., Jones, K.G., Wellings, K., Johnson, A.M., Graham, C.A., Datta, J., & Mercer, C. (2015). Estimating the prevalence of sexual function problems: The impact of morbidity criteria. *Journal of Sex Research, 53*(8), 955-967. doi:10.1080/00224499.2015.1089214

Nicholson, C., & McGuinness, T. (2014). Gender dysphoria and children. *Journal of Psychosocial Nursing, 52*(8), 27-30.

Petrosky, E., Bocchini Jr, J.A., Hariri, S., Chesson, H., Curtis, C.R., Saraiya, M., . . . Markowitz, L.E. (2015). Use of 9-valent human papillomavirus (HPV) vaccine: Updated HPV vaccination recommendations of the advisory committee on immunization practices. *Morbidity and Mortality Weekly Report, 64*(11), 300-304. Retrieved from http://www.cdc.gov/mmwr/preview/mmwrhtml/mm6411a3.htm

Ploderl, M., Wagenmakers, E.J., Tremblay, P., Ramsay, R., Kralovec, K., Fartacek, C., & Fartacek, R. (2013). Suicide risk and sexual orientation: A critical review. *Archives of Sexual Behavior, 42*(5), 715-727.

Robins, L.N., Helzer, J.E., Weissman, M.M., Orvaschel, H., Gruenberg, E., Burke, J.D., & Regier, D.A. (1984). Lifetime prevalence of specific psychiatric disorders in three sites. *Archives of General Psychiatry, 41*(10), 949-958.

Sadock, B.J., Sadock V.A., & Ruiz, P. (2015). *Synopsis of psychiatry: Behavioral sciences/clinical psychiatry* (11th ed.). Philadelphia: Lippincott Williams & Wilkins.

Stroumsa, D. (2014). The state of transgender health care: Policy, law, and medical frameworks. *American Journal of Public Health, 104*(3), 31-37.

Vallerand, A., Sanoski, C.A., & Deglin, J. (2016). *Davis drug guide for nurses* (15th ed.). Philadelphia: F.A. Davis.

Waldinger, M. (2016). Premature ejaculation, In S. Levine, C. Risen, & S. Althof (Eds.), *Handbook of clinical sexuality for mental health professionals* (3rd ed., pp. 134-149). New York: Routledge.

Wisse, B. (2015). *Prolactinoma.* Retrieved from https://www.nlm.nih.gov/medlineplus/ency/article/000336.htm

Classical References

Masters, W.H., & Johnson, V.E. (1966). *Human sexual response.* Boston: Little, Brown.

Masters, W.H., & Johnson, V.E. (1970). *Human sexual inadequacy.* Boston: Little, Brown.

Masters, W.H., Johnson, V.E., & Kolodny, R.C. (1995). *Human sexuality* (5th ed.). New York: Addison-Wesley Longman.

Eating Disorders

31

CORE CONCEPTS

Anorexia

Body Image

Bulimia

KEY TERMS

amenorrhea	binging	lanugo
anorexia nervosa	bulimia nervosa	obesity
binge eating disorder	emaciated	purging

OBJECTIVES
After reading this chapter, the student will be able to:

1. Identify and differentiate among several eating disorders.
2. Discuss epidemiological statistics related to eating disorders.
3. Describe symptomatology associated with anorexia nervosa, bulimia nervosa, and obesity, and use the information in client assessment.
4. Identify predisposing factors in the development of eating disorders.
5. Formulate nursing diagnoses and outcomes of care for clients with eating disorders.
6. Describe appropriate interventions for behaviors associated with eating disorders.
7. Identify topics for client and family teaching relevant to eating disorders.
8. Evaluate the nursing care of clients with eating disorders.
9. Discuss various modalities relevant to treatment of eating disorders.

HOMEWORK ASSIGNMENT
Please read the chapter and answer the following questions:

1. Anorexia nervosa may be associated with a primary dysfunction of which brain structure?
2. What is the level of body mass index (BMI) that is associated with the definition of obesity?
3. Individuals with anorexia nervosa have a "distorted body image." What does this mean?
4. What physiological signs may be associated with the excessive vomiting of the purging syndrome?

Nutrition is required to sustain life, and most individuals acquire nutrients from eating food; however, nutrition and life sustenance are not the only reasons most people eat food. Indeed, in an affluent culture, life sustenance may not even be a consideration. It is sometimes difficult to remember that many people in the affluent American culture, as well as all over the world, are starving from lack of food.

The hypothalamus contains the appetite regulation center within the brain. This complex neural system regulates the body's ability to recognize when it is hungry and when it has been sated. Some studies have shown evidence of serotonin and norepinephrine dysfunction in individuals with eating disorders. These neurotransmitters both play a role in regulating eating behavior (Sadock, Sadock, & Ruiz, 2015).

Society and culture also have substantial influence on eating behaviors. Eating is a social activity; seldom does an event of any social significance occur without the presence of food. Yet society and culture also influence how people, especially women, should look. History reveals regular fluctuation in what society has considered desirable in the human female body. Archives and historical paintings from the 16th and 17th centuries reveal that plump, full-figured women were considered fashionable and desirable. In the Victorian era, beauty was characterized by a slender, wan appearance that continued through the flapper era of the 1920s. During the Depression era and World War II, the full-bodied woman was again admired, only to be superseded in the late 1960s by the image of the superthin models propagated by the media, which remains the ideal of today. As it has been said, "A woman can't be too rich or too thin." Eating disorders, as we know them, can refute this concept.

This chapter explores the disorders associated with undereating and overeating. Because psychological or behavioral factors play a potential role in the presentation of these disorders, they fall well within the realm of psychiatry and psychiatric nursing. Epidemiological statistics are presented along with factors that have been implicated in the etiology of anorexia nervosa, bulimia nervosa, and binge eating disorder. An explanation of the symptomatology is presented as background knowledge for assessing the client with an eating disorder. Nursing care is described in the context of the nursing process. Various treatment modalities are explored.

Epidemiological Factors

Reports have indicated that the prevalence of **anorexia nervosa** has increased since the mid-20th century, both in the United States and in Western Europe. Studies indicate a prevalence rate for anorexia nervosa among young women in the United States of approximately 1 percent (Black & Andreasen, 2014). The disorder occurs predominantly in females 12 to 30 years of age. Fewer than 10 percent of cases are male, but this percentage may be underestimated due to a biased view of anorexia nervosa as solely a female disorder. See the Real People, Real Stories feature for Vic's perspective about his experience with having an eating disorder.

Social interests may also play a role in the prevalence of eating disorders. Among females, ballet training carries a seven times greater risk of developing anorexia

nervosa, and among males, the evidence of eating disorders is more prevalent among those participating in wrestling sports; a minority continue to have symptoms beyond their involvement in the sport (Sadock et al., 2015). Anorexia nervosa was once believed to be more prevalent in the higher socioeconomic classes, but evidence is lacking to support this hypothesis.

Bulimia nervosa is more prevalent than anorexia nervosa, with estimates up to 4 percent of young women (Black & Andreasen, 2014). Onset of bulimia nervosa occurs in late adolescence or early adulthood. Among college women, about 20 percent experience transient bulimic symptoms during the college years (Sadock et al., 2015). Cross-cultural research suggests that bulimia nervosa occurs primarily in societies that place emphasis on thinness as the model of attractiveness for women and where an abundance of food is available.

Binge eating disorder is defined in the *Diagnostic and Statistical Manual of Mental Disorders, Fifth Edition (DSM-5)* as recurrent episodes of eating significantly more than most people would eat in a similar time period under similar circumstances (APA, 2013). These episodes occur at least once a week for at least 3 months. This is the most common eating disorder and affects women twice as often as men (Sadock et al., 2015), with prevalence estimated at 4 percent of the U.S. population (Balodis, Grilo, & Potenza, 2015). Weight gain leading to obesity is a major health risk associated with this disorder. It is estimated that approximately 50 to 75 percent of people seeking medical attention for severe obesity have a binge eating disorder (Sadock et al., 2015).

Obesity has been defined as a body mass index (BMI) (weight/height^2) of 30 or greater. In the United States, statistics indicate that among adults 20 years of age and older, 69 percent are overweight, 35 percent of whom fall in the obese range (Centers for Disease Control and Prevention [CDC], 2015). The percentage of obese individuals is higher in African Americans and Latino Americans than among the white population (CDC, 2015). There is a correlation between low income and obesity in women, but most obese adults are not in the low-income group. Among women, there is a correlation between lower level of education and obesity, but no such correlation exists among men (CDC, 2015). Interestingly, the *DSM-5* does not include obesity as a mental disorder, stating the rationale that "a range of genetic, physiological, behavioral, and environmental factors that vary across individuals contributes to the development of obesity; thus obesity is not considered a mental disorder" (APA, 2013, p. 329). The *DSM-5* also notes, however, that obesity is a significant problem in several mental disorders (at least in part related to side effects of psychotropic

Real People, Real Stories: Living With an Eating Disorder

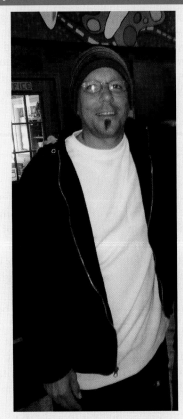

(Following is an excerpt of our conversation.)

Karyn: First of all, I appreciate your willingness to share your story.

Vic: I want to talk about this because there is such a stigma associated with being a guy and having an eating disorder. And it's hard for guys to find a support group of people who really "get it."

Karyn: What has your experience been with encountering stigma?

Vic: Well, my weight has sometimes been really high and sometimes very low. I fluctuate between anorexia and bulimia. So when my weight is really low, people have presumed I have AIDS. And in general, because eating disorders are presumed to be a female disorder, people have assumed I was gay. In high school, I was very heavy and the guys on the football team teased me a lot. I talked to my girlfriend at the time, and she suggested I try purging. I was using food and alcohol for comfort, but then I had to purge. I started working out a lot, and when I started getting compliments on my appearance, I began binging and purging every day and drinking alcohol. It was a stress relief for a while, but then it just wasn't working anymore and I still hated my appearance. To this day, there's not one thing I like about my appearance even though my physician is happy with my current weight. I was hiding it from my family for some time: wearing baggy clothes and two sets of clothes so people wouldn't see my flaws. The behaviors are very isolating. When I tried to talk to my dad. he just told me to be a man . . . but there was a lot of physical and emotional abuse from him, so I didn't get support there.

Karyn: Where have you found support?

Vic: My mom and my fiancée are my biggest supports, but it's a struggle to find support with other guys who have eating disorders, and I feel like they would really understand. I tried to start a support group on Facebook, and no one responded. I have an individual counselor who knows a lot about eating disorders, and I have a family practice physician, and they are both helpful. It's just not the same as having the support of others who are having the same experiences that you are.

Karyn: Have you ever been engaged in group treatment specifically for eating disorders?

Vic: I tried, at one point, but most insurances don't cover eating disorder treatment, or the treatment program doesn't take insurance. I went into treatment in 2009 for alcohol rehabilitation, and they didn't address the eating disorder. In fact, they kind of force you to eat and tell you that you'll probably gain weight as you go through rehab, so the bulimia kicked in again for me because I didn't want to get fat like the other people in recovery. But I've been sober since 2009, and I take Vivitrol injections (to manage alcohol dependence) once a month; it blocks the pleasure centers.

Karyn: And has that been effective?

Vic: Oh yes, definitely. And my AA buddies are very supportive, but they don't see food as a similar issue to alcohol, so they don't really see a need to discuss that. Plus, you can't abstain from food like you can from alcohol. And society itself can be a trigger: television, all the messages that you need to be a certain way, picnics, going out to eat, grocery stores, talking about food, et cetera. And I think I have an element of "people pleasing" in my personality, so I'm always worried about what other people are thinking about me.

Karyn: It's not uncommon for people with eating disorders to also have depression and sometimes have suicide thoughts. Have you ever been in that place?

Vic: Yeah, once last year I took an overdose of pills with some alcohol, but I called some friends and they got me in to get help.

Karyn: Do you still have times when you have those thoughts?

Vic: No. I'm doing really well right now. I still dabble from time to time with "the behavior" [Vic described this as his term for binging/purging or calorie restriction, stating that sometimes using the words can be a trigger for him], but not like before when I was taking up to 20 laxatives a day and my whole day was preoccupied with planning "the behaviors." I'm working in a setting that treats dual diagnosis clients, and I am hopeful that there may be opportunities to establish peer support groups for men with eating disorders, much like what exists in AA for alcohol recovery. As a guy, you just can't go to a group that is all women and talk

Continued

Real People, Real Stories: Living With an Eating Disorder—cont'd

about this stuff, especially what's going on with your body. And I don't want to be accused of "thirteen-steppin'."

Karyn: "Thirteen steppin'"?

Vic: Yeah, that's the "thirteenth step" in the twelve-step program. It's the guys that go to AA meetings to pick up girls who are in recovery because they know they are more vulnerable when they're trying to stay sober. [Chuckles]

Karyn: [Chuckles] I didn't know that was a thing. But I understand what you're saying about the difficulty of finding support with other men who understand and are willing to acknowledge their eating disorder. I hope the peer support group works out, and in the meantime, I'm glad to hear that you are accessing resources to support your own health.

---

medications) and that obesity may be a risk factor for the development of illnesses such as depression. Binge eating disorder, which *is* identified as a mental illness, carries a high risk for weight gain and obesity.

Application of the Nursing Process

Background Assessment Data: Anorexia Nervosa

> **CORE CONCEPT**
> **Anorexia**
> Prolonged loss of appetite.

> **CORE CONCEPT**
> **Body Image**
> A subjective concept of one's physical appearance based on the personal perceptions of self and the reactions of others.

Anorexia nervosa is characterized by a morbid fear of obesity. Symptoms include gross distortion of body image, preoccupation with food, and refusal to eat. The term *anorexia* is actually a misnomer. It was initially believed that individuals with anorexia nervosa did not experience sensations of hunger. However, research indicates that they do indeed suffer from pangs of hunger, and it is only with food intake of less than 200 calories per day that hunger sensations cease.

The distorted body image is manifested by the individual's perception of being "fat" when he or she is obviously underweight or even **emaciated** (excessively thin). Weight loss is usually accomplished by reduction in food intake and often extensive exercising. Self-induced vomiting and the abuse of laxatives or diuretics may occur.

Weight loss is excessive, with some individuals who present for health-care services weighing less than

85 percent of expected weight. Other symptoms include hypothermia, bradycardia, hypotension with orthostatic changes, peripheral edema, **lanugo** (fine, neonatal-like hair growth), and a variety of metabolic changes. **Amenorrhea** (absence of menstruation) usually follows weight loss, but sometimes it happens early in the disorder before severe weight loss has occurred.

Individuals with anorexia nervosa may be obsessed with food. For example, they may hoard or conceal food, talk about food and recipes at great length, or prepare elaborate meals for others, only to restrict themselves to limited low-calorie food intake. Compulsive behaviors such as hand washing may also be present.

Age at onset is usually early to late adolescence, and psychosexual development is often delayed. Feelings of depression and anxiety often accompany the disorder. In fact, some studies have suggested a possible interrelationship between eating disorders and affective disorders. Box 31–1 outlines the *DSM-5* diagnostic criteria for anorexia nervosa.

Background Assessment Data: Bulimia Nervosa

> **CORE CONCEPT**
> **Bulimia**
> Excessive, insatiable appetite.

Bulimia nervosa is an episodic, uncontrolled, compulsive, rapid ingestion of large quantities of food over a short period of time **(binging),** followed by inappropriate compensatory behaviors to rid the body of the excess calories. The food consumed during a binge often has high caloric content, a sweet taste, and a soft or smooth texture that can be eaten rapidly, sometimes even without being chewed (Sadock et al., 2015). The binging episodes often occur in secret and are usually terminated only by abdominal discomfort,

BOX 31-1 Diagnostic Criteria for Anorexia Nervosa

A. Restriction of energy intake relative to requirements leading to a significantly low body weight in the context of age, sex, developmental trajectory, and physical health. *Significantly low weight* is defined as a weight that is less than minimally normal, or, for children and adolescents, less than that minimally expected.

B. Intense fear of gaining weight or becoming fat, or persistent behavior that interferes with weight gain, even though at a significantly low weight.

C. Disturbance in the way in which one's body weight or shape is experienced, undue influence of body weight or shape on self-evaluation, or persistent lack of recognition of the seriousness of the current low body weight.

Specify whether:

Restricting Type: During the last 3 months, the individual has not engaged in recurrent episodes of binge eating or purging behavior (i.e., self-induced vomiting or the misuse of laxatives, diuretics, or enemas). This subtype describes presentations in which weight loss is accomplished primarily through dieting, fasting, and/or excessive exercise.

Binge-Eating/Purging Type: During the last 3 months, the individual has engaged in recurrent episodes of binge eating or purging behavior (i.e., self-induced vomiting or the misuse of laxatives, diuretics, or enemas).

Specify if:

In partial remission

In full remission

Specify current severity:

Mild: BMI ≥ 17 kg/m²   **Severe:** BMI 15–15.99 kg/m²
Moderate: BMI 16–16.99 kg/m²   **Extreme:** BMI < 15 kg/m²

Reprinted with permission from the Diagnostic and Statistical Manual of Mental Disorders, Fifth Edition *(Copyright 2013). American Psychiatric Association.*

sleep, social interruption, or self-induced vomiting. Although the eating binges may bring pleasure while they are occurring, self-degradation and depressed mood commonly follow.

To rid the body of the excessive calories, the individual engages in **purging** behaviors (self-induced vomiting or the misuse of laxatives, diuretics, or enemas) or other inappropriate compensatory behaviors, such as fasting or excessive exercise. Among these individuals, there is a persistent overconcern with personal appearance, particularly regarding how they believe others perceive them. Weight fluctuations are common because of the alternating binges and fasts. However, most individuals with bulimia are within a normal weight range—some slightly underweight, some slightly overweight.

Excessive vomiting and laxative or diuretic abuse may lead to problems with dehydration and electrolyte imbalance. Gastric acid in the vomitus also contributes to the erosion of tooth enamel. In rare instances, the individual may experience tears in the gastric or esophageal mucosa. Some individuals develop calluses on the dorsal surface of their hands, typically on knuckles, secondary to long-term self-induced vomiting. This feature is called *Russell's sign* after the British psychiatrist who first described it. It cannot be a reliable diagnostic symptom, however, since many individuals with purging behavior are able to induce vomiting without using their hands.

Common comorbidities include mood disorders, anxiety disorders, or substance abuse, most frequently involving central nervous central (CNS) stimulants or alcohol. About 50 percent of those with bulimia nervosa have had a history of anorexia nervosa (Sadock et al., 2015). The *DSM*-5 diagnostic criteria for bulimia nervosa are presented in Box 31–2.

Background Assessment Data: Binge Eating Disorder

Individuals with binge eating disorder have episodes of binge eating that may be similar to those with bulimia nervosa; however, binge eating disorder is absent of compensatory purging. As a result, this client is at risk for substantial weight gain. The episodes of eating are considered binges when they occur over a defined period of time, usually less than 2 hours (APA, 2013). Food consumption not only is rapid but often continues to the point that the individual feels uncomfortably full. Interpersonal stressors, low self-esteem, and boredom are identified as possible triggers. Typically, clients describe their eating as out of control. There is often accompanying guilt and depression. As many as 50 percent of individuals with binge eating disorder have a history of depression (Jaret, 2010). Another difference between bulimia nervosa and binge eating disorder is that rates of improvement are consistently higher among individuals with binge eating disorder than among those with bulimia nervosa

BOX 31–2 Diagnostic Criteria for Bulimia Nervosa

A. Recurrent episodes of binge eating. An episode of binge eating is characterized by both of the following:

1. Eating, in a discrete period of time (e.g., within any 2-hour period) an amount of food that is definitely larger than most individuals would eat during a similar period of time and under similar circumstances.
2. A sense of lack of control over eating during the episode (e.g., a feeling that one cannot stop eating or control what or how much one is eating).

B. Recurrent inappropriate compensatory behaviors in order to prevent weight gain, such as self-induced vomiting; misuse of laxatives, diuretics, or other medications; fasting; or excessive exercise.

C. The binge eating and inappropriate compensatory behaviors both occur, on average, at least once a week for 3 months.

D. Self-evaluation is unduly influenced by body shape and weight.

E. The disturbance does not occur exclusively during episodes of anorexia nervosa.

Specify if:

In partial remission

In full remission

Specify current severity:

Mild: An average of 1–3 episodes of inappropriate compensatory behaviors per week.

Moderate: An average of 4–7 episodes of inappropriate compensatory behaviors per week.

Severe: An average of 8–13 episodes of inappropriate compensatory behaviors per week.

Extreme: An average of 14 or more episodes of inappropriate compensatory behaviors per week.

Reprinted with permission from the Diagnostic and Statistical Manual of Mental Disorders, Fifth Edition *(Copyright 2013). American Psychiatric Association.*

(APA, 2013). The *DSM-5* diagnostic criteria for binge eating disorder are presented in Box 31–3.

Predisposing Factors and Theories of Etiology Associated With Anorexia Nervosa, Bulimia Nervosa, and Binge Eating Disorder

Biological Influences

Genetics A hereditary predisposition to eating disorders has been hypothesized on the basis of family histories and an apparent association with other disorders for which the likelihood of genetic influences exists. Some studies identify higher concordance rates in monozygotic than in dizygotic twins (Sadock et al, 2015). Anorexia nervosa is more common among sisters of those with the disorder than among the general population, but social factors such as modeling and mimicking may influence these relationships. Several studies have reported a higher than expected frequency of mood and substance use disorders among first-degree biological relatives of individuals with eating disorders (Puri & Treasaden, 2011).

Neuroendocrine Abnormalities Some speculation has occurred regarding a primary hypothalamic dysfunction in anorexia nervosa. Support for this hypothesis is gathered from the fact that many people with anorexia experience amenorrhea before the onset of starvation and significant weight loss.

Neurochemical Influences Neurochemical influences in bulimia may be associated with the neurotransmitters serotonin and norepinephrine. This hypothesis has been supported by the positive response these individuals have shown to therapy with the selective serotonin reuptake inhibitors (SSRIs). Some evidence also exists to indicate that low levels of the neurotransmitter serotonin (5-hydroxytryptamine [5-HT]) may play a role in compulsive eating (Uçeyler et al., 2010). Studies have found high levels of endogenous opioids in the spinal fluid of clients with anorexia, promoting the speculation that these chemicals may contribute to denial of hunger (Sadock et al., 2015). Some of these individuals have been shown to gain weight when given naloxone, an opioid antagonist. Questions still remain as to whether neurochemical changes are causal or are an outcome of the body's reaction to changes in nutrition and mood.

The etiology of binge eating disorder is unknown. Brain imaging studies of people with binge eating disorders reveal increased activity in the orbitofrontal cortex, the centers associated with reward and pleasure responses such as those seen in response to substances of abuse (Balodis et al., 2015). This has supported the hypothesis that binge eating disorder may be an illness of addiction.

Psychodynamic Influences

Psychodynamic theories suggest that the development of an eating disorder is rooted in an unfulfilled sense of separation-individuation. When events occur that threaten the vulnerable ego, feelings of lack of control over one's body (self) emerge. Behaviors associated with food and eating provide feelings of control over one's life.

BOX 31–3 **Diagnostic Criteria for Binge Eating Disorder**

A. Recurrent episodes of binge eating. An episode of binge eating is characterized by both of the following:
  1. Eating, in a discrete period of time (e.g., within any 2-hour period), an amount of food that is definitely larger than what most people would eat in a similar period of time under similar circumstances
  2. A sense of lack of control over eating during the episode (e.g., a feeling that one cannot stop eating or control what or how much one is eating)
B. The binge eating episodes are associated with 3 (or more) of the following:
  1. Eating much more rapidly than normal
  2. Eating until feeling uncomfortably full
  3. Eating large amounts of food when not feeling physically hungry
  4. Eating alone because of feeling embarrassed by how much one is eating
  5. Feeling disgusted with oneself, depressed, or very guilty after overeating
C. Marked distress regarding binge eating is present.
D. The binge eating occurs, on average, at least once a week for 3 months.
E. The binge eating is not associated with the recurrent use of inappropriate compensatory behavior as in bulimia nervosa and does not occur exclusively during the course of bulimia nervosa or anorexia nervosa.

Specify if:

In partial remission

In full remission

Specify current severity:

Mild: 1–3 binge eating episodes per week

Moderate: 4–7 binge eating episodes per week

Severe: 8–13 binge eating episodes per week

Extreme: 14 or more binge eating episodes per week

Reprinted with permission from the Diagnostic and Statistical Manual of Mental Disorders, Fifth Edition *(Copyright 2013). American Psychiatric Association.*

Family Influences

Historically, parents of children with eating disorders have been presumed to be overcontrolling and perfectionistic, causing pathology in their children. This theory has been problematic, at least in part because not all siblings in the same family develop eating disorders. There is not sufficient evidence to support these claims, and they may have contributed to a resistance toward seeking health care based on parents' fear that they will be judged as the cause of the problem. The American Academy for Eating Disorders has published a position statement (2009) that includes the following:

> The AED stands firmly against any model of eating disorders in which family influences are seen as the primary cause of eating disorders, condemns statements that blame families for their child's illness, and recommends that families be included in the treatment of younger patients, unless this is clearly ill-advised on clinical grounds.

Both perfectionistic and depressive tendencies do appear to be common in clients with anorexia nervosa, but Sadock and associates (2015) offer this explanation:

> Many anorectic patients feel that oral desires are greedy and unacceptable; therefore these desires are projectively disavowed . . . parents respond to the refusal to eat by becoming frantic about whether

the patient is actually eating. The patient can then view the parents as the ones who have unacceptable desires and can projectively disavow them.

Certainly conflicts arise in a family when a child is starving himself or herself, but it has become clear that family members need to be involved in treatment rather than shunned or blamed. Family-based approaches such as the Maudsley approach are supported by clinical evidence.

Background Assessment Data: Body Mass Index

Assessment for the presence of an eating disorder requires an understanding of the measurements for BMI. The following formula is used to determine an individual's BMI:

$$\text{Body mass index} = \frac{\text{Weight (kg)}}{\text{Height (m)}^2}$$

The BMI range for normal weight is 20 to 24.9. Studies by the National Center for Health Statistics indicate that *overweight* is defined as a BMI of 25.0 to 29.9 (based on U.S. Dietary Guidelines for Americans). Based on criteria of the World Health Organization, *obesity* is defined as a BMI of 30.0 or greater. These guidelines, which were released by the National Heart,

Lung, and Blood Institute in July 1998, markedly increased the number of Americans considered overweight. The average American woman has a BMI of 26, and fashion models typically have BMIs of 18. Anorexia nervosa is characterized by a BMI of 17 or lower. In extreme anorexia nervosa the BMI may be less than 15. Table 31–1 presents an example of some BMIs based on weight (in pounds) and height (in inches).

Diagnosis and Outcome Identification

Nursing diagnoses are formulated from the data gathered during the assessment phase and with background knowledge regarding predisposing factors to the disorder. Table 31–2 presents a list of client behaviors and the NANDA-I nursing diagnoses that correspond to those behaviors, which may be used in planning care for clients with eating disorders.

Outcome Criteria

The following criteria may be used for measurement of outcomes in the care of the client with eating disorders:

The client:

- Has achieved and maintained an expected BMI for age with consideration for body build, weight history, and any physiological disturbances (APA, 2013, p. 340)
- Has vital signs, blood pressure, and laboratory serum studies within normal limits
- Verbalizes importance of adequate nutrition
- Verbalizes knowledge regarding consequences of fluid loss caused by self-induced vomiting (or laxative/diuretic abuse) and importance of adequate fluid intake (anorexia nervosa, bulimia nervosa)
- Verbalizes events that precipitate anxiety and demonstrates techniques for its reduction
- Verbalizes ways in which he or she may gain more control of the environment and thereby reduce feelings of powerlessness
- Expresses less preoccupation with own appearance (anorexia nervosa, bulimia nervosa)
- Demonstrates ability to take control of own life without resorting to maladaptive eating behaviors (anorexia nervosa, bulimia nervosa, binge eating disorder)
- Has established a healthy pattern of eating for weight control, and weight loss toward a desired goal is progressing (binge eating disorder)
- Verbalizes plans for maintenance of weight control and relapse prevention (binge eating disorder)

Planning and Implementation

In most instances, individuals with eating disorders are treated on an outpatient basis, but in some cases hospitalization becomes necessary. Assessment findings that may necessitate hospitalization include the following:

- **Malnutrition:** Twenty percent below expected weight for height recommended for inpatient treatment; 30 percent below expected weight for height recommended for long-term intensive treatment (Sadock et al., 2015)
- **Dehydration:** Assessment includes thirst, orthostatic hypotension, tachycardia, elevated sodium levels, and other symptoms
- **Severe electrolyte imbalance:** Potassium levels below 3 mmol/L, phosphate levels below 3 mg/dL, magnesium levels below 1.4 mEq/L
- **Cardiac arrhythmia:** ST segment and T wave changes usually related to electrolyte imbalances
- **Severe bradycardia:** Below 50 beats per minute
- **Hypothermia:** Body temperature below 96.8
- **Hypotension:** A pattern of low blood pressure or orthostatic hypotension (20 mm Hg or greater drop in systolic blood pressure with positional changes and pulse rate increase by 20 or more beats)
- **Suicidal ideation** (see Chapter 17, Suicide Prevention, for an in-depth discussion of suicide risk assessment)

In addition to the physical assessment parameters listed previously, when an eating disorder is suspected, a general assessment includes asking patients about their eating patterns and body image, their dieting patterns, whether or not they feel driven to be thin, exercise patterns, and any use of substances including diet pills, laxatives, or diuretics (Micula-Gondek & Lackamp, 2011). Evidence of calluses on the dorsum of the hands, parotid enlargement, mouth ulcers, dental caries, and edema may also be assessment findings in the patient with purging behaviors.

The following section presents a group of selected nursing diagnoses, with short- and long-term goals and nursing interventions for each.

Imbalanced Nutrition: Less Than Body Requirements/Deficient Fluid Volume (Risk for or Actual)

Imbalanced nutrition: less than body requirements is defined as "intake of nutrients insufficient to meet metabolic needs" (Herdman & Kamitsuru, 2014, p. 161). *Deficient fluid volume* is defined as "decreased intravascular, interstitial, and/or intracellular fluid" (p. 177). Table 31–3 presents these nursing diagnoses in care plan format.

Client Goals

Outcome criteria include short- and long-term goals. Time lines are individually determined.

TABLE 31–1 Body Mass Index (BMI) Chart

BMI	19	20	21	22	23	24	25	26	27	28	29	30	31	32	33	34	35	36	37	38	39	40
HEIGHT (INCHES)											**BODY WEIGHT (POUNDS)**											
58	91	96	100	105	110	115	119	124	129	134	138	143	148	153	158	162	167	172	177	181	186	191
59	94	99	104	109	114	119	124	128	133	138	143	148	153	158	163	168	173	178	183	188	193	198
60	97	102	107	112	118	123	128	133	138	143	148	153	158	163	168	174	179	184	189	194	199	204
61	100	106	111	116	122	127	132	137	143	148	153	158	164	169	174	180	185	190	195	201	206	211
62	104	109	115	120	126	131	136	142	147	153	158	164	169	175	180	186	191	196	202	207	213	218
63	107	113	118	124	130	135	141	146	152	158	163	169	175	180	186	191	197	203	208	214	220	225
64	110	116	122	128	134	140	145	151	157	163	169	174	180	186	192	197	204	209	215	221	227	232
65	114	120	126	132	138	144	150	156	162	168	174	180	186	192	198	204	210	216	222	228	234	240
66	118	124	130	136	142	148	155	161	167	173	179	186	192	198	204	210	216	223	229	235	241	247
67	121	127	134	140	146	153	159	166	172	178	185	191	198	204	211	217	223	230	236	242	249	255
68	125	131	138	144	151	158	164	171	177	184	190	197	203	210	216	223	230	236	243	249	256	262
69	128	135	142	149	155	162	169	176	182	189	196	203	209	216	223	230	236	243	250	257	263	270
70	132	139	146	153	160	167	174	181	188	195	202	209	216	222	229	236	243	250	257	264	271	278
71	136	143	150	157	165	172	179	186	193	200	208	215	222	229	236	243	250	257	265	272	279	286
72	140	147	154	162	169	177	184	191	199	206	213	221	228	235	242	250	258	265	272	279	287	294
73	144	151	159	166	174	182	189	197	204	212	219	227	235	242	250	257	265	272	280	288	295	302
74	148	155	163	171	179	186	194	202	210	218	225	233	241	249	256	264	272	280	287	295	303	311
75	152	160	168	176	184	192	200	208	216	224	232	240	248	256	264	272	279	287	295	303	311	319
76	156	164	172	180	189	197	205	213	221	230	238	246	254	263	271	279	287	295	304	312	320	328

SOURCE: National Heart, Lung, and Blood Institute. (2013). Clinical guidelines on the identification, evaluation, and treatment of overweight and obesity in adults: Body mass index tables. Retrieved from www.nhlbi.nih.gov/guidelines/obesity/bmi_tbl.htm

TABLE 31–2 Assigning Nursing Diagnoses to Behaviors Commonly Associated With Eating Disorders

BEHAVIORS	NURSING DIAGNOSES
Refusal to eat; abuse of laxatives, diuretics, and/or diet pills; loss of 15 percent of expected body weight; pale conjunctiva and mucous membranes; poor muscle tone; amenorrhea; poor skin turgor; electrolyte imbalances; hypothermia; bradycardia; hypotension; cardiac irregularities; edema	Imbalanced nutrition: Less than body requirements
Decreased fluid intake; abnormal fluid loss caused by self-induced vomiting; excessive use of laxatives, enemas, or diuretics; electrolyte imbalance; decreased urine output; increased urine concentration; elevated hematocrit; decreased blood pressure; increased pulse rate; dry skin; decreased skin turgor; weakness	Deficient fluid volume
Minimizes symptoms; unable to admit impact of disease on life pattern; does not perceive personal relevance of symptoms; does not perceive personal relevance of danger	Denial
Compulsive eating; excessive intake in relation to metabolic needs; sedentary lifestyle; weight 20 percent over ideal for height and frame; BMI of 30 or more	Obesity
Distorted body image; views self as fat, even in the presence of normal body weight or severe emaciation; denies that problem with low body weight exists; difficulty accepting positive reinforcement; self-destructive behavior (self-induced vomiting, abuse of laxatives or diuretics, refusal to eat); preoccupation with appearance and how others perceive it *(anorexia nervosa, bulimia nervosa)* Verbalization of negative feelings about the way he or she looks and the desire to lose weight *(obesity)* Lack of eye contact; depressed mood *(all)*	Disturbed body image/Low self-esteem
Increased tension; increased helplessness; overexcited; apprehensive; fearful; restlessness; poor eye contact; increased difficulty taking oral nourishment; inability to learn	Anxiety (moderate to severe)

Table 31–3 | CARE PLAN FOR CLIENT WITH EATING DISORDERS: ANOREXIA NERVOSA AND BULIMIA NERVOSA

NURSING DIAGNOSES: IMBALANCED NUTRITION: LESS THAN BODY REQUIREMENTS/DEFICIENT FLUID VOLUME (RISK FOR OR ACTUAL)

RELATED TO: Refusal to eat/drink; self-induced vomiting; abuse of laxatives/diuretics

EVIDENCED BY: Loss of weight; poor muscle tone and skin turgor; lanugo; bradycardia; hypotension; cardiac arrhythmias; pale, dry mucous membranes

OUTCOME CRITERIA	NURSING INTERVENTIONS	RATIONALE
Short-Term Goals: • Client will gain *x* pounds per week (amount to be established by client, nurse, and dietitian) • Client will drink 125 mL of fluid each hour during waking hours. Long-Term Goal: • By time of discharge from treatment, client will exhibit no signs or symptoms of malnutrition or dehydration.	1. For the client who is emaciated and is unable or unwilling to maintain an adequate oral intake, the physician may order a liquid diet to be administered via nasogastric tube. Nursing care of the individual receiving tube feedings should be administered according to established hospital protocol. 2. For the client who is able and willing to consume an oral diet, the dietitian will determine	1. Without adequate nutrition, a life-threatening situation exists. 2. Adequate calories are required to allow a weight gain of 2–3 pounds per week.

Table 31–3 | CARE PLAN FOR CLIENT WITH EATING DISORDERS: ANOREXIA NERVOSA AND BULIMIA NERVOSA—cont'd

OUTCOME CRITERIA	NURSING INTERVENTIONS	RATIONALE
	the appropriate number of calories required to provide adequate nutrition and realistic weight gain.	
	3. Explain to the client that privileges and restrictions will be based on compliance with treatment and direct weight gain. Do not focus on food and eating.	3. The real issues have little to do with food or eating patterns. Focus on the control issues that have precipitated these behaviors.
	4. Weigh client daily (without the client observing the numbers on the scale) immediately upon arising and following first voiding. Always use same scale, if possible. Keep strict record of intake and output. Assess skin turgor and integrity regularly. Assess moistness and color of oral mucous membranes.	4. These assessments are important measurements of nutritional status and provide guidelines for treatment.
	5. Stay with client during established time for meals (usually 30 min) and for at least 1 hour following meals.	5. Lengthy mealtimes put excessive focus on food and eating and provide client with attention and reinforcement. The hour following meals may be used to discard food stashed from tray or to engage in self-induced vomiting.
	6. If weight loss occurs, enforce restrictions.	6. Restrictions and limits must be established and carried out consistently to avoid power struggles, to encourage client compliance with therapy, and to ensure client safety.
	7. Ensure that the client and family understand that if nutritional status deteriorates, tube feedings will be initiated. This is implemented in a matter-of-fact, nonpunitive way.	7. This intervention is carried out for the client's safety and protection from a life-threatening condition.
	8. Encourage the client to explore and identify the true feelings and fears that contribute to maladaptive eating behaviors.	8. Emotional issues must be resolved if these maladaptive responses are to be eliminated.

Short-term goals

■ The client will gain ___ pounds per week (amount to be established by client, nurse, and dietitian).

■ The client will drink 125 mL of fluid each hour during waking hours.

Long-term goal

■ By time of discharge from treatment, the client will exhibit no signs or symptoms of malnutrition or dehydration.

Interventions

■ For the client who is emaciated and is unable or unwilling to maintain an adequate oral intake, the physician may order a liquid diet to be administered via nasogastric tube. Without adequate nutrition, a life-threatening situation exists. Nursing care of the individual receiving tube feedings should be administered according to established hospital procedures.

■ For the client who is able and willing to consume an oral diet, the dietitian should determine the appropriate number of calories required to provide adequate nutrition and realistic (according to body structure and height) weight gain.

■ Explain the program of behavior modification to client and family. Explain that privileges and restrictions will be based on compliance with treatment and direct weight gain.

■ Do not focus on food and eating specifically. Instead, focus on the emotional issues that have precipitated these behaviors.

■ Do not discuss food or eating with the client once protocol has been established. Do, however, offer support and positive reinforcement for obvious improvements in eating behaviors.

■ Keep a strict record of intake and output. Weigh the client daily immediately on arising and following first voiding. Always use the same scale, if possible. Weighing a client in such a way that the client cannot see the numbers on a scale may be beneficial in reducing his or her focus on daily weight fluctuations or evidence of weight gain.

■ Assess vital signs, including blood pressure with positional changes to evaluate for orthostatic hypotension and pulse to evaluate for bradycardia. Bradycardia may be more pronounced at rest, so regular assessment during these times is especially important.

■ Assess skin turgor and integrity regularly. Assess moistness and color of oral mucous membranes. The condition of the skin and mucous membranes provides valuable data regarding client hydration. Discourage the client from bathing every day if the skin is very dry.

■ Sit with the client during mealtimes for support and to observe the amount ingested. A limit (usually 30 minutes) should be imposed on time allotted for meals. Without a time limit, meals can become lengthy, drawn-out sessions, providing the client with attention based on food and eating.

■ The client should be observed for at least 1 hour following meals. The client may use this time to discard food that has been stashed from the food tray or to engage in self-induced vomiting. He or she may need to be accompanied to the bathroom if self-induced vomiting is suspected.

■ If weight loss occurs, enforce restrictions. Restrictions and limits must be established and carried out consistently to avoid power struggles and encourage client compliance with therapy.

■ Ensure that the client and family understand that if nutritional status deteriorates, tube feedings will be initiated. This is implemented in a matter-of-fact, nonpunitive way, for the client's safety and protection from a life-threatening condition.

■ Encourage the client to explore and identify the true feelings and fears that contribute to maladaptive eating behaviors. Emotional issues must be resolved if these maladaptive responses are to be eliminated.

Denial

Denial is defined as a "conscious or unconscious attempt to disavow the knowledge or meaning of an event to reduce anxiety and/or fear, leading to the detriment of health" (Herdman & Kamitsuru, p. 335).

Client Goals

Outcome criteria include short- and long-term goals. Time lines are individually determined.

Short-term goal

■ The client will verbalize understanding of the correlation between emotional issues and maladaptive eating behaviors (within time deemed appropriate for individual client).

Long-term goal

■ By time of discharge from treatment, the client will demonstrate the ability to discontinue use of maladaptive eating behaviors and to cope with emotional issues in a more adaptive manner.

Interventions

■ Establish a trusting relationship with the client by being honest, accepting, and available and by keeping all promises. Convey unconditional positive regard.

■ Acknowledge the client's anger at feelings of loss of control brought about by the established eating regimen associated with the program of behavior modification. Anger is a normal human response and should be expressed in an appropriate manner. Feelings that are not expressed remain unresolved and add an additional component to an already serious situation.

■ Avoid arguing or bargaining with the client who is resistant to treatment. State matter-of-factly which behaviors are unacceptable and how privileges will be restricted for noncompliance. It is essential that all staff members are consistent with this intervention.

■ Encourage the client to verbalize feelings regarding his or her role within the family and issues related to dependence/independence, the intense need for achievement, and sexuality. Help the client recognize how maladaptive eating behaviors may be related to these emotional issues. Discuss ways in which he or she can gain control over these problematic areas of life without resorting to maladaptive eating behaviors.

Obesity

Obesity is defined as a condition in which an individual accumulates abnormal or excessive fat for age and gender that exceeds overweight (Herdman & Kamitsuru, p. 163).

Client Goals

Outcome criteria include short- and long-term goals. Time lines are individually determined.

Short-term goal

■ Client will verbalize understanding of what must be done to lose weight.

Long-term goal

■ Client will demonstrate a change in eating patterns that results in a steady weight loss.

Interventions

■ Encourage the client to keep a diary of food intake. A food diary provides the opportunity for the client to gain a realistic picture of the amount of food ingested and provides a database on which to tailor the dietary program.

■ Discuss feelings and emotions associated with eating. This helps to identify when the client is eating to satisfy an emotional need rather than a physiological one.

■ With input from the client, formulate an eating plan that includes food from the required food groups with emphasis on low-fat intake. It is helpful to keep the plan as similar as possible to the client's usual eating pattern. The diet must eliminate calories while maintaining adequate nutrition. The client is more likely to stay on the eating plan if he or she is able to participate in its creation and it deviates as little as possible from usual types of foods.

■ Identify realistic incremental goals for weekly weight loss. Reasonable weight loss (1 to 2 pounds per week) results in more lasting effects. Excessive, rapid weight loss may result in fatigue and irritability and ultimately lead to failure in meeting goals for weight loss. Motivation is more easily sustained by meeting "stair-step" goals.

■ Plan a progressive exercise program tailored to individual goals and choice. Exercise may enhance weight loss by burning calories and reducing appetite, increasing energy, toning muscles, and enhancing sense of well-being and accomplishment. Walking is an excellent choice for overweight individuals.

■ Discuss the probability of reaching plateaus when weight remains stable for extended periods. The client should know this is likely to happen as changes in metabolism occur. Plateaus cause frustration, and the client may need additional support during these times to remain on the weight-loss program.

■ Provide instruction about medications to assist with weight loss if ordered by the physician. Appetite-suppressant drugs and others that have weight loss as a side effect may be helpful to someone who is severely overweight. They should be used for this purpose for only a short period while the individual attempts to adjust to the new pattern of eating.

Disturbed Body Image/Low Self-Esteem

Disturbed body image is defined as "confusion in mental picture of one's physical self" (Herdman & Kamitsuru 2014, p. 275). *Low self-esteem* is defined as "negative self-evaluating/feelings about self or self-capabilities" (p. 271).

Client Goals (for the Client With Anorexia Nervosa or Bulimia Nervosa)

Outcome criteria include short- and long-term goals. Time lines are individually determined.

Short-term goal

■ The client will verbally acknowledge misperception of body image as "fat" within specified time (depending on severity and chronicity of condition).

Long-term goal

■ By the time of discharge from treatment, the client will demonstrate an increase in self-esteem as manifested by verbalizing positive aspects of self and exhibiting less preoccupation with own appearance as a more realistic body image is developed.

Client Goals (for the Client With Binge Eating Disorder and Associated Obesity)

Outcome criteria include short- and long-term goals. Time lines are individually determined.

Short-term goal

■ The client will begin to accept self based on self-attributes rather than on appearance.

Long-term goal

■ The client will pursue loss of weight as desired.

Interventions

For the client with anorexia nervosa or bulimia nervosa:

■ Help the client develop a realistic perception of body image and relationship with food. Compare specific measurement of the client's body with the client's perceived calculations. There may be a large discrepancy between the actual body size and the client's perception of his or her body size. The client needs to recognize that the misperception of body image is unhealthy and that maintaining control through maladaptive eating behaviors is dangerous—even life threatening.

■ Promote feelings of control within the environment through participation and independent decision-making. Through positive feedback, help the client learn to accept self as is, including weaknesses as well as strengths. The client must come to understand that he or she is a capable, autonomous individual who can perform outside the family unit and is not expected to be perfect. Control of his or her life must be achieved in other ways besides dieting and weight loss.

■ Help the client realize that perfection is unrealistic, and explore this need with him or her. As the client begins to feel better about self, identifies positive self-attributes, and develops the ability to accept certain personal inadequacies, the need for unrealistic achievement should diminish.

For the client with binge eating disorder and associated obesity:

■ Assess the client's feelings and attitudes about overeating and obesity. Obesity and compulsive eating behaviors may have deep-rooted psychological implications, such as compensation for lack of love and nurturing or a defense against intimacy.

■ Ensure that the client has privacy during self-care activities. The obese individual may be sensitive or self-conscious about his or her body.

■ Have the client recall coping patterns related to food in family of origin, and explore how these may affect current situation. Parents are role models for their children. Maladaptive eating behaviors may have been learned within the family system and are supported through positive reinforcement. Food may be substituted by the parent for affection and love, and eating is associated with a feeling of satisfaction, becoming the primary defense.

■ Determine the client's motivation for developing healthier patterns of eating. O'Melia (2014) stresses that traditional obesity management strategies, which typically include diets and food restriction, are less effective with binge eating disorder because the primary concern is developing healthier approaches to eating and reducing or eliminating binging behavior. Weight loss would be a secondary outcome. The individual may harbor repressed feelings of hostility that may be expressed inwardly on the self. Because of a poor self-concept, the person often has difficulty with relationships. When the motivation is to lose weight for someone else, healthier eating is less likely to be sustainable.

■ Help the client identify positive self-attributes. Focus on strengths and past accomplishments unrelated to physical appearance. It is important that self-esteem not be tied solely to size of the body. The client needs to recognize that obesity need not interfere with positive feelings regarding self-concept and self-worth.

■ Refer the client to a support or therapy group. Support groups can provide companionship, increase motivation, decrease loneliness and social ostracism, and give practical solutions to common problems. Group therapy can be helpful in dealing with underlying psychological concerns.

Concept Care Mapping

The concept map care plan (see Chapter 9, The Nursing Process in Psychiatric-Mental Health Nursing) is a diagrammatic teaching and learning strategy that allows visualization of interrelationships between medical diagnoses, nursing diagnoses, assessment data, and treatments. Examples of concept map care plans for clients with eating disorders are presented in Figures 31–1 and 31–2.

Client and Family Education

The role of client teacher is important in the psychiatric area, as it is in all areas of nursing. It is essential to include the family in education and treatment unless there are overriding reasons not to do so. A list of topics for client and family education relevant to eating disorders is presented in Box 31–4.

Evaluation

Evaluation of the client with an eating disorder requires a reassessment of the behaviors for which the client

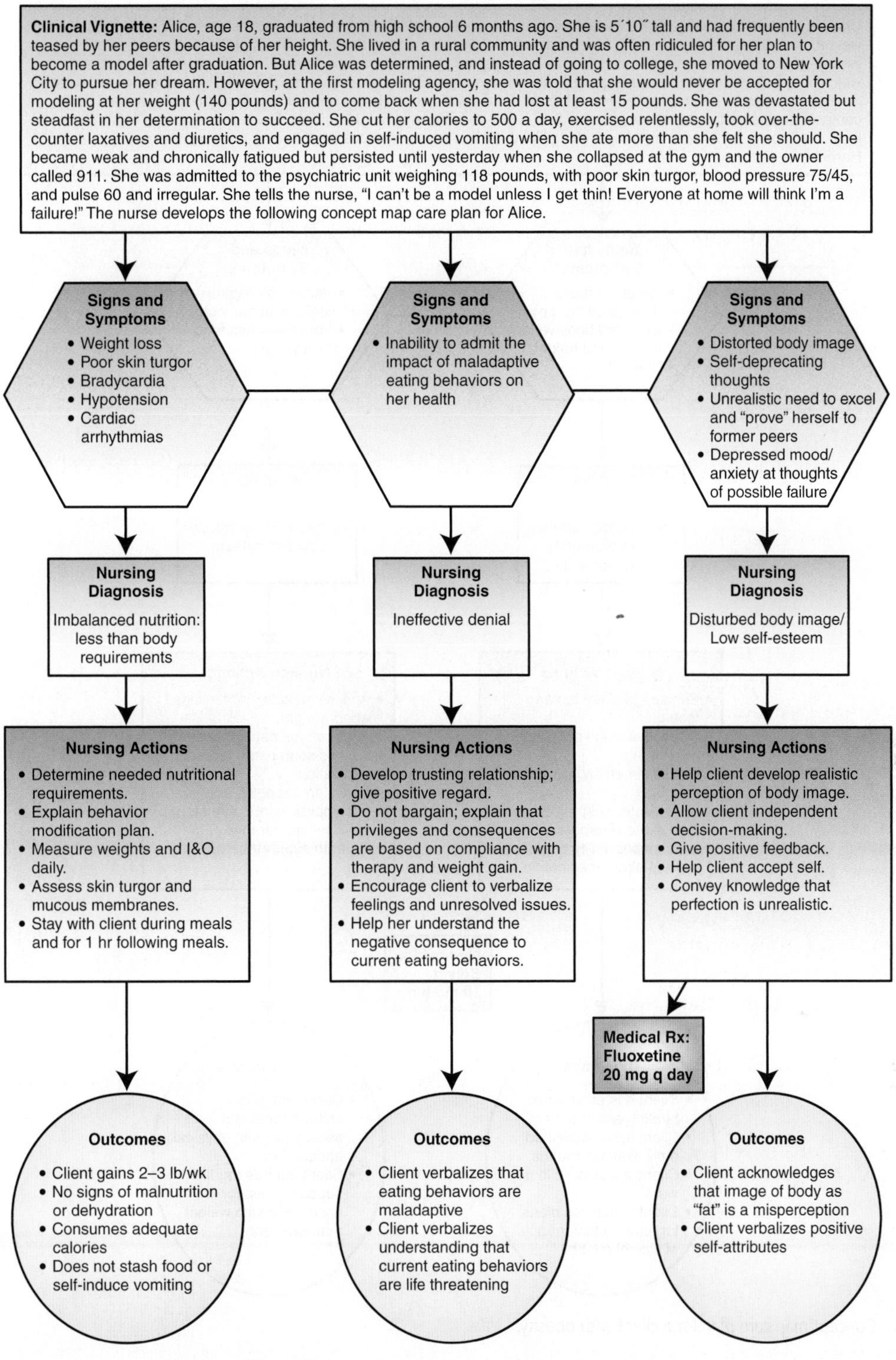

Clinical Vignette: Alice, age 18, graduated from high school 6 months ago. She is 5´10˝ tall and had frequently been teased by her peers because of her height. She lived in a rural community and was often ridiculed for her plan to become a model after graduation. But Alice was determined, and instead of going to college, she moved to New York City to pursue her dream. However, at the first modeling agency, she was told that she would never be accepted for modeling at her weight (140 pounds) and to come back when she had lost at least 15 pounds. She was devastated but steadfast in her determination to succeed. She cut her calories to 500 a day, exercised relentlessly, took over-the-counter laxatives and diuretics, and engaged in self-induced vomiting when she ate more than she felt she should. She became weak and chronically fatigued but persisted until yesterday when she collapsed at the gym and the owner called 911. She was admitted to the psychiatric unit weighing 118 pounds, with poor skin turgor, blood pressure 75/45, and pulse 60 and irregular. She tells the nurse, "I can't be a model unless I get thin! Everyone at home will think I'm a failure!" The nurse develops the following concept map care plan for Alice.

FIGURE 31–1 Concept map care plan for a client with anorexia nervosa.

sought treatment. Behavioral change will be required on the part of both the client and family members. The following types of questions may provide assistance in gathering data required for evaluating whether the nursing interventions have been effective in achieving the goals of therapy.

For the client with anorexia nervosa or bulimia nervosa:

■ Has the client steadily gained 2 to 3 pounds per week to at least 80 percent of expected body weight for age and size?
■ Is the client free of signs and symptoms of malnutrition and dehydration?

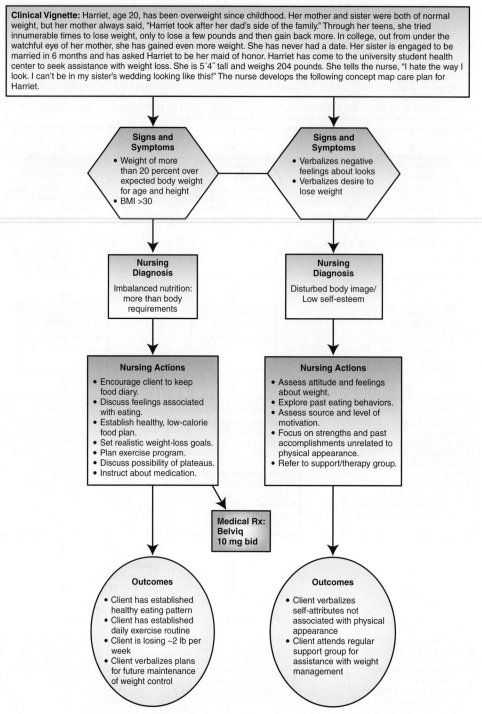

Clinical Vignette: Harriet, age 20, has been overweight since childhood. Her mother and sister were both of normal weight, but her mother always said, "Harriet took after her dad's side of the family." Through her teens, she tried innumerable times to lose weight, only to lose a few pounds and then gain back more. In college, out from under the watchful eye of her mother, she has gained even more weight. She has never had a date. Her sister is engaged to be married in 6 months and has asked Harriet to be her maid of honor. Harriet has come to the university student health center to seek assistance with weight loss. She is 5′4″ tall and weighs 204 pounds. She tells the nurse, "I hate the way I look. I can't be in my sister's wedding looking like this!" The nurse develops the following concept map care plan for Harriet.

Signs and Symptoms
- Weight of more than 20 percent over expected body weight for age and height
- BMI >30

Signs and Symptoms
- Verbalizes negative feelings about looks
- Verbalizes desire to lose weight

Nursing Diagnosis
Imbalanced nutrition: more than body requirements

Nursing Diagnosis
Disturbed body image/ Low self-esteem

Nursing Actions
- Encourage client to keep food diary.
- Discuss feelings associated with eating.
- Establish healthy, low-calorie food plan.
- Set realistic weight-loss goals.
- Plan exercise program.
- Discuss possibility of plateaus.
- Instruct about medication.

Nursing Actions
- Assess attitude and feelings about weight.
- Explore past eating behaviors.
- Assess source and level of motivation.
- Focus on strengths and past accomplishments unrelated to physical appearance.
- Refer to support/therapy group.

Medical Rx: Belviq 10 mg bid

Outcomes
- Client has established healthy eating pattern
- Client has established daily exercise routine
- Client is losing ~2 lb per week
- Client verbalizes plans for future maintenance of weight control

Outcomes
- Client verbalizes self-attributes not associated with physical appearance
- Client attends regular support group for assistance with weight management

FIGURE 31–2 Concept map care plan for a client with obesity.

■ Does the client consume adequate calories as determined by the dietitian?

■ Have there been any attempts to stash food from the tray to discard later?

■ Have there been any attempts to self-induce vomiting?

■ Has the client admitted that a problem exists and that eating behaviors are maladaptive?

■ Have behaviors aimed at manipulating the environment been discontinued?

■ Is the client willing to discuss the real issues concerning family roles, sexuality, dependence/ independence, and the need for achievement?

■ Does the client understand how he or she has used maladaptive eating behaviors in an effort to achieve a feeling of some control over life events?

BOX 31–4 Topics for Client/Family Education Related to Eating Disorders

NATURE OF THE ILLNESS

1. Symptoms of anorexia nervosa
2. Symptoms of bulimia nervosa
3. Symptoms of binge eating disorder
4. What constitutes obesity
5. Causes of eating disorders
6. Effects of the illness or condition on the body
7. Behaviors that may reinforce unhealthy responses such as television and social media, peer focus on clothing sizes, eating, and weight. Internet sources have become a means for sharing information among people with anorexia about how the individual can distract parents and health-care providers from recognizing the extent of weight loss. Family members can learn more about some of these behaviors to look out for and may want to monitor their child's use of Internet and social media resources.

MANAGEMENT OF THE ILLNESS

1. Principles of nutrition (foods for maintenance of wellness)
2. Ways client may feel in control of life (aside from eating)
3. Importance of expressing fears and feelings, rather than holding them inside
4. Alternative coping strategies (to maladaptive eating behaviors)
5. For the obese client:
    a. How to plan a reduced-calorie, nutritious diet
    b. How to read food content labels
    c. How to establish a realistic weight loss plan
    d. How to establish a planned program of physical activity
6. Correct administration of prescribed medications
7. Indication for and side effects of prescribed medications
8. Relaxation techniques
9. Problem-solving skills
10. Discuss the Maudsley approach for treatment of anorexia nervosa as an evidence-based option for family involvement in the recovery program

SUPPORT SERVICES

1. Weight Watchers International
2. Overeaters Anonymous
3. National Association of Anorexia Nervosa and Associated Disorders (ANAD)

    800 East Diehl Road #160

    Naperville, IL 60563

    (630) 577-1330

    www.anad.org
4. National Eating Disorders Association

    165 West 46th Street

    New York, NY 10036

    (212) 575-6200

    www.nationaleatingdisorders.org

Reprinted with permission from the Diagnostic and Statistical Manual of Mental Disorders, Fifth Edition *(Copyright 2013). American Psychiatric Association.*

■ Has the client acknowledged that perception of body image as "fat" is incorrect?

For the client with binge eating disorder and associated obesity:

■ Has the client shown a steady weight loss since starting the new eating plan?
■ Does the client verbalize a relapse prevention plan to avoid triggers and abstain from binging?

■ Does the client verbalize positive self-attributes not associated with body size or appearance?

For the client with anorexia, bulimia, or binge eating disorder and associated obesity:

■ Has the client been able to develop a more realistic perception of body image?
■ Has the client acknowledged that past self-expectations may have been unrealistic?

■ Does client accept self as less than perfect?
■ Has the client developed adaptive coping strategies to deal with stress without resorting to maladaptive eating behaviors?

Quality and Safety Education for Nurses (QSEN)

The Institute of Medicine (IOM) (now the National Academy of Medicine), in its 2003 report *Health Professions Education: A Bridge to Quality,* challenged faculties of medicine, nursing, and other health professions to ensure that their graduates have achieved a core set of competencies in order to meet the needs of the 21st-century health-care system. These competencies include *providing patient-centered care, maintaining safety, working in interdisciplinary teams, employing evidence-based practice, applying quality improvement,* and *utilizing informatics.* A QSEN teaching strategy is included in Box 31–5. The use of this type of activity is intended to arm the instructor and the student with guidelines for attaining the knowledge, skills, and attitudes necessary for achievement of quality and safety competencies in nursing.

Treatment Modalities

The immediate aim of treatment in eating disorders is to restore the client's nutritional status. Complications of emaciation, dehydration, and electrolyte imbalance can lead to death. Once the physical condition is no longer life threatening, other treatment modalities may be initiated.

Behavior Modification

Efforts to change the maladaptive eating behaviors of clients with anorexia nervosa and bulimia nervosa have become the widely accepted treatment. The importance of instituting a behavior modification program with these clients is to ensure that the program does not "control" them. Issues of control are central in these disorders, so for the program to be successful, the client must perceive that he or she is

---

BOX 31–5 QSEN TEACHING STRATEGY

Assignment: Using Evidence to Address Clinical Problems
Intervention With a Client Who Fears Gaining Weight (Anorexia Nervosa)
Competency Domain: Evidence-Based Practice

Learning Objectives: Student will:
• Differentiate clinical opinion from research and evidence summaries.
• Explain the role of evidence in determining the best clinical practice for intervening with clients who do not want to eat.
• Identify gaps between what is observed in the treatment setting to what has been identified as best practice.
• Discriminate between valid and invalid reasons for modifying evidence-based clinical practice based on clinical expertise or other reasons.
• Participate effectively in appropriate data collection and other research activities.
• Acknowledge own limitations in knowledge and clinical expertise before determining when to deviate from evidence-based best practices.

Strategy Overview:
1. Investigate the research related to intervening with a client who does not want to eat.
2. Identify best practices described in the literature. How were these best practices determined?
3. Compare and contrast staff intervention with best practices described in the literature.
4. Investigate staff perceptions related to intervening with a client who is refusing to eat.
5. How has the client developed these perceptions?
6. Do staff members view any problems associated with their practice versus best practice described in the literature? If so, how would they like to see the problem addressed?
7. Describe ethical issues associated with intervening with a client who does not want to eat.
8. What is your personal perception regarding the best evidence available to date related to intervening with a client who has anorexia nervosa? Are there situations that you can think of when you might deviate from the best practice model?
9. What questions do you have about intervening with a client who has anorexia nervosa that are not being addressed by current researchers?

Adapted from teaching strategy submitted by Pamela M. Ironside, Associate Professor, Indiana University School of Nursing, Indianapolis, IN. © 2009 QSEN; http://qsen.org. With permission.

in control of the treatment. The Maudsley approach, an evidence-based program for the treatment of adolescents with anorexia nervosa, modifies this concept in that the first phase of treatment is designed to encourage parental control of eating, with control returned to the adolescent once he or she demonstrates readiness and ability to establish control in healthier ways.

Successes have been observed when the client with anorexia nervosa is allowed to contract for privileges based on weight gain. The client has input into the care plan and can clearly see what the treatment choices are. The client has control over eating, over the amount of exercise pursued, and even over whether or not to induce vomiting. Goals of therapy, along with the responsibilities of each for goal achievement, are agreed on by client and staff.

Staff and client also agree on a system of rewards and privileges that can be earned by the client, who is given ultimate control. He or she has a choice of whether or not to abide by the contract, a choice of whether or not to gain weight, and a choice of whether or not to earn the desired privilege.

This method of treatment gives a great deal of autonomy to the client. It must be understood, however, that these behavior modification techniques are helpful for weight restoration only. Adjunctive individual psychotherapy and/or family psychoeducation may be required to prevent or reduce further morbidity. Cognitive-behavioral therapy (CBT) and dialectical behavior therapy (DBT) have demonstrated benefits in clients with anorexia, bulimia, and binge eating disorders (Black & Andreasen, 2014; O'Melia, 2014; Wright, Thase, & Beck, 2008).

By confronting irrational thinking patterns and associated feelings, CBT and DBT strive to eliminate the emotional components associated with unhealthy eating patterns.

Individual Therapy

Although individual psychotherapy is not the therapy of choice for eating disorders, it may be an adjunct to a comprehensive, multifaceted treatment approach when underlying comorbid psychological problems are contributing to the maladaptive behaviors. In supportive psychotherapy, the therapist encourages the client to explore unresolved conflicts and recognize the maladaptive eating behaviors as defense mechanisms to ease emotional pain. The goals are to resolve personal issues and establish more adaptive coping strategies for dealing with stressful situations.

Family Treatment: The Maudsley Approach

The Maudsley approach is one of the few evidence-based treatment approaches for teens with anorexia nervosa. This approach actively involves the family in each step of the process. In some of the first controlled studies of this method, 90 percent of clients showed improvement compared to 36 percent of those in individual therapies (Le Grange, 2005). The treatment program is conducted in an intensive outpatient program and involves three phases of treatment. Phase I is focused on weight restoration, and in this phase the parents are actively engaged in establishing the rules and guidelines around eating. Parents often need substantial support during this phase because they typically encounter frequent power struggles with their child. When the client accepts parental demands for increased food intake, demonstrates steady weight gain, and there is a change in the mood of the family (i.e., relief at having taken charge of the eating disorder; both adolescents and their parents identify reduced anxiety), phase II is ready to begin (LeGrange & Lock, no date). In this phase, control of maintaining weight gain is returned to the adolescent. Once he or she demonstrates ability to maintain above 95 percent of ideal weight, the shift to phase III focuses on assisting the adolescent to develop a healthy self-identity. This includes incorporating CBT and DBT skills, which have demonstrated effectiveness in treating this condition.

Psychopharmacology

Research has not yet identified a medication that results in definitive improvement of anorexia nervosa (Sadock et al., 2015). Trials of fluoxetine (Prozac) have shown some evidence of weight gain and, in general, SSRIs may be beneficial in the treatment of comorbid depression, but they also carry a black-box warning about risk of increasing suicide ideation in adolescents. The anticholinergic side effects of tricyclic antidepressants, including orthostatic hypotension, may be problematic for patients who are already at risk for these symptoms. It is important to recognize that depression and other mood and cognitive symptoms can be a symptom of malnutrition and starvation. When nutrition is restored those symptoms often improve.

Fluoxetine has been found useful in the treatment of bulimia nervosa (Schatzberg, Cole, & DeBattista, 2010). A dosage of 60 mg/day (triple the usual antidepressant dosage) was found to be most effective. It is possible that fluoxetine, an SSRI, may decrease the craving for carbohydrates, thereby decreasing the incidence of binge eating, which is often associated with consumption of large amounts of carbohydrates. Other antidepressants, such as imipramine (Tofranil), desipramine (Norpramin), amitriptyline (Elavil), nortriptyline (Aventyl), and phenelzine

(Nardil), also have been shown effective in controlled treatment studies (Sadock et al., 2015)

High-dose SSRIs have demonstrated some efficacy in promoting weight loss for clients with binge eating disorder, but the weight loss was temporary and weight *gain* typically occurred after the medication was discontinued (Sadock et al., 2015). Remember, too, that weight loss is a secondary symptom of binge eating disorder. An effective medication needs to also manage the symptom of binging. Two medications, topiramate and lisdexamfetamine (a dopamine-norepinephrine reuptake inhibitor, originally used in the treatment of attention-deficit/hyperactivity disorder) have demonstrated benefits in reducing incidents of both binge eating and weight loss (Balodis et al., 2015). Most studies reveal that medication in combination with CBT is more beneficial than medication alone (Sadock et al., 2015).

CASE STUDY AND SAMPLE CARE PLAN

NURSING HISTORY AND ASSESSMENT

When Katie fainted in history class, she was taken to the university health center by her roommate, Ashley. Ashley told the nurse that Katie has been taking a lot of over-the-counter laxatives and diuretics. She also said that Katie often self-induced vomiting when she felt that she had eaten too much. After an initial physical assessment, the nurse in the university health center referred Katie to the mental health clinic.

At the mental health clinic, Katie weighed 110 pounds and measured 5 feet 6 inches. She admitted to the psychiatric nurse that she tried to keep her weight down by dieting, but sometimes she got so hungry that she would overeat, and then she felt the need to self-induce vomiting to get rid of the calories. "I really don't like doing it, but lots of the girls do. In fact, that is where I got the idea. I always thought I was too fat in high school, but the competition wasn't so great there. Here all the girls are so pretty—and so thin! It's the only way I can keep my weight down!"

Katie also admitted that she hoards food in her dorm room and that she eats when she is feeling particularly anxious and depressed (often during the night). She admitted to having eaten several bags of potato chips and whole packages of cookies in a single sitting. She sometimes drives to the local hamburger stand in the middle of the night, orders several hamburgers, fries, and milkshakes, and consumes them as she sits in her car alone. She stated that she feels so much better while she is eating these foods but then feels panicky after they have been consumed. That is when she self-induces vomiting. "Then I feel more depressed, and the only thing that helps is eating! I feel so out of control!"

NURSING DIAGNOSES AND OUTCOME IDENTIFICATION

From the assessment data, the nurse develops the following nursing diagnosis for Katie:

Ineffective coping related to feelings of helplessness, low self-esteem, and lack of control in life situation.

■ **Short-Term Goal:** Client will identify and discuss fears and anxieties with the nurse.
■ **Long-Term Goal:** Client will identify adaptive coping strategies that can be realistically incorporated into her lifestyle, thereby eliminating binging and purging in response to anxiety.

PLANNING AND IMPLEMENTATION

INEFFECTIVE COPING

The following nursing interventions have been identified for Katie.

■ Establish a trusting relationship with Katie. Be honest and accepting. Show unconditional positive regard.
■ Help Katie identify the situations that produce anxiety and discuss how she coped with these situations before she began binging and purging.
■ Help Katie identify the emotions that precipitate binging (e.g., fear, boredom, anger, loneliness).
■ Once these high-risk situations have been identified, help her identify alternate behaviors, such as exercise, a hobby, or a warm bath.
■ Encourage Katie to express feelings that have been suppressed because they were considered unacceptable. Help her identify healthier ways to express those feelings.
■ Use role-play with Katie to deal with feelings and experiment with new behaviors.
■ Explore the dynamics of Katie's family and encourage family involvement for support with Katie's consent.
■ Teach the concepts of good nutrition, and the importance of healthy eating patterns in overall wellness.
■ Consult with the physician about a prescription for fluoxetine for Katie.
■ Help Katie find a support group for individuals with eating disorders. Encourage regular attendance in this group.

EVALUATION

The outcome criteria for Katie have been met. She discussed with the nurse the feelings that triggered binging episodes and the situations that precipitated those feelings. She has joined a support group of individuals with eating disorders and now has a "buddy" that she may call (even in the middle of the night) when she is feeling like binging. She has started riding her bicycle regularly and goes to the fitness center when she is feeling especially anxious. She still sees the mental health nurse weekly and continues to discuss her fears and anxieties. The urges to binge at stressful times have not disappeared completely. However, they have decreased in frequency, and Katie is now able to choose more adaptive strategies for dealing with stress.

Summary and Key Points

■ The incidence of eating disorders has continued to increase since the middle of the 20th century.

■ Individuals with anorexia nervosa, a disorder characterized by a morbid fear of obesity and a gross distortion of body image, literally can starve themselves to death.

■ The individual with anorexia nervosa believes he or she is fat even when emaciated. The disorder is commonly accompanied by depression and anxiety.

■ Bulimia nervosa is an eating disorder characterized by the consumption of huge amounts of food, usually in a short period of time and often in secret.

■ With bulimia nervosa, tension is relieved and pleasure felt during the time of the binge but is soon followed by feelings of guilt and depression.

■ Individuals with bulimia nervosa "purge" themselves of the excessive intake with self-induced vomiting or the misuse of laxatives, diuretics, or enemas. They also are subject to mood and anxiety disorders.

■ Binge eating disorder is characterized by the consumption of huge amounts of food by an individual who feels a lack of control over the eating behavior. It differs from bulimia nervosa in that the individual does not engage in behaviors to rid the body of the excess calories.

■ Compulsive eating can result in obesity, which is defined by the National Institutes of Health as a BMI of 30.

■ Obesity predisposes the individual to many health concerns, and at the morbid level (a BMI of 40), the weight alone can contribute to increases in morbidity and mortality.

■ Predisposing factors to eating disorders include genetics, physiological factors, family dynamics, and environmental and lifestyle factors.

■ Treatment modalities for eating disorders include behavior modification, individual psychotherapy, cognitive-behavioral therapy, family treatment (such as the Maudsley approach), and psychopharmacology.

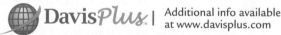 **DavisPlus** | Additional info available at www.davisplus.com

Review Questions
Self-Examination/Learning Exercise

Select the answer that is most appropriate for each of the following questions.

1. Some obese individuals take amphetamines to suppress appetite and help them lose weight. Which of the following is an adverse effect associated with use of amphetamines that makes this practice undesirable?
   a. Bradycardia
   b. Amenorrhea
   c. Tolerance
   d. Convulsions

2. The Maudsley approach to treatment of adolescents with anorexia nervosa advances which of the following fundamental concepts?
   a. Family should be actively involved in each phase of treatment.
   b. Parents should be prohibited from involvement in helping their child eat more, since there are often control issues.
   c. Adolescents need to work on developing healthy self-identities before they can begin to gain weight.
   d. Individual psychotherapy is the most effective treatment for adolescents with anorexia nervosa.

3. John has sought help for his concern that he is binge eating and feels like it has "gotten out of control." He asks the nurse what can be done to help him. Which of these is the most accurate response?
   a. Nothing can be done.
   b. Some medications and psychological treatments have demonstrated effectiveness in reducing binge eating behaviors.
   c. The primary problem is obesity. I can help you set up a calorie-restricted diet.
   d. Medications can help with weight loss, but there are no medications effective for reducing binge eating.

Continued

Review Questions—cont'd
Self-Examination/Learning Exercise

4. Emma, age 14, has just been admitted to the psychiatric unit for anorexia nervosa. She is emaciated and refusing to eat. What is the primary nursing diagnosis for Emma?
   a. Complicated grieving
   b. Imbalanced nutrition: Less than body requirements.
   c. Interrupted family processes
   d. Anxiety (severe)

5. Which of the following physical manifestations would you expect to assess in a client suffering from anorexia nervosa?
   a. Tachycardia, hypertension, hyperthermia
   b. Bradycardia, hypertension, hyperthermia
   c. Bradycardia, hypotension, hypothermia
   d. Tachycardia, hypotension, hypothermia

6. The nurse is caring for a client who has been hospitalized with anorexia nervosa and is severely malnourished. The client continues to refuse to eat. What is the most appropriate response by the nurse?
   a. "You know that if you don't eat, you will die."
   b. "If you continue to refuse to take food orally, you will be fed through a nasogastric tube."
   c. "You might as well leave if you are not going to follow your therapy regimen."
   d. "You don't have to eat if you don't want to. It is your choice."

7. Which medication has been used with some success in clients with anorexia nervosa?
   a. Lorcaserin (Belviq)
   b. Diazepam (Valium)
   c. Fluoxetine (Prozac)
   d. Carbamazepine (Tegretol)

8. Marissa is hospitalized on the psychiatric unit. She has a history and current diagnosis of bulimia nervosa. Which of the following symptoms would be congruent with Marissa's diagnosis?
   a. Binging, purging, obesity, hyperkalemia
   b. Binging, purging, normal weight, hypokalemia
   c. Binging, laxative abuse, amenorrhea, severe weight loss
   d. Binging, purging, severe weight loss, hyperkalemia

9. A hospitalized client with bulimia nervosa has stopped vomiting in the hospital and tells the nurse she is afraid she is going to gain weight. Which is the most appropriate response by the nurse?
   a. "Don't worry. The dietitian will ensure you don't get too many calories in your diet."
   b. "Don't worry about your weight. We are going to work on other problems while you are in the hospital."
   c. "I understand that you are concerned about your weight, and we will talk about the importance of good nutrition, but for now I want you to tell me about your recent invitation to join the National Honor Society. That's quite an accomplishment."
   d. "You are not fat, and the staff will ensure that you do not gain weight while you are in the hospital, because we know that is important to you."

10. Mandy presents in the emergency department with complaints of suicidal ideation. The following data is collected by the nurse. Which of these assessment findings suggests that bulimia nervosa might be a health problem? (Select all that apply.)
    a. Mandy's parotid glands appear enlarged.
    b. Mandy's teeth have a "moth eaten" pattern of tooth decay.
    c. Mandy reports that she takes laxatives daily.
    d. Mandy's weight is within the expected range.

MOVIE CONNECTIONS

The Best Little Girl in the World (anorexia nervosa)
• *Kate's Secret* (bulimia nervosa) • *For the Love of Nancy* (anorexia nervosa) • *Super Size Me* (obesity)

IMPLICATIONS OF RESEARCH FOR EVIDENCE-BASED PRACTICE

Waller, T., Lampman, C., & Lupfer-Johnson, G. (2012). Assessing bias against overweight individuals among nursing and psychology students: An implicit association test. *Journal of Clinical Nursing, 21*(23-24), 3504-3512. doi:10.1111/j.1365-2702.2012.04226.x

DESCRIPTION OF THE STUDY: Almost 69 percent of adults in the United States are overweight, and more than 35 percent of those are within the range of obesity. Obesity has become a leading health concern that impacts both physical and psychological health. Because attitudes can affect behaviors negatively, the authors undertook this study to determine the implicit or unconscious attitudes of nursing and psychology students toward overweight individuals in medical and nonmedical contexts. Study participants included 90 students in upper division nursing and psychology programs at the University of Alaska Anchorage. Mean age was 25 years. The majority were white. Others reported their race as Alaska Native or American Indian, African American, Asian, Hispanic, and Filipino. Attitudes were measured using an implicit association test (IAT) that measures how readily a target concept and an attribute are associated by analyzing reaction times. Participants sat at computers with dominant hand on response pad with the following instructions: "Please press the *blue* key as quickly as possible if you see a *thin* or *normal weight* person, or if you see a *positive* attribute used to describe a person. Please press the *yellow* key if you see an *overweight* person, or if you see a *negative* attribute used to describe a person." Attitudes were measured according to rapidity of response time in relation to associating images of overweight individuals with positive words and normal-weight or thin individuals with negative words (the inconsistent stereotype) as compared to associating positive words with thin or normal-weight individuals and negative words with obese or overweight individuals (the consistent stereotype). Scenarios exhibited individuals in both medical settings (patients) and nonmedical settings.

RESULTS OF THE STUDY: Students enrolled in a social psychology class analyzed the data for a class assignment. Results indicated a statistically significant implicit bias toward overweight individuals by both the nursing students and the psychology students. A stronger weight bias was noted when the target stimulus in the scenario was female than when the target stimulus was male. No significant differences in degree of bias toward weight were found between nursing and psychology students or between subjects in medical versus nonmedical settings.

IMPLICATIONS FOR NURSING PRACTICE: The authors suggest:

Providing education and support to overweight individuals is central to nursing practice in a society struggling to manage obesity. Negative stereotypes or beliefs about these individuals may result in poor patient care. Therefore, nurses and other healthcare professionals must be aware of personal biases and work to develop methods to address weight-related issues in a therapeutic manner. (p. 3504)

TEST YOUR CRITICAL THINKING SKILLS

Janice, a high school sophomore, wanted desperately to become a cheerleader. She practiced endlessly before tryouts, but she was not selected. A week later, her boyfriend, Roy, broke up with her to date another girl. Janice, who was 5 feet 3 inches tall and, at that time, weighed 110 pounds, decided it was because she was too fat. She began to exercise at every possible moment. She skipped meals and tried to keep her daily consumption to no more than 300 calories. She lost a great deal of weight but became very weak. She felt cold all of the time and wore sweaters in the warm weather. She collapsed during her physical education class at school and was rushed to the emergency department. On admission, she weighed 90 pounds. She was emaciated and anemic. The physician admitted her with a diagnosis of anorexia nervosa.

Answer the following questions about Janice:

1. What will be the *primary* consideration in her care?
2. How will treatment be directed toward helping her gain weight?
3. How will the nurse know if Janice is using self-induced vomiting to rid herself of food consumed at meals?

Communication Exercises

1. Helena was admitted to the psychiatric unit with a diagnosis of severe anorexia nervosa. After completing a meal, she asks the nurse to be excused so she can use the restroom. How would the nurse respond to Helena's request?

2. John has been seeking counseling for a binge eating disorder. When the nurse is weighing him, John states, "I hate myself. I should never have let myself get like this. I'm completely out of control." What would be the most empathic response by the nurse?

References

American Academy for Eating Disorders. (2009). Position statement: The role of the family in eating disorders. Retrieved from www.aedweb.org/index.php/23-get-involved/position-statements/88-the-role-of-the-family-in-eating-disorders

American Psychiatric Association. (2013). *Diagnostic and statistical manual of mental disorders* (5th ed.). Washington, DC: American Psychiatric Publishing.

Balodis, I.M., Grilo, C.M., & Potenza, M.N. (2015). Neurobiological underpinnings of obesity and addiction: A focus on binge eating disorder and implications for treatment. *Psychiatric Times.* Retrieved from www.psychiatrictimes.com/cme/neurobiological-underpinnings-obesity-and-addiction-focus-binge-eating-disorder-and-implications/page/0/2#sthash.D9vZ5Ijs.dpuf

Black, D.W., & Andreasen, N.C. (2014). *Introductory textbook of psychiatry* (6th ed.). Washington, DC: American Psychiatric Publishing.

Centers for Disease Control and Prevention. (2015). Adult overweight and obesity. Retrieved from www.cdc.gov/obesity/adult/index.html

Herdman, T.H., & Kamitsuru, S. (Eds.). (2014). *NANDA-I nursing diagnoses: Definitions and classification, 2015–2017.* Oxford: Wiley Blackwell.

Institute of Medicine. (2003). *Health professions education: A bridge to quality.* Washington, DC: Author.

Jaret, P. (2010). Eating disorders and depression. Retrieved from www.webmd.com/depression/features/eating-disorders

LeGrange, D. (2005). The Maudsley family-based treatment for adolescent anorexia nervosa. *World Psychiatry, 4*(3), 142-146.

LeGrange, D., & Lock, J. (no date). Family-based treatment of adolescent anorexia nervosa: The Maudsley approach. Retrieved from www.maudsleyparents.org/whatismaudsley.html

Micula-Gondek, W., & Lackamp, J. (2011). The ABCDEs of identifying eating disorders. *Current Psychiatry, 10*(7). Retrieved from www.currentpsychiatry.com/?id=22161&tx_ttnews[tt_news]=176106&cHash=677d188397e2489fe656c33f5b5d8801

National Heart, Lung, and Blood Institute. (2013). Clinical guidelines on the identification, evaluation, and treatment of overweight and obesity in adults: Body mass index tables. Retrieved from www.nhlbi.nih.gov/guidelines/obesity/bmi_tbl.htm

O'Melia, A.M. (2014). Binge eating disorder. *Current Psychiatry, 13*(4). Retrieved from www.currentpsychiatry.com/specialty-focus/eating-disorders/article/binge-eating-disorder/1e566fd65698cb7b06e0d2b355284392.html

Puri, B.K., & Treasaden, I.H. (2011). *Textbook of psychiatry* (3rd ed.). Philadelphia: Churchill Livingstone Elsevier.

Sadock, B.J., Sadock, V.A., & Ruiz, P. (2015). *Synopsis of psychiatry: Behavioral sciences/clinical psychiatry* (11th ed.). Philadelphia: Lippincott Williams & Wilkins.

Schatzberg, A.F., Cole, J.O., & DeBattista, C. (2010). *Manual of clinical psychopharmacology* (7th ed.). Washington, DC: American Psychiatric Publishing.

Uçeyler, N., Schutt, M., Palm, F., Vogel, C., Meier, M., Schmitt, A., . . . & Sommer, C. (2010). Lack of serotonin transporter in mice reduces locomotor activity and leads to gender-dependent late onset obesity. *International Journal of Obesity, 34*(4), 701-711. doi:10.1038/ijo.2009.289

Waller, T., Lampman, C., & Lupfer-Johnson, G. (2012). Assessing bias against overweight individuals among nursing and psychology students: An implicit association test. *Journal of Clinical Nursing, 21*(23-24), 3504-3512. doi:10.1111/j.1365-2702.2012.04226.x

Wright, J.H., Thase, M.E., & Beck, A. T. (2008). Cognitive therapy. In R.E. Hales, S.C. Yudofsky, & G.O. Gabbard (Eds.), *Textbook of psychiatry* (5th ed., pp. 1211-1256). Washington, DC: American Psychiatric Publishing.

Personality Disorders

32

CORE CONCEPT

Personality

KEY TERMS

antisocial personality disorder

avoidant personality disorder

borderline personality disorder

dependent personality
    disorder

histrionic personality disorder

narcissistic personality disorder

object constancy

obsessive-compulsive
    personality disorder

paranoid personality disorder

schizoid personality disorder

schizotypal personality
    disorder

splitting

OBJECTIVES
After reading this chapter, the student will be able to:

1. Define *personality*.
2. Compare stages of personality development according to Sullivan, Erikson, and Mahler.
3. Identify various types of personality disorders.
4. Discuss historical and epidemiological statistics related to various personality disorders.
5. Describe symptomatology associated with borderline personality disorder and antisocial personality disorder, and use these data in client assessment.
6. Identify predisposing factors for borderline personality disorder and antisocial personality disorder.

7. Formulate nursing diagnoses and goals of care for clients with borderline personality disorder and antisocial personality disorder.
8. Describe appropriate nursing interventions for behaviors associated with borderline personality disorder and antisocial personality disorder.
9. Evaluate nursing care of clients with borderline personality disorder and antisocial personality disorder.
10. Discuss various modalities relevant to treatment of personality disorders.

HOMEWORK ASSIGNMENT
Please read the chapter and answer the following questions:

1. What are the primary psychosocial predisposing factors to avoidant personality disorder?
2. How should a nurse care for the self-inflicted wounds of a client with borderline personality disorder?

3. What are some of the types of family dynamics that may predispose a person to antisocial personality disorder?

CORE CONCEPT

Personality

The totality of emotional and behavioral characteristics that are particular to a specific person and that remain somewhat stable and predictable over time.

The word *personality* is derived from the Greek term *persona*. It was originally used to describe the theatrical mask worn by some dramatic actors at the time. Over the years, it lost its connotation of pretense and illusion and came to represent the person behind the mask—the "real" person.

Personality *traits* may be defined as characteristics with which an individual is born or develops early in life. They influence the way he or she perceives and relates to the environment and remain stable over time. Personality *disorders* occur when these traits deviate markedly from the expectations of the individual's culture, become rigid and inflexible, contribute to maladaptive patterns of behavior or impairment in functioning, and lead to distress (American Psychiatric Association [APA], 2013). The most common symptoms occurring in personality disorders are impairment in interpersonal relationship functions (41%), dysfunctions in cognition (30%), affect (18%), and impulse control (6%) (Bornstein et al., 2014). In specific types of personality disorders, such as paranoid and schizotypal personality disorders, cognitive symptoms may appear more prominently. In other types, such as borderline personality and antisocial personality disorders, interpersonal dysfunctions may predominate (Bornstein et al., 2014). Virtually all individuals exhibit some behaviors associated with the various personality disorders from time to time. As previously stated, it is only when significant functional impairment occurs in response to these personality characteristics that the individual is thought to have a personality disorder.

Personality development occurs in response to a number of biological and psychological influences. These variables include (but are not limited to) heredity, temperament, experiential learning, and social interaction. A number of theorists have attempted to provide information about personality development. Most suggest that it occurs in an orderly, stepwise fashion. These stages overlap, however, as maturation occurs at different rates in different individuals. The theories of Sullivan (1953), Erikson (1963), and Mahler (Mahler, Pine, & Bergman, 1975) are presented at length in the chapter Theoretical Models of Personality Development available online at DavisPlus. The stages of personality development according to these three theorists are compared in Table 32–1. The nurse should understand "normal" personality development before learning about what is considered maladaptive.

Historical and epidemiological aspects of personality disorders are discussed in this chapter. Predisposing

TABLE 32–1 Comparison of Personality Development—Sullivan, Erikson, and Mahler

MAJOR DEVELOPMENTAL TASKS AND DESIGNATED AGES

SULLIVAN	ERIKSON	MAHLER
Birth to 18 months: Relief from anxiety through oral gratification of needs	Birth to 18 months: To develop a basic trust in the mothering figure and be able to generalize it to others	Birth to 1 month: Fulfillment of basic needs for survival and comfort
18 months to 6 years: Learning to experience a delay in personal gratification without undue anxiety	18 months to 3 years: To gain some self-control and independence within the environment	1 to 5 months: Developing awareness of external source of need fulfillment
6 to 9 years: Learning to form satisfactory peer relationships	3 to 6 years: To develop a sense of purpose and the ability to initiate and direct own activities	5 to 10 months: Commencement of a primary recognition of separateness from the mothering figure
9 to 12 years: Learning to form satisfactory relationships with persons of the same gender; the initiation of feelings of affection for another person	6 to 12 years: To achieve a sense of self-confidence by learning, competing, performing successfully, and receiving recognition from significant others, peers, and acquaintances	10 to 16 months: Increased independence through locomotor functioning; increased sense of separateness of self
12 to 14 years: Learning to form satisfactory relationships with persons of the opposite gender; developing a sense of identity	12 to 20 years: To integrate the tasks mastered in the previous stages into a secure sense of self	16 to 24 months: Acute awareness of separateness of self; learning to seek "emotional refueling" from mothering figure to maintain feeling of security

TABLE 32–1 **Comparison of Personality Development–Sullivan, Erikson, and Mahler–cont'd**		
MAJOR DEVELOPMENTAL TASKS AND DESIGNATED AGES		
SULLIVAN	**ERIKSON**	**MAHLER**
14 to 21 years: Establishing self-identity; experiences satisfying relationships; working to develop a lasting, intimate opposite-gender relationship	20 to 30 years: To form an intense, lasting relationship or a commitment to another person, a cause, an institution, or a creative effort	24 to 36 months: Sense of separateness established; on the way to object constancy: able to internalize a sustained image of loved object/person when it is out of sight; resolution of separation anxiety
	30 to 65 years: To achieve the life goals established for oneself, while also considering the welfare of future generations	
	65 years to death: To review one's life and derive meaning from both positive and negative events, while achieving a positive sense of self-worth In late, older adulthood (80 years and beyond) an additional stage of development, *transcendence*, refers to a period in which one develops a broader sense of one's meaning and spirituality that transcends themselves.	

factors that have been implicated in the etiology of personality disorders are presented. Symptomatology is explained to provide background knowledge for assessing clients with personality disorders.

Individuals with personality disorders are not often treated in acute care settings for the personality disorder as their primary psychiatric diagnosis. However, many clients with other psychiatric and medical diagnoses manifest symptoms of personality disorders. Nurses are likely to encounter clients with these personality characteristics in all health-care settings.

Nurses working in psychiatric settings are likely to encounter clients with borderline and antisocial personality characteristics. The behavior of clients with **borderline personality disorder** (BPD) is very unstable, and hospitalization is often required as a result of attempts at self-injury. The client with antisocial personality disorder may enter the psychiatric arena as a result of judicially ordered evaluation. Psychiatric intervention may be an alternative to imprisonment for antisocial behavior if it is deemed potentially helpful.

Nursing care of clients with BPD or antisocial personality disorder is presented in this chapter in the context of the nursing process. Various medical treatment modalities for personality disorders are explored.

Historical Aspects

In the fourth century BC, Hippocrates concluded that all disease stemmed from an excess of or imbalance among four bodily humors: yellow bile, black bile, blood, and phlegm. Hippocrates identified four fundamental personality styles that he concluded stemmed from excesses in the four humors: the irritable and hostile choleric (yellow bile), the pessimistic melancholic (black bile), the overly optimistic and extraverted sanguine (blood), and the apathetic phlegmatic (phlegm).

In 1801, the medical profession first recognized that personality disorders, apart from psychosis, were cause for their own special concern with the realization that an individual can behave irrationally even when the powers of intellect are intact. Nineteenth-century psychiatrists embraced the term *moral insanity*, the concept of which defines what we know today as personality disorders.

Historically, individuals with personality disorders have been labeled as "bad" or "immoral" and as deviants in the range of normal personality dimensions. The events and sequences that result in pathology of the personality are complicated and difficult to unravel. Continued study is needed to facilitate understanding of this complex behavioral phenomenon.

A major difficulty for psychiatrists has been the establishment of a classification of personality disorders. Ten specific types of personality disorders are identified in the *Diagnostic and Statistical Manual of Mental Disorders, Fifth Edition (DSM-5)* (APA, 2013). The APA has proposed a new, complex diagnostic system to identify impairments in personality functioning specifically related to the dimensions of *self* and *interpersonal relations* and to personality *trait domains and facets*. This system is very specific and addresses symptoms that may differ not only among personality disorders but also among individuals with the same personality disorder. This trait-specific diagnostic methodology is described in the *DSM-5* as an alternative approach to diagnosis of personality disorder and is recommended for further study.

The current diagnostic system classifies the personality disorders into three clusters according to description of personality traits. These include the following:

1. **Cluster A:** Behaviors described as odd or eccentric
   a. Paranoid personality disorder
   b. Schizoid personality disorder
   c. Schizotypal personality disorder
2. **Cluster B:** Behaviors described as dramatic, emotional, or erratic
   a. Antisocial personality disorder
   b. Borderline personality disorder
   c. Histrionic personality disorder
   d. Narcissistic personality disorder
3. **Cluster C:** Behaviors described as anxious or fearful
   a. Avoidant personality disorder
   b. Dependent personality disorder
   c. Obsessive-compulsive personality disorder

Types of Personality Disorders

Paranoid Personality Disorder

Definition and Epidemiological Statistics

Paranoid personality disorder is defined as a pattern of pervasive mistrust and suspiciousness of others, and misinterpretation of others' motives as malevolent (APA, 2013, p. 649). This pattern begins by early adulthood and remains present in a variety of contexts. Prevalence has been estimated at 1 to 4 percent of the general population, and often is diagnosed only when the individual seeks treatment for a mood or anxiety disorder (Black & Andreasen, 2014). The disorder is more commonly diagnosed in men than in women.

Clinical Picture

Individuals with paranoid personality disorder are constantly on guard, hypervigilant, and ready for any real or imagined threat. They appear tense and irritable. They have developed a hard exterior and become immune or insensitive to the feelings of others. They avoid interactions with other people lest they be forced to relinquish some of their own power. They always feel that others plan to take advantage of them.

They are extremely oversensitive and tend to misinterpret even minute cues within the environment, magnifying and distorting them into thoughts of trickery and deception. Because they trust no one, they are constantly "testing" the honesty of others. Their intimidating manner provokes exasperation and anger in almost everyone with whom they come in contact.

Individuals with paranoid personality disorder maintain their self-esteem by attributing their shortcomings to others. They do not accept responsibility for their own behaviors and feelings and project this responsibility onto others. They are envious and hostile toward those who are highly successful and believe the only reason they are not as successful is because they have been treated unfairly. People who are paranoid are extremely vulnerable and constantly on the defensive. Any real or imagined threat can release hostility and anger fueled by animosities from the past. The desire for reprisal and vindication is so intense that a possible loss of control can result in aggression and violence. These outbursts are usually brief, and the paranoid person soon regains the external control, rationalizes the behavior, and reconstructs the defenses central to his or her personality pattern.

The *DSM-5* diagnostic criteria for paranoid personality disorder are presented in Box 32–1.

BOX 32–1 **Diagnostic Criteria for Paranoid Personality Disorder**

A. A pervasive distrust and suspiciousness of others such that their motives are interpreted as malevolent, beginning by early adulthood and present in a variety of contexts, as indicated by four (or more) of the following:
   1. Suspects, without sufficient basis, that others are exploiting, harming, or deceiving him or her
   2. Is preoccupied with unjustified doubts about the loyalty or trustworthiness of friends or associates
   3. Is reluctant to confide in others because of unwarranted fear that the information will be used maliciously against him or her
   4. Reads hidden demeaning or threatening meanings into benign remarks or events
   5. Persistently bears grudges (i.e., is unforgiving of insults, injuries, or slights)
   6. Perceives attacks on his or her character or reputation that are not apparent to others and is quick to react angrily or to counterattack
   7. Has recurrent suspicions, without justification, regarding fidelity of spouse or sexual partner
B. Does not occur exclusively during the course of schizophrenia, a bipolar disorder or depressive disorder with psychotic features, or another psychotic disorder and is not attributable to the physiological effects of another medical condition.

Reprinted with permission from the Diagnostic and Statistical Manual of Mental Disorders, Fifth Edition *(Copyright 2013). American Psychiatric Association.*

Predisposing Factors

Research has indicated a possible hereditary link in paranoid personality disorder. Studies have revealed a higher incidence of paranoid personality disorder among relatives of clients with schizophrenia than among control subjects (Sadock, Sadock, & Ruiz, 2015).

Psychological predisposing factors, as is the case with many personality disorders, include a history of childhood trauma including neglect. People with paranoid personality disorder may have been subjected to parental antagonism and harassment. They learned to perceive the world as harsh and unkind, a place calling for protective vigilance and mistrust. They entered the world with a "chip-on-the-shoulder" attitude and were met with many rebuffs and rejections from others. Anticipating humiliation and betrayal by others, they learned to defend themselves by attacking first.

Schizoid Personality Disorder

Definition and Epidemiological Statistics

Schizoid personality disorder is characterized primarily by a profound defect in the ability to form personal relationships. People with this condition are often seen by others as eccentric, isolated, or lonely (Sadock et al., 2015). These individuals display a lifelong pattern of social withdrawal, and their discomfort with human interaction is apparent. The prevalence of schizoid personality disorder is difficult to determine because, as with many other personality disorders, it may go undiagnosed unless it is recognized when the individual seeks health care for other reasons. Estimates within the general population vary between 3 and 5 percent. Many people with the disorder are never observed in a clinical setting. Gender ratio of the disorder is unknown, although it is diagnosed more frequently in men.

Clinical Picture

People with schizoid personality disorder appear cold, aloof, and indifferent to others. They typically have a long-standing history of engaging in primarily solitary activities or engaging more with animals than people. They prefer to work in isolation and are unsociable, with little need or desire for emotional ties. They are able to invest enormous affective energy in intellectual pursuits.

In the presence of others, they appear shy, anxious, or uneasy. They are inappropriately serious about everything and have difficulty acting in a lighthearted manner. Their behavior and conversation exhibit little or no spontaneity. Typically, they are unable to experience pleasure, and their affect is commonly bland and constricted.

The *DSM-5* diagnostic criteria for schizoid personality disorder are presented in Box 32–2.

Predisposing Factors

Although the role of heredity in the etiology of schizoid personality disorder is unclear, introversion appears to be a highly inheritable characteristic. Further studies are required before definitive statements can be made. Psychosocially, the development of schizoid personality is probably influenced by early interactional patterns that the person found cold and unsatisfying. The childhoods of these individuals have often been characterized as bleak, cold, and lacking empathy and nurturing. A child brought up with this type of parenting may develop schizoid personality traits if that child possesses a temperamental disposition that is shy, anxious, and introverted.

Schizotypal Personality Disorder

Definition and Epidemiological Statistics

Individuals with **schizotypal personality disorder** were once described as "latent schizophrenics." Their

---

BOX 32–2 **Diagnostic Criteria for Schizoid Personality Disorder**

A. A pervasive pattern of detachment from social relationships and a restricted range of expression of emotions in interpersonal settings, beginning by early adulthood and present in a variety of contexts, as indicated by four (or more) of the following:
   1. Neither desires nor enjoys close relationships, including being part of a family
   2. Almost always chooses solitary activities
   3. Has little, if any, interest in having sexual experiences with another person
   4. Takes pleasure in few, if any, activities
   5. Lacks close friends or confidants other than first-degree relatives
   6. Appears indifferent to the praise or criticism of others
   7. Shows emotional coldness, detachment, or flattened affectivity
B. Does not occur exclusively during the course of schizophrenia, a bipolar disorder or depressive disorder with psychotic features, another psychotic disorder, or autism spectrum disorder and is not attributable to the physiological effects of another medical condition.

---

behavior is odd and eccentric but does not decompensate to the level of schizophrenia. Schizotypal personality is marked by symptoms that are closer to those of schizophrenia than those in schizoid personality. The former individuals show significant peculiarities in thinking, behavior, and appearance. Studies indicate that schizotypal personality disorder has a prevalence of around 3 percent (Sadock et al., 2015).

Clinical Picture

Individuals with schizotypal personality disorder are aloof and isolated and behave in a bland and apathetic manner. Magical thinking, ideas of reference, illusions, and depersonalization are part of their everyday world. Examples include superstitiousness; belief in clairvoyance, telepathy, or "sixth sense"; as well as beliefs that "others can feel my feelings."

The speech pattern is sometimes bizarre. People with this disorder often cannot orient their thoughts logically and become lost in personal irrelevancies and tangential asides that seem vague and digress from the topic at hand. This feature only further alienates them from others.

Under stress, these individuals may decompensate and demonstrate psychotic symptoms, such as delusional thoughts, hallucinations, or bizarre behaviors, but these are usually of brief duration (Sadock et al., 2015). They often talk or gesture to themselves, as if "living in their own world." Their affect is bland or inappropriate, such as laughing at their own problems or at a situation that most people would consider sad.

The *DSM-5* diagnostic criteria for schizotypal personality disorder are presented in Box 32–3.

Predisposing Factors

Evidence suggests that schizotypal personality disorder is more common among the first-degree biological relatives of people with schizophrenia than among the general population. It is now considered part of the genetic spectrum of schizophrenia (APA, 2013). Twin studies reveal a higher incidence in monozygotic twins than dizygotic twins (Sadock et al., 2015).

Psychological and environmental factors may also interact with genetic vulnerability in the development of schizotypal personality traits. One recent study (Hur et al., 2016) found that individuals with schizotypal personality disorder demonstrated reduced activation of brain areas responsive to motion perception and executive control of perception. These findings may explain a biological basis for the peculiar ways that individuals with schizotypal personality disorder behave in social situations. Affective blandness, peculiar behaviors, and discomfort with interpersonal relationships may provoke other children to avoid relationships with them, or worse, engage in bullying, which reinforces their withdrawal from others. Having failed repeatedly to cope with these adversities, they withdraw and reduce contact with individuals and situations that evoked sadness and humiliation. Their new inner world provides them with a more significant and potentially rewarding existence than the one experienced in reality.

Antisocial Personality Disorder

Definition and Epidemiological Statistics

Antisocial personality disorder is a pattern of socially irresponsible, exploitative, and guiltless behavior that reflects a general disregard for the rights of others.

BOX 32–3 Diagnostic Criteria for Schizotypal Personality Disorder

A. A pervasive pattern of social and interpersonal deficits marked by acute discomfort with, and reduced capacity for, close relationships as well as by cognitive or perceptual distortions and eccentricities of behavior, beginning by early adulthood and present in a variety of contexts, as indicated by five (or more) of the following:
  1. Ideas of reference (excluding delusions of reference)
  2. Odd beliefs or magical thinking that influences behavior and is inconsistent with subcultural norms (e.g., superstitiousness, belief in clairvoyance, telepathy, or "sixth sense;" in children and adolescents, bizarre fantasies or preoccupations)
  3. Unusual perceptual experiences, including bodily illusions
  4. Odd thinking and speech (e.g., vague, circumstantial, metaphorical, overelaborate, or stereotyped)
  5. Suspiciousness or paranoid ideation
  6. Inappropriate or constricted affect
  7. Behavior or appearance that is odd, eccentric, or peculiar
  8. Lack of close friends or confidants other than first-degree relatives
  9. Excessive social anxiety that does not diminish with familiarity and tends to be associated with paranoid fears rather than negative judgments about self
B. Does not occur exclusively during the course of schizophrenia, a bipolar disorder or depressive disorder with psychotic features, another psychotic disorder, or autism spectrum disorder.

These individuals exploit and manipulate others for personal gain and are unconcerned with obeying the law. They have difficulty sustaining consistent employment and developing stable relationships. This is one of the oldest and best-researched personality disorders and has been included in all editions of the *Diagnostic and Statistical Manual of Mental Disorders*. In the United States, prevalence is estimated to be about 3 percent in the general population, but in prison populations, the prevalence is 50 percent or higher (Hatchett, 2015). It is more common in men than in women, among the lower socioeconomic classes, and especially among highly mobile inhabitants of impoverished urban areas. The *DSM-5* currently identifies antisocial personality and psychopathy as synonymous terms, but recent research reveals that these are better understood as distinct disorders (Hatchett, 2015; Thompson, Ramos, & Willett, 2014). Substance use disorder is commonly identified as a comorbid disorder.

The clinical picture, predisposing factors, nursing diagnoses, and interventions for care of clients with antisocial personality disorder are presented later in this chapter.

Borderline Personality Disorder
Definition and Epidemiological Statistics

BPD is characterized by a pattern of intense and chaotic relationships, with affective instability and fluctuating attitudes toward other people. These individuals are impulsive, are directly and indirectly self-destructive, and lack a clear sense of identity. Prevalence of BPD is estimated at 1 to 2 percent of the population. It is generally estimated to be twice as common in women than in men (Sadock et al., 2015), and some have identified female-to-male ratios as high as 4 to 1 (Lubit, 2016).

The clinical picture, predisposing factors, nursing diagnoses, and interventions for care of clients with BPD are presented later in this chapter.

Histrionic Personality Disorder
Definition and Epidemiological Statistics

Histrionic personality disorder is characterized by colorful, dramatic, and extroverted behavior in excitable, emotional people. They have difficulty maintaining long-lasting relationships, although they require constant affirmation of approval and acceptance from others. This often gives rise to seductive, flirtatious behavior in efforts to reassure themselves of their attractiveness and gain approval. Prevalence of the disorder is thought to be about 2 to 3 percent, and it is more common in women than in men.

Clinical Picture

People with histrionic personality disorder tend to be self-dramatizing, attention-seeking, overly gregarious, and seductive. They use manipulative and exhibitionistic behaviors in their demands to be the center of attention. People with histrionic personality disorder often demonstrate, to an extreme, what our society tends to foster and admire in its members: to be well liked, successful, popular, extroverted, attractive, and sociable. However, beneath these surface characteristics is a driven quality—an all-consuming need for approval and a desperate striving to be conspicuous and evoke affection or attract attention at all costs. Failure to evoke the attention and approval they seek often results in feelings of dejection and anxiety.

Individuals with this disorder are highly distractible and flighty by nature. They have difficulty paying attention to detail. They can portray themselves as carefree and sophisticated on the one hand and as inhibited and naive on the other. They tend to be highly suggestible, impressionable, and easily influenced by others. They are strongly dependent.

Interpersonal relationships are fleeting and superficial. The person with histrionic personality disorder, having failed throughout life to develop the richness of inner feelings and without resources from which to draw, lacks the ability to provide another with genuinely sustained affection. Somatic complaints are not uncommon in these individuals, and fleeting episodes of psychosis may occur during periods of extreme stress.

The *DSM-5* diagnostic criteria for histrionic personality disorder are presented in Box 32–4.

Predisposing Factors

Heredity may be a factor because the disorder is apparently more common among first-degree biological relatives of people with the disorder than in the general population. Some traits may be inherited, whereas others are related to a combination of genetic predisposition and childhood experiences. But at present, the cause or causes are unknown.

From a psychosocial perspective, learning experiences may contribute to the development of histrionic personality disorder. The child may have learned that positive reinforcement was contingent on the ability to perform parentally approved and admired behaviors. It is likely that the child rarely received either positive or negative feedback. Parental acceptance and approval came inconsistently and only when the behaviors met parental expectations.

Narcissistic Personality Disorder
Definition and Epidemiological Statistics

Persons with **narcissistic personality disorder** have an exaggerated sense of self-worth. They lack empathy and are hypersensitive to the evaluation of others. They believe that they have the inalienable right to receive special consideration and that their desire is sufficient justification for possessing whatever they seek.

BOX 32–4 Diagnostic Criteria for Histrionic Personality Disorder

A pervasive pattern of excessive emotionality and attention seeking, beginning by early adulthood and present in a variety of contexts, as indicated by five (or more) of the following:

1. Is uncomfortable in situations in which he or she is not the center of attention
2. Interaction with others is often characterized by inappropriate sexually seductive or provocative behavior
3. Displays rapidly shifting and shallow expression of emotions
4. Consistently uses physical appearance to draw attention to self
5. Has a style of speech that is excessively impressionistic and lacking in detail
6. Shows self-dramatization, theatricality, and exaggerated expression of emotion
7. Is suggestible (i.e., easily influenced by others or circumstances)
8. Considers relationships to be more intimate than they actually are

---

Reprinted with permission from the Diagnostic and Statistical Manual of Mental Disorders, Fifth Edition *(Copyright 2013). American Psychiatric Association.*

This diagnosis appeared for the first time in the third edition of the *Diagnostic and Statistical Manual of Mental Disorders*. However, the concept of narcissism has its roots in the 19th century. It was viewed by early psychoanalysts as a normal phase of psychosexual development. The prevalence of narcissistic personality disorder is estimated at 1 to 6 percent (Sadock et al., 2015). It is diagnosed more often in men than in women.

Clinical Picture

Individuals with narcissistic personality disorder appear to lack humility, be overly self-centered, and exploit others to fulfill their own desires. They often do not conceive of their behavior as being inappropriate or objectionable. Because they view themselves as "superior" beings, they believe they are entitled to special rights and privileges.

Although often grounded in grandiose distortions of reality, their moods are usually optimistic, relaxed, cheerful, and carefree. This can easily change, however, because of fragile self-esteem. If they do not meet self-expectations, do not receive the positive feedback they expect from others, or draw criticism from others, they may respond with rage, shame, humiliation, or dejection. They may turn inward and fantasize rationalizations that convince them of their continued stature and perfection.

The exploitation of others for self-gratification results in impaired interpersonal relationships. In selecting a mate, narcissistic individuals frequently choose a person who will provide them with the praise and positive feedback that they require and who will not ask much from their partner in return.

The *DSM-5* diagnostic criteria for narcissistic personality disorder are presented in Box 32–5.

Predisposing Factors

Although the causes are unknown, psychodynamic theories have suggested that narcissistic personality disorder evolves from a parent-child dynamic of either excessive pampering or excessive criticism

---

BOX 32–5 Diagnostic Criteria for Narcissistic Personality Disorder

A pervasive pattern of grandiosity (in fantasy or behavior), need for admiration, and lack of empathy, beginning by early adulthood and present in a variety of contexts, as indicated by five (or more) of the following:

1. Has a grandiose sense of self-importance (e.g., exaggerates achievements and talents, expects to be recognized as superior without commensurate achievements)
2. Is preoccupied with fantasies of unlimited success, power, brilliance, beauty, or ideal love
3. Believes that he or she is "special" and unique and can only be understood by, or should associate with, other special or high-status people (or institutions)
4. Requires excessive admiration
5. Has a sense of entitlement (i.e., unreasonable expectations of especially favorable treatment or automatic compliance with his or her expectations)
6. Is interpersonally exploitative (i.e., takes advantage of others to achieve his or her own ends)
7. Lacks empathy: is unwilling to recognize or identify with the feelings and needs of others
8. Is often envious of others or believes that others are envious of him or her
9. Shows arrogant, haughty behaviors or attitudes

Reprinted with permission from the Diagnostic and Statistical Manual of Mental Disorders, Fifth Edition *(Copyright 2013). American Psychiatric Association.*

(Mayo Clinic, 2014). Children may then grow to project an image of invulnerability and self-sufficiency that conceals their true sense of emptiness and contributes to their inability to feel deep emotion.

Sadock and associates (2015) identify the propensity for an increase in narcissistic personality disorders among children whose parents had the disorder. Children may evolve into adults with narcissistic personality disorder through role modeling parent behavior, or as Sadock and associates suggest, these traits may be caused by a narcissistic parent's imparting an unrealistic omnipotence, grandiosity, beauty, and talent to their children.

Narcissism may also develop from an environment in which parents attempt to live their lives vicariously through their child. They expect the child to achieve the things they did not achieve, possess that which they did not possess, and have life better and easier than they did. The child is not subjected to the requirements and restrictions that may have dominated the parents' lives and thereby grows up believing he or she is above that which is required for everyone else.

Genetics and environment may both have a role in the development of narcissistic personality disorder. Research has identified a decreased volume of gray matter in areas of the brain responsible for empathy, emotional regulation, compassion, and cognitive functions (Gregory, 2016).

Avoidant Personality Disorder

Definition and Epidemiological Statistics

The individual with **avoidant personality disorder** is extremely sensitive to rejection and thus may lead a very socially withdrawn life. It is not that he or she is asocial; in fact, there may be a strong desire for companionship. The extreme shyness and fear of rejection, however, create the need for unusually strong assurances of unconditional acceptance. Prevalence of the disorder in the general population is about 2 to 3 percent, and it appears to be equally common in men and women.

Clinical Picture

Individuals with this disorder are awkward and uncomfortable in social situations. From a distance, others may perceive them as timid, withdrawn, or perhaps cold and strange. Those who have closer relationships with them, however, soon learn of their sensitivities, touchiness, evasiveness, and mistrustful qualities.

Their speech is usually slow and constrained, with frequent hesitations, fragmentary thought sequences, and occasional confused and irrelevant digressions. They are often lonely and express feelings of being unwanted. They view others as critical, betraying, and humiliating. They desire to have close relationships but avoid connecting with others because of their fear of being rejected. Depression, anxiety, and anger at oneself for failing to develop social relations are commonly experienced.

The *DSM-5* diagnostic criteria for avoidant personality disorder are presented in Box 32–6.

Predisposing Factors

There is no clear cause of avoidant personality disorder. Contributing factors are most likely a combination of biological, genetic, and psychosocial influences. Some infants who exhibit traits of hyperirritability, crankiness, tension, and withdrawal behaviors may possess a temperamental disposition toward an avoidant pattern later in life.

Psychosocial influences may include childhood trauma or neglect leading to fears of abandonment or views of the world as a hostile and dangerous place.

Dependent Personality Disorder

Definition and Epidemiological Statistics

Dependent personality disorder is characterized by lack of self-confidence and extreme reliance on others to take responsibility for them, sometimes to the point

---

BOX 32–6 **Diagnostic Criteria for Avoidant Personality Disorder**

A pervasive pattern of social inhibition, feelings of inadequacy, and hypersensitivity to negative evaluation, beginning by early adulthood and present in a variety of contexts, as indicated by four (or more) of the following:

1. Avoids occupational activities that involve significant interpersonal contact, because of fears of criticism, disapproval, or rejection
2. Is unwilling to get involved with people unless certain of being liked
3. Shows restraint within intimate relationships because of the fear of being shamed or ridiculed
4. Is preoccupied with being criticized or rejected in social situations
5. Is inhibited in new interpersonal situations because of feelings of inadequacy
6. Views self as socially inept, personally unappealing, or inferior to others
7. Is unusually reluctant to take personal risks or to engage in any new activities because they may prove embarrassing

of intense discomfort with being alone for even a brief period (Sadock et al., 2015). This mode of behavior is evident in the tendencies to allow others to make decisions, feel helpless when alone, act submissively, subordinate needs to others, tolerate mistreatment by others, demean oneself to gain acceptance, and fail to function adequately in situations that require assertive or dominant behavior.

Clinical Picture

Individuals with dependent personality disorder have a notable lack of self-confidence that is often apparent in their posture, voice, and mannerisms. They are typically passive and acquiescent to the desires of others. They are overly generous and thoughtful and underplay their own attractiveness and achievements. They may appear to others to "see the world through rose-colored glasses," but when alone, they may feel pessimistic, discouraged, and dejected. Others are not made aware of these feelings; their "suffering" is done in silence.

Individuals with dependent personality disorder assume the passive and submissive role in relationships. They are willing to let others make their important decisions. Should a dependent relationship end, they feel fearful and vulnerable because they lack confidence in their ability to care for themselves. They may hastily and indiscriminately attempt to establish another relationship with someone they believe can provide them with the nurturance and guidance they need.

They avoid positions of responsibility and become anxious when forced into them. They have feelings of low self-worth and are easily hurt by criticism and disapproval. They will do almost anything, even if it is unpleasant or demeaning, to earn the acceptance of others.

The *DSM-5* diagnostic criteria for dependent personality disorder are presented in Box 32–7.

Predisposing Factors

An infant may be genetically predisposed to a dependent temperament. Twin studies measuring submissiveness have shown a higher correlation between identical twins than fraternal twins.

Psychosocially, dependency is fostered in infancy when stimulation and nurturance are experienced exclusively from one source. The infant becomes attached to one source to the exclusion of all others. If this exclusive attachment continues as the child grows, the dependency is nurtured. A problem may arise when parents become overprotective and discourage independent behaviors on the part of the child. Parents who make new experiences unnecessarily easy for the child and refuse to allow him or her to learn by experience encourage their child to give up efforts at achieving autonomy. Dependent behaviors may be subtly rewarded in this environment, and the child may come to fear a loss of love or attachment from the parental figure if independent behaviors are attempted.

Obsessive-Compulsive Personality Disorder

Definition and Epidemiological Statistics

Individuals with **obsessive-compulsive personality disorder** are very serious and formal and have difficulty expressing emotions. They are overly disciplined, perfectionistic, and preoccupied with rules. They are inflexible about the way in which things must be done and have a devotion to productivity to the exclusion of personal pleasure. An intense fear of making mistakes leads to difficulty with decision-making. The disorder is relatively common and occurs more often in men than in women. Within the family constellation, it appears to be most common in oldest children. Recurrent obsessions and compulsions are absent in this personality disorder; if the client presents with

---

BOX 32–7 Diagnostic Criteria for Dependent Personality Disorder

A pervasive and excessive need to be taken care of that leads to submissive and clinging behavior and fears of separation, beginning by early adulthood and present in a variety of contexts, as indicated by five (or more) of the following:

1. Has difficulty making everyday decisions without an excessive amount of advice and reassurance from others
2. Needs others to assume responsibility for most major areas of his or her life
3. Has difficulty expressing disagreement with others because of fear of loss of support or approval (*Note:* Do not include realistic fears of retribution.)
4. Has difficulty initiating projects or doing things on his or her own (because of a lack of self-confidence in judgment or abilities rather than a lack of motivation or energy)
5. Goes to excessive lengths to obtain nurturance and support from others, to the point of volunteering to do things that are unpleasant
6. Feels uncomfortable or helpless when alone because of exaggerated fears of being unable to care for himself or herself
7. Urgently seeks another relationship as a source of care and support when a close relationship ends
8. Is unrealistically preoccupied with fears of being left to take care of himself or herself

such symptoms, they are diagnosed with obsessive-compulsive *disorder* rather than obsessive compulsive *personality* disorder (Sadock et al., 2015). Prevalence is estimated at anywhere from 2 to 8 percent.

Clinical Picture

Individuals with obsessive-compulsive personality disorder are inflexible and lack spontaneity. They are meticulous and work diligently and patiently at tasks that require accuracy and discipline. They are especially concerned with matters of organization and efficiency and tend to be rigid and unbending about rules and procedures.

Social behavior tends to be polite and formal. They are very "rank conscious," a characteristic that is reflected in their contrasting behaviors with "superiors" as opposed to "inferiors." They tend to be very solicitous to and ingratiating with authority figures. With subordinates, however, the compulsive person can become quite autocratic and condemnatory, often appearing pompous and self-righteous.

People with obsessive-compulsive personality disorder typify the "bureaucratic personality," the so-called company man. They see themselves as conscientious, loyal, dependable, and responsible and are contemptuous of people whose behavior they consider frivolous and impulsive. Emotional behavior is considered immature and irresponsible.

Although on the surface these individuals appear to be calm and controlled, underneath this exterior lies a great deal of ambivalence, conflict, and hostility. Individuals with this disorder commonly use the defense mechanism of reaction formation. Not daring to expose their true feelings of defiance and anger, they withhold these feelings so strongly that the opposite feelings come forth. The defenses of isolation, intellectualization, rationalization, and undoing are also commonly evident.

The *DSM-5* diagnostic criteria for obsessive-compulsive personality disorder are presented in Box 32–8.

Predisposing Factors

Genetic vulnerability may be a predisposing factor, since it is noted to occur more frequently in first-degree biological relatives than in the general population (Sadock et al., 2015). In the psychoanalytical view, the individual with obsessive-compulsive personality disorder was reared in an overly controlled environment. These parents expect their children to live up to imposed standards of conduct and condemn them if they do not. Praise for positive behaviors is bestowed on the child with much less frequency than punishment for undesirable behaviors. In this environment, individuals become experts in learning what they must *not* do to avoid punishment and condemnation rather than what they *can* do to achieve attention and praise. They learn to heed rigid restrictions and rules. Positive achievements are expected, taken for granted, and only occasionally acknowledged by their parents, whose comments and judgments are limited to pointing out transgressions and infractions of rules.

Application of the Nursing Process

Borderline Personality Disorder (Background Assessment Data)

Historically, there have been clients who did not classically conform to the standard categories of neuroses or psychoses. The designation "borderline"

BOX 32–8 Diagnostic Criteria for Obsessive-Compulsive Personality Disorder

A pervasive pattern of preoccupation with orderliness, perfectionism, and mental and interpersonal control, at the expense of flexibility, openness, and efficiency, beginning by early adulthood and present in a variety of contexts, as indicated by four (or more) of the following:

1. Is preoccupied with details, rules, lists, order, organization, or schedules to the extent that the major point of the activity is lost
2. Shows perfectionism that interferes with task completion (e.g., is unable to complete a project because his or her own overly strict standards are not met)
3. Is excessively devoted to work and productivity to the exclusion of leisure activities and friendships (not accounted for by obvious economic necessity)
4. Is overconscientious, scrupulous, and inflexible about matters of morality, ethics, or values (not accounted for by cultural or religious identification)
5. Is unable to discard worn-out or worthless objects even when they have no sentimental value
6. Is reluctant to delegate tasks or to work with others unless they submit to exactly his or her way of doing things
7. Adopts a miserly spending style toward both self and others; money is viewed as something to be hoarded for future catastrophes
8. Shows rigidity and stubbornness

Reprinted with permission from the Diagnostic and Statistical Manual of Mental Disorders, Fifth Edition *(Copyright 2013). American Psychiatric Association.*

was introduced to identify clients who seem to fall on the border between the two categories. Other terminology that has been used in an attempt to identify this disorder includes *ambulatory schizophrenia, pseudoneurotic schizophrenia,* and *emotionally unstable personality.* When the term *borderline* was first proposed for inclusion in the third edition of the *DSM,* some psychiatrists feared it might be used as a "wastebasket" diagnosis for difficult-to-treat clients. However, a specific set of criteria, listed in Box 32–9, has been established for diagnosing what has been described as "a consistent and stable course of unstable behavior."

Clinical Picture

Individuals with BPD always seem to be in a state of crisis and have frequent mood swings (although there may also be comorbid bipolar disorder). Their affect is one of extreme intensity, and their behavior reflects frequent changeability, within days, hours, or even minutes. They are sometimes described as "thriving on chaos," since they frequently generate chaos, particularly in interpersonal relationships. Often these individuals exhibit a single, dominant affective tone, such as depression, which may give way periodically to anxious agitation or inappropriate outbursts of anger.

Chronic Depression

Depression is so common in clients with this disorder that before the inclusion of BPD in the *DSM,* many of these clients were diagnosed with depressive disorder. Depression may be rooted in feelings of abandonment by the mother in early childhood (see "Predisposing Factors"). Underlying the depression is a sense of rage that is sporadically turned inward on the self

and externally on the environment. Seldom is the individual aware of the true source of these feelings until well into long-term therapy.

Inability to Be Alone

Because of this chronic fear of abandonment, clients with BPD have little tolerance for being alone. They prefer a frantic search for companionship, no matter how unsatisfactory, to sitting with feelings of loneliness, emptiness, and boredom (Sadock et al., 2015).

Patterns of Interaction

Clinging and Distancing

The client with BPD commonly exhibits a pattern of interaction with others characterized by clinging and distancing behaviors. When clients are clinging to another individual, they may exhibit helpless, dependent, or even childlike behaviors. They want to spend all their time with this person and express a frequent need to talk with and often seek constant reassurance from him or her. Impulsive behaviors, even self-mutilation, may result when they cannot be with this chosen individual. Distancing behaviors are characterized by hostility, anger, and devaluation of others, arising from a feeling of discomfort with closeness. Distancing behaviors also occur in response to separations, confrontations, or attempts to limit certain behaviors. Devaluation of others is manifested by discrediting or undermining their strengths and personal significance.

Splitting

Splitting is a primitive ego defense mechanism common in people with BPD. It arises from their lack of achievement of **object constancy** and is manifested by

---

BOX 32–9 Diagnostic Criteria for Borderline Personality Disorder

A pervasive pattern of instability of interpersonal relationships, self-image, and affects, and marked impulsivity beginning by early adulthood and present in a variety of contexts, as indicated by five (or more) of the following:

1. Frantic efforts to avoid real or imagined abandonment (*Note:* Do not include suicidal or self-mutilating behavior covered in criterion 5.)
2. A pattern of unstable and intense interpersonal relationships characterized by alternating between extremes of idealization and devaluation
3. Identity disturbance: markedly and persistently unstable self-image or sense of self
4. Impulsivity in at least two areas that are potentially self-damaging (e.g., spending, sex, substance abuse, reckless driving, binge eating) (*Note:* Do not include suicidal or self-mutilating behavior covered in criterion 5.)
5. Recurrent suicidal behavior, gestures, or threats, or self-mutilating behavior
6. Affective instability due to marked reactivity of mood (e.g., intense episodic dysphoria, irritability, or anxiety, usually lasting a few hours and only rarely more than a few days)
7. Chronic feelings of emptiness
8. Inappropriate, intense anger or difficulty controlling anger (e.g., frequent displays of temper, constant anger, recurrent physical fights)
9. Transient, stress-related paranoid ideation or severe dissociative symptoms

---

Reprinted with permission from the Diagnostic and Statistical Manual of Mental Disorders, Fifth Edition *(Copyright 2013). American Psychiatric Association.*

an inability to integrate and accept both positive and negative feelings. In their view, people—including themselves—and life situations are either all good or all bad. For example, a nurse-patient relationship may be perceived as very intense and overvalued (e.g., "no one else in the world can help me the way you do") until the individual with BPD feels threatened in any way, the cause of which could be as simple as a perception that the nurse looked at him or her with a different expression or was not immediately available to spend time with the individual. Because this individual also struggles with emotional regulation, suddenly the nurse is devalued, valuing is shifted to another nurse, and the image of the former nurse changes from beneficent caregiver to hateful and cruel persecutor. These shifting allegiances and valuing/devaluing responses can generate conflict, anger, and frustration in staff members (or in any interpersonal relationships) unless this dynamic is clearly understood and managed appropriately.

Manipulation

In their efforts to prevent the separation they so desperately fear, clients with this disorder become masters of manipulation. Virtually any behavior becomes an acceptable means of achieving the desired result: relief from separation anxiety. Playing one individual against another is a common ploy to allay these fears of abandonment.

Self-Destructive Behaviors

Repetitive self-mutilating behaviors are classic manifestations of BPD. About 75 percent of individuals with BPD have a history of at least one deliberate act of self-harm and the prevalence rate for completed suicides is around 9 percent (Lubit, 2016). Although these acts can be fatal, most commonly they are manipulative gestures designed to elicit a rescue response from significant others. Suicide attempts are quite common and result from feelings of abandonment following separation from a significant other. The endeavor is often attempted, however, with a measure of "safety," such as swallowing pills in an area where the person will surely be discovered by others or swallowing pills and making a phone call to report the deed to someone.

Other types of destructive behaviors include cutting, scratching, and burning. Various theories abound regarding why these individuals are able to inflict pain on themselves. One hypothesis suggests they may have higher levels of endorphins in their bodies than most people, thereby increasing their threshold for pain. Another theory relates to the individual's personal identity disturbance. It proposes that since many of the self-mutilating behaviors take place when the individual is in a state of depersonalization and derealization, he or she does not initially feel the pain. The mutilation continues until pain is felt in an attempt to counteract the feelings of unreality. Some clients with BPD have reported that "to feel pain is better than to feel nothing." The pain validates their existence.

Impulsivity

Individuals with BPD have poor impulse control based on primary process functioning. Impulsive behaviors associated with BPD include substance abuse, gambling, promiscuity, reckless driving, and binging and purging. Many times these behaviors occur in response to real or perceived feelings of abandonment.

Predisposing Factors to Borderline Personality Disorder

Biological Influences

BPD, once thought an entirely psychodynamic illness, has been the focus of much current research revealing a wealth of information about the neurobiological underpinnings of this illness. Current research clearly identifies that BPD evolves through a complex interplay of environmental factors, brain anatomy and function, genetics, and epigenetics (Pier et al., 2016).

Biochemical Clients with BPD have a high incidence of major depressive episodes, and antidepressants have demonstrated benefits in some cases (Sadock et al., 2015). This fact and supporting information from brain imaging studies have led to the hypothesis that serotonin and/or norepinephrine dysregulation may contribute to the development of BPD. As stated elsewhere, questions remain about whether these dysfunctions contribute to the development of such disorders or whether they are a neurochemical response to intense emotional states.

Genetic An increased prevalence of major depression and substance use disorders in first-degree relatives of individuals with BPD suggests that there are complex genetic vulnerabilities as well as environmental influences (Sadock et al., 2015). Clients with BPD are five times more likely to have a first-degree relative with BPD, and many studies have shown personality traits such as impulsivity, affect lability, and neuroticism to be heritable (MacIntosh, Godbout, & Dubash, 2015). Epigenetic studies have identified changes to the oxytocin system (related to being a carrier of a specific allele) as associated with negative perceptions of others, increased stress markers, decreased empathy, confidence, and positivity (Pier et al., 2016). Treatment with oxytocin has demonstrated some benefits but requires more research.

Neurobiological Magnetic resonance imaging studies to assess anatomical and functional activities in the brain have identified several factors associated with BPD. Decreases in the volume of the left amygdala and right hippocampus are apparent. The left amygdala, left hippocampus, and posterior cingulate cortex show heightened activation, and the prefrontal cortex shows decreased activation during the processing of negative emotions (Pier et al., 2016).

Psychosocial Influences

Childhood Trauma   Research about specific *types* of trauma that predispose one to the development of BPD is inconsistent, but there is clear and strong evidence that they are linked (MacIntosh et al., 2015). In some instances, this disorder has been likened to posttraumatic stress disorder (PTSD) in response to childhood trauma and abuse. In fact, BPD has been considered a controversial diagnosis because of the many apparent overlaps with PTSD, but, as MacIntosh and associates (2015) cite, other research (Hodges et al., 2013) demonstrates that the complexity of symptoms seen in BPD does not fit with general profiles of PTSD sufferers. Ford and Courtois (2014) cite several studies identifying a 30 to 40 percent comorbidity of PTSD and BPD and indicating that about 85 percent of those diagnosed with BPD were initially diagnosed with PTSD. In these cases, the BPD symptoms persisted after remission of PTSD symptoms. Comorbid substance use disorders may also complicate the differentiation of symptoms and treatment needs. Thorough assessment to identify the multiple psychosocial influences in BPD is clearly essential.

Developmental Factors

Theory of Object Relations   According to Mahler's theory of object relations (Mahler et al., 1975), infants pass through six phases from birth to 36 months, when a sense of separateness from the parenting figure is finally established. Between the ages of 16 to 24 months (phase 5, the rapprochement phase), children become acutely aware of their separateness, and because this is frightening, they look to the mother for "emotional refueling" and to maintain a sense of security while at the same time beginning to explore their separateness and independence. (See Table 32–1 for a more detailed outline of Mahler's theory.)

According to object relations theorists, the individual with BPD becomes fixed in the rapprochement phase of development. This occurs when the child shows increasing separation and autonomy. The mother, who feels secure in the relationship as long as the child is dependent, begins to feel threatened by the child's increasing independence. The mother may be experiencing her own fears of abandonment. In response to separation behaviors, the mother withdraws the emotional support or "refueling" that is so vitally needed during this phase for the child to feel secure. Instead, the mother rewards clinging, dependent behaviors and punishes (withholding emotional support) independent behaviors. With his or her sense

of emotional survival at stake, the child learns to behave in a manner that satisfies the parental wishes. The child develops an internal conflict based on fear of abandonment. He or she wants to achieve independence common to this stage of development but fears that the mother will withdraw emotional support as a result. This unresolved fear of abandonment remains with the child into adulthood. Unresolved grief for the nurturing they failed to receive results in internalized rage that manifests in the depression so common in people with BPD.

Other research looking at attachment issues in childhood suggest that childhood maltreatment, particularly neglect, may be associated with reactive attachment disorder, which results in the development of neurocognitive deficits, particularly temporal limbic dysfunction; the symptoms of BPD with regard to unhealthy attachment in relationships may be related, at least in part, to these neurocognitive deficits rooted in childhood development disruptions (Minzenberg, Poole, & Vinogradov, 2008; Pier et al., 2016).

Diagnosis and Outcome Identification

Nursing diagnoses are formulated from the data gathered during the assessment phase and with background knowledge regarding predisposing factors to the disorder. Table 32–2 presents a list of client behaviors and the NANDA-I nursing diagnoses that correspond to these behaviors, which may be used in planning care for clients with BPD.

Outcome Criteria

The following criteria may be used for measurement of outcomes in the care of clients with BPD.

The client:

■ Has not harmed self
■ Seeks out staff when desire for self-mutilation is strong
■ Is able to identify true source of anger
■ Expresses anger appropriately
■ Relates to more than one staff member
■ Completes activities of daily living independently
■ Does not manipulate one staff member against the other in order to fulfill own desires

Planning and Implementation

The following section presents a group of selected nursing diagnoses common to clients with BPD, with short- and long-term goals and nursing interventions for each.

Risk for Self-Mutilation/Risk for Self-Directed or Other-Directed Violence

Risk for self-mutilation is defined as "vulnerable to deliberate self-injurious behavior causing tissue damage with

TABLE 32–2 Assigning Nursing Diagnoses to Behaviors Commonly Associated With Borderline Personality Disorder

BEHAVIORS	NURSING DIAGNOSES
Risk factors: History of self-injurious behavior; history of inability to plan solutions; impulsivity; irresistible urge to damage self; feels threatened with loss of significant relationship	Risk for self-mutilation
Risk factors: History of suicide attempts; suicidal ideation; suicidal plan; impulsiveness; childhood abuse; fears of abandonment; internalized rage	Risk for self-directed violence; Risk for suicide
Risk factors: Body language (e.g., rigid posture, clenching of fists and jaw, hyperactivity, pacing, breathlessness, threatening stances); history of childhood abuse; impulsivity; transient psychotic symptomatology	Risk for other-directed violence
Depression; persistent emotional distress; rumination; separation distress; traumatic distress; verbalizes feeling empty; inappropriate expression of anger	Complicated grieving
Alternating clinging and distancing behaviors; staff splitting; manipulation	Impaired social interaction
Feelings of depersonalization and derealization	Disturbed personal identity
Transient psychotic symptoms (disorganized thinking; misinterpretation of the environment); increased tension; decreased perceptual field	Anxiety (severe to panic)
Dependent on others; excessively seeks reassurance; manipulation of others; inability to tolerate being alone	Chronic low self-esteem

the intent of causing nonfatal injury to attain relief of tension" (Herdman & Kamitsuru, 2014, p. 414). *Risk for self-directed or other-directed violence* is defined as "vulnerable to behaviors in which an individual demonstrates that he or she can be physically, emotionally, and/or sexually harmful to self or others" (pp. 410–411).

Client Goals

Outcome criteria include short- and long-term goals. Time lines are individually determined.

Short-term goals

■ The client will seek out a staff member if feelings of harming self or others emerge.
■ The client will not harm self or others.

Long-term goal

■ The client will not harm self or others.

Interventions

■ Observe the client's behavior frequently. Do this through routine activities and interactions; avoid appearing watchful and suspicious. Close observation is required so that intervention can occur if required to ensure the client's (and others') safety.
■ Encourage the client to seek out a staff member when the urge for self-mutilation is experienced. Discussing feelings of self-harm with a trusted individual provides some relief to the client. An attitude of acceptance of the client as a worthwhile individual is conveyed.

■ If self-mutilation occurs, care for the client's wounds in a matter-of-fact manner. Do not give positive reinforcement to this behavior by offering sympathy or additional attention. Lack of attention to the maladaptive behavior may decrease repetition of its use.
■ Encourage the client to talk about feelings he or she was having just before this behavior occurred. To problem-solve the situation with the client, knowledge of the precipitating factors is important.
■ Act as a role model for the appropriate expression of angry feelings, and give positive reinforcement to the client when attempts to appropriately express anger are made. It is vital that the client expresses angry feelings because suicide and other self-destructive behaviors are often viewed as a result of anger turned inward on the self.
■ Remove all dangerous objects from the client's environment so that he or she may not purposefully or inadvertently use them to inflict harm to self or others.
■ Try to redirect violent behavior with physical outlets for the client's anxiety (e.g., punching bag, jogging). Physical exercise is a safe and effective way of relieving pent-up tension.
■ Have sufficient staff available to indicate a show of strength to the client if it becomes necessary. This conveys to the client evidence of control over the situation and provides some physical security for staff.
■ Administer tranquilizing medications as ordered by the physician, or obtain an order if necessary.

Monitor the client for effectiveness of the medication and for the appearance of adverse side effects. Some patients show disinhibition with this class of drugs (Sadock et al., 2015). Tranquilizing medications such as anxiolytics or antipsychotics may have a calming effect on the client and thus prevent aggressive behaviors.

■ If the client is not calmed by "talking down" or by medication, use of mechanical restraints may be necessary. The avenue of the "least restrictive alternative" must be selected when planning interventions for a violent client. Restraints should be used only as a last resort, after all other interventions have been unsuccessful, and the client is clearly at risk of harm to self or others. Trauma-informed care should always be the foundation for decisions about appropriate intervention.

■ If restraint is deemed necessary, ensure that sufficient staff is available to assist. Follow protocol established by the institution. As agitation decreases, assess the client's readiness for restraint removal or reduction. Remove one restraint at a time while assessing the client's response. This minimizes the risk of injury to client and staff.

■ If warranted by high acuity of the situation, staff may need to be assigned on a one-to-one basis. Because of their extreme fear of abandonment, clients with BPD should not be left alone at a stressful time, as it may cause an acute rise in anxiety and agitation levels.

Complicated Grieving

Complicated grieving is defined as "a disorder that occurs after the death of a significant other [or any other loss of significance to the individual], in which the experience of distress accompanying bereavement fails to follow normative expectations and manifests in functional impairment" (Herdman & Kamitsuru, p. 339). Table 32–3 presents this nursing diagnosis in care plan format.

Table 32–3 | CARE PLAN FOR THE CLIENT WITH BORDERLINE PERSONALITY DISORDER

NURSING DIAGNOSIS: COMPLICATED GRIEVING

RELATED TO: Maternal deprivation during rapprochement phase of development (internalized as a loss, with fixation in anger stage of grieving process); possible childhood physical or sexual abuse

EVIDENCED BY: Depressed mood, acting-out behaviors

OUTCOME CRITERIA	NURSING INTERVENTIONS	RATIONALE
Short-Term Goal • Within 5 days, the client discusses with nurse or therapist maladaptive patterns of expressing anger. **Long-Term Goal** • By time of discharge from treatment, the client is able to identify the true source of angry feelings, accept ownership of these feelings, and express them in a socially acceptable manner, in an effort to satisfactorily progress through the grieving process.	1. Convey an accepting attitude—one that creates a nonthreatening environment for client to express feelings. Be honest and keep all promises. 2. Identify the function that anger, frustration, and rage serve for client. Allow him or her to express these feelings within reason. 3. Encourage client to discharge pent-up anger through participation in large motor activities (e.g., brisk walks, jogging, physical exercises, volleyball, punching bag, exercise bike). 4. Explore with client the true source of the anger. This is a painful therapy that often leads to regression as client deals with the feelings of early abandonment or issues of abuse.	1. An accepting attitude conveys to client that you believe he or she is a worthwhile person. Trust is enhanced. 2. Verbalization of feelings in a nonthreatening environment may help client come to terms with unresolved issues. 3. Physical exercise provides a safe and effective method for discharging pent-up tension. 4. Reconciliation of the feelings associated with this stage is necessary before progression through the grieving process can continue.

Table 32–3 | CARE PLAN FOR THE CLIENT WITH BORDERLINE PERSONALITY DISORDER–cont'd

OUTCOME CRITERIA	NURSING INTERVENTIONS	RATIONALE
	5. As anger is displaced onto the nurse or therapist, caution must be taken to guard against the negative effects of countertransference. These are very difficult clients who have the capacity for eliciting a whole array of negative feelings from the therapist.	5. The existence of negative feelings by the nurse or therapist must be acknowledged, but they must not be allowed to interfere with the therapeutic process.
	6. Explain the behaviors associated with the normal grieving process. Help client recognize his or her position in this process.	6. Knowledge of the acceptability of the feelings associated with normal grieving may help to relieve some of the guilt that these responses generate.
	7. Help client understand appropriate ways to express anger. Give positive reinforcement for behaviors used to express anger appropriately. Act as a role model. It is important to let client know when he or she has done something that has generated angry feelings in you.	7. Positive reinforcement enhances self-esteem and encourages repetition of desirable behaviors. Role-modeling ways to express anger in an appropriate manner is a powerful learning tool.
	8. Set limits on acting-out behaviors and explain consequences of violation of those limits. Be supportive, yet consistent and firm, in caring for this client.	8. Client lacks sufficient self-control to limit maladaptive behaviors, so assistance is required. Without consistency on the part of all staff members working with this client, a positive outcome will not be achieved.

Client Goals

Outcome criteria include short- and long-term goals. Time lines are individually determined.

Short-term goal

■ Within 5 days, the client will discuss with nurse or therapist maladaptive patterns of expressing anger.

Long-term goal

■ By the time of discharge from treatment, the client will be able to identify the true source of angry feelings, accept ownership of these feelings, and express them in a socially acceptable manner, in an effort to satisfactorily progress through the grieving process.

Interventions

■ Convey an accepting attitude—one that creates a nonthreatening environment for the client to express feelings. Be honest and keep all promises. An accepting attitude conveys to the client that you believe he or she is a worthwhile person. Trust is enhanced.

■ Identify the function that anger, frustration, and rage serve for the client. Allow him or her to express these feelings within reason. Verbalization of feelings in a nonthreatening environment may help the client come to terms with unresolved issues.

■ Encourage the client to discharge pent-up anger through participation in large motor activities (e.g., brisk walks, jogging, physical exercises, volleyball, punching bag, exercise bike). Physical exercise provides a safe and effective method for discharging pent-up tension.

■ Explore with the client the true source of anger. This is painful therapy that often leads to regression as the client deals with feelings of early abandonment or abuse. It seems that sometimes the client must "get worse before he or she can get better." Reconciliation of the feelings associated with this stage is necessary before progression through the grieving process can continue.

■ As anger is displaced onto the nurse or therapist, caution must be taken to guard against the negative effects of countertransference. These behaviors have the capacity to elicit an array of negative feelings from the caregiver. The existence of negative feelings by the nurse or therapist must be acknowledged but must not be allowed to interfere with the therapeutic process.

■ Explain the behaviors associated with the normal grieving process. Help the client recognize his or her position in this process. Knowledge of the acceptability of the feelings associated with normal grieving may help to relieve some of the guilt that these responses generate.

■ Help the client understand appropriate ways of expressing anger. Give positive reinforcement for behaviors used to express anger appropriately. Act as a role model. It is appropriate to let the client know when he or she has done something that has generated angry feelings in you. Role-modeling ways to express anger in an appropriate manner is a powerful learning tool.

■ Clearly identify expected behaviors within the milieu and set limits on behaviors that are in violation of stated expectations with clearly stated consequences. For example, the nurse states clearly to the patient on admission that physical contact among patients is not permitted. When the patient is noticed putting her arm around a male patient, the nurse clarifies the limit, indicates that this is not acceptable behavior, and communicates that if the behavior continues, the patient will not be permitted to continue participating in the current activity. Be supportive, yet consistent and firm, in caring for this client. The client lacks sufficient self-control to limit maladaptive behaviors, so assistance is required. Without consistency on the part of all staff members working with this client, a positive outcome will not be achieved.

Impaired Social Interaction

Impaired social interaction is defined as "insufficient or excessive quantity or ineffective quality of social exchange" (Herdman & Kamitsuru, 2014, p. 301).

Client Goals

Outcome criteria include short- and long-term goals. Time lines are individually determined.

Short-term goal

■ Within 5 days, the client will discuss with the nurse or therapist behaviors that impede the development of satisfactory interpersonal relationships.

Long-term goal

■ By the time of discharge from treatment, the client will interact appropriately with others in the therapy setting in both social and therapeutic activities (evidencing a discontinuation of splitting and clinging and distancing behaviors).

Interventions

■ Encourage the client to examine these behaviors and associated feelings (to recognize that they are occurring). He or she may be unaware of splitting or of clinging and distancing patterns of interaction with others. Recognition must take place before change can occur. For example, when a client begins to recognize that he or she feels less anxious when engaging in disruptive behaviors, a foundation is laid for exploring healthier strategies for anxiety reduction.

■ Help the client understand that you will be available, without reinforcing dependent behaviors. Knowledge of your availability may provide needed security.

■ Rotate staff members who work with the client to avoid the development of dependence on particular individuals. The client must learn to relate to more than one staff member in an effort to decrease the use of splitting and diminish fears of abandonment. Communication and consistency among the staff team members in adherence to the established plan of care is essential to minimize opportunities for the client to successfully manipulate or split staff members.

■ With the client, explore feelings that relate to fears of abandonment and engulfment. Help him or her understand that clinging and distancing behaviors are engendered by these fears. Exploration of feelings with a trusted individual may help the client come to terms with unresolved issues.

■ Help the client understand how these behaviors interfere with satisfactory relationships. He or she may be unaware of how others perceive these behaviors and why they are not acceptable.

■ Help the client work toward achievement of object constancy. Be available without promoting dependency. Give positive reinforcement for independent behaviors. The client must resolve fears of abandonment to establish satisfactory intimate relationships.

■ Provide education, support, and referral resources for family members and significant others who may also experience anger and frustration at failed attempts to navigate interpersonal relationships with the client. Research has shown that family members of these clients often report feeling excluded and discriminated against by health-care providers (Lawn, Diped, & McMahon, 2015).

> **CLINICAL PEARL** Recognize when the client is playing one staff member against another. Remember that splitting is the primary defense mechanism of individuals with BPD, and the impressions they have of others as either "all good" or "all bad" are a manifestation of this defense. Do not engage the client in discussions that are attempts to degrade other staff members. Suggest instead that the client discuss problems directly with the staff person involved.

Concept Care Mapping

The concept map care plan is an innovative approach to planning and organizing nursing care (see Chapter 9, The Nursing Process in Psychiatric-Mental Health Nursing). It is a diagrammatic teaching and learning strategy that allows visualization of interrelationships between medical diagnoses, nursing diagnoses, assessment data, and treatments. An example of a concept map care plan for a client with BPD is presented in Figure 32–1.

Evaluation

Reassessment is conducted to determine if the nursing actions have been successful in achieving the objectives of care. Evaluation of the nursing actions for the client with BPD may be facilitated by gathering information using the following types of questions:

- Has the client been able to seek out staff when feeling the desire for self-harm?
- Has the client avoided self-harm?
- Can the client correlate times of desire for self-harm to times of elevation in level of anxiety?
- Can the client discuss feelings with staff (particularly feelings of depression and anger)?
- Can the client identify the true source toward which the anger is directed?
- Can the client verbalize understanding of the basis for his or her anger?
- Can the client express anger appropriately?
- Can the client function independently?
- Can the client relate to more than one staff member?
- Can the client verbalize the knowledge that the staff members will return and are not abandoning him or her when leaving for the day?
- Can the client separate from the staff in an appropriate manner?
- Can the client delay gratification and refrain from manipulating others in order to fulfill own desires?
- Can the client verbalize resources within the community from whom he or she may seek assistance in times of extreme stress?

NOTE: The client with BPD is at high risk for stigmatization, even among health-care professionals (Black, Pfhol, & Blum, 2011; McNee, Donogue, & Coppola, 2014; Weight & Kendal, 2013; Westwood & Baker, 2010). Client behaviors such as manipulating, lying, and splitting violate the nurse's sense of success in establishing a trusting relationship with this individual and may culminate in negative or distancing behaviors from the nurse. The following guidelines are helpful in decreasing negative attitudes and stigmatization of this client:

- Understand the disorder and the impact of childhood trauma on the dynamics of the client's behavior to develop an approach of compassion and convey hopefulness that this is a treatable condition.
- Recognize that even brief encounters with a client during short hospital stays provide an opportunity to convey connectedness and a sense that they are valued. This is particularly important since the client with BPD is interpersonally hypersensitive, fears abandonment, and has had a history of instability in interpersonal relationships (Helleman et al., 2014).
- Frequently reflect on your feelings in response to client behavior. For example, self-harming behaviors by the client frequently generate feelings of anger and frustration in nurses when the behavior seems to be manipulative rather than a sign of true distress. These feelings may culminate in the nurse distancing themselves from the client (Westwood & Baker, 2010). Indeed, self-harming behaviors may be used as a tool for manipulating others *and* they are a sign of true distress.
- Develop a clear model of communication and intervention among team members for the hospitalized client with BPD. Consistency in intervention helps to model healthy interpersonal skills for the client and may minimize successful efforts at splitting staff members. In addition, when health-care team members develop strong communication skills with each other, it provides a foundation for discussing and confronting negative attitudes toward the client and promotes culture change. For example, McNee and associates (2014) developed a commitment among team members that they would avoid using phrases like "acting out" or "attention-seeking" since these reinforced a culture of negativity toward the client.

Antisocial Personality Disorder (Background Assessment Data)

In the *DSM-I,* antisocial behavior was categorized as a "sociopathic or psychopathic" reaction that could be symptomatic of any of several underlying personality disorders. The *DSM-II* represented it as a separate personality type, a distinction that has been retained in

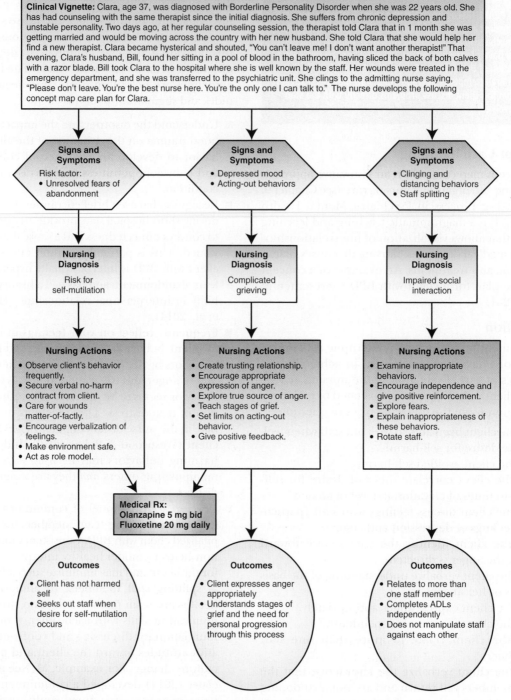

FIGURE 32–1 Concept map care plan for a client with borderline personality disorder.

subsequent editions. The *DSM-5* diagnostic criteria for antisocial personality disorder are presented in Box 32–10.

Individuals with antisocial personality disorder are seldom seen in most clinical settings, and when they are, it is commonly a way to avoid legal consequences. Sometimes they are admitted to the health-care system by court order for psychological evaluation. Most frequently, however, these individuals are encountered in prisons, jails, and rehabilitation services.

Although the *DSM-5* continues to identify antisocial personality disorder as synonymous with psychopathy, recent evidence is beginning to distinguish these as separate entities (Anderson et al., 2014; APA, 2013; Thompson et al., 2014; Verona & Patrick, 2015). Antisocial personality disorder as a distinct

> ### BOX 32–10 **Diagnostic Criteria for Antisocial Personality Disorder**
>
> A. A pervasive pattern of disregard for and violation of the rights of others occurring since age 15 years, as indicated by three (or more) of the following:
> 1. Failure to conform to social norms with respect to lawful behaviors as indicated by repeatedly performing acts that are grounds for arrest
> 2. Deceitfulness, as indicated by repeated lying, use of aliases, or conning others for personal profit or pleasure
> 3. Impulsivity or failure to plan ahead
> 4. Irritability and aggressiveness, as indicated by repeated physical fights or assaults
> 5. Reckless disregard for safety of self or others
> 6. Consistent irresponsibility, as indicated by repeated failure to sustain consistent work behavior or honor financial obligations
> 7. Lack of remorse, as indicated by being indifferent to or rationalizing having hurt, mistreated, or stolen from another
> B. Individual is at least 18 years.
> C. There is evidence of conduct disorder with onset before age 15 years.
> D. The occurrence of antisocial behavior is not exclusively during the course of schizophrenia or bipolar disorder.

Reprinted with permission from the Diagnostic and Statistical Manual of Mental Disorders, Fifth Edition *(Copyright 2013). American Psychiatric Association.*

entity is identified as characterized by *behaviors* that are reactive to perceived threats, control, and a negative affect; psychopathy is described as *personality traits* that include low fear, low empathy, domination, callous cruelty, and emotional insensitivity (Thompson et al, 2014; Verona & Patrick, 2015). Those with either diagnosis may be considered prone to violence, but with different etiologies and potentially different responses in treatment. For the purpose of this text, they are discussed together as antisocial personality disorder.

Clinical Picture

Antisocial personality disorder is a pattern of socially irresponsible, exploitative, and guiltless behavior that reflects a general disregard for the rights of others. Individuals with antisocial personality disorder exploit and manipulate others for personal gain and are unconcerned with obeying the law. They have difficulty sustaining consistent employment and developing stable relationships. They appear cold and callous, often intimidating others with their brusque and belligerent manner. They tend to be argumentative and, at times, cruel and malicious. They lack warmth and compassion and are often suspicious of these qualities in others.

Individuals with antisocial personality have a very low tolerance for frustration, act impulsively, and are unable to delay gratification. They are restless and easily bored, often taking chances and seeking thrills as if they were immune to danger. Their pattern of impulsivity may be manifested in failure to plan ahead culminating in sudden job, residence, or relationship changes (APA, 2013).

When things go their way, individuals with this disorder act cheerful, even gracious and charming. But because of their low tolerance for frustration, this pleasant exterior can change very quickly. When momentary desires are challenged, they are likely to become furious and vindictive. Easily provoked to attack, their first inclination is to demean and dominate. They believe that "good guys finish last," and they show contempt for the weak and underprivileged. They exploit others to fulfill their own desires, showing no trace of shame or guilt for their behavior.

Individuals with antisocial personalities see themselves as victims, using projection, devaluing, and denial as primary ego defense mechanisms. They do not accept responsibility for the consequences of their behavior. Instead, the perception of victimization by others justifies their malicious behavior, lest they be the recipient of unjust persecution and hostility from others. Physical attacks or other acts of aggression are not uncommon.

Satisfying interpersonal relationships are not possible because individuals with antisocial personalities have learned to trust only themselves. They have a philosophy that "it's every man for himself" and that one should stop at nothing to avoid being manipulated by others. They may disregard their safety and that of others through reckless sexual activity, substance use, reckless driving, or child neglect (APA, 2013).

One of the most distinctive characteristics of individuals with antisocial personality is their tendency to ignore conventional authority and rules. They act as though established social norms and guidelines for self-discipline and cooperative behavior do not apply to them. They are flagrant in their disrespect for the law and for the rights of others.

Predisposing Factors to Antisocial Personality Disorder
Biological Influences

Antisocial personality is more common among first-degree biological relatives of those with the disorder than among the general population. Twin and adoptive studies have implicated the role of genetics in antisocial personality disorder, especially for the personality traits of callousness and unemotional responses, which may be more definitive of psychopathy (Thompson et al., 2014). Interestingly, other antisocial behaviors among twins seemed to be more environmentally influenced, so based on current evidence, this is a complex disorder with both genetic and environmental influences. Recent research has suggested that a particular gene, *MAOA,* may be moderated after exposure to violence such as child maltreatment, physical abuse, or sexual abuse (Oullett-Morin et al., 2016). Moderation of this gene is believed to be associated with the eventual development of differential features of antisocial personality, although the authors note that more research is needed. Nonetheless, it lends support to the idea that a complex interaction of genetics and environment is involved in the development of antisocial personality disorder.

Characteristics associated with temperament in the newborn may be significant in the predisposition to antisocial personality disorder. Parents who bring children with behavior disorders to clinics often report that the child displayed temper tantrums from infancy and would become furious when awaiting a bottle or a diaper change. As these children mature, they commonly develop a bullying attitude toward other children. Parents report that they are undaunted by punishment and generally quite unmanageable.

The likelihood of developing antisocial personality disorder is increased if the individual had attention-deficit/hyperactivity disorder and conduct disorder as a child (APA, 2013). Other brain imaging studies have identified deficits in prefrontal cortex gray matter, which regulates cognitive control and inhibition, and decreased activity in the amygdala, which is responsible for modulating fearful or threatening stimuli. Still other studies have identified dysregulation of neurotransmitters (dopamine and serotonin), and endocrine abnormalities (testosterone and cortisol) in individuals with antisocial personality disorder, which may be related to the symptoms of impulsivity (Thompson et al., 2014). Neuropsychological studies have demonstrated an increased reactivity to environmental irritants and cues that may be triggers for disinhibition (Verona & Patrick, 2015).

Family Dynamics

Antisocial personality disorder frequently arises from a chaotic home environment. Parental deprivation during the first 5 years of life appears to be a critical predisposing factor in the development of antisocial personality disorder. Separation due to parental delinquency appears to be more highly correlated with the disorder than is parental loss from other causes.

Studies have shown that antisocial personality disorder in adulthood is highly associated with physical abuse and neglect, teasing, and lack of parental bonding in childhood (Krastins et al., 2014; Kolla et al., 2013). Severe physical abuse was particularly correlated to violent offending, triggering the development of a pattern of reactive aggression that is persistent over one's lifetime (Kolla et al., 2013). The abuse also contributes to the development of antisocial behavior in that it provides a model for behavior and may result in injury to the child's central nervous system, thereby impairing the child's ability to function appropriately. Although a diagnosis of antisocial personality disorder is only made when the client is at least 18 years old, these behavioral patterns are often seen earlier in childhood and adolescence. When they are identified in children and adolescents, the diagnosis is *conduct disorder,* and the common symptoms are bullying, fighting, physical cruelty to animals, destruction of property and theft, and others (APA, 2013). Whether better identification and early intervention might prevent more dangerous behavior in adulthood is yet to be determined through ongoing research.

Diagnosis and Outcome Identification

Nursing diagnoses are formulated from the data gathered during the assessment phase and with background knowledge regarding predisposing factors to the disorder. Table 32–4 presents a list of client behaviors and the NANDA-I nursing diagnoses that correspond to those behaviors, which may be used in planning care for clients with antisocial personality disorder.

Outcome Criteria

The following criteria may be used for measurement of outcomes in the care of the client with antisocial personality disorder.

The client:

■ Discusses angry feelings with staff and in group sessions
■ Has not harmed self or others
■ Can rechannel hostility into socially acceptable behaviors
■ Follows rules and regulations of the therapy environment
■ Can verbalize which of his or her behaviors are not acceptable
■ Shows regard for the rights of others by delaying gratification of own desires when appropriate

---

TABLE 32–4 Assigning Nursing Diagnoses to Behaviors Commonly Associated With Antisocial Personality Disorder

BEHAVIORS	NURSING DIAGNOSES
Risk factors: Body language (e.g., rigid posture, clenching of fists and jaw, hyperactivity, pacing, breathlessness, threatening stances); cruelty to animals; rage reactions; history of childhood abuse; history of violence against others; impulsivity; substance abuse; negative role-modeling; inability to tolerate frustration	Risk for other-directed violence
Disregard for societal norms and laws; absence of guilty feelings; inability to delay gratification; denial of obvious problems; grandiosity; hostile laughter; projection of blame and responsibility; ridicule of others; superior attitude toward others	Defensive coping
Manipulation of others to fulfill own desires; inability to form close, personal relationships; frequent lack of success in life events; passive-aggressiveness; overt aggressiveness (hiding feelings of low self-esteem)	Chronic low self-esteem
Inability to form a satisfactory, enduring, intimate relationship with another; dysfunctional interaction with others; use of unsuccessful social interaction behaviors	Impaired social interaction
Demonstration of inability to take responsibility for meeting basic health practices; history of lack of health-seeking behavior; demonstrated lack of knowledge regarding basic health practices; lack of expressed interest in improving health behaviors	Ineffective health maintenance

---

- Does not manipulate others in an attempt to increase feelings of self-worth
- Verbalizes understanding of knowledge required to maintain basic health needs

Planning and Implementation

The following section presents a group of selected nursing diagnoses common to clients with antisocial personality disorder, with short- and long-term goals and nursing interventions for each.

Risk for Other-Directed Violence

Risk for other-directed violence is defined as "vulnerable to behaviors in which an individual demonstrates that he or she can be physically, emotionally, and/or sexually harmful to others" (Herdman & Kamitsuru, 2014, p. 410).

Client Goals

Outcome criteria include short- and long-term goals. Time lines are individually determined.

Short-term goals

- Within 3 days, the client will discuss angry feelings and situations that precipitate hostility.
- The client will not harm others.

Long-term goal

- The client will not harm others.

Interventions

- Convey an accepting attitude toward this client. Feelings of rejection are undoubtedly familiar to him or her. Work on development of trust. Be honest, keep all promises, and convey the message to the client that it is not *him* or *her* but the *behavior* that is unacceptable. An attitude of acceptance promotes feelings of self-worth. Trust is the basis of a therapeutic relationship. Be alert, however, to the tendency of this client to manipulate others. Do not misconstrue charm or compliments as indicative of mutual trust. Maintaining clear, professional boundaries is essential.
- Maintain a low level of stimuli in the client's environment (low lighting, few people, simple decor, low noise level). A stimulating environment may increase agitation and promote aggressive behavior.
- Observe the client's behavior frequently through routine activities and interactions; avoid appearing watchful and suspicious. Close observation is required so that intervention can occur if needed to ensure the client's (and others') safety.
- Remove all dangerous objects from the client's environment so that he or she may not purposefully or inadvertently use them to inflict harm to self or others.
- Help the client identify the true object of his or her hostility (e.g., "You seem to be upset with . . ."). Because of weak ego development, the client may misuse the defense mechanism of displacement. Helping him or her recognize this in a nonthreatening manner may help reveal unresolved issues so that they may be confronted.
- Encourage the client to gradually verbalize hostile feelings. Verbalization of feelings in a nonthreatening environment may help the client come to terms with unresolved issues.

- Explore with the client alternative ways of handling frustration (e.g., large motor skills that channel hostile energy into socially acceptable behavior). Physically demanding activities help to relieve pent-up tension.
- The staff should maintain and convey a calm attitude toward the client. Anxiety is contagious and can be transferred from staff to client. A calm attitude provides the client with a feeling of safety and security.
- Have sufficient staff available to present a show of strength to the client if necessary. This conveys to the client evidence of control over the situation and provides some physical security for the staff.
- Administer tranquilizing medications as ordered by the physician or obtain an order if necessary. Monitor the client for effectiveness of the medication as well as for appearance of adverse side effects. Antianxiety agents (e.g., lorazepam, chlordiazepoxide, oxazepam) produce a calming effect and may help to allay hostile behaviors. (NOTE: Medications are not often prescribed for clients with antisocial personality disorder because of these individuals' strong susceptibility to addictions.)
- If the client is not calmed by "talking down" or by medication, use of mechanical restraints may be necessary. The avenue of the "least restrictive alternative" must be selected when planning interventions for a violent client. Restraints should be used only as a last resort, after all other interventions have been unsuccessful, and when the client is clearly at risk of harm to self or others.
- If restraint is deemed necessary, ensure that sufficient staff is available to assist. Follow protocol established by the institution.
- As agitation decreases, assess the client's readiness for restraint removal or reduction. Remove one restraint at a time while assessing the client's response. This minimizes the risk of injury to client and staff.

Defensive Coping

Defensive coping is defined as "repeated projection of falsely positive self-evaluation based on a self-protective pattern that defends against underlying perceived threats to positive self-regard" (Herdman & Kamitsuru, 2014, p. 324).

Client Goals

Outcome criteria include short- and long-term goals. Time lines are individually determined.

Short-term goals

- Within 24 hours after admission, the client will verbalize understanding of treatment setting rules and regulations and the consequences for violation.

- The client will verbalize personal responsibility for difficulties experienced in interpersonal relationships within (time period reasonable for client).

Long-term goals

- By the time of discharge from treatment, the client will be able to cope more adaptively by delaying gratification of own desires and following rules and regulations of the treatment setting.
- By the time of discharge from treatment, the client will demonstrate ability to interact with others without becoming defensive, rationalizing behaviors, or expressing grandiose ideas.

Interventions

- From the onset, the client should be made aware of which behaviors are acceptable and which are not. Explain consequences of violation of the limits. A consequence must involve something of value to the client. All staff must be consistent in enforcing these limits. Consequences should be administered in a matter-of-fact manner immediately following the infraction. Because the client cannot (or will not) impose own limits on maladaptive behaviors, these behaviors must be delineated and enforced by staff. Undesirable consequences may help to decrease repetition of these behaviors.
- The ideal goal would be for this client to eventually internalize societal norms, beginning with a step-by-step, "either/or" approach on the unit (*either* you do [don't do] this, *or* this will occur). Explanations must be concise, concrete, and clear, with little or no capacity for misinterpretation.

> **CLINICAL PEARL**
>
> Do not attempt to coax or convince the client to do the "right thing." Do not use the words "You should (or shouldn't) . . ."; instead, use the words "You will be expected to. . . ."

- Provide positive feedback or reward for acceptable behaviors. Positive reinforcement enhances self-esteem and encourages repetition of desirable behaviors.
- In an attempt to assist the client to delay gratification, increase the length of time requirement for acceptable behavior in order to achieve the reward. For example, 2 hours of acceptable behavior may be exchanged for a phone call; 4 hours of acceptable behavior for 2 hours of television; 1 day of acceptable behavior for a recreational therapy bowling activity; 5 days of acceptable behavior for a weekend pass.
- A milieu unit provides the appropriate environment for the client with antisocial personality. The

democratic approach, with specific rules and regulations, community meetings, and group therapy sessions, emulates the type of societal situation in which the client must learn to live. Feedback from peers is often more effective than confrontation from an authority figure. The client learns to follow the rules of the group as a positive step in the progression toward internalizing the rules of society.

■ Help the client gain insight into his or her own behavior. Often, these individuals deny that their behavior is inappropriate. For example, rationalizing may be reflected in statements such as, "The owner of this store has so much money, he'll never miss the little bit I take. He has everything, and I have nothing. It's not fair! I deserve to have some of what he has." The client must come to understand that certain behaviors will not be tolerated within society and that severe consequences are imposed on those individuals who refuse to comply. The client must *want* to change behavior before he or she can be helped. One of the difficulties posed in interventions for personality disorders is that often the behaviors are ego-syntonic; in other words, the client may not perceive these behaviors as requiring change.

■ Talk about past behaviors with the client. Discuss which are acceptable by societal norms and which are not. Help the client identify ways in which he or she has exploited others and the benefits versus consequences of previous behavior. Explore the client's insight into feelings associated with his or her behavior. An attempt may be made to enlighten the client to the sensitivity of others by promoting self-awareness in an effort to help the client gain insight into his or her own behavior.

■ Throughout the relationship with the client, maintain an attitude of "It is not *you*, but *your behavior*, that is unacceptable." An attitude of acceptance promotes feelings of dignity and self-worth.

Concept Care Mapping

The concept map care plan care (see Chapter 9) is a diagrammatic teaching and learning strategy that allows visualization of interrelationships between medical diagnoses, nursing diagnoses, assessment data, and treatments. An example of a concept map care plan for a client with antisocial personality disorder is presented in Figure 32–2.

Evaluation

Reassessment is conducted to determine if the nursing actions have been successful in achieving the objectives of care. Evaluation of the nursing actions for the client with antisocial personality disorder may be facilitated by gathering information using the following types of questions:

■ Does the client recognize when anger is getting out of control?
■ Can the client seek out staff instead of expressing anger in an inappropriate manner?
■ Can the client use other sources for rechanneling anger (e.g., physical activities)?
■ Has harm to others been avoided?
■ Can the client follow rules and regulations of the therapeutic milieu with little or no reminding?
■ Can the client verbalize which behaviors are appropriate and which are not?
■ Does the client express a desire to change?
■ Can the client delay gratification of own desires in deference to those of others when appropriate?
■ Does the client refrain from manipulating others to fulfill own desires?
■ Does the client fulfill activities of daily living willingly and independently?
■ Can the client verbalize methods of achieving and maintaining optimal wellness?
■ Can the client verbalize community resources from which he or she can seek assistance with daily living and health-care needs when required?

Treatment Modalities

Few would argue that treatment of individuals with personality disorders is difficult and may even seem impossible. Personality characteristics are learned very early in life and may be genetically influenced. Many of the symptoms of a personality disorder are viewed by the individual as ego-syntonic, so there may be little motivation to seek treatment or to explore change. It is not surprising, then, that these enduring patterns of behavior may take years to change, if change occurs. The main treatment modalities for personality disorders are psychosocial and pharmacological, but most of the available evidence comes from studies of borderline and antisocial personality disorders.

Comorbid conditions are common in most personality disorders, and there is evidence that treating these conditions may have positive outcomes. For example, Hatchett (2015) identifies that, in a review of the literature, psychosocial interventions for clients with antisocial personality disorder lack both treatment efficacy and clinical utility; however, treatment of comorbid substance use disorder has demonstrated positive outcomes. Further, when individuals with antisocial personality disorder have comorbid depression, they are more likely to persevere with treatment. This may be related to the fact that symptoms

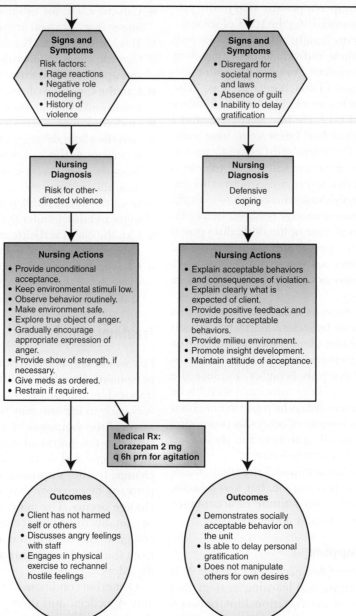

Clinical Vignette: Hank, age 32, is the oldest of five children of a single mother, each of whom had a different father. He was physically abused by his mother's boyfriends, did not attend school regularly, and eventually dropped out in 10th grade. He has a history of violence, always carries a weapon (gun or knife) on his person, and threatens to use it if he is challenged in his attempts to fulfill his own desires. He has had numerous skirmishes with the law: shoplifting, auto theft, possession and sale of heroin and cocaine, and, most recently, armed robbery of a liquor store. He was identified by his image on the store's surveillance camera. Because of his long history of criminal behavior, the judge has ordered that Hank undergo psychological testing before he is sentenced. On the psychiatric unit, he says to the nurse, "Why am I here? I'm not crazy! And I've never hurt anybody! I don't belong in this loony bin!" The nurse develops the following concept map care plan for Hank.

Signs and Symptoms

Risk factors:
• Rage reactions
• Negative role modeling
• History of violence

Signs and Symptoms

• Disregard for societal norms and laws
• Absence of guilt
• Inability to delay gratification

Nursing Diagnosis

Risk for other-directed violence

Nursing Diagnosis

Defensive coping

Nursing Actions

• Provide unconditional acceptance.
• Keep environmental stimuli low.
• Observe behavior routinely.
• Make environment safe.
• Explore true object of anger.
• Gradually encourage appropriate expression of anger.
• Provide show of strength, if necessary.
• Give meds as ordered.
• Restrain if required.

Nursing Actions

• Explain acceptable behaviors and consequences of violation.
• Explain clearly what is expected of client.
• Provide positive feedback and rewards for acceptable behaviors.
• Provide milieu environment.
• Promote insight development.
• Maintain attitude of acceptance.

Medical Rx: Lorazepam 2 mg q 6h prn for agitation

Outcomes

• Client has not harmed self or others
• Discusses angry feelings with staff
• Engages in physical exercise to rechannel hostile feelings

Outcomes

• Demonstrates socially acceptable behavior on the unit
• Is able to delay personal gratification
• Does not manipulate others for own desires

FIGURE 32–2 Concept map care plan for a client with antisocial personality disorder.

of depression are considered undesirable (not ego-syntonic) and therefore may promote interest in improvement. He notes that this review should not be interpreted as meaning that a client's personality disorder is untreatable. Instead, Hatchett cites the conclusion of Skeem and associates (2011) that this client should be identified as "high risk" and requiring intensive treatment to maximize public safety.

Whereas Hatchett (2015) reviewed the literature specifically related to treatment for antisocial personality disorders, other literature reviews identify that, for personality disorders in general, there is strong evidence of the effectiveness of psychotherapeutic interventions (Papaioannou, Brazier, & Parry, 2013, Stoffers et al., 2012); again, the bulk of research focuses on borderline and antisocial personality disorders

(Bateman, 2014). Still other researchers identify that treatment focused on tackling the defense mechanisms associated with each personality disorder may be a more effective way to mediate improvement (Perry, Presniak, & Olson, 2013). For example, therapy focused on exploring the dissociation common in patients with BPD or exploring the defense mechanism of devaluing others, as seen in clients with antisocial personality, may promote overall improvement in symptoms. There is general agreement that all treatment modalities for personality disorders require intensive long-term plans of care. Selection of intervention is generally based on the area of greatest dysfunction, such as cognition, affect, behavior, or interpersonal relations. Following is a brief description of various types of therapies and the disorders to which they are customarily suited.

Individual Psychotherapy

Depending on the therapeutic goals, psychotherapy with personality disorders may be time-limited interpersonal psychotherapy or may involve long-term psychoanalytic therapy. Interpersonal psychotherapy may be particularly appropriate because personality disorders largely reflect problems in interpersonal relationship skills.

Long-term psychotherapy attempts to understand and modify the maladjusted behaviors, cognition, and affects of clients with personality disorders that dominate their personal lives and relationships.

Milieu or Group Therapy

This treatment is especially appropriate for individuals with antisocial personality disorder, who respond more adaptively to support and feedback from peers. In milieu or group therapy, feedback from peers is more effective than one-to-one interaction with a therapist.

Group therapy—particularly homogenous supportive groups that emphasize the development of social skills—may also be helpful in overcoming social anxiety and developing interpersonal trust and rapport in clients with avoidant personality disorder.

Cognitive-Behavioral Therapy

Behavioral strategies offer reinforcement for positive change. Social skills training and assertiveness training teach alternative ways to deal with frustration. Cognitive strategies help the client recognize and correct distorted and irrational thinking patterns. Davidson and associates (2009) found that the addition of cognitive-behavioral therapy to usual treatment for clients with antisocial personality disorders afforded a reduction in both verbal and physical aggression. There is also limited evidence that cognitive therapy is beneficial for clients with schizotypal personality disorder (Bateman, 2014).

Dialectical Behavior Therapy

Dialectical behavior therapy (DBT) is a type of psychotherapy originally developed by Marsha Linehan, PhD, specifically as a treatment for the chronic self-injurious and parasuicidal behavior of clients with BPD (Sadock et al., 2015). Rooted in a belief that the primary problem for this client is emotional dysregulation (a kind of emotional reactivity to perceived threats), DBT has become a well-established treatment for clients with BPD. It is a complex, eclectic treatment that combines the concepts of cognitive, behavioral, and interpersonal therapies with Eastern mindfulness practices. The four primary modes of treatment in DBT include the following:

1. **Group skills training:** In these groups, clients are taught skills relevant to the problems experienced by people with BPD, such as core mindfulness skills, interpersonal effectiveness skills, emotion modulation skills, and distress tolerance skills (Kiehn & Swales, 2013).
2. **Individual psychotherapy:** Weekly sessions address dysfunctional behavioral patterns, personal motivation, and skills strengthening.
3. **Telephone contact:.** The therapist is available to the client by telephone, according to limits set by the therapist but usually for 24 hours a day. Kiehn and Swales (2013) state, "Telephone contact is to give the patient help and support in applying the skills that she is learning to her real life situation between sessions and to help her find ways of avoiding self-injury."
4. **Therapist consultation/team meeting:** Therapists meet regularly to review their work with their clients. These meetings are focused specifically on providing support for each other, keeping the therapists motivated, and providing effective treatment to their clients. DBT has been well studied, and the evidence supports the benefits of this treatment for clients with BPD. O'Connell and Dowling (2014), citing a review of seven studies (Binks et al., 2006), report:

> Despite the difficulty in treating people with BPD, if the person with BPD engaged in their treatment plan, there was a reduction in anxiety levels, depression, self-harm, hospital admission, and the use of prescribed medication. (p. 522)

This method of treatment is now being used with other disorders, including substance use disorders, eating disorders, schizophrenia, and PTSD (Sadock et al., 2015). Bateman (2014) cautions, however, that of the many interventions specialized for the treatment of personality disorders, improvement is more often evidenced by symptom reduction rather than significant improvements in social functioning.

Psychopharmacology

Psychopharmacology may be helpful in some instances. Although these drugs have no effect in the direct treatment of the disorder itself, some symptomatic relief can be achieved. Among the cluster A disorders, there has been limited evidence of the benefits of antipsychotic medication in the treatment of schizotypal personality disorder, but the risk to benefit ratio is unclear (Bateman, 2014).

For the treatment of BPD, symptom-targeted pharmacotherapy has been identified as an important adjunct. Antipsychotic medications show benefit in treating cognitive-perceptual symptoms, selective serotonin reuptake inhibitors show some benefit in treating emotional dysregulation, and mood-stabilizing agents have shown some benefit in treating emotional dysregulation and impulsive and aggressive symptoms (Bateman, 2014). As mentioned previously, some current research identifies the benefits of adjunctive oxytocin therapy (Pier et al., 2016).

For antisocial personality disorder, pharmacotherapy is generally not recommended unless it is being used to treat a comorbid condition. Among the cluster C group of personality disorders, no randomized trials have been published that support pharmacological treatment for these disorders (Bateman, 2014).

Caution must be given to prescribing medications outside of a structured setting because of the high risk for substance abuse by these individuals.

CASE STUDY AND SAMPLE CARE PLAN

NURSING HISTORY AND ASSESSMENT

Anthony, age 34, has been admitted to the psychiatric unit with a diagnosis of antisocial personality disorder. He was recently arrested and convicted for armed robbery of a convenience store and attempted murder of the store clerk. Due to the actions of the store clerk, who quickly alerted police, and to the store surveillance camera, Anthony was identified and apprehended within hours of the crime. The judge has ordered physical, neurological, and psychiatric evaluations before sentencing Anthony.

Anthony was physically and psychologically abused as a child by his alcoholic father. He was suspended from high school because of failing grades and habitual truancy. He has a long history of arrests, beginning with shoplifting at age 7, progressing in adolescence to burglary, auto theft, and sexual assault, and finally to armed robbery and attempted murder. He was on probation when he committed his latest crime.

On the psychiatric unit, Anthony is loud, belligerent, and uncooperative. When Julie, his admitting nurse, arrives to work the evening shift on Anthony's second hospital day, he says to her, "I'm so glad you are finally here. You are the best nurse on the unit. I can't talk to anyone but you. These people are nothing but a bunch of loonies around here—and that includes staff as well as patients! Maybe you and I could walk down to the coffee shop together later. Are you married? I'd sure like to get to know you better after I get out of this nut house!"

NURSING DIAGNOSES AND OUTCOME IDENTIFICATION

From the assessment data, the nurse develops the following nursing diagnoses for Anthony:

A. **Risk for other-directed violence** related to history of violence against others and history of childhood abuse.
   a. **Short-Term Goals:** Client will discuss angry feelings and situations that precipitate hostility. Client will not harm others.
   b. **Long-Term Goal:** Client will not harm others.

B. **Defensive coping** related to low self-esteem, dysfunctional nuclear family, underdeveloped ego and superego, evidenced by absence of guilt feelings, disregard for societal laws and norms, inability to delay gratification, superior attitude toward others, denial of problems, and projection of blame and responsibility.
   a. **Short-Term Goal:** Client will verbalize understanding of unit rules and regulations and consequences for violation of them.
   b. **Long-Term Goals:** Client will be able to delay gratification and follow rules and regulations of the unit. Client will verbalize personal responsibility for own actions and behaviors.

PLANNING AND IMPLEMENTATION

RISK FOR OTHER-DIRECTED VIOLENCE
The following nursing interventions have been identified for Anthony.

1. Develop a trusting relationship with Anthony by conveying an accepting attitude. Ensure that he understands it is not him but his behavior that is unacceptable.
2. Try to keep excess stimuli out of the environment. Speak to Anthony in a calm, quiet voice.
3. Observe Anthony's behavior regularly through routine activity so that he does not become suspicious and angry about being watched. This is important so that if hostile and aggressive behaviors are observed, intervention may prevent harm to Anthony, staff members, and/or other patients.
4. Sit with Anthony and encourage him to talk about his anger and hostile feelings. Help him understand where these feelings originate and who is the true target of the hostility.
5. Help him develop adaptive ways of dealing with frustration, such as exercise and other physical activities.
6. Administer tranquilizing medication as ordered by the physician.

CASE STUDY AND SAMPLE CARE PLAN—cont'd

7. If Anthony should become out of control and mechanical restraints become necessary, ensure that sufficient staff is available to intervene. Do not use restraints as a punishment, but only as a last resort, protective measure for Anthony and the other patients.

DEFENSIVE COPING
The following nursing interventions have been identified for Anthony.

1. Explain to Anthony which of his behaviors are acceptable on the unit and which are not. Simply state that unacceptable behaviors will not be tolerated.
2. Determine appropriate consequences for violation of these limits (e.g., no TV or movies; no phone calls; time-out room). Ensure that all staff members follow through with these consequences.
3. Do not be taken in by Anthony's attempts to flatter or "charm" staff members. Compliments from Anthony are another form of manipulative behavior. Explain to Anthony that you will not accept these types of comments from him, and if they continue, impose consequences.
4. Encourage Anthony to talk about his past misdeeds. Try to help him understand how he would feel if someone treated him in the manner that he has treated others.

EVALUATION

The outcome criteria for Anthony have only partially been met. Personality characteristics such as those of Anthony's are deep rooted and enduring. He is not likely to change. Unless testing reveals a serious, treatable medical problem, Anthony will probably continue to suffer legal consequences and prison sentences until he develops insight and willingness to engage in behavior change. During his time on the psychiatric unit, harm to self and others has been avoided. He has discussed his anger and hostile feelings with Julie and other staff members. He continues to become belligerent when told that he cannot smoke on the unit and must wait for someone to escort him to the smoking area. He yells at the other patients and calls them "nut cases." He refuses to take responsibility for his actions and blames negative behavioral outcomes on others. He has begun a regular exercise program in the fitness room and receives positive feedback from the staff for this attempt to integrate healthier coping strategies.

Summary and Key Points

- Clients with personality disorders are undoubtedly some of the most difficult individuals health-care workers are likely to encounter.
- Personality characteristics are formed very early in life and are difficult, if not impossible, to change. In fact, some clinicians believe the therapeutic approach is not to try to change the characteristics but rather to decrease the inflexibility of the maladaptive traits and reduce their interference with everyday functioning and meaningful relationships.
- The concept of a personality disorder has been present throughout the history of medicine. Problems have arisen in the attempt to establish a classification system for these disorders.
- The *DSM-5* identifies 10 individual personality disorders: antisocial, avoidant, borderline, histrionic, dependent, narcissistic, obsessive-compulsive, paranoid, schizoid, and schizotypal.
- Nursing care of the client with a personality disorder is accomplished using the steps of the nursing process.

- Other treatment modalities include interpersonal psychotherapy, psychoanalytical psychotherapy, milieu or group therapy, cognitive-behavioral therapy, dialectical behavior therapy, and psychopharmacology.
- Individuals with BPD may enter the health-care system because of their instability and frequent attempts at self-destructive behavior.
- The individual with antisocial personality disorder may become part of the health-care system to avoid legal consequences or because of a court order for psychological evaluation.
- Nurses who work in all types of clinical settings should be familiar with the characteristics associated with personality disorders.
- Nurses working in psychiatry must be knowledgeable about appropriate intervention with these clients, for it is unlikely that they will encounter a greater professional challenge than these clients present.

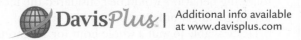

Review Questions
Self-Examination/Learning Exercise

Select the answer that is most appropriate for each of the following questions.

1. Kim has a diagnosis of borderline personality disorder. She often exhibits alternating clinging and distancing behaviors. The most appropriate nursing intervention with this type of behavior would be to:
   a. Encourage Kim to establish trust in one staff person, with whom all therapeutic interaction should take place.
   b. Secure a verbal contract from Kim that she will discontinue these behaviors.
   c. Withdraw attention if these behaviors continue.
   d. Rotate staff members who work with Kim so that she will learn to relate to more than one person.

2. Kim, a client diagnosed with borderline personality disorder, manipulates the staff in an effort to fulfill her own desires. All of the following may be examples of manipulative behaviors in the borderline client *except:*
   a. Refusal to stay in room alone, stating, "It's so lonely."
   b. Asking Nurse Jones for cigarettes after 30 minutes, knowing the assigned nurse has explained she must wait 1 hour.
   c. Stating to Nurse Jones, "I really like having you for my nurse. You're the best one around here."
   d. Cutting arms with razor blade after discussing dismissal plans with physician.

3. "Splitting" by the client with BPD denotes:
   a. Evidence of precocious development.
   b. A primitive defense mechanism in which the client sees objects as all good or all bad.
   c. A brief psychotic episode in which the client loses contact with reality.
   d. Two distinct personalities within the borderline client.

4. According to Margaret Mahler, predisposition to BPD occurs when developmental tasks go unfulfilled in which of the following phases?
   a. Autistic phase, during which the child's needs for security and comfort go unfulfilled.
   b. Symbiotic phase, during which the child fails to bond with the mother.
   c. Differentiation phase, during which the child fails to recognize a separateness between self and mother.
   d. Rapprochement phase, during which the mother withdraws emotional support in response to the child's increasing independence.

5. Jack is a new client on the psychiatric unit with a diagnosis of antisocial personality disorder. Which of the following characteristics would you expect to assess in Jack?
   a. Lack of guilt for wrongdoing
   b. Insight into his own behavior
   c. Ability to learn from past experiences
   d. Compliance with authority

6. Milieu therapy is a good choice for clients with antisocial personality disorder because it:
   a. Provides a system of punishment and rewards for behavior modification.
   b. Emulates a social community in which the client may learn to live harmoniously with others.
   c. Provides mostly one-to-one interaction between the client and therapist.
   d. Provides a very structured setting in which the clients have very little input into the planning of their care.

7. In evaluating the progress of Jack, a client diagnosed with antisocial personality disorder, which of the following behaviors would be considered the most significant indication of positive change?
   a. Jack got angry only once in group this week.
   b. Jack was able to wait a whole hour for a cigarette without verbally abusing the staff.
   c. On his own initiative, Jack sent a note of apology to a man he had injured in a recent fight.
   d. Jack stated that he would no longer start any more fights.

Review Questions—cont'd
Self-Examination/Learning Exercise

8. Which of the following behavioral patterns is characteristic of individuals with narcissistic personality disorder?
   a. Overly self-centered and exploitative of others
   b. Suspicious and mistrustful of others
   c. Rule conscious and disapproving of change
   b. Anxious and socially isolated

9. Jessica is a nurse who was floated to the psychiatric unit to cover for a staff nurse who called out sick. She encounters a patient diagnosed with BPD, and the patient states, "Thank goodness they sent you to the unit. No one else here has taken the time to listen to my concerns." This may be an example of which symptom common in BPD?
   a. Impulsivity
   b. Self-harming behaviors
   c. Dissociation
   d. Splitting

10. Which of the following behavioral patterns is characteristic of individuals with schizotypal personality disorder?
   a. Belittling themselves and their abilities
   b. A lifelong pattern of social withdrawal
   c. Suspicious and mistrustful of others
   b. Overreacting inappropriately to minor stimuli

IMPLICATIONS OF RESEARCH FOR EVIDENCE-BASED PRACTICE

Brook, J., Lee. J.Y., Rubenstone, E., Brook, D., & Finch, S. (2014). Triple comorbid trajectories of tobacco, alcohol, and marijuana use as predictors of antisocial personality disorder and generalized anxiety disorder among urban adults. *American Journal of Public Health, 104*(8), 1413-1420. doi:10.2105/AJPH.2014.301880

DESCRIPTION OF THE STUDY: As part of the Harlem longitudinal development study, 816 urban youth of African American and Puerto Rican heritage were studied from the age of 19 until 32 years of age to evaluate the likelihood that those who were multi-substance users (alcohol, tobacco, and marijuana) were at greater risk for developing antisocial personality disorder (ASPD) and/or generalized anxiety disorder (GAD) in adulthood. The authors note that previous research has supported a relationship between multi-substance use and the development of ASPD. Evidence has also shown that psychosocial outcomes are worse when there is multi-substance abuse versus use of only one substance.

RESULTS OF THE STUDY: The concomitant use of tobacco, alcohol, and marijuana did significantly increase the likelihood of developing antisocial personality disorder in adulthood. A surprising finding was that, contrary to other research studies, this population did not show a decline in substance use after the mid-20s (as is typical of other populations), suggesting that these co-occurring problems may be more persistent for this population. The authors hypothesize that this may be related to less conventional ties (such as family or institutions) and more exposure to deviant peers, drug abusers, and antisocial behavior.

IMPLICATIONS FOR NURSING PRACTICE: Understanding the evidence base for treatment issues relevant to specific cultural and ethnic groups provides the nurse with a foundation for providing culturally sensitive and informed care. This study highlights risks for African American and Puerto Rican youth in urban settings, and the findings suggest that earlier intervention and treatment of comorbid substance use disorders may be effective in decreasing the likelihood of antisocial personality disorders in adulthood as well as decreasing their risk for longer-standing substance use disorders. Nursing assessment, particularly among adolescents, should include assessment for multi-substance use as well as for evidence of conduct disorder behavior and treatment should focus on addressing all substances.

TEST YOUR CRITICAL THINKING SKILLS

Dana, age 32, was diagnosed with borderline personality disorder when she was 26 years old. Her husband took her to the emergency department when he walked into the bathroom and found her cutting her legs with a razor blade. At that time, assessment revealed that Dana had a long history of self-mutilation, which she had carefully hidden from her husband and others. Dana began long-term psychoanalytical psychotherapy on an outpatient basis. Therapy revealed that Dana had been physically and sexually abused as a child by both her mother and her father, both now deceased. She admitted to having chronic depression, and her husband related episodes of rage reactions. Dana has been hospitalized on the psychiatric unit for a week because of suicidal ideations. After making a no-suicide contract with the staff, she is allowed to leave the unit on pass to keep a dental appointment that she made a number of weeks ago. She has just returned to the unit and says to her nurse, "I just took 20 Desyrel while I was sitting in my car in the parking lot."

Answer the following questions related to Lana:

1. The nurse is well acquainted with Dana and believes this is a manipulative gesture. How should the nurse handle this situation?
2. What is the priority nursing diagnosis for Dana?
3. Dana likes to "split" the staff into "good guys" and "bad guys." What is the most important intervention for splitting by a person with borderline personality disorder?

💬 Communication Exercises

1. Nathan, age 37, has been admitted to the hospital for a psychiatric evaluation after being arrested for armed robbery of a convenience store. He has a history of encounters with law enforcement since early adolescence. He has been diagnosed with antisocial personality disorder. Nathan says to the nurse, "Hey pretty lady! Where have you been all my life?"
   - How would the nurse respond appropriately to this statement by Nathan?
2. "I really got a bum rap! I had no intentions of hurting anyone. The gun only had one bullet in it! I just wanted to scare that clerk into giving me a few bucks! Just my bad luck an off-duty cop had to walk in about that time."
   - How would the nurse respond appropriately to this statement by Nathan?
3. "You're really cute. Are you married? I'm pretty sure my lawyer can get me out of this rap, and I'll be a free man! Why don't you give me your phone number and I'll call you sometime. We could go out and have some fun!"
   - How would the nurse respond appropriately to this statement by Nathan?

MOVIE CONNECTIONS

Taxi Driver (schizoid personality) • *One Flew Over the Cuckoo's Nest* (antisocial) • *The Boston Strangler* (antisocial) • *Just Cause* (antisocial) • *The Dream Team* (antisocial) • *Goodfellas* (antisocial) • *Fatal Attraction* (borderline) • *Play Misty for Me* (borderline) • *Girl, Interrupted* (borderline) • *Gone With the Wind* (histrionic) • *Wall Street* (narcissistic) • *The Odd Couple* (obsessive-compulsive)

References

American Psychiatric Association (APA). (2013). *Diagnostic and statistical manual of mental disorders* (5th ed.). Washington, DC: APA.

Anderson, J.L., Sellbom, M., Wygant, D.B., Salekin, R.T., & Krueger, R.F. (2014). Examining the association between *DSM-5* section III antisocial personality traits and psychopathy in community and university samples. *Journal of Personality Disorders, 28*(5), 675-697. doi:10.1521/pedi_2014_28_134

Bateman, A.W., Gunderson, J., & Mulder, R. (2015). Treatment of personality disorder. *www.lancet.com, 385*(9969), 735-743. doi:10.1016/S0140-6736(14)61394-5

Binks, C., Fenton, M., McCarthy, L., Lee, T., Adams, C. & Duggan, C. (2006). Psychological therapies for people with borderline personality disorders (review). *Cochrane Database of Systematic Reviews, 1.* doi:10.1002/14651858.CD005652

Black, D.W., & Andreasen, N.C. (2014). *Introductory textbook of psychiatry* (6th ed.). Washington, DC: American Psychiatric Publishing.

Black, D., Pfhol, B., & Blum, M. (2011). Attitudes towards borderline personality disorder: A survey of 706 mental health clinicians. *CNS Spectrums, 16*(3), 67-74. doi:10.1017/S109285291200020X

Bornstein, R.F., Bianucci, V., Fishman, D.P., & Biars, J.W. (2104). Toward a firmer foundation for *DSM-5.1*: Domains of impairment in *DSM IV/DSM-5* personality disorders. *Journal of Personality Disorders, 28*(2), 212-224. doi:10.1521/pedi_2013_27_116

Brook, J., Lee., J.Y., Rubenstone, E., Brook, D., & Finch, S. (2014). Triple comorbid trajectories of tobacco, alcohol, and marijuana use as predictors of antisocial personality disorder and generalized anxiety disorder among urban adults. *American Journal of Public Health, 104*(8), 1413-1420. doi:10.2105/AJPH. 2014.301880

Davidson, K.M., Tyrer, P., Tata, P., Cook, D., Gumely, A., Ford, I., . . . Crowford, M.J. (2009). Cognitive behaviour therapy for violent men with antisocial personality disorder in the community: An exploratory randomized controlled trial. *Psychological Medicine, 39*(4), 569-577. doi:10.1017/S00332910708004066

Ford, J.D., & Courtois, C.A. (2014). Complex PTSD, affect dysregulation, and borderline personality disorder. *Borderline Personality Disorder and Emotion Dysregulation, 1*(9), 1-7. doi:10.1186/2051-6673-1-9

Gregory, C. (2016). Narcissistic personality disorder: A guide to signs, diagnosis, and treatment. Retrieved from https://www.psycom.net/personality-disorders/narcissistic

Hatchett, G. (2015). Treatment guidelines for clients with antisocial personality disorder. *Journal of Mental Health Counseling, 37*(1), 15-27. doi:http://dx.doi.org/10.17744/mehc.37.1. 52g325w385556315

Helleman, M., Goossens, P.J., Kaasenbrood, A., & Van Achterberg, T. (2014). Experiences of patients with borderline personality disorder with the brief admission intervention: A phenomenological study. *International Journal of Mental Health Nursing, 23*(5), 442-450. doi:10.1111/inm.12074

Herdman, T.H., & Kamitsuru, S. (Eds.). (2014). *NANDA-I nursing diagnoses: Definitions and classification, 2015–2017.* Chichester, UK: Wiley Blackwell.

Hodges, M., Godbout, N., Briere, J., Lanktree, C., Gilbert, A., & Kletzka, N.T. (2013). Cumulative trauma and symptom complexity in children: A path analysis. *Child Abuse and Neglect, 37*(11), 891-898. doi:10.1016/j.chiabu.2013.04.001

Hur, J.W., Blake, R., Cho, K.I.K., Kim, J., Kim, S.Y., Choi, S., . . . Kwon, J.S. (2016). Biological motion perception, brain responses, and schizotypal personality disorder. *JAMA Psychiatry, 73*(3), 260-267. doi:10.1001/jamapsychiatry.2015.2985

Kiehn, B., & Swales, M. (2013). An overview of dialectical behaviour therapy in the treatment of borderline personality disorder. *Psychiatry Online.* Retrieved from http://www.priory.com/dbt.htm

Kolla, N.J., Malcolm, C., Attard, S., Arenovich, T., Blackwood, N., & Hodgins, S. (2013). Childhood maltreatment and aggressive behavior in violent offenders with psychopathy. *Canadian Journal of Psychiatry, 58*(8), 487-494. doi:10.1177/070674371305800808

Krastins, A., Francis, A.J., Field, A.M., & Carr, S.N. (2014). Childhood predictors of adult antisocial personality disorder symptomatology. *Australian Psychologist 49*(3), 142-150. doi:10.1111/ap.12048

Lawn, S., Diped, B.A., & McMahon, J. (2015). Experience of family carers of people diagnosed with borderline personality disorder. *Journal of Psychiatric and Mental Health Nursing, 22*(4), 234-243. doi:10.1111/jpm.12193

Lubit, R.H. (2016). Borderline personality disorder. *eMedicine Psychiatry.* Retrieved from http://emedicine.medscape.com/article/913575-overview

MacIntosh, H.B., Godbout, N., & Dubash, N. (2015). Borderline personality disorder: Disorder of trauma or personality, a review of the empirical literature. *Canadian Psychology, 56*(2), 227-241. doi:10.1037/cap0000028

Mayo Clinic. (2014). Narcissistic personality disorder: Risk factors. Retrieved from http://www.mayoclinic.org/diseases-conditions/narcissistic-personality-disorder/basics/risk-factors/con-20025568

McNee, L., Donogue, C., & Coppola, A.M. (2014). A team approach to borderline personality disorder. *Mental Health Practice, 17*(10), 33-35. doi:http://dx.doi.org/10.7748/mhp.17.10.33.e887

Minzenberg, M.J., Poole, J.H., & Vinogradov, S. (2008). A neurocognitive model of borderline personality disorder: Effects of childhood sexual abuse and relationship to adult social attachment disturbance. *Development and Psychopathology, 20*(1), 341-68. doi:10.1017/S0954579408000163.

O'Connell, B., & Dowling, M. (2014). Dialectical behavior therapy (DBT) in the treatment of borderline personality disorder. *Journal of Psychiatric and Mental Health Nursing, 21*(6), 518-525. doi:10.1111/jpm.12116

Ouellet-Morin, I., Côté, S.M., Vitaro, F., Hébert, M., Carbonneau, R., Lacourse, E., & Tremblay, R.E. (2016). Effects of the MAOA gene and levels of exposure to violence on antisocial outcomes. *British Journal of Psychiatry, 208*(1), 42-48. doi:10.1192/bjp.bp.114.162081

Papaioannou, D., Brazier, J., & Parry, G. (2013). How to measure quality of life for cost effectiveness analyses or personality disorders: A systematic review. *Journal of Personality Disorders, 27*(3), 383-401. doi:10.1521/pedi_2013_27_075

Perry, J.C., Presniak, M.D., & Olson, T.R. (2013). Defense mechanisms in schizotypal, borderline, antisocial, and narcissistic personality disorders. *Psychiatry, 76*(1), 32-52. doi:10.1521/psyc.2013.76.1.32

Pier, K., Marin, L.K., Wilsnack, J., & Goodman, M. (2016). The neurobiology of borderline personality disorder. *Psychiatric Times.* Retrieved from www.psychiatrictimes.com/special-reports/neurobiology-borderline-personality-disorder/page/0/1

Sadock, B.J., Sadock, V.A., & Ruiz, P. (2015). *Synopsis of psychiatry: Behavioral sciences/clinical psychiatry* (11th ed.). Philadelphia: Lippincott Williams & Wilkins.

Skeem, J.L., Polaschek, D.L., Patrick, C.J., & Lilienfeld, S.O. (2011). Psychopathic personality: Bridging the gap between scientific evidence and public policy. *Psychological Science in the Public Interest, 12*(3), 95-162. doi:10.1177/1529100611426706

Stoffers, J.M., Vollm, B., Rucker, G., Timmer, A., Huband, N., & Lieb, K. (2012). Psychological therapies for people with borderline personality disorders (review). *Cochrane Database of Systematic Reviews.* doi:10.1002/14651858.CD005652.pub2

Thompson, D.F., Ramos, C.L., & Willett, J.K. (2014). Psychopathy: Clinical features, developmental basis, and therapeutic challenges. *Journal of Clinical Pharmacology and Therapeutics, 39,* 485-495. doi:10.1111/jcpt.12182

Verona, E., & Patrick, C.J. (2015). Psychobiological aspects of antisocial personality disorder, psychopathy, and violence. *Psychiatric Times.* Retrieved from www.psychiatrictimes.com/special-reports/psychobiological-aspects-antisocial-personality-disorder-psychopathy-and-violence

Weight, J., & Kendal, S. (2013). Staff attitudes towards inpatients with borderline personality disorder. *Mental Health Practice, 17*(3), 35-38. doi:http://dx.doi.org/10.7748/mhp2013.11.17.3.34.e827

Westwood, I., & Baker, J. (2010). Attitudes and perceptions of mental health nurses towards borderline personality disorder clients in acute mental health settings: A review of the literature. *Journal of Psychiatric and Mental Health Nursing, 17*(7), 657-662. doi:10.1111/j.1365-2850.2010.01579.x

Classical References

Erikson, E. (1963). *Childhood and society* (2nd ed.). New York: WW Norton.

Mahler, M., Pine, F., & Bergman, A. (1975). *The psychological birth of the human infant.* New York: Basic Books.

Sullivan, H.S. (1953). *The interpersonal theory of psychiatry.* New York: WW Norton.

Psychiatric Mental Health Nursing of Special Populations

33

Children and Adolescents

KEY TERMS

aggression	echolalia	negativism
clinging	impulsivity	palilalia

OBJECTIVES

After reading this chapter, the student will be able to:

1. Identify psychiatric disorders that commonly have their onset in infancy, childhood, or adolescence.
2. Discuss predisposing factors implicated in the etiology of intellectual disability, autism spectrum disorder, attention-deficit/hyperactivity disorder, conduct disorder, oppositional defiant disorder, Tourette's disorder, and separation anxiety disorder.
3. Identify symptomatology and use the information in the assessment of clients with the aforementioned disorders.

4. Identify nursing diagnoses common to clients with these disorders and select appropriate nursing interventions for each.
5. Discuss relevant criteria for evaluating nursing care of clients with selected infant, childhood, and adolescent psychiatric disorders.
6. Describe treatment modalities relevant to selected disorders of infancy, childhood, and adolescence.

HOMEWORK ASSIGNMENT

Please read the chapter and answer the following questions:

1. What maternal prenatal activity has been associated with attention-deficit/hyperactivity disorder (ADHD) in children?
2. What antidepressant medication has been used with some success in treating ADHD?

3. Neuroimaging brain studies in children with Tourette's disorder have consistently found dysfunction in what area of the brain?
4. What are some family behaviors that have been implicated as influential in the development of separation anxiety disorder?

This chapter examines various disorders in which symptoms usually first become evident during infancy, childhood, or adolescence. However, some of the disorders discussed in this chapter may appear later in life, and symptoms associated with other disorders, such as major depressive disorder or bipolar disorder, may appear in childhood or adolescence.

All nurses working with children or adolescents should be knowledgeable about "normal" stages of growth and development. Theoretical Models of Personality Development, a bonus chapter available online at DavisPlus, discusses this topic. At best, the developmental process is one that is fraught with challenges. Behavioral responses are individual and idiosyncratic. They are, indeed, *human* responses.

Whether or not a child's behavior indicates emotional problems is often difficult to determine. Guidelines for making such a determination should consider appropriateness of the behavior regarding age and cultural norms and whether the behavior interferes with adaptive functioning. This chapter focuses on the nursing process in care of clients with intellectual disability, autism spectrum disorder (ASD), attention-deficit/hyperactivity disorder (ADHD), conduct disorder, oppositional defiant disorder (ODD), Tourette's disorder, and separation anxiety disorder. Additional treatment modalities are included.

Neurodevelopmental Disorders

Intellectual Disability (Intellectual Developmental Disorder)

The *Diagnostic and Statistical Manual of Mental Disorders, Fifth Edition (DSM-5)* defines intellectual disability as a "disorder with onset during the developmental period that includes both intellectual and adaptive functioning deficits in conceptual, social, and practical domains" (American Psychiatric Association [APA], 2013, p. 33). The incidence rate in the general population is about 1 percent (APA, 2013). Onset of intellectual and adaptive deficits occurs during the developmental period. Level of severity (mild, moderate, severe, or profound) is based on adaptive functioning within the three domains. General intellectual functioning is measured by both clinical assessment and an individual's performance on intelligence quotient (IQ) tests. Adaptive functioning refers to the person's ability to adapt to the requirements of daily living and the expectations of his or her age and cultural group. The *DSM-5* diagnostic criteria for intellectual disability are presented in Box 33–1.

Predisposing Factors

The etiology of intellectual disability may be primarily biological, primarily psychosocial, a combination of

> ## BOX 33–1 Diagnostic Criteria for Intellectual Disability (Intellectual Developmental Disorder)
>
> Intellectual disability (intellectual developmental disorder) is a disorder with onset during the developmental period that includes both intellectual and adaptive functioning deficits in conceptual, social, and practical domains. The following three criteria must be met:
>
> A. Deficits in intellectual functions, such as reasoning, problem-solving, planning, abstract thinking, judgment, academic learning, and learning from experience, confirmed by both clinical assessment and individualized, standardized intelligence testing.
> B. Deficits in adaptive functioning that result in failure to meet developmental and sociocultural standards for personal independence and social responsibility. Without ongoing support the adaptive deficits limit functioning in one or more activities of daily life, such as communication, social participation, and independent living, across multiple environments, such as home, school, work, and community.
> C. Onset of intellectual and adaptive deficits during the developmental period.
>
> *Specify* current severity:
>
> **Mild**
>
> **Moderate**
>
> **Severe**
>
> **Profound**

Reprinted with permission from the Diagnostic and Statistical Manual of Mental Disorders, Fifth Edition *(Copyright 2013). American Psychiatric Association.*

both, or in some instances unknown. Regardless of etiology, the common factors are significant impairments in intellectual functions and social adaptation.

Genetic Factors

Genetic factors are implicated as the cause of intellectual disability in approximately 5 percent of cases. These factors include inborn errors of metabolism, such as Tay-Sachs disease, phenylketonuria, and hyperglycinemia. Also included are chromosomal disorders, such as Down syndrome and Klinefelter's syndrome, and single-gene abnormalities, such as fragile X syndrome, tuberous sclerosis, and neurofibromatosis.

Disruptions in Embryonic Development

Conditions that result in early alterations in embryonic development account for approximately 30 percent of intellectual disability cases. Damages may occur in response to toxicity associated with maternal ingestion of alcohol or other drugs. For example, fetal alcohol syndrome has been identified as one of the leading preventable causes of intellectual disability. Maternal illnesses and infections during pregnancy (e.g., rubella, cytomegalovirus) and complications of pregnancy (e.g., toxemia, uncontrolled diabetes) also can result in congenital intellectual disability (Sadock, Sadock, & Ruiz, 2015).

Pregnancy and Perinatal Factors

Approximately 10 percent of cases of intellectual disability are the result of circumstances that occur during pregnancy (e.g., fetal malnutrition, viral and other infections, and prematurity) or during the birth process. Examples of the latter include trauma to the head incurred during the process of birth, placenta previa or premature separation of the placenta, and prolapse of the umbilical cord.

General Medical Conditions Acquired in Infancy or Childhood

General medical conditions acquired during infancy or childhood account for approximately 5 percent of cases of intellectual disability. They include infections, such as meningitis and encephalitis; poisonings, such as from insecticides, medications, and lead; and physical trauma, such as head injuries, asphyxiation, and hyperpyrexia (Sadock et al., 2015).

Sociocultural Factors and Other Mental Disorders

Between 15 and 20 percent of cases of intellectual disability may be attributed to deprivation of nurturance and social stimulation and to impoverished environments associated with poor prenatal and perinatal care and inadequate nutrition. Additionally, other mental disorders, such as ASD, can result in intellectual disability.

Recognition of the cause and period of inception provides information regarding what to expect in terms of behavior and potential. However, each child is different, and consideration must be given on an individual basis.

Application of the Nursing Process to Intellectual Disability

Background Assessment Data (Symptomatology)

The degree of severity of intellectual disability may be measured by the client's IQ level. Four levels have been delineated: mild, moderate, severe, and profound. The various behavioral manifestations and abilities associated with each of these levels of severity are outlined in Table 33–1.

Nurses should assess and focus on each client's strengths and individual abilities. Knowledge regarding level of independence in the performance of self-care activities is essential to the development of an adequate plan for nursing care.

Nursing Diagnosis

Selection of appropriate nursing diagnoses for the client with intellectual disability depends largely on the degree of severity of the condition and the client's capabilities. Possible nursing diagnoses include the following:

- Risk for injury related to altered physical mobility or aggressive behavior
- Self-care deficit related to altered physical mobility or lack of maturity
- Impaired verbal communication related to developmental alteration
- Impaired social interaction related to speech deficiencies or difficulty adhering to conventional social behavior
- Delayed growth and development related to isolation from significant others, inadequate environmental stimulation, genetic factors
- Anxiety (moderate to severe) related to hospitalization and absence of familiar surroundings
- Defensive coping related to feelings of powerlessness and threat to self-esteem
- Ineffective coping related to inadequate coping skills secondary to developmental delay

Outcome Identification

Outcome criteria include short- and long-term goals. Time lines are individually determined. The following criteria may be used for measurement of outcomes in the care of the client with intellectual disability.

The client:

- Has experienced no physical harm
- Has had self-care needs fulfilled
- Interacts with others in a socially appropriate manner
- Has maintained anxiety at a manageable level
- Is able to accept direction without becoming defensive
- Demonstrates adaptive coping skills in response to stressful situations

Planning and Implementation

Table 33–2 provides a plan of care for the child with intellectual disability using selected nursing diagnoses, outcome criteria, and appropriate nursing interventions and rationales.

Although this plan of care is directed toward the individual client, it is essential that family members or primary caregivers participate in the ongoing care of the client with intellectual disability. They need to receive information regarding the scope of the condition, realistic expectations and client potentials, methods for modifying behavior as required, and community resources from which they may seek assistance and support.

TABLE 33–1 Developmental Characteristics of Intellectual Developmental Disorder by Degree of Severity

LEVEL (IQ)	ABILITY TO PERFORM SELF-CARE ACTIVITIES	COGNITIVE/EDUCATIONAL CAPABILITIES	SOCIAL/COMMUNICATION CAPABILITIES	PSYCHOMOTOR CAPABILITIES
Mild (50–70)	Capable of independent living with assistance during times of stress.	Capable of academic skills to sixth-grade level. As adult can achieve vocational skills for minimum self-support.	Capable of developing social skills. Functions well in a structured, sheltered setting.	Psychomotor skills usually not affected, although may have some slight problems with coordination.
Moderate (35–49)	Can perform some activities independently. Requires supervision.	Capable of academic skill to second-grade level. As adult may be able to contribute to own support in sheltered workshop.	May experience some limitation in speech communication. Difficulty adhering to social convention may interfere with peer relationships.	Motor development is fair. Vocational capabilities may be limited to unskilled gross motor activities.
Severe (20–34)	May be trained in elementary hygiene skills. Requires complete supervision.	Unable to benefit from academic or vocational training. Profits from systematic habit training.	Minimal verbal skills. Wants and needs often communicated by acting-out behaviors.	Poor psychomotor development. Able to perform only simple tasks under close supervision.
Profound (below 20)	No capacity for independent functioning. Requires constant aid and supervision.	Unable to profit from academic or vocational training. May respond to minimal training in self-help if presented in the close context of a one-to-one relationship.	Little, if any, speech development. No capacity for socialization skills.	Lack of ability for both fine and gross motor movements. Requires constant supervision and care. May be associated with other physical disorders.

SOURCES: Adapted from Black, D.W., & Andreasen, N.C. (2014). *Introductory textbook of psychiatry* (6th ed.). Washington, DC: American Psychiatric Publishing; Sadock, B.J., Sadock, V.A., & Ruiz, P. (2015). *Synopsis of psychiatry: Behavioral sciences/clinical psychiatry* (11th ed.). Philadelphia: Lippincott Williams & Wilkins.

Table 33–2 | CARE PLAN FOR THE CHILD WITH INTELLECTUAL DISABILITY

NURSING DIAGNOSIS: RISK FOR INJURY

RELATED TO: Altered physical mobility or aggressive behavior

OUTCOME CRITERIA	NURSING INTERVENTIONS	RATIONALE
Short- and Long-Term Goal • Client does not experience injury.	1. Create a safe environment for client. 2. Ensure that small items are removed from area where client will be ambulating and that sharp items are out of reach. 3. Store items that client uses frequently within easy reach. 4. Pad side rails and headboard of client with history of seizures. 5. Prevent physical aggression and acting out behaviors by learning to recognize signs that client is becoming agitated.	1–5. Client safety is a nursing priority.

Continued

Table 33–2 | CARE PLAN FOR THE CHILD WITH INTELLECTUAL DISABILITY—cont'd

NURSING DIAGNOSIS: SELF-CARE DEFICIT

RELATED TO: Altered physical mobility or lack of maturity

OUTCOME CRITERIA	NURSING INTERVENTIONS	RATIONALE
Short-Term Goal • Client is able to participate in aspects of self-care. Long-Term Goal • Client has all self-care needs met.	1. Identify aspects of self-care that may be within client's capabilities. Work on one aspect of self-care at a time. Provide simple, concrete explanations. Offer positive feedback for efforts. 2. When one aspect of self-care has been mastered to the best of client's ability, move on to another. Encourage independence but intervene when client is unable to perform.	1. Positive reinforcement enhances self-esteem and encourages repetition of desirable behaviors. 2. Client comfort and safety are nursing priorities.

NURSING DIAGNOSIS: IMPAIRED VERBAL COMMUNICATION

RELATED TO: Developmental alteration

OUTCOME CRITERIA	NURSING INTERVENTIONS	RATIONALE
Short-Term Goal • Client establishes trust with caregiver and a means of communication of needs. Long-Term Goal • Client's needs are being met through established means of communication. • If client cannot speak or communicate by other means, needs are met by caregiver's anticipation of client's needs.	1. Maintain consistency of staff assignment over time. 2. Anticipate and fulfill client's needs until satisfactory communication patterns are established. Learn (from family, if possible) special words client uses that are different from the norm. Identify nonverbal gestures or signals that client may use to convey needs if verbal communication is absent. Practice these communications skills repeatedly.	1. Consistency of staff assignments facilitates trust and the ability to understand client's actions and communications. 2. Some children with intellectual disability, particularly at the severe level, can learn only by systematic habit training.

NURSING DIAGNOSIS: IMPAIRED SOCIAL INTERACTION

RELATED TO: Speech deficiencies or difficulty adhering to conventional social behavior

OUTCOME CRITERIA	NURSING INTERVENTIONS	RATIONALE
Short-Term Goal • Client attempts to interact with others in the presence of trusted caregiver. Long-Term Goal • Client is able to interact with others using behaviors that are socially acceptable and appropriate to developmental level.	1. Remain with client during initial interactions with others on the unit. 2. Explain to other clients the meaning behind some of client's nonverbal gestures and signals. Use simple language to explain to client which behaviors are acceptable and which are not. Establish a procedure for behavior modification with rewards for appropriate behaviors and aversive reinforcement for inappropriate behaviors.	1. Presence of a trusted individual provides a feeling of security. 2. Positive, negative, and aversive reinforcements can contribute to desired changes in behavior. These privileges and penalties are individually determined as staff learns client's likes and dislikes.

Evaluation

Evaluation of care given to the client with intellectual disability should reflect positive behavioral changes. Evaluation is accomplished by determining if the goals of care (as identified previously) have been met through implementation of the nursing actions selected. The nurse reassesses the plan and makes changes as required. Reassessment data may include information gathered by asking the following questions:

■ Have nursing actions providing for the client's safety been sufficient to prevent injury?

■ Have all of the client's self-care needs been fulfilled? Can he or she fulfill some of these needs independently?

■ Has the client been able to communicate needs and desires so that he or she can be understood?

■ Has the client learned to interact appropriately with others?

■ When regressive behaviors surface, can the client accept constructive feedback and discontinue the inappropriate behavior?

■ Has anxiety been maintained at a manageable level?

■ Has the client learned new coping skills through behavior modification? Does the client demonstrate evidence of increased self-esteem because of the accomplishment of these new skills and adaptive behaviors?

■ Have primary caregivers been taught realistic expectations of the client's behavior and methods for attempting to modify unacceptable behaviors?

■ Have primary caregivers been given information regarding various resources from which they can seek assistance and support within the community?

CORE CONCEPT

Autism Spectrum Disorder

A heterogenous group of neurodevelopmental syndromes characterized by a wide range of communication impairments and restricted, repetitive behaviors (Sadock et al., 2015).

Autism Spectrum Disorder

Clinical Findings

In the *Diagnostic and Statistical Manual of Mental Disorders, Fourth Edition, Text Revision* (APA, 2000), the category of autism spectrum disorder (ASD) encompasses a broad spectrum of associated diagnoses that included autistic disorder, Rett's disorder, childhood disintegrative disorder, pervasive developmental disorder not otherwise specified, and Asperger's disorder. The *DSM-5* groups these disorders into a single diagnostic category—autism spectrum disorder. The diagnosis is adapted to each individual by clinical specifiers (e.g., level of severity, verbal abilities) and associated features (e.g., known genetic disorders, epilepsy, intellectual disability) (APA, 2013). ASD is characterized by a withdrawal of the child into an internal fantasy world of his or her own creation. The child has abnormal or impaired development in social interaction and communication and a restricted repertoire of activity and interests, some of which may be considered somewhat bizarre.

Epidemiology and Course

The Autism and Developmental Disabilities Monitoring (ADDM) Network estimates that 1 in 68 children in the United States is identified with ASD and reports that this number has increased 123 percent since 2002 (Centers for Disease Control and Prevention [CDC], 2016a). ASD occurs about five times more often in boys than in girls. Almost half (46%) of individuals with ASD have an average or above average IQ. Onset of the disorder occurs in early childhood, and in most cases it runs a chronic course, with symptoms persisting into adulthood.

Predisposing Factors

Neurological Implications

Imaging studies have revealed a number of alterations in major brain structures of individuals with ASD. Total brain volume, the size of the amygdala, and the size of the striatum have all been identified as enlarged in about 9 to16 percent of children younger than age 4 with ASD. There is also evidence of a decrease in size over time (Hazlett et al., 2011; Kranjac, 2016; Sadock et al., 2015). Sadock and associates identify that this pattern of change in total brain volume over time lends support for the hypothesis that there are critical periods in the brain's plasticity that, when disrupted, may contribute to the development of ASD. These findings related to brain plasticity also support that early recognition and intervention can be meaningful in improving functional abilities over time. Recent in vitro stem cell reprogramming research is beginning to identify the cellular mechanisms responsible for early brain overgrowth and the subsequent disruptions in neural connectivity that may yield valuable information about causes and treatment options (Marchetto et al., 2016).

Genetics

Research has revealed strong evidence that genetic factors play a significant role in the etiology of ASD. About 15 percent of ASD cases are related to a known genetic mutation; in most cases, its expression is related to multiple genes (Sadock et al., 2015). Genetic studies have identified genes that are linked to both autism and schizophrenia, suggesting the two conditions are related (Gilman et al., 2012), although researchers identify that the mutations that occur in each disease lead to functional differences. Kranjac (2016) reports that rare genetic variants such as copy number variations increase the risk for autism by 20 to 60 percent. Familial and twin studies have also supported genetic influences. DNA studies have implicated areas on several chromosomes containing genes that may contribute to the development of ASD. Genetic studies have also identified disruptions in serotonin (5-HT). Because 5-HT is important in brain development, changes in 5-HT may be associated with enlargement in the brain (Sadock et al., 2015).

Prenatal and Perinatal Influences

Some of the prenatal risk factors associated with development of ASD include advanced parental age, fetal exposure to valproate, gestational diabetes, and gestational bleeding (APA, 2013; Sadock et al., 2015). Perinatal influences include low birth weight, obstetrical complications (particularly those associated with neonatal hypoxia), hyperbilirubinemia, congenital malformation, and ABO or Rh factor incompatibilities (Sadock et al., 2015). Exposure to environmental toxins, including air pollution and pesticides, showed the strongest links to ASD when it occurred during preconception, gestational, and early childhood stages (Rossignol & Frye, 2016).

Application of the Nursing Process to Autism Spectrum Disorder

Background Assessment Data (Symptomatology)

The symptomatology presented here is common among children with ASD, but it is important to understand these disorders along a spectrum with varying levels of functionality. Some individuals who meet criteria for ASD may be highly functional and highly intelligent despite communication impairments and repetitive or restrictive behaviors. The dramatic increase in prevalence of ASD has led to research focused on differential and common features along the continuum as well on etiological factors. This information is important in creating an accurate plan of care for the client. Because ASD is a *spectrum* disorder, the symptomatology described here should be understood on a continuum ranging from mild to severe.

Impairment in Social Interaction Children with ASD have difficulty forming interpersonal relationships with others. They show little interest in people and often do not respond to others' attempts at interaction. As infants, they may have an aversion to affection and physical contact. As toddlers, the attachment to a significant adult may be either absent or manifested as exaggerated adherence behaviors. In childhood, a lack of spontaneity is manifested in less cooperative play, less imaginative play, and fewer friendships. Those children with minimal handicaps may progress to the point of recognizing other children as part of their environment, but they struggle, nonetheless, in interpersonal relationships. Social interaction is further impaired by deficits in ability to accurately process others' feelings or affect. Higher-functioning children may recognize their difficulty with social skills even though they may desire friendship. In one study (Strunz et al., 2015), researchers noted that as these relational struggles unfold into adulthood, it is difficult at times to distinguish ASD from personality disorders because there are disruptions in interpersonal relationships within both groups. They found that the differential features in ASD were less extroversion, less openness to experience, increased inhibition, and increased compulsivity than among those with personality disorders.

Impairment in Communication and Imaginative Activity Both verbal and nonverbal skills are affected. In more severe ASD, language may be totally absent or characterized by immature structure or idiosyncratic utterances whose meaning is clear only to those who are familiar with the child's past experiences. Nonverbal communication, such as facial expression or gestures, may be absent or socially inappropriate. Sometimes children with ASD are misinterpreted as being deaf as a result of their lack of response to sounds, while other children may overreact to sound or other stimuli. In some cases, children with ASD demonstrate special abilities, such as fluent reading skills while still in preschool (Sadock et al., 2015). The pattern of play is often restricted and repetitive.

Restricted Activities and Interests Even minor changes in the environment are often met with resistance or sometimes with agitated irritability. Attachment to or extreme fascination with objects that move or spin (e.g., fans) is common. Stereotyped body movements (hand-clapping, rocking, whole-body swaying) and verbalizations (repetition of words or phrases) are typical. Diet abnormalities may include eating only a few specific foods or consuming an excessive amount of fluids. Self-injurious behaviors, such as head banging or biting the hands or arms, may be evident. Harrop and associates (2014) studied children with ASD compared to children without this disorder and found that all children demonstrated some repetitive behaviors as part of their development of skill mastery, but children with ASD displayed a wider range of repetitive behaviors in many different circumstances.

The *DSM-5* diagnostic criteria for ASD are presented in Box 33–2. The criteria specify a range of behaviors, with varying levels of severity, thus addressing the spectrum of symptomatology associated with this diagnosis.

Nursing Diagnosis

Based on data collected during the nursing assessment, possible nursing diagnoses for the client with ASD include the following:

■ Risk for self-mutilation or self injury related to neurological, cognitive, or social deficits
■ Impaired social interaction related to inability to trust; neurological alterations, evidenced by lack of responsiveness to, or interest in, people
■ Impaired verbal communication related to withdrawal into the self; neurological alterations, evidenced by inability or unwillingness to speak; lack of nonverbal expression
■ Disturbed personal identity related to neurological alterations; delayed developmental stage, evidenced by difficulty separating own physiological and emotional needs and personal boundaries from those of others

Outcome Identification

Outcome criteria include short- and long-term goals. Time lines are individually determined. The following criteria may be used for measurement of outcomes in the care of the client with ASD.

BOX 33–2 Diagnostic Criteria for Autism Spectrum Disorder

A. Persistent deficits in social communication and social interaction across multiple contexts, as manifested by the following, currently or by history (examples are illustrative, not exhaustive):
  1. Deficits in social-emotional reciprocity, ranging, for example, from abnormal social approach and failure of normal back-and-forth conversation; to reduced sharing of interests, emotions, or affect; to failure to initiate or respond to social interactions.
  2. Deficits in nonverbal communicative behaviors used for social interaction, ranging, for example, from poorly integrated verbal and nonverbal communication; to abnormalities in eye contact and body language or deficits in understanding and use of gestures; to a total lack of facial expressions and nonverbal communication.
  3. Deficits in developing, maintaining, and understanding relationships, ranging, for example, from difficulties adjusting behavior to suit various social contexts; to difficulties in sharing imaginative play or in making friends; to absence of interest in peers.

Specify current severity:

Severity is based on social communication impairments and restricted, repetitive patterns of behavior.

B. Restricted, repetitive patterns of behavior, interests, or activities, as manifested by at least two of the following, currently or by history (examples are illustrative, not exhaustive):
  1. Stereotyped or repetitive motor movements, use of objects, or speech (e.g., simple motor stereotypies, lining up toys or flipping objects, echolalia, idiosyncratic phrases).
  2. Insistence on sameness, inflexible adherence to routines, or ritualized patterns of verbal or nonverbal behavior (e.g., extreme distress at small changes, difficulties with transitions, rigid thinking patterns, greeting rituals, need to take same route or eat same food every day).
  3. Highly restricted, fixated interests that are abnormal in intensity or focus (e.g., strong attachment to or preoccupation with unusual objects, excessively circumscribed or perseverative interests).
  4. Hyper- or hypo-reactivity to sensory input or unusual interest in sensory aspects of environment (e.g., apparent indifference to pain/temperature, adverse response to specific sounds or textures, excessive smelling or touching of objects, visual fascination with lights or movement).

Specify current severity:

Severity is based on social communication impairments and restricted, repetitive patterns of behavior.

C. Symptoms must be present in the early developmental period (but may not become fully manifest until social demands exceed limited capacities, or may be masked by learned strategies in later life).
D. Symptoms cause clinically significant impairment in social, occupational, or other important areas of current functioning.
E. These disturbances are not better explained by intellectual disability (intellectual developmental disorder) or global developmental delay. Intellectual disability and autism spectrum disorder frequently co-occur; to make comorbid diagnoses of autism spectrum disorder and intellectual disability, social communication should be below that expected for general developmental level.

Specify if:

With or without accompanying intellectual impairment
With or without accompanying language impairment
Associated with a known medical or genetic condition or environmental factor
Associated with another neurodevelopmental, mental, or behavioral disorder
With catatonia

The client:

■ Exhibits no evidence of self-harm
■ Interacts appropriately with at least one staff member
■ Demonstrates trust in at least one staff member
■ Is able to communicate so that he or she can be understood by at least one staff member
■ Demonstrates behaviors that indicate he or she has begun the separation/individuation process

Planning and Implementation

Table 33–3 provides a plan of care for the child with ASD, including selected nursing diagnoses, outcome criteria, and appropriate nursing interventions and rationales.

Evaluation

Evaluation of care for the child with ASD reflects whether the nursing actions have been effective in

Table 33–3 | CARE PLAN FOR THE CHILD WITH AUTISM SPECTRUM DISORDER

NURSING DIAGNOSIS: RISK FOR SELF-MUTILATION

RELATED TO: Neurological alterations; history of self-mutilative behaviors; hysterical reactions to changes in the environment

OUTCOME CRITERIA	NURSING INTERVENTIONS	RATIONALE
Short-Term Goal • Client demonstrates alternative behavior (e.g., initiating interaction between self and nurse) in response to anxiety within specified time. (Length of time required for this objective will depend on severity and chronicity of the disorder.) **Long-Term Goal** • Client does not harm self.	1. Work with child on a one-to-one basis. 2. Try to determine if the self-mutilative behavior occurs in response to increasing anxiety, and if so, to what the anxiety may be attributed. 3. Try to intervene with diversion or replacement activities and offer self to child as anxiety level starts to rise. 4. Protect child when self-mutilative behaviors occur. Devices such as a helmet, padded hand mitts, or arm covers may provide protection when the risk for self-harm exists.	1. One-to-one interaction facilitates trust. 2. Mutilative behaviors may be averted if the cause can be determined and alleviated. 3. Diversion and replacement activities may provide needed feelings of security and substitute for self-mutilative behaviors. 4. Client safety is a priority nursing intervention.

NURSING DIAGNOSIS: IMPAIRED SOCIAL INTERACTION

RELATED TO: Inability to trust; neurological alterations

EVIDENCED BY: Lack of responsiveness to, or interest in, people

OUTCOME CRITERIA	NURSING INTERVENTIONS	RATIONALE
Short-Term Goal • Client demonstrates trust in one caregiver (as evidenced by facial responsiveness and eye contract) within specified time (depending on severity and chronicity of disorder). **Long-Term Goal** • Client initiates social interactions (physical, verbal, nonverbal) with caregiver by time of discharge from treatment.	1. Assign a limited number of caregivers to child. Ensure that warmth, acceptance, and availability are conveyed. 2. Provide child with familiar objects, such as familiar toys or a blanket. Support child's attempts to interact with others. 3. Give positive reinforcement for eye contact with something acceptable to child (e.g., food, familiar object). Gradually replace with social reinforcement (e.g., touch, smiling, hugging).	1. Warmth, acceptance, and availability, along with consistency of assignment, enhance the establishment and maintenance of a trusting relationship. 2. Familiar objects and presence of a trusted individual provide security during times of distress. 3. Being able to establish eye contact is essential to child's ability to form satisfactory interpersonal relationships.

Table 33–3 | CARE PLAN FOR THE CHILD WITH AUTISM SPECTRUM DISORDER–cont'd

NURSING DIAGNOSIS: IMPAIRED VERBAL COMMUNICATION

RELATED TO: Withdrawal into the self; neurological alterations

EVIDENCED BY: Inability or unwillingness to speak; lack of nonverbal expression

OUTCOME CRITERIA	NURSING INTERVENTIONS	RATIONALE
Short-Term Goal • Client establishes trust with one caregiver (as evidenced by facial responsiveness and eye contact) by specified time (depending on severity and chronicity of disorder). **Long-Term Goal** • Client establishes a means of communicating needs and desires to others.	1. Maintain consistency in assignment of caregivers. 2. Anticipate and fulfill child's needs until communication can be established. 3. Seek clarification and validation. 4. Give positive reinforcement when eye contact is used to convey nonverbal expressions.	1. Consistency facilitates trust and enhances the caregiver's ability to understand child's attempts to communicate. 2. Anticipating needs helps to minimize frustration while child is learning communication skills. 3. Validation ensures that the intended message has been conveyed. 4. Positive reinforcement increases self-esteem and encourages repetition.

NURSING DIAGNOSIS: DISTURBED PERSONAL IDENTITY

RELATED TO: Neurological alterations; delayed developmental stage

EVIDENCED BY: Difficulty separating own physiological and emotional needs and personal boundaries from those of others

OUTCOME CRITERIA	NURSING INTERVENTIONS	RATIONALE
Short-Term Goal • Client names own body parts as separate and individual from those of others. **Long-Term Goal** • Client develops ego identity (evidenced by ability to recognize physical and emotional self as separate from others) by time of discharge from treatment.	1. Assist child to recognize separateness during self-care activities, such as dressing and feeding. 2. Assist child in learning to name own body parts. This can be facilitated by the use of mirrors, drawings, and pictures of the child. Encourage appropriate touching of, and being touched by, others.	1. Recognition of body parts during dressing and feeding increases child's awareness of self as separate from others. 2. All of these activities may help increase child's awareness of self as separate from others.

achieving the established goals. The nursing process calls for reassessment of the plan. Questions for gathering reassessment data may include the following:

■ Has the child been able to establish trust with at least *one* caregiver?

■ Have the nursing actions directed toward preventing mutilative behaviors or other injury been effective in protecting the client from self-harm?

■ Has the child attempted to interact with others? Has he or she received positive reinforcement for these efforts?

■ Has eye contact improved?

■ Has the child established a means of communicating his or her needs and desires to others? Have all self-care needs been met?

■ Does the child demonstrate an awareness of self as separate from others? Can he or she name own body parts and body parts of caregiver?

■ Can he or she accept touch from others? Does he or she willingly and appropriately touch others?

Psychopharmacological Intervention for ASD

Pharmacological interventions are directed toward relief of targeted irritability symptoms such as aggression, hyperactivity self-harm, impulsivity, and temper tantrums. There are no medications that treat the core symptoms of ASD. The U.S. Food and Drug Administration (FDA) has approved two medications for the treatment of irritability associated with ASD: risperidone (Risperdal; in children and adolescents 5 to 16 years) and aripiprazole (Abilify; in children and adolescents 6 to 17 years). When administering risperidone, caution must be maintained concerning uncommon but serious possible side effects, including neuroleptic malignant syndrome, tardive dyskinesia, hyperglycemia, and diabetes.

In clinical studies with aripiprazole, the most frequently reported adverse events included sedation, fatigue, weight gain, vomiting, somnolence, and tremor. The most common reasons for discontinuation of aripiprazole were sedation, drooling, tremor, vomiting, and extrapyramidal disorder.

CORE CONCEPT

Hyperactivity

Excessive psychomotor activity that may be purposeful or aimless, accompanied by physical movements and verbal utterances that are usually more rapid than normal. Inattention and distractibility are common with hyperactive behavior.

Attention-Deficit/Hyperactivity Disorder

Clinical Findings, Epidemiology, and Course

The essential behavior pattern of a child with ADHD is one of inattention and/or hyperactivity and **impulsivity.** These children are highly distractible and unable to contain stimuli. Motor activity is excessive, and movements are random and impulsive. Onset of the disorder is difficult to diagnose in children younger than age 4 years because their characteristic behavior is much more variable than that of older children. Frequently, the disorder is not recognized until the child enters school. It is more common in boys (14.1%) than girls (6.2%), and the overall prevalence among school-age children is 10.2 percent (CDC, 2016b). In about 60 to 70 percent of the cases, ADHD persists into young adulthood, and about 25 percent will subsequently meet the criteria for antisocial personality disorder as adults (Black & Andreasen, 2014).

In diagnosing ADHD, the *DSM-5* criteria are further specified according to current clinical presentation. These subtypes include a combined presentation (meeting the criteria for both inattention and hyperactivity/impulsivity), a predominantly inattentive presentation, and a predominantly hyperactive/impulsive presentation.

CORE CONCEPT

Impulsiveness

The trait of acting without reflection and without thought to the consequences of the behavior. An abrupt inclination to act (and the inability to resist acting) on certain behavioral urges.

Predisposing Factors

Biological Influences

Genetics A number of studies have revealed supportive evidence of genetic influences in the etiology of ADHD. Twin studies show an increased risk for monozygotic twins and a risk of two to eight times for siblings and parents of a child with ADHD (Sadock et al., 2015). Adoption studies reveal that biological parents of children with ADHD more often display psychopathology than do the adoptive parents.

Studies of genetic evidence for ADHD have found genetic variants and mutations such as copy number variants on a specific region of chromosome 16 (Acosta et al., 2016; Williams et al., 2010). The researchers also found that copy number variants overlap with chromosomal regions previously linked to ASD and schizophrenia.

Biochemical Theory Although it is believed that certain neurotransmitters—particularly dopamine, norepinephrine, and possibly serotonin—are involved in producing the symptoms associated with ADHD, their involvement is still under investigation. Hypotheses about the impact of neurotransmitters are largely based on benefits associated with taking stimulant medications, which are known to affect dopamine and norepinephrine levels (see Fig. 33–1).

Anatomical Influences Some studies have implicated alterations in specific areas of the brain in individuals with ADHD. Brain imaging studies show decreased volume and activity in the prefrontal cortex, anterior cingulated, globus pallidus, caudate, thalamus, and cerebellum (Sadock et al., 2015).

Prenatal, Perinatal, and Postnatal Factors Maternal smoking during pregnancy has been linked to hyperkinetic-impulsive behavior in offspring (ADHD Institute, 2016; Froehlich et al., 2009). Intrauterine exposure to toxic substances, including alcohol, can produce effects on behavior. Fetal alcohol syndrome includes hyperactivity, impulsivity, and inattention, as well as physical anomalies. Maternal infections during pregnancy have also been associated with higher risks for ADHD.

Perinatal and postnatal influences that may contribute to ADHD are low birth weight, trauma, early infancy infections, or other insults to the brain during

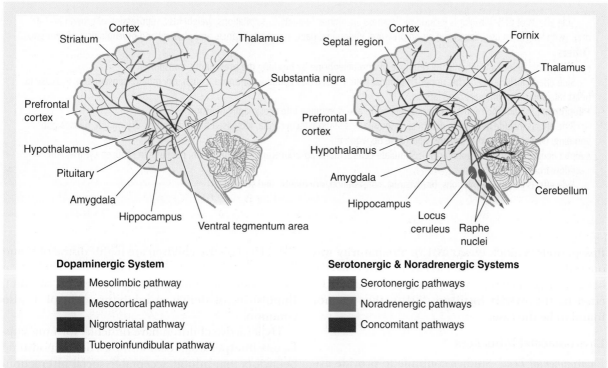

FIGURE 33–1 Neurobiology of Attention-Deficit/Hyperactivity Disorder.

NEUROTRANSMITTERS

The major neurotransmitters implicated in the pathophysiology of ADHD are dopamine, norepinephrine, and possibly serotonin. Dopamine and norepinephrine appear to be depleted in ADHD. Serotonin in ADHD has been studied less extensively, but recent evidence suggests that it also is reduced in children with ADHD.

NEUROTRANSMITTER FUNCTIONS

- Norepinephrine is thought to play a role in the ability to perform executive functions, such as analysis and reasoning, and in the cognitive alertness essential for processing stimuli and sustaining attention and thought.
- Dopamine is thought to play a role in sensory filtering, memory, concentration, controlling emotions, locomotor activity, and reasoning.
- Deficits in norepinephrine and dopamine have both been implicated in the inattention, impulsiveness, and hyperactivity associated with ADHD.
- Serotonin appears to play a role in ADHD, although possibly a less significant role than norepinephrine and dopamine. It has been suggested that alterations in serotonin may be related to the disinhibition and impulsivity observed in children with ADHD. It may play a role in mood disorders, particularly depression, which is a common comorbid disorder associated with ADHD.

FUNCTIONAL AREAS OF THE BRAIN AFFECTED

- **Prefrontal cortex:** Associated with maintaining attention, organization, and executive function. Also serves to modulate behavior inhibition, with serotonin as the predominant central inhibiting neurotransmitter for this function.
- **Basal ganglia** (particularly the caudate nucleus and globus pallidus): Involved in the regulation of high-level movements. In association with its connecting circuits to the prefrontal cortex, may also be important in cognition. Interruptions in these circuits may result in inattention or impulsivity.
- **Hippocampus:** Plays an important role in learning and memory.
- **Limbic System** (composed of the amygdala, hippocampus, mammillary body, hypothalamus, thalamus, fornix, cingulate gyrus, and septum pellucidum): Regulation of emotions. A neurotransmitter deficiency in this area may result in restlessness, inattention, or emotional volatility.
- **Reticular activating system** (composed of the reticular formation [located in the brainstem] and its connections): It is the major relay system among the many pathways that enter and leave the brain. It is thought to be the center of arousal and motivation and is crucial for maintaining a state of consciousness.

MEDICATIONS FOR ADHD

CNS Stimulants

- Amphetamines (dextroamphetamine, lisdexamfetamine, methamphetamine, and mixtures): Cause the release of norepinephrine from central noradrenergic neurons. At higher doses, dopamine may be released in the mesolimbic system.
- Methylphenidate and dexmethylphenidate: Block the reuptake of norepinephrine and dopamine into the presynaptic neuron and increase the release of these monoamines into the extraneuronal space.

Continued

Side effects of CNS stimulants include restlessness, insomnia, headache, palpitations, weight loss, suppression of growth in children (with long-term use), increased blood pressure, abdominal pain, anxiety, tolerance, and physical and psychological dependence.

Others

• Atomoxetine: Selectively inhibits the reuptake of norepinephrine by blocking the presynaptic transporter.

Side effects include headache, upper abdominal pain, nausea and vomiting, anorexia, cough, dry mouth, constipation, increase in heart rate and blood pressure, and fatigue.

• Bupropion: Inhibits the reuptake of norepinephrine and dopamine into presynaptic neurons.

Side effects include headache, dizziness, insomnia or sedation, tachycardia, increased blood pressure, dry mouth, nausea and vomiting, weight gain or loss, seizures and (dose dependent).

• Alpha agonists (clonidine, guanfacine): Stimulate central alpha-adrenoreceptors in the brain, resulting in reduced sympathetic outflow from the CNS.

Side effects include palpitations, bradycardia, constipation, dry mouth, and sedation.

this period (Sadock et al., 2015). Prematurity was once identified as posing an increased risk for ADHD, but in a large research study (Heinonen et al., 2010) cited by the ADHD Institute (2016), this was not found to be the case.

Environmental Influences

Environmental Lead Studies continue to provide evidence of the adverse effects of elevated body levels of lead on cognitive and behavioral development in children (Froehlich et al., 2009; Rossignol & Frye, 2016). Froehlich and associates' research showed a direct link to ADHD. The government has placed tighter restrictions on the substance in recent years, making exposure to toxic levels less prevalent than it once was. However, reports indicate that at least 4 million households in the United States include children who are being exposed to lead and that approximately 500,000 U.S. children ages 1 to 5 have blood lead levels above 5 micrograms per deciliter, the reference level at which the initiation of public health actions is recommended (CDC, 2016c).

Diet Factors The possible link between food dyes and additives, such as artificial flavorings, preservatives, and sugar, was introduced in the mid-1970s. Studies on these possibilities have failed to confirm a clear link.

Psychosocial Influences

Disorganized or chaotic environments or a disruption in family equilibrium may contribute to ADHD in some individuals. Galéra and associates (2011) identified several psychosocial influences associated with the development of ADHD, including non-intact family, young maternal age at birth of the target child, paternal history of antisocial behavior, and maternal depression.

Application of the Nursing Process to ADHD

Background Assessment Data (Symptomatology)

A major portion of the hyperactive child's problems relate to difficulties in performing age-appropriate tasks. Hyperactive children are highly distractible and have extremely limited attention spans. They often shift from one uncompleted activity to another. Impulsivity, or deficit in inhibitory control, is also common.

Hyperactive children have difficulty forming satisfactory interpersonal relationships. They demonstrate behaviors that inhibit acceptable social interaction. They are disruptive and intrusive in group endeavors. They have difficulty complying with social norms. Some children with ADHD are very aggressive or oppositional, whereas others exhibit more regressive and immature behaviors. Low frustration tolerance and outbursts of temper are common.

Children with ADHD have boundless energy, exhibiting excessive levels of activity, restlessness, and fidgeting. They have been described as "perpetual motion machines," continuously running, jumping, wiggling, or squirming. They experience a greater than average number of accidents, from minor mishaps to more serious incidents that may lead to physical injury or the destruction of property. The *DSM-5* diagnostic criteria for ADHD are presented in Box 33–3.

Comorbidity The prevalence of comorbid psychiatric disorders with ADHD is common, with up to 30 percent demonstrating comorbid depression and 20 percent demonstrating comorbid anxiety (Sherman & Tarnow, 2013). The APA (2013) reports that in children with ADHD who have both symptoms of inattention and hyperactivity/impulsivity, ODD co-occurs about 50 percent of the time. They further identify that most children and adolescents with disruptive mood dysregulation disorder also meet criteria for ADHD. Other comorbidities include conduct disorder, specific learning disorder, and intermittent explosive disorder. Sadock and associates (2015) identify that although bipolar mania and ADHD share many core features, such as distractibility, excessive talking, and hyperactivity, children with

BOX 33-3 Diagnostic Criteria for Attention-Deficit/Hyperactivity Disorder

A. A persistent pattern of inattention and/or hyperactivity-impulsivity that interferes with functioning or development, as characterized by (1) and/or (2):

1. **Inattention:** Six (or more) of the following symptoms have persisted for at least 6 months to a degree that is inconsistent with developmental level and that negatively impacts directly on social and academic/occupational activities. *Note:* The symptoms are not solely a manifestation of oppositional behavior, defiance, hostility, or failure to understand tasks or instructions. For older adolescents and adults (age 17 and older), at least five symptoms are required.

   a. Often fails to give close attention to details or makes careless mistakes in schoolwork, at work, or during other activities (e.g., overlooks or misses details, work is inaccurate).

   b. Often has difficulty sustaining attention in tasks or play activities (e.g., has difficulty remaining focused during lectures, conversations, or reading lengthy reading).

   c. Often does not seem to listen when spoken to directly (e.g., mind seems elsewhere, even in the absence of any obvious distraction).

   d. Often does not follow through on instructions and fails to finish schoolwork, chores, or duties in the workplace (e.g., starts tasks but quickly loses focus and is easily sidetracked).

   e. Often has difficulty organizing tasks and activities (e.g., difficulty managing sequential tasks; difficulty keeping materials and belongings in order; messy, disorganized, work; has poor time management; fails to meet deadlines).

   f. Often avoids, dislikes, or is reluctant to engage in tasks that require sustained mental effort (e.g., schoolwork or homework; for older adolescents and adults, preparing reports, completing forms, reviewing lengthy papers).

   g. Often loses things necessary for tasks or activities (e.g., school materials, pencils, books, tools, wallets, keys, paperwork, eyeglasses, or mobile telephones).

   h. Is often easily distracted by extraneous stimuli (for older adolescents and adults, may include unrelated thoughts).

   i. Is often forgetful in daily activities (e.g., chores, running errands; for older adolescents and adults, returning calls, paying bills, keeping appointments).

2. **Hyperactivity and Impulsivity:** Six (or more) of the following symptoms have persisted for at least 6 months to a degree that is inconsistent with developmental level and that negatively impacts directly on social and academic/occupational activities. *Note:* The symptoms are not solely a manifestation of oppositional behavior, defiance, hostility, or a failure to understand tasks or instructions. For older adolescents and adults (age 17 and older), at least five symptoms are required.

   a. Often fidgets with or taps hands or feet or squirms in seat.

   b. Often leaves seat in situations when remaining seated is expected (e.g., leaves his or her place in the classroom, in the office or other workplace, or in other situations that require remaining in place).

   c. Often runs about or climbs in situations where it is inappropriate. (*Note:* In adolescents or adults, may be limited to feeling restless.)

   d. Often unable to play or engage in leisure activities quietly.

   e. Is often "on the go," acting as if "driven by a motor" (e.g., is unable to be or uncomfortable being still for extended time, as in restaurants, meetings; may be experienced by others as being restless and difficult to keep up with).

   f. Often talks excessively.

   g. Often blurts out an answer before a question has been completed (e.g., completes people's sentences; cannot wait for turn in conversation).

   h. Often has difficulty waiting his or her turn (e.g., while waiting in line).

   i. Often interrupts or intrudes on others (e.g., butts into conversations, games, or activities; may start using other people's things without asking or receiving permission; for adolescents or adults, may intrude into or take over what others are doing).

B. Several inattentive or hyperactive-impulsive symptoms were present prior to age 12 years.

C. Several inattentive or hyperactive-impulsive symptoms are present in two or more settings (e.g., at home, school or work; with friends or relatives; in other activities).

D. There is clear evidence that the symptoms interfere with or reduce the quality of social, academic, or occupational functioning.

E. The symptoms do not occur exclusively during the course of schizophrenia or another psychotic disorder and are not better explained by another mental disorder (e.g., mood disorder, anxiety disorder, dissociative disorder, personality disorder, substance intoxication or withdrawal).

Specify whether:

1. **Combined presentation:** If both Criterion A1 (inattention) and Criterion A2 (hyperactivity-impulsivity) are met for the past 6 months.

2. **Predominantly inattentive presentation:** If Criterion A1 (inattention) is met but Criterion A2 (hyperactivity-impulsivity) is not met for the past 6 months.

3. **Predominantly hyperactive/impulsive presentation:** If Criterion A2 (hyperactivity-impulsivity) is met and Criterion A1 (inattention) is not met for the past 6 months.

Specify if: **In partial remission**
Specify current severity: **Mild, Moderate, Severe**

bipolar I disorder exhibit symptoms that wax and wane, whereas children with ADHD have more persistent, continuous symptoms. They note that bipolar disorder and ADHD can coexist and that when certain features of ADHD occur, they appear to predict future mania. Sherman and Tarnow (2013) identify that the prevalence of comorbid bipolar disorder and ADHD is around 20 percent. These authors also note that because ADHD is associated with frontal lobe abnormalities, it is not a surprise that 89.4 percent of children with frontal lobe epilepsy also had comorbid ADHD.

Nursing Diagnosis

Based on the data collected during the nursing assessment, possible nursing diagnoses for the child with ADHD include the following:

- Risk for injury related to impulsive and accident-prone behavior and the inability to perceive self-harm
- Impaired social interaction related to intrusive and immature behavior
- Low self-esteem related to dysfunctional family system and negative feedback
- Noncompliance with task expectations related to low frustration tolerance and short attention span

Outcome Identification

Outcome criteria include short- and long-term goals. Time lines are individually determined. The following criteria may be used for measurement of outcomes in the care of the child with ADHD.

The client:

- Has experienced no physical harm
- Interacts with others appropriately
- Verbalizes positive aspects about self
- Demonstrates fewer demanding behaviors
- Cooperatives with staff in an effort to complete assigned tasks

Planning and Implementation

Table 33–4 provides a plan of care for the child with ADHD using nursing diagnoses common to the disorder, outcome criteria, and appropriate nursing interventions and rationales.

Concept Care Mapping

The concept map care plan is an innovative approach to planning and organizing nursing care (see Chapter 9, The Nursing Process in Psychiatric-Mental Health Nursing). It is a diagrammatic teaching and learning strategy that allows visualization of

---

Table 33–4 | CARE PLAN FOR THE CHILD WITH ATTENTION-DEFICIT/HYPERACTIVITY DISORDER

NURSING DIAGNOSIS: RISK FOR INJURY

RELATED TO: Impulsive and accident-prone behavior and the inability to perceive self-harm

OUTCOME CRITERIA	NURSING INTERVENTIONS	RATIONALE
Short- and Long-Term Goal • Client is free of injury.	1. Ensure that client has a safe environment. Remove objects from immediate area on which client could injure self as a result of random, hyperactive movements.	1. Objects that are appropriate to the normal living situation can be hazardous to child whose motor activities are out of control.
	2. Identify deliberate behaviors that put child at risk for injury. Institute consequences for repetition of this behavior.	2. Behavior can be modified with aversive reinforcement.
	3. If there is risk of injury associated with specific therapeutic activities, provide adequate supervision and assistance, or limit client's participation if adequate supervision is not possible.	3. Client safety is a nursing priority.

Table 33–4 | CARE PLAN FOR THE CHILD WITH ATTENTION-DEFICIT/HYPERACTIVITY DISORDER–cont'd

NURSING DIAGNOSIS: IMPAIRED SOCIAL INTERACTION

RELATED TO: Intrusive and immature behavior

OUTCOME CRITERIA	NURSING INTERVENTIONS	RATIONALE
Short-Term Goal • Client interacts in age-appropriate manner with nurse in one-to-one relationship within 1 week. **Long-Term Goal** • Client observes limits set on intrusive behavior and demonstrates ability to interact appropriately with others.	1. Develop a trusting relationship with child. Convey acceptance of child separate from the unacceptable behavior. 2. Discuss with client those behaviors that are and are not acceptable. Describe in a matter-of-fact manner the consequences of unacceptable behavior. Follow through. 3. Provide group situations for client.	1. Unconditional acceptance increases feelings of self-worth. 2. Aversive reinforcement can alter undesirable behaviors. 3. Appropriate social behavior is often learned from the positive and negative feedback of peers.

NURSING DIAGNOSIS: LOW SELF-ESTEEM

RELATED TO: Dysfunctional family system and negative feedback

OUTCOME CRITERIA	NURSING INTERVENTIONS	RATIONALE
Short-Term Goal • Client independently directs own care and activities of daily living within 1 week. **Long-Term Goal** • Client demonstrates increased feelings of self-worth by verbalizing positive statements about self and exhibiting fewer demanding behaviors.	1. Ensure that goals are realistic. 2. Plan activities that provide opportunities for success. 3. Convey unconditional acceptance and positive regard. 4. Offer recognition of successful endeavors and positive reinforcement for attempts made. Give immediate positive feedback for acceptable behavior.	1. Unrealistic goals set client up for failure, which diminishes self-esteem. 2. Success enhances self-esteem. 3. Affirmation of client as worthwhile human being may increase self-esteem. 4. Positive reinforcement enhances self-esteem and may increase the desired behaviors.

NURSING DIAGNOSIS: NONCOMPLIANCE (WITH TASK EXPECTATIONS)

RELATED TO: Low frustration tolerance and short attention span

OUTCOME CRITERIA	NURSING INTERVENTIONS	RATIONALE
Short-Term Goal • Client participates in and cooperates during therapeutic activities. **Long-Term Goal** • Client is able to complete assigned tasks independently or with a minimum of assistance.	1. Provide an environment for task efforts that is as free of distractions as possible. 2. Provide assistance on a one-to-one basis, beginning with simple, concrete instructions.	1. Client is highly distractible and is unable to perform in the presence of even minimal stimulation. 2. Client lacks the ability to assimilate information that is complicated or has abstract meaning.

Continued

Table 33–4 | CARE PLAN FOR THE CHILD WITH ATTENTION-DEFICIT/HYPERACTIVITY DISORDER–cont'd

OUTCOME CRITERIA	NURSING INTERVENTIONS	RATIONALE
	3. Ask client to repeat instructions to you.	3. Repetition of the instructions helps to determine client's level of comprehension.
	4. Establish goals that allow client to complete a part of the task, rewarding each step-completion with a break for physical activity.	4. Short-term goals are not so overwhelming to one with such a short attention span. The positive reinforcement (physical activity) increases self-esteem and provides incentive for client to pursue the task to completion.
	5. Gradually decrease the amount of assistance given while assuring client that assistance is still available if deemed necessary.	5. This encourages client to perform independently while providing a feeling of security with the presence of a trusted individual.

interrelationships between medical diagnoses, nursing diagnoses, assessment data, and treatments. An example of a concept map care plan for a client with ADHD is presented in Figure 33–2.

Evaluation

Evaluation of the care of a client with ADHD involves examining client behaviors following implementation of the nursing actions to determine if the goals of therapy have been achieved. Collecting data by using the following types of questions may provide appropriate information for evaluation.

■ Have the nursing actions directed at client safety been effective in protecting the child from injury?
■ Has the child been able to establish a trusting relationship with the primary caregiver?
■ Is the client responding to limits set on unacceptable behaviors?
■ Is the client able to interact appropriately with others?
■ Is the client able to verbalize positive statements about self?
■ Is the client able to complete tasks independently or with a minimum of assistance? Can he or she follow through after listening to simple instructions?
■ Is the client able to apply self-control to decrease motor activity?

Psychopharmacological Intervention for ADHD

Indications

Pharmacological intervention, particularly stimulants, are considered the first line of treatment for ADHD

(Sadock et al., 2015). For a list of agents used to treat ADHD, see Table 33–5. The mechanism of action is unclear, but since these drugs are known to elevate dopamine and norepinephrine levels, it is hypothesized that their effectiveness is in response to neurotransmitter dysregulation. They have generally mild side effects but are contraindicated in anyone with cardiac problems or risks for cardiac problems.

One study (Van Den Ban et al., 2014) explored whether use of stimulants had an impact on reducing injuries and hospital admissions for children with ADHD. This topic is relevant because this population has a high incidence of injury and hospital admissions related to hyperactivity and impulsivity. About 60 percent show suboptimal motor performance, which may also increase their risks for injury. The researchers found that children taking ADHD drugs (mostly stimulants) had a twofold higher risk of injury-related hospital admissions than among those not treated with ADHD drugs. They also found that children who were on ADHD drugs and psychotropic drugs such as antipsychotics and benzodiazepines had five times increased risk for injuries and hospital admissions than those who were on ADHD medication alone. The severity of ADHD in children on medication may, in part, account for these findings, but it is significant that while mediating other core symptoms of ADHD, medication may not reduce risks for injury. Amphetamines have been a common substance of abuse and demonstrate a high risk for dependence, and similar concerns have been identified for clients with ADHD. The recent FDA approval of Adzenys XR-ODT, a

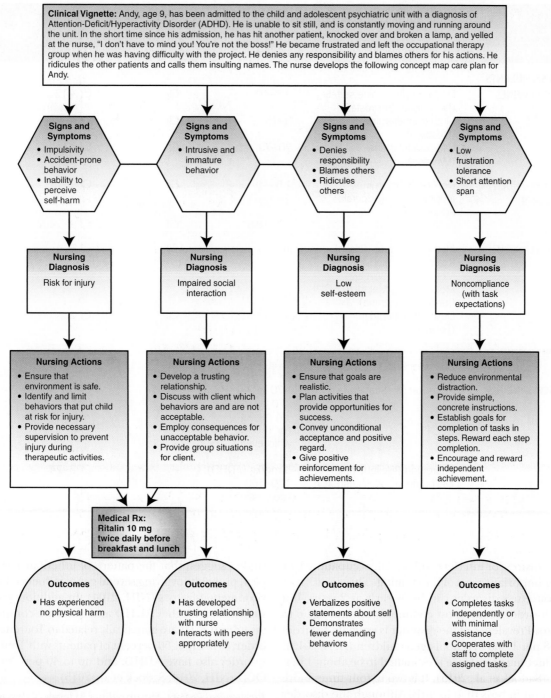

Clinical Vignette: Andy, age 9, has been admitted to the child and adolescent psychiatric unit with a diagnosis of Attention-Deficit/Hyperactivity Disorder (ADHD). He is unable to sit still, and is constantly moving and running around the unit. In the short time since his admission, he has hit another patient, knocked over and broken a lamp, and yelled at the nurse, "I don't have to mind you! You're not the boss!" He became frustrated and left the occupational therapy group when he was having difficulty with the project. He denies any responsibility and blames others for his actions. He ridicules the other patients and calls them insulting names. The nurse develops the following concept map care plan for Andy.

Signs and Symptoms
- Impulsivity
- Accident-prone behavior
- Inability to perceive self-harm

Signs and Symptoms
- Intrusive and immature behavior

Signs and Symptoms
- Denies responsibility
- Blames others
- Ridicules others

Signs and Symptoms
- Low frustration tolerance
- Short attention span

Nursing Diagnosis
Risk for injury

Nursing Diagnosis
Impaired social interaction

Nursing Diagnosis
Low self-esteem

Nursing Diagnosis
Noncompliance (with task expectations)

Nursing Actions
- Ensure that environment is safe.
- Identify and limit behaviors that put child at risk for injury.
- Provide necessary supervision to prevent injury during therapeutic activities.

Nursing Actions
- Develop a trusting relationship.
- Discuss with client which behaviors are and are not acceptable.
- Employ consequences for unacceptable behavior.
- Provide group situations for client.

Nursing Actions
- Ensure that goals are realistic.
- Plan activities that provide opportunities for success.
- Convey unconditional acceptance and positive regard.
- Give positive reinforcement for achievements.

Nursing Actions
- Reduce environmental distraction.
- Provide simple, concrete instructions.
- Establish goals for completion of tasks in steps. Reward each step completion.
- Encourage and reward independent achievement.

Medical Rx:
Ritalin 10 mg twice daily before breakfast and lunch

Outcomes
- Has experienced no physical harm

Outcomes
- Has developed trusting relationship with nurse
- Interacts with peers appropriately

Outcomes
- Verbalizes positive statements about self
- Demonstrates fewer demanding behaviors

Outcomes
- Completes tasks independently or with minimal assistance
- Cooperates with staff to complete assigned tasks

FIGURE 33–2 Concept map care plan for a client with attention deficit/hyperactivity disorder.

flavored, chewable amphetamine mixture tablet, has raised concerns that it might be a recipe for increased medication use in children and become a gateway drug (Grohol, 2016). See Chapter 4, Psychopharmacology, for a complete discussion of the medications used in the treatment of ADHD, including safety and education issues.

Tourette's Disorder

Clinical Findings, Epidemiology, and Course

Tourette's disorder is characterized by the presence of multiple motor tics and one or more vocal tics, which may appear simultaneously or at different periods during the illness (APA, 2013). The disturbance may

TABLE 33–5 Medications for Attention-Deficit/Hyperactivity Disorder

CHEMICAL CLASS	GENERIC (TRADE) NAME	DAILY DOSAGE RANGE (mg)	CONTROLLED CATEGORIES	PREGNANCY CATEGORIES/ HALF-LIFE (hr)
CNS STIMULANTS				
AMPHETAMINES	Dextroamphetamine sulfate (Dexedrine; Dextrostat)	2.5–40	CII	C/ ~12
	Methamphetamine (Desoxyn)	5–25	CII	C/ 4–5
	Lisdexamfetamine (Vyvanse)	20–70	CII	C/ <1
AMPHETAMINE MIXTURES	Dextroamphetamine/ amphetamine (Adderall; Adderall XR)	2.5–40	CII	C/ 9–13
	Adzenys XR-ODT	6.3–18.8	CII	C/ 9–14
MISCELLANEOUS	Methylphenidate (Ritalin; Ritalin-SR; Ritalin LA; Methylin; Methylin ER; Metadate ER; Metadate CD; Concerta; Daytrana)	10–60	CII	C/ 2–4
	Dexmethylphenidate (Focalin)	5–20	CII	C/ 2.2
ALPHA AGONISTS	Clonidine (Catapres)	0.05–0.3	—	C/ 12–16
	Guanfacine (Tenex; Intuniv)	1–4	—	B/ 10–30
MISCELLANEOUS	Atomoxetine (Strattera)	>70 kg: 40–100; ≤70 kg: 0.5– 1.4 mg/kg (or 100 mg, whichever is less)	—	C/ 5.2 (metabolites 6–8)
	Bupropion (Wellbutrin; Wellbutrin SR; Wellbutrin XL)	3 mg/kg (ADHD); 100–300 (depression)	—	C/ 8–24

cause distress or interfere with social, occupational, or other important areas of functioning. The age at onset of Tourette's disorder can be as early as 2 years, but the disorder occurs most commonly around age 6 to 7 years. Prevalence of the disorder is estimated at from 3 to 8 per 1,000 in school-aged children (APA, 2013). The lifetime prevalence is estimated to be about 1 percent (Sadock et al., 2015). It is two to four times more common in boys than in girls. Although the disorder can be lifelong, most people with this condition experience the worst tic symptoms in their early teens with gradual improvement thereafter (National Institutes of Health [NIH], 2014).

Predisposing Factors

Biological Factors

Genetics Various genetic studies, including twin studies and adoption studies, support a genetic basis for this neurological disorder (Sadock et al., 2015). Although evidence supports that it is an inherited disorder, recent studies suggest that the pattern of inheritance is complex, probably involving several genes influenced by environmental factors (NIH, 2104). In addition, genetic studies suggest that ADHD and obsessive-compulsive disorder (OCD) are genetically related to Tourette's disorder; as many as 50 percent of patients with Tourette's disorder also have ADHD, and up to 40 percent have OCD (NIH, 2014; Sadock et al., 2015).

Biochemical Factors Abnormalities in levels of dopamine, choline, *N*-acetylaspartate, creatine, myoinositol, and norepinephrine have all been demonstrated in neuroimaging studies. The effectiveness of antipsychotic medication (particularly haloperidol and fluphenazine) in suppressing tics also supports neurotransmitter involvement in Tourette's disorder (Sadock et al., 2015). However, Sadock and associates add that there is variability in response to antipsychotic medications, and sometimes Tourette's disorder has emerged in clients being treated with antipsychotics. Based on current evidence, while there appear to be several biochemical influences in this disorder, these are complex interactions and are not well understood.

Structural Factors Neuroimaging brain studies have been consistent in finding dysfunction in the basal ganglia. The frontal lobes, the cortex, and abnormalities in the circuits that connect these regions have also been implicated in the pathology of this disorder (NIH, 2014). Although many influences have been identified, the direct cause is still unknown. It is probably a complex interaction of genetics, biochemistry, and environmental influences.

Environmental Factors

Some studies have shown that environmental influences such as maternal alcohol use during pregnancy, low birth weight, complications during childbirth, and infection may be associated with the development of Tourette's disorder (CDC, 2016d). Further research is needed to confirm these influences. Sadock and associates (2015) report that studies inferring beta-hemolytic streptococcal infections as a mechanism in Tourette's disorder have been "conflicting and controversial, and this mechanism appears to be unlikely as an etiology of Tourette's disorder in most cases" (p. 1198).

Application of the Nursing Process to Tourette's Disorder

Background Assessment Data (Symptomatology)

The motor tics of Tourette's disorder may involve the head, torso, and upper and lower limbs. Initial symptoms may begin with a single motor tic, most commonly eye blinking, or with multiple symptoms. Tics tend to first occur in the face and neck and progress downward to the torso and lower limbs over time (Sadock et al., 2015). Simple motor tics include movements such as eye blinking, neck jerking, shoulder shrugging, and facial grimacing. The more complex motor tics include squatting, hopping, skipping, tapping, and retracing steps.

Vocal tics include various words or sounds such as squeaks, grunts, barks, sniffs, snorts, coughs, and, in rare instances, a complex vocal tic involving the uttering of obscenities. Vocal tics may include repeating certain words or phrases out of context, repeating one's own sounds or words **(palilalia),** or repeating what others say **(echolalia).**

The movements and vocalizations are experienced as compulsive and irresistible but can be suppressed for varying lengths of time. Many report a buildup of tension as they attempt to suppress tics to the point where they feel the tic must be expressed against their will. Tics are often worse during periods of stress or excitement and better during periods of calm, focused activity (NIH, 2014). In most cases, tics are diminished during sleep. Neurobehavioral disorders that are common in conjunction with Tourette's disorder (and may be more troublesome than the tics themselves) are inattention, hyperactivity and impulsivity as is seen in ADHD, OCD, depression, and anxiety. Many children with Tourette's disorder also manifest difficulty with reading, writing, and arithmetic (NIH, 2014). The *DSM-5* diagnostic criteria for Tourette's disorder are presented in Box 33–4.

Nursing Diagnosis

Based on data collected during the nursing assessment, possible nursing diagnoses for the client with Tourette's disorder include the following:

■ Risk for self-directed or other-directed violence related to low tolerance for frustration
■ Impaired social interaction related to impulsiveness and oppositional and aggressive behavior
■ Low self-esteem related to embarrassment associated with tic behaviors

Outcome Identification

Outcome criteria include short- and long-term goals. Time lines are individually determined. The following criteria may be used for measurement of outcomes in the care of the client with Tourette's disorder.

The client:

■ Has not harmed self or others
■ Interacts with staff and peers in an appropriate manner
■ Demonstrates self-control by managing tic behavior
■ Follows rules of the unit without becoming defensive
■ Verbalizes positive aspects about self

Planning and Implementation

Table 33–6 provides a plan of care for the child or adolescent with Tourette's disorder using selected

---

BOX 33–4 Diagnostic Criteria for Tourette's Disorder

A. Both multiple motor and one or more vocal tics have been present at some time during the illness, although not necessarily concurrently.
B. The tics may wax and wane in frequency but have persisted for more than 1 year since first tic onset.
C. Onset is before age 18 years.
D. The disturbance is not attributable to the physiological effects of a substance (e.g., cocaine) or another medical condition (e.g., Huntington's disease, postviral encephalitis).

Reprinted with permission from the Diagnostic and Statistical Manual of Mental Disorders, Fifth Edition *(Copyright 2013). American Psychiatric Association.*

Table 33–6 | CARE PLAN FOR THE CHILD OR ADOLESCENT WITH TOURETTE'S DISORDER

NURSING DIAGNOSIS: RISK FOR SELF-DIRECTED OR OTHER-DIRECTED VIOLENCE

RELATED TO: Low tolerance for frustration

OUTCOME CRITERIA	NURSING INTERVENTIONS	RATIONALE
Short-Term Goal • Client seeks out staff or support person at any time if thoughts of harming self or others should occur. **Long-Term Goal** • Client does not harm self or others.	1. Observe client's behavior frequently through routine activities and interactions. Become aware of behaviors that indicate a rise in agitation.	1. Stress commonly increases tic behaviors. Recognition of behaviors that precede the onset of aggression may provide the opportunity to intervene before violence occurs.
	2. Monitor for self-destructive behavior and impulses. A staff member may need to stay with client to prevent self-mutilation.	2. Client safety is a nursing priority.
	3. Provide hand coverings and other restraints that prevent client from self-mutilative behaviors.	3. For client's protection, provide immediate external controls against self-aggressive behaviors.
	4. Redirect violent behavior with physical outlets for frustration.	4. Excess energy is released through physical activities and a feeling of relaxation is induced.

NURSING DIAGNOSIS: IMPAIRED SOCIAL INTERACTION

RELATED TO: Impulsiveness; oppositional and aggressive behavior

OUTCOME CRITERIA	NURSING INTERVENTIONS	RATIONALE
Short-Term Goal • Client develops a one-to-one relationship with a nurse or support person within 1 week. **Long-Term Goal** • Client is able to interact with staff and peers using age-appropriate, acceptable behaviors.	1. Develop a trusting relationship with client. Convey acceptance of the person separate from the unacceptable behavior.	1. Unconditional acceptance increases feelings of self-worth.
	2. Discuss with client which behaviors are and are not acceptable. Describe in matter-of-fact manner the consequences of unacceptable behavior. Follow through.	2. Aversive reinforcement can alter undesirable behaviors.
	3. Provide group situations for client.	3. Appropriate social behavior is often learned from the positive and negative feedback of peers.

NURSING DIAGNOSIS: LOW SELF-ESTEEM

RELATED TO: Embarrassment associated with tic behaviors

OUTCOME CRITERIA	NURSING INTERVENTIONS	RATIONALE
Short-Term Goal • Client verbalizes positive aspects about self not associated with tic behaviors.	1. Convey unconditional acceptance and positive regard.	1. Communicating a perception of client as a worthwhile human being may increase self-esteem.

Table 33–6 | CARE PLAN FOR THE CHILD OR ADOLESCENT WITH TOURETTE'S DISORDER–cont'd

OUTCOME CRITERIA	NURSING INTERVENTIONS	RATIONALE
Long-Term Goal • Client exhibits increased feeling of self-worth as evidenced by verbal expression of positive aspects about self, past accomplishments, and future prospects.	2. Set limits on manipulative behavior. Take caution not to reinforce manipulative behaviors by providing desired attention. Identify the consequences of manipulation. Administer consequences matter-of-factly when manipulation occurs.	2. Aversive consequences may work to decrease unacceptable behaviors.
	3. Help client understand that he or she uses manipulation to try to increase own self-esteem. Interventions should reflect other actions to accomplish this goal.	3. When client feels better about self, the need to manipulate others will diminish.
	4. If client chooses to suppress tics in the presence of others, provide a specified "tic time" during which he or she "vents" tics, feelings, and behaviors (alone or with staff).	4. Allows for release of tics and assists in sense of control and management of symptoms.
	5. Ensure that client has regular one-to-one time with nursing staff.	5. One-to-one time gives the nurse the opportunity to provide client with information about the illness and healthy ways to manage it. Exploring feelings about the illness helps client incorporate the illness into a healthy sense of self.

nursing diagnoses, outcome criteria, and appropriate nursing interventions and rationales.

Evaluation

Evaluation of care for the child with Tourette's disorder reflects whether the nursing actions have been effective in achieving the established goals. The nursing process calls for reassessment of the plan. Questions for gathering reassessment data may include the following:

■ Has the client refrained from causing harm to self or others during times of increased tension?
■ Has the client developed adaptive coping strategies for dealing with frustration to prevent resorting to self-destruction or aggression to others?
■ Is the client able to interact appropriately with staff and peers?
■ Is the client able to suppress tic behaviors when he or she chooses to do so?

■ Does the client set a time for "release" of the suppressed tic behaviors?
■ Does the client verbalize positive aspects about self, particularly as they relate to his or her ability to manage the illness?
■ Does the client comply with treatment in a nondefensive manner?

Psychopharmacological Intervention for Tourette's Disorder

Systematic review of current evidence supports the efficacy of antipsychotic agents, both typical and atypical agents, and the use of alpha$_2$-adrenergic agonist agents (such as clonidine) in treating tics (Weisman et al., 2013). The researchers note that alpha$_2$ agonists are more effective in treating tics among patients with ADHD. Pharmacotherapy is most effective when combined with psychosocial therapy, such as behavioral therapy, individual counseling or psychotherapy, and/or family therapy. Medications that are used in the treatment of Tourette's disorder include antipsychotics and alpha agonists.

Antipsychotics

The conventional antipsychotics, haloperidol (Haldol) and pimozide (Orap), have been approved by the FDA for control of tics and vocal utterances associated with Tourette's disorder. These drugs have been widely investigated and proven highly effective in alleviating these symptoms. They are often not the first-line choice of therapy, however, because of their propensity for severe adverse effects such as extrapyramidal symptoms, neuroleptic malignant syndrome, tardive dyskinesia, and electrocardiographic changes. Haloperidol is not recommended for children younger than 3 years of age, and pimozide should not be administered to children younger than 12 years.

Although not presently approved by the FDA for use in Tourette's disorder, some clinicians prefer to prescribe the atypical antipsychotics, such as risperidone (Risperdal), olanzapine (Zyprexa), or ziprasidone (Geodon), because of their more favorable side-effect profiles. Sadock and associates (2015) identify risperidone as the most well-studied atypical antipsychotic for the treatment of tics and report that there is considerable evidence for its efficacy. These medications have a lower incidence of neurological side effects than the typical antipsychotics, although extrapyramidal symptoms have been observed with risperidone. Common side effects include weight gain, metabolic side effects, and hyperprolactinemia (Sadock et al., 2015). Ziprasidone has been associated with increased risk of QTc interval prolongation. Hyperglycemia has also been reported in some patients taking atypical antipsychotics.

Alpha Agonists

Clonidine (Catapres) and guanfacine (Tenex, Intuniv) are alpha-adrenergic agonists that are approved for use as antihypertensive agents. The extended-release forms have been approved by the FDA for the treatment of ADHD. These medications may be used for treatment of Tourette's disorder because of their favorable side-effect profile and because they are often effective for comorbid symptoms of ADHD, anxiety, and insomnia. Common side effects include dry mouth, sedation, headaches, fatigue, and dizziness or postural hypotension. Guanfacine is longer lasting and less sedating than clonidine, but its efficacy in reducing tics is controversial (Sadock et al., 2015). Alpha agonists should not be prescribed for children and adolescents with preexisting cardiac or vascular disease. They should not be discontinued abruptly; to do so could result in

symptoms of nervousness, agitation, tremor, and a rapid rise in blood pressure.

Disruptive Behavior Disorders

Oppositional Defiant Disorder
Clinical Findings, Epidemiology, and Course

ODD is characterized by a persistent pattern of angry mood and defiant behavior that occurs more frequently than is usually observed in individuals of comparable age and developmental level and interferes with social, educational, occupational, or other important areas of functioning (APA, 2013). It must be understood as distinct, pervasive, and more disruptive than the sometimes negativistic and oppositional behavior that is typical in children and adolescents. The disorder typically begins by 8 years of age and usually not later than early adolescence. Prevalence estimates range from 2 to 16 percent, and common comorbid disorders include ADHD, anxiety, major depressive disorder, conduct disorder, and substance use disorders (APA, 2013). It is more prevalent in boys than in girls before puberty, but the rates are more closely equal after puberty. The *DSM-5* identifies that ODD often precedes conduct disorder, especially in children with onset of conduct disorder prior to 10 years of age (APA, 2013).

Predisposing Factors
Biological Influences

The role, if any, that genetics, temperament, or biochemical alterations play in the etiology of ODD is still unclear. Some studies have identified genetic influences in the establishment of a child's temperament, but there is not clear evidence of this connection in ODD. However, having a temperament in which the child has difficulty regulating emotions and has low frustration tolerance is an identified risk factor for ODD (Mayo Clinic, 2016).

Family Influences

Opposition during various developmental stages is both normal and healthy. Children first exhibit oppositional behaviors at around 10 or 11 months of age, again as toddlers between 18 and 36 months of age, and finally during adolescence. Pathology is considered only when the developmental phase is prolonged or when there is overreaction in the child's environment to his or her behavior.

Some children exhibit these behaviors in a more intense form than others. Sadock and associates (2015) report, "Epidemiological studies of negativistic traits in nonclinical populations found such behavior in 16 to 22 percent of school-age children" (p. 1245).

Some parents interpret average or increased level of developmental oppositional behavior as hostility and a deliberate effort on the part of the child to be in control. If power and control are issues for parents or if they exercise authority for their own needs, a power struggle can be established between the parents and the child that sets the stage for the development of ODD. Lubit (2015) suggests the following pattern of family dynamics:

■ There is the combination of a strong-willed child with a reactive and high-energy temperament and parents who are authoritarian rather than authoritative.
■ The parents become frustrated with the strong-willed child who does not obey and increase their attempts to enforce authority.
■ The child reacts to the excessive parental control with anger and increased self-assertion.

Lubit (2015) states:

These patterns develop when parents inadvertently reinforce disruptive and deviant behaviors in a child by giving those behaviors a significant amount of negative attention. At the same time, the parents, who are often exhausted by the struggle to obtain compliance with simple requests, usually fail to provide positive attention; often, the parents have infrequent positive interactions with their children. The pattern of negative interactions evolves quickly as the result of repeated, ineffective, emotionally expressed commands and comments; ineffective harsh punishments; and insufficient attention and modeling of appropriate behaviors.

Application of the Nursing Process to ODD

Background Assessment Data (Symptomatology)

ODD is characterized by passive-aggressive behaviors such as stubbornness, procrastination, disobedience, carelessness, **negativism,** testing of limits, resistance to directions, deliberately ignoring the communication of others, and unwillingness to compromise. Other symptoms that may be evident are running away, school avoidance, school underachievement, temper tantrums, fighting, and argumentativeness.

Initially, the oppositional attitude is directed toward the parents, but in time, relationships with peers and teachers become affected. These impairments in social interaction often lead to depression, anxiety, and additional problematic behavior (Lubit, 2015).

Usually these children do not see themselves as being oppositional but believe the problem is caused by the unreasonable demands of others. These children are often friendless, perceiving human relationships as negative and unsatisfactory. School performance is usually poor because of their refusal to participate and their resistance to external demands.

The *DSM-5* diagnostic criteria for ODD are presented in Box 33–5.

Nursing Diagnosis

Based on the data collected during the nursing assessment, possible nursing diagnoses for the client with ODD include the following:

■ Noncompliance with therapy related to negative temperament, denial of problems, underlying hostility
■ Defensive coping related to retarded ego development, low self-esteem, unsatisfactory parent/child relationship
■ Low self-esteem related to lack of positive feedback, retarded ego development
■ Impaired social interaction related to negative temperament, underlying hostility, manipulation of others

Outcome Identification

Outcome criteria include short- and long-term goals. Time lines are individually determined. The following criteria may be used for measurement of outcomes in the care of the client with ODD.

The client:

■ Complies with treatment by participating in therapies without negativism
■ Accepts responsibility for his or her part in the problem
■ Takes direction from staff without becoming defensive
■ Does not manipulate other people
■ Verbalizes positive aspects about self
■ Interacts with others in an appropriate manner

Planning and Implementation

Table 33–7 provides a plan of care for the child with ODD using nursing diagnoses common to the disorder, outcome criteria, and appropriate nursing interventions and rationales.

Evaluation

The evaluation step of the nursing process calls for reassessment of the plan of care to determine if the nursing actions have been effective in achieving the goals of therapy. The following questions can be used with the child or adolescent with ODD to gather information for the evaluation.

■ Is the client cooperating with schedule of therapeutic activities? Is level of participation adequate?
■ Is the client's attitude toward therapy less negative?
■ Is the client accepting responsibility for problem behavior?
■ Is the client verbalizing the unacceptability of his or her passive-aggressive behavior?

BOX 33–5 Diagnostic Criteria for Oppositional Defiant Disorder

A. A pattern of angry/irritable mood, argumentative/defiant behavior, or vindictiveness lasting at least 6 months as evidenced by at least four symptoms from any of the following categories, and exhibited during interaction with at least one individual that is not a sibling.

ANGRY/IRRITABLE MOOD
1. Often loses temper.
2. Is often touchy or easily annoyed.
3. Is often angry and resentful.

ARGUMENTATIVE/DEFIANT BEHAVIOR
4. Often argues with authority figures or, for children and adolescents, with adults.
5. Often actively defies or refuses to comply with requests from authority figures or with rules.
6. Often deliberately annoys others.
7. Often blames others for his or her mistakes or misbehavior.

VINDICTIVENESS
8. Has been spiteful or vindictive at least twice within the past 6 months.

   Note: The persistence and frequency of these behaviors should be used to distinguish a behavior that is within normal limits from a behavior that is symptomatic. For children younger than 5 years, the behavior should occur on most days for a period of at least 6 months unless otherwise noted

(Criterion A8). For individuals 5 years or older, the behavior should occur at least once per week for at least 6 months, unless otherwise noted (Criterion A8). While these frequency criteria provide guidance on a minimal level of frequency to define symptoms, other factors should also be considered, such as whether the frequency and intensity of the behaviors are outside a range that is normative for the individual's developmental level, gender, and culture.

B. The disturbance in behavior is associated with distress in the individual or others in his or her immediate social context (e.g., family, peer group, work colleagues), or it impacts negatively on social, educational, occupational, or other important areas of functioning.

C. The behaviors do not occur exclusively during the course of a psychotic, substance use, depressive, or bipolar disorder. Also, the criteria are not met for disruptive mood dysregulation disorder.

Specify current severity:

Mild: Symptoms are confined to only one setting (e.g., at home, at school, at work, with peers).

Moderate: Some symptoms are present in at least two settings.

Severe: Some symptoms are present in three or more settings.

Reprinted with permission from the Diagnostic and Statistical Manual of Mental Disorders, Fifth Edition *(Copyright 2013). American Psychiatric Association.*

Table 33–7 | CARE PLAN FOR THE CHILD/ADOLESCENT WITH OPPOSITIONAL DEFIANT DISORDER

NURSING DIAGNOSIS: NONCOMPLIANCE WITH THERAPY
RELATED TO: Negative temperament; denial of problems; underlying hostility

OUTCOME CRITERIA	NURSING INTERVENTIONS	RATIONALE
Short-Term Goal • Client participates in and cooperates during therapeutic activities. Long-Term Goal • Client completes assigned tasks willingly and independently or with a minimum of assistance.	1. Set forth a structured plan of therapeutic activities. Start with minimum expectations and increase as client begins to manifest evidence of compliance.	1. Structure provides security and one or two activities may not seem as overwhelming as the whole schedule of activities presented at one time.
	2. Establish a system of rewards for compliance with therapy and consequences for noncompliance. Ensure that the rewards and consequences are concepts of value to client.	2. Positive, negative, and aversive reinforcements can contribute to desired changes in behavior.
	3. Convey acceptance of client separate from the undesirable behaviors being exhibited. ("It is not *you,* but your *behavior,* that is unacceptable.")	3. Unconditional acceptance enhances self-worth and may contribute to a decrease in the need for passive-aggression toward others.

Table 33–7 | CARE PLAN FOR THE CHILD/ADOLESCENT WITH OPPOSITIONAL DEFIANT DISORDER–cont'd

NURSING DIAGNOSIS: DEFENSIVE COPING

RELATED TO: Retarded ego development; low self-esteem; unsatisfactory parent/child relationship

OUTCOME CRITERIA	NURSING INTERVENTIONS	RATIONALE
Short-Term Goal • Client verbalizes personal responsibility for difficulties experienced in interpersonal relationships within (time period reasonable for client). **Long-Term Goal** • Client accepts responsibility for own behaviors and interacts with others without becoming defensive.	1. Help client recognize that feelings of inadequacy provoke defensive behaviors, such as blaming others for problems, and the need to "get even." 2. Provide immediate, nonthreatening feedback for passive-aggressive behavior. 3. Help identify situations that provoke defensiveness, and practice through role-play more appropriate responses. 4. Provide immediate positive feedback for acceptable behaviors.	1. Recognition of the problem is the first step toward initiating change. 2. Because client denies responsibility for problems, he or she is denying the inappropriateness of behavior. 3. Role-playing provides confidence to deal with difficult situations when they actually occur. 4. Positive feedback encourages repetition, and immediacy is significant for these children who respond to immediate gratification.

NURSING DIAGNOSIS: LOW SELF-ESTEEM

RELATED TO: Lack of positive feedback; retarded ego development

OUTCOME CRITERIA	NURSING INTERVENTIONS	RATIONALE
Short-Term Goal • Client participates in own self-care and discusses with nurse aspects of self about which he or she feels good. **Long-Term Goal** • Client demonstrates increased feelings of self-worth by verbalizing positive statements about self and exhibiting fewer manipulative behaviors.	1. Ensure that goals are realistic. 2. Plan activities that provide opportunities for success. 3. Convey unconditional acceptance and positive regard. 4. Set limits on manipulative behavior. Take caution not to reinforce manipulative behaviors by providing desired attention. Identify the consequences of manipulation. Administer consequences matter-of-factly when manipulation occurs. 5. Help client understand that he or she uses this behavior to try to increase own self-esteem. Interventions should reflect other actions to accomplish this goal.	1. Unrealistic goals set client up for failure, which diminishes self-esteem. 2. Success enhances self-esteem. 3. Affirmation of client as a worthwhile human being may increase self-esteem. 4. Aversive reinforcement may work to decrease unacceptable behaviors. 5. When client feels better about self, the need to manipulate others will diminish.

Continued

Table 33–7 | CARE PLAN FOR THE CHILD/ADOLESCENT WITH OPPOSITIONAL DEFIANT DISORDER—cont'd

NURSING DIAGNOSIS: IMPAIRED SOCIAL INTERACTION

RELATED TO: Negative temperament; underlying hostility; manipulation of others

OUTCOME CRITERIA	NURSING INTERVENTIONS	RATIONALE
Short-Term Goal • Client interacts in age-appropriate manner with nurse in one-to-one relationship within 1 week. **Long-Term Goal** • Client is able to interact with staff and peers using age-appropriate, acceptable behaviors.	1. Develop a trusting relationship with client. Convey acceptance of the person separate from the unacceptable behavior.	1. Unconditional acceptance increases feelings of self-worth and may serve to diminish feelings of rejection that have accumulated over a long period.
	2. Explain to client about passive-aggressive behavior. Explain how these behaviors are perceived by others. Describe which behaviors are not acceptable and role-play more adaptive responses. Give positive feedback for acceptable behaviors.	2. Role-playing is a way to practice behaviors that do not come readily to client, making it easier when the situation actually occurs. Positive feedback enhances repetition of desirable behaviors.
	3. Provide peer group situations for client.	3. Appropriate social behavior is often learned from the positive and negative feedback of peers. Groups also provide an atmosphere for using the behaviors rehearsed in role-play.

■ Is he or she able to identify which behaviors are unacceptable and substitute more adaptive behaviors?

■ Is the client able to interact with staff and peers without defending behavior in an angry manner?

■ Is the client able to verbalize positive statements about self?

■ Is increased self-worth evident with fewer manifestations of manipulation?

■ Is the client able to make compromises with others when issues of control emerge?

■ Is anger and hostility expressed in an appropriate manner? Can the client verbalize ways of releasing anger adaptively?

■ Is he or she able to verbalize true feelings instead of allowing them to emerge through use of passive-aggressive behaviors?

Conduct Disorder

Clinical Findings, Epidemiology, and Course

With conduct disorder, there is a repetitive and persistent pattern of behavior in which the basic rights of others or major age-appropriate societal norms or rules are violated (APA, 2013). Physical **aggression** is common, and peer relationships are disturbed. Conduct disorder is one of the most frequent reasons that children and adolescents are referred for psychiatric intervention (Sadock et al., 2015). Prevalence estimates range from 2 percent to more than 10 percent, rises from childhood to adolescence, and is more common in males than females (APA, 2013). There is a higher male predominance among those with the childhood-onset subtype. A number of comorbidities are common with conduct disorder, including ADHD, mood disorders, learning disorders, and substance use disorders. When the disorder begins in childhood, there is more likely to be a history of ODD and a greater likelihood of antisocial personality disorder in adulthood than if the disorder is diagnosed in adolescence. Black and Andreasen (2014) report that an estimated 40 percent of boys and 25 percent of girls with conduct disorder will develop adult antisocial personality disorder.

CORE CONCEPT

Temperament

Personality characteristics that define an individual's mood and behavioral tendencies. The sum of physical, emotional, and intellectual components that affect or determine a person's actions and reactions.

Predisposing Factors

Biological Influences

Genetics Family, twin, and adoptive studies have revealed a significantly higher number of individuals with conduct disorder among those who have family members with the disorder (Black & Andreasen, 2014). Although genetic factors appear to be involved in the etiology of conduct disorder, little is yet known about the actual mechanisms involved in genetic transmission. There is some evidence, however, of the distinction between behaviors that appear to be genetic versus environmental risk factors. In a large study of male twins ($N = 2,769$), researchers attempted to determine the structure of genetic and environmental influences in conduct disorder and found the familial risk to conduct disorder is composed of two discrete dimensions of genetic risk, rule-breaking (such as truancy), and overt aggression (harming other people), and one dimension of shared environmental risk, reflecting covert delinquency (such as stealing and hurting animals) (Kendler, Aggen, & Patrick, 2013). Studies such as these support a complex dynamic of both genetic and environmental factors in the development of conduct disorder.

Temperament The term *temperament* refers to personality traits that become evident very early in life and may be present at birth. Children who show signs of an irritable temperament, poor compliance, inattentiveness, and impulsivity as early as age 2 may show signs of conduct disorder at later ages (Bernstein, 2014). Bernstein adds that children with severe temperamental disturbances, including poor attachment, may develop ODD and conduct disorder despite good parental intervention. More commonly, however, these children come from unstable families, with frequent changes in residence and economic stress. Evidence suggests a genetic influence in temperament and an association between temperament and behavioral problems later in life.

Neurobiological Factors Sadock and associates (2015) identify three neurobiological findings relevant to conduct disorders. First, neuroimaging studies identify decreased gray matter in limbic structures, bilateral insula (an area of the cortex that plays a role connecting emotional responses to pain), and the left amygdala. Second, studies have found high plasma concentration of serotonin and low levels in cerebrospinal fluid, both of which are correlated with aggression and violence. The third finding was that aggressive children had "significantly greater relative right frontal brain activity at rest than healthy controls" (p. 1250).

Psychosocial Influences

Peer Relationships Poor academic performance and social maladaptation often lead to affiliations with a deviant peer group. "Considerable research indicates that the deviant peer group provides training in criminal and delinquent behavior including substance abuse" (Bernstein, 2014). In addition to evidence that engaging in risk-taking behaviors can yield reinforcement on a social level (acceptance within a peer group), Bernstein notes that "studies of neural processing show that risk-taking may be associated with reward-related brain activation."

Family Influences

The following factors related to family dynamics have been implicated as contributors in the predisposition to conduct disorder and typically combine to create a pattern of chaotic disruption in family life (Bernstein, 2014; Mayo Clinic, 2016; Sadock et al., 2015):

- Parental rejection, neglect, or severe physical and verbal aggression
- Inconsistent or harsh, punitive discipline
- Parental sociopathy
- Lack of parental supervision
- Frequent changes in residence
- Economic stressors
- Parents with antisocial personality disorder, severe psychopathology, and/or alcohol/other substance dependence
- Marital conflict and divorce (particularly with persistent hostility)

Application of the Nursing Process to Conduct Disorder

Background Assessment Data (Symptomatology)

The classic characteristic of conduct disorder is the use of physical aggression to violate the rights of others. The behavior pattern manifests itself in virtually all areas of the child's life (home, school, with peers, and in the community). Stealing, lying, and truancy are common problems. The child lacks feelings of guilt or remorse.

The use of tobacco, liquor, or nonprescribed drugs, as well as the participation in sexual activities, occurs earlier than at the expected age for the peer group. Projection is a common defense mechanism.

Low self-esteem is manifested by a "tough guy" image. Characteristics include poor frustration tolerance, irritability, and frequent temper outbursts. Symptoms of anxiety and depression are not uncommon.

Level of academic achievement may be low in relation to age and IQ. Manifestations associated with ADHD (e.g., attention difficulties, impulsiveness, and hyperactivity) are common in children with conduct disorder.

The *DSM-5* diagnostic criteria for conduct disorder are presented in Box 33–6.

Nursing Diagnosis

Based on the data collected during the nursing assessment, possible nursing diagnoses for the client with conduct disorder include the following:

- Risk for other-directed violence related to characteristics of temperament, peer rejection, negative parental role models, dysfunctional family dynamics
- Impaired social interaction related to negative parental role models, impaired peer relations leading to inappropriate social behaviors
- Defensive coping related to low self-esteem and dysfunctional family system
- Low self-esteem related to lack of positive feedback and unsatisfactory parent-child relationship

Outcome Identification

Outcome criteria include short- and long-term goals. Time lines are individually determined. The following criteria may be used for measurement of outcomes in the care of the client with conduct disorder.

The client:

- Has not harmed self or others
- Interacts with others in a socially appropriate manner
- Accepts direction without becoming defensive
- Demonstrates evidence of increased self-esteem by discontinuing exploitative and demanding behaviors toward others

Planning and Implementation

Table 33–8 provides a plan of care for the child with conduct disorder using nursing diagnoses common to the disorder, outcome criteria, and appropriate nursing interventions and rationales.

BOX 33–6 Diagnostic Criteria for Conduct Disorder

A. A repetitive and persistent pattern of behavior in which the basic rights of others or major age-appropriate societal norms or rules are violated, as manifested by the presence of at least three of the following 15 criteria in the past 12 months from any of the categories below, with at least one criterion present in the past 6 months:

AGGRESSION TO PEOPLE AND ANIMALS

1. Often bullies, threatens, or intimidates others.
2. Often initiates physical fights.
3. Has used a weapon that can cause serious physical harm to others (e.g., a bat, brick, broken bottle, knife, gun).
4. Has been physically cruel to people.
5. Has been physically cruel to animals.
6. Has stolen while confronting a victim (e.g., mugging, purse snatching, extortion, armed robbery).
7. Has forced someone into sexual activity.

DESTRUCTION OF PROPERTY

8. Has deliberately engaged in fire setting with the intention of causing serious damage.
9. Has deliberately destroyed others' property (other than by fire setting).

DECEITFULNESS OR THEFT

10. Has broken into someone else's house, building, or car.
11. Often lies to obtain goods or favors or to avoid obligations (i.e., "cons" others).
12. Has stolen items of nontrivial value without confronting a victim (e.g., shoplifting, but without breaking and entering; forgery).

SERIOUS VIOLATIONS OF RULES

13. Often stays out at night despite parental prohibitions, beginning before age 13 years.

14. Has run away from home overnight at least twice while living in parental or parental surrogate home, or once without returning for a lengthy period.
15. Is often truant from school, beginning before age 13 years.

B. The disturbance in behavior causes clinically significant impairment in social, academic, or occupational functioning.
C. If the individual is age 18 years or older, criteria are not met for antisocial personality disorder.

Specify whether:

Childhood-Onset Type: Individuals show at least one symptom characteristic of conduct disorder prior to age 10 years.

Adolescent-Onset Type: Individuals show no symptom characteristic of conduct disorder prior to age 10 years.

Unspecified Onset: Criteria for a diagnosis of conduct disorder are met, but there is not enough information available to determine whether the onset of the first symptom was before or after age 10 years.

Specify if:

With limited prosocial emotions

Specify current severity:

Mild

Moderate

Severe

Table 33–8 | CARE PLAN FOR CHILD/ADOLESCENT WITH CONDUCT DISORDER

NURSING DIAGNOSIS: RISK FOR OTHER-DIRECTED VIOLENCE

RELATED TO: Characteristics of temperament, peer rejection, negative parental role models, dysfunctional family dynamics

OUTCOME CRITERIA	NURSING INTERVENTIONS	RATIONALE
Short-Term Goal • Client discusses feelings of anger with nurse or therapist. Long-Term Goal • Client does not harm others or others' property.	1. Observe client's behavior frequently through routine activities and interactions. Become aware of behaviors that indicate a rise in agitation. 2. Redirect violent behavior with physical outlets for suppressed anger and frustration. 3. Encourage client to express anger, and act as a role model for appropriate expression of anger. Explore child's perceptions and feelings about contributing factors and triggers for anger and violent behavior. 4. Ensure that a sufficient number of staff is available to indicate a show of strength if necessary. 5. Administer tranquilizing medication, if ordered, or use mechanical restraints or isolation room only if situation cannot be controlled with less restrictive means.	1. Recognition of behaviors that precede the onset of aggression may provide the opportunity to intervene before violence occurs. 2. Excess energy is released through physical activities, inducing a feeling of relaxation. 3. Discussion of situations that create anger may lead to more effective ways of dealing with them. 4. This conveys evidence of control over the situation and provides physical security for staff and others. 5. It is client's right to expect the use of techniques that ensure safety of client and others by the least restrictive means.

NURSING DIAGNOSIS: IMPAIRED SOCIAL INTERACTION

RELATED TO: Negative parental role models; impaired peer relations leading to inappropriate social behavior

OUTCOME CRITERIA	NURSING INTERVENTIONS	RATIONALE
Short-Term Goal • Client interacts in age-appropriate manner with nurse in one-to-one relationship within 1 week. Long-Term Goal • Client is able to interact with staff and peers using age-appropriate, acceptable behaviors.	1. Develop a trusting relationship with client. Convey acceptance of the person separate from the unacceptable behavior. 2. Discuss with client which behaviors are and are not acceptable. Describe in matter-of-fact manner the consequence of unacceptable behavior. Follow through. 3. Provide group situations for client.	1. Unconditional acceptance increases feeling of self-worth. 2. Aversive reinforcement can alter or extinguish undesirable behaviors. 3. Appropriate social behavior is often learned from the positive and negative feedback of peers.

Continued

Table 33–8 | CARE PLAN FOR CHILD/ADOLESCENT WITH CONDUCT DISORDER–cont'd

NURSING DIAGNOSIS: DEFENSIVE COPING

RELATED TO: Low self-esteem and dysfunctional family system

OUTCOME CRITERIA	NURSING INTERVENTIONS	RATIONALE
Short-Term Goal • Client verbalizes personal responsibility for difficulties experienced in interpersonal relationships within a time period reasonable for client.	1. Explain to client the correlation between feelings of inadequacy and the need for acceptance from others and how these feelings provoke defensive behaviors, such as blaming others for own behaviors.	1. Recognition of the problem is the first step in the change process toward resolution.
Long-Term Goal • Client accepts responsibility for own behaviors and interacts with others without becoming defensive.	2. Provide immediate, matter-of-fact, nonthreatening feedback for unacceptable behaviors.	2. Client may not realize how these behaviors are being perceived by others.
	3. Help identify situations that provoke defensiveness, and practice through role-play more appropriate responses.	3. Role-playing provides confidence to deal with difficult situations when they actually occur.
	4. Provide immediate positive feedback for acceptable behaviors.	4. Positive feedback encourages repetition, and immediacy is significant for these children, who respond to immediate gratification.

NURSING DIAGNOSIS: LOW SELF-ESTEEM

RELATED TO: Lack of positive feedback and unsatisfactory parent/child relationship

OUTCOME CRITERIA	NURSING INTERVENTIONS	RATIONALE
Short-Term Goal • Client participates in own self-care and discusses with nurse aspects of self about which he or she feels good.	1. Ensure that goals are realistic.	1. Unrealistic goals set client up for failure, which diminishes self-esteem.
Long-Term Goal • Client demonstrates increased feelings of self-worth by verbalizing positive statements about self and exhibiting fewer manipulative behaviors.	2. Plan activities that provide opportunities for success.	2. Success enhances self-esteem.
	3. Convey unconditional acceptance and positive regard.	3. Communicating that client is a worthwhile human being helps to increase self-esteem.
	4. Set limits on manipulative behavior. Take caution not to reinforce manipulative behaviors by providing desired attention. Identify the consequences of manipulation. Administer consequences matter-of-factly when manipulation occurs.	4. Aversive consequences may work to decrease unacceptable behaviors.
	5. Help client understand that he or she uses this behavior in order to try to increase own self-esteem. Interventions should reflect other actions to accomplish this goal.	5. When client feels better about self, the need to manipulate others will diminish.

Evaluation

Following the planning and implementation of care, evaluation is made of the behavioral changes in the child with conduct disorder. This is accomplished by determining if the goals of therapy have been achieved. Reassessment, the next step in the nursing process, may be initiated by gathering information using the following questions:

■ Have the nursing actions directed toward managing the client's aggressive behavior been effective?

■ Have interventions prevented harm to others or others' property?

■ Is the client able to express anger in an appropriate manner?

■ Has the client developed more adaptive coping strategies to deal with anger and feelings of aggression?

■ Does the client demonstrate the ability to trust others? Is he or she able to interact with staff and peers in an appropriate manner?

■ Is the client able to accept responsibility for his or her own behavior? Is there less blaming of others?

■ Is the client able to accept feedback from others without becoming defensive?

■ Is the client able to verbalize positive statements about self?

■ Is the client able to interact with others without engaging in manipulation?

Anxiety Disorders

Separation Anxiety Disorder
Clinical Findings, Epidemiology, and Course

Separation anxiety disorder is characterized by excessive fear or anxiety concerning separation from those to whom the individual is attached (APA, 2013). The anxiety is beyond that which would be expected for the individual's developmental level and interferes with social, academic, occupational, or others areas of functioning. Onset may occur any time before age 18 years but is most commonly diagnosed around age 5 or 6, when the child goes to school. Diagnosis at this time may be related to the surfacing of symptoms when the child is faced with new stressors and the recognition of symptoms by school counselors and teachers. It is estimated that about 1 percent of children age 2 to 5 already show symptoms of anxiety disorders. In this age group, these signs may be a reflection of anxiety that they are mimicking from their parents. Assessment of the child and the family is important in assuring accurate diagnosis. Prevalence estimates for the disorder average about 4 percent in children and young adults, and it is more common in girls than in boys. Most children grow out of it, but in some instances the symptoms can persist into adulthood. Separation anxiety disorder can be a precursor to adult panic disorder (Black & Andreasen, 2014).

Predisposing Factors
Biological Influences

Genetics A greater number of children with relatives who manifest anxiety problems develop anxiety disorders than do children with no such family patterns. The results are significant enough to speculate that there is a hereditary influence in the development of separation anxiety disorder, but the mode of genetic transmission has not been determined. Sadock and associates (2015) state:

> Current consensus on the genetics of anxiety disorders suggests that what is inherited is a general predisposition toward anxiety, with resulting heightened levels of arousability, emotional reactivity, and increased negative affect, all of which increase the risk for the development of separation anxiety disorder [and other anxiety disorders]. (p. 1255)

Temperament It is well established that children differ in temperament from one another starting at birth or shortly thereafter. "The temperamental traits of shyness and withdrawal in unfamiliar situations, have been shown to be associated with a higher risk of developing separation anxiety disorder [as well as other anxiety disorders]" (Sadock et al., 2015, p. 1255).

Environmental Influences

Stressful Life Events Studies have shown a relationship between life events and the development of anxiety disorders. Significant change or loss often coincides with the development of the disorder (Sadock et al., 2015). Children of mothers who were stressed during pregnancy also appear to be at greater risk for developing separation anxiety disorder (Dryden-Edwards, 2015).

Family Influences

Various theories expound on the idea that anxiety disorders in children are related to an attachment issue with the mother. Three family influences that have demonstrated an increased risk for anxiety disorders in children include parental overprotection, insecure parent-child attachment, and maternal depression (Sadock et al., 2015).

Some parents may also transfer their fears and anxieties to their children through role-modeling. For example, a parent who becomes significantly fearful and apprehensive when confronted with unfamiliar circumstances, such as a job or residence change, teaches the child that this is an appropriate response.

Application of the Nursing Process to Separation Anxiety Disorder

Background Assessment Data (Symptomatology)

Onset of this disorder may occur as early as preschool age; it rarely begins as late as adolescence. In most cases, the child has difficulty separating from the mother. Occasionally, the separation reluctance is directed toward the father, siblings, or other significant individual to whom the child is attached. Anticipation of separation may result in tantrums, crying, screaming, complaints of physical problems, and **clinging** behaviors.

Reluctance or refusal to attend school occurs in the majority of these children. Up to 80 percent of children with school refusal meet criteria for separation anxiety disorder (Dryden-Edwards, 2015). Younger children may "shadow" or follow around the person from whom they are afraid to be separated. During middle childhood or adolescence, they may refuse to sleep away from home (e.g., at a friend's house or at camp). Interpersonal peer relationships are usually not a problem with these children. They are generally well liked by their peers and are reasonably socially skilled.

Worrying is common and relates to the possibility of harm coming to self or to the attachment figure. Younger children may even have nightmares to this effect. Specific phobias are not uncommon (e.g., fear of the dark, ghosts, animals). Depressed mood is frequently present and often precedes the onset of the anxiety symptoms, which commonly occur following a major stressor. The *DSM-5* diagnostic criteria for separation anxiety disorder are presented in Box 33–7.

Nursing Diagnosis

Based on the data collected during the nursing assessment, possible nursing diagnoses for the client with separation anxiety disorder include the following:

- Anxiety (severe) related to family history, temperament, overattachment to parent, negative role modeling
- Ineffective coping related to unresolved separation conflicts and inadequate coping skills evidenced by numerous somatic complaints
- Impaired social interaction related to reluctance to be away from attachment figure

Outcome Identification

Outcome criteria include short- and long-term goals. Time lines are individually determined. The following criteria may be used for measurement of outcomes in the care of the client with separation anxiety disorder.

The client:

- Is able to maintain anxiety at manageable level
- Demonstrates adaptive coping strategies for dealing with anxiety when separation from attachment figure is anticipated

---

BOX 33–7 Diagnostic Criteria for Separation Anxiety Disorder

A. Developmentally inappropriate and excessive fear or anxiety concerning separation from those to whom the individual is attached, as evidenced by at least three of the following:
  1. Recurrent excessive distress when anticipating or experiencing separation from home or major attachment figures.
  2. Persistent and excessive worry about losing major attachment figures or about possible harm to them, such as illness, injury, disasters, or death.
  3. Persistent and excessive worry about experiencing an untoward event (e.g., getting lost, being kidnapped, having an accident, becoming ill) that causes separation from a major attachment figure.
  4. Persistent reluctance or refusal to go out, away from home, to school, to work, or elsewhere because of fear of separation.
  5. Persistent and excessive fear of or reluctance about being alone or without major attachment figures at home or in other settings.
  6. Persistent reluctance or refusal to sleep away from home or to go to sleep without being near a major attachment figure.
  7. Repeated nightmares involving the theme of separation.
  8. Repeated complaints of physical symptoms (e.g., headaches, stomachaches, nausea, vomiting) when separation from major attachment figures occurs or is anticipated.
B. The fear, anxiety, or avoidance is persistent, lasting at least 4 weeks in children and adolescents and typically 6 months or more in adults.
C. The disturbance causes clinically significant distress or impairment in social, academic, occupational, or other important areas of functioning.
D. The disturbance is not better accounted for by another mental disorder, such as refusing to leave home because of excessive resistance to change in autism spectrum disorder; delusions or hallucinations concerning separation in psychotic disorders; refusal to go outside without a trusted companion in agoraphobia; worries about ill health or other harm befalling significant others in generalized anxiety disorder; or concerns about having an illness in illness anxiety disorder.

Reprinted with permission from the Diagnostic and Statistical Manual of Mental Disorders, Fifth Edition *(Copyright 2013). American Psychiatric Association.*

■ Interacts appropriately with others and spends time away from attachment figure to do so

Planning and Implementation

Table 33–9 provides a plan of care for the child or adolescent with separation anxiety, using nursing diagnoses common to this disorder, outcome criteria, and appropriate nursing interventions and rationales.

Evaluation

Evaluation of the child or adolescent with separation anxiety disorder requires reassessment of the behaviors for which the family sought treatment. Both the client and the family members will have to change their behavior. The following types of questions may provide assistance in gathering data required for evaluating whether the nursing interventions have been effective in achieving the goals of therapy.

■ Is the client able to maintain anxiety at a manageable level (i.e., without temper tantrums, screaming, or clinging)?

■ Have complaints of physical symptoms diminished?

■ Has the client demonstrated the ability to cope in more adaptive ways in the face of escalating anxiety?

■ Have the parents identified their role in the separation conflict? Are they able to discuss more adaptive coping strategies?

■ Does the client verbalize an intention to return to school?

■ Have nightmares and fears of the dark subsided?

■ Is the client able to interact with others away from the attachment figure?

■ Has the precipitating stressor been identified? Have strategies for coping more adaptively to similar stressors in the future been established?

Quality and Safety Education for Nurses (QSEN)

The Institute of Medicine (now the National Academy of Medicine), in its 2003 report *Health Professions Education: A Bridge to Quality*, challenged faculties of

---

Table 33–9 | CARE PLAN FOR THE CLIENT WITH SEPARATION ANXIETY DISORDER

NURSING DIAGNOSIS: ANXIETY (SEVERE)

RELATED TO: Family history; temperament; overattachment to parent; negative role modeling

OUTCOME CRITERIA	NURSING INTERVENTIONS	RATIONALE
Short-Term Goal • Client discusses fears of separation with trusted individual. Long-Term Goal • Client maintains anxiety at no higher than moderate level in the face of events that formerly have precipitated panic.	1. Establish an atmosphere of calmness, trust, and genuine positive regard.	1. Trust and unconditional acceptance are necessary for satisfactory nurse-client relationship. Calmness is important because anxiety is easily transmitted from one person to another.
	2. Assure client of his or her safety and security.	2. Symptoms of panic anxiety are very frightening.
	3. Explore child's or adolescent's fears of separating from the parents. Explore with parents possible fears they may have of separation from child.	3. Some parents may have an underlying fear of separation from the child, of which they are unaware and which they are unconsciously transferring to child.
	4. Help parents and child initiate realistic goals (e.g., child to stay with sitter for 2 hours with minimal anxiety; or, child to stay at friend's house without parents until 9 p.m. without experiencing panic anxiety).	4. Parents may be so frustrated with child's clinging and demanding behaviors that assistance with problem-solving may be required.
	5. Give, and encourage parents to give, positive reinforcement for desired behaviors.	5. Positive reinforcement encourages repetition of desirable behaviors.

Continued

Table 33–9 | CARE PLAN FOR THE CLIENT WITH SEPARATION ANXIETY DISORDER—cont'd

NURSING DIAGNOSIS: INEFFECTIVE COPING

RELATED TO: Unresolved separation conflicts and inadequate coping skills

EVIDENCED BY: Numerous somatic complaints

OUTCOME CRITERIA	NURSING INTERVENTIONS	RATIONALE
Short-Term Goal • Client verbalizes correlation of somatic symptoms to fear of separation. **Long-Term Goal** • Client demonstrates use of more adaptive coping strategies (rather than physical symptoms) in response to stressful situations.	1. Encourage child or adolescent to discuss specific situations in life that produce the most distress and describe his or her response to these situations. Include parents in the discussion. 2. Help child or adolescent who is perfectionistic to recognize that self-expectations may be unrealistic. Connect times of unmet self-expectations to the exacerbation of physical symptoms. 3. Encourage parents and child to identify more adaptive coping strategies that child could use in the face of anxiety that feels overwhelming. Practice through role-play.	1. Client and family may be unaware of the correlation between stressful situations and the exacerbation of physical symptoms. 2. Recognition of maladaptive patterns is the first step in the change process. 3. Practice facilitates the use of the desired behavior when the individual is actually faced with the stressful situation.

NURSING DIAGNOSIS: IMPAIRED SOCIAL INTERACTION

RELATED TO: Reluctance to be away from attachment figure

OUTCOME CRITERIA	NURSING INTERVENTIONS	RATIONALE
Short-Term Goal • Client spends time with staff or other support person, without presence of attachment figure, without excessive anxiety. **Long-Term Goal** • Client is able to spend time with others (without presence of attachment figure) without excessive anxiety.	1. Develop a trusting relationship with client. 2. Attend groups with child and support efforts to interact with others. Give positive feedback. 3. Convey to child the acceptability of his or her not participating in group in the beginning. Gradually encourage small contributions until client is able to participate more fully. 4. Help client set small personal goals (e.g., "Today I will speak to one person I don't know").	1. This is the first step in helping client learn to interact with others. 2. Presence of a trusted individual provides security during times of distress. Positive feedback encourages repetition. 3. Small successes will gradually increase self-confidence and decrease self-consciousness, so that client will feel less anxious in the group situation. 4. Simple, realistic goals provide opportunities for success that increase self-confidence and may encourage client to attempt more difficult objectives in the future.

medicine, nursing, and other health professions to ensure that their graduates have achieved a core set of competencies in order to meet the needs of the 21st-century health-care system. These competencies include *providing patient-centered care, working in interdisciplinary teams, maintaining safety, employing evidence-based practice, applying quality improvement,* and *utilizing informatics.* A QSEN teaching strategy is presented in Box 33–8. The use of this type of activity is intended to arm the instructor and student with guidelines for attaining the knowledge, skills, and attitudes necessary for achievement of quality and safety competencies in nursing.

General Therapeutic Approaches

Treatment for neurodevelopmental disorders, disruptive behavior disorders, and anxiety disorders poses many challenges and requires a comprehensive treatment plan that may include individual, group, and family therapies; family education; pharmacotherapy; and psychotherapeutic interventions specifically designed for the unique clinical issues presented in each disorder. General therapeutic approaches are described in the next sections.

Behavior Therapy

Behavior therapy is based on the concepts of classical conditioning and operant conditioning and is a common and effective treatment with disruptive behavior disorders such as ADHD, ODD, and conduct disorder. With this approach, rewards are given for appropriate behaviors and withheld when behaviors are disruptive or otherwise inappropriate. The principle behind behavior therapy is that positive reinforcements encourage repetition of desirable behaviors and aversive reinforcements (punishments) discourage repetition of undesirable behaviors. Behavior modification techniques—the system of rewards and consequences—can be taught to parents to be used in the home environment. Consistency is an essential component.

In the treatment setting, individualized behavior modification programs are designed for each client.

Family Therapy

Children cannot be separated from their family. Therapy for children and adolescents must involve the entire family if problems are to be resolved. Parents should be involved in designing and implementing the treatment plan for the child and all other aspects of the treatment process.

The genogram can be used to identify problem areas between family members. It provides an overall picture of the family life over several generations, including roles that various family members play and emotional distance between specific individuals. Areas for change can be easily identified.

The impact of family dynamics on disruptive behavior disorders has been identified. The impact of disruptive behavior on family dynamics cannot be ignored. Family coping can become severely compromised by the chronic stress of dealing with a child with a behavior disorder. It is therefore imperative that the treatment plan for the identified client be instituted within the context of family-centered care.

BOX 33–8 QSEN TEACHING STRATEGY

Assignment: Patient-Centered Care: Kleinman's Mini-Ethnography
Interviewing Families of Children With Psychiatric Disorders

Competency Domain: Patient-Centered Care

Learning Objectives: Student will:
• Demonstrate skills in hearing patients' and family members' stories of living with the disorder.
• Identify his or her own explanatory models of the disorder.
• Demonstrate attitudes that reflect a desire to cultivate cultural humility and cultural competence in nursing practice.

Strategy Overview:
1. Read "Anthropology in the Clinic: The Problem of Cultural Competency and How to Fix It," by A. Kleinman and P. Benson. The article is available online at www.plosmedicine.org/article/info:doi/10.1371/journal.pmed.0030294
2. Based on the mini-ethnography described by Kleinman and Benson, interview a family member of a child with a psychiatric disorder and elicit a narrative of his or her experience in living with the disorder.
3. Drawing on notes from the interview, write one paper that is the narrative of the illness from the perspective of the interviewee and another paper that describes the student's own explanatory model.

Source: Adapted from teaching strategy submitted by Lisa Day, Assistant Clinical Professor, UCSF, School of Nursing, San Francisco, CA. © 2009 QSEN; http://qsen.org. With permission.

Group Therapy

Group therapy provides children and adolescents with the opportunity to interact within an association of their peers. This experience can be both gratifying and overwhelming, depending on the child.

Group therapy provides a number of benefits. Appropriate social behavior often is learned from the positive and negative feedback of peers. Opportunity is provided to learn to tolerate and accept differences in others, learn that it is acceptable to disagree, offer and receive support from others, and practice these new skills in a safe environment. It is also a way to learn from the experiences of others.

Group therapy with children and adolescents can take several forms. Music therapy groups allow clients to express feelings through music, often when they are unable to express themselves in any other way. Art and activity/craft therapy groups allow individual expression through artistic means.

Group play therapy is the treatment of choice for many children between the ages of 3 and 9 years, and evidence supports its effectiveness for many different childhood problems. The Association for Play Therapy (2016) states:

> Play therapy builds on the natural way that children learn about themselves and their relationships in the world around them. Through play therapy, children learn to communicate with others, express feelings, modify behavior, develop problem-solving skills, and learn a variety of ways of relating to others. Play provides a safe psychological distance from their problems and allows expression of thoughts and feelings appropriate to their development.

Psychoeducational groups are very beneficial for adolescents. The only drawback to this type of group is that it works best when the group is closed-ended; that is, once the group has been formed, no one is allowed to join until the group has reached its preestablished closure. Members are allowed to propose topics for discussion. The leader serves as teacher much of the time and facilitates discussion of the proposed topic. Members may from time to time be presenters and serve as discussion leaders. Sometimes, psychoeducation groups evolve into traditional therapy discussion groups.

Psychopharmacology

Several of the disorders presented in this chapter are treated with medications. The appropriate pharmacology was presented in the section in which the disorder was discussed. Medication should never be the sole method of treatment. It is undeniable that medication can and does improve quality of life for families of children and adolescents with these disorders.

However, research has indicated that medication alone is not as effective as a combination of medication and psychosocial therapy. It is important for families to understand that there is no way to "give him a pill and make him well." The importance of the psychosocial therapies cannot be overstressed. Some clinicians will not prescribe medications for a client unless he or she also participates in concomitant psychotherapy sessions. The beneficial effects of the medications promote improved coping ability, which in turn enhances the intent of the psychosocial therapy.

Summary and Key Points

- Intellectual disability is defined by deficits in general intellectual functioning and adaptive functioning.
- Four levels of intellectual disability—mild, moderate, severe, and profound—are associated with various behavioral manifestations and abilities.
- ASD is characterized by a withdrawal of the child into the self and into a fantasy world of his or her own creation.
- It is generally accepted that ASD is caused by abnormalities in brain structures or functions. Genetic factors are also thought to play a significant role in ASD.
- Children with ADHD may exhibit symptoms of inattention or hyperactivity and impulsiveness or a combination of the two.
- Genetics plays a role in the etiology of ADHD. Neurotransmitters that have been implicated include dopamine, norepinephrine, and serotonin. Maternal smoking during pregnancy has been linked to hyperactive behavior in offspring.
- CNS stimulants, alpha agonists, atomoxetine, and bupropion are commonly used to treat ADHD.
- The essential feature of Tourette's disorder is the presence of multiple motor tics and one or more vocal tics.
- Common medications used with Tourette's disorder include haloperidol, pimozide, clonidine, guanfacine, and atypical antipsychotics such as risperidone, olanzapine, and ziprasidone.
- Oppositional defiant disorder is characterized by a pattern of negativistic, defiant, disobedient, and hostile behavior toward authority figures that occurs more frequently than is usually observed in individuals of comparable age and developmental level.
- With conduct disorder, there is a repetitive and persistent pattern of behavior in which the basic rights of others or major age-appropriate societal norms or rules are violated.
- The essential feature of separation anxiety disorder is excessive anxiety concerning separation from the

home or from those to whom the person is attached.

■ Children with separation anxiety disorder may have temperamental characteristics present at birth that predispose them to the disorder.

■ General therapeutic approaches for child and adolescent psychiatric disorders include behavior therapy, family therapy, group therapies (including music, art, crafts, play, and psychoeducation), and psychopharmacology.

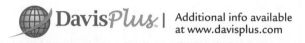

DavisPlus. | Additional info available at www.davisplus.com

Review Questions
Self-Examination/Learning Exercise

Select the answer that is most appropriate for each of the following questions.

1. In an effort to help the child with mild to moderate intellectual developmental disorder develop satisfying relationships with others, which of the following nursing interventions is most appropriate?
   a. Interpret the child's behavior for others.
   b. Set limits on behavior that is socially inappropriate.
   c. Allow the child to behave spontaneously, for he or she has no concept of right or wrong.
   d. This child is not capable of forming social relationships.

2. The child with autism spectrum disorder has difficulty with trust. With this in mind, which of the following nursing actions would be most appropriate?
   a. Encourage all staff to hold the child as often as possible, conveying trust through touch.
   b. Assign a different staff member each day so the child will learn that everyone can be trusted.
   c. Assign the same staff person as often as possible to promote feelings of security and trust.
   d. Avoid eye contact because it is extremely uncomfortable for the child and may even discourage trust.

3. Which of the following nursing diagnoses would be considered the *priority* in planning care for the child with severe autism spectrum disorder?
   a. Risk for self-mutilation evidenced by banging head against wall
   b. Impaired social interaction evidenced by unresponsiveness to people
   c. Impaired verbal communication evidenced by absence of verbal expression
   d. Disturbed personal identity evidenced by inability to differentiate self from others

4. Which of the following activities would be most appropriate for the child with attention-deficit/hyperactivity disorder?
   a. Monopoly
   b. Volleyball
   c. Pool
   d. Checkers

5. Which of the following groups is most commonly used for drug management of the child with attention-deficit/hyperactivity disorder?
   a. CNS depressants (e.g., diazepam [Valium])
   b. CNS stimulants (e.g., methylphenidate [Ritalin])
   c. Anticonvulsants (e.g., phenytoin [Dilantin])
   d. Major tranquilizers (e.g., haloperidol [Haldol])

6. The child with attention-deficit/hyperactivity disorder has a nursing diagnosis of impaired social interaction. Which of the following nursing interventions are appropriate for this child? (Select all that apply.)
   a. Socially isolate the child when interactions with others are inappropriate.
   b. Set limits with consequences on inappropriate behaviors.
   c. Provide rewards for appropriate behaviors.
   d. Provide group situations for the child.

Continued

Review Questions—cont'd
Self-Examination/Learning Exercise

7. The nursing history and assessment of an adolescent with a conduct disorder might reveal all of the following behaviors *except:*
   a. Manipulation of others for fulfillment of own desires.
   b. Chronic violation of rules.
   c. Feelings of guilt associated with the exploitation of others.
   d. Inability to form close peer relationships.

8. Certain family dynamics often predispose adolescents to the development of conduct disorder. Which of the following patterns is thought to be a contributing factor?
   a. Parents who are overprotective
   b. Parents who have high expectations for their children
   c. Parents who consistently set limits on their children's behavior
   d. Parents who are alcohol dependent

9. Which of the following is *least* likely to predispose a child to Tourette's disorder?
   a. Absence of parental bonding
   b. Family history of the disorder
   c. Abnormalities of brain neurotransmitters
   d. Structural abnormalities of the brain

10. Which of the following medications is used to treat Tourette's disorder?
    a. Methylphenidate (Ritalin)
    b. Haloperidol (Haldol)
    c. Imipramine (Tofranil)
    d. Phenytoin (Dilantin)

IMPLICATIONS OF RESEARCH FOR EVIDENCE-BASED PRACTICE

Melagari, M.G., Nanni, V., Lucidi, F., Russo, P., Donfrancesco, R., & Cloninger, C.R. (2015). Temperamental and character profiles of preschool children with ODD, ADHD, & anxiety disorders. *Comprehensive Psychiatry, 58,* 94-101. doi:10.1016/j.comppsych.2015.01.001

DESCRIPTION OF THE STUDY: This study evaluated the reports of 120 parents of preschool children with ADHD, ODD, or anxiety disorders to identify whether their reports of child temperament and character accurately predicted their child's diagnostic picture using a specific assessment inventory (the Preschool Temperament and Character Inventory).

RESULTS OF THE STUDY: The researchers found that three dimensions of temperament (harm avoidance, novelty seeking, and persistence) enabled correct identification of ADHD, ODD, or anxiety disorders 75 percent of the time.

Specifically, children with ADHD showed high scores on novelty-seeking and low scores on reward dependence and persistence; children with anxiety disorders showed high scores on harm avoidance; and children with ODD had higher scores on novelty-seeking, persistence, and harm avoidance.

IMPLICATIONS FOR NURSING PRACTICE: This study has implications for nurses who work with children, and particularly those who work in schools. Early identification of these childhood disorders enables intensive and comprehensive intervention to be initiated at the earliest signs of a developing disorder. If temperament profiles can accurately differentiate among these disorders, then screening as early as preschool is justified and may help to mediate longer-term consequences of these disorders by enabling targeted intervention.

TEST YOUR CRITICAL THINKING SKILLS

Jimmy, age 9, has been admitted to the child psychiatric unit with a diagnosis of attention-deficit/hyperactivity disorder. He has been unmanageable at school and at home and has had several suspensions from school for continuous disruption of his class. He refuses to sit in his chair or do his work. He yells out in class, interrupts the teacher and the other students, and lately has become physically aggressive when he cannot have his way. Most recently, he was suspended after hitting his teacher when she asked him to return to his seat.

Jimmy's mother describes him as a restless and demanding baby who grew into a restless and demanding toddler. He has never gotten along well with his peers. Even as a small child, he would take his friends' toys away from them or bite them if they tried to hold their own with him. His 5-year-old sister is afraid of him and refuses to be alone with him.

During the nurse's intake assessment, Jimmy paced the room or rocked in his chair. He talked incessantly on a superficial level and jumped from topic to topic. He told the nurse that he did not know why he was there. He acknowledged that he had some problems at school but said that it was only because the other kids picked on him and the teacher did not like him. He said he got into trouble at home sometimes but that it was because his parents liked his little sister better than they liked him.

The physician has ordered methylphenidate 5 mg twice a day for Jimmy. His response to this order is, "I'm not going to take drugs. I'm not sick!"

Answer the following questions related to Jimmy:

1. What are the pertinent assessment data to be noted by the nurse?
2. What is the primary nursing diagnosis for Jimmy?
3. Aside from client safety, to what problems would the nurse want to direct intervention with Jimmy?

MOVIE CONNECTIONS

Bill (intellectual disability) • *Bill, On His Own* (intellectual disability) • *Sling Blade* (intellectual disability) • *Forrest Gump* (intellectual disability) • *Rain Man* (autism spectrum disorder [ASD]) • *Mercury Rising* (ASD) • *Niagara, Niagara* (Tourette's disorder) • *Toughlove* (conduct disorder)

References

Acosta, M.T., Swanson, J., Stehli, A., Molina, B., Martinez, A.F., Arcos-Burgos, . . . MTA Team. (2016). ADGRL3 (LPHN3) variants are associated with a refined phenotype of ADHD in the MTA study. *Molecular Genetics and Genomic Medicine, 4*(5), 540-547. doi:10.1002/mgg3.230

ADHD Institute. (2016). Environmental risk factors. Retrieved from www.adhd-institute.com/burden-of-adhd/aetiology/environmental-risk-factors

American Psychiatric Association. (2000). *Diagnostic and statistical manual of mental disorders* (4th ed., text rev.). Washington, DC: American Psychiatric Publishing.

American Psychiatric Association. (2013). *Diagnostic and statistical manual of mental disorders* (5th ed.). Washington, DC: American Psychiatric Publishing.

Association for Play Therapy. (2016). Play therapy makes a difference. Retrieved from www.a4pt.org/?page=PTMakesADifference

Bernstein, B.E. (2014). Conduct disorder. Retrieved from http://emedicine.medscape.com/article/918213-overview#a3

Black, D.W., & Andreasen, N.C. (2014). *Introductory textbook of psychiatry* (6th ed.). Washington, DC: American Psychiatric Publishing.

Centers for Disease Control and Prevention. (2016a). Autism Spectrum Disorders Autism and Developmental Disabilities Monitoring Network. Retrieved from www.cdc.gov/ncbddd/autism/addm.html

Centers for Disease Control and Prevention. (2016b). FastStats: Attention deficit hyperactivity disorder (ADHD). Retrieved from www.cdc.gov/nchs/fastats/adhd.htm

Centers for Disease Control and Prevention. (2016c). Childhood lead poisoning data, statistics, and surveillance. Retrieved from www.cdc.gov/nceh/lead

Centers for Disease Control and Prevention. (2016d). Tourette syndrome: Risk factors and causes. Retrieved from www.cdc.gov/ncbddd/tourette/riskfactors.html

Dryden-Edwards, R. (2015). Separation anxiety. Retrieved from www.medicinenet.com/separation_anxiety/page4.htm

Froehlich T.E., Lanphear B.P., Auinger P., Hornung, R., Epstein, J.N., Braun, J., & Kahn, R.S. (2009). Association of tobacco and lead exposures with attention-deficit/hyperactivity disorder. *Pediatrics, 124*(6), 1054-1063. doi:10.1542/peds.2009-0738

Galéra, C., Côté, S.M., Bouvard, M.P., Pingault, J.B., Melchior, M., Michel, G., . . . Tremblay, R.E. (2011). Early risk factors for hyperactivity-impulsivity and inattention trajectories from age 17 months to 8 years. *Archives of General Psychiatry, 68*(12), 1267-1275. doi:10.1001/archgenpsychiatry.2011.138

Gilman, S.R., Chang, J., Xu, B., Bawa, T.S., Gogos, J.A., Karayiorgou, M., & Vitkup, D. (2012). Diverse types of genetic variation converge on functional gene networks involved in schizophrenia. *Nature Neuroscience, 15*(12), 1723–1728. doi:10.1038/nn.3261

Grohol, J. (2016). New chewable ADHD medication, Adzenys, has some worried. *Psych Central.* Retrieved from http://psychcentral.com/news/2016/05/31/new-chewable-adhd-medication-adzenys-has-some-worried/104077.html

Harrop, C., McConachie, H., Emsly, R., Leadbitter, K., Green, J., & the PACT Consortium. (2014). Restricted and repetitive behaviors in autism spectrum disorders and typical development: Cross-sectional and longitudinal comparisons. *Journal of Autism and Developmental Disorders, 44*(5), 1207-1219. doi:10.1007/s10803-13-1986-5

Hazlett, H.C., Poe, M.D., Gerig, G., Styner, M., Chappell, C., Smith, R.G., . . . Piven, J. (2011). Early brain overgrowth in autism associated with an increase in cortical surface area before age 2 years. *Archives of General Psychiatry, 68*(5), 467-476. doi:10.1001/archgenpsychiatry.2011.39

Heinonen K., Raikkonen K., Pesonen A.K., Andersson, S., Kajnatie, E., Eriksson, J.G., . . . Lano, A. (2010). Behavioural symptoms of attention deficit/hyperactivity disorder in preterm and term children born small appropriate for gestational age: A longitudinal study. *BMC Pediatrics, 10*(1), 91. doi:10.1186/1471-2431-10-91

Institute of Medicine. (2003). *Health professions education: A bridge to quality.* Washington, DC: Institute of Medicine.

Kendler, K.S., Aggen, S.H., & Patrick, C.J. (2013). Familial influences on conduct disorder reflect 2 genetic factors and 1 shared environmental factor. *JAMA Psychiatry, 70*(1), 78-86. doi:10.1001/jamapsychiatry.2013.267

Kranjac, D. (2016). In vitro modeling of early brain overgrowth in autism. Retrieved from www.psychiatryadvisor.com/neurodevelopmental-disorder/modeling-early-brain-overgrowth-in-autism/article/508852/

Lubit, R.H. (2015). Oppositional defiant disorder. Retrieved from http://emedicine.medscape.com/article/918095-overview

Marchetto, M.C., Belinson, H., Tian, Y., Freitas, B.C., Fu, C., Vadodaria, K.C. . . . Muotri, A.R. (2016). Altered proliferation and networks in neural cells derived from idiopathic autistic individuals. *Molecular Psychiatry.* doi:10.1038/mp.2016.95

Mayo Clinic. (2016). Oppositional defiant disorder. Retrieved from www.mayoclinic.org/diseases-conditions/oppositional-defiant-disorder/basics/risk-factors/con-20024559

Melagari, M.G., Nanni, V., Lucidi, F., Russo, P., Donfrancesco, R., & Cloninger, C.R. (2015). Temperamental and character profiles of preschool children with ODD, ADHD, & anxiety disorders. *Comprehensive Psychiatry, 58,* 94-101. doi:10.1016/j.comppsych.2015.01.001

National Institutes of Health. (2014). Tourette's syndrome fact sheet. Retrieved from www.ninds.nih.gov/disorders/tourette/detail_tourette.htm#3231_1

Rossignol, D.A., & Frye, R.E. (2016). Environmental toxicants and autism spectrum disorder. Retrieved from www.psychiatrictimes.com/special-reports/environmental-toxicants-and-autism-spectrum-disorder

Sadock, B.J., Sadock, V.A., & Ruiz, P. (2015). *Synopsis of psychiatry: Behavioral sciences/clinical psychiatry* (11th ed.). Philadelphia: Lippincott Williams & Wilkins.

Sherman, J., & Tarnow, J. (2013). What are common comorbidities in ADHD? *Psychiatric Times.* Retrieved from www.psychiatrictimes.com/adhd/what-are-common-comorbidities-in-adhd

Strunz, S., Westphal, L., Ritter, K., Heuser, I., Dziobek, I., & Roepke, S. (2015). Personality pathology of adults with autism spectrum disorder without accompanying intellectual impairment in comparison to adults with personality disorders. *Journal of Autism and Developmental Disorders, 45,* 4026-4038. doi:10.1007/s10803-14-2183-x

Van Den Ban, E., Souverein, P., Meijer, W., Van Engeland, H., Swaab, H., Egber, T., & Heerdinle, E. (2014). Association between ADHD drug use and injuries among children and adolescents. *European Child and Adolescent Psychiatry, 23,* 95-102. doi:10.1007/s00787-013-0432-8

Weisman, H., Qureshi, I.A., Leckman, J.F., Scahill, L., & Bloch, M.H. (2013). Systematic review: Pharmacological treatment of tic disorders—efficacy of antipsychotic and alpha-2 adrenergic agonist agents. *Neuroscience and Biobehavioral Reviews, 37*(6), 1162-1171. doi:10.1016/j.neubiorev.2012.09.008

Williams, N.M., Zaharieva, I., Martin, A., Langley, K., Mantripragada, K., Holmans, P., . . . Gudmundsson, O.O. (2010). Rare chromosomal deletions and duplications in attention-deficit hyperactivity disorder: A genome-wide analysis. *Lancet, 376*(9750), 1401-1408. doi:10.1016/S0140-6736(10)61109-9

The Aging Individual

34

KEY TERMS

attachment

bereavement overload

disengagement theory

geriatrics

gerontology

geropsychiatry

granny-dumping

long-term memory

Medicaid

Medicare

menopause

osteoporosis

reminiscence therapy

short-term memory

transcendence

OBJECTIVES
After reading this chapter, the student will be able to:

1. Discuss societal perspectives on aging.
2. Describe an epidemiological profile of aging in the United States.
3. Discuss various theories of aging.
4. Describe biological, psychological, sociocultural, and sexual aspects of the normal aging process.
5. Discuss retirement as a special concern to the aging individual.
6. Explain personal and sociological perspectives of long-term care of the aging individual.
7. Describe the problem of elder abuse as it exists in today's society.
8. Discuss the implications of the increasing number of suicides among the elderly population.
9. Apply the steps of the nursing process to the care of aging individuals.

HOMEWORK ASSIGNMENT
Please read the chapter and answer the following questions:

1. Which theory of aging postulates that life span and longevity changes are predetermined?
2. How is the ability to learn affected by aging?
3. What is the most common cause of psychopathology in the elderly?
4. What are some factors that are thought to contribute to elder abuse?

What is it like to grow old? It is not likely that many people in the American culture would state that it is something they want to do. Most would agree, however, that it is "better than the alternative."

Roberts (1991) recounts the tale of Supreme Court Justice Oliver Wendell Holmes Jr. In the year before he retired at age 91 as the oldest justice ever to sit on the Supreme Court of the United States, Holmes and his close friend Justice Louis Brandeis, then a mere 74 years old, were out for one of their frequent walks on Washington's Capitol Hill. On this particular day, the justices spotted a very attractive young woman approaching them. As she passed, Holmes paused, sighed, and said to Brandeis, "Oh, to be 70 again!" Obviously, being old is relative to the individual experiencing it.

Growing old has not historically been desirable among the youth-oriented American culture. However, with 66 million baby boomers reaching their 65th birthdays by the year 2030, greater emphasis is being placed on the needs of an aging population. The disciplines of **gerontology** (the study of the aging process), **geriatrics** (the branch of clinical medicine specializing in problems of the elderly), and **geropsychiatry** (the branch of clinical medicine specializing in psychopathology of the elderly population) are expanding rapidly in response to this demand.

Growing old in a society that has been obsessed with youth may have a critical impact on the mental health of many people. This situation has serious implications for psychiatric nursing.

What is it like to grow old? More and more people will be able to answer this question as the 21st century progresses. Perhaps they will also be asking the question that Roberts (1991) asks: "How did I get here so fast?"

This chapter focuses on physical and psychological changes associated with the aging process, as well as special concerns of the elderly population, such as retirement, long-term care, elder abuse, and high suicide rates. The nursing process is presented as the vehicle for delivery of nursing care to elderly individuals.

How Old Is *Old*?

The concept of "old" has changed drastically over the years. Our prehistoric ancestors probably had a life span of 40 years, with the average individual living around 18 years. As civilization developed, mortality rates remained high as a result of periodic famine and frequent malnutrition. An improvement in the standard of living was not truly evident until about the middle of the 17th century. Since that time, assured food supply, changes in food production, better

housing conditions, and more progressive medical and sanitation facilities have contributed to population growth, declining mortality rates, and substantial increases in longevity.

In 1900, the average life expectancy in the United States was 47 years, and only 4 percent of the population was age 65 or older. By 2014, the average life expectancy at birth was 78.8 years (76.4 years for men and 81.2 years for women) (National Center for Health Statistics, 2016).

The U.S. Census Bureau has created a system for classification of older Americans:

■ Older: 55 through 64 years
■ Elderly: 65 through 74 years
■ Aged: 75 through 84 years
■ Very old: 85 years and older

Some gerontologists have elected to use a simpler classification system:

■ Young old: 60 through 74 years
■ Middle old: 75 through 84 years
■ Old old: 85 years and older

So how old is *old?* Obviously, the term cannot be defined by a number. Myths and stereotypes of aging have long obscured our understanding of the aged and the process of aging. Ideas that all elderly individuals are sick, depressed, obsessed with death, senile, and incapable of change affect the way elderly people are treated. They even shape the pattern of aging for people who believe them by becoming self-fulfilling prophecies—people start to believe they should behave in certain ways and therefore act according to those beliefs. Generalized assumptions can be demeaning and can interfere with the quality of life for older individuals.

Just as there are many differences in individual adaptation at earlier stages of development, so it is in the elderly population. Erikson (1963) has suggested that the mentally healthy older person possesses a sense of ego integrity and self-acceptance that will help in adapting to the ambiguities of the future with a sense of security and optimism.

Murray, Zentner, and Yakimo (2009) stated:

> [Having accomplished the earlier developmental tasks], the person accepts life as his or her own and as the only life for the self. He or she would wish for none other and would defend the meaning and the dignity of the lifestyle. The person has further refined the characteristics of maturity described for the middle-aged adult, achieving both wisdom and an enriched perspective about life and people. (p. 662)

Everyone, particularly health-care workers, should see aging people as individuals, each with specific needs and abilities, rather than as a stereotypical group. Some individuals may seem "old" at 40, whereas others may not seem "old" at 70. Variables such as attitude, mental health, physical health, and degree of independence strongly influence how an individual perceives himself or herself. Surely, in the final analysis, whether one is considered "old" must be self-determined.

Epidemiological Statistics

The Population

In 1980, Americans 65 years of age and older numbered 25.5 million. By 2014, this number increased to 46.2 million and is expected to double by 2060 to 98 million (Administration on Aging [AoA], 2016). In 2015, that number represented 14.5 percent of the population, and it is projected that by 2040 the number of Americans older than age 65 will represent 21.7 percent of the population. The population of those 85 years of age and older is expected to triple by the year 2040. As of 2014, 0.2 percent of the population was older than 100 (AoA, 2016).

Marital Status

In 2015, of individuals age 65 and older, 70 percent of men and 45 percent of women were married (AoA, 2016). Thirty-four percent of all women in this age group were widowed. There were three times as many widows as widowers, which is consistent with the longer life expectancy for women.

Living Arrangements

The majority of individuals age 65 or older live alone, with a spouse, or with relatives. In 2014, 2.2 million adults older than 65 were living in a household with a grandchild present, and 554,579 of these grandparents had primary responsibility for the grandchild living with them (AoA, 2016). This trend continues to grow and has significant implications for the changing complexion of older adult life. At any one time, fewer than 5 percent of people in this age group live in institutions. This percentage increases dramatically with age, ranging from 1 percent for persons 65 to 74 years, to 3 percent for persons 75 to 84 years, to 10 percent for persons 85 and older. See Figure 34–1 for a distribution of living arrangements for persons age 65 and older.

Economic Status

More than 4.5 million (10%) individuals aged 65 or older were below the poverty level in 2014. When the U.S Census Bureau figures adjusted for regional variations in cost of housing, other benefits, and out-of-pocket expenses such as for medical care, the

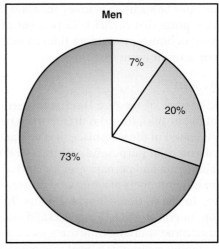

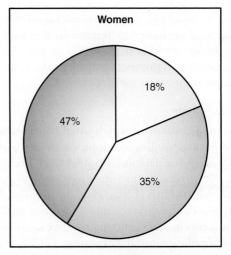

FIGURE 34–1 Living arrangements of noninstitutionalized persons aged 65 and older (Source: Administration on Aging, Aging statistics, 2016, retrieved from https://www.giaging.org/documents/A_Profile_of_Older_Americans__2016.pdf

percentage of those living below the poverty level rose to 14.4 percent (AoA, 2016). These statistics are higher than those from 2012 and 2013, suggesting a trend toward increasing numbers of older adults living below the poverty level. Older women had a higher poverty rate than older men, and older Hispanic women living alone had the highest poverty rate. Poor people who have worked all their lives can expect to become poorer in old age, and others will become poor only after becoming old. However, there is a substantial number of affluent and middle-income older persons.

Of individuals in this age group, 81 percent owned their own homes in 2013 (AoA, 2016). However, the housing of this population of Americans is usually older and less adequate than that of the younger population; therefore, a higher percentage of income must be spent on maintenance and repairs. The AoA reports that in 2013, 45 percent of older adults living in houses spent more than 25 percent of their income on housing costs.

Employment

With the passage of the Age Discrimination in Employment Act in 1967, forced retirement has been virtually eliminated in the workplace. It is well accepted that involvement in purposeful activity is vital to successful adaptation and perhaps even to survival at any age. Increasing numbers of adults over 65 are remaining active in employment environments. In 2015, 8.8 million Americans (18.8 %) aged 65 and older were in the labor force (working or actively seeking work), and that number represents a steady increase for both men and women since around the year 2000 (AoA, 2016). This increase is particularly apparent in the 65- to 69-year-old age group. The data does not clarify whether this tendency to remain in the workforce during older adulthood is related to the desire to remain active and productive through the labor force or is based in necessity for income.

Health Status

The number of days in which usual activities are restricted because of illness or injury increases with age. The Centers for Disease Control and Prevention (CDC, 2015) reports that approximately 80 percent of older adults have at least one chronic condition, and 50 percent have two or more chronic conditions. The most commonly occurring conditions among the elderly population are hypertension (71%), arthritis (49%), heart disease (30%), cancer (24%), and diabetes (21%) (AoA, 2016).

Emotional and mental illnesses increase over the life cycle. Depression is particularly prevalent, and suicide is a serious problem among elderly Americans. Prevalence of major depression is estimated at between 1 and 5 percent for the general population of older adults but may rise to as high as 13.5 percent for older adults requiring hospitalization or home health care (CDC, 2015). The CDC adds that depression in this age group is particularly underdiagnosed and undertreated by both health-care providers and older adults themselves, perhaps related to a misperception that this is a normal part of aging or a natural reaction to illnesses. Neurocognitive disorders increase dramatically in old age.

Theories of Aging

A number of theories related to the aging process have been described. These theories are grouped into two broad categories: biological and psychosocial.

Biological Theories

Biological theories attempt to explain the physical process of aging, including molecular and cellular changes in the major organ systems and the body's ability to function adequately and resist disease. They also attempt to explain why people age differently and what factors affect longevity and the body's ability to resist disease.

Genetic Theory

According to one genetic theory, aging is an involuntarily inherited process that operates over time to alter cellular or tissue structures. This theory suggests that life-span and longevity changes are predetermined. This is supported by the finding that identical twins have similar life spans and children of parents with a long life span tend to live for a long time as well (Guarente, 2016).

A second genetic theory identifies aging as a process of genetic mutations that essentially create errors in transmission of information, causing molecules to become dysfunctional. Epigenetics, which involves the study of changes in the way genes are expressed in the absence of changes in the sequence of nucleic acids (Venes, 2014), has confirmed fascinating findings that have implications for aging and illness. First, it was discovered that DNA methylation (the addition of a methyl group to a DNA base) is a mechanism responsible for gene regulation. Genome studies of aging cells and tissues have shown a variable "DNA methylation drift," which creates changes in aging stem cells that culminates in reduced stem cell plasticity, stem cell exhaustion, and focal defects that can lead to illnesses such as cancer (Issa, 2014). Issa describes that "aging pathologies in turn accelerate methylation drift by promoting chronic inflammation and uncontrolled proliferation which creates a vicious cycle that may explain why some illnesses increase . . . exponentially . . . with age" (p.28).

With ongoing research, we may discover what aging will look like for an individual and what his or her disease risks are. If epigenetic drift can be prevented, it may be possible to prevent diseases associated with aging.

Wear-and-Tear Theory

Proponents of this theory believe that the body wears out on a scheduled basis. Since animals have some ability to repair themselves, this theory does not seem to fit what we know about biological systems (Guarente, 2016). A related theory suggests that free radicals, the waste products of metabolism, accumulate and cause damage to important biological structures. Free radicals are molecules with unpaired electrons that exist normally in the body; they also are produced by ionizing radiation, ozone, and chemical toxins. According to this theory, these free radicals cause DNA damage, cross-linkage of collagen, and the accumulation of age pigments.

Environmental Theory

According to this theory, factors in the environment (e.g., industrial carcinogens, sunlight, trauma, and infection) bring about changes in the aging process. Although these factors are known to accelerate aging, the impact of the environment is a secondary rather than a primary factor in aging. Science is only beginning to uncover the many environmental factors that affect aging.

Autoimmune Theory

The autoimmune theory describes an age-related decline in the immune system. As people age, their ability to defend against foreign organisms decreases, resulting in susceptibility to infection and diseases such as cancer. A rise in the body's autoimmune response occurs in which aging cells can no longer distinguish foreign bodies and instead begin to attack themselves. This leads to the development of autoimmune diseases such as rheumatoid arthritis and allergies to food and environmental agents. However, this theory is based on clinical rather than experimental evidence (Guarente, 2016).

Neuroendocrine Theory

The neuroendocrine theory was first developed in 1954 by Vladimir Dilman, MD, who subsequently worked with another physician, Ward Dean, to update this theory in the early 1990s. The theory suggests that as humans age, the hypothalamus declines in its ability to regulate hormones and becomes less sensitive to their effects. Consequently, hormone secretion and effectiveness declines. Dilman identified several hypotheses about why this decrease in sensitivity occurs, including reduced neurotransmitter levels (serotonin in particular), decline in the secretion of pineal gland hormones, reduced glucose utilization and fat accumulation, neuronal lesions caused by chronically elevated cortisol levels secondary to stress, and accumulation of cholesterol in plasma membranes of neurons (Ward, 2015). Some believe that hormone replacements impacted by the hypothalamus may be a future treatment to counter the effects of aging, but more research is needed.

Psychosocial Theories

Psychosocial theories focus on social and psychological changes that accompany advancing age, as opposed to the biological implications of anatomic deterioration. Several theories have attempted to describe how attitudes and behavior in the early phases of life affect people's reactions during the late phase. This work is called the process of "successful aging."

Personality Theory

Personality theories address aspects of psychological growth without delineating specific tasks or expectations for older adults. Some evidence suggests that personality characteristics in old age are highly correlated with early life characteristics. Murray and associates (2009) state:

> No specific personality changes occur as a result of aging. The older person becomes more of what he or she was. The older person continues to develop emotionally and in personality and adds on characteristics instead of making drastic changes. (p. 663)

However, people in extreme old age show greater similarity with one another in certain characteristics, possibly related to similar changes in physical functioning and social roles.

In one study of personality traits, Srivastava and associates (2003) examined the Big Five personality trait dimensions in a large sample to determine how personality changes over the life span, including conscientiousness, agreeableness, neuroticism, openness, and extraversion. The participants ranged in age from 21 to 60. The researchers found that conscientiousness (being organized and disciplined) increased throughout the age range studied, with the biggest increases during the 20s. Agreeableness (being warm, generous, and helpful) increased most during a person's 30s. Neuroticism (being anxious and emotionally labile) declined with age for women but did not decline for men. Openness (being accepting of new experiences) showed small declines with age for both men and women. Extroversion (being outwardly expressive and interested in the environment) declined for women but did not show changes in men. This study contradicts the view that personality traits tend to stop changing in early adulthood. These researchers suggest that personality traits change gradually but systematically throughout the life span. Their research was foundational in understanding the adult population, though the elderly were not evaluated in that study.

In a review of the research on personality and aging that studied people between 60 and 80 years of age, Srivastava and Das (2013) identify support for the premise that personality traits are relatively stable but change somewhat over the long term with age and possibly in response to intervention. The personality trait of conscientiousness, for example, was found to be relatively stable when viewed over the course of a lifetime.

As the population of older adults continues to grow, research has focused not only on what constitutes aging but more specifically what constitutes successful aging. Srivastava and Das stress that personality is undeniably influential in successful aging (they note that the term "successful aging" is often but is controversial to some). Rowe and Kahn (1997) provide the classic paradigm for successful aging, identifying three criteria that must be met: (a) absence of disease, disability, and risk factors; (b) maintaining physical and mental functioning, and; (c) active engagement in life.

So what role do personality factors play in these aspects of successful aging? The research of Kern and Friedman (2008) has identified the personality trait of conscientiousness as most linked to health-promoting behaviors. Even more recent research (Terracciano et al., 2010) studied the genetic underpinnings of each of the Big Five personality traits and, among other findings, identified a gene associated with the trait of conscientiousness. They found that this personality trait gene was associated with the same gene that has been linked to some neurodegenerative diseases, including Alzheimer's disease. Could personality traits unravel the mysteries of aging and age-related illnesses? What all of this means for intervening upon and possibly improving the aging process is still unknown. Future research may begin to unfold the intricate interaction between genetic and environmental influences such that personality traits might become alterable to promote healthier, more successful aging.

Developmental Task Theory

In contrast to the personality theories of aging, which discuss a largely stable process that continues into old age, developmental task theory holds that there are activities and challenges that one must accomplish at predictable, changing stages in life to achieve successful aging. Erikson (1963) described the primary task of old age as being able to see one's life as having been lived with integrity. In the absence of achieving that sense of having lived well, the older adult is at risk for becoming preoccupied with feelings of regret or despair. As noted previously, the life span was significantly shorter when Erikson's developmental tasks and stages were first identified. In the late 1990s, Erikson expanded the concept of **transcendence** as an additional stage that occurs after the stage of integrity versus despair (Erikson & Erikson, 1997). McCarthy, Ling, and Carini (2013) identify transcendence as a concept within the spiritual domain, and they cite McCarthy and Bockweg's (2012) definition:

> Transcendence [is] an inherent developmental process, resulting in a shift from a rational, materialistic view to a wider world view characterized by broadened personal boundaries, within interpersonal, intrapersonal, transpersonal, and temporal dimensions resulting in an increased sense of meaning in life, well-being, and life satisfaction. (p. 180)

McCarthy and associates' research on transcendence supported that this concept is a significant contributor to successful aging.

Disengagement Theory

Disengagement theory describes the process of withdrawal by older adults from societal roles and responsibilities. According to the theory, this withdrawal process is predictable, systematic, inevitable, and necessary for the proper functioning of a growing society. Older adults were believed to be happy when social contacts diminished and responsibilities were assumed by a younger generation, providing time for reflecting on life's accomplishments and coming to terms with unfulfilled expectations. For society, the benefit is an orderly transfer of power from old to young.

There have been many critics of this theory, and the postulates have been challenged. For many healthy and productive older individuals, the prospect of a slower pace and fewer responsibilities is undesirable.

Activity Theory

In direct opposition to the disengagement theory is the activity theory of aging, which holds that the way to age successfully is to stay active. Sadock, Sadock, and Ruiz (2015) report that growing evidence supports the importance of remaining socially active for both physical and emotional well-being. Cultural expectations are influential, and as older Americans increasingly reap the benefits of physical and social activity, cultural expectations begin to shift. Many fitness classes, for example, are now finding a membership of people in their 80s and beyond.

Continuity Theory

This theory, also known as the *developmental theory*, is a follow-up to the disengagement and activity theories. It emphasizes the individual's previously established coping abilities and personal character traits as a basis for predicting how the person will adjust to the changes of aging. Basic lifestyle characteristics are likely to remain stable in old age, barring physical or other types of complications that necessitate change. A person who has enjoyed the company of others and an active social life will continue to enjoy this lifestyle into old age. One who has preferred solitude and a limited number of activities will probably find satisfaction in a continuation of this lifestyle.

Maintenance of internal continuity is motivated by the need for preservation of self-esteem, ego integrity, cognitive function, and social support. As they age, individuals maintain self-concept by reinterpreting current experiences so that old values can take on new meanings in keeping with present circumstances. Internal self-concepts and beliefs are not readily vulnerable to environmental change, and external continuity in skills, activities, roles, and relationship styles can remain remarkably stable into the 70s and beyond.

The Normal Aging Process

Biological Aspects of Aging

Individuals are unique in their physical and psychological aging processes, as influenced by their predisposition or resistance to illness; the effects of their external environment and behaviors; their exposure to trauma, infections, and past diseases; and the health and illness practices they have adopted during their life spans. As the individual ages, a quantitative loss of cells and changes in many of the enzymatic activities within cells results in a diminished responsiveness to biological demands made on the body. Age-related changes occur at different rates for different individuals, although in actuality, when growth stops, aging begins. This section presents a brief overview of the normal biological changes that occur with the aging process.

Skin

One of the most dramatic changes that occurs in aging is the loss of elastin in the skin. This effect, along with changes in collagen, causes aged skin to wrinkle and sag. Excessive exposure to sunlight compounds these changes and increases the risk of developing skin cancer.

Fat redistribution results in a loss of the subcutaneous cushion of adipose tissue. Thus, older people lose "insulation," the skin appears thinner, and they are more sensitive to extremes of ambient temperature than are younger people. A diminished supply of blood vessels to the skin results in a slower rate of healing.

Cardiovascular System

The age-related decline in the cardiovascular system is thought to be the major determinant of decreased tolerance for exercise, loss of conditioning, and the overall decline in energy reserve. The aging heart is characterized by modest hypertrophy and loss of pacemaker cells, resulting in a decrease in maximal heart rate and diminished cardiac output (Blair, 2012). This results in a decrease in response to work demands and some diminishment of blood flow to the brain, kidneys, liver, and muscles. Heart rate also slows with time. If arteriosclerosis is present, cardiac function is further compromised.

Respiratory System

Thoracic expansion is diminished by an increase in fibrous tissue and loss of elastin. Pulmonary vital capacity decreases and the amount of residual air increases. Scattered areas of fibrosis in the alveolar septa interfere with exchange of oxygen and carbon dioxide. These changes are accelerated by the use of cigarettes or other inhaled substances. Cough and laryngeal reflexes are reduced, causing decreased ability to defend the airway. Decreased pulmonary blood flow and diffusion ability result in reduced efficiency in responding to sudden respiratory demands.

Musculoskeletal System

Skeletal aging involving the bones, muscles, ligaments, and tendons probably generates the most frequent limitations on activities of daily living for aging individuals. Loss of muscle mass is significant, although this occurs more slowly in men than in women. Demineralization of the bones occurs at a rate of about 1 percent per year throughout the life span in both men and women. However, this increases to approximately 10 percent in women around **menopause,** making them particularly vulnerable to **osteoporosis.**

Individual muscle fibers become thinner and less elastic with age. Muscles become less flexible following disuse. Diminished storage of muscle glycogen results in loss of energy reserve for increased activity. These changes are accelerated by nutritional deficiencies and inactivity.

Gastrointestinal System

In the oral cavity, the teeth show a reduction in dentine production, shrinkage and fibrosis of root pulp, gingival retraction, and loss of bone density in the alveolar ridges. There is some loss of peristalsis in the stomach and intestines, and gastric acid production decreases. Levels of intrinsic factor may also decrease, resulting in vitamin B_{12} malabsorption in some aging individuals. A significant decrease in absorptive surface area of the small intestine may be associated with some decline in nutrient absorption. Motility slowdown of the large intestine, combined with poor dietary habits, dehydration, lack of exercise, and some medications, may give rise to problems with constipation.

A modest decrease in size and weight of the liver results in losses in enzyme activity required to deactivate certain medications by the liver. These age-related changes can influence the metabolism and excretion of these medications. These changes, along with the pharmacokinetics of the drug, must be considered when giving medications to aging individuals.

Endocrine System

A decreased level of thyroid hormones causes a lowered basal metabolic rate. Decreased amounts of adrenocorticotropic hormone may result in less efficient stress response.

Impairments in glucose tolerance are evident in aging individuals. Studies of glucose challenges show that insulin levels are equivalent to or slightly higher than those from younger challenged individuals, although peripheral insulin resistance appears to play a significant role in carbohydrate intolerance. The observed glucose clearance abnormalities and insulin resistance in older people may be related to many factors other than biological aging (e.g., obesity, family history of diabetes) and may be influenced substantially by diet or exercise.

Genitourinary System

Age-related declines in renal function occur because of a steady attrition of nephrons and sclerosis within the glomeruli over time. Vascular changes affect blood flow to the kidneys, which results in reduced glomerular filtration and tubular function. Elderly people are prone to develop inappropriate antidiuretic hormone secretion, causing slight elevation in levels of blood urea nitrogen and creatinine. The overall decline in renal function has serious implications for physicians who prescribe medications for elderly individuals.

In men, enlargement of the prostate gland is common as aging occurs. Prostatic hypertrophy is associated with an increased risk for urinary retention and may also be a cause of urinary incontinence (Johnston, Harper, & Landefeld, 2013). Loss of muscle and sphincter control, as well as the use of some medications, may cause urinary incontinence in women. Not only is this problem a cause of social stigma, but it increases the risk of urinary tract infection and local skin irritation if left untreated. Normal changes in the genitalia are discussed in the section "Sexual Aspects of Aging."

Immune System

Aging results in changes in both cell-mediated and antibody-mediated immune responses. The size of the thymus gland declines continuously beginning just after puberty, reaching about 15 percent of its original size at age 50. The consequences of these changes include a greater susceptibility to infections and a diminished inflammatory response that results in delayed healing. There is also evidence of an increase in various autoantibodies as a person ages, increasing the risk of autoimmune disorders such as rheumatoid arthritis (National Institutes of Health, 2014). Because of the overall decrease in efficiency of the immune system, the proliferation of abnormal cells is facilitated in the elderly individual. Cancer is the best example of aberrant cells allowed to proliferate due to the ineffectiveness of the immune system.

Nervous System

With aging, an absolute loss of neurons correlates with decrease in brain weight of about 10 percent by age 90 (Murray et al., 2009). Gross morphological examination reveals gyral atrophy in the frontal, temporal, and parietal lobes; widening of the sulci; and ventricular enlargement. These changes have been identified in careful study of adults with normal intellectual function.

The brain has enormous reserve, and little cerebral function is lost over time, although greater functional decline is noted in the periphery. There appears to be a disproportionately greater loss of cells in the cerebellum, the locus ceruleus, the substantia nigra, and olfactory bulbs, accounting for some of the more characteristic aging behaviors such as mild gait disturbances, sleep disruptions, and decreased smell and taste perception.

Some of the age-related changes within the nervous system may be caused by alterations in neurotransmitter release, uptake, turnover, catabolism, or receptor functions (Beers & Jones, 2006; Blair, 2012). A great deal of attention is being given to brain biochemistry and in particular to the neurotransmitters acetylcholine, dopamine, norepinephrine, and epinephrine. These biochemical changes may be responsible for the altered responses of many older persons to stressful events and some biological treatments.

Sensory Systems
Vision

Visual acuity begins to decrease in midlife. Presbyopia (blurred near vision) is the standard marker of aging of the eye. It is caused by a loss of elasticity of the crystalline lens and results in compromised accommodation.

Cataract development is inevitable if the individual lives long enough for vision changes to occur. Cataracts occur when the lens of the eye becomes less resilient due to compression of fibers and increasingly opaque as proteins lump together, ultimately resulting in a loss of visual acuity.

The color in the iris may fade, and the pupil may become irregular in shape. A decrease in production of secretions by the lacrimal glands may cause dryness and result in increased irritation and infection. The pupil may become constricted, requiring an increase in the amount of light needed for reading.

Hearing

Hearing changes significantly with the aging process. Gradually, the ear loses its sensitivity to discriminate sounds because of damage to the hair cells of the cochlea. The most dramatic decline appears to be in perception of high-frequency sounds.

Age-related hearing loss, called *presbycusis,* is common and affects more than half of all adults by age 75 years (Blevins, 2015). It occurs more frequently in men than in women, a fact that may be related to differences in levels of lifetime noise exposure.

Taste and Smell

Beyond 70 years of age, taste sensitivity begins to decline related to atrophy and loss of taste buds (Shock, 2015). Taste discrimination decreases, and bitter taste sensations predominate. Sensitivity to sweet and salty tastes is diminished.

The deterioration of the olfactory bulbs is accompanied by loss of smell acuity. The effect of aging on sense of smell has not been precisely identified and is difficult to evaluate because so many environmental factors influence sensitivity to smell (Shock, 2015). However, some decreased sensitivity may be related to loss of nerve endings in the nose and decreased mucus production (MedlinePlus, 2014).

Touch and Pain

Although the primary sensory changes related to aging are in hearing and vision, sensitivity to touch and pain may also decline or change because of decreased blood flow to nerve endings, in the spinal cord, or to the brain (MedlinePlus, 2014). These changes have critical implications for the elderly in their potential inability to use sensory warnings to escape serious injury.

Psychological Aspects of Aging

Memory Functioning

Age-related memory deficiencies and slower response times have been extensively reported in the literature. Although **short-term memory** seems to deteriorate with age, perhaps because of poorer sorting strategies, **long-term memory** does not show similar changes. However, in nearly every instance, well-educated, mentally active people do not exhibit the same decline in memory functioning as their peers who lack similar opportunities to flex their minds. Nevertheless, with few exceptions, the time required for memory scanning is longer for both recent and remote recall among older people. This can sometimes be attributed to social or

health factors (e.g., stress, fatigue, illness), but it can also occur because of certain normal physical changes associated with aging (e.g., decreased blood flow to the brain).

Intellectual Functioning

There appears to be a high degree of regularity in intellectual functioning across the adult age span. Crystallized abilities, or knowledge acquired in the course of the socialization process, tend to remain stable over the adult life span. Fluid abilities, or abilities involved in solving novel problems, tend to decline gradually from youth to old age. In other words, intellectual abilities of older people do not decline but do become obsolete. The age of their formal educational experiences is reflected in their intelligence scoring.

Learning Ability

The ability to learn is not diminished by age. Studies, however, have shown that some aspects of learning do change with age. The ordinary slowing of reaction time with age for nearly all tasks or the overarousal of the central nervous system may account for lower performance levels on tests requiring rapid responses. Under conditions that allow for self-pacing by the participant, differences in accuracy of performance diminish. Ability to learn continues throughout life, although it is strongly influenced by interests, activity, motivation, health, and experience. Adjustments need to be made in teaching methodology and time allowed for learning.

Adaptation to the Tasks of Aging

Loss and Grief

Individuals experience losses from the very beginning of life. By the time individuals reach their 60s and 70s, they have experienced numerous losses, and mourning has become a lifelong process. Unfortunately, with the aging process comes a convergence of losses, the timing of which makes it impossible for the aging individual to complete the grief process in response to one loss before another occurs. Because grief is cumulative, this can result in **bereavement overload,** which has been implicated in the predisposition to depression in the elderly.

Attachment to Others

Many studies have confirmed the importance of interpersonal relationships at all stages in the life cycle. Murray and associates (2009) state:

> [Social networks] contribute to well-being of the elder by (a) promoting socialization and companionship, (b) elevating morale and life satisfaction, (c) buffering the effects of stressful events, (d) providing a confidant, and (e) facilitating coping skills and mastery. (p. 620)

This need for **attachment** is consistent with the activity theory of aging that correlates the importance of social integration with successful adaptation in later life. Evidence supports that in addition to the psychosocial benefits, social engagement is also correlated with physical and cognitive health in older adulthood (Thomas, 2011).

Maintenance of Self-Identity

Maintaining a positive self-concept and identity is important in successful aging. Individuals who tend toward a rigid self-identity and a negative self-concept will no doubt struggle with any changes and adaptations faced in the aging process. For example, someone whose identity centers entirely around his job may struggle more with identity in retirement than someone whose identity includes job, family, travel, and hobbies. Researchers in one study found that maintaining a youthful age identity and positive perceptions and experiences related to aging had a self-enhancing function for self-esteem and identity (Westerhof, Whitbourne, & Freeman, 2012). The authors compared citizens in the United States with those in the Netherlands and found that for the former, this self-enhancing function was stronger than for those from the latter. They concluded that factors influencing self-identity and self-concept in older age need to be considered within the cultural context.

Dealing With Death

Death anxiety is a universal phenomenon, and attitudes about death are a result of cumulative life experiences (Lehto & Stein, 2009). As average life span has increased, there has been a resurgence of interest in research about death anxiety. Lehto and Stein conducted an extensive review of the research to lay a foundation for an emerging understanding of this concept. Kübler-Ross's (1969) pioneering research on attitudes about death and the experience of dying paved the way for discussions of this issue, but as Lehto and Stein identify in their review, death anxiety is largely denied or repressed. They cite several studies confirming that religious beliefs reduced death anxiety and suggest that such beliefs are beneficial because they provide a context for meaning about life and death. Positive self-esteem mediates death anxiety or at least "assists in preventing overt manifestations of death anxiety" (Lehto & Stein, p. 27). Other researchers similarly found that fear of the dying process among elderly individuals in care institutions was correlated with low self-esteem, feelings of purposelessness, and poor mental health (Missler et al., 2012). These authors also found that death anxiety was more strongly correlated with fears for significant others than fear of the unknown.

Interestingly, death anxiety seems to be the highest during middle age and stabilizes by later adulthood. But as Lehto and Stein (2009) identified, maladaptive consequences of death anxiety include mental illnesses such as depression and anxiety disorders, so assessing and intervening with regard to death anxiety may be beneficial in preventing longer-term consequences. Self-esteem interventions, for example, may be beneficial in preventing older adult depression secondary to death anxiety. Some research has shown that death education is beneficial in reducing anxiety associated with fear of death (McClatchey & King, 2015). Addressing these issues with middle-aged clients may be in the interest of primary or secondary prevention in the aging process.

Psychiatric Disorders in Later Life

Cognitive disorders, depressive disorders, phobias, and alcohol use disorders are among the most common psychiatric illnesses in later life (Sadock et al., 2015). Recent attention is focused on the growing opiate addiction problem in the older adult population. Many factors influence symptomatology, including medical conditions and medications. One should never assume that psychiatric symptoms are a usual part of aging. For example, as Sadock and colleagues identify, "Age itself is not a risk factor for depression but being widowed and having a chronic medical illness are associated with vulnerability to depressive disorders" (p. 1346). A thorough assessment is essential to distinguish the multiple factors that may be concurrently influencing symptomatology.

Neurocognitive Disorder

Neurocognitive disorders (NCDs) are the most common causes of psychopathology in the elderly. About half of these disorders are of the Alzheimer's type, characterized by an insidious onset and a gradually progressive course of cognitive impairment. No curative treatment is currently available. Symptomatic treatments, including pharmacological interventions, attention to the environment, and family support, can help to maximize the client's level of functioning.

Delirium

Delirium is one of the most common and critical forms of psychopathology in later life. A number of factors have been identified that predispose elderly people to delirium, including structural brain disease, reduced capacity for homeostatic regulation, impaired vision and hearing, a high prevalence of chronic disease, reduced resistance to acute stress, and age-related changes in the pharmacokinetic and pharmacodynamics of drugs. Delirium needs to be recognized and the underlying condition treated as soon as possible. A high mortality rate is associated with this condition.

Depression

Depressive disorders are the most common affective illnesses occurring after the middle years. The incidence of increased depression among elderly people is influenced by the variables of physical illness, functional disability, cognitive impairment, and loss of a spouse (Lang, 2012). Somatic symptoms are common in the depressed elderly. Symptomatology often mimics that of NCD, a condition called *pseudodementia*. (See Chapter 22, Neurocognitive Disorders, Table 22-1 for a comparison of the symptoms of NCD and pseudodementia.) Suicide is prevalent in the elderly, with declining health and decreased economic status considered important influencing factors. Treatment of depression in the elderly individual may include psychotropic medications or electroconvulsive therapy. Tricyclic antidepressants pose a risk for orthostatic hypotension and other anticholinergic effects, and selective serotonin reuptake inhibitors pose a higher risk for hyponatremia in the elderly, so risks and benefits of medication use should be carefully reviewed.

Schizophrenia

Schizophrenia typically begins in young adulthood. In most instances, individuals who manifest psychotic disorders early in life show a decline in psychopathology as they age. Late-onset schizophrenia (after age 60) is rare, and when it does occur, it is more common in women and is often characterized by paranoid delusions or hallucinations. Antipsychotic agents may be beneficial but should be used judiciously and at lower than usual doses (Sadock et al., 2015).

Anxiety Disorders

Most anxiety disorders begin in early to middle adulthood, but some appear for the first time after age 60. Because the autonomic nervous system is more fragile in older persons, the response to a major stressor is often quite intense. The presence of physical disability frequently compounds the situation, resulting in a more severe posttraumatic stress response than is commonly observed in younger persons. In older adults, symptoms of anxiety and depression often accompany each other, making it difficult to determine which disorder is dominant.

Personality Disorders

Personality disorders are uncommon in the elderly population. The incidence of personality disorders among individuals older than age 65 is less than 5 percent. Most elderly people with personality disorder have likely manifested the symptomatology for many years.

Sleep Disorders

Sleep disorders are very common in the aging individual. Roughly 50 percent of older adults report difficulty initiating or maintaining sleep (Crowley, 2011), and these disorders may contribute to cognitive changes. Contributing factors include medical conditions, medications, age-related changes in circadian rhythms, sleep-disordered breathing, and restless leg syndrome (Crowley, 2011; Roepke & Ancoli-Israel, 2010). Sedative-hypnotics, along with nonpharmacological approaches, are often used as sleep aids for the elderly. Changes associated with metabolism and elimination must be considered when maintenance medications are administered for chronic insomnia in the aging client.

Sociocultural Aspects of Aging

Old age brings many important socially induced changes, some of which have the potential for negative effects on both the physical and mental well-being of older persons. In American society, old age is defined arbitrarily as 65 years or older because that is when most people are able to retire with full Social Security and other pension benefits. Recent legislation has increased the age beyond 65 years for full Social Security benefits. Currently, the age increases yearly (based on year of birth) until 2027, when the age for full benefits will be 67 for all individuals.

Elderly people in virtually all cultures share some basic needs and interests. There is little doubt that most individuals choose to live the most satisfying life possible for as long as possible. They want protection from hazards and release from the weariness of everyday tasks. They want to be treated with the respect and dignity that individuals who have reached this pinnacle in life deserve, and they want to die with the same respect and dignity.

Historically, the aged have had special status in society. Even today, in some cultures the aged are the most powerful, the most engaged, and the most respected members. This has not been the case in modern industrial societies, although trends in the status of the aged differ widely between one industrialized country and another. For example, the status and integration of the aged in Japan have remained relatively high when compared with other industrialized nations, including the United States. There are subcultures in the United States, including Latino American, African American, and Asian American, in which the elderly have a higher degree of status than they receive in the mainstream population. The aged are awarded a position of honor in cultures that place emphasis on family cohesiveness. In these cultures, the aged are revered for their knowledge and wisdom gained through their years of life experiences (Purnell, 2013).

Many negative stereotypes color the perspective on aging in the United States. Views of elderly individuals as always tired or sick, slow and forgetful, isolated and lonely, unproductive, and angry determine the way younger individuals relate to the elderly in this society. Increasing disregard for the elderly has resulted in a type of segregation as aging individuals voluntarily seek out or are involuntarily placed in special residences for older adults.

Assisted living centers, retirement apartment complexes, and even entire retirement communities intended solely for individuals over age 50 are becoming increasingly common. In 2014, 63 percent of persons age 65 and older lived in 14 states, with the largest numbers in California, Florida, Texas, New York, and Pennsylvania (AoA, 2016). It is important for elderly individuals to feel part of an integrated group, and they are migrating to these areas in an effort to achieve this integration. This phenomenon provides additional corroboration for the activity theory of aging and the importance of attachment to others.

Employment is another area in which the elderly experience discrimination. Although compulsory retirement has been virtually eliminated, discrimination still exists in hiring and promotion practices. Many employers are reluctant to retain or hire older workers. It is difficult to determine how much of the failure to hire and promote results from discrimination based on age alone and how much of it is related to a realistic and fair appraisal of the aged employee's ability and efficiency. It is true that some elderly individuals may perform at lower levels than younger workers do, but there are many who likely can do a *better* job than their younger counterparts if given the opportunity. Nevertheless, surveys have shown that some employers accept the negative stereotypes about elderly individuals and believe that older workers are hard to please, set in their ways, less productive, frequently absent, and involved in more accidents.

The status of the elderly may improve with time and as their numbers increase with the aging of the baby boomers. As older individuals gain political power, the benefits and privileges designed for the elderly will increase. There is power in numbers, and the 21st century promises power for people age 65 and older.

Sexual Aspects of Aging

Sexuality and the sexual needs of elderly people are frequently misunderstood, condemned, stereotyped, ridiculed, repressed, and ignored. Americans have grown up in a society that has liberated sexual expression for all other age groups but still retains certain Victorian standards regarding sexual expression by the elderly. Negative stereotyped notions concerning

sexual interest and activity among the elderly are common. Some of these include ideas that older people have no sexual interests or desires, that they are sexually undesirable, or that they are too fragile or too ill to engage in sexual activity. Some people even believe it is disgusting or comical to consider elderly individuals as sexual beings.

These cultural stereotypes undoubtedly play a large part in the misperception many people hold regarding sexuality of the aged, and they may be reinforced by the common tendency of the young to deny the inevitability of aging. With reasonably good health and an interesting and interested partner, there is no inherent reason why individuals should not enjoy an active sexual life well into late adulthood (King & Regan, 2013).

Physical Changes Associated With Sexuality

Many of the changes in sexuality that occur in later years are related to the physical changes that take place at that time of life.

Changes in Women

Menopause may begin anytime during the 40s or early 50s. During this time, there is a gradual decline in ovary function and the subsequent production of estrogen, which results in a number of changes. The walls of the vagina become thin and inelastic, the vagina itself shrinks in both width and length, and the amount of vaginal lubrication noticeably decreases. Orgastic uterine contractions may become spastic. All of these changes can result in painful penetration, vaginal burning, pelvic aching, or irritation on urination. In some women, the discomfort may be severe enough to result in avoidance of intercourse. Paradoxically, these symptoms are more likely to occur with infrequent intercourse (once a month or less). Regular and more frequent sexual activity results in a greater capacity for sexual performance (King & Regan, 2013). Other symptoms associated with menopause in some women include hot flashes, night sweats, sleeplessness, irritability, mood swings, migraine headaches, urinary incontinence, and weight gain.

Some menopausal women elect to take hormone replacement therapy (HRT) for relief of these symptoms. With estrogen therapy, the symptoms of menopause are minimized or eliminated, but this treatment is associated with increased risk for breast and endometrial cancer. To combat this latter effect, many women also take a second hormone, progesterone. Taken for 7 to 10 days during the month, progesterone decreases the risk of estrogen-induced endometrial cancer. Some physicians prescribe a low dose of progesterone that is taken along with estrogen for the entire month. A combination pill taken in this manner is also available.

Results of the Women's Health Initiative reported in the *Journal of the American Medical Association* indicated that the combination pill is associated with an increased risk of cardiovascular disease and breast cancer. Benefits related to colon cancer and osteoporosis were reported; however, investigators stopped this arm of the study and suggested discontinuation of this treatment. In a 3-year follow-up study of the participants, the results showed that the increased risk for cardiovascular disease dissipated with discontinuation of the hormone therapy (Heiss et al., 2008).

Other studies have indicated that HRT may have a *cardioprotective* effect, but Yang and Reckelhoff's review of the literature (2011) did not substantiate that finding. Their review cites other studies that suggest the cardiovascular risks versus benefits may be associated with the age at which HRT is initiated. A more recent Women's Health Initiative study reported that their findings do not support use of HRT for chronic disease prevention but indicate that it may be beneficial in some management of menopause symptoms (Manson et al., 2013). Controversies about HRT and conflicting study findings continue to highlight the need for ongoing research on this topic.

Changes in Men

Testosterone production declines gradually over the years, beginning between ages 40 and 60. A major change resulting from this hormone reduction is that erections occur more slowly and require more direct genital stimulation to achieve. There may also be a modest decrease in the firmness of the erection in men older than age 60. Erectile dysfunction is more common as men grow older but it can often be managed and sometimes reversed (National Institute on Aging, 2016). The refractory period lengthens with age, increasing the amount of time following orgasm before the man may achieve another erection. The volume of ejaculate gradually decreases, and the force of ejaculation lessens. The testes become somewhat smaller, but most men continue to produce viable sperm well into old age. Prolonged control over ejaculation in middle-aged and elderly men may bring increased sexual satisfaction for both partners.

Sexual Behavior in the Elderly

Coital frequency in early marriage and the overall quantity of sexual activity between ages 20 and 40 correlate significantly with frequency patterns of sexual activity during aging (Masters, Johnson, & Kolodny,

1995). Although sexual interest and behavior do appear to decline somewhat with age, studies show that significant numbers of elderly men and women have active and satisfying sex lives well into their 80s. A survey commissioned by the American Association of Retired Persons provided some revealing information regarding the sexual attitudes and behavior of senior citizens. Some statistics from the survey are summarized in Table 34–1. The information from this survey clearly indicates that sexual activity can and does continue well past the 70s for healthy, active individuals who have regular opportunities for sexual expression. King and Regan (2013) identify that if an individual has healthy attitudes about sexuality and healthy sexual relationships in younger adulthood, those will probably continue into older adulthood.

Special Concerns of the Elderly Population

Retirement

Statistics reflect that a larger percentage of Americans are living longer and many of them are retiring earlier. Reasons often given for the increasing pattern of early retirement include health problems, Social Security and other pension benefits, attractive "early-out" packages offered by companies, and long-held plans (e.g., turning a hobby into a money-making situation). The Bureau of Labor Statistics' Current Population Surveys indicated a gradual increase, between 2004 and 2014, in the percentage of adults aged 65 and older who have delayed retirement (Hipple, 2015). Although many choose early retirement, the overall trend appears to be that more older adults keep working.

Studies show that 10 to 20 percent of individuals reenter the workforce following retirement (Cahill, Giandrea, & Quinn, 2011). Reentry is more common among men than women and among individuals who are younger and in good health at the time of retirement. Reasons people give for returning to work include negative reactions to being retired, feelings of being unproductive, economic hardship, and loneliness. Recent downturns in economic conditions have forced many retired people to seek employment to augment dwindling retirement resources.

Retirement has both social and economic implications for elderly individuals. The role is fraught with ambiguity and requires many adaptations on the part of those involved.

Social Implications

Retirement is often anticipated as an achievement, in principle, but is met with many mixed feelings when it actually occurs. Our society places a great deal of importance on productivity, making as much money

TABLE 34–1 Sexuality at Midlife and Beyond

	AGES	MEN (%)	WOMEN (%)
Have sex at least once a week	45–49	50	26
	50–59	41	32
	60–69	24	24
	70+	15	5
Report very satisfied with physical relationship	45–49	60	48
	50–59	50	40
	60–69	52	41
	70+	26	27
Report very satisfied with emotional relationship	45–49	26	37
	50–59	32	23
	60–69	28	29
	70+	20	24
Report sexual activity is important to their overall quality of life	45–49	69	33
	50–59	65	28
	60–69	55	33
	70+	46	12
Believe nonmarital sex is okay	45–49	88	86
	50–59	91	75
	60–69	80	71
	70+	68	61
Describe their partners as physically attractive	45–49	50	60
	50–59	53	48
	60–69	58	58
	70+	51	48
Report always or usually having an orgasm with sexual intercourse	45–49	95	70
	50–59	88	64
	60–69	91	59
	70+	82	61
Report being impotent	45–49	6	
	50–59	16	
	60–69	29	
	70+	48	
Report having used medicine, hormones, or other treatments to improve sexual functioning	45–49	7	9
	50–59	12	16
	60–69	14	14
	70+	13	13
What would most improve your sex life?	All	Better health for self; partner initiates sex more often; less stress	Less stress; better health for self and partner; finding a partner

Adapted from the 2010 May AARP Research Survey on Sex, Romance, and Relationships: AARP Survey of Midlife and Older Adults by Linda Fisher with the Assistance of Gretchen Anderson, Matrika Chapagain, Xenia Montenegro, James Smoot, Amishi Takalkar. Copyright 2010 AARP. All rights reserved.

as possible, and doing it at as young an age as possible. These types of values contribute to the ambiguity associated with retirement. Although leisure has been acknowledged as a legitimate reward for workers, leisure during retirement historically has lacked the same social value. Adjustment to this life-cycle event

becomes more difficult in the face of societal values that are in direct conflict with the new lifestyle.

Historically, many women have derived substantial self-esteem from their families—birthing them, rearing them, and being a "good mother." Likewise, many men have achieved self-esteem through work-related activities—creativity, productivity, and earning money. With the termination of these activities may come a loss of self-worth, resulting in depression in some individuals who are unable to adapt satisfactorily. Well-being in retirement is linked to factors such as stable health status and access to health-care services, adequate income, the ability to pursue new goals or activities, extended social network of family and friends, and satisfaction with current living arrangements (Murray et al., 2009).

American society often identifies an individual by his or her occupation. This is reflected in the conversations of people meeting each other for the first time. Undoubtedly, most everyone has either asked or been asked at some point in time, "What do you do?" or "Where do you work?" Occupation determines status, and retirement represents a significant change in status. The basic ambiguity of retirement occurs in an individual's or society's definition of this change. Is it undertaken voluntarily or involuntarily? Is it desirable or undesirable? Is one's status made better or worse by the change? With the population of older adults growing, retirement versus remaining in the workforce will continue to be an important issue for this age group. Clearly, this is a major life event that requires planning and realistic expectations of life changes.

Economic Implications

Because retirement is generally associated with a 20 to 40 percent reduction in personal income, the standard of living after retirement may be adversely affected. Most older adults derive postretirement income from a combination of Social Security benefits, public and private pensions, and income from savings or investments.

The Social Security Act of 1935 promised assistance with financial security for the elderly. Since then, the original legislation has been modified, yet the basic philosophy remains intact. Its effectiveness, however, is now in question. Faced with deficits, the program is forced to pay benefits to the currently retired from both the reserve funds and monies being collected at present. There is genuine concern about future generations, when there may be no reserve funds from which to draw. Because many of the programs that benefit older adults depend on contributions from the younger population, the growing ratio of older Americans to younger people may affect society's ability to supply the goods and services necessary to meet this expanding demand.

Medicare and **Medicaid** were established by the government to provide medical care benefits for elderly and indigent Americans. The Medicaid program is jointly funded by state and federal governments, and coverage varies significantly from state to state. Medicare covers only a percentage of health-care costs; therefore, to reduce risk related to out-of-pocket expenditures, many older adults purchase private "medigap" policies designed to cover charges in excess of those approved by Medicare.

The magnitude of retirement earnings depends almost entirely on preretirement income. The poor will remain poor and the wealthy are unlikely to lower their status during retirement; however, for many in the middle classes, the relatively fixed income sources may be inadequate, possibly forcing them to face financial hardship for the first time in their lives.

Long-Term Care

Long-term care facilities are defined by the level of care they provide. They may be skilled nursing facilities, intermediate care facilities, or a combination of the two. Some institutions provide convalescent care for individuals recovering from acute illness or injury, some provide long-term care for individuals with chronic illness or disabilities, and still others provide both types of assistance.

Most elderly individuals prefer to remain in their own homes or in the homes of family members for as long as this is possible without deterioration of family or social patterns. Many elderly individuals are placed in institutions as a last resort only after heroic efforts have been made to keep them in their own or a relative's home. The increasing emphasis on home health care has extended the period of independence for aging individuals.

Fewer than 4 percent of the population ages 65 and older live in nursing homes. The percentage increases dramatically with age, ranging from 1 percent for persons aged 65 to 74 and 3 percent for persons aged 75 to 84 to 10 percent for persons aged 85 and older (AoA, 2016). A profile of the "typical" elderly nursing home resident is about 80 years of age, white, female, and widowed, with multiple chronic health conditions.

Risk Factors for Institutionalization

In determining who in our society will need long-term care, several factors have been identified that appear to place people at risk. The following risk factors are taken into consideration to predict potential need for services and to estimate future costs.

Age

Because people grow older in very different ways and the range of differences becomes greater with the passage of time, age is becoming a less relevant characteristic than it once was. However, because of the high prevalence of chronic health conditions and disabilities and the greater chance of diminishing social supports associated with advancing age, the 65-and-older population is often viewed as an important long-term care target group.

Health

Level of functioning, as determined by ability to perform various behaviors or activities—such as bathing, eating, mobility, meal preparation, handling finances, judgment, and memory—is a measurable risk factor. The need for ongoing assistance from another person is critical in determining the need for long-term care.

Mental Health Status

Mental health problems are risk factors in assessing need for long-term care. Many symptoms associated with certain mental disorders (especially neurocognitive disorders), such as memory loss, impaired judgment, impaired intellect, and disorientation, would render the individual incapable of meeting the demands of daily living independently.

Socioeconomic and Demographic Factors

Low income generally is associated with greater physical and mental health problems among the elderly. Because many elderly individuals have limited finances, they are less able to purchase care resources available outside of institutions (e.g., home health care), although Medicare and Medicaid now contribute a limited amount to this type of noninstitutionalized care.

Women are at greater risk of being institutionalized than men, not because they are less healthy but because they tend to live longer and thus reach the age at which more functional and cognitive impairments occur. They are also more likely to be widowed. Whites have a higher rate of institutionalization than nonwhites. This may be related to cultural and financial influences.

Marital Status, Living Arrangement, and the Informal Support Network

Individuals who are married and live with a spouse are the least likely of all disabled people to be institutionalized. Those who live alone without resources for home care and with few or no relatives living nearby to provide informal care are at higher risk for institutionalization.

Attitudinal Factors

Many people dread the thought of even visiting a nursing home, let alone moving to one or placing a relative in one. Negative perceptions exist of nursing homes as "places to go to die." The media picture and subsequent reputation of nursing homes has not been positive. Stories of substandard care and patient abuse have scarred the industry, making it difficult for those facilities that are clean, well managed, and provide innovative, quality care to their residents to rise above the stigma.

State and national licensing boards perform periodic inspections to ensure that standards set forth by the federal government are met. These standards address quality of patient care as well as adequacy of the nursing home facility. Yet many elderly individuals and their families still perceive nursing homes as a place to go to die, and the fact that many of these institutions are poorly equipped, understaffed, and disorganized keeps this societal perception alive. There are, however, many excellent nursing homes that strive to go beyond the minimum federal regulations for Medicaid and Medicare reimbursement. In addition to medical, nursing, rehabilitation, and dental services, social and recreational services are provided to increase the quality of life for elderly people living in nursing homes. These activities include playing cards, bingo, and other games; parties; church activities; books; television; movies; and arts, crafts, and other classes. Some nursing homes provide occupational and professional counseling. These facilities strive to enhance opportunities for improving quality of life and for becoming "places to live" rather than "places to die."

Elder Abuse

Abuse of elderly individuals is a serious form of family violence. Statistics regarding the prevalence of elder abuse are difficult to determine. It is estimated that annually up to 2 million older adults in the United States are victims of abuse (Stark, 2012). However, the data suggest that only about 84 percent of these cases are reported to authorities. The abuser is often a relative who lives with the elderly person and may be the assigned caregiver. Typical caregivers who are likely to be abusers of the elderly were described by Murray and associates (2009) as those under economic stress, substance abusers, those who themselves have been victims of previous family violence, and those who are exhausted and frustrated by the caregiver role. Identified risk factors for victims of abuse include being a white female aged 70 or older, mental or physical impairment, inability to meet daily self-care needs, and having care needs that exceed the caretaker's ability.

Abuse of elderly individuals may be psychological, physical, or financial. Neglect may be intentional or unintentional. Psychological abuse includes yelling, insulting, harsh commands, threats, silence, and social isolation. Physical abuse is described as striking, shoving, beating, or restraint. Financial abuse refers to misuse or theft of finances, property, or material possessions. Neglect implies failure to fulfill the physical needs of an individual who cannot do so independently. Unintentional neglect is inadvertent, whereas intentional neglect is deliberate. In addition, elderly individuals may be the victims of sexual abuse, which is sexual intimacy between two persons that occurs without the consent of one of the persons involved. Another type of abuse, called **granny-dumping** by the media, involves abandoning elderly individuals at emergency departments, nursing homes, or other facilities—literally leaving them in the hands of others when the strain of caregiving becomes intolerable. Types of elder abuse are summarized in Box 34–1.

Elder victims often minimize the abuse or deny that it has occurred. The elderly person may be unwilling to disclose information because of fear of retaliation, embarrassment about the existence of abuse in the family, protectiveness toward a family member, or unwillingness to institute legal action. Adding to this unwillingness to report is that infirm elders are often isolated, so their mistreatment is less likely to be noticed by those who might be alert to symptoms of abuse. For these reasons, detection of abuse in the elderly is difficult at best.

Factors That Contribute to Abuse

A number of contributing factors have been implicated in the abuse of elderly individuals.

Longer Life

The 65-and-older age group has become the fastest growing segment of the population. Within this segment, the number of elderly older than age 75 has increased most rapidly. This trend is expected to continue well into the 21st century. The 75-and-older age group is the one most likely to be physically or mentally impaired, requiring assistance and care from family members. This group also is the most vulnerable to abuse from caregivers.

Dependency

Dependency appears to be the most common precondition in domestic abuse. Changes associated with normal aging or induced by chronic illness often result in loss of self-sufficiency in the elderly person, requiring that he or she become dependent on another for assistance with daily functioning. Long life may also consume finances to the point that the elderly individual becomes financially dependent on another. This type of dependency also increases the elderly person's vulnerability to abuse.

Stress

The stress inherent in the caregiver role is a factor in most abuse cases. Some clinicians believe that elder abuse results from individual or family psychopathology. Others suggest that even psychologically healthy family members can become abusive as a result of the exhaustion and acute stress caused by overwhelming caregiving responsibilities. This is compounded in an age group that has been dubbed the "sandwich generation"—those individuals who

---

BOX 34–1 **Examples of Elder Abuse**

PHYSICAL ABUSE
Striking, hitting, beating
Shoving
Bruising
Cutting
Restraining

PSYCHOLOGICAL ABUSE
Yelling
Insulting, name-calling
Harsh commands
Threats
Ignoring, silence, social isolation
Withholding of affection

NEGLECT (INTENTIONAL OR UNINTENTIONAL)
Withholding food and water
Inadequate heating

Unclean clothes and bedding
Lack of needed medication
Lack of eyeglasses, hearing aids, false teeth

FINANCIAL ABUSE OR EXPLOITATION
Misuse of the elderly person's income by the caregiver
Forcing the elderly person to sign over financial affairs to another person against his or her will or without sufficient knowledge about the transaction

SEXUAL ABUSE
Sexual molestation; rape
Any type of sexual intimacy against the elderly person's will

SOURCES: Murray, R.B., Zentner, J.P., & Yakimo, R. (2009). *Health promotion strategies through the life span (8th ed.). Upper Saddle River, NJ: Prentice Hall;* Sadock, B.J., Sadock, V.A., & Ruiz, P. (2015). *Synopsis of psychiatry: Behavioral sciences/clinical psychiatry (11th ed.). Philadelphia: Lippincott Williams & Wilkins.*

elected to delay childbearing so that they are now at a point in their lives when they are "sandwiched" between providing care for their children and providing care for their aging parents.

Learned Violence

Children who have been abused or have witnessed abusive and violent parents are more likely to evolve into abusive adults. In some families, abusive behavior is the normal response to tension or conflict, and this type of behavior can be transmitted from one generation to another. There may be unresolved family conflicts or retaliation for previous maltreatment that foster and promote abuse of the elderly person.

Identifying Elder Abuse

Because so many elderly individuals are reluctant to report personal abuse, health-care workers must be able to detect signs of mistreatment when they are in a position to do so. Box 34–1 listed a number of *types* of elder abuse. The following *manifestations* of the various categories of abuse have been identified (Koop, 2012; Murray et al., 2009):

■ Indicators of psychological abuse include a broad range of behaviors such as the symptoms associated with depression, withdrawal, anxiety, sleep disorders, and increased confusion or agitation.

■ Indicators of physical abuse may include bruises, welts, lacerations, burns, punctures, evidence of hair pulling, and skeletal dislocations and fractures.

■ Neglect may be manifested as consistent hunger, poor hygiene, inappropriate dress, consistent lack of supervision, consistent fatigue or listlessness, unattended physical problems or medical needs, or abandonment.

■ Sexual abuse may be suspected when the elderly person is presented with pain or itching in the genital area; bruising or bleeding in external genitalia, vaginal, or anal areas; or unexplained sexually transmitted disease.

■ Financial abuse may be occurring when there is an obvious disparity between assets and satisfactory living conditions or when the elderly person complains of a sudden lack of sufficient funds for daily living expenses.

Health-care workers often feel intimidated when confronted with cases of elder abuse. In these instances, referral to an individual experienced in management of victims of such abuse may be the most effective approach to evaluation and intervention. Health-care workers are responsible for reporting suspicions of elder abuse. An investigation is then conducted by regulatory agencies, whose job it is to determine if the suspicions are corroborated. Every effort must be made to ensure the client's safety, but it is important to remember that a competent elderly person has the right to choose his or her health-care options. As inappropriate as it may seem, some elderly individuals choose to return to the abusive situation. In this instance, he or she should be provided with names and phone numbers to call for assistance if needed. A follow-up visit by an adult protective services representative should be conducted.

Increased efforts need to be made to ensure that health-care providers have comprehensive training in the detection of and intervention in elder abuse. More research is needed to increase knowledge and understanding of the phenomenon of elder abuse and ultimately to effect more sophisticated strategies for prevention, intervention, and treatment.

Suicide

Although persons aged 65 and older comprise only 14.1 percent of the population, they represent a disproportionately high percentage of individuals who die by suicide. The highest number of suicides (19.3%) occurred among those 85 years of age and older (American Foundation for Suicide Prevention, 2016). The group especially at risk appears to be white men older than age 65, who are at five times greater risk for suicide than the general population (Sadock et al., 2015). Predisposing factors include loneliness, financial problems, physical illness, loss, and depression.

Increased social isolation may be a contributing factor to suicide among the elderly. The number of elderly individuals who are divorced, widowed, or otherwise living alone has increased, and being a widow is associated with higher risk for depression and suicide (Sadock et al., 2015).

Many elderly individuals express symptoms associated with depression that are never recognized as such, particularly somatic symptoms. Any sign of helplessness or hopelessness should prompt an assessment for suicide risk using clear and often closed-ended questions to elicit a specific response. These include:

■ Have you thought of hurting yourself or taking your own life?
■ Do you have a plan for hurting yourself?
■ Have you ever acted on that plan?
■ Have you ever attempted suicide?

Components of intervention with a suicidal elderly person should include demonstrations of genuine concern, interest, and caring; indications of empathy for his or her fears and concerns; and help in identifying, clarifying, and formulating a plan of action to deal with the unresolved issue. If the elderly person's behavior seems particularly lethal, additional family or staff coverage and contact should be arranged to prevent isolation.

Application of the Nursing Process

Assessment

Assessment of the elderly individual may follow the same framework used for all adults, but with consideration of the possible biological, psychological, sociocultural, and sexual changes that occur in the normal aging process described previously in this chapter. In no other area of nursing is it more important to practice holistic nursing than with the elderly. Older adults are likely to have multiple physical problems that contribute to problems in other areas of their lives. Obviously, these components cannot be addressed as separate entities. Nursing the elderly is a multifaceted, challenging process because of the multiple changes occurring at this time in the life cycle and the way in which each change affects every aspect of the individual.

Several considerations are unique to assessment of the elderly. Assessment of the older person's thought processes is a primary responsibility. Knowledge about the presence and extent of disorientation or confusion will influence the way in which the nurse approaches elder care.

Information about sensory capabilities is also extremely important. Because hearing loss is common, the nurse should lower the pitch and loudness of his or her voice when addressing the older person. Looking directly into the face of the older person when talking facilitates communication. Questions that require a declarative sentence in response should be asked; in this way, the nurse is able to assess the client's ability to use words correctly. Visual acuity can be determined by assessing adaptation to the dark, color matching, and the perception of color contrast. Knowledge about these aspects of sensory functioning is essential in the development of an effective care plan.

The nurse should be familiar with the normal physical changes associated with the aging process. Following are examples of some of these changes:

■ Less effective response to changes in environmental temperature, resulting in hypothermia
■ Decreases in oxygen use and the amount of blood pumped by the heart, resulting in cerebral anoxia or hypoxia
■ Skeletal muscle wasting and weakness, resulting in difficulty in physical mobility
■ Limited cough and laryngeal reflexes, resulting in risk of aspiration
■ Demineralization of bones, resulting in spontaneous fracturing
■ Decrease in gastrointestinal motility, resulting in constipation
■ Decrease in the ability to interpret painful stimuli, resulting in risk of injury

Common psychosocial changes associated with aging include the following:

■ Prolonged and exaggerated grief, resulting in depression
■ Physical changes, resulting in disturbed body image
■ Changes in status, resulting in loss of self-worth

This list is by no means exhaustive. The nurse should consider many other alterations in his or her assessment of the client. Knowledge of the client's functional capabilities is essential for determining the physiological, psychological, and sociological needs of the elderly individual. Age alone does not preclude the occurrence of all these changes. The aging process progresses at a wide range of variance, and each client must be assessed as a unique individual.

Diagnosis and Outcome Identification

Virtually any nursing diagnosis may be applicable to the aging client, depending on individual needs for assistance. Based on normal changes that occur in the elderly, the following nursing diagnoses may be considered:

Physiologically related diagnoses

■ Risk for trauma related to confusion, disorientation, muscular weakness, spontaneous fractures, and falls
■ Hypothermia related to loss of adipose tissue under the skin, evidenced by increased sensitivity to cold and body temperature below 98.6°F
■ Decreased cardiac output related to decreased myocardial efficiency secondary to age-related changes, evidenced by decreased tolerance for activity and decline in energy reserve
■ Ineffective breathing pattern related to increase in fibrous tissue and loss of elasticity in lung tissue, evidenced by dyspnea and activity intolerance
■ Risk for aspiration related to diminished cough and laryngeal reflexes
■ Impaired physical mobility related to muscular wasting and weakness, evidenced by need for assistance in ambulation
■ Imbalanced nutrition less than body requirements, related to inefficient absorption from gastrointestinal tract, difficulty chewing and swallowing, anorexia, and difficulty in feeding self, evidenced by wasting syndrome, anemia, and weight loss
■ Constipation related to decreased motility; inadequate diet; insufficient activity or exercise, evidenced by decreased bowel sounds; hard, formed stools; or straining at stool
■ Stress urinary incontinence related to degenerative changes in pelvic muscles and structural supports associated with increased age, evidenced by

reported or observed dribbling with increased abdominal pressure or urinary frequency
- Urinary retention related to prostatic enlargement, evidenced by bladder distention, frequent voiding of small amounts, dribbling, or overflow incontinence
- Disturbed sensory perception related to age-related alterations in sensory transmission, evidenced by decreased visual acuity, hearing loss, diminished sensitivity to taste and smell, or increased touch threshold (This diagnosis has been retired by NANDA-I but retained in this text because of its appropriateness to the specific behaviors described.)
- Insomnia related to age-related cognitive decline, decrease in ability to sleep ("sleep decay"), or medications, evidenced by interrupted sleep, early awakening, or falling asleep during the day
- Chronic pain related to degenerative changes in joints, evidenced by verbalization of pain or hesitation to use weight-bearing joints
- Self-care deficit (specify) related to weakness, confusion, or disorientation, evidenced by inability to feed self, maintain hygiene, dress or groom self, or use the toilet without assistance
- Risk for impaired skin integrity related to alterations in nutritional state, circulation, sensation, or mobility

Psychosocially related diagnoses

- Disturbed thought processes related to age-related changes that result in cerebral anoxia, evidenced by short-term memory loss, confusion, or disorientation (This diagnosis has been retired by NANDA-I but retained in this text because of its appropriateness to the specific behaviors described.)
- Complicated grieving related to bereavement overload, evidenced by symptoms of depression
- Risk for suicide related to depressed mood and feelings of low self-worth
- Powerlessness related to lifestyle of helplessness and dependency on others, evidenced by depressed mood, apathy, or verbal expressions of having no control or influence over life situation
- Low self-esteem related to loss of preretirement status, evidenced by verbalization of negative feelings about self and life
- Fear related to nursing home placement, evidenced by symptoms of severe anxiety and statements such as, "Nursing homes are places to go to die"
- Disturbed body image related to age-related changes in skin, hair, and fat distribution, evidenced by verbalization of negative feelings about body
- Ineffective sexuality pattern related to pain associated with vaginal dryness, evidenced by reported dissatisfaction with decrease in frequency of sexual intercourse

- Sexual dysfunction related to medications (e.g., antihypertensives) evidenced by inability to achieve an erection
- Social isolation related to total dependence on others, evidenced by expression of inadequacy in or absence of significant purpose in life
- Risk for trauma (elder abuse) related to caregiver role strain
- Caregiver role strain related to severity and duration of the care receiver's illness; lack of respite and recreation for the caregiver, evidenced by feelings of stress in relationship with care receiver; feelings of depression and anger; or family conflict around issues of providing care

Outcome Criteria

The following criteria may be used for measurement of outcomes in the care of the elderly client.

The client:

- Has not experienced injury
- Maintains reality orientation consistent with cognitive level of functioning
- Manages own self-care with assistance
- Expresses positive feelings about self, past accomplishments, and hope for the future
- Compensates adaptively for diminished sensory perception

Caregivers:

- Can problem-solve effectively regarding care of the elderly client
- Demonstrate adaptive coping strategies for dealing with stress of caregiver role
- Openly express feelings
- Express desire to join a support group of other caregivers

Planning and Implementation

In Table 34–2, selected nursing diagnoses are presented for the elderly client. Outcome criteria are included, along with appropriate nursing interventions and rationale for each.

Reminiscence therapy is especially helpful with elderly clients. This therapeutic intervention is highlighted in Box 34–2.

Evaluation

Reassessment is conducted to determine if the nursing actions have been successful in achieving the objectives of care. Evaluation of nursing actions for the elderly client may be facilitated by gathering information using the following types of questions:

- Has the client escaped injury from falls, burns, or other means to which he or she is vulnerable because of age?

(Text continued on page 798)

Table 34–2 | CARE PLAN FOR THE ELDERLY CLIENT

NURSING DIAGNOSIS: RISK FOR TRAUMA

RELATED TO: Confusion, disorientation, muscular weakness, spontaneous fractures, falls

OUTCOME CRITERIA	NURSING INTERVENTIONS	RATIONALE

Short-Term Goals:
• Client calls for assistance when ambulating or carrying out other activities.
• Client does not experience injury.
Long-Term Goal:
• Client does not experience injury.
	1. The following measures may be instituted:
	  a. Arrange furniture and other items in the room to accommodate client's disabilities.
	  b. Store frequently used items within easy access.
	  c. Keep bed in unelevated position. Pad side rails and headboard if client has history of seizures. Keep bedrails up when client is in bed (if permitted by institutional policy).
	  d. Assign room near nurses' station; observe frequently.
	  e. Assist client with ambulation.
	  f. Keep a dim light on at night.
	  g. If client is a smoker, cigarettes and lighter or matches should be kept at the nurses' station and dispensed only when someone is available to stay with client while he or she is smoking.
	  h. Frequently orient client to place, time, and situation.
	  i. Soft restraints may be required if client is very disoriented and hyperactive.
		1. To ensure client safety.

NURSING DIAGNOSIS: DISTURBED THOUGHT PROCESSES

RELATED TO: Age-related changes that result in cerebral anoxia

EVIDENCED BY: Short-term memory loss, confusion, or disorientation

OUTCOME CRITERIA	NURSING INTERVENTIONS	RATIONALE
Short-Term Goal: • Client accepts explanations of inaccurate interpretations of the environment within (time to be determined based on client condition). **Long-Term Goal:** • Client interprets the environment accurately and maintains reality orientation to the best of his or her cognitive ability.	1. Frequently orient client to reality. Use clocks and calendars with large numbers that are easy to read. Notes and large, bold signs may be useful as reminders. Allow client to have personal belongings. 2. Keep explanations simple. Use face-to-face interaction. Speak slowly and do not shout. 3. Discourage rumination on delusional thoughts. Talk about real events and real people.	1. To help maintain orientation and aid in memory and recognition. 2. To facilitate comprehension. Shouting may create discomfort and, in some instances, may provoke anger. 3. Rumination promotes disorientation. Reality orientation increases sense of self-worth and personal dignity.

Continued

Table 34–2 | CARE PLAN FOR THE ELDERLY CLIENT—cont'd

OUTCOME CRITERIA	NURSING INTERVENTIONS	RATIONALE
	4. Monitor for medication side effects.	4. Physiological changes in the elderly can alter the body's response to certain medications. Toxic effects may intensify altered thought processes.

NURSING DIAGNOSIS: SELF-CARE DEFICIT (SPECIFY)

RELATED TO: Weakness, disorientation, confusion, or memory deficits

EVIDENCED BY: Inability to fulfill activities of daily living (ADLs)

OUTCOME CRITERIA	NURSING INTERVENTIONS	RATIONALE
Short-Term Goal: • Client participates in ADLs with assistance from caregiver. Long-Term Goals: • Client accomplishes ADLs to the best of his or her ability. • Unfulfilled needs are met by caregivers.	1. Provide a simple, structured environment: a. Identify self-care deficits and provide assistance as required. Promote independent actions as able. b. Allow plenty of time for client to perform tasks. c. Provide guidance and support for independent actions by talking client through the task one step at a time. d. Provide a structured schedule of activities that does not change from day to day. e. ADLs should follow home routine as closely as possible. f. Allow consistency in assignment of daily caregivers.	1. To minimize confusion.

NRSING DIAGNOSIS: CAREGIVER ROLE STRAIN

RELATED TO: Severity and duration of the care receiver's illness; lack of respite and recreation for the caregiver

EVIDENCED BY: Feelings of stress in relationship with care receiver; feelings of depression and anger; family conflict around issues of providing care

OUTCOME CRITERIA	NURSING INTERVENTIONS	RATIONALE
Short-Term Goal: • Caregivers verbalize understanding of ways to facilitate the caregiver role. Long-Term Goal: • Caregivers achieve effective problem-solving skills and develop adaptive coping mechanisms to regain equilibrium.	1. Assess prospective caregivers' ability to anticipate and fulfill client's unmet needs. Provide information to assist caregivers with this responsibility. Ensure that caregivers are aware of available community support systems from which they can seek assistance when required. Examples include adult day-care centers, housekeeping and homemaker services, respite care services, or a local	1. Caregivers require relief from the pressures and strain of providing 24-hour care for their loved one. Studies have shown that elder abuse arises out of caregiving situations that place overwhelming stress on the caregivers.

Table 34–2 | CARE PLAN FOR THE ELDERLY CLIENT–cont'd

OUTCOME CRITERIA	NURSING INTERVENTIONS	RATIONALE
	chapter of the Alzheimer's Association. This organization sponsors a nationwide 24-hour hotline to provide information and link families who need assistance with nearby chapters and affiliates: 800-272-3900.	
	2. Encourage caregivers to express feelings, particularly anger.	2. Release of these emotions can serve to prevent psychopathology, such as depression or psychophysiological disorders, from occurring.
	3. Encourage participation in support groups composed of members with similar life situations.	3. Hearing others who are experiencing the same problems discuss ways in which they have coped may help caregiver adopt more adaptive strategies. Individuals with similar life experiences provide empathy and support for each other.

NURSING DIAGNOSIS: LOW SELF-ESTEEM

RELATED TO: Loss of preretirement status; early stages of cognitive decline

EVIDENCED BY: Verbalization of negative feelings about self and life

OUTCOME CRITERIA	NURSING INTERVENTIONS	RATIONALE
Short-Term Goal: • Client verbalizes positive aspects of self and past accomplishments. Long-Term Goal: • Client participates in group activities in which he or she can experience a feeling of enjoyment and accomplishment (to the best of his or her ability).	1. Encourage client to express honest feelings in relation to loss of prior status. Acknowledge pain of loss. Support client through process of grieving. Assess for depression and warning signs of risk for suicide. 2. If lapses in memory are occurring, devise methods for assisting client with memory deficit. Examples: a. Name sign on door identifying client's room b. Identifying sign on outside of dining room door c. Identifying sign on outside of restroom door d. Large clock, with oversized numbers and hands, appropriately placed e. Large calendar, indicating one day at a time, with month, day, and year in bold print f. Printed, structured daily schedule, with one copy for client and one posted on unit wall g. "News board" on unit wall where current news of national and local interest may be posted	1. Client may be fixed in anger stage of grieving process, which is turned inward on the self, resulting in diminished self-esteem. 2. These aids may assist client to function more independently, thereby increasing self-esteem.

Continued

Table 34–2 | CARE PLAN FOR THE ELDERLY CLIENT–cont'd

OUTCOME CRITERIA	NURSING INTERVENTIONS	RATIONALE
	3. Encourage client's attempts to communicate. If verbalizations are not understandable, express to client what you think he or she intended to say. It may be necessary to reorient client frequently.	3. The ability to communicate effectively with others may enhance self-esteem.
	4. Encourage reminiscence and discussion of life review (see Box 34–2). Sharing picture albums, if possible, is especially good. Also discuss present-day events.	4. Reminiscence and life review help client resume progression through the grief process associated with disappointing life events and increase self-esteem as successes are reviewed.
	5. Encourage participation in group activities. May need to accompany client at first until he or she feels secure that the group members will be accepting, regardless of limitations in verbal communication.	5. Positive feedback from group members increases self-esteem.
	6. Encourage client to be as independent as possible in self-care activities. Provide written schedule of tasks to be performed. Intervene in areas where client requires assistance.	6. The ability to perform independently preserves self-esteem.

NURSING DIAGNOSIS: DISTURBED SENSORY PERCEPTION

RELATED TO: Age-related alterations in sensory transmission

EVIDENCED BY: Decreased visual acuity, hearing loss, diminished sensitivity to taste and smell, and increased touch threshold

OUTCOME CRITERIA	NURSING INTERVENTIONS*	RATIONALE
Short-Term Goal: • Client does not experience injury due to diminished sensory perception. Long-Term Goals: • Client attains optimal level of sensory stimulation. • Client does not experience injury due to diminished sensory perception.	1. The following nursing strategies are indicated: a. Provide meaningful sensory stimulation to all special senses through conversation, touch, music, or pleasant smells. b. Encourage wearing of glasses, hearing aids, prostheses, and other adaptive devices. c. Use bright, contrasting colors in the environment. d. Provide large-print reading materials, such as books, clocks, calendars, and educational materials. e. Maintain room lighting that distinguishes day from night and that is free of shadows and glare.	1. To assist client with diminished sensory perception and because client safety is a nursing priority.

Table 34–2 | CARE PLAN FOR THE ELDERLY CLIENT–cont'd

OUTCOME CRITERIA	NURSING INTERVENTIONS	RATIONALE
	f. Teach client to scan the environment to locate objects.	
	g. Help client to locate food on plate using "clock" system, and describe food if client is unable to visualize; assist with feeding as needed.	
	h. Arrange physical environment to maximize functional vision.	
	i. Place personal items and call light within client's field of vision.	
	j. Teach client to watch the person who is speaking.	
	k. Reinforce wearing of hearing aid; if client does not have an aid, may consider a communication device (e.g., amplifier).	
	l. Communicate clearly, distinctly, and slowly, using a low-pitched voice and facing client; avoid overarticulation.	
	m. Remove as much unnecessary background noise as possible.	
	n. Do not use slang or extraneous words.	
	o. As speaker, position self at eye level and no farther than 6 feet away.	
	p. Get the client's attention before speaking.	
	q. Avoid speaking directly into the client's ear.	
	r. If the client does not understand what is being said, rephrase the statement rather than simply repeating it.	
	s. Help client select foods from the menu that will ensure discrimination between various tastes and smells.	
	t. Ensure that food has been properly cooled so that client with diminished pain threshold is not burned.	
	u. Ensure that bath or shower water is appropriate temperature.	
	v. Use backrubs and massage as therapeutic touch to stimulate sensory receptors.	

*The interventions for this nursing diagnosis were adapted from Rogers-Seidl, F.F. (1997). *Geriatric nursing care plans* (2nd ed.). St. Louis: Mosby Year Book.

BOX 34–2 Reminiscence Therapy and Life Review With the Elderly

Studies have indicated that *reminiscence,* or thinking about the past and reflecting on it, may promote better mental health in old age. *Life review* is related to reminiscence but differs in that it is a more guided or directed cognitive process that constructs a history or story in an autobiographical way (Murray et al., 2009).

Elderly individuals who spend time thinking about the past experience an increase in self-esteem and are less likely to suffer depression. Some psychologists believe that life review may help some people adjust to memories of an unhappy past. Others view reminiscence and life review as ways to bolster feelings of well-being, particularly in older people who can no longer remain active.

Reminiscence therapy can take place on a one-to-one basis or in a group setting. In reminiscence groups, elderly individuals share significant past events with peers. The nurse leader facilitates the discussion of topics that deal with specific life transitions, such as childhood, adolescence, marriage, childbearing, grandparenthood, and retirement. Members share both positive and negative aspects, including personal feelings, about these life cycle events.

Reminiscence on a one-to-one basis can provide a way for elderly individuals to work through unresolved issues from the past. Painful issues may be too difficult to discuss in the group setting. As the individual reviews his or her life process,

the nurse can validate feelings and help the elderly client come to terms with painful issues that may have been long suppressed. This process is necessary if the elderly individual is to maintain (or attain) a sense of positive identity and self-esteem and ultimately achieve the goal of ego integrity as described by Erikson (1963).

A number of creative measures can be used to facilitate life review with the elderly individual. Having the client keep a journal for sharing may be a way to stimulate discussion (as well as providing a permanent record of past events for significant others). Pets, music, and special foods have a way of provoking memories from the client's past. Photographs of family members and past significant events are an excellent way of guiding the elderly client through his or her autobiographical review.

Care must be taken in the life review to assist clients to work through unresolved issues. Anxiety, guilt, depression, and despair may result if the individual is unable to work through the problems and accept them. Life review can work in a negative way if the individual comes to believe that his or her life was meaningless. However, it can be a very positive experience for the person who can take pride in past accomplishments and feel satisfied with his or her life, resulting in a sense of serenity and inner peace in the older adult.

■ Can caregivers verbalize means of providing a safe environment for the client?

■ Does the client maintain reality orientation at an optimum for his or her cognitive functioning?

■ Can the client distinguish between reality-based and non-reality-based thinking?

■ Can caregivers verbalize ways in which to orient client to reality as needed?

■ Is the client able to accomplish self-care activities independently to his or her optimum level of functioning?

■ Does the client seek assistance for aspects of self-care that he or she is unable to perform independently?

■ Does the client express positive feelings about himself or herself?

■ Does the client reminisce about accomplishments that have occurred in his or her life?

■ Does the client express some hope for the future?

■ Does the client wear eyeglasses or a hearing aid if needed to compensate for sensory deficits?

■ Does the client consistently look others in the face to facilitate hearing when they are talking to him or her?

■ Does the client use helpful aids, such as signs identifying various rooms, to help maintain orientation?

■ Can the caregivers work through problems and make decisions regarding care of the elderly client?

■ Do the caregivers include the elderly client in the decision-making process, if appropriate?

■ Can the caregivers demonstrate adaptive coping strategies for dealing with the strain of long-term caregiving?

■ Are the caregivers open and honest in expression of feelings?

■ Can the caregivers verbalize community resources to which they can go for assistance with their caregiving responsibilities?

■ Have the caregivers joined a support group?

Summary and Key Points

■ Care of the aging individual presents one of the greatest challenges for nursing.

■ The growing population of individuals aged 65 and older suggests that the trend will progress well into the 21st century.

■ America is a youth-oriented society. It is not desirable to be old in mainstream American culture.

■ In some cultures, the elderly are revered and hold a special place of honor within the society, but in highly industrialized countries such as the

United States, status declines with the decrease in productivity and participation in the mainstream of society.

■ Individuals experience many changes as they age. Physical changes occur in virtually every body system.

■ Psychologically, there may be age-related memory deficiencies, particularly for recent events.

■ Intellectual functioning does not decline with age, but length of time required for learning increases.

■ Aging individuals experience many losses, potentially leading to bereavement overload. They are vulnerable to depression and to feelings of low self-worth.

■ The elderly population represents a disproportionately high percentage of individuals who die by suicide.

■ Neurocognitive disorders are the most frequent causes of psychopathology in the elderly. Sleep disorders are very common.

■ The need for sexual expression by the elderly is often misunderstood within our society. Although many physical changes occur at this time of life that alter an individual's sexuality, if he or she has reasonably good health and a willing partner, sexual activity can continue well past the 70s for most people.

■ Retirement has both social and economic implications for elderly individuals. Society often equates an individual's status with occupation, and loss of employment may result in the need for adjustment in the standard of living because retirement income may be reduced by 20 to 40 percent of preretirement earnings.

■ Less than 4 percent of the population aged 65 and older live in nursing homes. A profile of the typical elderly nursing home resident is a white woman about 80 years old, widowed, with multiple chronic health conditions. Much stigma is attached to what some still call "rest homes" or "old age homes," and many elderly people still equate them with a "place to go to die."

■ The strain of the caregiver role has become a major dilemma in our society. Elder abuse is sometimes inflicted by caregivers for whom the role has become overwhelming and intolerable. There is an intense need to find assistance for these people, who must provide care for their loved ones on a 24-hour basis. Home health care, respite care, support groups, and financial assistance are needed to ease the burden of this role strain.

■ Caring for elderly individuals requires a special kind of inner strength and compassion. The poem that follows conveys a vital message for nurses.

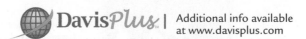

DavisPlus | Additional info available at www.davisplus.com

What Do You See, Nurse?

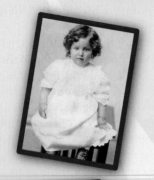

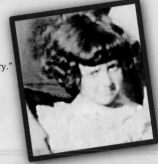

What do you see, nurse, what do you see?
　　What are you thinking when you look at me?
A crabbed old woman, not very wise.
　　Uncertain of habit, with faraway eyes.
Who dribbles her food and makes no reply
　　When you say in a loud voice, "I do wish you'd try."
Who seems not to notice the things that you do
　　And forever is losing a stocking or shoe.
Who unresisting or not, lets you do as you will
　　With bathing and feeding, the long day to fill.
Is that what you're thinking, is that what you see?
　　Then open your eyes, you're not looking at me.
I'll tell you who I am as I sit there so still.
　　As I move at your bidding, as I eat at your will.
I'm a small child of ten with a father and a mother,
　　Brothers and sisters who love one another.

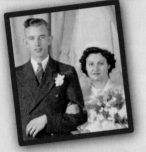

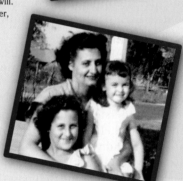

A young girl at sixteen with wings on her feet
　　Dreaming that soon now a lover she'll meet.
A bride soon at twenty—my heart gives a leap
　　Remembering the vows that I promised to keep.
At twenty-five, now, I have young of my own
　　Who need me to build a secure happy home.
A woman of thirty, my young now grow fast
　　Bound to each other with ties that should last.

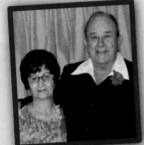

At forty my young will now soon be gone,
　　But my man stays beside me to see I don't mourn.
At fifty once more babies play round my knee.
　　Again we know children, my loved one and me.

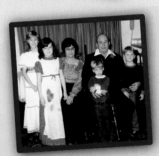

Dark days are upon me, my husband is dead.
　　I look at the future, I shudder with dread.
For my young are all busy rearing young of their own.
　　And I think of the years and the love I have known.

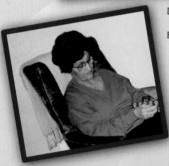

I'm an old woman now and nature is cruel.
　　Tis her jest to make old age look like a fool.
The body it crumbles, grace and vigor depart.
　　There is now just a stone where I once had a heart.
But inside this old carcass a young girl still dwells.
　　And now and again my battered heart swells.

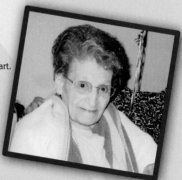

I remember the joys, I remember the pain.
　　And I'm loving and living life all over again.
I think of the years all too few—gone so fast.
　　And accept the stark fact that nothing can last.
So open your eyes, nurse, open and see.
　　Not a crabbed old woman—look closer—SEE ME.

Author Unknown

Review Questions
Self-Examination/Learning Exercise

Select the answer that is most appropriate for each of the following questions.

1. Stanley, age 72, is admitted to the hospital for depression. His son reports that he has periods of confusion and forgetfulness. In her admission assessment, the nurse notices an open sore on Stanley's arm. When she questions him about it, he says, "I scraped it on the fence two weeks ago. It's smaller than it was." How might the nurse analyze these data?
   a. Consider that Stanley may have been attempting self-harm.
   b. The delay in healing may indicate that Stanley has developed skin cancer.
   c. A diminished inflammatory response in the elderly increases healing time.
   d. Age-related skin changes and distribution of adipose tissue delay healing in the elderly.

2. What is the most appropriate way to communicate with an elderly person who is deaf in his right ear?
   a. Speak loudly into his left ear.
   b. Speak to him from a position on his left side.
   c. Speak face-to-face in a high-pitched voice.
   d. Speak face-to-face in a low-pitched voice.

3. Why is it important for the nurse to check the temperature of the water before an elderly individual gets into the shower?
   a. The client may catch a cold if the water temperature is too low.
   b. The client may burn himself because of a higher pain threshold.
   c. Elderly clients have difficulty discriminating between hot and cold.
   d. The water must be exactly 98.6°F.

4. Mr. B., age 79, is admitted to the psychiatric unit for depression. He has lost weight and become socially isolated. His wife died 5 years ago, and his son tells the nurse, "He did very well when Mom died. He didn't even cry." Which would be the priority nursing diagnosis for Mr. B.?
   a. Complicated grieving
   b. Imbalanced nutrition: less than body requirements
   c. Social isolation
   d. Risk for injury

5. Mr. B., age 79, is admitted to the psychiatric unit for depression. He has lost weight and has become socially isolated. His wife died 5 years ago, and he lives alone. A suicide assessment is conducted. Why is Mr. B. at high risk for suicide?
   a. All depressed people are at high risk for suicide.
   b. Mr. B. is in the age group in which the highest percentage of suicides occur.
   c. Mr. B. is a white man, recently bereaved, living alone.
   d. His son reports that Mr. B. owns a gun.

6. Mr. B., age 79, is admitted to the psychiatric unit for depression. He has lost weight and has become socially isolated. His wife died 5 years ago, and his son tells the nurse, "He did very well when Mom died. He didn't even cry." Which would be the priority nursing intervention for Mr. B.?
   a. Take blood pressure once each shift.
   b. Ensure that Mr. B. attends group activities.
   c. Encourage Mr. B. to eat all of the food on his food tray.
   d. Encourage Mr. B. to talk about his wife's death.

7. In group exercise, Mr. B., a 79-year-old man with major depression, becomes tired and short of breath very quickly. This is most likely due to:
   a. Age-related changes in the cardiovascular system.
   b. A sedentary lifestyle.
   c. The effects of pathological depression.
   d. Medication the physician has prescribed for depression.

Continued

Review Questions—cont'd
Self-Examination/Learning Exercise

8. Clara, an 80-year-old woman, says to the nurse, "I'm all alone now. My husband is gone. My best friend is gone. My daughter is busy with her work and family. I might as well just go, too." Which is the best response by the nurse?
   a. "Are you thinking that you want to die, Clara?"
   b. "You have lots to live for, Clara."
   c. "Cheer up, Clara. You have so much to be thankful for."
   d. "Tell me about your family, Clara."

9. An elderly client says to the nurse, "I don't want to go to that crafts class. I'm too old to learn anything." Based on knowledge of the aging process, which of the following is a true statement?
   a. Memory functioning in the elderly most likely reflects loss of long-term memories of remote events.
   b. Intellectual functioning declines with advancing age.
   c. Learning ability remains intact, but time required for learning increases with age.
   d. Cognitive functioning is rarely affected in aging individuals.

10. According to the literature, which of the following is most important for individuals to maintain a healthy, adaptive old age?
    a. To remain socially interactive
    b. To disengage slowly in preparation of the last stage of life
    c. To move in with family
    d. To maintain total independence and accept no help from anyone

IMPLICATIONS OF RESEARCH FOR EVIDENCE-BASED PRACTICE

Turvey, C.L., Conwell, Y., Jones, M.P., Phillips, C., Simonsick, E., Pearson, J.L., & Wallace, R. (2002). Risk factors for late-life suicide: A prospective, community-based study. *American Journal of Geriatric Psychiatry, 10*(4), 398-406. doi:10.1097/00019442-200207000-00006

DESCRIPTION OF THE STUDY: Studies have suggested that a negative or depressive mental outlook, being widowed or divorced, sleeping more than 9 hours per day, and drinking more than three alcoholic beverages per day are risk factors for late-life suicide. The primary aim of this study was to examine the relationship between completed suicide in late life and physical health, disability, and social support. The participants were 14,456 individuals selected from a general population of elderly subjects age 65 and older. Control subjects were a group of 420 individuals who were matched by age and sex. This 10-year longitudinal study began in 1981. Variables were assessed at baseline, year 3, and year 6, with a 10-year mortality follow-up. Baseline variables included sleep quality, social support, alcohol use, medical illness, physical impairment, cognitive impairment, and depressive symptoms.

RESULTS OF THE STUDY: The 10-year mortality follow-up indicated that 75 percent of the control subjects had died, but none had died from suicide. Twenty-one of the

14,456 participants died by suicide within the follow-up period. Twenty of the 21 suicide victims were male. Average age was 78.6 years, with a range from 67 to 90 years. The most common means was gunshot. Other means included hanging, cutting, overdose, drowning, and carbon monoxide inhalation, and one participant jumped to his death. In this study, presence of friends or relatives to confide in was negatively associated with suicide. Likewise, regular church attendance was more common in control subjects than in the participant sample, indicating an even wider range of community support. Those who died by suicide had reported more depressive symptoms than those who did not, but they did not consume more alcohol (inconsistent with previous studies). Poor sleep quality was positively correlated with suicide in this study, but no specific physical illness was identified as a predisposition. The authors identify the small suicide sample as a limitation of this study.

IMPLICATIONS FOR NURSING PRACTICE: This study identified depression, poor sleep quality, and limited social support as important variables in the potential for elderly suicide. Sleep disturbance may be an important indicator of depression, whereas limited social support may be a contributing factor. The study provides reinforcement for the U.S. Department of Health and Human Services (USDHHS) recommendation

IMPLICATIONS OF RESEARCH FOR EVIDENCE-BASED PRACTICE—cont'd

in *National Strategy for Suicide Prevention: Goals and Objectives for Action* (2001). The USDHHS recommends detection and treatment of depression as a strategy to prevent late-life suicide. The authors stated, "Because both depression and social support are amenable to intervention, this study provides further evidence for the possible

effectiveness of such strategies to reduce suicides among older adults." Nurses can become actively involved in assessing for these risk factors, as well as planning, implementing, and evaluating the effectiveness of strategies for preventing suicide in the elderly population.

IMPLICATIONS OF RESEARCH FOR EVIDENCE-BASED PRACTICE

Jeste, D.V., Savla, G.N., Thompson, W.K., Vahia, I.V., Glorioso, D.K., Martin, A.S., . . . Kraemer, H.C. (2013). Association between older age and successful aging: Critical role of resilience and depression. *American Journal of Psychiatry, 170*(2), 188-196. doi:10.1176/appi.ajp.2012. 12030386

DESCRIPTION OF THE STUDY: This study was a Successful AGing Evaluation (SAGE) study of 1,006 community-dwelling adults between 55 and 99 years of age. The mean age of respondents was 77.3 years of age. Telephone interviews were conducted for 25 minutes followed by a comprehensive mail-in survey in which physical, cognitive, and psychological domains were assessed. In addition, participants completed a self-reported rating of successful aging.

RESULTS OF THE STUDY: Contrary to the researchers' hypothesis, older age was associated with higher reported ratings of successful aging in spite of worsening physical and cognitive functions. The two factors contributing most to successful aging were higher scores on resilience and lower scores on depression. These were similar in strength to physical disability as an influential factor in successful aging. The authors identify, therefore, that interventions

focused on increasing resilience and decreasing depression might be factors as strong as decreasing physical disability in contributing to successful aging. They add that the study highlighted the benefits of self-measurement tools. This is supported by the fact that when people were asked about their own perceptions, information was revealed that was contrary to what was expected.

IMPLICATIONS FOR NURSING PRACTICE: First, this study underscores the importance of thorough assessment to rule out depression in the elderly and to initiate intervention as soon as possible when it is identified. Historically, depression has been underrecognized and undertreated in this population, and we are learning that reducing depression may have a significant impact on successful aging. Second, nurses can play an active role in assessing, educating, and initiating other interventions to promote resilience in the elderly. Finally, as the authors suggest, using self-reporting measures provides a valuable tool for identifying the abilities and needs of this population. Stated more simply, when health-care providers listen to what the client has to say, there is much to be learned and it lays the foundation for patient-centered care.

TEST YOUR CRITICAL THINKING SKILLS

Mrs. M., age 76, is seeing her primary physician for her regular 6-month physical examination. Mrs. M.'s husband died 2 years ago, at which time she sold her home in Kansas and came to live in California with her only child, a daughter. The daughter is married and has three children (one in college and two teenagers at home). The daughter reports that her mother is becoming increasingly withdrawn, stays in her room, and eats very little. She has lost 13 pounds since her last 6-month visit. The primary physician refers Mrs. M. to a psychiatrist, who hospitalizes her for evaluation. He diagnoses Mrs. M. with major depressive disorder.

Mrs. M. tells the nurse, "I didn't want to leave my home, but my daughter insisted. I would have been all right. I miss my friends and my church. Back home I drove my car everywhere. But there's too

much traffic out here. They sold my car and I have to depend on my daughter or grandkids to take me places. I hate being so dependent! I miss my husband so much. I just sit and think about him and our past life all the time. I don't have any interest in meeting new people. I want to go home!"

Mrs. M. admits to having some thoughts of dying, although she denies feeling suicidal. She denies having a plan or means for taking her life. "I really don't want to die, but I just can't see much reason for living. My daughter and her family are so busy with their own lives. They don't need me—or even have time for me!"

Answer the following questions about Mrs. M.:

1. What would be the *primary* nursing diagnosis for Mrs. M.?
2. Formulate a short-term goal for Mrs. M.
3. From the assessment data, identify the major problem that may be a long-term focus of care for Mrs. M.

MOVIE CONNECTIONS

The Hiding Place • *On Golden Pond* • *To Dance With the White Dog*

References

American Foundation for Suicide Prevention. (2016). Facts and figures. Retrieved from www.afsp.org/understanding-suicide/facts-and-figures

Administration on Aging. (2016). Profile of older Americans: 2016. Retrieved from https://www.giaging.org/documents/A_Profile_of_Older_Americans__2016.pdf

American Association of Retired Persons (AARP). (2010). *Sex, romance, and relationships: AARP survey of midlife and older adults.* Washington, DC: AARP.

Beers, M.H., & Jones, T.V. (Eds.). (2006). *The Merck Manual of Health & Aging.* New York, NY: Ballantine Books

Blair, K. (2012). Assessing the older adult: What's different? In J.W. Lange (Ed.), *The nurse's role in promoting optimal health of older adults* (pp. 149-160). Philadelphia: F.A. Davis.

Blevins, N.H. (2015). Presbycusis. *Wolters Kluwer Health.* Retrieved from www.uptodate.com/contents/presbycusis.

Cahill, K.E., Giandrea, M.D., & Quinn, J.F. (2011). Reentering the labor force after retirement. *Monthly Labor Review, 134*(6), 34-42.

Centers for Disease Control and Prevention. (2015). Depression is not a normal part of growing older. Retrieved from www.cdc.gov/aging/mentalhealth/depression.htm

Crowley, K. (2011). Sleep and sleep disorders in older adults. *Neuropsychology Review, 21*(1), 41-53. doi:10.1007/s11065-010-9154-6

Guarente, L.P. (2016). Aging: Life process. Retrieved from www.britannica.com/science/aging-life-process

Heiss, G., Wallace, R., Anderson, G.L., Aragak, A., Beresford, S.A.A., Brzyski, R., . . . Stefanick, M.L. (2008). Health risks and benefits three years after stopping randomized treatment with estrogen and progestin. *Journal of the American Medical Association, 299*(9), 1036-1045. doi:10.1001/jama.299.9.1036

Hipple, S.F. (2015). People who are not in the labor force: Why aren't they working?, *Numbers, 4*(15). Retrieved from www.bls.gov/opub/btn/volume-4/people-who-are-not-in-the-labor-force-why-arent-they-working.htm

Issa, J.P. (2014). Aging and epigenetic drift: A vicious cycle. *Journal of Clinical Investigation, 124*(1), 24-29. doi:10.1172/JCI69735

Jeste, D.V., Savla, G.N., Thompson, W.K., Vahia, I.V., Glorioso, D.K., Martin, A.S., . . . Kraemer, H.C. (2013). Association between older age and successful aging: Critical role of resilience and depression. *American Journal of Psychiatry, 170*(2), 188-196. doi:10.1176/appi.ajp.2012. 12030386

Johnston, C.B., Harper, G.M., & Landefeld, C.S. (2013). Geriatric disorders. In S.J. McPhee & M.A. Papadakis (Eds.), *Current medical diagnosis and treatment* (pp. 57-73). New York: McGraw Hill Medical.

Kern, M.L., & Friedman, H.S. (2008). Do conscientious individuals live longer? A quantitative review. *Health Psychology, 27*(5), 505-512. doi:10.1037/0278-6133.27.5.505.

King, B.M., & Regan, P.(2013). *Human sexuality today* (8th ed.). Upper Saddle River, NJ: Pearson Prentice Hall.

Koop, P.M. (2012). Older adults as caregivers and care recipients. In J.W. Lange (Ed.), *The nurse's role in promoting optimal health of older adults* (pp. 295-305). Philadelphia: F.A. Davis.

Lang, R. (2012). Challenges to mental wellness. In J.W. Lange (Ed.), *The nurse's role in promoting optimal health of older adults* (pp. 339-370). Philadelphia: F.A. Davis.

Lehto, R.H. & Stein, K. I. (2009). Death anxiety: An analysis of an evolving concept. *Research and Theory for Nursing Practice, 23*(1), 23-41. doi:10.1891/1541-6577.23.1.23

Manson, A.E., Chlebowski, R.T., Stefanick, M.L., Aragaki, A.K., Rossouw, J.E., Prentice, R.L., . . . Wallace, R.B. (2013). Menopausal hormone therapy and health outcomes during the intervention and extended poststopping phases of the women's health initiative randomized trials. *Journal of the American Medical Association, 310*(13), 1353-1368. doi:10.1001/jama.2013.278040

McCarthy, V.L., & Bockweg, M. (2012). The role of transcendence in a holistic view of successful aging: A concept analysis and model of transcendence in maturation and aging. *Journal of Holistic Nursing, 31*(2), 84-92. doi:10.1177/0898010112463492

McCarthy, V.L., Ling, J., & Carini, R.M. (2013). The role of self-transcendence: A missing variable in the pursuit of successful aging? *Research in Gerontological Nursing, 6*(3), 178-186. doi:10.3928/19404921-20130508-01

McClatchey, I.S., & King, S. (2015). The impact of death education on fear of death and death anxiety among human services students. *Omega(Westport), 71*(4), 343-361. doi:10.1177/0030222815572606

MedlinePlus. (2014). Aging changes in the senses. Retrieved from https://www.nlm.nih.gov/medlineplus/ency/article/004013.htm

Missler, M., Stroebe, M., Geurtsen, L., Mastenbroek, M., Chmoun, S., & van der Houwen, K. (2012). Exploring death anxiety among elderly people: A literature review and empirical investigation. *Omega (Westport), 64*(4), 357-379. doi:10.2190/OM.64.4.e

Murray, R.B., Zentner, J.P., & Yakimo, R. (2009). *Health promotion strategies through the life span* (8th ed.). Upper Saddle River, NJ: Prentice Hall.

National Center for Health Statistics. (2016). Health, United States, 2015: With special feature on racial and ethnic health disparities. Retrieved from www.cdc.gov/nchs/data/hus/hus15.pdf#015

National Institutes of Health. (2014). Aging changes in immunity. Retrieved from https://www.nlm.nih.gov/medlineplus/ency/article/004008.htm

National Institute on Aging. (2016). Sexuality in later life. Retrieved from https://www.nia.nih.gov/health/publication/sexuality-later-life

Purnell, L.D. (2013). *Transcultural health care: A culturally competent approach* (4th ed.). Philadelphia: F.A. Davis.

Roepke, I.S., & Ancoli-Israel, S. (2010). Sleep disorders in the elderly. *Indian Journal of Medical Research, 131*(2), 302-310.

Sadock, B.J., Sadock, V.A., & Ruiz, P. (2015). *Synopsis of psychiatry: Behavioral sciences/clinical psychiatry* (11th ed.). Philadelphia: Lippincott Williams & Wilkins.

Shock, N.W. (2015). Human aging: Physiology and sociology. Retrieved www.britannica.com/science/human-aging

Srivastava, S., & Das, R.C. (2013). Personality pathways of successful ageing. *Industrial Psychiatry Journal, 22*(1), 1-3. doi:10.4103/0972-6748.123584

Srivastava, S., John, O.P., Gosling, S.D., & Potter, J. (2003). Development of personality in early and middle adulthood: Set like plaster or persistent change? *Journal of Personality and Social Psychology, 84*(5), 1041-1053. doi:10.1037/0022-3514.84.5.1041

Stark, S. (2012). Elder abuse: Screening, intervention, and prevention. *Nursing 2012, 42*(10), 24-29. doi:10.1097/01.NURSE.0000421438.66790.c8

Terracciano, A., Sanna, S., Uda, M., Deiana, B., Usala, G., Busonero, F., . . . Costa, P.T. (2010). Genome-wide association scan for five major dimensions of personality. *Molecular Psychiatry, 15*(6), 647-656. doi:10.1038/mp.2008.113

Thomas, P.A. (2011). Trajectories of social engagement and limitations in late life. *Journal of Health and Social Behavior, 52*(4), 430-443. doi:10.1177/0022146511411922

Turvey, C.L., Conwell, Y., Jones, M.P., Phillips, C., Simonsick, E., Pearson, J.L., & Wallace, R. (2002). Risk factors for late-life suicide: A prospective, community-based study. *American Journal of Geriatric Psychiatry, 10*(4), 398-406. doi:10.1097/00019442-200207000-00006

Ward, D. (2015). Neuroendocrine theory of aging: Chapter 1. Retrieved from http://warddeanmd.com/articles/neuroendocrine-theory-of-aging-chapter-1

Westerhof, G.J., Whitbourne, S.K., & Freeman, J.P. (2012). The aging self in a cultural context: The relation of conceptions of aging to identity processes and self-esteem in the United States and the Netherlands. *The Journals of Gerontology. Series B, Psychological Sciences and Social Sciences, 67B*(1), 52-56. doi:10.1093/geronb/gbr075

Venes, D. (Ed.). (2014). *Taber's cyclopedic medical dictionary.* Philadelphia, PA: F.A. Davis.

Yang, X., & Reckelhoff, J.F. (2011). Estrogen, hormonal replacement therapy and cardiovascular disease. *Current Opinion in Nephrology and Hypertension, 20*(2), 133-138. doi:10.1097/MNH.0b013e3283431921

Classical References

Erikson, E.H. (1963). *Childhood and society* (2nd ed.). New York: WW Norton.

Erikson, E.H., & Erikson, J.M. (1997). *The life cycle completed: Extended version with new chapters on the ninth stage of development.* New York: WW Norton.

Kübler-Ross, E. (1969). *On death and dying.* New York: Macmillan.

Masters, W.H., Johnson, V.E., & Kolodny, R.C. (1995). *Human sexuality* (5th ed.). New York: Addison-Wesley Longman.

Roberts, C.M. (1991). *How did I get here so fast?* New York: Warner Books.

Rogers-Seidl, F.F. (1997). *Geriatric nursing care plans* (2nd ed.). St. Louis: Mosby Year.

Rowe, J.W., & Kahn, R.L. (1997). Successful aging. *Gerontology, 37*(4), 433-440. doi:10.1093/geront/37.4.433

35

Survivors of Abuse or Neglect

CHAPTER OUTLINE

KEY TERMS

acquaintance rape

child sexual abuse

compounded rape reaction

controlled response pattern

cycle of battering

date rape

emotional abuse

emotional neglect

expressed response pattern

intimate partner violence

marital rape

physical neglect

rape trauma syndrome

safe house or shelter

sexual exploitation of a child

silent rape reaction

statutory rape

OBJECTIVES
After reading this chapter, the student will be able to:

1. Describe epidemiological statistics associated with intimate partner violence, child abuse, and sexual assault.
2. Discuss characteristics of victims and victimizers.
3. Identify predisposing factors to abusive behaviors.
4. Describe physical and psychological effects on the survivors of intimate partner violence, child abuse, and sexual assault.

5. Identify nursing diagnoses, goals of care, and appropriate nursing interventions for care of survivors of intimate partner violence, child abuse, and sexual assault.
6. Evaluate nursing care of survivors of intimate partner violence, child abuse, and sexual assault.
7. Discuss modalities relevant to treatment of survivors of abuse.

HOMEWORK ASSIGNMENT
Please read the chapter and answer the following questions:

1. What neurotransmitters have been implicated in the etiology of aggression and violence?
2. What is the most common reason that women give for staying in an abusive relationship?

3. Describe a compounded rape reaction.
4. What are some adult manifestations of childhood sexual abuse?

Abuse is a significant and frightening public health problem. Books, newspapers, movies, and television inundate their readers and viewers with stories of "man's inhumanity to man" (no gender bias intended).

More than 1 in 3 women (35.6%) and more than 1 in 4 men (28%) experience rape, physical violence, and/or stalking by an intimate partner during their lives (Centers for Disease Control and Prevention [CDC], 2016a).

Rape is vastly underreported in the United States. Because many of these attacks go unreported and unrecognized, sexual assault is often considered a silent, violent epidemic. In the United States, 1 in 5 women and 1 in 71 men report having been raped at some time in their lives (CDC, 2016b). The CDC also reports that rape often occurs before 25 years of age; 42 percent of reported rapes occurred before 18 years of age. This crime is often committed by someone known to the victim.

Child abuse and related fatalities continue to be a significant health concern, although most recent statistics identify an overall decline for the period from 2009 to 2013 (U.S. Department of Health and Human Services [USDHHS], 2015). During the same time period, the number of children seen by child protective services agencies has increased. Public awareness, better screening tools with differential response systems, and funding for prevention programs have all been identified as possible contributing factors for changes in these current trends. Based on the 2013 statistics (USDHHS, 2015), 9.1 in 1,000 children (679,000) were victimized; 79.5 percent of those were neglected, 18 percent were physically abused, 9 percent were sexually abused, and 8.7 percent were victims of psychological maltreatment. Human trafficking, which includes sex trafficking, is defined by federal law as "a commercial sex act [that] is induced by force, fraud, or coercion, or in which the person induced to perform such act has not attained 18 years of age" (U.S. Department of Education, 2013). Prevalence statistics are difficult to compile, but sex trafficking of children has been reported in all 50 U.S. states, and traffickers have been known to prey on children as young as 9 years of age. An estimated 1,520 children died from causes related to abuse or neglect in 2013.

Elder abuse and neglect is also a significant problem. The CDC (2016c) estimates that 1 in 10 people older than age 60 and living at home are victims of abuse, neglect, and/or financial exploitation. There is general agreement that these statistics underestimate the scope of the problem. Despite mandatory reporting laws in most states and the recent trend toward more reporting of abuse, adult protective services vary markedly among states. One study found that for every case that came to the attention of these agencies, 24 had not been reported (National Center on Elder Abuse, 2015).

Abuse affects all populations equally. It occurs among all races, religions, economic classes, ages, and educational backgrounds. The phenomenon is cyclical in that many abusers were themselves victims of abuse as children.

Family violence is not a new problem; in fact, it is probably as old as humankind and has been documented as far back as biblical times. Child abuse became a mandatory reportable occurrence in the United States in 1968. Responsibility for the protection of elders from abuse rests primarily with the states. In 1987, Congress passed amendments to the Older Americans Act of 1965 that provide for state Area Agencies on Aging to assess the need for elder abuse prevention services. These laws have made it possible for individuals who once felt powerless to stop the abuse against them to come forward and seek advice, support, and protection.

This chapter discusses intimate partner violence, child abuse (including neglect), and sexual violence. Elder abuse is discussed in more detail in Chapter 34, The Aging Individual. Factors that predispose individuals to commit acts of abuse against others, as well as the physical and psychological effects on the survivors, are examined.

Nursing of individuals who have experienced abusive behavior from others is presented within the context of the nursing process. Various treatment modalities are described.

Predisposing Factors

What predisposes individuals to be abusive? Although no one really knows for sure, several theories have been espoused. As researchers have sought to better understand aggression and violence, two distinct forms of aggression have been identified: reactive aggression, which is associated with impulsivity and is more common among people who have a history of being abused, and proactive aggression, which is initiated rather than provoked and is more common in psychopathy (Rosell & Siever, 2015). Most research is associated with reactive aggression. The following is a brief discussion of current evidence associated with biological, psychological, and sociocultural influences.

Biological Theories

Neurophysiological Influences

Research demonstrates consistently that lower amygdala volume plays a role in aggression (Rosell & Siever, 2015). The amygdala, which is responsible for impulse control and affective processing, appears to be less well modulated in people with aggression, and responses to fear are reduced. The limbic prefrontal cortex also has a primary role in aggression; smaller volumes of left-sided gray matter and greater right-sided volume have been noted in people with aggressive traits. Evidence has also demonstrated lowered connectivity between the amygdala and the prefrontal cortex as associated with increased aggression. The striatum, an area of the brain that plays a critical role in selection and inhibition of affective, cognitive, and motor responses, has been identified as dysfunctional in aggression (Rosell & Siever, 2015).

Biochemical Influences

Studies have associated increased dopamine release with aggression, and low levels of striatal serotonin have been associated with increases in impulsivity and aggression (Rosell & Siever, 2015). Evidence supports that high plasma (and low cerebrospinal fluid) concentrations of 5-hydroxyindoleacetic acid (5-HIAA) serotonin are associated with aggression (Sadock, Sadock, & Ruiz, 2015). Finally, research shows that a complex interaction between testosterone and cortisol levels is associated with aggression (Batrinos, 2012). Research is ongoing to explore these mechanisms, their interactions in the brain, and the influence of environmental factors. An explanation of these biochemical influences on violent behavior is presented in Figure 35–1.

Genetic Influences

Various genetic components related to aggressive behavior have been investigated. Studies have found a potential role for the X-linked monoamine oxidase A gene in the etiology of antisocial behaviors (Sadock et al., 2015). This gene may have implications for impulsivity and aggression, but further research is needed. Human and animal genetics studies show a strong role for 5-hydroxytryptamine (5-HT) transporter genes in aggression.

Disorders of the Brain

Organic brain syndromes associated with various cerebral disorders have been implicated in the predisposition to aggressive and violent behavior (Sadock et al., 2015). Brain tumors, particularly in the areas of the limbic system and the temporal lobes; trauma to the brain, resulting in cerebral changes; and diseases, such as encephalitis (or medications that may affect this syndrome) and epilepsy, particularly temporal lobe epilepsy, have all been implicated.

Psychological Theories

Psychodynamic Theory

The psychodynamic theorists imply that unmet needs for satisfaction and security result in an underdeveloped ego and a weak superego. It is thought that when frustration occurs, aggression and violence supply this individual with a dose of power and prestige that boosts self-image and validates a significance to his or her life that is lacking. The immature ego cannot prevent dominant id behaviors from occurring, and the weak superego is unable to produce feelings of guilt.

Learning Theory

Children learn to behave by imitating their role models, usually their parents. Models are more likely to be imitated when they are perceived as prestigious or influential or when the behavior is followed by positive reinforcement. Children may have an idealistic perception of their parents during the very early developmental stages, but as they mature, they often begin to imitate the behavior patterns of their teachers, friends, and others. Individuals who were abused as children or who witnessed domestic violence as a child are more likely to manifest reactive aggression as adults (Rosell & Siever, 2015).

Adults and children alike model many behaviors after individuals they observe on television and in movies. Unfortunately, modeling can result in maladaptive as well as adaptive behavior, particularly when children view heroes triumphing over villains by using violence. Individuals who have a biological predisposition toward aggressive behavior may be more susceptible to negative role modeling.

Sociocultural Theories

Societal Influences

Although they agree that biological and psychological aspects are influential, social scientists believe that aggressive behavior is primarily a product of one's culture and social structure.

American society essentially was founded on a general acceptance of violence as a means of solving problems. The concept of relative deprivation (lack of necessities for life in comparison to another individual or group) has been shown to have a profound effect on collective violence within a society. Poverty, prolonged unemployment, family breakdown, and exposure to violence in the community and in the family have all been linked to increases in aggression (American Psychological Association, 2016; Sullivan, 2009).

One's culture also influences the manner in which violence and aggression is expressed; in American culture, violence is more often expressed in physical aggression, and in Japanese culture,

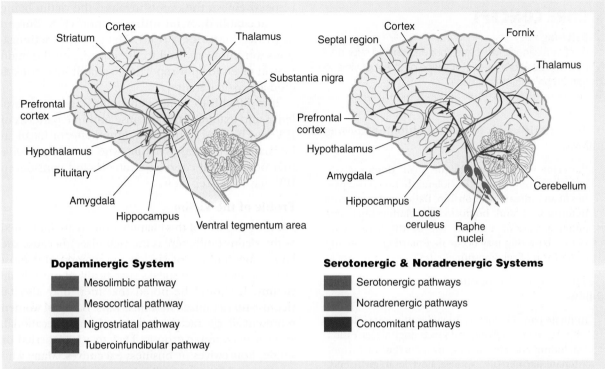

FIGURE 35–1 Neurobiology of violence.

NEUROTRANSMITTERS

Neurotransmitters that have been implicated in the etiology of aggression and violence include decreases in striatal serotonin and increases in norepinephrine and dopamine.

ASSOCIATED AREAS OF THE BRAIN

• Limbic structures: Emotional alterations
• Prefrontal and frontal cortices: Modulation of social judgment
• Amygdala: Anxiety, rage, fear
• Hypothalamus: Stimulates sympathetic nervous system in fight-or-flight response
• Hippocampus: Learning and memory

MEDICATIONS USED TO MODULATE AGGRESSION

1. Studies have suggested that selective serotonin reuptake inhibitors (SSRIs) may reduce irritability and aggression consistent with the hypothesis of reduced serotonergic activity in aggression.
2. Mood stabilizers that dampen limbic irritability may be important in reducing the susceptibility to react to provocation or threatening stimuli by overactivation of limbic system structures such as the amygdala (Rosell & Siever, 2015). Carbamazepine (Tegretol), phenytoin (Dilantin), and divalproex sodium (Depakote) have yielded positive results. Lithium has also been used effectively in violent individuals (Schatzberg, Cole, & DeBattista, 2015).
3. Antiadrenergic agents such as beta blockers (e.g., propranolol) have been shown to reduce aggression in some individuals, presumably by dampening excessive noradrenergic activity (Schatzberg et al., 2015).
4. In their ability to modulate excessive dopaminergic activity, antipsychotics—both typical and atypical—have been helpful in the control of aggression and violence, particularly in individuals with comorbid psychosis.

aggression is expressed more often by verbal means (Sullivan, 2009).

Application of the Nursing Process

Background Assessment Data

Data related to **intimate partner violence,** child abuse and neglect, and sexual assault are presented in this section. Characteristics of both victim and abuser are addressed. This information may be used as background knowledge in designing plans of care for these clients.

Intimate Partner Violence

Various terms are used to describe the pattern of violence between intimate partners, including intimate partner violence (IPV), domestic violence, and battering.

CORE CONCEPT
Battering
A pattern of coercive control founded on and supported by physical and/or sexual violence or threat of violence toward an intimate partner.

Tracy (2016) adds to the definition of *battering* as follows:

Battering is also known by the term "domestic violence" and refers to acts of violence between two parties in an intimate relationship. Battering happens in heterosexual and homosexual relationships and either a male or a female can be the batterer or victim. Battering may occur in a marriage or in any other form of relationship.

The CDC (2015) defines *intimate partner violence* as follows:

Intimate partner violence includes physical violence, sexual violence, stalking and psychological aggression (including coercive tactics) by a current or former intimate partner (i.e., spouse, boyfriend/girlfriend, dating partner, or ongoing sexual partner). An intimate partner is a person with whom one has a close personal relationship that may be characterized by the partners' emotional connectedness, regular contact, ongoing physical contact and sexual behavior, identity as a couple, and familiarity and knowledge about each other's lives. The relationship need not involve all of these dimensions.

The U.S. Department of Justice (2012) defines *intimate partner violence* as:

A pattern of abusive behavior that is used by an intimate partner to gain or maintain power and control over the other intimate partner. [Intimate partner] violence can be physical, sexual, emotional, economic, or psychological actions or threats of actions that influence another person. This includes any behaviors that intimidate, manipulate, humiliate, isolate, frighten, terrorize, coerce, threaten, blame, hurt, injure, or wound someone.

Physical abuse between domestic partners may be known as spousal abuse, domestic or family violence, wife or husband battering, or IPV. Data from the U.S. Bureau of Justice Statistics (2012) reflect that over the period from 1993 to 2010, 82 percent of victims of intimate partner violence were women, women aged 25 to 34 experienced the highest per capita rates of intimate violence, and intimate partners committed 2 percent of the nonfatal violence against men. Two-thirds of IPV events for both men and women involved physical attack, 8 percent of IPV events for women involved sexual violence, and between 4 percent and 8 percent (for women and men

respectively) of the events involved the victim being shot at, stabbed, or hit with a weapon (U.S. Bureau of Justice Statistics, 2014a). Many of the victimizations were not reported to the police, and the main reason given for not reporting is that it was "considered a personal matter."

It is difficult to completely understand the prevalence and extent of IPV because multiple patterns of IPV may be used to threaten, intimidate, or harm an intimate partner, and victims who do not perceive that nonphysical coercive strategies are considered IPV may never report it.

Profile of the Victim

For the purposes of this chapter, women are identified as the victim (and men as the victimizer) because the largest percentage of victims are women and most of the available data speaks specifically about female victims. It should be noted that men may also be victims and victimized in similar ways. Battered women represent all age, racial, religious, cultural, educational, and socioeconomic groups. They may be married or single, housewives or business executives. Many who are battered have low self-esteem, commonly adhere to feminine sex-role stereotypes, and often accept the blame for the batterer's actions. Feelings of guilt, anger, fear, and shame are common. They may be isolated from family and support systems.

Some women in violent relationships grew up in abusive homes and may have left those homes, even gotten married, at a very young age in order to escape the abuse. The battered woman views her relationship as male dominant, and as the battering continues, her ability to see the options available and make decisions concerning her life (and possibly those of her children) decreases. The phenomenon of *learned helplessness* may be applied to the woman's progressing inability to act on her own behalf. Learned helplessness occurs when an individual comes to understand that regardless of his or her behavior, the outcome is unpredictable and usually undesirable.

Profile of the Victimizer

Men who batter usually are characterized as persons with low self-esteem. Pathologically jealous, they present a "dual personality," one to the partner and one to the rest of the world (Meskill & Conner, 2013). They are often under a great deal of stress with which they have a limited ability to cope. The typical abuser is very possessive and perceives his spouse as a possession. He becomes threatened when she shows any sign of independence or attempts to share herself and her time with others. Small children are often ignored by the abuser; however, they may also become the targets of abuse as they grow older, particularly if they attempt to protect their mother from abuse. The abuser also may use threats of taking the children away as a tactic of emotional abuse.

The abusing man typically wages a continuous campaign of degradation against his female partner. He insults and humiliates her and everything she does at every opportunity. He strives to keep her isolated from others and totally dependent on him. He demands to know where she is at every moment, and when she tells him, he challenges her honesty. He achieves power and control through intimidation.

The Cycle of Battering

In her classic studies of battered women and their relationships, Walker (1979) identified a cycle of predictable behaviors that are repeated over time. The behaviors can be divided into three distinct phases that vary in time and intensity both within the same relationship and among different couples. Figure 35–2 depicts a graphic representation of the **cycle of battering.**

Phase I. The Tension-Building Phase During this phase, the woman senses that the man's tolerance for frustration is declining. He becomes angry with little provocation, but after lashing out at her may be quick to apologize. The woman may become very nurturing and compliant, anticipating his every whim in an effort to prevent his anger from escalating. She may just try to stay out of his way.

Minor battering incidents may occur during this phase, and in a desperate effort to avoid more serious confrontations, the woman accepts the abuse as legitimately directed toward her. She denies her anger and rationalizes his behavior (e.g., "I need to do better," "He's under so much stress at work," "It's the alcohol. If only he didn't drink"). She assumes the guilt for the abuse, even reasoning that perhaps she *did* deserve the abuse, just as her aggressor suggests.

The minor battering incidents continue, and the tension mounts as the woman waits for the impending explosion. The abuser begins to fear that his partner will leave him. His jealousy and possessiveness increase, and he uses threats and brutality to keep her in his captivity. Battering incidents become more intense, after which the woman becomes less and less psychologically capable of restoring equilibrium. She withdraws from him, which he misinterprets as rejection, further escalating his anger toward her. Phase I may last from a few weeks to many months or even years.

Phase II. The Acute Battering Incident This phase is the most violent and the shortest, usually lasting up to 24 hours. It most often begins with the batterer justifying his behavior to himself. By the end of the incident, however, he cannot understand what has happened, only that in his rage he has lost control over his behavior.

This incident may begin with the batterer wanting to "just teach her a lesson." In some instances, the woman may intentionally provoke the behavior. Having come to a point in phase I in which the tension is unbearable, long-term battered women know that once the acute phase is behind them, things will be better.

During phase II, women feel their only option is to find a safe place to hide from the batterer. The beating is severe, and many women can describe the violence in great detail, almost as if dissociation from their bodies had occurred. The batterer generally minimizes the severity of the abuse. Help is usually sought only in the event of severe injury or if the woman fears for her life or those of her children.

Phase III. Calm, Loving, Respite ("Honeymoon") Phase In this phase, the batterer becomes extremely loving, kind, and contrite. He promises that the abuse will never recur and begs her forgiveness. He is afraid she will leave him and uses every bit of charm he can muster to ensure this does not happen. He believes he can now control his behavior, and because he has "taught her a lesson," he believes she will not "act up" again.

He plays on her feelings of guilt, and she desperately wants to believe him. She wants to believe that he *can* change and that she will no longer have to suffer abuse. During this phase, the woman relives her original dream of ideal love and chooses to believe that *this* is what her partner is *really* like.

This loving phase becomes the focus of the woman's perception of the relationship. She bases her reason for remaining in the relationship on this "magical" ideal phase and hopes against hope that the previous phases will not be repeated. This hope is evident even in those women who have lived through a number of horrendous cycles.

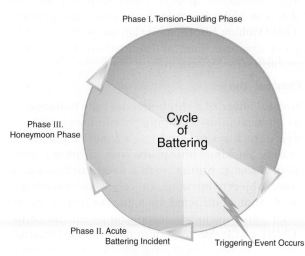

FIGURE 35–2 The cycle of battering.

Although phase III usually lasts somewhere between the lengths of time associated with phases I and II, it can be so short as to almost pass undetected. In most instances, the cycle soon begins again with renewed tensions and minor battering incidents. In an effort to "steal" a few precious moments of the phase III kind of love, the battered woman becomes a collaborator in her own abusive lifestyle. Victim and batterer become locked together in an intense, symbiotic relationship.

Why Do They Stay?

Probably the most common response that battered women give for staying is that they fear for their life and/or the lives of their children. As the battering progresses, the man gains power and control through intimidation and fear, with threats such as, "I'll kill you and the kids if you try to leave." Challenged by these threats and compounded by her low self-esteem and sense of powerlessness, the woman sees no way out. In fact, she may try to leave only to return when confronted by her partner and the psychological power he holds over her.

Victims have been known to stay in an abusive relationship for many reasons, some of which include the following (Dockterman, 2014; Malkin, 2013; Meskill & Conner, 2013):

■ **Fear of retaliation:** A woman may have been threatened with murder of herself and her children. Other acts Dockterman (2014) describes as psychological terrorism, such as sleep deprivation, blackmail, and murdering pets, may be used to increase fear of retaliation. In the lesbian, gay, bisexual, and transgender community, fear of being outed is sometimes used to manipulate the victim.

■ **Fear of losing custody of children:** Women are sometimes threatened by the spouse that he or she will take away the children. There may have been attempts to convince the woman that she is an unfit mother.

■ **Physical or financial dependence:** Victims may fear they are unable to care for themselves without the victimizer. Victims with disabilities may also be physically dependent on the victimizer for caregiving and physical support.

■ **Lack of a support network:** The victim may be under pressure from family members to stay in the marriage and try to work things out. In addition, the victimizer may have isolated the victim from family and friends.

■ **Cultural/religious reasons:** Cultural or religious convictions against divorce may dictate trying to save the marriage at all costs.

■ **Hopefulness:** The victim remembers good times and love in the relationship and has hope that her partner will change his behavior and they can have good times again.

■ **Lack of attention to the danger:** Malkin (2013) describes the dissociation that accompanies posttraumatic stress disorder (PTSD), which may contribute to the victim's numbness or lack of awareness of the reality of the situation. Or, as Leslie Morgan Steiner poignantly states in a Ted talk (cited by Dockterman, 2014):

> Why did I stay? I didn't know he was abusing me. Even though he held those loaded guns to my head, pushed me down stairs, threatened to kill our dog, pulled the key out of the car ignition as I drove down the highway, poured coffee grinds on my head as I dressed for a job interview, I never once thought of myself as a battered wife. Instead I was a very strong woman in love with a deeply troubled man, and I was the only person on earth who could help [him] face his demons.

It is important to recognize that when a victim leaves an abusive relationship, he or she is at a 75 percent greater risk of being killed by the partner, and the abuse often does not stop once a person has left (Colorado Bar Association, 2016). Clients should be empowered to make that decision and provided with resources and referrals to maximize their safety if they choose to leave, but, nonetheless, the decision must be theirs to make.

Child Abuse

Erik Erikson (1963) stated, "The worst sin is the mutilation of a child's spirit." Children are vulnerable and relatively powerless, and the effects of maltreatment are infinitely deep and long-lasting. Child maltreatment typically includes physical or emotional injury, physical or emotional neglect, or sexual acts inflicted upon a child by a caregiver. The Child Abuse Prevention and Treatment Act (CAPTA), as amended and reauthorized in 2010, identifies a minimum set of acts or behaviors that characterize maltreatment (Child Welfare Information Gateway [CWIG], 2013). States may use these as foundations on which to establish state legislation.

Physical Abuse

Physical abuse of a child includes "any nonaccidental physical injury (ranging from minor bruises to severe fractures or death) as a result of punching, beating, kicking, biting, shaking, throwing, stabbing, choking, hitting (with a hand, stick, strap, or other object), burning, or otherwise harming a child, that is inflicted by a parent, caregiver, or other person who has responsibility for the child" (CWIG, 2013). Maltreatment is considered whether or not the caretaker intended to cause harm or even if the injury resulted from overdiscipline or physical punishment. The most obvious way to detect this type of abuse is by outward physical signs. However, behavioral indicators also may be evident.

Signs of Physical Abuse Indicators of physical abuse may include any of the following (CWIG, 2013). The child:

- Has unexplained burns, bites, bruises, broken bones, or black eyes
- Has fading bruises or other marks noticeable after an absence from school
- Seems frightened of the parents and protests or cries when it is time to go home
- Shrinks at the approach of adults
- Reports injury by a parent or another adult caregiver
- Abuses animals or pets

Physical abuse may be suspected when the parent or other adult caregiver (CWIG, 2013):

- Offers conflicting, unconvincing, or no explanation for the child's injury
- Describes the child as "evil" or in some other very negative way
- Uses harsh physical discipline with the child
- Has a history of abuse as a child
- Has a history of abusing animals or pets

Emotional Abuse

Emotional abuse involves a pattern of behavior on the part of the parent or caretaker that results in serious impairment of the child's social, emotional, or intellectual functioning. Examples of emotional injury include belittling or rejecting the child, ignoring the child, blaming the child for things over which he or she has no control, isolating the child from normal social experiences, and using harsh and inconsistent discipline. Behavioral indicators of emotional maltreatment may include (CWIG, 2013):

- Extremes in behavior, such as overly compliant or demanding behavior, extreme passivity, or aggression
- Inappropriately adult (e.g., parenting other children) or inappropriately infantile (e.g., frequently rocking or head-banging) behavior
- Delays in physical or emotional development
- Suicide attempts
- Lack of attachment to the parent

Emotional abuse may be suspected when the parent or other adult caregiver (CWIG, 2013):

- Constantly blames, belittles, or berates the child
- Is unconcerned about the child and refuses to consider offers of help for the child's problems
- Overtly rejects the child

Physical and Emotional Neglect

> ## CORE CONCEPT
> ### Neglect
> **Physical neglect** of a child includes refusal of or delay in seeking health care, abandonment, expulsion from the home or refusal to allow a runaway to return home, and inadequate supervision.
>
> **Emotional neglect** refers to a chronic failure by the parent or caretaker to provide the child with the hope, love, and support necessary for the development of a sound, healthy personality.

Indicators of Neglect The possibility of neglect may be considered when the child (CWIG, 2013):

- Is frequently absent from school
- Begs or steals food or money
- Lacks needed medical or dental care, immunizations, or glasses
- Is consistently dirty and has severe body odor
- Lacks sufficient clothing for the weather
- Abuses alcohol or other drugs
- States that there is no one at home to provide care

The possibility of neglect may be considered when the parent or other adult caregiver (CWIG, 2013):

- Appears to be indifferent to the child
- Seems apathetic or depressed
- Behaves irrationally or in a bizarre manner
- Is abusing alcohol or other drugs

Sexual Abuse of a Child

Various definitions of **child sexual abuse** are available in the literature. CAPTA defines *sexual abuse* as:

> Employment, use, persuasion, inducement, enticement, or coercion of any child to engage in, or assist any other person to engage in, any sexually explicit conduct or simulation of such conduct for the purpose of producing any visual depiction of such conduct; or the rape, and in cases of caretaker or inter-familial relationships, statutory rape, molestation, prostitution, or other form of sexual exploitation of children, or incest with children. (CWIG, 2013)

Included in the definition is **sexual exploitation of a child,** in which a child is induced or coerced into engaging in sexually explicit conduct for the purpose of promoting any performance, and child sexual abuse, in which a child is being used for the sexual pleasure of an adult (parent or caretaker) or any other person.

CORE CONCEPT

Incest

The occurrence of sexual contacts or interaction between, or sexual exploitation of, close relatives, or between participants who are related to each other by a kinship bond that is regarded as a prohibition to sexual relations (e.g., caretakers, stepparents, stepsiblings) (Sadock et al., 2015).

Indicators of Sexual Abuse Child abuse may be considered a possibility when the child (CWIG, 2013):

- Has difficulty walking or sitting
- Suddenly refuses to change for gym or to participate in physical activities
- Reports nightmares or bedwetting
- Experiences a sudden change in appetite
- Demonstrates bizarre, sophisticated, or unusual sexual knowledge or behavior
- Becomes pregnant or contracts a venereal disease, particularly if younger than age 14
- Runs away
- Reports sexual abuse by a parent or another adult caregiver
- Attaches very quickly to strangers or new adults in their environment

Sexual abuse may be considered a possibility when the parent or other adult caregiver (CWIG, 2013):

- Is unduly protective of the child or severely limits the child's contact with other children, especially of the opposite sex
- Is secretive and isolated
- Is jealous or controlling with family members

Characteristics of the Abuser

A number of factors have been associated with adults who abuse or neglect their children. Sadock and associates (2015) report that parents who abuse their children were often victims of abuse in their own early lives and have impaired attachment with their child. Substance use disorders increase the risk of child abuse and neglect. Hosier (2015) identifies additional characteristics that may be associated with an abusive parent:

- Isolated with little support from family and friends
- Expects that the child should fulfill their emotional needs
- Prone to depression
- Frequent outbursts, anger and rage
- Low frustration tolerance

Flaherty and Stirling (2010) identify a number of factors that place a child at risk for maltreatment. They cite certain characteristics of the child, the parent, and the environment. These characteristics are presented in Box 35–1. When multiple factors coexist, the risk of child abuse increases.

The Incestuous Relationship

A great deal of attention has been given to the study of father-daughter incest. In these cases, there is usually an impaired sexual relationship between the parents. Communication between the parents is ineffective, which prevents them from correcting their problems. Typically, the father is domineering, impulsive, and physically abusive, while the mother is passive and submissive and denigrates her role as wife and mother. She is often aware of, or at least strongly

---

BOX 35–1 Factors and Characteristics That Place a Child at Risk for Maltreatment

Child	Parent	Environment (Community and Society)
Emotional/behavioral difficulties	Low self-esteem	Social isolation
Chronic illness	Poor impulse control	Poverty
Physical disabilities	Substance abuse/alcohol abuse	Unemployment
Developmental disabilities	Young maternal or paternal age	Low educational achievement
Preterm birth	Abused as a child	Single-parent home
Unwanted	Depression or other mental illness	Non-biologically related male living in the home
Unplanned	Poor knowledge of child development or unrealistic expectations of the child	Family or intimate partner violence
	Negative perception of normal child behavior	

SOURCE: Flaherty, E.G., Stirling, J., & Committee on Child Abuse and Neglect. (2010). Clinical report—The pediatrician's role in child maltreatment prevention. Pediatrics, 126(4), 833-841. Reprinted with permission.

suspects, the incestuous behavior between the father and daughter but may believe in or fear her husband's absolute authority over the family. She may deny that her daughter is being harmed and may actually be grateful that her husband's sexual demands are being met by someone other than herself.

Onset of the incestuous relationship typically occurs when the daughter is 8 to 10 years of age and commonly begins with genital touching and fondling. In the beginning, the child may accept the sexual advances from her father as signs of affection. As the incestuous behavior continues and progresses, the daughter usually becomes more bewildered, confused, and frightened, never knowing whether her father will be paternal or sexual in his interactions with her.

The relationship may become a love-hate situation on the part of the daughter. She continues to strive for the ideal father-daughter relationship but is fearful and hateful of the sexual demands he places on her. The mother may be alternately caring and competitive as she witnesses her husband's possessiveness and affections directed toward her daughter. Out of fear that his daughter may expose their relationship, the father may attempt to interfere with her normal peer relationships (Sadock et al., 2015).

Although the oldest daughter in a family is most vulnerable to becoming a participant in father-daughter incest, some fathers form sequential relationships with several daughters. If incest has been reported with one daughter, it should be suspected with all of the other daughters.

The Adult Survivor of Incest

Several common characteristics have been identified in adults who have experienced childhood incest, most notably a fundamental lack of trust resulting from an unsatisfactory parent-child relationship. This causes low self-esteem and a poor sense of identity. Children of incest often feel trapped, for they have been admonished not to talk about the experience and may even fear for their lives if they are exposed. If they do muster the courage to report the incest, often to the mother, they sometimes are not believed. This is confusing to the child, who is left with a sense of self-doubt and the inability to trust his or her own feelings. The child develops feelings of guilt with the realization over the years that the parents are using him or her in an attempt to solve their own problems.

Childhood sexual abuse commonly disrupts the development of a normal association of pleasure with sexual activity. Peer relationships are often delayed, altered, inhibited, or perverted. In some instances, individuals who were sexually abused as children completely retreat from sexual activity and avoid all close

interpersonal relationships throughout life, while others engage in high-risk and frequent sexual activity. Other adult manifestations of childhood sexual abuse in women include diminished libido, pain/penetration disorder, nymphomania, and promiscuity. In male survivors of childhood sexual abuse, erectile disorder, premature ejaculation, exhibitionistic disorder, and compulsive sexual conquests may occur. Sadock and associates (2015) report that child maltreatment, including repeated sexual abuse, causes changes in a child's brain that are evident on magnetic resonance imaging in adult survivors. They add that a robust finding from 20 studies indicates that childhood maltreatment culminates in future increased levels of C-reactive protein, fibrinogen, and pro-inflammatory cytokines. These inflammatory markers increase the adult survivor's risk for multiple physical illnesses. Depression, anxiety, substance use, eating disorders, suicidal behaviors, and a pattern of unstable relationships are also identified as increased risks from a history of child maltreatment (Sadock et al., 2015).

The conflicts associated with pain (either physical or emotional) and sexual pleasure experienced by children who are sexually abused are commonly manifested symbolically in adult relationships. Women who were abused as children often enter into relationships with men who abuse them physically, sexually, or emotionally. Berman (2013) describes this pattern as "repetition compulsion," a reliving of trauma in adult relationships rooted in subconscious efforts to "fix" situations they were unable to fix in childhood. The outcome is a repetitive cycle of unhealthy and often dangerous relationships. Berman adds that about a third of children who were abused or neglected in childhood become perpetrators of the same kinds of abuse as parents.

Adult survivors of incest who come forward with their stories usually are estranged from nuclear family members, blamed for disclosing the "family secret," and often accused of overreacting to the incest. Frequently, the estrangement becomes permanent when family members continue to deny the behavior and the individual is accused of lying. Many survivors choose to make the disclosure only after the death of their parents. Revelation of these past activities can be one way of contributing to the healing process for which incest survivors so desperately strive.

Sexual Violence

Sexual violence is often equated with rape, but that is only one type of sexual assault. It is important for nurses and other health-care providers to be aware that sexual violence includes any act of sexual coercion, including penetration, unwanted sexual contact, and noncontact unwanted sexual experiences (CDC, 2016a). All of these experiences can result in trauma, and assessment for history of these events is foundational to providing trauma-informed care. Read about Bridget's experiences in this chapter's "Real People, Real Stories" feature.

CORE CONCEPT

Rape

The expression of power and dominance by means of sexual violence, most commonly by men over women, although men may also be rape victims.

Sexual assault is any type of sexual act in which an individual is threatened or coerced, or forced, to submit against his or her will. Rape, a type of sexual assault, occurs over a broad spectrum of experiences ranging from the surprise attack by a stranger to insistence on sexual intercourse by an acquaintance or spouse. Regardless of the defining source, one common theme always emerges: rape is an act of aggression, not one of passion.

Acquaintance rape (called **date rape** if the encounter occurs during a social engagement agreed to by the victim) is a term applied to situations in which the rapist is acquainted with the victim. They may be

Real People, Real Stories: Bridget's Journey

This individual wished to remain anonymous. Bridget is not her real name. Her story is a poignant lesson in the various ways that one can be victimized, the long-term impact of such experiences on one's sense of self-esteem and personal safety, and the importance of nurses' understanding of trauma-informed care.

Karyn: I appreciate your willingness to talk about your experiences. If at any time you become uncomfortable discussing these events we don't need to continue. All right?

Bridget: I've had a lot of therapy, and I feel like it's important to tell and keep on telling so that, hopefully, something good will come out of it. When I was 6 years old, I had a crush on my best friend's brother. He was 12 years old, and when he started giving me attention, I thought he liked me; until he took me into a room, took my clothes off, and was touching me. He wanted me to take his clothes off, and I said no. I told my mom, and she intervened with his parents, but when a second incident occurred, my mother stopped me from going to my friend's house. I felt a lot of shame and embarrassment, but I never really talked about my feelings. For a long time, I carried around the belief that it was somehow my fault because I had a crush on him. I found out later that there were several other children who he molested and that his mom had implied they were "making it up."

When I was around 8 years old, I was in a toy store and a man came up from behind me and rubbed my rear end under my dress. I ran to get my father, but the perpetrator ran out of the store, and my parents decided not to call the police. They felt like I'd been scared enough. As an adult, I can understand that. But as a child, I felt like someone did a bad thing to me, and I wished that someone had defended me. As a middle schooler, one of the neighborhood girls wanted to play Truth or Dare. I think she did this with a lot of girls. The dare was to take off my clothes after which she put her hands on me. I said no but felt paralyzed with fear when she touched me anyway. She

was a year older, and again, I remember feeling powerless and thinking I didn't know what to do.

In another incident in middle school, one of the boys jumped out in front of me in the school hallway and grabbed my breasts. A teacher saw him do it and was going to send him to the principal's office, but the boy looked scared and I somehow thought it must be my job to protect him . . . or maybe I was trying to act like it was no big deal, so I told the teacher to just let him go. I didn't want to get the boy in trouble, and I was so embarrassed and humiliated, I just wanted it to go away. Part of me wishes the teacher hadn't listened to me, though. I don't think that boy had any idea how much he hurt me and how awful it was.

Karyn: I think that may be a common reaction by girls or women; even though someone has offended against us, we don't want to hurt them in return. And it minimizes the fact that *we* have been hurt.

Bridget: Yes, and my parents were knee deep in the Catholic training that if someone hurts you, you should just walk away or turn the other cheek. That influenced my own thinking, that you don't defend yourself—you should just walk away and avoid conflict. But that's a misunderstanding of the "turn the other cheek" teaching, which is really about showing forgiveness when people demonstrate remorse. It doesn't mean letting people hurt you without consequences. Around this time, I started putting on a lot of weight. I've always felt it was, in part, a reaction meant to keep people at a distance, so they couldn't hurt me.

Karyn: I've heard other people share a similar coping or defense mechanism; doing something simply to keep people away. Was that effective?

Bridget: It only added to my self-esteem issues. I struggled with the question of why these things were happening to me. I felt like *I* must be doing *something* wrong. As a teenager, I struggled with anxiety and depression, and I was sent to a psychiatrist, but it wasn't helpful. Then when I moved to New York City for college, there were a couple of incidents on the subway. One was a frail-looking elderly

Real People, Real Stories: Bridget's Journey—cont'd

man who stuck his hand between my legs, and when I turned around to confront him, he was laughing at me. I felt very powerless. I thought about kicking him, but, again, I didn't want to injure this shriveled-up old man, and I also didn't know if he had a knife, a gun. . . . So there's the fear, the powerlessness, and the anger that someone was touching me and *laughing* at me, and I could do nothing. I wondered if I was sending out some vibe—i.e., it must be my fault. My friend told me I needed to learn how to put on an angry face and carry an umbrella to better defend myself. I knew I had anxiety and self-esteem issues, and that's when I decided I needed therapy.

Karyn: That took a lot of courage to identify what you needed to do to take some control back. What has been most helpful about that process?

Bridget: I explored the underpinnings of my self-esteem issues and identified coping skills, but nonetheless, as an adult many things can trigger the feelings of vulnerability, anxiety, and low self-esteem: news stories about rape or abuse, or times when women or children are demeaned in the media, especially from people manipulating their power or authority. That brings up a lot of "stuff" for me. When my counselor challenged me to identify what was in the way of being able to set all this stuff aside—that's when I had the insight that I just wanted to know something good could come out of all this pain.

Karyn: One of the things you've told me is that you've been able to teach your daughters how to respond in such situations.

Bridget: Yes, that was important and felt like a victory. I'm better able to identify potentially harmful situations. I've taught them to listen to that inner voice, where you get that "bad feeling" you can get that warns you when you're in a situation that may require defending or protecting yourself, and I taught my daughters how to be prepared. I've told them that if someone tries to touch them, it's okay to fight back. It's okay to tell me, school officials, tell *anyone,* and to keep telling until someone believes them and responds. I want them to know that it's safe to talk to me about their feelings and that they are not powerless.

Karyn: I think that's an important message for health-care professionals as well: to listen, to not brush off someone's experiences but rather to explore the events, thoughts, and feelings and identify coping strategies.

Bridget: Yes, I think sometimes adults who thought it was less traumatizing for me to walk away or try to forget

about it thought they were helping, but that's not the answer. Even now, after all these years, I wasn't sure if you would think my story was important enough to tell, I mean, to some people, it might not seem so bad. I wasn't raped, it wasn't a family member—but it still left me feeling awful.

Karyn: I think your story is very important to tell. You are taking the opportunity to teach others that victimization can occur in a variety of ways, that it can have long-term effects on self-esteem, and that it is important to find ways to regain a sense of control and self-worth. I really appreciate your sharing this. What do you think are the most important things that nurses need to know about your and others' experience with victimization and trauma?

Bridget: First of all, that 40 years later, those incidents still affect me. I saw a picture of the boy who molested me on a friend's Facebook page, and I felt sick and afraid all over again. And I beat myself up for still letting it get to me. Nurses need to know that even events that happened years ago can influence one's emotional responses in the present.

Second, the idea of "getting closure," even so many years later, is a misnomer. Certain things can trigger those memories and anxieties, and when they come back, all you can do is drag them out and talk about them again and again and again. It's another version of "you tell and you tell and you don't stop telling" until you remember that you survived it, that it wasn't your fault, and that you don't need to feel ashamed or embarrassed or humiliated (even if part of you still does).

Third, I want nurses to know that they are the front lines, and no matter what clinical area they practice in, a history of sexual trauma or abuse can affect how their patients experience and receive health care. I had a lot of trouble as an adult fertility patient, having to dress and undress so many times and deal with so many invasive procedures. It was important to tell my health-care providers why my heart was pounding, why I seemed so nervous, why I hated mammographies and regular GYN exams a little bit more than the average woman. . . . That, as always, a nurse's ability to care and offer compassion can make the biggest difference, and it all begins with trust and helping your patient to "tell." And I wanted to say thank you for the times those nurses held my hand, and squeezed tight, and told me that I would be okay.

---

out on a first date, have been dating for a number of months, or merely be acquaintances or schoolmates. College campuses are the location for a staggering number of these types of rapes, a great many of which go unreported. An increasing number of colleges and universities are establishing programs for rape prevention and counseling for survivors of rape.

Marital rape, which has been recognized only in recent years as a legal category, occurs when a spouse is liable for sexual abuse directed at a marital partner against that person's will. Historically, with societal acceptance of the concept of women as marital property, the legal definition of rape held an exemption within the marriage relationship. In 1993, marital rape became a crime in all 50 states, under at least one section of the sexual offenses code. In 17 states and the District of Columbia, there are no exemptions from rape prosecution granted to husbands. However, in 33 states, there are still some exemptions given to husbands from rape prosecution, and in all states where husbands can be prosecuted, the criteria for proving marital rape are very stringent.

Statutory rape is unlawful intercourse between a person who is over the age of consent and a person who is under the age of consent. The legal age of consent varies from state to state, ranging from age 14 to 18 (King & Regan, 2014). An adult who has intercourse with a person who is younger than the age of consent can be arrested for statutory rape, even if the interaction occurred between consenting individuals.

Profile of the Victimizer

It is difficult to profile a rapist because rapists comprise a heterogenous group and are not distinguished by looks or intelligence. They tend to score normally on psychological tests with the exception of higher scores on expressing anger (St. Petersburg College, 2016). Sadock and associates (2015) identify that the underlying motives of rape perpetrators can be classified into four groups: sexual sadists who are aroused by inflicting pain, exploitative predators who are using the victim to gratify needs such as dominance and power, inadequate men who are obsessed with fantasies of sex they believe cannot be achieved without force, and those who are displacing anger and rage. They add that victims of childhood abuse show increased likelihood of perpetrating violence of all kinds in adulthood.

The majority of rapes are premeditated. Behavioral characteristics that have been associated with premeditation include seeking out a victim who appears to be vulnerable (capable of being overpowered or isolated from others), violating or ignoring others' rights (sometimes in a way that informs whether a potential victim is passive or tolerant of those behaviors), or generally lacking skills of empathy. But again, while these behaviors might be observed more commonly, they do not define the complete profile of these perpetrators. A feminist view suggests that rape is most common in societies that encourage aggressiveness in males, that have distinct gender roles, and in which men regard women's roles as inferior (King & Regan, 2014). Male aggressiveness as a cultural norm, however, does not explain why some men become perpetrators of criminal aggression and violence while others do not.

Statistics show that most rapists are between the ages of 25 and 44. Fifty-four percent are white, 32 percent are African American, and the remainder are of other races, mixed race, or unknown race (U.S. Bureau of Justice Statistics, 2011). In 80 percent of rape and sexual assault cases, the offender was known to the victim, and 1 in 10 rapes involved the use of a weapon (U.S. Bureau of Justice Statistics, 2014b). Statistics such as these help describe aspects of the problem, but understanding the essence of the perpetrator of aggression and violence is the subject of ongoing research.

The Victim

Rape can occur at any age, but the most recent statistics suggest that the highest-risk age group is females younger than age 34, those with lower income, and those living in rural areas (U.S. Bureau of Justice Statistics, 2014b). Most sexual assault victims are single women, and the attack frequently occurs in or close to the victim's own neighborhood.

Although women are at highest risk for rape perpetrated by males, males may also be victimized by women or other men. Sadock and associates (2015) describe the dynamics as identical and state that in all cases:

> the crime enables the rapist to discharge aggression and aggrandize himself [or herself]. The victim is usually smaller than the rapist, perceived as passive . . . and is used as an object. (p. 826)

Rape survivors who present themselves for care shortly after the crime has occurred likely are experiencing an overwhelming sense of violation and helplessness that began with the powerlessness and intimidation experienced during the rape. Burgess (1974), who has classically defined what has been described as **rape trauma syndrome,** identified two emotional patterns of response that may occur within hours after a rape and with which health-care workers may be confronted in the emergency department or rape crisis center. In the **expressed response pattern,** the survivor expresses feelings of fear, anger, and anxiety through such behaviors as crying, sobbing, restlessness, and tension. In the **controlled response pattern,** the feelings are masked or hidden, and a calm, composed, or subdued affect is seen.

The following manifestations may be evident in the days and weeks after the attack (Burgess, 2010):

- Contusions and abrasions about various parts of the body
- Headaches, fatigue, sleep pattern disturbances
- Stomach pains, nausea and vomiting
- Vaginal discharge and itching, burning upon urination, rectal bleeding and pain
- Rage, humiliation, embarrassment, desire for revenge, and self-blame
- Fear of physical violence and death

The long-term effects of sexual assault depend largely on the individual's ego strength, social support system, and the way he or she was treated as a victim (Burgess, 2010). Various long-term effects include increased restlessness, dreams and nightmares, and phobias (particularly those having to do with sexual interaction). Some women report that it takes years to get over the experience; they describe a sense of vulnerability and a loss of control over their own lives during this period. They feel defiled and unable to wash themselves clean, and some women are unable to remain living alone in their home or apartment.

Some survivors develop a **compounded rape reaction,** in which additional symptoms such as depression and suicide, substance abuse, and even psychotic behaviors may be noted (Burgess, 2010). Another variation has been called the **silent rape reaction,** in which the survivor tells no one about the assault. Anxiety is suppressed and the emotional burden may become overwhelming. The unresolved sexual trauma may not be revealed until the woman is forced to face another sexual crisis in her life that reactivates the previously unresolved feelings.

Diagnosis and Outcome Identification

Nursing diagnoses are formulated from the data gathered during the assessment phase and with background knowledge regarding predisposing factors to the situation. Some common nursing diagnoses for survivors of abuse include:

- Rape-trauma syndrome related to sexual assault evidenced by verbalizations of the attack; bruises and lacerations over areas of body; severe anxiety
- Powerlessness related to cycle of battering evidenced by verbalizations of abuse; bruises and lacerations over areas of body; fear for her safety and that of her children; verbalizations of no way to get out of the relationship
- Risk for delayed development related to abusive family situation

Outcome Criteria

The following criteria may be used to measure outcomes in the care of abuse survivors:

The client who has been sexually assaulted:

- Is no longer experiencing panic anxiety
- Demonstrates a degree of trust in the primary nurse
- Has received immediate attention to physical injuries
- Has initiated behaviors consistent with the grief response

The client who has been physically battered:

- Has received immediate attention to physical injuries

- Verbalizes assurance of his or her immediate safety
- Discusses life situation with primary nurse
- Can verbalize choices from which he or she may receive assistance

The child who has been abused:

- Has received immediate attention to physical injuries
- Demonstrates trust in primary nurse by discussing abuse through the use of play therapy
- Is demonstrating a decrease in regressive behaviors

Planning and Implementation

Table 35–1 provides a plan of care for the client who is a survivor of abuse. Nursing diagnoses are presented, along with outcome criteria, appropriate nursing interventions, and rationales for each.

Concept Care Mapping

The concept map care plan (see Chapter 9, The Nursing Process in Psychiatric-Mental Health Nursing) is a diagrammatic teaching and learning strategy that allows visualization of interrelationships between medical diagnoses, nursing diagnoses, assessment data, and treatments. An example of a concept map care plan for a client who is a survivor of abuse is presented in Figure 35–3.

Evaluation

Evaluation of nursing actions to assist survivors of abuse must be considered on both a short- and a long-term basis.

Short-term evaluation may be facilitated by gathering information using the following types of questions:

- Has the individual been reassured of his or her safety?
- Is this evidenced by a decrease in panic anxiety?
- Have wounds been properly cared for and provision made for follow-up care?
- Have emotional needs been attended to?
- Has trust been established with at least one person to whom the client feels comfortable relating the abusive incident?
- Have available support systems been identified and notified?
- Have options for immediate circumstances been presented?

Long-term evaluation may be conducted by health-care workers who have contact with the individual long after the immediate crisis has passed.

- Is the individual able to conduct activities of daily living satisfactorily?
- Have physical wounds healed properly?

Table 35–1 | CARE PLAN FOR SURVIVORS OF ABUSE

NURSING DIAGNOSIS: RAPE-TRAUMA SYNDROME

RELATED TO: Sexual assault

EVIDENCED BY: Verbalizations of the attack; bruises and lacerations over areas of body; severe anxiety

OUTCOME CRITERIA	NURSING INTERVENTIONS	RATIONALE
Short-Term Goal: • Client's physical wounds heal without complication. **Long-Term Goal:** • Client begins a healthy grief resolution, initiating the process of physical and psychological healing (time to be individually determined).	1. It is important to communicate the following to the individual who has been sexually assaulted: • You are safe here. • I'm sorry that it happened. • I'm glad you survived. • It's not your fault. No one deserves to be treated this way. • You did the best that you could.	1. The woman who has been sexually assaulted fears for her life and must be reassured of her safety. She may also be overwhelmed with self-doubt and self-blame, and these statements instill trust and validate self-worth.
	2. Explain every assessment procedure that will be conducted and why it is being conducted. Ensure that data collection is conducted in a caring, nonjudgmental manner. Engage the services of a sexual assault nurse examiner, where available, to facilitate evidence collection and client advocacy (See bonus chapter, Forensic Nursing, for further discussion; available on-line at DavisPlus.com)	2. This may serve to decrease fear/anxiety and increase trust.
	3. Ensure that client has adequate privacy for all immediate postcrisis interventions. Try to have as few people as possible providing the immediate care or collecting immediate evidence.	3. The posttrauma client is extremely vulnerable. Additional people in the environment increase this feeling of vulnerability and serve to escalate anxiety.
	4. Encourage client to give an account of the assault. Listen, but do not probe.	4. Nonjudgmental listening provides an avenue for catharsis that client needs to begin healing. A detailed account may be required for legal follow-up, and a caring nurse, as client advocate, may help to lessen the trauma of evidence collection.
	5. Discuss with client whom to call for support or assistance. Provide information about referrals for aftercare.	5. Because of severe anxiety and fear, the client may need assistance from others during immediate postcrisis period. Provide referral information in writing for later reference (e.g., psychotherapist, mental health clinic, community advocacy group).

Table 35–1 | CARE PLAN FOR SURVIVORS OF ABUSE–cont'd

NURSING DIAGNOSIS: POWERLESSNESS

RELATED TO: Cycle of battering

EVIDENCED BY: Verbalizations of abuse; bruises and lacerations over areas of body; fear for own safety and that of children; verbalizations of no way to get out of the relationship

OUTCOME CRITERIA	NURSING INTERVENTIONS	RATIONALE
Short-Term Goal: • Client recognizes and verbalizes choices available, thereby perceiving some control over life situation. Long-Term Goal: • Client exhibits control over life situation by making decision about what to do regarding living with cycle of abuse.	1. In collaboration with physician, ensure that all physical wounds, fractures, and burns receive immediate attention. Take photographs if client permits.	1. Client safety is a nursing priority. Photographs may be called as evidence if charges are filed.
	2. Take client to a private area to do the interview.	2. If client is accompanied by the person who did the battering, she is not likely to be truthful about the injuries.
	3. If she has come alone or with her children, assure her of her safety. Encourage her to discuss the battering incident. Ask questions about whether this has happened before, whether the abuser takes drugs, whether the woman has a safe place to go, and whether she is interested in pressing charges.	3. Some women will attempt to keep secret how their injuries occurred in an effort to protect the partner or because they are fearful that the partner will kill them if they tell.
	4. Ensure that "rescue" efforts are not attempted by the nurse. Offer support, but remember that the final decision must be made by client.	4. Making her own decision gives client a sense of control over her life situation. Imposing judgments and giving advice are nontherapeutic.
	5. Stress to client the importance of safety. She must be made aware of the variety of resources that are available to her. These may include crisis hot lines, community groups for women who have been abused, shelters, counseling services, and information regarding the victim's rights in the civil and criminal justice system. Following a discussion of these available resources, the woman may choose for herself. If her decision is to return to the marriage and home, this choice also must be respected.	5. Knowledge of available choices decreases the individual's sense of powerlessness, but true empowerment comes only when she chooses to use that knowledge for her own benefit.

Continued

Table 35–1 | CARE PLAN FOR SURVIVORS OF ABUSE–cont'd

NURSING DIAGNOSIS: RISK FOR DELAYED DEVELOPMENT
RELATED TO: Child abuse

OUTCOME CRITERIA	NURSING INTERVENTIONS	RATIONALE
Short-Term Goal: • Client develops trusting relationship with nurse and reports how evident injuries were sustained. **Long-Term Goal:** • Client demonstrates behaviors consistent with age-appropriate growth and development.	1. Perform complete physical assessment of the child. Take particular note of bruises (in various stages of healing), lacerations, and client complaints of pain in specific areas. Do not overlook or discount the possibility of sexual abuse. Assess for nonverbal signs of abuse: aggressive conduct, excessive fears, extreme hyperactivity, apathy, withdrawal, age-inappropriate behaviors.	1. An accurate and thorough physical assessment is required to provide appropriate care for client.
	2. Conduct an in-depth interview with the parent or adult who accompanies the child. Consider: If the injury is being reported as an accident, is the explanation reasonable? Is the injury consistent with the explanation? Is the injury consistent with the child's developmental capabilities?	2. Fear of imprisonment or loss of child custody may place the abusive parent on the defensive. Discrepancies may be evident in the description of the incident, and lying to cover up involvement is a common defense that may be detectable in an in-depth interview.
	3. Use games or play therapy to gain child's trust. Use these techniques to assist in describing his or her side of the story.	3. Establishing a trusting relationship with an abused child is extremely difficult. He or she may not even want to be touched. These types of play activities can provide a nonthreatening environment that may enhance the child's attempt to discuss these painful issues.

- Is the client appropriately progressing through the behaviors of grieving?
- Is the client free of sleep disturbances (nightmares, insomnia), psychosomatic symptoms (headaches, stomach pains, nausea/vomiting), regressive behaviors (enuresis, thumb sucking, phobias), and psychosexual disturbances?
- Is the individual free from problems with interpersonal relationships?
- Has the individual considered the alternatives for change in his or her personal life?
- Has a decision been made relative to the choices available?
- Is he or she satisfied with the decision that has been made?

Treatment Modalities

Crisis Intervention

The focus of the initial interview and follow-up with the client who has been sexually assaulted is on the rape incident alone. Problems not associated with the rape are not dealt with at this time. The goal of crisis intervention is to help survivors return to their previous lifestyle as quickly as possible.

The client should be involved in the intervention from the beginning. This promotes a sense of competency, control, and decision-making. Because an overwhelming sense of powerlessness accompanies the rape experience, active involvement by the survivor is both a validation of personal worth and the beginning

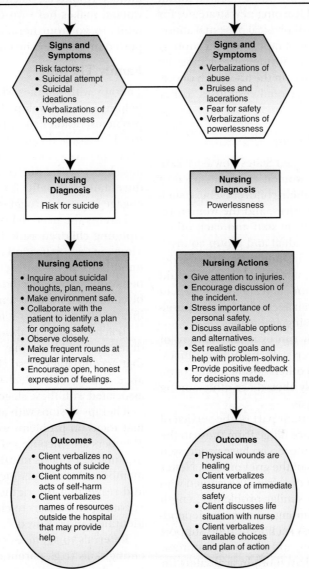

Clinical Vignette: Annette and Charles, both 21, have been dating for 2 years. Charles has always been jealous and gets very angry when Annette even talks to another man. He has hit her several times, hard enough to produce bruises, but never on her face, and she is able to hide the abuse from others. Tonight at a party, Annette danced with another man, and Charles became violent. He punched the man in the face and dragged Annette out to the parking lot. She yelled at him, "This is it! We are through! I don't ever want to see you again!" He started beating her around the face and upper body, and yelled, "You can't break up with me! I won't allow it! You belong to me, and no one else!" He left her lying in the parking lot. She felt powerless and, in her despondency, opened her purse and swallowed half a bottle of acetaminophen. When she told her girlfriend, Dana, what had happened, Dana called 911, and Annette was taken to the hospital. She was treated for the overdose, and her wounds were cleaned and dressed. Following physical stability, she was transferred to the psychiatric unit. She tells the nurse, "I can't live like this. He won't let me go! I don't know what to do!" The nurse develops the following concept map care plan for Annette.

Signs and Symptoms

Risk factors:
- Suicidal attempt
- Suicidal ideations
- Verbalizations of hopelessness

Signs and Symptoms

- Verbalizations of abuse
- Bruises and lacerations
- Fear for safety
- Verbalizations of powerlessness

Nursing Diagnosis

Risk for suicide

Nursing Diagnosis

Powerlessness

Nursing Actions

- Inquire about suicidal thoughts, plan, means.
- Make environment safe.
- Collaborate with the patient to identify a plan for ongoing safety.
- Observe closely.
- Make frequent rounds at irregular intervals.
- Encourage open, honest expression of feelings.

Nursing Actions

- Give attention to injuries.
- Encourage discussion of the incident.
- Stress importance of personal safety.
- Discuss available options and alternatives.
- Set realistic goals and help with problem-solving.
- Provide positive feedback for decisions made.

Outcomes

- Client verbalizes no thoughts of suicide
- Client commits no acts of self-harm
- Client verbalizes names of resources outside the hospital that may provide help

Outcomes

- Physical wounds are healing
- Client verbalizes assurance of immediate safety
- Client discusses life situation with nurse
- Client verbalizes available choices and plan of action

FIGURE 35–3 Concept map care plan for a client with physical abuse.

of the recovery process. Crisis intervention is time limited, usually 6 to 8 weeks. If problems resurface beyond this time, the individual is referred for assistance from other agencies (e.g., long-term psychotherapy from a psychiatrist or mental health clinic).

During the crisis period, attention is given to coping strategies for dealing with the symptoms common to the posttrauma client. Initially, the individual undergoes a period of disorganization during which

there is difficulty making decisions, extreme or irrational fears, and general mistrust. Observable manifestations may range from stark hysteria to expression of anger and rage to silence and withdrawal. Guilt and feelings of responsibility for the rape, as well as numerous physical manifestations, are common. The crisis counselor attempts to help the individual draw upon previous successful coping strategies to regain control over his or her life.

If the client is a victim of domestic violence, the counselor ensures that various resources and options are made known to the individual so that she may make a personal decision about moving forward with her life. Discussing strategies for minimizing the dangers of leaving (sometimes called an escape plan) may be helpful if the client is considering leaving the relationship. Support groups provide a valuable forum for reducing isolation and learning new strategies for coping with the aftermath of physical or sexual abuse. Particularly for the survivor of rape, the peer support group provides a therapeutic forum for reducing the sense of isolation she may feel in the aftermath of predictable social and interpersonal responses to her experience.

The Safe House or Shelter

Most major cities in the United States now have **safe houses** or **shelters** where women can be assured of protection for them and their children. These shelters provide a variety of services, and the women receive emotional support from staff and each other. Most shelters provide individual and group counseling; help with bureaucratic institutions such as the police, legal representation, and social services; child care and children's programs; and aid for the woman in making future plans, such as employment counseling and linkages with housing authorities.

The shelters are usually run by a combination of professional and volunteer staff, including nurses, psychologists, lawyers, and others. Women who themselves have been previously abused are often among the volunteer staff members.

Group work is an important part of the service of shelters. Women in residence range from those in the immediate crisis phase to those who have progressed through a variety of phases of the grief process. Newer members can learn a great deal from the women who have successfully resolved similar problems. Length of stay varies a great deal among individuals, depending on a number of factors such as outside support network, financial situation, and personal resources.

The shelter provides a haven of physical safety for the battered woman and promotes expression of the intense emotions she may be experiencing regarding her situation. A woman often exhibits depression, extreme fear, or even violent expressions of anger and rage. In the shelter, she learns that these feelings are normal and that others have experienced these same emotions in similar situations. She is allowed to grieve for what has been lost and for what was expected but not achieved. Help is provided in overcoming the tremendous guilt associated with self-blame. This is a difficult step for someone who has accepted responsibility for another's behavior over a long period.

New arrivals at the shelter are given time to experience the relief from the safety and security provided. Making decisions is discouraged during the period of immediate crisis and disorganization. Once the woman's emotions have become more stable, planning for the future begins. Through information from staff and peers, she learns about available community resources. Feedback is provided, but the woman makes her own decision about "where she wants to go from here." She is accepted and supported in whatever she chooses to do.

Family Therapy

Therapy with families who use violence focuses on helping them develop democratic ways of solving problems. Studies show that the more a family uses the democratic means of conflict resolution, the less likely they are to engage in physical violence. Families must learn to deal with problems in ways that can produce mutual benefits for all concerned rather than engage in power struggles among family members.

Parents also need to learn effective methods of disciplining children aside from physical punishment. Time-out techniques and methods that emphasize the importance of positive reinforcement for acceptable behavior can be very effective. Family members must be committed to consistent use of this behavior modification technique for it to be successful.

Teaching parents about expectations for various developmental levels may alleviate some of the stress that accompanies these changes. Anticipatory guidance is needed to deal with the crises commonly associated with these stages.

Therapy sessions with all family members together may focus on problems with family communication. Members are encouraged to express honest feelings in a manner that is nonthreatening to other family members. Active listening, assertiveness techniques, and respecting the rights of others are taught and encouraged. Barriers to effective communication are identified and resolved.

Referrals to agencies that promote effective parenting skills (e.g., parent effectiveness training) may be made. Alternative agencies that may relieve the stress of parenting (e.g., Mom's Day Out programs, sitter-sharing organizations, and day-care institutions) also may be considered. Support groups for abusive parents may also be helpful, and assistance in locating or initiating such a group may be provided.

Summary and Key Points

■ Abuse is the maltreatment of one person by another.
■ Intimate partner violence, child abuse, and sexual assault are widespread, and all populations are equally affected.

- Various factors have been theorized as influential in the predisposition to violent behavior. Physiological and biochemical influences within the brain have been suggested, as has the possibility of a direct genetic link.
- Organic brain syndromes associated with various cerebral disorders and traumatic brain injury have been implicated in the predisposition to aggressive and violent behavior.
- Psychoanalytical theorists relate the predisposition to violent behavior to underdeveloped ego and a poor self-concept.
- Learning theorists suggest that children imitate the abusive behavior of their parents. This theory has been substantiated by studies that show that individuals who were abused as children or whose parents disciplined them with physical punishment are more likely to be abusive as adults.
- Societal influences, such as acceptance of violence as a means of solving problems, also have been implicated.
- Women who are battered often take blame for their situations. They may have been reared in abusive families and thus expect this type of behavior.
- Battered women commonly see no way out of their present situation and may be encouraged by their social support network to remain in the abusive relationship.

- Child abuse includes physical and emotional abuse, physical and emotional neglect, and sexual abuse of a child.
- A child may experience many years of abuse without reporting it because of fear of retaliation by the abuser.
- Some children report incest experiences to their mothers, only to be rebuffed by her and told to remain secretive about the abuse.
- Adult survivors of incest often experience physical and emotional manifestations as a result of the incestuous relationship.
- Sexual assault is identified as an act of aggression, not passion.
- A history of abuse and neglect in childhood increase one's risk of perpetrating abuse and neglect upon others in adulthood. Rape is a traumatic experience, and many women experience flashbacks, nightmares, rage, physical symptoms, depression, and thoughts of suicide for many years after the occurrence.
- Treatment modalities for survivors of abuse include crisis intervention with the sexual assault victim, safe shelter for battered women, and therapy for families who use violence.

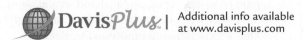 *DavisPlus* | Additional info available at www.davisplus.com

Review Questions
Self-Examination/Learning Exercise

Select the answer that is most appropriate for each of the following questions.

1. Sharon, a woman with multiple cuts and abrasions, arrives at the emergency department with her three small children. She tells the nurse her husband inflicted the wounds. She says, "I didn't want to come. I'm really okay. He only does this when he has too much to drink. I just shouldn't have yelled at him." The best response by the nurse is:
   a. "How often does he drink too much?"
   b. "It is not your fault. You did the right thing by coming here."
   c. "How many times has he done this to you?"
   d. "He is not a good husband. You have to leave him before he kills you."

2. Sharon, a woman with multiple cuts and abrasions, arrives at the emergency department with her three small children. She tells the nurse her husband inflicted the wounds. In the interview, Sharon tells the nurse, "He's been getting more and more violent lately. He's been under a lot of stress at work the last few weeks, so he drinks a lot when he gets home. He always gets mean when he drinks. I was getting scared. So I just finally told him I was going to take the kids and leave. He got furious when I said that and began beating me with his fists." With knowledge about the cycle of battering, what does this situation represent?
   a. Phase I. Sharon was desperately trying to stay out of his way and keep everything calm.
   b. Phase I. A minor battering incident for which Sharon assumes all the blame.
   c. Phase II. The acute battering incident that Sharon provoked with her threat to leave.
   d. Phase III. The honeymoon phase where the husband believes that he has "taught her a lesson and she won't act up again."

Continued

Review Questions—cont'd
Self-Examination/Learning Exercise

3. A battered woman presents to the emergency department with multiple cuts and abrasions. Her right eye is swollen shut. She says that her husband did this to her. What is the *priority* nursing intervention?
   a. Tending to the immediate care of her wounds
   b. Providing her with information about a safe place to stay
   c. Administering the prn tranquilizer ordered by the physician
   d. Explaining how she may go about bringing charges against her husband

4. A woman who has a long history of being battered by her husband is staying at the woman's shelter. She has received emotional support from staff and peers and has been made aware of the alternatives open to her. Nevertheless, she decides to return to her home and marriage. The best response by the nurse to the woman's decision is:
   a. "I just can't believe you have decided to go back to that horrible man."
   b. "I'm just afraid he will kill you or the children when you go back."
   c. "What makes you think things have changed with him?"
   d. "I hope you have made the right decision. Call this number if you need help."

5. Jana, age 5, is sent to the school nurse's office with an upset stomach. She has vomited and soiled her blouse. When the nurse removes her blouse, she notices that Jana has numerous bruises on her arms and torso in various stages of healing. She also notices some small scars. Jana's abdomen protrudes on her small, thin frame. From the objective physical assessment, the nurse suspects that:
   a. Jana is experiencing physical and sexual abuse.
   b. Jana is experiencing physical abuse and neglect.
   c. Jana is experiencing emotional neglect.
   d. Jana is experiencing sexual and emotional abuse.

6. A school nurse notices bruises and scars on a child's body, but the child refuses to say how she received them. Another way in which the nurse can get information from the child is to:
   a. Have her evaluated by the school psychologist.
   b. Tell her she may select a "treat" from the treat box (e.g., sucker, balloon, junk jewelry) if she answers the nurse's questions.
   c. Explain to her that if she answers the questions, she may stay in the nurse's office and not have to go back to class.
   d. Use a "family" of dolls to role-play the child's family with her.

7. A school nurse notices bruises and scars on a child's body. The nurse suspects that the child is being physically abused. How should the nurse proceed with this information?
   a. As a health-care worker, report the suspicion to child protective services.
   b. Check the child again in a week and see if there are any new bruises.
   c. Meet with the child's parents and ask them how she got the bruises.
   d. Initiate paperwork to have the child placed in foster care.

Review Questions—cont'd
Self-Examination/Learning Exercise

8. Kate is an 18-year-old freshman at the state university. She was extremely flattered when Don, a senior star football player, invited her to a party. On the way home, he parked the car in a secluded area by the lake. He became angry when she refused his sexual advances. He began to beat her and finally raped her. She tried to fight him, but his physical strength overpowered her. He dumped her in the dorm parking lot and left. The dorm supervisor rushed Kate to the emergency department. Kate says to the nurse, "It's all my fault. I shouldn't have allowed him to stop at the lake." The nurse's best response is:

   a. "Yes, you're right. You put yourself in a very vulnerable position when you allowed him to stop at the lake."

   b. "You are not to blame for his behavior. You obviously made some right decisions, because you survived the attack."

   c. "There's no sense looking back now. Just look forward, and make sure you don't put yourself in the same situation again."

   d. "You'll just have to see that he is arrested so he won't do this to anyone else."

9. A young woman who has just undergone a sexual assault is brought into the emergency department by a friend. What is the *priority* nursing intervention?

   a. Help her to bathe and clean herself up.

   b. Provide physical and emotional support during evidence collection.

   c. Provide her with a written list of community resources for survivors of rape.

   d. Discuss the importance of a follow-up visit to evaluate for sexually transmitted diseases.

10. A woman who was sexually assaulted 6 months ago by a male acquaintance has been attending a support group for survivors of rape. From this group, she has learned that the most likely reason the man raped her was that:

   a. Because he had been drinking, he was not in control of his actions.

   b. He had not had sexual relations with a girl in many months.

   c. He was predisposed to become a rapist by virtue of the poverty conditions under which he was reared.

   d. He was expressing power and dominance by means of sexual aggression and violence.

IMPLICATIONS OF RESEARCH FOR EVIDENCE-BASED PRACTICE

Bowland, S., Edmond, T., & Fallot, R.D. (2012). Evaluation of a spiritually focused intervention with older trauma survivors. *Social Work, 57*(1), 73-82.

DESCRIPTION OF THE STUDY: The purpose of this study was to evaluate a spiritually focused group intervention for a sample of women trauma survivors older than age 55 years (*n* = 21, control group *n* = 22). The authors cite research supporting that older women value spirituality more than men or younger adults, and often this was correlated to personal growth, well-being, and involvement in creative activities. They also cited research linking personal violation (trauma) to spiritual crisis. Inclusion criteria sought a homogenous group of participants

who all had a background in Christian tradition. They randomly assigned participants into treatment and control groups, and they chose a treatment intervention that was a "manualized, psychoeducational, cognitive restructuring and skill building approach to addressing spiritual struggles in recovery." They evaluated for changes in symptoms of depression, anxiety, PTSD, and physical symptoms.

RESULTS OF THE STUDY: The treatment group in this study was found to have fewer symptoms of depression, anxiety, and PTSD and fewer physical symptoms than the control group at the completion of the intervention. These gains were still evident at 3-month follow-up.

Continued

IMPLICATIONS OF RESEARCH FOR EVIDENCE-BASED PRACTICE—cont'd

IMPLICATIONS FOR NURSING PRACTICE: Holistic nursing practice includes addressing the spiritual needs of clients in recovery, particularly since spiritual crisis has been identified as a risk for trauma survivors. This study supported that interventions focused on spiritual needs can have an impact on symptom reduction for several disorders common to this population. Use of structured interventions, consideration for homogeneity of belief traditions, and individual assessment of the client's interest in such interventions are important variables to consider.

IMPLICATIONS OF RESEARCH FOR EVIDENCE-BASED PRACTICE

McClean, C.P., Morris, S.H., Conklin, P., Jayawickreme, N., & Foa, E.B. (2014). Trauma characteristics and posttraumatic stress disorder among adolescent survivors of childhood sexual abuse. *Journal of Family Violence, 29*(5), 559-566. doi:10.1007/s10896-014-9613-6

DESCRIPTION OF THE STUDY: This study examined the relationship between specific characteristics of childhood sexual abuse and the severity of consequent PTSD, depression, suicide ideation, and substance use symptoms. The risk for illness subsequent to trauma is well documented in the literature, but these researchers wanted to know if specific characteristics such as the relationship of the perpetrator to the victim, the duration or frequency of abuse, and the type of abuse could predict the severity of future PTSD or other symptoms. The participants ($N = 83$) were a culturally diverse sample of female adolescents who were already seeking treatment. The researchers note that there have been conflicting findings in existing research about these relationships in previous studies of adolescents.

RESULTS OF THE STUDY: One significant finding in this study was that the frequency of sexual abuse victimization was correlated with an increase in suicide ideation. Contrary to what the researchers expected to find, the type of trauma, the relationship of the perpetrator, and the duration of victimization did not predict severity of other future illness symptoms, including depression, PTSD, and substance use. They acknowledge that two influential variables are that (1) all participants in their sample had already identified themselves as having moderate to high PTSD, and (2) the severity of symptoms may be more distinctive in adulthood, so the relationships that are not clear in a study of adolescents may become clearer as the adolescent moves through adulthood.

IMPLICATIONS FOR NURSING PRACTICE: The finding that frequency of victimization was linked to increased suicide ideation suggests that nurses who conduct victim assessment should assess for suicide ideation and evaluate risks for suicide attempts, especially in adolescents who have sustained frequent sexual abuse victimization.

The other findings of this research (including their review of studies with conflicting results) highlight that it is important for nurses to explore the bulk of available research on any issue to increase confidence in their clinical judgments.

TEST YOUR CRITICAL THINKING SKILLS

Sandy is a psychiatric registered nurse who works at a safe house for battered women. Lisa has just been admitted with her two small children after she was treated in the emergency department. She was beaten severely by her husband while he was intoxicated last night. She escaped with her children after he passed out in their bedroom.

In her initial assessment, Sandy learns from Lisa that she has been battered by her husband for 5 years, beginning shortly after their marriage. She explained that she "knew he drank quite a lot before we were married, but thought he would stop after we had kids." Instead, the drinking has increased. Sometimes he does not even get home from work until midnight, after stopping to drink at the bar with his buddies.

Lately, he has begun to express jealousy and a lack of trust in Lisa, accusing her of numerous infidelities and indiscretions, none of which are true. Lisa says, "If only he wasn't under so much stress on his job, then maybe he wouldn't drink so much. Maybe if I tried harder to make everything perfect for him at home—I don't know. What do you think I should do to keep him from acting this way?"

Answer the following questions related to Lisa:

1. What is an appropriate response to Lisa's question?
2. Identify the priority psychosocial nursing diagnosis for Lisa.
3. What must the nurse do to ensure that Lisa learns from this experience?

Communication Exercises

1. Sarah is being treated in the emergency department for wounds inflicted by her husband. She says to the nurse, "He's really not a bad person. He's just under so much stress right now. His company is laying people off, and he thinks he will be next. He drinks a lot when he comes home from work. I just need to make things easier for him at home. I shouldn't have asked him to mow the lawn."
   - How would the nurse respond appropriately to this statement by Sarah?
2. "I don't know what to do. I'm afraid he will hurt the kids."
   - How would the nurse respond appropriately to this statement by Sarah?
3. "I don't want to press charges. I just want to go home!"
   - How would the nurse respond appropriately to this statement by Sarah?

MOVIE CONNECTIONS

The Burning Bed (domestic violence) • *Life With Billy* (domestic violence) • *Two Story House* (child abuse) • *The Prince of Tides* (domestic violence) • *Radio Flyer* (child abuse) • *Flowers in the Attic* (child abuse) • *A Case of Rape* (sexual assault) • *The Accused* (sexual assault)

References

American Psychological Association. (2016). Violence and socioeconomic status. Retrieved from www.apa.org/pi/ses/resources/publications/violence.aspx

Batrinos, M.L. (2012). Testosterone and aggressive behavior in man. *International Journal of Endocrinology and Metabolism 10*(3), 563-568. doi:10.5812/ijem.3661

Berman, L. (2013). How childhood abuse can manifest in adult relationships. Retrieved from www.everydayhealth.com/sexual-health/dr-laura-berman-childhood-abuse-and-adult-relationships.aspx

Bowland, S., Edmond, T., & Fallot, R.D. (2012). Evaluation of a spiritually focused intervention with older trauma survivors. *Social Work, 57*(1), 73-82.

Burgess, A. (2010). Rape violence. Gannett Education Course #60025. Retrieved from http://ce.nurse.com/60025/Rape-Violence

Centers for Disease Control and Prevention. (2016a). Intimate partner violence: Data sources. Retrieved from https://www.cdc.gov/violenceprevention/intimatepartnerviolence/datasources.html

Centers for Disease Control and Prevention. (2016b). Rape prevention and education. Retrieved from www.cdc.gov/ViolencePrevention/RPE/index.html

Centers for Disease Control and Prevention. (2016c). Elder abuse prevention. Retrieved from www.cdc.gov/features/elderabuse

Centers for Disease Control and Prevention. (2015). Intimate partner violence surveillance: Uniform definitions and recommended data elements, version 2.0. Retrieved from https://www.cdc.gov/violenceprevention/pdf/intimatepartnerviolence.pdf

Child Welfare Information Gateway. (2013). What is child abuse and neglect? Recognizing the signs and symptoms. Retrieved from https://www.childwelfare.gov/pubs/factsheets/whatiscan

Colorado Bar Association. (2016). The challenges and effects of leaving an abusive situation. Retrieved from https://www.cobar.org/index.cfm/ID/21090

Dockterman, E. (2014). Why women stay: The paradox of abusive relationships. Retrieved from http://time.com/3309687/why-women-stay-in-abusive-relationships

Flaherty, E.G., Stirling, J., & Committee on Child Abuse and Neglect. (2010). The pediatrician's role in child maltreatment prevention. *Pediatrics, 126*(4), 833-841. doi:10.1542/peds.2010-2087

Hosier, D. (2015). Characteristics of abusive mothers. Retrieved from http://childhoodtraumarecovery.com/2015/10/21/characteristics-of-abusive-mothers

King, B.M., & Regan, P. (2014). *Human sexuality today* (8th ed.). Upper Saddle River, NJ: Prentice Hall.

Malkin, C. (2013). Why do people stay in abusive relationships? Retrieved from https://www.psychologytoday.com/blog/romance-redux/201303/why-do-people-stay-in-abusive-relationships

McClean, C.P., Morris, S.H., Conklin, P., Jayawickreme, N., & Foa, E.B. (2014). Trauma characteristics and posttraumatic stress disorder among adolescent survivors of childhood sexual abuse. *Journal of Family Violence, 29*(5), 559–566. doi:10.1007/s10896-014-9613-6

Meskill, J., & Conner, M. (2013). Understanding and dealing with domestic violence against women. Retrieved from www.oregoncounseling.org/Handouts/DomesticViolenceWomen.htm

National Center on Elder Abuse. (2015). Elder abuse: The size of the problem. Department of Health and Human Services. Retrieved from www.ncea.aoa.gov/library/data/

Rosell, D.R., & Siever, L.J. (2015). The neurobiology of aggression and violence. *CNS Spectrum, 20*(3), 254-279. doi:10.1017/S109285291500019X

Sadock, B.J., Sadock, V.A., & Ruiz, P. (2015). *Synopsis of psychiatry: Behavioral sciences/clinical psychiatry* (11th ed.). Philadelphia: Lippincott Williams & Wilkins.

Schatzberg, A.F., Cole, J.O., & DeBattista, C. (2015). *Manual of clinical psychopharmacology* (8th ed.). Washington, DC: American Psychiatric Publishing.

St. Petersburg College. (2016). Sexual misconduct: Profile of a rapist. Retrieved from https://www.spcollege.edu/pages/pb_3col.aspx?pageid=8801

Sullivan, L.E. (Ed.). (2009). *The SAGE glossary of social and behavioral sciences*. Los Angeles: Sage Publications.

Tracy, N. (2016). What is battering? Retrieved from www.healthyplace.com/abuse/domestic-violence/what-is-battering

U.S. Bureau of Justice Statistics. (2011). Criminal victimization in the United States—Statistical tables index. Retrieved from http://bjs.ojp.usdoj.gov/content/pub/html/cvus/index.cfm

U.S Bureau of Justice Statistics. (2012). Intimate partner violence, 1993–2010. Retrieved from www.bjs.gov/index.cfm?ty=pbdetail&iid=4536

U.S. Bureau of Justice Statistics. (2014a). Intimate partner violence: Attributes of victimization, 1999–2011. Retrieved from www.bjs.gov/index.cfm?ty=pbdetail&iid=4801

U.S. Bureau of Justice Statistics. (2014b). Rape and sexual assault among college-ag females, 1995–2013. Retrieved from www.bjs.gov/index.cfm?ty=pbdetail&iid=5176

U.S. Department of Education. (2013). Human trafficking of children in the United States. Retrieved from www2.ed.gov/about/offices/list/oese/oshs/factsheet.html

U.S. Department of Health and Human Services, Administration for Children and Families, Administration on Children, Youth and Families, Children's Bureau. (2015). Child maltreatment 2013. Retrieved from www.acf.hhs.gov/programs/cb/research-data-technology/statistics-research/child-maltreatment

U.S. Department of Justice. (2012). Areas of focus. Retrieved from www.ovw.usdoj.gov/areas-focus.html

Classical References

Burgess, A. W., & Holmström, L. L. (1974). Rape trauma syndrome. *American Journal of Psychiatry, 131*(9), 981-986.doi: 10.1176/appi.ajp.131.9.981.

Erikson, E.H. (1963). *Childhood and society* (2nd ed.). New York: WW Norton.

Walker, L.E. (1979). *The battered woman.* New York: Harper & Row.

Community Mental Health Nursing

36

CORE CONCEPTS

Community

Primary Prevention

Secondary Prevention

Tertiary Prevention

KEY TERMS

case management

case manager

deinstitutionalization

diagnosis-related groups (DRGs)

mobile outreach units

prospective payment

shelters

storefront clinics

OBJECTIVES

After reading this chapter, the student will be able to:

1. Discuss the changing focus of care in the field of mental health.
2. Define the concepts of care associated with the public health model.
3. Discuss primary prevention of mental illness within the community.
4. Identify populations at risk for mental illness within the community.
5. Discuss nursing intervention in primary prevention of mental illness within the community.
6. Discuss secondary prevention of mental illness within the community.
7. Describe treatment alternatives related to secondary prevention within the community.
8. Discuss tertiary prevention of mental illness within the community as it relates to the seriously mentally ill and homeless mentally ill.
9. Relate historical and epidemiological factors associated with caring for the seriously mentally ill and homeless mentally ill within the community.
10. Identify treatment alternatives for care of the seriously mentally ill and homeless mentally ill within the community.
11. Apply steps of the nursing process to care of the seriously mentally ill and homeless mentally ill within the community.

HOMEWORK ASSIGNMENT

Please read the chapter and answer the following questions:

1. What are *diagnosis-related groups* (DRGs)?
2. Describe and differentiate how interventions at the primary, secondary, and tertiary prevention levels are implemented.
3. Name three common client populations that benefit from psychiatric home health nursing.
4. What is the most common psychiatric diagnosis among homeless people with mental illness?

This chapter explores the concepts of primary and secondary prevention of mental illness within communities. Additional focus is placed on tertiary prevention of mental illness: treatment with community resources of those who suffer from severe and persistent mental illness, including homeless persons with mental illness. Emphasis is given to the role of the psychiatric nurse in the various treatment alternatives within the community setting.

The Changing Focus of Care

Before 1840, there was no known treatment for individuals with mental illness. Because mental illness was perceived as incurable, the only "reasonable" intervention was thought to be removing these individuals from the community to a place where they would do no harm to themselves or others.

In 1841, Dorothea Dix, a former schoolteacher, began a personal crusade on behalf of institutionalized individuals with mental illness. Her efforts resulted in more humane treatment of these clients and the establishment of a number of psychiatric hospitals across the country.

After the movement initiated by Dix, the number of hospitals for persons with mental illness increased, although unfortunately not as rapidly as did the population with mental illness. Hospitals became overcrowded and understaffed, with conditions that would have sorely distressed Dix.

The community mental health movement had its impetus in the 1940s. With establishment of the National Mental Health Act of 1946, the U.S. government awarded grants to the states to develop mental health programs outside of state hospitals. Outpatient clinics and psychiatric units in general hospitals were inaugurated. Then, in 1949, as an outgrowth of the National Mental Health Act, the National Institute of Mental Health (NIMH) was established. The U.S. government has charged this agency with the responsibility for mental health in the United States.

In 1955, the Joint Commission on Mental Health and Illness was established by Congress to identify the nation's mental health needs and make recommendations for improvement in psychiatric care. In 1961, the Joint Commission published the report *Action for Mental Health* in which recommendations were made for treatment of clients with mental illness, training for caregivers, and improvements in education and research on mental illness. With consideration given to these recommendations, Congress passed the Mental Retardation Facilities and Community Mental Health Centers Construction Act (often called the *Community Mental Health Centers Act*) of 1963. This act called for the construction of comprehensive community mental health centers, the cost of which would be shared by federal and state governments. The **deinstitutionalization** movement (the closing of state mental hospitals and discharging of individuals with mental illness) had begun.

Unfortunately, many state governments did not have the capability to match the federal funds required for the establishment of these mental health centers. Some communities found it difficult to follow the rigid requirements for services required by the legislation that provided the grant.

In 1980, the Community Mental Health Systems Act, which would have a major role in renovation of mental health care, was established. Funding was authorized for community mental health centers, services to high-risk populations, and rape research and services. Approval was also granted for the appointment of an associate director for minority concerns at NIMH. However, before this plan could be enacted, the newly inaugurated administration set forth its intention to diminish federal involvement. Budget cuts reduced the number of mandated services, and federal funding for community mental health centers was terminated in 1984.

Meanwhile, costs of care for hospitalized psychiatric clients continued to rise. The problem of the "revolving door" began to intensify. Individuals with severe and persistent mental illness had no place to go when their symptoms exacerbated except back to the hospital. Individuals without support systems remained in the hospital for extended periods because of lack of appropriate community services. Hospital services were paid for by cost-based, retrospective reimbursement: Medicaid, Medicare, and private health insurance. Retrospective reimbursement encouraged hospital expenditure; the more services provided, the more payment received.

This system of health-care delivery was interrupted in 1983 with the advent of **prospective payment**—the Reagan administration's proposal of cost containment. It was directed at control of Medicare costs by setting forth preestablished amounts that would be reimbursed for specific diagnoses, or **diagnosis-related groups (DRGs).** Since that time, prospective payment has also been integrated by the states (Medicaid) and by some private insurance companies, drastically affecting the amount of reimbursement for health-care services.

Under prospective payment, general hospital services to psychiatric clients have been severely restricted. Clients who present with acute symptoms, such as acute psychosis, suicidal ideations or attempts, or manic exacerbations, constitute the largest segment of the psychiatric hospital census. Clients with less serious illnesses (e.g., moderate depression or adjustment disorders) may be hospitalized, but length of stay has been shortened considerably by the reimbursement guidelines. Clients are being discharged from the hospital with a greater need for aftercare than in the past, when hospital stays were longer. A positive outgrowth of these struggles with costly hospital stays and restricted reimbursement has been the development of a broader continuum of outpatient treatment options than what has been available historically. In the past, individuals who needed psychiatric treatment saw an outpatient therapist or were hospitalized, but today there are partial hospitalization programs, intensive outpatient programs, aftercare programs, and a host of other community-based services available to clients with mental health disorders.

Deinstitutionalization continues to impact mental health care in the United States. Care for the client in the hospital has become cost prohibitive, whereas care for the client in the community is considered cost effective. However, the community mental health movement has also been criticized for being a continuation of an "overly narrow biomedical model" (Vanderplasschen et al., 2013). Ironically, the prison populations of homeless and mentally ill persons has risen dramatically during this same time period, one of the problems that Dorothea Dix fought so adamantly against in the first place. The reality of the provision of health-care services today is often more of a political and funding issue than providers would care to admit. Decisions about how to treat are rarely made without consideration of cost and method of payment.

The recovery model (see Chapter 21, The Recovery Model) promises the hope of integrating the support of community mental health services, peer support, and client empowerment to improve interventions and outcomes as we look to the future. We must serve the consumer by working collaboratively to provide the essential services for health promotion, for early intervention, and to promote improvement in quality of life for this population.

The Public Health Model

The premise of the model of public health is based largely on the concepts set forth by Gerald Caplan (1964) during the initial community mental health movement. They include primary prevention, secondary prevention, and tertiary prevention. These concepts have expanded beyond mental health treatment and are now widely accepted as guiding principles in clinical and community settings over a wide range of medical and nursing specialties.

CORE CONCEPT

Primary Prevention

Services aimed at reducing the incidence of mental disorders within the population.

Primary prevention targets both individuals and the environment. Emphasis is twofold:

1. Assisting individuals to increase their ability to cope effectively with stress
2. Targeting and diminishing harmful forces (stressors) within the environment

Nursing in primary prevention is focused on the targeting of groups at risk and the provision of educational programs. Examples include:

■ Teaching parenting skills and child development to prospective new parents
■ Teaching physical and psychosocial effects of alcohol/drugs to elementary school students
■ Teaching techniques of stress management to virtually anyone who desires to learn
■ Teaching groups of individuals ways to cope with the changes associated with various maturational stages
■ Teaching concepts of mental health to various groups within the community
■ Providing education and support to unemployed or homeless individuals
■ Providing education and support to other individuals in various transitional periods (e.g., widows and widowers, new retirees, and women entering the work force in middle life)

These are only a few examples of the types of services nurses provide in primary prevention. Such services can be offered in a variety of convenient public settings (e.g., churches, schools, colleges, community centers, YMCAs and YWCAs, workplaces of employee organizations, meetings of women's groups, or civic or social organizations such as parent-teacher associations, health fairs, and community shelters).

CORE CONCEPT

Secondary Prevention

Interventions aimed at minimizing early symptoms of psychiatric illness and directed toward reducing the prevalence and duration of the illness.

Secondary prevention is accomplished through early identification of problems and prompt initiation of effective treatment. Nursing in secondary prevention focuses on recognition of symptoms and provision of or referral for treatment. Examples include:

■ Ongoing assessment of individuals at high risk for illness exacerbation (e.g., during home visits, day care, community health centers, or in any setting where screening of high-risk individuals might occur)

■ Provision of care for individuals in whom illness symptoms have been assessed (e.g., individual or group counseling, medication administration, education and support during period of increased stress [crisis intervention], staffing rape crisis centers, suicide hotlines, homeless shelters, shelters for abused persons, or mobile mental health units)

■ Referral for treatment of individuals in whom illness symptoms have been assessed. Referrals may come from support groups, community mental health centers, emergency services, psychiatrists or psychologists, and day or partial hospitalization. Inpatient therapy on a psychiatric unit of a general hospital or in a private psychiatric hospital may be necessary. Psychopharmacology and various adjunct therapies may be initiated as part of the treatment.

Secondary prevention is addressed extensively in Unit 4, Nursing Care of Clients With Alterations in Psychosocial Adaptation, of this text. Nursing assessment, diagnosis and outcome identification, planning and implementation, and evaluation are discussed for many of the mental illnesses identified in the *Diagnostic and Statistical Manual of Mental Disorders, Fifth Edition* (DSM-5) (American Psychiatric Association [APA], 2013). These concepts may be applied in any setting where nursing is practiced.

CORE CONCEPT

Tertiary Prevention

Services aimed at reducing the residual defects that are associated with severe and persistent mental illness.

Tertiary prevention is accomplished in two ways:

1. Preventing complications of the illness
2. Promoting rehabilitation directed toward achievement of each individual's maximum level of functioning

Historically, individuals with severe and persistent mental illness often experienced long hospitalizations that resulted in loss of social skills and increased dependency. With deinstitutionalization, many of these individuals may never have experienced hospitalization, but they still do not possess adequate skills to live productive lives within the community.

Nursing in tertiary prevention focuses on helping clients learn or relearn socially appropriate behaviors so that they may achieve a satisfying role within the community. Examples include:

■ Consideration of the rehabilitation process at the time of initial diagnosis and treatment planning

■ Teaching the client daily living skills and encouraging independence to his or her maximum ability

■ Referring clients for various aftercare services (e.g., support groups, day treatment programs, partial hospitalization programs, psychosocial rehabilitation programs, group home, or other transitional housing)

■ Monitoring effectiveness of aftercare services (e.g., through home health visits or follow-up appointments in community mental health centers)

■ Making referrals for support services when required (e.g., some communities have programs linking individuals with serious mental disorders to volunteers who develop friendships with the individuals and may assist with household chores, shopping, and other activities of daily living with which the individual is having difficulty, in addition to participating in social activities with the individual)

Nursing care at the tertiary level of prevention can be administered on an individual or group basis and in a variety of settings, such as inpatient hospitalization, day or partial hospitalization, group home or halfway house, shelters, home health care, nursing homes, and community mental health centers.

The Community as Client

Primary Prevention

CORE CONCEPT

Community

A group, population, or cluster of people with at least one common characteristic, such as geographic location, occupation, ethnicity, or health concern.

Primary prevention within communities encompasses the twofold emphasis defined earlier in this chapter:

1. Identifying stressful life events that precipitate crises and targeting the relevant populations at high risk
2. Intervening with these high-risk populations to prevent or minimize harmful consequences

Populations at Risk

One way to view populations at risk is to focus on types of crises that individuals experience in their lives. Two broad categories are maturational crises and situational crises.

Maturational Crises

Maturational crises are crucial experiences associated with various stages of growth and development. Erikson

(1963) described eight stages of the life cycle during which individuals struggle with developmental "tasks." Crises can occur during any of these stages, although several developmental periods and life-cycle events have been recognized as having increased crisis potential: adolescence, marriage, parenthood, midlife, and retirement.

Adolescence The task for adolescence according to Erikson (1963) is *identity versus role confusion*. This is the time in life when individuals ask questions such as "Who am I?," "Where am I going?," and "What is life all about?"

Adolescence is a transition into young adulthood. It is a very volatile time in most families. Commonly, conflict arises over issues of control. Parents sometimes have difficulty relinquishing even a minimal amount of the control they have had throughout their child's infancy, toddlerhood, and school-aged years at this time when the adolescent is seeking increased independence. It may seem that the adolescent is 25 years old one day and 5 years old the next. An often-quoted definition of an adolescent, by an anonymous author, is: "A toddler with hormones and wheels."

At this time, adolescents are "trying out their wings," although they possess an essential need to know that the parents (or surrogate parents) are available if support is required. In fact, it is believed that the most frequent immediate precipitant to adolescent suicide is loss of or threat of loss or abandonment by parents or closest peer relationship.

Adolescents have many issues to deal with and many choices to make. Some of these include issues that relate to self-esteem and body image (in a body that is undergoing rapid changes), peer relationships (with both genders), education and career selection, establishing a set of values and ideals, sexuality and sexual experimentation (including issues of birth control and prevention of sexually transmitted infections), drug and alcohol use, and physical appearance.

Nursing interventions with adolescents at the primary level of prevention focus on providing support and accurate information to ease the difficult transition they are undergoing. Educational offerings can be presented in schools, churches, youth centers, or any location in which groups of teenagers gather. Types of programs may include, but are not limited to, the following:

■ Alateen groups for adolescents with alcoholic parent(s)
■ Other support groups for teenagers who are in need of assistance to cope with stressful situations (e.g., children dealing with divorce of their parents, pregnant teenagers, teenagers coping with abortion, adolescents coping with the death of a parent)

■ Educational programs that inform about and validate bodily changes and emotions about which there may be some concerns
■ Educational programs that inform about positive self-esteem and resilience
■ Educational programs that inform about sexuality, pregnancy, contraception, and sexually transmitted infections
■ Educational programs that inform about the use of alcohol and other drugs

Marriage The "American dream" of the 1950s—especially that of the American woman—was to marry, have two or three children, buy a house in the suburbs, and drive a station wagon. To not be at least betrothed by their mid-20s caused many women to fear becoming an "old maid." Living together without the benefit of marriage was unacceptable and rarely considered an option.

Times have changed considerably since the middle of the 20th century. Today's young women are choosing to pursue careers before entering into marriage, to continue their careers after marriage, or to not marry at all. Many couples are deciding to live together without being married, and, as with most trends, the practice now receives more widespread societal acceptance than it once did. Although there are far more culturally accepted relationship and living arrangement choices in today's society, crises may develop related to conflicting values between generations within a family and related to the many factors influencing those choices, including economic concerns. Cultural changes such as the growth in individualism and self-realization have decreased interest in long-term commitments and childbearing, but economics and the reality of gender inequalities in the workplace have accentuated conflicts around choosing how to move forward at this stage of life (Kaakinen et al., 2015).

When young adults do decide to enter into marriage, crisis may develop associated with unrealistic or uninformed expectations about this institution. It is well understood that children raised in abusive, dysfunctional families are at higher risk for subconsciously choosing partners who perpetuate the experiences they had while growing up. Both of these circumstances can increase the risk for crisis within a marriage.

Nursing interventions at the primary level of prevention with individuals in this stage of development involve education about what to expect at various stages in the marriage. Many high schools offer courses in marriage and family living in which students role-play anticipatory marriage and family situations. Nurses could offer these kinds of classes within the community to individuals considering marriage. Educating young adults about factors to consider when choosing a spouse, particularly the risks associated with choosing a partner who perpetuates a cycle of violence, may provide the opportunity to provide primary prevention at the level of basic survival. Too many people enter marriage with the notion that, as sure as the depth of their love, their soon-to-be husband or wife will discontinue his or her "undesirable" traits and change into the perceived ideal spouse. Primary prevention with these individuals involves:

■ Encouraging honest communication
■ Determining what each person expects from the relationship
■ Discerning whether each individual can accept compromise

This type of intervention can be effective in individual or couple's therapy and in support or educational groups of couples experiencing similar circumstances.

Parenthood There is perhaps no developmental stage that creates an upheaval equal to that of the arrival of a child. Even when the child is desperately wanted and pleasurably anticipated, his or her arrival usually results in some degree of chaos within the family.

Because the family operates as a system, the addition of a new member influences all parts of the system as a whole. If it is a first child, the relationship between spouses is likely to be affected by the demands of caring for the infant on a 24-hour basis. If there are older children, they may resent the attention showered on the new arrival and show their resentment in a variety of creative ways.

The concept of having a child (particularly the first one) is often romanticized, with little or no consideration given to the realities and responsibilities that accompany this "bundle of joy." Many young parents are shocked to realize that such a tiny human can create so many changes in so many lives. It is unfortunate that although parenting is one of the most important positions an individual will hold in life, it is one for which he or she is often least prepared.

Nursing intervention at the primary level of prevention with those in the developmental stage of parenthood must begin long before the child is even born. How do we prepare individuals for parenthood? *Anticipatory guidance* is the term used to describe the interventions used to help new parents know what they might expect. Volumes have been written on the subject, but it is also important for expectant parents to have a support person or network with whom they can talk honestly and express feelings, excitement, and fears. Nurses can provide the following type of information to help ease the transition into parenthood (Kaakinen et al., 2015; Spock, 2012).

■ **Prepared childbirth classes:** These classes present what most couples can expect along with information about possible deviations from what is expected.

■ **Information about what to expect after the baby arrives:**
  ■ *Parent-infant bonding:* Expectant parents should know that it is common for parent-infant bonding not to occur immediately. The strong attachment will occur as parent and infant get to know each other.
  ■ *Changing communication patterns and relationship styles:* The couple should be encouraged to engage in open, honest communication with each other. Education should be offered about expected changes in communication patterns and the challenges of establishing communication with an infant as well as resources for referral if communication patterns are creating significant role strain. Frustrated attempts to adapt to these challenges can have consequences for the infant as well. In some cases, an infant's need may be neglected if the parents lack skills or resources to navigate communication challenges. "The most extreme example of an inability to adapt to communication patterns with an infant is shaken baby syndrome" (Kaakinen et al., 2015, p.363). Discuss strategies family members may use to maintain motivation and morale as well as provide for comfort, rest, and self-care for each member.
  ■ *Clothing and equipment:* Expectant parents need to know what is required to care for a newborn child. Financing childbearing and child rearing, arranging space for a child, and lifestyle should be considered.
  ■ *Feeding:* Advantages and disadvantages of breastfeeding and formula feeding should be presented. The couple should be supported in whatever method is chosen. Anticipatory guidance related to technique should be provided for one or both methods as the expectant parents request.
  ■ *Other expectations:* It is important for expectant parents to receive anticipatory guidance about the infant's sleeping and crying patterns, bathing the infant, care of the circumcision and cord, toys that provide stimulation of the newborn's senses, aspects of providing a safe environment, and when to call the physician.
■ **Stages of growth and development:** It is very important for parents to understand what behaviors should be expected at what stage of development. It is also important to know that their child may not necessarily follow the age guidelines associated with these stages. However, a substantial deviation from these guidelines should be reported to the pediatrician.

Midlife What is middle age? A colleague once remarked that upon turning 50 years of age, she stated, "'Now I can say I am officially middle aged' . . . until I began thinking about how few individuals I really knew who were 100!"

Midlife crises are not defined by a specific number. Various sources in the literature identify these conflicts as occurring anytime between ages 35 and 65.

What is a midlife crisis? It is very individual, but a number of patterns have been identified within three broad categories:

1. **An alteration in perception of the self:** One's perception of self may change slowly, or a person may suddenly become aware of being "old" or "middle aged." Other biological changes that occur naturally with the aging process may also affect the crises that occur at this time. In women, a gradual decrease in estrogen production initiates menopause, which results in a variety of physical and emotional symptoms. Some physical symptoms include hot flashes, vaginal dryness, cessation of menstruation, loss of reproductive ability, night sweats, insomnia, headaches, and minor memory disturbances. Emotional symptoms include anxiety, depression, crying for no reason, and temper outbursts.

   Some men experience hot flashes, sweating, chills, dizziness, and heart palpitations, while others may experience severe depression and an overall decline in physical vigor (Sadock, Sadock, & Ruiz, 2015). An alteration in sexual functioning is not uncommon.

2. **An alteration in perception of others:** A change in relationship with adult children requires a sensitive shift in caring. Wright and Leahey (2013) state:

   The family of origin must relinquish the primary roles of parent and child. They must adapt to the new roles of parent and adult child. This involves renegotiation of emotional and financial commitments. The key emotional process during this stage is for family members to deal with a multitude of exits from and entries into the family system. (p. 107)

   These experiences are particularly difficult when parents' values conflict with the relationships and types of lifestyles their children choose. An alteration in perception of one's parents also begins to occur during this time. Having always looked to parents for support and comfort, the middle-aged individual may suddenly find that the roles are beginning to reverse. Aging parents may look to their children for assistance with decisions regarding their everyday lives and chores they have previously accomplished independently. When parents die, middle-aged individuals must come to terms with their own mortality. The process of recognition and resolution of one's own finitude begins in earnest at this time.

3. **An alteration in perception of time:** Middle age has been defined as the end of youth and the beginning of old age. Individuals often experience a sense that time is running out: "I haven't done all I want to do or accomplished all I intended to accomplish!" Depression and a sense of loss may occur as individuals realize that some of the goals established in their youth may go unmet.

The term *empty nest syndrome* has been used to describe the adjustment period parents experience when the last child leaves home to establish an independent residence. The crisis is often more profound for the mother who has devoted her life to nurturing her family. As the last child leaves, she may perceive her future as uncertain and meaningless.

Some women who have devoted their lives to rearing their children decide to develop personal interests and pursue personal goals once the children are grown. This occurs at a time when many husbands have begun to decrease what may have been a compulsive drive for occupational security during the earlier years of their lives. This disparity in common goals may create conflict between husband and wife. At a time when she is experiencing more value in herself and her own life, he may begin to feel less valued. This may also relate to a decrease in the amount of time and support from the wife to which the husband has become accustomed. This type of role change will require numerous adaptations on the part of both spouses.

Finally, an alteration in one's perception of time may be related to the societal striving for eternal youth. The individual may try to delay the external changes that come with aging by the use of cosmetics, hormone creams, or even surgery. This yearning for youth may take the form of sexual promiscuity or extramarital affairs with much younger individuals, in an effort to prove that one "still has what it takes." Some individuals reach for the trappings of youth with regressive-type behaviors, such as the middle-aged man who buys a motorcycle and joins a motorcycle club, and the 50-year-old woman who wears miniskirts and flirts with her daughter's boyfriends. These individuals may be denying their own past and experience. With a negative view of self, they strongly desire to relive their youth.

Nursing intervention at the primary level of prevention with those in the developmental stage of midlife involves providing accurate information regarding changes that occur during this time of life and support for adapting to these changes effectively. These interventions might include:

■ Nutrition classes to inform individuals in this age group about the essentials of diet and exercise. Educational materials on how to avoid obesity and the importance of good nutrition can be included.
■ Assistance with ways to improve health (e.g., quit smoking, cease or reduce alcohol consumption, reduce fat intake).

- Discussions of the importance of having regular physical examinations, including Pap and breast examinations for women and prostate examinations for men. Monthly breast self-examinations should be taught and yearly mammograms encouraged.
- Classes on menopause should be given. Provide information about what to expect. Myths that abound regarding this topic should be expelled. Support groups for women (and men) undergoing the menopausal experience could be formed.
- Support and information related to physical changes occurring in the body during this time of life. Assist with the grief response that some individuals will experience in relation to loss of youth, empty nest, and sense of identity.
- Support and information related to care of aging parents should be given. Individuals should be referred to community resources for respite and assistance before strain of the caregiver role threatens to disrupt the family system.

Retirement Retirement, which is often anticipated as an achievement in principle, may be met with ambivalence when it actually occurs. Our society places profound importance on productivity and earning as much money as possible at as young an age as possible. These types of values contribute to the ambivalence associated with retirement. Although leisure has been acknowledged as a legitimate reward for workers, leisure during retirement has never been accorded the same social value. Adjustment to this life-cycle event becomes more difficult in the face of societal values that are in direct conflict with the new lifestyle.

Historically, many women have derived much of their self-esteem from having children, rearing children, and being "good mothers." Likewise, many men have achieved self-esteem through work-related activities—creativity, productivity, and earning money. Termination of these activities can result in a loss of self-worth, and individuals who are unable to adapt satisfactorily may become depressed.

It would appear that retirement is becoming, and will continue to become, more accepted by societal standards. With more and more individuals living longer, a growing number of aging persons will spend more time in retirement. At present, retirement has become more of an institutionalized expectation, with increasing acceptance as a social status.

Nursing intervention at the primary level of prevention with the developmental task of retirement involves providing information and support to individuals who have retired or are considering retirement. Support can be provided on a one-to-one basis to assist these individuals to sort out their feelings regarding retirement. Well-being in retirement is linked to factors such as stable health status, adequate income, the ability to pursue new goals or activities, extended social network of family and friends, and satisfaction with current living arrangements.

One hallmark of change for many older adults is the increasing numbers of grandparents who are caring for grandchildren and, in many cases, assuming primary responsibility for their care (Kaakinen et al., 2015). Nurses can promote primary prevention of crisis through education about resources for caregiving assistance and evidence-based information about this new role. In fact, evidence shows that in spite of grief and burdens associated with caregiving, many grandparents identify that this role revealed their inner strength and gave them a sense of accomplishment (Kaakinen et al., 2015).

Support can also be provided in a group environment. Support groups of individuals undergoing the same types of experiences can be extremely helpful. Nurses can form and lead groups to assist retiring individuals through this critical period. These groups can also serve to provide information about available resources that offer assistance to individuals in or nearing retirement, such as information concerning Medicare, Social Security, and Medicaid; information related to organizations that specialize in hiring retirees; and information regarding ways to use newly acquired free time constructively.

Situational Crises

Situational crises are acute responses that occur as a result of an external stressor. The number and types of situational stressors are limitless and may be real or exist only in the perception of the individual. Some types of situational crises that put individuals at risk for mental illness are discussed next.

Poverty A number of studies have identified poverty as a direct correlation to emotional illness. This may have to do with the direct consequences of poverty, such as inadequate and crowded living conditions, nutritional deficiencies, medical neglect, unemployment, and homelessness.

High Rate of Life-Change Events Many studies have found that changes in life patterns when a large number of significant events occur in close proximity tend to decrease a person's ability to deal with stress, sometimes resulting in physical or emotional illness (McLeod, 2010). These include events such as death of a loved one, divorce, being fired from a job, a change in living conditions, a change in place of employment or residence, physical illness, or a change in body image caused by the loss of a body part or function.

Environmental Conditions Environmental conditions can create situational crises. Tornados, floods, hurricanes, and earthquakes have wreaked devastation on thousands of individuals and families in recent years.

Trauma Individuals who have encountered traumatic experiences must be considered at risk for emotional illness. These include those considered outside the range of typical human experience, such as rape, war, physical attack, torture, or natural or manmade disaster.

Nursing intervention at the primary level of prevention with individuals experiencing situational crises is aimed at helping them maintain the highest possible level of functioning while offering support and assistance with problem-solving during the crisis period. Interventions for nursing of clients in crisis include the following:

■ Use a reality-oriented approach. The focus of the problem is on the here and now.

■ Remain with the individual who is experiencing panic anxiety.

■ Establish a rapid working relationship by showing unconditional acceptance, actively listening, and attending to immediate needs.

■ Discourage lengthy explanations or rationalizations of the situation; promote an atmosphere for verbalization of true feelings.

■ Set firm limits on aggressive, destructive behaviors. At high levels of anxiety, behavior is likely to be impulsive and regressive. Establish at the outset what is acceptable and what is not, and maintain consistency.

■ Clarify the problem the individual is facing. The nurse does this by describing his or her perception of the problem and comparing it with the individual's perception of the problem.

■ Help the individual determine what he or she believes precipitated the crisis.

■ Acknowledge feelings of anger, guilt, helplessness, and powerlessness, while taking care not to provide positive feedback for these feelings.

■ Guide the individual through a problem-solving process by which he or she may move in the direction of positive life change:
  ■ Help the individual confront the source of the problem that is creating the crisis response.
  ■ Encourage the individual to discuss changes he or she would like to make. Jointly determine whether desired changes are realistic.
  ■ Encourage exploration of feelings about aspects that cannot be changed, and explore alternative ways of coping more adaptively in these situations.
  ■ Discuss alternative strategies for creating change in situations that can realistically be changed.
  ■ Weigh benefits and consequences of each alternative.
  ■ Assist the individual to select alternative coping strategies that will help alleviate future crises.

■ Identify external support systems and new social networks from which the individual may seek assistance in times of stress.

Nursing at the level of primary prevention focuses largely on education of the consumer to prevent initiation or exacerbation of mental illness. An example of content that may be included in one type of primary prevention teaching plan is presented in Table 36-1.

Secondary Prevention
Populations at Risk

Secondary prevention within communities relates to early detection of and prompt intervention with individuals experiencing mental illness symptoms. The same maturational and situational crises presented in the previous section on primary prevention are used to discuss intervention at the secondary level of prevention.

Maturational Crises

Adolescence The need for intervention at the secondary level of prevention in adolescence occurs when disruptive and age-inappropriate behaviors become the norm, and the family can no longer cope adaptively with the situation. All levels of dysfunction are considered—from dysfunctional family coping to the need for hospitalization of the adolescent.

Nursing intervention with the adolescent at this level may occur in the community setting at community mental health centers, physician's offices, schools, public health departments, and crisis intervention centers. Nurses may work with families to problem-solve and improve coping and communication skills, or they may work on a one-to-one basis with the adolescent in an attempt to modify behavior patterns.

Adolescents may be hospitalized for a variety of problems, including (but not limited to) conduct disorders, adjustment disorders, eating disorders, substance-related disorders, depression, and anxiety disorders. Inpatient care is determined by severity of symptomatology. Nursing care of adolescents in the hospital setting focuses on problem identification and stabilizing a crisis situation. Once stability has been achieved, clients are commonly discharged to outpatient care. If an adolescent's home situation has been deemed unsatisfactory, the state may take custody and the child is then discharged to a group or foster home.

Marriage Problems that commonly disrupt a marriage relationship include substance abuse on the part of one or both partners and disagreements on issues of sex, money, children, gender roles, and infidelity, among others.

Nursing intervention at the secondary level of prevention with individuals encountering marriage problems may include one or more of the following:

■ Counseling with the couple or with one of the spouses on a one-to-one basis

TABLE 36–1 Client Education for Primary Prevention: Drugs of Abuse

CLASS OF DRUGS	EFFECTS	SYMPTOMS OF OVERDOSE	TRADE NAMES	COMMON NAMES	EFFECTS ON THE BODY (CHRONIC OR HIGH-DOSE USE)
CNS DEPRESSANTS Alcohol	Relaxation, loss of inhibitions, lack of concentration, drowsiness, slurred speech, sleep	Nausea, vomiting; shallow respirations; cold, clammy skin; weak, rapid pulse; coma; possible death	Ethyl alcohol, beer, gin, rum, vodka, bourbon, whiskey, liqueurs, wine, brandy, sherry, champagne	Booze, alcohol, liquor, drinks, cocktails, high-balls, nightcaps, moonshine, white lightning, firewater	Peripheral nerve damage, skeletal muscle wasting, encephalopathy, psychosis, cardiomyopathy, gastritis, esophagitis, pancreatitis, hepatitis, cirrhosis of the liver, leukopenia, thrombocytopenia, sexual dysfunction
Other (barbiturates and nonbarbiturates)	Same as alcohol	Anxiety, fever, agitation, hallucinations, disorientation, tremors, delirium, convulsions, possible death	Seconal Nembutal Amytal Valium Librium Chloral hydrate Miltown	Red birds Yellow birds Blue birds Blues/yellows Green & whites Mickies Downers	Decreased REM sleep, respiratory depression, hypotension, possible kidney or liver damage, sexual dysfunction
CNS STIMULANTS Amphetamines and related drugs	Hyperactivity, agitation, euphoria, insomnia, loss of appetite	Cardiac arrhythmias, headache, convulsions, hypertension, rapid heart rate, coma, possible death	Dexedrine, Didrex, Tenuate, Bontril, Ritalin, Focalin, Provigil	Uppers, pep pills, wakeups, bennies, eye-openers, speed, black beauties, sweet A's	Aggressive, compulsive behavior; paranoia; hallucinations; hypertension
Cocaine	Euphoria, hyperactivity, restlessness, talkativeness, increased pulse, dilated pupils	Hallucinations, convulsions, pulmonary edema, respiratory failure, coma, cardiac arrest, possible death	Cocaine hydrochloride	Coke, flake, snow, dust, happy dust, gold dust, girl, Cecil, C, toot, blow, crack	Pulmonary hemorrhage, myocardial infarction, ventricular fibrillation
Synthetic stimulants	Agitation, insomnia, irritability, dizziness, decreased ability to think clearly, increased heart rate, chest pains	Depression, paranoia, delusions, suicidal thoughts, seizures, panic attacks, nausea, vomiting, heart attack, stroke	Mephedrone, MDPV (3-4 methylenedioxypyrovalerone)	Bath salts, bliss, vanilla sky, ivory wave, purple wave	Increased heart rate, increased blood pressure, nosebleeds, hallucinations, aggressive behavior

Category	Drug	Street Names	Effects	Overdose	Other Effects
OPIOIDS	Heroin	Snow, stuff, H, Harry, horse	Euphoria, lethargy, drowsiness, lack of motivation, constricted pupils	Shallow breathing, slowed pulse, clammy skin, pulmonary edema, respiratory arrest, convulsions, coma, possible death	Respiratory depression, constipation, fecal impaction, hypotension, decreased libido, retarded ejaculation, impotence, orgasm failure
	Morphine	M, morph, Miss Emma			
	Codeine	Schoolboy			
	Dilaudid	Lords			
	Demerol	Doctors			
	Dolophine	Dollies			
	Percodan	Perkies			
	Talwin	T's			
	Opium	Big O, black stuff			
		U47700 (synthetic)			
HALLUCINOGENS	LSD	Acid, cube, big D	Visual hallucinations, disorientation, confusion, paranoid delusions, euphoria, anxiety, panic, increased pulse	Agitation, extreme hyperactivity, violence, hallucinations, psychosis, convulsions, possible death	Panic reaction, acute psychosis, flashbacks
	PCP	Angel dust, hog, peace pill			
	Mescaline	Mesc			
	DMT	Businessman's trip			
	STP, DOM	Serenity and peace			
	MDMA	Ecstasy, XTC			
	Ketamine	Special K, vitamin K, Kit Kat			
CANNABINOLS	Cannabis	Marijuana, pot, grass, joint, Mary Jane, MJ	Relaxation, talkativeness, lowered inhibitions, euphoria, mood swings	Fatigue, paranoia, delusions, hallucinations, possible psychosis	Tachycardia, orthostatic hypotension, chronic bronchitis, problems with infertility, amotivational syndrome
	Hashish	Hash, rope, sweet Lucy			

- Referral to a couples' support group
- Identification of the problem and possible solutions; support and guidance as changes are undertaken
- Referral to a sex therapist
- Referral to a financial advisor
- Referral to parental effectiveness training

When a marriage fails, individuals often experience a spectrum of troubling emotions including anger, mistrust, depression, and grief (even among individuals who initiate divorce). In community health settings, nurses can lead support groups for newly divorced individuals. They can also provide one-to-one counseling for individuals experiencing the emotional chaos engendered by the dissolution of a marriage relationship.

Divorce also has an impact on the children involved. Nurses can intervene with the children of divorce in an effort to prevent dysfunctional behaviors associated with the break-up of a marriage.

Parenthood Intervention at the secondary level of prevention with parents can be required for a number of reasons. A few of these include:

- Physical, emotional, or sexual abuse of a child
- Physical or emotional neglect of a child
- Birth of a child with special needs
- Diagnosis of a terminal illness in a child
- Death of a child

Nursing intervention at the secondary level of prevention includes recognition of the physical and behavioral signs that indicate possible abuse of a child. The child may be cared for in the emergency department or as an inpatient on the pediatric unit or child psychiatric unit of a general hospital.

Nursing intervention with parents may include teaching effective methods of disciplining children aside from physical punishment. Methods that emphasize the importance of positive reinforcement for acceptable behavior can be very effective. Family members must be committed to consistent use of this behavior modification technique for it to be successful.

Parents should also be informed about behavioral expectations at the various levels of development. Knowledge of what to expect from children at these various stages may provide needed anticipatory guidance to deal with the crises commonly associated with each stage.

Therapy sessions with all family members may focus on communication problems. Members are encouraged to express honest feelings in a manner that is nonthreatening to other family members. Active listening, assertiveness techniques, and respect for the rights of others are taught and encouraged. Barriers to effective communication are identified and resolved.

Referrals to agencies that promote effective parenting skills may be made (e.g., parent effectiveness training). Alternative agencies that may provide relief from the stress of parenting may also be considered (e.g., Mom's Day Out programs, sitter-sharing organizations, and day-care institutions). Support groups for abusive parents may also be helpful and assistance in locating or initiating such a group may be provided.

The nurse can assist parents who are grieving the loss of a child or the birth of a child with special needs by helping them express their true feelings associated with the loss. Feelings such as shock, denial, anger, guilt, powerlessness, and hopelessness must be expressed for the parents to progress through the grief response.

Home health-care assistance can be provided for the family of a child with special needs by making referrals to other professionals, such as speech, physical, and occupational therapists; medical social workers; psychologists; and nutritionists. If the child with special needs is hospitalized, the home health nurse can provide specific information to hospital staff that may be helpful in providing continuity of care for the client and in the transition for the family.

Nursing intervention also includes providing assistance in the location of and referral to support groups that deal with loss of a child or birth of a child with special needs. Some nurses may serve as leaders of these types of groups in the community.

Midlife Nursing care at the secondary level of prevention during midlife becomes necessary when the individual is unable to integrate all of the changes that are occurring during this period. An inability to accept the physical and biological changes, the changes in relationships between themselves and their adult children and aging parents, and the loss of the perception of youth may result in depression that help may be needed to resolve.

Retirement Retirement can also result in depression for individuals who are unable to satisfactorily grieve for the loss of this aspect of their lives. This is more likely to occur if the individuals have not planned for retirement or if they have derived most of their self-esteem from their employment.

Nursing intervention at the secondary level of prevention with depressed individuals takes place in both inpatient and outpatient settings. Severely depressed clients with suicidal ideations will need close observation in the hospital setting, whereas those with mild to moderate depression may be treated in the community. A plan of care for the client with depression is found in Chapter 25, Depressive Disorders. These concepts apply to the secondary level of prevention and may be used in all nursing care settings.

The physician may elect to use pharmacotherapy with antidepressants. Nurses may intervene by providing information to the client about what to expect from the medication, possible side effects, adverse effects, and how to self-administer the medication.

Situational Crises

Nursing care at the secondary level of prevention with clients undergoing situational crises occurs only if crisis intervention at the primary level failed and the individual is unable to function socially or occupationally. Exacerbation of mental illness symptoms requires intervention at the secondary level of prevention. These disorders were addressed extensively in Unit 4. Nursing assessment, diagnosis and outcome identification, planning, implementation, and evaluation were discussed for many of the mental illnesses identified in the *DSM-5* (APA, 2013). These skills may be applied in any setting where nursing is practiced.

A case study situation of nursing care at the secondary level of prevention in a community setting is presented in Box 36–1.

Tertiary Prevention

Individuals With Severe and Persistent Mental Illness

Severe and persistent mental illness is characterized by complex symptoms that reflect a biological phenomenon "causing marked changes in a person's ability to make choices based on consequences, to socialize, to access community supports, to identify what is real, and to organize thoughts (UNC Center of Excellence for Community Mental Health, 2015). Other definitions stress that severe mental illness is marked by severe functional impairment, substantially

---

BOX 36–1 Secondary Prevention Case Study: Parenthood

The identified patient was a petite, doll-like 4-year-old girl named Tanya. She was the older of two children. The other child was a boy named Joseph, aged 2. The mother was 5 months pregnant with their third child. The family had been referred to the nurse after Tanya was placed in foster care following a report to child protective services by her nursery school teacher that the child had marks on her body suspicious of child abuse.

The parents, Paulo and Annette, were in their mid-20s. Paulo had lost his job at an aircraft plant 3 months ago and had been unable to find work since. Annette brought in a few dollars from cleaning houses for other people, but the family was struggling to survive.

Paulo and Annette were angry at having to see the nurse. After all, "Parents have the right to discipline their children." The nurse did not focus on the *intent* of the behavior but instead looked at factors in the family's life that could be viewed as stressors. This family had multiple stressors: poverty, the father's unemployment, the age and spacing of the children, the mother's chronic fatigue from work at home and in other people's homes, and finally, having a child removed from the home against the parents' wishes.

During therapy with this family, the nurse discussed the behaviors associated with various developmental levels. She also discussed possible deviations from these norms and when they should be reported to the physician. The nurse and the family discussed Tanya's behavior and how it compared with the norms.

The parents also discussed their own childhoods. They were able to relate some of the same types of behaviors that they observed in Tanya, but they both admitted that they came from families whose main method of discipline was physical punishment. Annette had been the oldest child in her large family and had been expected to "keep the younger ones in line." When she had not done so, she was punished with her father's belt. She expressed anger toward her father, although she had never been allowed to express it at the time.

Paulo's father had died when he was a small boy, and Paulo had been expected to be the "man of the family." From the time he was very young, he worked at odd jobs to bring money into the home. Consequently, he had little time for the usual activities of childhood and adolescence. He held much resentment toward the young men who "had everything and never had to work for it."

Paulo and Annette had high expectations for Tanya. In effect, they expected her to behave in a manner well beyond her developmental level. These expectations were based on the reflections of their own childhoods. They were uncomfortable with the spontaneity and playfulness of childhood because they had had little personal experience with these behaviors. When Tanya balked and expressed the verbal assertions common to early childhood, Paulo and Annette interpreted these behaviors as defiance toward them and retaliated with anger in the manner in which they had been parented.

With the parents, the nurse explored feelings and behaviors from their past so that they were able to understand the correlation to their current behaviors. They learned to negotiate ways to deal with Tanya's age-appropriate behaviors. In combined therapy with Tanya, they learned how to relate to her childishness and even how to enjoy playing with both of their children.

The parents ceased blaming each other for the family's problems. Annette had spent a good deal of her time deprecating Paulo for his lack of support of his family, and Paulo blamed Annette for being "unable to control her daughter." Communication patterns were clarified, and life in the family became more peaceful.

Without a need to "prove himself" to his wife, Paulo's efforts to find employment met with success because he no longer felt the need to turn down jobs that he believed his wife would perceive to be beneath his capabilities. Annette no longer works outside the home, and both she and Paulo participate in the parenting chores. Tanya and her siblings continue to demonstrate age-appropriate developmental progression.

interfering with major life activities (National Institute of Mental Health [NIMH], 2015). These disorders are identified by criteria listed in the *DSM-5*. Diagnoses may include schizophrenia and related disorders, bipolar disorder, autism spectrum disorders, major depressive disorder, panic disorder, obsessive-compulsive disorder, posttraumatic stress disorder, borderline personality disorder, and attention-deficit/hyperactivity disorder. Based on 2014 statistics, severe mental illness affects about 4.2 percent of the population residing in communities in the United States (NIMH, 2015). The actual number may be significantly higher, since this research did not attempt to include the homeless or those who were in correctional facilities for the entire year.

Historical and Epidemiological Aspects

In 1955, more than half a million individuals resided in public mental hospitals, compared to fewer than 100,000 based on today's estimates.

Deinstitutionalization of persons with serious mental illness began in the 1960s as national policy change based on a strong belief in the individual's right to freedom. Other considerations included the deplorable conditions of some of the state asylums, the introduction of psychotropic medications, and the cost-effectiveness of caring for these individuals in the community setting.

Deinstitutionalization began to occur rapidly and without sufficient planning for the needs of these individuals as they reentered the community. Those who were fortunate enough to have support systems to provide assistance with living arrangements and sheltered employment experiences most often received the outpatient treatment they required. Those without adequate support, however, either managed to survive on a meager income or were forced to join the ranks of the homeless. Some ended up in nursing homes meant to provide care for individuals with physical disabilities.

Certain segments of our population with severe and persistent mental illness have been left untreated: the elderly, the working poor, the homeless, and those individuals previously covered by funds cut by various social reforms. These circumstances have promoted a greater number of crisis-oriented emergency department visits and hospital admissions for individuals with severe and persistent mental illness, as well as frequent confrontations with law enforcement officials.

In 2002, President George W. Bush established the New Freedom Commission on Mental Health, charged with conducting a comprehensive study of the United States mental health service delivery system. They were to identify unmet needs and barriers to services and recommend steps for improvement in services and support for individuals with serious mental illness. In July 2003, the commission presented its final report to the President (President's New Freedom Commission on Mental Health, 2003). The Commission identified the following five barriers:

1. **Fragmentation and gaps in care for children:** About 7 to 9 percent of all children (aged 9 to 17) have a serious emotional disturbance (SED). The Commission found that services for children are even more fragmented than those for adults, with more uncoordinated funding and differing eligibility requirements. Only a fraction of children with SED appear to have access to school-based or school-linked mental health services. Children with SED who are identified for special education services have higher levels of absenteeism, higher drop-out rates, and lower levels of academic achievement than students with other disabilities.

2. **Fragmentation and gaps in care for adults with serious mental illness:** The commission expressed concern that so many adults with serious mental illness are homeless, dependent on alcohol or drugs, unemployed, and untreated. According to the World Health Organization (WHO), mental and behavioral disorders account for 13.6 percent of the total Disability Adjusted Life Years (DALYs) lost due to all disease and injuries in the United States, with the majority of those being associated with major depressive disorder (US Burden of Disease Collaborators, 2013). The Commission identified public attitudes and the stigma associated with mental illness as major barriers to treatment. Stigma is often internalized by individuals with mental illness, leading to hopelessness, lower self-esteem, and isolation. Stigma deprives these individuals of the support they need to recover.

3. **High unemployment and disability for people with serious mental illness:** Undetected, untreated, and poorly treated mental disorders interrupt careers, leading many individuals into lives of disability, poverty, and long-term dependence. The Commission found a 90 percent unemployment rate among adults with serious mental illness—the worst level of employment of any group of people with disabilities. Some surveys have shown that many individuals with serious mental illness *want* to work and could do so with modest assistance. However, the largest "program" of assistance the United States has for people with mental illness is disability payments. Sadly, societal stigma is also reflected in employment discrimination against people with mental illness.

4. **Older adults with mental illnesses are not receiving care:** The Commission reported that about 5 to

10 percent of older adults have major depression, yet most cases are not properly recognized and treated. The report stated:

Older people are reluctant to get care from specialists. They feel more comfortable going to their primary care physician. Still, they are often more sensitive to the stigma of mental illness, and do not readily bring up their sadness and despair. If they acknowledge problems, they are more likely than young people to describe physical symptoms. Primary care doctors may see their suffering as "natural" aging, or treat their reported physical distress instead of the underlying mental disorder. What is often missed is the deep impact of depression on older people's capacity to function in ways that are seemingly effortless for others.

5. **Mental health and suicide prevention are not yet national priorities:** The failure of the United States to prioritize mental health puts many lives at stake. Families struggle to maintain equilibrium while communities strain (and often fail) to provide needed assistance for adults and children who suffer from mental illness. Over 30,000 lives are lost annually to suicide. About 90 percent of those who take their life have a mental disorder. Many individuals who die by suicide have not had care that would help them to affirm life in the months before their deaths. Both the American Psychiatric Association and the National Mental Health Association called on the U.S. Congress to pass parity legislation. In 2008, a federal law known as the Paul Wellstone and Pete Domenici Mental Health Parity and Addiction Equity Act was enacted that generally prevents group health plans and health insurance issuers that provide mental health or substance use disorder benefits from imposing less favorable benefit limitations on those benefits than on medical/surgical benefits. In 2010, the Affordable Care Act amended this legislation to include individual insurance plans, and in 2014, a final regulation clarified and expanded the parity law (Centers for Medicare and Medicaid Services [CMS], 2015a). Many recent national initiatives since the Commission's report have attempted to bridge the gaps, particularly with efforts to address the national suicide rates and the opiate overdose epidemic.

The Commission outlined the following goals and recommendations for mental health reform:

Goal 1. Americans will understand that mental health is essential to overall health.

Commission recommendations:

■ Advance and implement a national campaign to reduce the stigma of seeking care and a national strategy for suicide prevention.

■ Address mental health with the same urgency as physical health.

Goal 2. Mental health care will be consumer and family driven.

Commission recommendations:

■ Develop an individualized plan of care for every adult with a serious mental illness and child with a serious emotional disturbance.

■ Involve consumers and families fully in orienting the mental health system toward recovery.

■ Align relevant federal programs to improve access and accountability for mental health services.

■ Create a comprehensive state mental health plan.

■ Protect and enhance the rights of people with mental illness.

Goal 3. Disparities in mental health services will be eliminated.

Commission recommendations:

■ Improve access to quality care that is culturally competent.

■ Improve access to quality care in rural and geographically remote areas.

Goal 4. Early mental health screening, assessment, and referral to services will be common practice.

Commission recommendations:

■ Promote the mental health of young children.

■ Improve and expand school mental health programs.

■ Screen for co-occurring mental and substance use disorders and link with integrated treatment strategies.

■ Screen for mental disorders in primary health care across the life span and connect to treatment and supports.

Goal 5. Excellent mental health care will be delivered and research will be accelerated.

Commission recommendations:

■ Accelerate research to promote recovery and resilience, and ultimately to cure and prevent mental illnesses.

■ Advance evidence-based practices using dissemination and demonstration projects, and create a public-private partnership to guide their implementation.

■ Improve and expand the workforce providing evidence-based mental health services and supports.

■ Develop the knowledge base in four understudied areas: mental health disparities, long-term effects of medications, trauma, and acute care.

Goal 6. Technology will be used to access mental health care and information.

Commission recommendations:

■ Use health technology and telehealth to improve access and coordination of mental health care, especially for Americans in remote areas or in underserved populations.

■ Develop and implement integrated electronic health record and personal health information systems.

The Substance Abuse and Mental Health Services Administration (SAMHSA), in collaboration with a number of other federal agencies, currently identifies about 390 federal action agenda initiatives to address mental health issues for specific, underserved populations, suicide prevention, and a host of other community and public health concerns (SAMHSA, 2017). Most recently, the surgeon general released a landmark report in 2016 identifying substance abuse as a national health priority in response to the rising death toll from opiate overdoses.

Many nurse leaders see this period of health-care reform as an opportunity for nurses to expand their roles and assume key positions in education, prevention, assessment, and referral. Nurses are, and will continue to be, in key positions to help individuals with severe and persistent mental illness remain as independent as possible, manage their illnesses within the community setting, and minimize the number of hospitalizations required.

Treatment Alternatives

In the current *Scope and Standards of Practice: Psychiatric Mental Health Nursing* (American Nurses Association, American Psychiatric Nurses Association, & International Society of Psychiatric-Mental Health Nurses, 2014), community-based care is identified as within the scope of practice for psychiatric-mental health registered nurses. It defines community-based care as potentially including "care delivered in partnership with health care consumers in their homes, worksites, mental health clinics and programs, health maintenance organizations, shelters and clinics for the homeless, crisis centers, senior centers, group homes, and other community settings" (p. 24). It is clear that psychiatric nurses can and should play an active role in mental health care in the community.

Community Mental Health Centers The goal of community mental health centers in caring for individuals with severe and persistent mental illness is to improve coping ability and prevent exacerbation of acute symptoms. A major obstacle in meeting this goal has been the lack of advocacy or sponsorship for clients who require services from a variety of sources. This has placed responsibility for health care on individuals with mental illness who are often unable to cope with everyday life.

Case management (which was discussed in Chapter 9, The Nursing Process in Psychiatric-Mental Health Nursing, of this text) has become a recommended method of treatment for individuals with severe and persistent mental illness. Ling and Ruscin (2013) state:

> Nurses may be uniquely qualified to be case managers because of their holistic and broad-based background, understanding of health care, and role in patient education and referrals. Case management is an area of practice that offers nurses an opportunity to build on their clinical knowledge, communication, and nursing process skills to function in an expanded patient care role.

Ling and Ruscin (2013) identify six essential activities and nursing role functions that blend with the steps of the nursing process to form a framework for nursing case management:

1. **Assessment:** During the assessment process, the nurse gathers pertinent information about a client's situation and ability to function. Information may be obtained through physical examination, client interview, medical records, and reports from significant others. Ling and Ruscin state, "The case manager's goal is to obtain accurate information about the patient's status and identify factors that may significantly affect the patient's recovery and care."

2. **Planning:** A service care plan is devised with client participation. The plan should include mutually agreed-on goals, specific actions directed toward goal achievement, and selection of essential resources and services through collaboration among health-care professionals, the client, and the family or significant others.

3. **Implementation:** In this phase, the client receives the needed services from the appropriate providers. In some instances, the nursing **case manager** is also a provider of care, while in others, he or she is only the coordinator of care.

4. **Coordination:** The case manager organizes, secures, integrates, and modifies the resources necessary to accomplish the case management goals (Case Management Society of America [CMSA], 2016). This coordination effort involves the client, the physician, any other pertinent health-care providers, and family members or significant others concerned with the client's care. The case manager ensures that all tests and treatments are conducted according to schedule and maintains close communication with all health-care providers to ensure that client care is proceeding according to the plan.

5. **Monitoring:** The case manager monitors the effectiveness of the care plan by gathering pertinent information from various sources at regular intervals to determine the client's response and progress (CMSA, 2016). If problems are identified, immediate adjustments are made.

6. **Evaluation:** The case manager evaluates the client's responses to interventions and progress toward preestablished goals. Regular contact is maintained with client, family or significant others, and direct service providers. Ongoing coordination of care continues until outcomes have been achieved. If the expected outcomes are not achieved, the case manager reevaluates the plan to determine the reason and takes steps to intervene and modify the existing plan.

A case study of nursing case management within a community mental health center is presented in Box 36–2.

Assertive Community Treatment (ACT) The National Alliance on Mental Illness (NAMI, 2016) defines ACT as:

> a team-based treatment model that provides multidisciplinary, flexible treatment and support to people with mental illness 24/7. ACT is based around the idea that people receive better care when their mental health care providers work together. ACT team

members help the person address every aspect of their life, whether it be medication, therapy, social support, employment or housing.

This approach includes members from psychiatry, social work, nursing, and substance abuse and vocational rehabilitation. The ACT team provides these services 24 hours a day, 7 days a week, 365 days a year.

The ACT team provides treatment, rehabilitation, and support services to individuals with severe and persistent mental illness who are unable to receive treatment from a traditional model of case management. The team is usually able to provide most services with minimal referrals to other mental health programs or providers. Services are provided within community settings, such as a person's home, local restaurants, parks, nearby stores, and anywhere else the individual requires assistance with living skills. NAMI (2016) reports, "Studies have shown that ACT is more effective than traditional treatment for people experiencing mental illnesses such as schizophrenia and schizoaffective disorder and can reduce hospitalizations by 20%."

BOX 36–2 Nursing Case Management in the Community Mental Health Center: A Case Study

William is a 63-year-old man with chronic schizophrenia who came into the community mental health center upon the recommendation of a local church where he sometimes attends their meal program. The nurse begins a comprehensive assessment and assures William that she wants to collaborate with him to identify how to best meet his needs. She assesses his basic physical health, management of daily living, family involvement, work history, involvement with any other social agencies, finances, medications, and other concerns identified by William.

She determines that William has not been taking antipsychotic medication for at least 3 months. Prior to that, he had been living in a house with several other individuals, most of whom were abusing substances. They were helping him access medications from a community medication program but were often taking or reselling most of his prescription. When the house was raided by police, William became homeless. He is currently disorganized in his thinking and actively hallucinating.

He expresses desire to take medication but feels that finding a place to live is his most important priority. There is no family involvement, and William is unable to identify any support systems.

The nurse contacts the social worker for assistance with housing options and social resources such as food stamps, and contacts the physician to schedule an appointment for medication evaluation.

The nurse recommends that William attend the partial hospitalization program offered at the community mental health center, and he agrees but says he does not have transportation. The local church has offered to help William

in any way they can, so the nurse contacts them and asks about their availability to provide transportation. The church informs her that they can provide transportation on Tuesdays and Thursdays.

During the assessment, William identified that sometimes the "people start fighting" in his mind and when he starts to scream back someone nearby always calls the police because they "don't get that I'm just trying to defend myself."

The nurse then engages a peer support specialist who introduces William to Alfonzo, a 65-year-old man with chronic schizophrenia who is willing to provide support to William regarding symptom management. Alfonzo is also willing to provide transportation to the partial hospitalization program on the days when the church resources are not available.

The nurse notices that William has some open sores on his feet. She cleans and bandages his feet, orders bloodwork to assess for infection, and accesses socks and footwear from the clothes bank offered through the Salvation Army.

She continues to meet regularly with William once a month on a day that he attends PHP and administers the Prolixin injection ordered by the physician. During her reassessment, William identifies that he has been "hanging out" with Alfonzo and states "he really understands me." He expresses still hearing people fight sometimes in his head but is not as bothered by them. The social worker has facilitated group home placement, which is not available for another 3 months, but in the meantime the local homeless shelter has arranged for William to stay there. The local church has offered William a small stipend to help with stuffing envelopes, and when the nurse asks him how that job is going, William says, "They are nice people at the church, and they say I really help them, too."

Partial Hospitalization Programs Partial hospitalization programs, also called day or evening treatment programs, are designed to prevent institutionalization or to ease the transition from inpatient hospitalization to community living. Various types of treatment are offered. Many include therapeutic community (milieu) activities; individual, group, and family therapies; psychoeducation; alcohol and drug education; crisis intervention; therapeutic recreational activities; and occupational therapy. Many programs offer medication administration and monitoring as part of their care. Some programs have established medication clinics for individuals on long-term psychopharmacological therapy. These clinics may include educational classes and support groups for individuals with similar conditions and treatments.

Partial hospitalization programs generally offer a comprehensive treatment plan formulated by an interdisciplinary team of psychiatrists, psychologists, nurses, occupational and recreational therapists, and social workers. Nurses take a leading role in the administration of partial hospitalization programs. They lead groups, provide crisis intervention, conduct individual counseling, act as role models, and make necessary referrals for specialized treatment. Use of the nursing process provides continual evaluation of the program, and modifications can be made as necessary.

Partial hospitalization programs are an effective method of preventing hospitalization for many individuals with severe and persistent mental illness. They are a way of transitioning these individuals from the acute care setting back into the mainstream community. For some individuals who have been deinstitutionalized, they provide structure, support, opportunities for socialization, and an improvement in their overall quality of life.

Community Residential Facilities Community residential facilities for persons with severe and persistent mental illness are known by many names: group homes, halfway houses, foster homes, boarding homes, sheltered care facilities, transitional housing, independent living programs, social rehabilitation residences, and others. These facilities differ by the purpose for which they exist and the activities that they offer.

Some of these facilities provide food, shelter, housekeeping, and minimal supervision and assistance with activities of daily living. Others may also include a variety of therapies and serve as a transition between hospital and independent living. In addition to the basics, services might include individual and group counseling, medical care, job training or employment assistance, and leisure-time activities.

The concept of transitional housing for individuals with serious mental illness is sound and has often been a successful means of therapeutic support and intervention for maintaining them within the community. However, without guidance and planning, transition to the community can be futile. These individuals may be ridiculed and rejected by the community or be targets of unscrupulous individuals who take advantage of their inability to care for themselves. These occurrences may increase maladaptive responses to the demands of community living and exacerbate the mental illness. Some facilities have live-in professionals who are available at all times, some have professional staff who are on call for intervention during crisis situations, and some are staffed by volunteers and individuals with little knowledge or background for understanding and treating persons with severe and persistent mental illness. A period of structured reorientation to the community in a supervised living situation monitored by professionals is more likely to result in a successful transition for the individual with severe and persistent mental illness.

Psychiatric Home Health Care For the individual with serious mental illness who no longer lives in a structured, supervised setting, home health care may help him or her maintain independent living. To receive home health care, individuals must validate their homebound status for the prospective payer (Medicare, Medicaid, most insurance companies, and Department of Veterans Affairs [VA] benefits). An acute psychiatric diagnosis is not sufficient to qualify for the service. The client must show that he or she is unable to leave the home without considerable difficulty or the assistance of another person. The plan of treatment and subsequent charting must explain why the client's psychiatric disorder keeps him or her at home and justify the need for home services.

Homebound clients most often have a diagnosis of depressive disorder, neurocognitive disorder, anxiety disorder, bipolar disorder, or schizophrenia. Many elderly clients are homebound because of medical conditions that impair mobility and necessitate home care.

Nurses who provide psychiatric home care must have an in-depth knowledge of psychopathology, psychopharmacology, and how medical and physical problems can be influenced by psychiatric impairments. These nurses must be highly adept at performing biopsychosocial assessments. They must be sensitive to changes in behavior that signal that the client is decompensating psychiatrically or medically so that early intervention may be implemented.

Another important job of the psychiatric home health nurse is monitoring the client's adherence to the regimen of psychotropic medications. Some clients receiving injectable medications remain on home health care only until they can be placed on oral medications. Those clients receiving oral medications require close monitoring for adherence and assistance with the uncomfortable side effects of some of these drugs. Lack of adherence to the medication regimen is responsible for approximately two-thirds of psychiatric hospital readmissions. Home health nurses can assist clients with this problem by helping them see the relationship between control of their psychiatric symptoms and adherence to their medication regimen.

Client populations that benefit from psychiatric home health nursing include:

- **Elderly clients:** These individuals do not necessarily have a psychiatric diagnosis but may be experiencing emotional difficulties caused by medical, sociocultural, or developmental factors. Depressed mood and social isolation are common.
- **Persons with severe and persistent mental illness:** These individuals have a history of psychiatric illness and hospitalization. They require long-term medications and continual supportive care. Common diagnoses include recurrent major depressive disorder, schizophrenia, and bipolar disorder.
- **Individuals in acute crisis situations:** These individuals are in need of crisis intervention and/or short-term psychotherapy.

Medicare requires that psychiatric home nursing care be provided by "psychiatrically trained nurses," which CMS defines as "nurses who have special training and/or experience beyond the standard curriculum required for a registered nurse" (CMS, 2015b). The guidelines that cover psychiatric nursing services are not well defined by the CMS. This has presented reimbursement problems for psychiatric nurses in the past. The CMS statement regarding psychiatric nursing services is presented in Box 36–3.

BOX 36–3 **CMS Guidelines for Psychiatric Home Nursing Care**

PSYCHIATRIC EVALUATION, THERAPY, AND TEACHING

The evaluation, psychotherapy, and teaching needed by a patient suffering from a diagnosed psychiatric disorder that requires active treatment by a psychiatrically trained nurse and the costs of the psychiatric nurse's services may be covered as a skilled nursing service. Psychiatrically trained nurses are nurses who have special training and/or experience beyond the standard curriculum required for a registered nurse. The services of the psychiatric nurse are to be provided under a plan of care established and reviewed by a physician.

From Centers for Medicare & Medicaid Services. (2015b). Medicare Benefit Policy Manual. *Baltimore, MD: Author.*

Preparation for psychiatric home health nursing, in addition to the registered nurse licensure, should include several years of psychiatric inpatient treatment experience. It is also recommended that the nurse have medical-surgical nursing experience, because of common client physical comorbidity and the holistic nursing perspective. Additional training and experience in psychotherapy is viewed as an asset. However, psychotherapy is not the primary focus of psychiatric home nursing care. In fact, most reimbursement sources do not pay for exclusively insight-oriented therapy. Crisis intervention, client education, and hands-on care are common interventions in psychiatric home nursing care.

The psychiatric home health nurse provides comprehensive nursing care, incorporating interventions for physical and psychosocial problems into the treatment plan. The interventions are based on the client's mental and physical health status, cultural influences, and available resources. The nurse is accountable to the client at all times during the therapeutic relationship. Nursing interventions are carried out with appropriate knowledge and skill, and referrals are made when the need is outside the scope of nursing practice. Continued collaboration with other members of the health-care team (e.g., psychiatrist, social worker, psychologist, occupational therapist, and/or physical therapist) is essential for maintaining continuity of care.

A case study of psychiatric home health care and the nursing process is presented in Box 36–4. A plan of care for Mrs. C. (the client in the case study) is presented in Table 36–2. Nursing diagnoses are presented, along with outcome criteria, appropriate nursing interventions, and rationale for each.

Care for the Caregivers Psychiatric home health care also provides support and assistance to primary caregivers. When family is the provider of care on a 24/7 schedule for a loved one with a severe and persistent mental disorder, it can be very exhausting and very frustrating. A care plan for primary caregivers is presented in Table 36–3.

The Homeless Population

Historical and Epidemiological Aspects

In 1993, Dr. Richard Lamb, a recognized expert in the field of severe and persistent mental illness, wrote:

> Alec Guinness, in his memorable role as a British Army colonel in *Bridge on the River Kwai*, exclaims at the end of the film when he finally realizes he has been working to help the enemy, "What have I done?" As a vocal advocate and spokesman for deinstitutionalization and community treatment of severely mentally ill patients for well over two decades, I often find myself asking that same question. (p. 1209)

BOX 36–4 Psychiatric Home Health Care and the Nursing Process: A Case Study

ASSESSMENT

Mrs. C., age 76, has been living alone in her small apartment for 6 months since the death of her husband, to whom she had been married for 51 years. Mrs. C. was an elementary school teacher for 40 years, retiring at age 65 with an adequate pension. She and her husband had no children. A niece looks in on Mrs. C. regularly. It was she who contacted Mrs. C.'s physician when she observed that Mrs. C. was not eating properly, was losing weight, and seemed to be isolating herself more and more. She had not left her apartment in weeks. Her physician referred her to psychiatric home health care.

On her initial visit, Carol, the psychiatric home health nurse, conducted a preliminary assessment revealing the following information about Mrs. C.:

1. Blood pressure 90/60 mm Hg
2. Height 5'5"; weight 102 lb
3. Poor skin turgor; dehydration
4. Subjective report of occasional dizziness
5. Subjective report of loss of 20 pounds since the death of her husband
6. Oriented to time, place, person, and situation
7. Memory (remote and recent) intact
8. Flat affect
9. Mood is dysphoric and tearful at times, but client is cooperative
10. Denies thoughts to harm self, but states, "I feel so alone; so useless"
11. Subjective report of difficulty sleeping
12. Subjective report of constipation

DIAGNOSIS AND OUTCOME IDENTIFICATION

The following nursing diagnoses were formulated for Mrs. C.:

1. Complicated grieving related to death of husband evidenced by symptoms of depression such as withdrawal, anorexia, weight loss, difficulty sleeping, dysphoric/tearful mood
2. Risk for injury related to dizziness and weakness from lack of activity, low blood pressure, and poor nutritional status
3. Social isolation related to depressed mood and feelings of worthlessness, evidenced by staying home alone, refusing to leave her apartment

OUTCOME CRITERIA

The following criteria were selected as measurement of outcomes in the care of Mrs. C.:

1. Experiences no physical harm/injury
2. Is able to discuss feelings about husband's death with nurse

3. Sets realistic goals for self
4. Is able to participate in problem solving regarding her future
5. Eats a well-balanced diet with snacks to restore nutritional status and gain weight
6. Drinks adequate fluid daily
7. Sleeps at least 6 hours per night and verbalizes feeling well rested
8. Shows interest in personal appearance and hygiene, and is able to accomplish self-care independently
9. Seeks to renew contact with previous friends and acquaintances
10. Verbalizes interest in participating in social activities

PLANNING AND IMPLEMENTATION

A plan of care for Mrs. C. is presented in Table 36–2.

Evaluation

Mrs. C. started the second week taking trazodone (Desyrel) 150 mg at bedtime. Her sleep was enhanced, and within 2 weeks she showed a noticeable improvement in mood. She began to discuss how angry she felt about being all alone in the world. She admitted that she had felt anger toward her husband but experienced guilt and tried to suppress that anger. As she was assured that these feelings were normal, they became easier for her to express.

The nurse arranged for a local teenager to do some weekly grocery shopping for Mrs. C. and contacted the local Meals on Wheels program, which delivered her noon meal to her every day. Mrs. C. began to eat more and slowly gained a few pounds. She still has an occasional problem with constipation but verbalizes improvement with the addition of vegetables, fruit, and a daily stool softener prescribed by her physician.

Mrs. C. used her walker until she felt she was able to ambulate without assistance. She reports that she no longer experiences dizziness, and her blood pressure has stabilized at around 100/70 mm Hg.

Mrs. C. has joined a senior citizens group and attends activities weekly. She has renewed previous friendships and formed new acquaintances. She sees her physician monthly for medication management and visits a local adult day health center for regular blood pressure and weight checks. Her niece still visits regularly, but her favorite relationship is the one she has formed with her constant canine companion, Molly, whom Mrs. C. rescued from the local animal shelter and who continually demonstrates her unconditional love and gratitude.

The number of homeless individuals in the United States has been estimated at over 3.5 million (National Coalition for the Homeless [NCH], 2014). It is difficult to determine the true scope of the problem because even the statisticians who collect the data have difficulty defining homeless persons. They have sometimes been identified as "those people who sleep in shelters or public spaces." This approach results in

underestimates because available shelter services are insufficient to meet the numbers of homeless people (U.S. Conference of Mayors [USCM], 2014).

According to the Stewart B. McKinney Act, a person is considered homeless who:

lacks a fixed, regular, and adequate night-time residence; and . . . has a primary night-time residency that is: (A) a supervised publicly or privately operated

Table 36–2 | CARE PLAN FOR PSYCHIATRIC HOME HEALTH CARE OF DEPRESSED ELDERLY (MRS. C.)

NURSING DIAGNOSIS: COMPLICATED GRIEVING

RELATED TO: Death of husband

EVIDENCED BY: Symptoms of depression such as withdrawal, anorexia, weight loss, difficulty sleeping, and dysphoric/tearful mood

OUTCOME CRITERIA	NURSING INTERVENTIONS	RATIONALE
Short-Term Goal: • Mrs. C. discusses any angry feelings she has about the loss of her husband. **Long-Term Goal:** • Mrs. C. demonstrates adaptive grieving behaviors and evidence of progression toward resolution.	1. Assess Mrs. C.'s position in the grief process. 2. Develop a trusting relationship by showing empathy and caring. Be honest and keep all promises. Show genuine positive regard. 3. Explore feelings of anger and help Mrs. C. direct them toward the source. Help her understand it is appropriate and acceptable to have feelings of anger and guilt about her husband's death. 4. Encourage Mrs. C. to review honestly the relationship she had with her husband. With support and sensitivity, point out reality of the situation in areas where misrepresentations may be expressed. 5. Determine if Mrs. C. has spiritual needs that are going unfulfilled. If so, contact spiritual leader for intervention with Mrs. C. 6. Refer Mrs. C. to physician for medication evaluation.	1. Accurate baseline data are required to plan accurate care for Mrs. C. 2. These interventions provide the basis for a therapeutic relationship. 3. Knowledge of acceptability of the feelings associated with normal grieving may help to relieve some of the guilt that these responses generate. 4. Mrs. C. must give up an idealized perception of her husband. Only when she is able to see both positive and negative aspects about the relationship will the grieving process be complete. 5. Recovery may be blocked if spiritual distress is present and care is not provided. 6. Antidepressant therapy may help Mrs. C. to function while confronting the dynamics of her depression.

NURSING DIAGNOSIS: RISK FOR INJURY

RELATED TO: Dizziness and weakness from lack of activity, low blood pressure, and poor nutritional status

OUTCOME CRITERIA	NURSING INTERVENTIONS	RATIONALE
Short-Term Goals: • Mrs. C. uses walker when ambulating. • Mrs. C. does not experience physical harm or injury. **Long-Term Goal:** • Mrs. C. does not experience physical harm or injury.	1. Assess vital signs at every visit. Report to physician should they fall below baseline. 2. Encourage Mrs. C. to use walker until strength has returned. 3. Visit Mrs. C. during mealtimes and sit with her while she eats. Encourage her niece to do the same. Ensure that easy to prepare, nutritious foods for meals and snacks are available in the house and that they are items that Mrs. C. likes.	1. Client safety is a nursing priority. 2. The walker will help prevent Mrs. C. from falling. 3. She is more likely to eat what is convenient and what she enjoys.

Continued

Table 36–2 | CARE PLAN FOR PSYCHIATRIC HOME HEALTH CARE OF DEPRESSED ELDERLY (MRS. C.)—cont'd

OUTCOME CRITERIA	NURSING INTERVENTIONS	RATIONALE
	4. Contact local meal delivery service (e.g., Meals on Wheels) to deliver some of Mrs. C.'s meals.	4. This ensures that she receives at least one complete and nutritious meal each day.
	5. Weigh Mrs. C. each week.	5. Weight gain is a measurable, objective means of assessing whether Mrs. C. is eating.
	6. Ensure that diet contains sufficient fluid and fiber.	6. Adequate dietary fluid and fiber will help to alleviate constipation. She may also benefit from a daily stool softener.

NURSING DIAGNOSIS: SOCIAL ISOLATION

RELATED TO: Depressed mood and feelings of worthlessness

EVIDENCED BY: Staying home alone, refusing to leave apartment

OUTCOME CRITERIA	NURSING INTERVENTIONS	RATIONALE
Short-Term Goal: • Mrs. C. discusses with nurse feelings about past social relationships and those she may like to renew. Long-Term Goal: • Mrs. C. renews contact with friends and participates in social activities.	1. As nutritional status is improving and strength is gained, encourage Mrs. C. to become more active. Take walks with her; help her perform simple tasks around her house.	1. Increased activity enhances both physical and mental status.
	2. Assess lifelong patterns of relationships.	2. Basic personality characteristics will not change. Mrs. C. will very likely keep the same style of relationship development that she had in the past.
	3. Help her identify present relationships that are satisfying and activities that she considers interesting.	3. She is the person who truly knows what she likes, and these personal preferences will facilitate success in reversing social isolation.
	4. Consider the feasibility of a pet.	4. There are many documented studies of the benefits to elderly individuals of companion pets.
	5. Suggest possible alternatives that Mrs. C. may consider as she seeks to participate in social activities. These may include foster grandparent programs, senior citizens centers, church activities, craft groups, and volunteer activities. Help her to locate individuals with whom she may attend some of these activities.	5. She is more likely to attend and participate if she does not have to do so alone.

| **Table 36-3 \| CARE PLAN FOR PRIMARY CAREGIVER OF CLIENT WITH SEVERE AND PERSISTENT MENTAL ILLNESS** | | |

NURSING DIAGNOSIS: CAREGIVER ROLE STRAIN

RELATED TO: Severity and duration of the care receiver's illness and lack of respite and recreation for the caregiver

EVIDENCED BY: Feelings of stress in relationship with care receiver, feelings of depression and anger, family conflict around issues of providing care

OUTCOME CRITERIA	NURSING INTERVENTIONS	RATIONALE
Short-Term Goal: • Caregivers verbalize understanding of ways to facilitate the caregiver role. Long-Term Goal: • Caregivers demonstrate effective problem-solving skills and develop adaptive coping mechanisms to regain equilibrium.	1. Assess caregivers' abilities to anticipate and fulfill client's unmet needs. Provide information to assist caregivers with this responsibility. Ensure that caregivers encourage client to be as independent as possible.	1. Caregivers may be unaware of what the client can realistically accomplish. They may be unaware of the nature of the illness.
	2. Ensure that caregivers are aware of available community support systems from which they may seek assistance when required. Examples include respite care services, day treatment centers, and adult day-care centers.	2. Caregivers require relief from the pressures and strain of providing 24-hour care for their loved one. Studies have shown that abuse arises out of caregiving situations that place overwhelming stress on the caregivers.
	3. Encourage caregivers to express feelings, particularly anger.	3. Release of these emotions can serve to prevent psychopathology, such as depression or psychophysiological disorders, from occurring.
	4. Encourage participation in support groups comprised of members with similar life situations. Provide information about support groups that may be helpful: a. National Alliance on Mental Illness (NAMI) (800) 950-NAMI b. American Association on Intellectual and Developmental Disabilities (AAIDD) (800) 424-3688 c. Alzheimer's Association (800) 272-3900	4. Hearing others who are experiencing the same problems discuss ways in which they have coped may help caregiver adopt more adaptive strategies. Individuals who are experiencing similar life situations provide empathy and support for each other.

shelter designed to provide temporary living accommodations, (B) an institution that provides a temporary residence for individuals intended to be institutionalized, or (C) a public or private place not designed for, or ordinarily used as, a regular sleeping accommodation for human beings. (NCH, 2009)

The National Alliance to End Homelessness (2015) reports that in ongoing recovery from the recession,

the homeless population decreased in 2014 by 2.3 percent. However, statistics are not reported for the subpopulation of those with severe mental illness. Federal and state assistance programs may be responsible for some of this decrease. Efforts to meet the needs of this population continue. In October 2016, amendments to the McKinney-Vento Act went into effect that include provisions for homeless children and young adults to receive adequate and accessible education.

Mental Illness and Homelessness

The prevalence of severe mental illness among the homeless population is difficult to clarify. SAMHSA (2016) provides the following demographics through statistics gathered from Projects for Assistance in Transition from Homelessness, (PATH), which is specifically established for funding services to people with severe mental illness (SMI). Thus, these statistics are based on the makeup of PATH clients:

Age Thirty-nine percent of clients with SMI are younger than age 30; individuals between the ages of 31 and 61 make up the bulk of this population at 70 percent; about 5 percent are older than age 61.

Gender Fifty-nine percent of homeless individuals are male, and 41 percent are female.

Ethnicity The homeless SMI population is estimated to be 57 percent Caucasian, 34 percent African American, 13 percent Hispanic, 3 percent of other single races/ethnic groups, and 5 percent of multiple races (SAMHSA, 2016). The ethnic makeup of homeless populations varies according to geographic location.

The USCM (2014) survey revealed that approximately 28 percent of the homeless population suffers from some form of mental illness. Who are these individuals, and why are they homeless? Some blame the deinstitutionalization movement. Persons with mental illness who were released from state and county mental hospitals and did not have families with whom they could reside sought residence in board-and-care homes of varying quality. Halfway houses and supportive group living arrangements were helpful but scarce. Many of those with families returned to their homes, but because families received little if any instruction or support, the environment was frequently turbulent, and individuals with mental illness often went on to leave these homes.

Types of Mental Illness Among the Homeless A number of studies have been conducted, primarily in large urban areas, that have addressed the most common types of mental illness among homeless individuals. Schizophrenia is frequently described as the most common diagnosis. Other prevalent disorders include bipolar disorder, substance addiction, depression, personality disorders, and neurocognitive disorders. Many exhibit psychotic symptoms, many are former residents of long-term care institutions for the mentally ill, and many have such a strong desire for independence that they isolate themselves in an effort to avoid identification by the mental health system. Many are clearly a danger to themselves or others, yet they often do not even see themselves as ill. SAMHSA (2016) identifies that in 2015, 53 percent of clients

receiving PATH services had a co-occurring substance use disorder.

Contributing Factors to Homelessness Among Individuals With Mental Illness

Deinstitutionalization As previously stated, deinstitutionalization is frequently implicated as a contributing factor to homelessness among individuals with mental illness. Deinstitutionalization began out of expressed concern by mental health professionals and others who described the "deplorable conditions" under which mentally ill individuals were housed.

The advent of psychotropic medications and the community mental health movement began a growing philosophical view that individuals with mental illness receive better and more humanitarian treatment in the community than in state hospitals far removed from their homes. It was believed that commitment and institutionalization in many ways deprived these individuals of their civil rights. Not the least of the motivating factors for deinstitutionalization was the financial burden these clients placed on state governments.

While the deinstitutionalization movement has prompted an expansion of community mental health resources, the number of people with mental illness incarcerated in correctional facilities has skyrocketed and is now estimated to be two to four times that of the general population (National Institute of Corrections, 2016). Supporters of the community mental health movement have argued that ongoing problems for those with severe mental illness are related to lack of compliance with medications, but critics have argued that the community mental health model is too narrowly focused on a biomedical approach and needs to revise and expand its services to meet the complex needs of this population going forward.

Deinstitutionalization has been criticized for contributing to both homelessness rates and criminalization of people with mental illnesses, but several other factors have been implicated as well.

Poverty Cuts in various government entitlement programs have depleted the allotments available for individuals with severe and persistent mental illness living in the community. The job market is prohibitive for individuals whose behavior is incomprehensible or even frightening to many. The stigma and discrimination associated with mental illness may be diminishing slowly but remains highly visible to those who suffer from its effects.

Scarcity of Affordable Housing Not only is there a scarcity of affordable housing but the number of single-room-occupancy (SRO) hotels has diminished drastically. SRO hotels provided a means of relatively inexpensive housing, and although some people believe that these facilities nurtured isolation, they provided adequate shelter from the elements for their occupants. So many individuals currently frequent the shelters of our cities that there is concern they are becoming mini-institutions for individuals with serious mental illness.

Other Factors Several other factors that may contribute to homelessness have been identified:

■ **Lack of affordable health care:** For families barely able to scrape together enough money to pay for day-to-day living, a catastrophic illness can create the level of poverty that starts the downward spiral to homelessness.

■ **Domestic violence:** The NCH (2014) reports that domestic violence is a primary cause of homelessness, with approximately 63 percent of homeless women having experienced domestic violence in their adult lives. Battered women are often forced to choose between an abusive relationship and homelessness.

■ **Addiction disorders:** Individuals with untreated alcohol or drug addictions are at increased risk for homelessness. The following have been cited as obstacles to addiction treatment for homeless persons: lack of health insurance, lack of documentation, waiting lists, scheduling difficulties, daily contact requirements, lack of transportation, ineffective treatment methods, lack of supportive services, and cultural insensitivity.

Community Resources for the Homeless

Interfering Factors Among the many issues that complicate service planning for homeless individuals with mental illness is this population's penchant for mobility. Frequent relocation confounds service delivery and interferes with providers' efforts to ensure appropriate care. Some individuals with serious mental illness may be affected by homelessness only temporarily or intermittently. These individuals are sometimes called the "episodically homeless." Others move around within neighborhoods or cities as needs and availability of services change. A large number of the homeless mentally ill population exhibits continuous unbounded movement over wide geographical areas.

Not all homeless individuals with mental illness are mobile. Some studies have indicated that a large percentage remain in the same location over a number of years. Health-care workers must identify movement patterns of homeless people in their area to at least try to bring the best care possible to this unique population. This may indeed mean delivering services to those individuals who do not seek out services on their own.

Health Issues Life as a homeless person can have severe consequences in terms of health. Exposure to the elements, poor diet, sleep deprivation, risk of violence, injuries, and lack of health care lead to a precarious state of health and exacerbate preexisting illnesses. It has been estimated that about 40 percent of homeless individuals abuse alcohol. Compared to other homeless individuals, those who abuse alcohol are at greater risk for neurological impairment, heart disease and hypertension, chronic lung disease, gastrointestinal disorders, hepatic dysfunction, and trauma.

Thermoregulation is a health problem for all homeless individuals because of their exposure to all kinds of weather. It is a compounded problem for the homeless alcoholic who spends much time in an altered level of consciousness.

It is difficult to determine whether mental illness is a cause or effect of homelessness. Some behaviors that seem deviant may in actuality be adaptations to life on the street. Homeless individuals may even seek hospitalization in psychiatric institutions in an attempt to get off the streets for a while.

Outbreaks of tuberculosis among homeless persons continue to challenge public control efforts (CDC, 2013). Crowded **shelters** provide ideal conditions for spread of respiratory infections among inhabitants. The risk of acquiring tuberculosis is also increased by the prevalence of alcoholism, drug addiction, HIV infection, and poor nutrition among homeless individuals.

Dietary deficiencies are a continuing problem for homeless individuals. Not only is the homeless person commonly in a poor nutritional state, but the condition itself exacerbates a number of other health problems. Homeless people suffer from higher mortality rates and a greater number of serious disorders than their counterparts in the general population.

Sexually transmitted infections (STIs), such as gonorrhea and syphilis, are a serious problem for the homeless. One of the most serious STIs prevalent among homeless individuals is HIV infection. Street life is precarious for individuals whose systems are immunosuppressed by HIV. Rummaged food scraps are often spoiled, and exposure to the elements is a continuous threat. Individuals with HIV who stay in shelters often are exposed to the infectious diseases of others, which can be life-threatening in this vulnerable condition.

Homeless children have special health needs. Children without a home are prone to higher rates of asthma, ear infections, stomach problems, and speech problems than their counterparts who are not homeless. They are also more likely to experience mental health problems, such as anxiety, depression, and withdrawal.

A growing problem that has captured national attention is the increasing number of hate crimes perpetrated against the homeless. These attacks do not appear to be specifically directed toward the mentally ill but rather reflect a primary bias against homeless people. Based on a report by NCH (2012), most of the victims (88%) are male, 72 percent are 40 years of age or older, 21 percent of the attacks are fatal, and at least 50 percent of the perpetrators are under the age of 20. The NCH highlights the problem more dramatically in the statement, "While this report provides alarming numbers, it is important to note that homeless people are so poorly treated by society that their attacks are often forgotten or unreported" (p. 10). Community mental health nurses have an opportunity and a responsibility to assess and intervene for homeless people who are a vulnerable population on so many levels.

Types of Resources Available

Homeless Shelters   Shelters for the homeless in the United States vary from converted warehouses that provide cots or floor space for overnight stays to significant operations that provide a multitude of social and health-care services. They are run by volunteers and paid professionals and sponsored by churches, community governments, and various social agencies.

It is impossible, then, to describe a "typical" shelter. One description is the provision of lodging, food, and clothing to individuals who are in need of these services. Some shelters also provide medical and psychiatric evaluations, first aid and other health-care services, and referral for case management services by nurses or social workers.

Individuals who seek services from the shelter are generally assigned a bed or cot, issued a set of clean linen, provided a place to shower, shown laundry facilities, and offered a meal in the shelter kitchen or dining hall. Most shelters attempt to separate dormitory areas for men and women, with various consequences for those who violate the rules.

Shelters cover expenses through private and corporate donations, church sponsorships, and government grants. From the outset, shelters were conceptualized as "temporary" accommodations for individuals who needed a place to spend the night. Realistically, they have become permanent lodging for homeless individuals with little hope for improving their situations. Some individuals even use their shelters' mailing address.

Shelters provide a safe and supportive environment for homeless individuals who have no other place to go. Some homeless people who inhabit shelters use the resources offered to improve their lot in life, whereas others become hopelessly dependent on the shelter's provisions. To a few, the availability of a shelter may mean the difference between life and death.

Health-Care Centers and Storefront Clinics   Some communities have established "street clinics" to serve the homeless population. Many are operated by nurse practitioners who work in consultation with physicians in the area. In recent years, some of these clinics have provided clinical sites for nursing students in community health rotations. Some have been staffed by nursing school faculties that have established group practices in the community setting.

A wide variety of services are offered at these clinics, including administering medications, assessing vital signs, screening for tuberculosis and other communicable diseases, giving immunizations and flu shots, changing dressings, and administering first aid. Physical and psychosocial assessments, health education, and supportive counseling are also frequent interventions.

Nursing in **storefront clinics** for the homeless provides many special challenges, not the least of which is poor working conditions. These clinics often operate under severe budgetary constraints with inadequate staffing, supplies, and equipment, in rundown facilities located in high-crime neighborhoods. Frustration is often high among nurses who work in these clinics, as they are seldom able to see measurable progress in their homeless clients. Maintenance of health management is virtually impossible for individuals who have no resources outside the health-care setting. If return appointments for preventive care are made, they are often missed.

Mobile Outreach Units   Outreach programs literally reach out to the homeless in their own environments in an effort to provide health care. Volunteers and paid professionals form teams to seek out homeless individuals who are in need of assistance. They offer coffee, sandwiches, and blankets in an effort to show concern and establish trust. Assistance can be provided at the site if possible. If not, every effort is made to ensure that the individual is linked with a source that can provide the necessary services.

Mobile outreach units provide assistance to homeless individuals who are in need of physical or psychological care. The emphasis of outreach programs is to accommodate the homeless who refuse to seek treatment elsewhere. Most target the mentally ill segment of the population. When trust has been established and the individual agrees to come to the team's office, medical and psychiatric treatment is initiated. Involuntary hospitalization is initiated when an individual is deemed harmful to self or others, or otherwise meets the criteria to be considered "gravely disabled."

The Homeless Client and the Nursing Process

A case study demonstrating nursing process with a homeless client is presented in Box 36–5.

BOX 36–5 Case Study: Nursing Process With a Homeless Client

ASSESSMENT

Joe, age 68, is brought to the Community Health Clinic by two of his peers, who report, "He just had a fit. He needs a drink bad!" Joe is dirty and unkempt, has visible tremors of the upper extremities, and is weak enough to require assistance when ambulating. He is cooperative as the nurse completes the intake assessment. He is coherent, although thought processes are slow. He is disoriented to time and place. He appears somewhat frightened as he scans the unfamiliar surroundings. He is unable to tell the nurse when he had his last drink. He reports no physical injury, and none is observable.

Joe carries a small bag with a few personal items inside, including a Department of Veterans Affairs (VA) benefit card, identifying him as a veteran of the Vietnam War. The nurse finds a cot for Joe, ensures that his vital signs are stable, and telephones the number on the VA card. The clinic nurse discovers that Joe is well known to the admissions personnel at the VA. He has a 35-year history of schizophrenia with numerous hospitalizations. At the time of his last discharge, he was taking fluphenazine (Prolixin) 10 mg twice a day. He told the clinic nurse that he took the medication for a few months after he got out of the hospital but then did not have the prescription refilled. He could not remember when he had last taken fluphenazine.

Joe also has a long history of alcohol-related disorders and has participated in the VA substance rehabilitation program three times. He has no home address and receives his VA disability benefit checks at a shelter address. He reports that he has no family. The nurse makes arrangements for VA personnel to drive Joe from the clinic to the VA hospital, where he is admitted for detoxification. She sets up a case management file for Joe and arranges with the hospital to have Joe return to the clinic after discharge.

DIAGNOSIS AND OUTCOME IDENTIFICATION

The following nursing diagnosis was formulated for Joe:

- Ineffective health maintenance related to ineffective coping skills evidenced by abuse of alcohol, lack of follow-through with antipsychotic medication, and lack of personal hygiene

Ongoing criteria were selected as outcomes for Joe:

- Follows the rules of the group home and maintains his residency status
- Attends weekly sessions of group therapy at the VA day treatment program
- Attends weekly sessions of Alcoholics Anonymous and maintains sobriety
- Reports regularly to the health clinic for injections of fluphenazine
- Volunteers at the VA hospital 3 days a week
- Secures and retains permanent employment

PLANNING AND IMPLEMENTATION

During Joe's hospitalization, the clinic nurse remained in contact with his case. Joe received complete physical and dental examinations and treatment during his hospital stay. The clinic nurse attended the treatment team meeting for Joe as his outpatient case manager. It was decided at the meeting to try giving Joe injections of fluphenazine decanoate because of his history of lack of adherence to his daily oral medication regimen. The clinic nurse would administer the injection every 4 weeks.

At Joe's follow-up clinic visit, the nurse explains to Joe that she has found a group home where he may live with others who have personal circumstances similar to his. At the group home, meals will be provided and the group home manager will ensure that Joe's basic needs are fulfilled. A criterion for remaining at the residence is for Joe to remain alcohol free. Joe is agreeable to these living arrangements.

With Joe's concurrence, the clinic nurse also performs the following interventions:

- Goes shopping with Joe to purchase some new clothing, allowing Joe to make decisions as independently as possible
- Helps Joe move into the group home and introduces him to the manager and residents
- Helps Joe change his address from the shelter to the group home so that he may continue to receive his VA benefits
- Enrolls Joe in the weekly group therapy sessions of the day treatment facility connected with the VA hospital
- Helps Joe locate the nearest Alcoholics Anonymous group and identifies a sponsor who will ensure that Joe gets to the meetings
- Sets up a clinic appointment for Joe to return in 4 weeks for his fluphenazine injection; telephones Joe 1 day in advance to remind him of his appointment
- Instructs Joe to return to or call the clinic if any of the following symptoms occur: sore throat, fever, nausea and vomiting, severe headache, difficulty urinating, tremors, skin rash, or yellow skin or eyes
- Assists Joe in securing transportation to and from appointments
- Encourages Joe to set realistic goals for his life and offers recognition for follow-through
- When Joe is ready, discusses employment alternatives with him; suggests the possibility of starting with a volunteer job (perhaps as a VA hospital volunteer)

EVALUATION

Evaluation of the nursing process with homeless individuals who have mental illness must be highly individualized. Statistics show that chances for relapse with this population are high. Therefore, it is extremely important that outcome criteria be realistic so as not to set the client up for failure.

Summary and Key Points

■ The focus of psychiatric care is shifting from inpatient hospitalization to outpatient care within the community. This trend is largely due to the need for greater cost effectiveness in providing medical care to the masses.

■ The community mental health movement began in the 1960s with the closing of state hospitals and the deinstitutionalization of many individuals with severe and persistent mental illness.

■ Mental health care within the community targets primary prevention (reducing the incidence of mental disorders within the population), secondary prevention (reducing the prevalence of psychiatric illness by shortening the course of the illness), and tertiary prevention (reducing the residual defects that are associated with severe and persistent mental illness).

■ Primary prevention focuses on identification of populations at risk for mental illness, increasing their ability to cope with stress, and targeting and diminishing harmful forces within the environment.

■ The focus of secondary prevention is accomplished through early identification of problems and prompt initiation of effective treatment.

■ Tertiary prevention focuses on preventing complications of the illness and promoting rehabilitation directed toward achievement of the individual's maximum level of functioning.

■ Registered nurses serve as providers of psychiatric-mental health care in the community setting.

■ Nurses provide outpatient care for individuals with severe and persistent mental illness in community mental health centers, in day and evening treatment programs, in partial hospitalization programs, in community residential facilities, and with psychiatric home health care.

■ Homeless persons with mental illness provide a special challenge for the community mental health nurse. Care is provided within homeless shelters, at health-care centers or storefront clinics, and through mobile outreach programs.

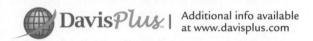 DavisPlus | Additional info available at www.davisplus.com

Review Questions
Self-Examination/Learning Exercise

Select the answer that is most appropriate for each of the following questions.

1. Which of the following represents a nursing intervention at the primary level of prevention?
   a. Teaching a class in parent effectiveness training
   b. Leading a group of adolescents in drug rehabilitation
   c. Referring a married couple for sex therapy
   d. Leading a support group for battered women

2. Which of the following represents a nursing intervention at the secondary level of prevention?
   a. Teaching a class about menopause to middle-aged women
   b. Providing support in the emergency room to a rape victim
   c. Leading a support group for women in transition
   d. Making monthly visits to the home of a client with schizophrenia to ensure medication compliance

3. Which of the following represents a nursing intervention at the tertiary level of prevention?
   a. Serving as case manager for a mentally ill homeless client
   b. Leading a support group for newly retired men
   c. Teaching prepared childbirth classes
   d. Caring for a depressed widow in the hospital

4. John, a homeless person, has just come to live in the shelter. The shelter nurse is assigned to his care. Which of the following is a *priority* intervention on the part of the nurse?
   a. Referring John to a social worker
   b. Developing a plan of care for John
   c. Conducting a behavioral and needs assessment on John
   d. Helping John apply for Social Security benefits

Review Questions—cont'd
Self-Examination/Learning Exercise

5. John, a homeless person, has a history of schizophrenia and nonadherence to his medication regimen. Which of the following medications might be the best choice for John?
   a. Haldol
   b. Navane
   c. Lithium carbonate
   d. Prolixin decanoate

6. Ann is a psychiatric home health nurse. She has just received an order to begin regular visits to Mrs. W., a 78-year-old widow who lives alone. Mrs. W.'s primary care physician has diagnosed her as depressed. Which of the following criteria would qualify Mrs. W. for home health visits?
   a. Mrs. W. never learned to drive and has to depend on others for her transportation.
   b. Mrs. W. is physically too weak to travel without risk of injury.
   c. Mrs. W. refuses to seek assistance as suggested by her physician, "because I don't have a psychiatric problem."
   d. Mrs. W. says she would rather have home visits than go to the physician's office.

7. Ann is a psychiatric home health nurse. She has just received an order to begin regular visits to Mrs. W., a 78-year-old widow who lives alone. Mrs. W.'s primary care physician has diagnosed her as depressed. Which of these potential problems is a priority to evaluate for during the first home visit?
   a. Complicated grieving
   b. Social isolation
   c. Risk for injury
   d. Sleep pattern disturbance

8. Mrs. W., a 78-year-old depressed widow, says to her home health nurse, "What's the use? I don't have anything to live for anymore." Which is the best response on the part of the nurse?
   a. "Of course you do, Mrs. W. Why would you say such a thing?"
   b. "You seem so sad. I'm going to do my best to cheer you up."
   c. "Let's talk about why you are feeling this way."
   d. "Are you having thoughts about harming yourself in any way?"

9. The physician orders trazadone (Desyrel), 150 mg to be taken at bedtime, for Mrs. W., a 78-year-old widow with depression. Which of the following statements about this medication would be appropriate for the home health nurse to make in teaching Mrs. W. about trazadone?
   a. "You may feel dizzy when you stand up, so go slowly when you get up from sitting or lying down."
   b. "You must not eat chocolate while you are taking this medicine."
   c. "We will need to draw a sample of blood to send to the lab every month while you are on this medication."
   d. "If you don't feel better right away with this medicine, the doctor can order a different kind for you."

10. Which of the following issues have been identified as contributing to the rise in the population of those who are homeless? (Select all that apply.)
   a. Poverty
   b. Lack of affordable health care
   c. Substance abuse
   d. Severe and persistent mental illness
   e. Growth in the number of family members living together

IMPLICATIONS OF RESEARCH FOR EVIDENCE-BASED PRACTICE

Ng, P., Chun, W.K., & Tsun, A. (2012). Recovering from hallucinations: A qualitative study of coping with voices hearing of people with schizophrenia in Hong Kong. *The Scientific World Journal, 2012*(5), 1-8. doi:10.1100/2012/232619

DESCRIPTION OF THE STUDY: This study involved in-depth interviews with 20 people who had schizophrenia and were hearing voices to learn more about their coping strategies. All of the participants were living in halfway houses, receiving Social Security assistance, and taking psychotropic medications. Most had been living with schizophrenia for 20 years or more. The authors note literature supporting that those who had coping strategies were better able to manage, whereas "non-copers" had more difficulty managing and perceived the voices as negative and aggressive. The most common coping strategies were social engagement (by talking with others, the voices were less pronounced) and manipulating the level of sensory stimulation (including selectively listening to the voices). They also cite the significance of exploring coping strategies, since auditory hallucinations often persisted in spite of psychotropic medication.

RESULTS OF THE STUDY: Several effective coping strategies were identified:

1. Changing social contacts through ignoring or justifying the voices

2. Manipulating and regulating the voices
3. Changing their perceptions about the meaning of the voices

IMPLICATIONS FOR NURSING PRACTICE: In a strictly biomedical approach, auditory hallucinations are a phenomenon that is to be treated and hopefully eliminated. Studies such as this encourage nurses to expand their understanding of this phenomenon and options for intervention. The authors summarize implications for practice that are relevant for nurses and other health-care providers:

1. We need to develop a respectful attitude toward voice-hearing experiences.
2. We need to understand voice hearing and coping strategies in a cultural context; some cultures prefer alternative strategies over medication for coping.
3. Specialized programs for coping with voice hearing will promote adjustment to community living.
4. Specialized training for professionals about how discussing hallucinations can be informative, particularly with regard for their propensity toward self-harm or violence.
5. Family education about auditory hallucinations and how some people cope may provide a foundation that allows for open discussion about hearing voices within a supportive context.

IMPLICATIONS OF RESEARCH FOR EVIDENCE-BASED PRACTICE

Corbiere, M., Samson, E., Villotti, P., & Pelletier, J.F. (2012). Strategies to fight stigma toward people with mental disorders: Perspectives from different stakeholders. *The Scientific World Journal, 2012*(3), 1-10. doi:10.1100/2012/516358

DESCRIPTION OF THE STUDY: The purpose of this survey was to identify perspectives of mental health professionals, clients with mental illness, family members, and other mental health care providers to identify a broad range of activities being used to combat stigma toward people with mental illness. The participants ($N = 253$) were delegates to a Canadian conference and were asked to identify specific practices used to reduce prejudice and stigma in this population.

RESULTS OF THE STUDY: Fifteen categories of activities were identified that fell under six main themes:

Education: Stigma may be reduced by providing factual knowledge about mental illnesses.

Contact: Direct interaction with affected persons may decrease negative attitudes.

Protestation: Protesting against bias and promoting advocacy may support culture change through personal protestation.

Person-centered: Incorporating an attitude of normalizing in interaction with clients and modifying elements that

contribute to the client being identifiable in the general population may promote social integration.

Working on recovery and social inclusion: Supporting, assisting, and encouraging clients to capitalize on their strengths promotes working on integration in the community.

Reflexive consciousness: Encouraging others to reflect on their attitudes about mental illness promotes insight and creates a foundation for change in attitudes.

IMPLICATIONS FOR NURSING PRACTICE: As the authors cite, the literature reports more than 40 negative consequences of stigma, the effects of which extend beyond the individual to family, friends, and health-care workers. Successful community mental health and recovery models must address reduction of the stigma associated with mental illness. Student nurses, as they begin to learn about this vulnerable and often disenfranchised population, are often confronted with their own attitudes and ask ,"What can I do?" A study such as this informs about central themes and activities for nurses to support patients with mental illness in any practice or community setting. The authors note that knowledge is helpful but does not necessarily translate to behavior change, so perhaps the more important question is, "What *will* you do?"

References

American Nurses Association (ANA), American Psychiatric Nurses Association, & International Society of Psychiatric-Mental Health Nurses. (2014). *Scope and standards of practice: Psychiatric-mental health nursing* (2nd ed.). Silver Spring, MD: ANA.

American Psychiatric Association. (2013). *Diagnostic and statistical manual of mental disorders* (5th ed.). Washington, DC: American Psychiatric Publishing.

Case Management Society of America (CMSA). (2016). *Standards of practice for case management.* Little Rock, AR: CMSA.

Centers for Disease Control and Prevention. (2013, March 22). Trends in tuberculosis—United States, 2012. *Morbidity and Mortality Weekly, 62*(11), 201-205.

Centers for Medicare & Medicaid Services. (2015a). The mental health parity and addiction equity act. Retrieved from https://www.cms.gov/CCIIO/Programs-and-Initiatives/Other-Insurance-Protections/mhpaea_factsheet.html

Centers for Medicare & Medicaid Services. (2015b). *Medicare Benefit Policy Manual.* Baltimore, MD: CMS.

Corbiere, M., Samson, E., Villotti, P., & Pelletier, J.F. (2012). Strategies to fight stigma toward people with mental disorders: Perspectives from different stakeholders. *The Scientific World Journal, 2012*(3), 1-10. doi:10.1100/2012/516358

Kaakinen, J.R., Coehlo, D.P., Steele, R., Tabacco, A., & Harmon Hanson, S.M.(2015). *Family health care nursing: Theory, practice, and research* (5th ed.). Philadelphia: F. A. Davis.

Ling, C., & Ruscin, C. (2013). Case management basics. Gannett Education Course #60102. Retrieved from http://ce.nurse.com/60102/Case-Management-Basics

McLeod, S.A. (2010). SRRS—Stress of life events. Retrieved from www.simplypsychology.org/SRRS.html

National Alliance on Mental Illness. (2016). Psychosocial treatments: Assertive community treatment. Retrieved from https://www.nami.org/Learn-More/Treatment/Psychosocial-Treatments

National Alliance to End Homelessness. (2015). *The state of homelessness in America 2015.* Retrieved from www.endhomelessness.org/library/entry/the-state-of-homelessness-in-america-2015

National Coalition for the Homeless. (2009). Who is homeless? Retrieved from www.nationalhomeless.org

National Coalition for the Homeless. (2012). Senseless violence: A survey of hate crimes/violence against the homeless in 2012. Retrieved from http://nationalhomeless.org/wp-content/uploads/2014/01/Hate-Crimes-Report-2012.pdf

National Coalition for the Homeless. (2014). *National Hunger and Homelessness Awareness Week 2014 manual.* Retrieved from http://nationalhomeless.org/wp-content/uploads/2014/09/Manual2014.pdf

National Institute of Corrections. (2016). What are we doing? Mentally ill persons in corrections. Retrieved from http://nicic.gov/mentalillness

National Institute of Mental Health. (2015). Serious mental illness (SMI) among U.S. adults. Retrieved from www.nimh.nih.gov/health/statistics/prevalence/serious-mental-illness-smi-among-us-adults.shtml

Ng, P., Chun, W.K., & Tsun, A. (2012). Recovering from hallucinations: A qualitative study of coping with voices hearing of people with schizophrenia in Hong Kong. *The Scientific World Journal, 2012*(5), 1-8. doi:10.1100/2012/232619

President's New Freedom Commission on Mental Health. (2003). *Achieving the promise: Transforming mental health care in America.* Retrieved from http://govinfo.library.unt.edu/mentalhealth commission/reports/reports.htm

Sadock, B.J., Sadock, V.A., & Ruiz, P. (2015). *Synopsis of psychiatry: Behavioral sciences/clinical psychiatry* (11th ed.). Philadelphia: Lippincott Williams & Wilkins.

Spock, B. (2012). *Baby and child care* (9th ed.). New York: Gallery Books.

Substance Abuse & Mental Health Services Administration. (2017). Federal action agenda (search). Retrieved from https://search.samhsa.gov/search?q=federal+action+agenda+initiatives&sort=date%3AD%3AL%3Ad1&output=xml_no_dtd&ie=UTF-8&oe=UTF-8&client=beta_frontend_drupal&proxystylesheet=beta_frontend_drupal&filter=1&site=data%7CSAMHSA_Beta_Drupal%7Cdefault_collection%7CNewsletter&collectionator=data%7CSAMHSA_Beta_Drupal%7Cdefault_collection%7CNewsletter

Substance Abuse and Mental Health Services Administration. (2016). Homelessness programs and resources. Retrieved from www.samhsa.gov/homelessness-programs-resources

US Burden of Disease Collaborators. (2013). The state of US health, 1990-2010: Burden of diseases, injuries, and risk factors. *Journal of the American Medical Association, 310*(6), 591-608. doi:10.1001/jama.279.21.1703

UNC Center for Excellence in Community Mental Health. (2015). Severe and persistent mental illness. Retrieved from www.med.unc.edu/psych/cecmh/patient-client-information/patient-client-information-and-resources/clients-and-families-resources/just-what-is-a-severe-and-persistent-mental-illness.

U.S. Conference of Mayors (USCM). (2014). *A status report on hunger and homelessness in America's cities: 2014.* Washington, DC: USCM.

Vanderplasschen, W., Rapp, R.C., Pearce, S., Vandevelde, S., & Broekaert, E. (2013). Mental health, recovery, and the community. *The Scientific World Journal, 2013*(4), 1-3. doi:http://dx.doi.org/10.1155/2013/926174

Wright, L.M., & Leahey, M. (2013). *Nurses and families: A guide to family assessment and intervention* (6th ed.). Philadelphia: F.A. Davis.

Classical References

Caplan, G. (1964). *Principles of preventive psychiatry.* New York: Basic Books.

Erikson, E. (1963). *Childhood and society* (2nd ed.). New York: WW Norton.

Lamb, H.R. (1993). Perspectives on effective advocacy for homeless mentally ill persons. *Hospital and Community Psychiatry, 43*(12), 1209-1212. doi:http://dx.doi.org/10.1176/ps.43.12.1209

37

The Bereaved Individual

CHAPTER OUTLINE

KEY TERMS

OBJECTIVES

After reading this chapter, the student will be able to:

1. Describe various types of loss that trigger the grief response in individuals.
2. Discuss theoretical perspectives of grieving as proposed by Elisabeth Kübler-Ross, John Bowlby, George Engel, and J. William Worden.
3. Differentiate between normal and maladaptive responses to loss.
4. Discuss grieving behaviors common to individuals at various stages across the life span.
5. Describe customs associated with grief in individuals of various cultures.
6. Formulate nursing diagnoses and goals of care for individuals experiencing the grief response.
7. Describe appropriate nursing interventions for individuals experiencing the grief response.
8. Identify relevant criteria for evaluating nursing care of individuals experiencing the grief response.
9. Describe the concept of hospice care for people who are dying and their families.
10. Discuss the use of advance directives for individuals to provide directions about their future medical care.

HOMEWORK ASSIGNMENT

Please read the chapter and answer the following questions:

1. What type of maladaptive response to loss occurs when an individual becomes fixed in the anger stage of grief? What clinical disorder is associated with this occurrence?
2. Describe the phenomenon of bereavement overload.
3. With what types of behaviors is grief manifested in school-aged children?
4. According to Engel, when is the grief response thought to be resolved?

CORE CONCEPT
Loss
The experience of separation from something of personal importance.

Loss is anything that is perceived as such by the individual. The separation from loved ones or the giving up of treasured possessions, for whatever reason; the experience of failure, either real or perceived; or life events that create change in a familiar pattern of existence—all can be experienced as loss, and all can trigger behaviors associated with the grieving process. Loss and bereavement are universal events encountered by all beings that experience emotions. Following are examples of some notable forms of loss:

- A significant other (person or pet), through death, divorce, or separation for any reason.
- Illness or debilitating conditions. Examples include (but are not limited to) diabetes, stroke, cancer, rheumatoid arthritis, multiple sclerosis, Alzheimer's disease, hearing or vision loss, and spinal cord or head injuries. Some of these conditions not only incur a loss of physical and/or emotional wellness but may also result in the loss of personal independence.
- Developmental/maturational changes or situations, such as menopause, andropause, infertility, "empty nest," aging, impotence, or hysterectomy.
- Real or perceived loss of hopes, dreams, and potential for specific accomplishments.
- Personal possessions that symbolize familiarity and security in a person's life. Separation from these familiar and personally valued external objects represents a loss of material extensions of the self.

CORE CONCEPT
Grief
Deep mental and emotional anguish that is a response to the subjective experience of loss of something significant.

Some texts differentiate the terms **mourning** and grief by describing mourning as the psychological process (or stages) through which the individual passes on the way to successful adaptation to the loss of a valued object. Grief may be viewed as the subjective states that accompany mourning or the emotional work involved in the mourning process. Similarly, **bereavement** is described as the period of grief and sadness that is the normal process of reacting to a loss and may include mental, physical, social, and emotional reactions (MedlinePlus, 2015). For purposes of this text, grief work, bereavement, and the process of mourning are collectively referred to as the *grief response*.

This chapter examines human responses to the experience of loss. Care of bereaved individuals is presented in the context of the nursing process.

Theoretical Perspectives on Loss and Bereavement

Stages of Grief

Behavior patterns associated with the grief response include many individual variations. However, sufficient similarities have been observed to warrant characterization of the grief response as a syndrome that has a predictable course with an expected resolution. Early theorists, including Kübler-Ross (1969), Bowlby (1961), and Engel (1964), described behavioral stages through which individuals advance in their progression toward resolution. A number of variables influence one's progression through the grief process, and it should be viewed as a dynamic rather than linear process. Some individuals may reach acceptance only to revert to an earlier stage, some may never complete the sequence, and some may never progress beyond the initial stage.

A more contemporary grief specialist, J. William Worden (2009), offers a set of tasks that must be processed in order to complete the grief response. He suggests that it is possible for a person to accomplish some of these tasks and not others, resulting in an incomplete bereavement that impairs further growth and development. A comparison of the similarities among these four models of the normal grief response is presented in Table 37–1.

Elisabeth Kübler-Ross

These well-known stages of the grief process were identified by Kübler-Ross in her extensive work with dying patients. Behaviors associated with each of these stages can be observed in individuals experiencing the loss of any concept of personal value.

- **Stage I: Denial.** In this stage, the individual has difficulty believing that the loss has occurred. He or she may say, "No, it can't be true!" or "It's just not possible." This stage may protect the individual against the psychological pain of reality.
- **Stage II: Anger.** This is the stage when reality sets in. Feelings associated with this stage include sadness, guilt, shame, helplessness, and hopelessness. Self-blame or blaming of others may lead to feelings of anger toward the self and others. The anxiety level may be elevated, and the individual may experience confusion and a decreased ability to function independently. He or she may be preoccupied with an idealized image of what has been lost. Numerous somatic complaints are common.

TABLE 37–1 **Stages and Tasks of the Normal Grief Response: A Comparison of Models by Elisabeth Kübler-Ross, John Bowlby, George Engel, and William Worden**

STAGES/TASKS				POSSIBLE TIME DIMENSION	BEHAVIORS
KÜBLER-ROSS	**BOWLBY**	**ENGEL**	**WORDEN**		
I. Denial	I. Numbness/ protest	I. Shock/ disbelief	I. Accepting the reality of the loss	Occurs immediately on experiencing the loss. Usually lasts no more than a few weeks.	Individual has difficulty believing that the loss has occurred.
II. Anger	II. Disequilibrium	II. Developing awareness		In most cases begins within hours of the loss. Peaks within a few weeks.	Anger is directed toward self or others. Ambivalence and guilt may be felt toward the lost entity.
III. Bargaining					The individual fervently seeks alternatives to improve current situation.
		III. Restitution			Attends to various rituals associated with the culture in which the loss has occurred.
IV. Depression	III. Disorganization and despair	IV. Resolution of the loss	II. Processing the pain of grief	Very individual. Commonly 6 to 12 months. Longer for some.	The actual work of grieving. Preoccupation with the lost entity. Feelings of helplessness and loneliness occur in response to realization of the loss. Feelings associated with the loss are confronted.
			III. Adjusting to a world without the lost entity	Ongoing.	How the environment changes depends on the roles the lost entity played in the life of the bereaved person. Adaptations will have to be made as the changes are presented in daily life. New coping skills will have to be developed.
V. Acceptance	IV. Reorganization	V. Recovery	IV. Finding an enduring connection with the lost entity in the midst of embarking on a new life		Resolution is complete. The bereaved person experiences a reinvestment in new relationships and new goals. The lost entity is not purged or replaced, but relocated in the life of the bereaved. At this stage, terminally ill persons express a readiness to die.

■ **Stage III: Bargaining.** At this stage in the grief response, the individual attempts to strike a bargain with God for a second chance or for more time. The person acknowledges the loss or impending loss but holds out hope for additional alternatives, as evidenced by statements such as, "If only I could. . ." or "If only I had. . . ."

■ **Stage IV: Depression.** In this stage, the individual mourns for that which has been or will be lost. This is a very painful stage when the individual must confront feelings associated with having lost someone or something of value (called *reactive* depression). An example is the individual who is mourning a change in body image. Feelings associated with an impending loss (called *preparatory* depression) are also confronted. Examples include permanent lifestyle changes related to the altered body image or even an impending loss of life itself. Regression, withdrawal, and social isolation may be observed behaviors with this stage. Therapeutic intervention should be available but not imposed, with guidelines for implementation based on client readiness.

■ **Stage V: Acceptance.** At this time, the individual has worked through the behaviors associated with the other stages and accepts or is resigned to the loss. Anxiety decreases and methods for coping with the loss have been established. The client is less preoccupied with what has been lost and increasingly interested in other aspects of the environment. If this is an impending death of self, the individual is ready to die. The person may become very quiet and withdrawn, seemingly devoid of feelings. These behaviors are an attempt to facilitate the passage by slowly disengaging from the environment.

John Bowlby

John Bowlby hypothesized four stages in the grief process. He suggests that these behaviors can be observed in all individuals who have experienced the loss of something or someone of value, even in babies as young as 6 months of age.

■ **Stage I: Numbness or protest.** This stage is characterized by a feeling of shock and disbelief that the loss has occurred. Reality of the loss is not acknowledged.

■ **Stage II: Disequilibrium.** During this stage, the individual has a profound urge to recover what has been lost. Behaviors associated with this stage include a preoccupation with the loss, intense weeping and expressions of anger toward the self and others, and feelings of ambivalence and guilt associated with the loss.

■ **Stage III: Disorganization and despair.** Feelings of despair occur in response to realization that the loss has occurred. Activities of daily living become increasingly disorganized, and behavior is characterized by restlessness and aimlessness. Efforts to regain productive patterns of behavior are ineffective, and the individual experiences fear, helplessness, and hopelessness. Somatic complaints are common. Perceptions of visualizing or being in the presence of that which has been lost may occur. Social isolation is common, and the individual may feel a great deal of loneliness.

■ **Stage IV: Reorganization.** The individual accepts or becomes resigned to the loss. New goals and patterns of organization are established. The individual begins a reinvestment in new relationships and indicates a readiness to move forward within the environment. Grief subsides and recedes into valued remembrances.

George Engel

■ **Stage I: Shock and disbelief.** The initial reaction to a loss is a stunned, numb feeling and refusal by the individual to acknowledge the reality of the loss. Engel states that this stage is an attempt by the individual to protect the self "against the effects of the overwhelming stress by raising the threshold against its recognition or against the painful feelings evoked thereby."

■ **Stage II: Developing awareness.** This stage begins within minutes to hours of the loss. Behaviors associated with this stage include excessive crying and regression to a state of helplessness and a childlike manner. Awareness of the loss creates feelings of emptiness, frustration, anguish, and despair. Anger may be directed toward the self or toward others in the environment who are held accountable for the loss.

■ **Stage III: Restitution.** In this stage, the various rituals associated with loss within a culture are performed. Examples include funerals, wakes, special attire, a gathering of friends and family, and religious practices customary to the spiritual beliefs of the bereaved. Participation in these rituals is thought to assist the individual to accept the reality of the loss and facilitate the recovery process.

■ **Stage IV: Resolution of the loss.** This stage is characterized by a preoccupation with the loss. The concept of the loss is idealized, and the individual may even imitate admired qualities of the lost entity. Preoccupation with the loss gradually decreases over a year or more, and the individual eventually begins to reinvest feelings in others.

■ **Stage V: Recovery.** Obsession with the loss has ended, and the individual is able to go on with his or her life.

J. William Worden

Worden views the bereaved person as active and self-determining rather than a passive participant in the grief process. He proposes that bereavement includes a set of tasks that must be reconciled in order to complete the grief process. Worden's four tasks of mourning include the following:

■ **Task I. Accepting the reality of the loss.** When something of value is lost, it is common for individuals to refuse to believe that the loss has occurred. Behaviors include misidentifying individuals in the environment for their lost loved one, retaining possessions of the lost loved one as though he or she has not died, and removing all reminders of the lost loved one so as not to have to face the reality of the loss. Worden (2009) stated:

Coming to an acceptance of the reality of the loss takes time since it involves not only an intellectual acceptance but also an emotional one. The bereaved person may be intellectually aware of the finality of the loss long before the emotions allow full acceptance of the information as true. (p. 42)

Belief and denial are intermittent while grappling with this task. It is thought that traditional rituals such as the funeral help some individuals move toward acceptance of the loss.

■ **Task II. Processing the pain of grief.** Pain associated with a loss includes both physical pain and emotional pain. This pain must be acknowledged and worked through. To avoid or suppress it serves only to delay or prolong the grieving process. People do this by refusing to allow themselves to think painful thoughts, by idealizing or avoiding reminders of lost entity, and by using alcohol or drugs. The intensity of the pain and the manner in which it is experienced are different for all individuals. However, the commonality is that it *must* be experienced. Failure to do so generally results in some form of depression that commonly requires therapy that focuses on working through the pain of grief that the individual failed to face at the time of the loss. In this very difficult Task II, individuals must "allow themselves to process the pain—to feel it and to know that one day it will pass" (p. 45).

■ **Task III. Adjusting to a world without the lost entity.** It usually takes a number of months for a bereaved person to realize what his or her world will be like without the lost entity. In the case of a lost loved one, how the environment changes will depend on the types of roles that person fulfilled in life. In the case of a changed lifestyle, the individual will be required to make adaptations to his or her environment in terms of the changes as they are presented in daily life. In addition, those individuals who had defined their identity through the lost entity will require an adjustment to their own sense of self. Worden states:

The coping strategy of redefining the loss in such a way that it can redound to the benefit of the survivor is often part of the successful completion of Task III. (p. 47)

If the bereaved person experiences failures in his or her attempt to adjust in an environment without the lost entity, feelings of low self-esteem may result. Regressed behaviors and feelings of helplessness and inadequacy are not uncommon. Worden states:

[Another] area of adjustment is to one's sense of the world. Loss through death can challenge one's fundamental life values and philosophical beliefs—beliefs that are influenced by our families, peers, education, and religion as well as life experiences. The bereaved person searches for meaning in the loss and its attendant life changes in order to make sense of it and to regain some control of his or her life. (pp. 48–49)

To be successful in Task III, bereaved individuals must develop new skills to cope and adapt to their new environment without the lost entity. Successful achievement of this task determines the outcome of the mourning process—that of continued growth or a state of arrested development.

■ **Task IV. Finding an enduring connection with the lost entity in the midst of embarking on a new life.** This task allows the bereaved person to identify a special place for the lost entity. Individuals need not purge from their history or find a replacement for that which has been lost. Instead, there is a continued presence of the lost entity that becomes *relocated* in the life of the bereaved. Successful completion of Task IV involves letting go of past attachments and forming new ones. However, there is also the recognition that although the relationship between the bereaved and what has been lost is changed, it is nonetheless still a relationship. Worden suggests that one never loses memories of a significant relationship. He states:

For many people, Task IV is the most difficult one to accomplish. They get stuck at this point in their grieving and later realize that their life in some way stopped at the point the loss occurred. (p. 52)

Worden relates the story of a teenaged girl who had a difficult time adjusting to the death of her father. After 2 years, when she began to finally fulfill some of the tasks associated with successful grieving, she wrote these words that express rather clearly what bereaved people in Task IV are struggling with: "There are other people to be loved, and it doesn't mean that I love Dad any less" (p. 52).

Length of the Grief Process

Stages of grief allow bereaved persons an orderly approach to the resolution of mourning. Each stage presents tasks that must be overcome through a painful experiential process. Engel (1964) stated that successful resolution of the grief response is thought to have occurred when a bereaved individual is able "to remember comfortably and realistically both the pleasures and disappointments of [that which is lost]." The length of the grief process depends on the individual and can last for a number of years without being maladaptive. The acute phase of normal grieving usually lasts about 6 to 8 weeks—longer in older adults—but complete resolution of the grief response may take much longer. Sadock, Sadock, and Ruiz (2015) stated:

> Ample evidence suggests that the bereavement process does not end within a prescribed interval; certain aspects persist indefinitely for many otherwise high-functioning, normal individuals. Common manifestations of protracted grief occur intermittently . . . most grief does not fully resolve or permanently disappear; rather grief becomes circumscribed and submerged only to reemerge in response to certain triggers. (p. 1355)

A number of factors influence the eventual outcome of the grief response. The grief response can be more difficult if:

■ The bereaved person was strongly dependent on or perceived the lost entity as an important means of physical and/or emotional support.
■ The relationship with the lost entity was highly ambivalent. A love–hate relationship may instill feelings of guilt that can interfere with the grief work.
■ The individual has experienced a number of recent losses. Grief tends to be cumulative, and if previous losses have not been resolved, each succeeding grief response becomes more difficult.
■ The loss is that of a young person. Grief over loss of a child is often more intense than that over the loss of an elderly person. Traumatic death in general increases the likelihood of abnormal grief, but when a child dies a sudden or violent death, evidence supports an increased incidence of posttraumatic stress disorder (PTSD) in parents (Kearns, 2014). One study found PTSD symptoms in more than 25 percent of the mothers up to 5 years after the death (Parris, 2011). The state of the person's physical or psychological health is unstable at the time of the loss.
■ The bereaved person perceives (whether real or imagined) some responsibility for the loss.
■ The loss is secondary to suicide.
■ The loss is a traumatic death such as murder.

The grief response may be facilitated if:

■ The individual has the support of significant others to assist him or her through the mourning process.
■ The individual has the opportunity to prepare for the loss. Grief work is more intense when the loss is sudden and unexpected. The experience of *anticipatory grieving* is thought to facilitate the grief response that occurs at the time of the actual loss.

Worden (2009) states:

> There is a sense in which mourning can be finished, when people regain an interest in life, feel more hopeful, experience gratification again, and adapt to new roles. There is also a sense in which mourning is never finished. [People must understand] that mourning is a long-term process and that the culmination will not be a pre-grief state. (p. 77)

Anticipatory Grief

Anticipatory grieving is the experiencing of the feelings and emotions associated with the normal grief response before the loss actually occurs. One dissimilar aspect relates to the fact that conventional grief tends to diminish in intensity with the passage of time. Anticipatory grief can become more intense as the expected loss becomes imminent.

Although anticipatory grief is thought to facilitate the actual mourning process following the loss, there may be some problems. In the case of a dying person, difficulties can arise when the family members complete the process of anticipatory grief and detachment from the dying person occurs prematurely. The person who is dying experiences feelings of loneliness and isolation as the psychological pain of imminent death is faced without family support. Another example of difficulty associated with premature completion of the grief response is the reaction that can occur on the return of persons long absent and presumed dead (e.g., soldiers missing in action or prisoners of war). In this instance, resumption of the previous relationship may be difficult for the bereaved person.

Anticipatory grieving may serve as a defense for some individuals to ease the burden of loss when it actually occurs. It may prove to be less functional for others who, because of interpersonal, psychological, or sociocultural variables, are unable in advance of the actual loss to express the intense feelings that accompany the grief response.

One qualitative study examined the unique process of grief for family caregivers of a relative who has dementia. One common theme was that in addition to anticipatory grief related to the final loss, these family members were, at the same time, grieving actual losses throughout the journey of their family member's illness (Peacock, Hammond-Collins, & Ford, 2014).

These included grieving the loss of the ill person's personality, companionship, social self, and cognition as the disease progressed. The grief reactions of these active caregivers were similar to those of bereaved caregivers, although their family member was still alive. This study highlights the multiplicity of factors that can influence the grieving process.

Maladaptive Responses to Loss

When, then, is the grieving response considered to be maladaptive? Three types of pathological grief reactions have been described: delayed or inhibited grief, an exaggerated or distorted grief response, and chronic or prolonged grief.

Delayed or Inhibited Grief

Delayed or inhibited grief refers to the absence of evidence of grief when it ordinarily would be expected. Many times, cultural influences, such as the expectation to keep a "stiff upper lip," contribute to the delayed response.

Delayed or inhibited grief is potentially pathological because the person is simply not dealing with the reality of the loss. He or she remains fixed in the denial stage of the grief process, sometimes for many years. When this occurs, the grief response may be triggered, sometimes many years later, when the individual experiences a subsequent loss. Sometimes the grief process is triggered spontaneously or in response to a seemingly insignificant event. Overreaction to another person's loss may be one manifestation of **delayed grief.**

The recognition of delayed grief is critical because, depending on the profoundness of the loss, the failure of the mourning process may prevent assimilation of the loss and thereby delay a return to satisfying living. Without the learnings that the grief process can provide, subsequent losses may be compounded by previously unresolved grief work. Delayed grieving most commonly occurs because of ambivalent feelings toward the lost entity, outside pressure to resume normal function, or perceived lack of internal and external resources to cope with a profound loss.

Distorted (Exaggerated) Grief Response

In the distorted grief reaction, all of the symptoms associated with normal grieving are exaggerated. Feelings of sadness, helplessness, hopelessness, powerlessness, anger, and guilt, as well as numerous somatic complaints, render the individual dysfunctional in terms of management of daily living. Morrow (2016) describes this as a state of feeling "trapped" in one's grief during which the grief response either stays the same or intensifies over a prolonged period.

When the exaggerated grief reaction occurs, the individual remains fixed in the anger stage of the grief response. This anger may be directed toward others in the environment to whom the individual may be attributing the loss. However, many times the anger is turned inward on the self. When this occurs, depression is the result. Depressive mood disorder is a type of exaggerated grief reaction. This should be distinguished, though, from the depression that is considered part of the normal grieving process. (See Table 37–2.)

Chronic or Prolonged Grieving

Some authors have discussed a chronic or prolonged grief response as a type of maladaptive grief response. Care must be taken in making this determination because, as stated previously, length of the grief response depends on the individual. An adaptive response may take years for some people. A prolonged process may be considered maladaptive when certain behaviors are exhibited. Prolonged grief may be a problem when behaviors such as those that prevent the bereaved from adaptively performing activities of daily living are in evidence. An example is of a widow who refused to participate in family gatherings following the death of her husband. For many years until her own death, she took a sandwich to the cemetery on holidays, sat on the tombstone, and ate her "holiday meal" with her husband. Whether one's behaviors constitute prolonged or chronic grieving must consider cultural context. In some cultures, establishing a memorial ritual to the deceased is the norm, whereas in other cultures, it might be perceived as prolonged grieving.

Normal versus Maladaptive Grieving

Several authors have identified one crucial difference between normal and maladaptive grieving: the loss of self-esteem. Marked feelings of worthlessness are indicative of depression rather than uncomplicated bereavement. Corr and Corr (2013) state, "Normal grief reactions do not include the loss of self-esteem commonly found in most clinical depression" (p. 241). Pies (2013) affirmed:

> Unlike the person with [major depressive disorder] MDD, most recently bereaved individuals are usually not preoccupied with feelings of worthlessness, hopelessness, or unremitting gloom; rather, self-esteem is usually preserved; the bereaved person can envision a "better day;" and positive thoughts and feelings are often interspersed with negative ones.

Hensley and Clayton (2013) add that when clinically depressed inpatients were compared to individuals experiencing depression associated with bereavement, four symptoms were absent in the bereavement population: suicidal thoughts, feeling like they were a burden to others, feeling like they would rather be dead, and psychomotor retardation. These may be considered associated symptoms of low self-esteem and feelings of worthlessness. The presence of suicide ideation automatically indicates an abnormal grief reaction and requires careful assessment and immediate intervention to prevent the risk for completed suicide.

It is thought that this major difference between normal grieving and a maladaptive grieving response (the feeling of worthlessness or low self-esteem) ultimately precipitates depression, which can be a progressive situation for some individuals. Studies have identified the incidence of major depressive disorder among the bereaved to be at around 35 percent at 1 month following a loss. While this tends to decrease over time, 8 to 11 percent develop chronic depression (Hensley & Clayton, 2013). The authors add that factors such as poor physical health, poor mental health, and substance use disorders prior to a loss increase the risk for chronic depression following loss. A summary of differences between normal grieving and clinical depression is presented in Table 37–2.

Application of the Nursing Process

Background Assessment Data: Concepts of Death—Developmental Issues

All individuals have their own unique concept of death, which is influenced by past experiences with death as well as age and level of emotional development. This section addresses the various perceptions of death according to developmental age.

Children
Birth to Age 2

Infants are unable to recognize and understand death, but they can experience the feelings of loss and separation. Infants who are separated from their mother may become quiet, lose weight, and sleep less. Children at this age will likely sense changes in the atmosphere of the home where a death has occurred. They often react to the emotions of adults by becoming more irritable and crying more.

Ages 3 to 5

Preschoolers and kindergartners have some understanding about death but often have difficulty distinguishing between fantasy and reality. They believe death is reversible, and their thoughts about death may include magical thinking. For example, they may believe that their thoughts or behaviors caused a person to become sick or to die.

Children of this age are capable of understanding at least some of what they see and hear from adult conversations or media reports. They become frightened if they feel a threat to themselves or their loved ones. They are concerned with safety issues and require a great deal of personal reassurance that they will be protected. Regressive behaviors, such as loss of bladder or bowel control, thumb sucking, and temper tantrums are common. Changes in eating and sleeping patterns may also occur.

TABLE 37–2 Normal Grief Reactions versus Symptoms of Clinical Depression

NORMAL GRIEF	CLINICAL DEPRESSION
Self-esteem intact	Self-esteem is disturbed
May openly express anger	Usually does not directly express anger
Experiences a mixture of "good and bad days"	Persistent state of dysphoria
Able to experience moments of pleasure	Anhedonia is prevalent
Accepts comfort and support from others	Does not respond to social interaction and support from others
Maintains feeling of hope	Feelings of hopelessness prevail
May express guilt feelings over some aspect of the loss	Has generalized feelings of guilt
Relates feelings of depression to specific loss experienced	Does not relate feelings to a particular experience
May experience transient physical symptoms	Expresses chronic physical complaints

SOURCES: Corr, C.A., & Corr, D.M. (2013). *Death and dying: Life & living* (7th ed.). Belmont, CA: Wadsworth; Pies, R.W. (2013). Grief and depression: The sages knew the difference. *Psychiatric Times*, April 29, 2013. Retrieved from www.psychiatrictimes.com/display/article/10168/2140230; Sadock, B.J., Sadock, V.A., & Ruiz, P. (2015). *Synopsis of psychiatry: Behavioral sciences/clinical psychiatry* (11th ed.). Philadelphia: Lippincott Williams & Wilkins.

Ages 6 to 9

Children at this age are beginning to understand the finality of death. They are able to understand a more detailed explanation of why or how a person died, although the concept of death is often associated with old age or with accidents. They may believe that death is contagious and avoid association with individuals who have experienced a loss by death. Death is often personified, in the form of a "bogey man" or a monster—someone who takes people away or someone whom they can avoid if they try hard enough. It is difficult for them to perceive their own death. Normal grief reactions at this age include regressive and aggressive behaviors, withdrawal, school phobias, somatic symptoms, and clinging behaviors.

Ages 10 to 12

Preadolescent children are able to understand that death is final and eventually affects everyone, including themselves. They are interested in the physical aspects of dying and the final disposition of the body. They may ask questions about how the death will affect them personally. Feelings of anger, guilt, and depression are common. Peer relationships and school performance may be disrupted. There may be a preoccupation with the loss and a withdrawal into the self. Adams (2014) states that evidence supports that young people who are bereaved are more likely to be poor school attenders, change schools, be excluded, and less likely to be involved in activities both in and out of school, which puts them at higher risk for underperformance, health problems, and feelings of hopelessness. They will require support, flexibility in management of anger responses, and reassurance of their own safety and self-worth.

Adolescents

Adolescents are usually able to view death on an adult level. They understand death to be universal and inevitable; however, they have difficulty tolerating the intense feelings associated with the death of a loved one. They may or may not cry. They may withdraw into themselves or attempt to go about usual activities in an effort to avoid dealing with the pain of the loss. Some teens exhibit acting-out behaviors, such as aggression and defiance. It is often easier for adolescents to discuss their feelings with peers than with their parents or other adults. Some adolescents may show regressive behaviors, whereas others react by trying to take care of their loved ones who are also grieving. In general, individuals of this age group have an attitude of immortality. Although they understand

that their own death is inevitable, the concept is so far-reaching as to be imperceptible.

Adults

The adult's concept of death is influenced by experiential, cultural, and religious backgrounds. Behaviors associated with grieving in the adult were discussed in the section "Theoretical Perspectives on Loss and Bereavement."

Older Adults

Philosophers and poets have described late adulthood as the "season of loss." By the time individuals reach their 60s and 70s, they have experienced numerous losses, and mourning has become a life-long process. Those who are most successful at adapting earlier in life will similarly cope better with the losses and grief inherent in aging. Unfortunately, with the aging process comes a convergence of losses, the timing of which makes it impossible for the aging individual to complete the grief process in response to one loss before another occurs. Because grief is cumulative, this can result in **bereavement overload,** in which the person is less able to adapt and reintegrate, complicated grief responses ensue, and mental and physical health may be jeopardized (Tousley, 2013). Bereavement overload has been implicated as a predisposing factor in the development of depressive disorder in older adults.

Some believe that bereavement among elderly couples is also associated with increased risk for mortality. While many variables influence mortality in this population, evidence suggests that, in cases where the loss is anticipated, there is not an increased risk for mortality, but when the loss was unexpected, there was indeed an increased risk (King et al., 2013, Shah et al., 2013). This research highlights the need for additional assessment and support during the bereavement period when loss, particularly of a spouse, is unexpected.

Background Assessment Data: Bereavement Risk Assessment

Several tools have been developed to assess the risk for maladaptive grief responses. They incorporate many of the issues previously discussed and are framed to identify multiple risk factors commonly associated with complicated grief reactions that may require additional resources and intervention. Some of the factors commonly assessed as indicators of increased risk for maladaptive grief follow:

- Additional financial problems posed by the loss
- Lack of coping skills or lack of experience in responding to loss

- Emotional or physical dependence on the lost person or item
- History of mental illness or substance abuse
- History of trauma, including abuse
- Multiple losses within a short time frame

While formalized tools are more often used in palliative care settings, they constitute an important aspect of assessment for all nurses responding to the needs of the bereaved client.

Background Assessment Data: Concepts of Death—Cultural Issues

As previously stated, bereavement practices are greatly influenced by cultural and religious backgrounds. It is important for health-care professionals to have an understanding of these individual differences to provide culturally sensitive care to their clients. Clinicians must be able to identify and appreciate what is culturally expected or required, because failure to carry out expected rituals may hinder the grief process and result in unresolved grief for some bereaved individuals. Box 37–1 provides a set of guidelines for assessing culturally specific death rituals. Following is a discussion of selected culturally specific death rituals.

African Americans

Customs of bereaved African Americans are similar to those of the dominant American culture of the same religion and social class, with a blending of cultural practices from the African heritage. Most African American Christians are affiliated with the Baptist and Methodist denominations.

Funeral services may differ from the traditional European American service with ceremonies and rituals modified by the musical rhythms and patterns of speech and worship that are unique to African Americans. Often, feelings are expressed openly and publicly at the funeral, and some view eulogies as extremely important. Services usually conclude with a viewing of the body and burial at a cemetery. Burial rather than cremation is usually chosen (Hazell, 2016).

Many African Americans attempt to maintain a strong connection with their loved ones who have died. This connection may take the form of communication with the deceased's spirit through mediums who are believed to possess this special capability.

Asian Americans

Chinese Americans

Death and bereavement in the Chinese tradition are centered on ancestor worship. Chinese people have an intuitive fear of death and avoid references to it. Tsai (2013) states:

> Many Chinese are hesitant to purchase life insurance because of their fear that it is inviting death. The color white is associated with death and is considered bad luck. Black is also a bad luck color. (p. 189)

In the traditional Chinese culture, people often do not express their emotions openly. Mourners are recognized by black armbands and white strips of cloth tied around their heads (Tsai, 2013). The dead are honored by placing food, money for the person's spirit, or articles made of paper around the coffin. The purpose of these rituals is based on the belief that one must help the dead to live a comfortable and rich afterlife (Chang, 2017). Suicide is culturally prohibited since traditional Chinese teaching stresses that life is given by one's parents and no one has the right to take it away (Chang, 2017). While this might serve as a protective factor against suicide for traditional Chinese Americans, it also adds another dimension to the grief process when suicide does occur.

Japanese Americans

The dominant religion among the Japanese is Buddhism. On death of a loved one, the body is prepared by close family members. This is followed by a 2-day period of visitation by family and friends, during which there is prayer, burning of incense, and presentation of gifts. Funeral ceremonies are held at the Buddhist temple, and cremation is common. The mourning period is 49 days, the end of which is marked by a family prayer service and the serving of special rice dishes. It is believed that at this time, the departed has joined those already in the hereafter. Perpetual prayers may be donated through a gift to the temple (Ito & Hattori, 2013).

BOX 37–1 Guidelines for Assessing Culturally Specific Death Rituals

DEATH RITUALS AND EXPECTATIONS
1. Identify culturally specific death rituals and expectations.
2. Explain death rituals and mourning practices.
3. What are specific burial practices, such as cremation?

RESPONSES TO DEATH AND GRIEF
4. Identify cultural responses to death and grief.
5. Explore the meaning of death, dying, and the afterlife.

SOURCE: Adapted from Purnell, L.D. (2013). The Purnell model for cultural competence. In L.D. Purnell (Ed.), Transcultural health care: A culturally competent approach (4th ed.). Philadelphia: F.A. Davis.

Vietnamese Americans

Buddhism is the predominant religion among the Vietnamese. Attitudes toward death are influenced by the Buddhist emphasis on cyclic continuity and reincarnation. Many Vietnamese people believe that birth and death are predestined.

Most Vietnamese people prefer to die at home, and most do not approve of autopsy. Cremation is common. The final moments before the funeral procession are a time of prayer for the immediate family. Individuals in mourning wear white clothing for 14 days. During the following year, men wear black armbands and women wear white headbands (Mattson, 2013). The 1-year anniversary of an individual's death is commemorated. Clergy should be called to visit the sick only at the request of the client or family and is usually associated with last rites, especially by Vietnamese people who practice Catholicism. For this reason, hospital visitation by clergy may be very upsetting to clients. Receiving flowers also may be distressing, as flowers usually are reserved for the rites of the dead (Appel, 2017).

Filipino Americans

Following a death in the Filipino community, a wake is held with family and friends. This wake usually takes place in the home of the deceased and lasts up to a week before the funeral. A large proportion of Filipinos are Catholic. Munoz (2013) states:

> Among Catholics, 9 days of novenas are held in the home or in the church. These special prayers ask God's blessing for the deceased. Depending upon the economic resources of the family, food and refreshments are served after each prayer day. Sometimes the last day of the novena takes on the atmosphere of a *fiesta* or a celebration. Filipino families in the United States follow variations of this ritual according to their social and economic circumstances. (p. 242)

Most follow the traditional custom of wearing dark clothing—black armbands for men and black dresses for women—for 1 year after the death, at which time ritualistic mourning officially ends. Emotional outbursts of uncontrolled crying are common expressions of grief. Fainting as a bereavement practice is not uncommon (Munoz, 2013). Burial of the body is most common, but cremation is acceptable.

Jewish Americans

Traditional Judaism believes in an afterlife where the soul continues to flourish, although today many dispute this interpretation (Selekman, 2013). However, most Jewish people show little concern about life after death, and focus is concentrated more on how one conducts one's present life. Taking one's own life is forbidden, and orthodox Jewish people may deny the person full burial honors; however, the more liberal view is to emphasize the needs of the survivors.

A dying person is never left alone. At death, the face is covered with a cloth, and the body is treated with respect. Autopsy is not allowed by Orthodox Jews unless it is required by law, the deceased person has requested it, or it may save the life of another (Bralock & Padgham, 2017).

For the funeral, the body is wrapped in a shroud and placed in a wooden, unadorned casket. No wake and no viewing are part of a Jewish funeral. Cremation is prohibited. Selekman (2013) states:

> After the funeral, mourners are welcomed to the home of the closest relative. Water to wash one's hands before entering is outside the front door, symbolic of cleansing the impurities associated with contact with the dead. The water is not passed from person to person, just as it is hoped that the tragedy is not passed. At the home, a meal is served to all the guests. This "meal of condolence" or "meal of consolation" is traditionally provided by the neighbors and friends. (p. 350)

The 7-day period beginning with the burial is called *shiva.* During this time, mourners do not work, and no activity is permitted that diverts attention from thinking about the deceased. Mourning lasts 30 days for a relative and 1 year for a parent, at which time a tombstone is erected and a graveside service is held (Selekman, 2013).

Mexican Americans

Most Mexican Americans view death as a natural part of life. The predominant religion is Catholic, and many of the death rituals are a reflection of these religious beliefs. A vigil by family members is kept over the sick or dying person. Following the death, large numbers of family and friends gather for a *velorio,* a festive watch over the body of the deceased person (Zoucha & Zamarripa, 2013). Mexican American culture values strong family ties and maintaining an ongoing connection with a deceased family member may be manifested in dreams, storytelling, ongoing rituals, and pictorial memorials (McMurry et al., 2017).

Mourning is called *luto* and is symbolized by wearing black, black and white, or dark clothing and by subdued behavior. Often the bereaved refrain from attending movies or social events and from listening to radio or watching television. For middle-aged or elderly Mexican Americans, the period of bereavement may last for 2 years or more. These mourning behaviors do not indicate a sign of respect for the dead; instead, they demonstrate evidence that the individual is grieving for a loved one. Burial is more common than cremation, and often the body is buried within 24 hours of death, which is required by law in Mexico (Zoucha & Zamarripa, 2013).

American Indian/Alaska Native

More than 500 American Indian/Alaska Native tribes are now recognized by the U.S. government. Although many of the tribal traditions have been modified throughout the years, some of their traditional values have been preserved.

The Navajo of the Southwest, the largest American Indian tribe in the United States, do not bury the body of a deceased person for 4 days after death. Beliefs require that a cleansing ceremony take place before burial to prevent the spirit of the dead person from trying to assume control of someone else's spirit (Purnell, 2014). The dead are buried with their shoes on the wrong feet and rings on their index fingers. The Navajo generally do not express their grief openly and are reluctant to touch the body of a dead person. Purnell (2014) states:

> One death taboo involves talking with clients concerning a fatal disease or illness. Effective discussions require that the issue be presented in the third person, as if the illness or disorder occurred with someone else. Never suggest that the patient is dying. To do so would imply that the provider wishes the patient dead. If the patient does die, it would imply that the provider might have evil powers. (p. 70)

Nursing Diagnosis and Outcome Identification

From analysis of the assessment data, appropriate nursing diagnoses are formulated for the client and family experiencing grief and loss. From these identified diagnoses, accurate planning of nursing care is executed. Possible nursing diagnoses for grieving persons include:

- Risk for complicated grieving related to loss of a valued entity/concept; loss of a loved one
- Risk for spiritual distress related to complicated grief process

The following criteria may be used for measurement of outcomes in the care of the grieving client:

The client:

- Acknowledges awareness of the loss
- Is able to express feelings about the loss
- Verbalizes stages of the grief process and behaviors associated with each
- Expresses personal satisfaction and support from spiritual practices

Planning and Implementation

Table 37–3 provides a plan of care for the grieving person. Selected nursing diagnoses are presented, along with outcome criteria, appropriate nursing interventions, and rationales for each.

Evaluation

In the final step of the nursing process, a reassessment is conducted to determine if the nursing actions have been successful in achieving the objectives of care. Evaluation of the nursing actions for the grieving

---

Table 37–3 | CARE PLAN FOR THE GRIEVING PERSON

NURSING DIAGNOSIS: RISK FOR COMPLICATED GRIEVING
RELATED TO: Loss of a valued entity/concept; loss of a loved one

OUTCOME CRITERIA	NURSING INTERVENTIONS	RATIONALE
Short-Term Goals: • Client acknowledges awareness of the loss. • Client expresses feelings about the loss. • Client verbalizes own position in the grief process. Long-Term Goal: • Client progresses through the grief process in a healthful manner toward resolution.	1. Assess client's stage in the grief process. Assess for bereavement risk factors. 2. Develop trust. Show empathy, concern, and unconditional positive regard. 3. Help client actualize the loss by talking about it. "When did it happen? How did it happen?" and so forth. 4. Help client identify and express feelings. Some of the more problematic feelings include: a. *Anger.* The anger may be directed at the deceased, at	1. Accurate baseline data are required to provide appropriate assistance. 2. Developing trust provides the basis for a therapeutic relationship. 3. Reviewing the events of the loss can help client come to full awareness of the loss. 4. Until client can recognize and accept personal feelings regarding the loss, grief work cannot progress. a. Many people will not admit to angry feelings, believing it

Continued

Table 37–3 | CARE PLAN FOR THE GRIEVING PERSON—cont'd

OUTCOME CRITERIA	NURSING INTERVENTIONS	RATIONALE
	God, displaced onto others, or retroflected inward on the self. Encourage client to examine this anger and validate the appropriateness of this feeling. b. *Guilt.* Client may feel that he or she did not do enough to prevent the loss. Help client by reviewing the circumstances of the loss and the reality that it could not be prevented. c. *Anxiety and helplessness.* Help client to recognize the way that life was managed before the loss. Help client to put the feelings of helplessness into perspective by pointing out ways that he or she managed situations effectively without help from others. Role-play life events and assist with decision-making situations.	is inappropriate and unjustified. Expression of this emotion is necessary to prevent fixation in this stage of grief. b. Feelings of guilt prolong resolution of the grief process. c. Client may have fears that he or she may not be able to carry on alone.
	5. Interpret normal behaviors associated with grieving, and provide client with adequate time to grieve.	5. Understanding of the grief process will help prevent feelings of guilt generated by these responses. Individuals need adequate time to adjust to the loss and all its ramifications. This involves getting past birthdays and anniversaries of which the deceased was a part.
	6. Provide continuing support. If this is not possible by the nurse, then offer referrals to support groups. Support groups of individuals going through the same experiences can be very helpful for the grieving individual.	6. The availability of emotional support systems facilitates the grief process.
	7. Identify pathological defenses that client may be using (e.g., drug/alcohol use, somatic complaints, social isolation). Assist client in understanding why these are not healthy defenses and how they delay the process of grieving.	7. The bereavement process is impaired by behaviors that mask the pain of the loss.
	8. Encourage client to make an honest review of the relationship with the lost entity. Journal keeping is a facilitative tool with this intervention.	8. Only when client is able to see both positive and negative aspects related to the loss will the grieving process be complete.

Table 37–3 | CARE PLAN FOR THE GRIEVING PERSON–cont'd

NURSING DIAGNOSIS: RISK FOR SPIRITUAL DISTRESS

RELATED TO: Complicated grief process

OUTCOME CRITERIA	NURSING INTERVENTIONS	RATIONALE
Short-Term Goal: • Client identifies meaning and purpose in life, moving forward with hope for the future. Long-Term Goal: • Client expresses achievement of support and personal satisfaction from spiritual practices.	1. Be accepting and nonjudgmental when client expresses anger and bitterness (toward God, the universe, etc.). Stay with client. 2. Encourage client to ventilate feelings related to meaning of own existence in the face of current loss. 3. Encourage client as part of grief work to reach out to previously used religious practices for support. Encourage client to discuss these practices and how they provided support in the past. 4. Assure client that he or she is not alone when feeling inadequate in the search for life's answers. 5. Contact spiritual leader of client's choice, if he or she requests.	1. The nurse's presence and non-judgmental attitude increase client's feelings of self-worth and promote trust in the relationship. 2. Client may believe he or she cannot go on living without lost object. Catharsis can provide relief and put life back into realistic perspective. 3. Client may find comfort in religious rituals with which he or she is familiar. 4. Validation of client's feelings and assurance that they are shared by others offer encouragement and an affirmation of acceptability. 5. These individuals serve to provide relief from spiritual distress and often can do so when other support persons cannot.

client may be facilitated by gathering information using the following types of questions:

■ Has the client discussed the recent loss with staff and family members?

■ Is the client able to verbalize feelings and behaviors associated with each stage of the grieving process and recognize his or her own position in the process?

■ Has obsession with and idealization of the lost entity subsided?

■ Is anger toward the loss expressed appropriately?

■ Is the client able to participate in usual religious practices and feel satisfaction and support from them?

■ Is the client seeking out interaction with others in an appropriate manner?

■ Is the client able to verbalize positive aspects about his or her life, past relationships, and prospects for the future?

Additional Assistance

Hospice

Hospice is a program that provides palliative and supportive care to meet the special needs of people who

are dying and their families. Hospice care provides physical, psychological, spiritual, and social care for the person for whom aggressive treatment is no longer appropriate. Various models of hospice exist, including freestanding institutions that provide both inpatient and home care, those affiliated with hospitals and nursing homes in which hospice services are provided within the institutional setting, and hospice organizations that provide home care only. Historically, the hospice movement in the United States has evolved mainly as a system of home-based care.

Hospice helps clients achieve physical and emotional comfort so that they can concentrate on living life as fully as possible. Clients are urged to stay active for as long as they are able—to take part in activities they enjoy and to focus on the quality of life.

Hospice follows an interdisciplinary team approach to provide care for the terminally ill individual in the familiar surroundings of the home environment. The interdisciplinary team consists of nurses, attendants (homemakers, home health aides), physicians, social workers, volunteers, and health-care workers from other disciplines as required for individual clients.

The hospice approach is based on seven components: the interdisciplinary team, pain and symptom management, emotional support to client and family, pastoral and spiritual care, bereavement counseling, 24-hour on-call nurse/counselor, and staff support. These are the ideal, and not all hospice programs may include all of these services. The National Hospice and Palliative Care Organization (NHPCO) is an organization that publishes standards of care based on principles that are directed at the hospice program concept.

Interdisciplinary Team

Nurses

A registered nurse usually acts as case manager for care of hospice clients. The nurse assesses the client's and family's needs, establishes the goals of care, supervises and assists caregivers, evaluates care, serves as client advocate, and provides educational information as needed to client, family, and caregivers. He or she also provides physical care when needed, including IV therapy.

Attendants

These individuals are usually the members of the team who spend the most time with the client. They assist with personal care and all activities of daily living. Without these daily attendants, many individuals would be unable to spend their remaining days in their home. Attendants may be noncertified and provide basic housekeeping services; they may be certified nursing assistants who assist with personal care; or they may be licensed vocational or practical nurses who provide more specialized care, such as dressing changes or tube feedings.

Physicians

The client's primary physician and the hospice medical consultant have input into the care of the hospice client. Orders may continue to come from the primary physician, whereas pain and symptom management may come from the hospice consultant. Ideally, these physicians attend weekly client care conferences and provide in-service education for hospice staff as well as others in the medical community.

Social Workers

The social worker assists the client and family members with psychosocial issues, including those associated with the client's condition, financial issues, legal needs, and bereavement concerns. The social worker provides information on community resources from which client and family may receive support and assistance. Some of the functions of the nurse and social worker may overlap at times.

Trained Volunteers

Volunteers are vital to the hospice concept. They provide services that may otherwise be financially impossible. They are specially selected and extensively trained, and they provide services such as transportation, companionship, respite care, recreational activities, light housekeeping, and sensitivity to the needs of families in stressful situations.

Rehabilitation Therapists

Physical therapists may assist hospice clients in an effort to minimize physical disability. They may assist with strengthening exercises and provide assistance with special equipment needs. Occupational therapists may help the debilitated client learn to accomplish activities of daily living as independently as possible. Other consultants, such as speech therapists, may be called upon for the client with special needs.

Dietitian

A nutritional consultant may be helpful to the hospice client who is experiencing nausea and vomiting, diarrhea, anorexia, and weight loss. A nutritionist can ensure that the client is receiving the proper balance of calories and nutrients.

Counseling Services

The hospice client may require the services of a psychiatrist or psychologist if there is a history of mental illness or if neurocognitive disorder or depression has become a problem. Other types of counseling services are available to provide assistance in dealing with the special needs of each client.

Pain and Symptom Management

Improved quality of life at all times is a primary goal of hospice care. Thus, a major intervention for all caregivers is to ensure that the client is as comfortable as possible, whether experiencing pain or other types of symptoms common in the terminal stages of an illness.

Emotional Support

Members of the hospice team encourage clients and families to discuss the eventual outcome of the disease process. Some individuals find discussing issues associated with death and dying uncomfortable, and if so, their decision is respected. However, honest discussion of these issues provides a sense of relief for some people, and they are more realistically prepared for the future. It may even draw some clients and families closer together during this stressful time.

Pastoral and Spiritual Care

Hospice philosophy supports the individual's right to seek guidance or comfort in the spiritual practices most suited to that person. The hospice team members help the client obtain the spiritual support and guidance for which he or she expresses a preference.

Bereavement Counseling

Hospice provides a service to surviving family members or significant others after the death of their loved one. This is usually provided by a bereavement counselor, but when one is not available, volunteers with special training in bereavement care may be of service. A grief support group may be helpful for the bereaved and provide a safe place for them to discuss their own fears and concerns about the death of a loved one.

24-Hour On-Call

The standards of care set forth by NHPCO state that care shall be available 24 hours a day, 7 days a week. A nurse or counselor is usually available by phone or for home visits around the clock. The knowledge that emotional or physical support is available at any time should it be required provides considerable support and comfort to significant others or family caregivers.

Staff Support

Team members (all who work closely and frequently with the client) often experience emotions similar to those of the client or their family and/or significant others. They may experience anger, frustration, or fears of death and dying—all of which must be addressed through staff support groups, team conferences, time off, and adequate and effective supervision. Burnout is a common problem among hospice staff. Stress can be reduced, trust enhanced, and team functioning more effective if lines of communication are kept open among all members (medical director through volunteer), if information is readily accessible through staff conferences and in-service education, and if staff know they are appreciated and feel good about what they are doing.

Advance Directives

The term **advance directive** refers to either a living will or a durable power of attorney for health care (also called a health-care proxy). Either document allows an individual to provide directions about his or her future medical care.

A living will is a written document made by a competent individual that provides instructions that should be used when that individual is no longer able to express his or her wishes for health-care treatment. The durable power of attorney for health care is a written form that gives another person legal power to make decisions regarding health care when an individual is no longer capable of making such decisions. Some states have adopted forms that combine the intent of the durable power of attorney for health care (i.e., to have a proxy) and the intent of the living will (i.e., to state choices for end-of-life medical treatment).

Doctors usually follow clearly stated directives. It is important that the physician be informed that an advance directive exists and what the specific wishes of the client are. Advance directives are legally binding in all 50 states in the United States (Sadock et al., 2015). In 1991, the U.S. Congress passed the *Patient Self-Determination Act*. This legislation requires that all health-care facilities must advise clients of their rights to refuse treatment, to make advance directives available to clients on admission, and to keep records of whether a client has an advance directive or a designated health-care proxy (Sadock et al., 2015). State laws also define how and under what circumstances individuals can refuse life-sustaining medical interventions. These are generally referred to as natural death acts. Nurses need to be aware of both federal law and the applicable state laws in the state where they practice nursing.

In spite of the laws allowing for an advance directive document, many people have not established this document for themselves—and even when advance directives exist, they may not be honored when circumstances are confusing or unclear. In emergency situations, treatment decisions sometimes must be made before information about an advanced directive is available. Catalano and Catalano (2015) identify additional reasons why advance directives are sometimes not honored:

■ Advance directives that were formulated long before their implementation may call into question whether the client understood the ramifications of their decisions for future medical problems and interventions at that time.

■ In general, the language used in standard living will documents is not specific enough to cover all health-care circumstances. Consequently, health-care providers may lack clarity about how to proceed because the advance directive lacks clarity.

■ Since state laws vary, when a client is in a state other than the one where the advance directive was established, it may raise questions about the document's legality.

Advance directives are designed to allow the client to be in control of decisions about his or her right to live or die. It is also a way to spare family and loved ones the burden of making choices without knowing the wishes of the person who is dying. Nurses can play an active role in discussing advance directives within a culturally sensitive framework and encouraging clients who have advance directives to review and update them periodically to assure that their wishes remain clear.

Summary and Key Points

- Loss is the experience of separation from something of personal importance.

- Loss is anything that is perceived as such by the individual.

- Loss of any concept of value to an individual can trigger the grief response.

- Elisabeth Kübler-Ross identified five stages that individuals pass through on their way to resolution of a loss: denial, anger, bargaining, depression, and acceptance.

- John Bowlby described similar stages: stage I, numbness or protest; stage II, disequilibrium; stage III, disorganization and despair; and stage IV, reorganization.

- George Engel's stages include shock and disbelief, developing awareness, restitution, resolution of the loss, and recovery.

- J. William Worden, a more contemporary clinician, has proposed that bereaved individuals must accomplish a set of four tasks in order to complete the grief process: accepting the reality of the loss, processing the pain of grief, adjusting to a world without the lost entity, and finding an enduring connection with the lost entity in the midst of embarking on a new life.

- The length of the grief process is highly individual and can last for a number of years without being maladaptive.

- The acute stage of the grief process typically lasts a couple of months, but resolution usually takes much longer.

- Anticipatory grieving is the experiencing of the feelings and emotions associated with the normal grief process in response to anticipation of the loss.

- Anticipatory grieving is thought to facilitate the grief process when the actual loss occurs.

- Three types of pathological grief reactions have been described:
  1. Delayed or inhibited grief in which there is absence of grief when it ordinarily would be expected
  2. Distorted or exaggerated grief response in which the individual remains fixed in the anger stage of the grief process and the symptoms associated with normal grieving are exaggerated

  3. Chronic or prolonged grieving in which the individual is unable to let go of grieving behaviors after an extended period of time and in which behaviors indicate that he or she is not accepting that the loss has occurred

- Several authors have identified one crucial difference between normal and maladaptive grieving: the loss of self-esteem.

- Feelings of worthlessness, feeling that one is a burden to others, suicidal ideation, and psychomotor retardation are indicative of clinical depression rather than uncomplicated bereavement.

- Very young children do not understand death but often react to the emotions of adults by becoming more irritable and crying more frequently. They often believe death is reversible.

- School-aged children understand the finality of death. Grief behaviors may reflect regression or aggression, school phobias, or sometimes a withdrawal into the self.

- Adolescents are usually able to view death on an adult level. Grieving behaviors may include withdrawal or acting out. Although they understand that their own death is inevitable, the concept is so far-reaching as to be imperceptible.

- By the time a person reaches the 60s or 70s, he or she has experienced numerous losses. Because grief is cumulative, this can result in bereavement overload. Depression is a common response.

- Nurses must be aware of the death rituals and grief behaviors common to various cultures. Some of these rituals associated with African Americans, Asian Americans, Filipino Americans, Jewish Americans, Mexican Americans, and Native Americans were presented in this chapter.

- Hospice is a program that provides palliative and supportive care to meet the special needs of people who are dying and their families.

- The term *advance directive* refers to either a living will or a durable power of attorney for health care. Advance directives allow clients to be in control of decisions at the end of life and spare family and loved ones the burden of making choices without knowing what is most important to the person who is dying.

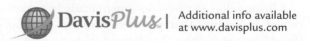

DavisPlus | Additional info available at www.davisplus.com

Review Questions
Self-Examination/Learning Exercise

Select the answer that is most appropriate for each of the following questions.

1. Which of the following is most likely to initiate a grief response in an individual? (Select all that apply.)
   a. Death of a pet dog
   b. Being told by her doctor that she has begun menopause
   c. Failing an exam
   d. Losing a spouse through divorce

2. Nancy, who is dying of cancer, says to the nurse, "I just want to see my new grandbaby. If only God will let me live until she is born, then I'll be ready to go." This is an example of which of Kübler-Ross's stages of grief?
   a. Denial
   b. Anger
   c. Bargaining
   d. Acceptance

3. Gloria, a recent widow, states, "I'm going to have to learn to pay all the bills. Hank always did that. I don't know if I can handle all of that." This is an example of which of the tasks described by Worden?
   a. Task I: Accepting the reality of the loss
   b. Task II: Processing the pain of grief
   c. Task III: Adjusting to a world without the lost entity
   d. Task IV: Finding an enduring connection with the lost entity in the midst of embarking on a new life

4. Engel identifies which of the following as successful resolution of the grief process?
   a. When the bereaved person can talk about the loss without crying
   b. When the bereaved person no longer talks about the lost entity
   c. When the bereaved person puts all remembrances of the loss out of sight
   d. When the bereaved person can discuss both positive and negative aspects about the lost entity

5. Which of the following is thought to facilitate the grief process?
   a. The ability to grieve in anticipation of the loss
   b. The ability to grieve alone without interference from others
   c. Having recently grieved for another loss
   d. Taking personal responsibility for the loss

6. When Frank's wife of 34 years dies, he is very stoic, handles all the funeral arrangements, does not cry or appear sad, and comforts all of the other family members in their grief. Two years later, when Frank's best friend dies, Frank has sleep disturbances, difficulty concentrating, loss of weight, and difficulty performing on his job. This is an example of which of the following maladaptive responses to loss?
   a. Delayed grieving
   b. Distorted grieving
   c. Prolonged grieving
   d. Exaggerated grieving

7. A major difference between normal and maladaptive grieving has been identified by which of the following?
   a. There are no feelings of depression in normal grieving.
   b. There is no loss of self-esteem in normal grieving.
   c. Normal grieving lasts no longer than 1 year.
   d. In normal grief the person does not show anger toward the loss.

Continued

Review Questions—cont'd
Self-Examination/Learning Exercise

8. Which grief reaction can the nurse anticipate in a 10-year-old child?
   a. Statements that the deceased person will soon return
   b. Regressive behaviors, such as loss of bladder control
   c. A preoccupation with the loss
   d. Thinking that they may have done something to cause the death

9. Which of the following is a correct statement when attempting to distinguish normal grief from clinical depression?
   a. In clinical depression, anhedonia is prevalent.
   b. In normal grieving, the person has generalized feelings of guilt.
   c. The person who is clinically depressed relates feelings of depression to a specific loss.
   d. In normal grieving, there is a persistent state of dysphoria.

10. Which of the following is *not* true regarding grieving by an adolescent?
    a. Adolescents may not show their true feelings about the death.
    b. Adolescents tend to have an immortal attitude.
    c. Adolescents do not perceive death as inevitable.
    d. Adolescents may exhibit acting out behaviors as part of their grief.

IMPLICATIONS OF RESEARCH FOR EVIDENCE-BASED PRACTICE

Moriarty, J., Maguire, A., O'Reilly, D., & McCann, M. (2015). Bereavement after informal caregiving: Assessing mental health burden using linked population data. *American Journal of Public Health, 105*(8), 1630-1637. doi:10.2105/AJPH. 2015.302597

DESCRIPTION OF THE STUDY: The researchers linked prescription records for antidepressant and antianxiety medications to characteristics and life event data for members of a longitudinal study in Northern Ireland to assess comparative mental health burdens for nonprofessional (family/household) bereaved caregivers, bereaved non-caregivers, and non-bereaved caregivers ($N = 317{,}264$). Their expressed intent was to identify who suffers most after the death of someone close to them so that resources for intervention can be targeted appropriately.

RESULTS OF THE STUDY: The first significant finding was that both caregivers and bereaved individuals were at 20 to 50 times greater risk for mental health problems than non-caregivers in similar circumstances. Another significant finding was that among working-aged people who were bereaved caregivers, mental health issues were greater than those of other caregivers; the greater the hours of caregiving, the greater their risks for sustained mental health issues in bereavement. The researchers identify that this finding was contrary to other studies that have found increased resilience among bereaved caregivers. This has been thought to be, among other things, a positive outcome of anticipatory grief. The idea that bereavement might provide a relief of sorts from the caregiving burden was found to be untrue for working-aged adults. Older adult bereaved caregivers, by contrast, seemed to recover more quickly from caregiver bereavement.

IMPLICATIONS FOR NURSING PRACTICE: The bereavement process for caregivers of an ill family member may carry additional risk for mental health problems in the bereavement process, but this study highlights the particular burden of working-aged caregivers and the potential impact on bereavement and their mental health. The researchers suggest that this prolonged risk may be related to disrupted work schedules, employability, and disrupted social networks. For nurses working with bereaved caregivers, these findings suggest the importance of assessing for mental health issues during bereavement, particularly for working-age adults. Education and provision of resources for ongoing support may be beneficial in reducing long-term, sustained mental health problems for this subgroup.

IMPLICATIONS OF RESEARCH FOR EVIDENCE-BASED PRACTICE

Sealey, M., Breen, L.J., O'Connor, M., & Aoun, J.M. (2015). A scoping review of bereavement risk assessment measures: Implications for palliative care. *Palliative Medicine, 29*(7), 577-589. doi:10.1177/0269216315576262

DESCRIPTION OF THE STUDY: This study attempts to address the concern that while palliative care standards and policies recommend bereavement support to family caregivers, there is uncertainty about whether interventions are being appropriately aligned with bereavement support needs. The authors conducted a scoping review of literature ($N = 3,142$) from 1982 to 2014 to identify the use and appropriateness of bereavement risk assessment tools.

RESULTS OF THE STUDY: The researchers identified 19 different measures used to assess bereavement risks: some for before the patient's death ($n = 5$), some for after the patient's death ($n = 10$), and some for screening for prolonged or complex grief ($n = 4$). Their analysis found that the majority had acceptable psychometric properties, but their feasibility for use in palliative care varied widely.

The authors note that while their primary aim was to identify those at risk for poor bereavement outcomes, the complexities and variables of the grief process make this a difficult challenge and that this study is a first step in an attempt to understand future needs.

IMPLICATIONS FOR NURSING PRACTICE: The researchers identify implications for practice that are relevant to nurses working with bereaved clients and in palliative care:

1. Risk assessment is an essential step for provision of bereavement support according to need.
2. These findings will help guide palliative care services toward evidence-based assessment and intervention and will inform palliative care standards and policies.

In general, nurses who work with currently bereaved clients or who are anticipating needs of future bereaved clients must be knowledgeable about identified risks associated with maladaptive or prolonged grieving. Systematic assessment will promote targeted intervention with the goal of facilitating the bereavement process toward adaptive outcomes.

Communication Exercises

1. Jane's husband has been hospitalized for several days in end-stage congestive heart failure, and Jane has just been told that he has died. She begins sobbing and screams at the nurse, "You killed my husband! I should have never brought him to the hospital!"
   • What would be an appropriate, empathic response by the nurse?
2. The doctor has shared with John test results revealing that his terminal cancer has not responded to treatment. John looks to the nurse and asks, "Am I dying?"
   • What would be an appropriate response by the nurse?
3. Nancy has been told that she has a terminal illness. She says to the nurse, "Why would God do this to me?"
   • What response by the nurse would demonstrate sensitivity to Nancy's spiritual distress?

References

Adams, J. (2014). Death and bereavement: A whole-school approach. *Community Practitioner, 87*(8), 35-36. doi:10.12968/bjsn.2012.7.9.450

Appel, S.J. (2017). Vietnamese Americans. In J.N. Giger (Ed.), *Transcultural nursing: Assessment and intervention* (7th ed., pp. 430-465). St. Louis, MO: Mosby.

Bralock, A.R., & Padgham, C.S. (2017). Jewish Americans. In J.N. Giger (Ed.), *Transcultural nursing: Assessment and intervention* (7th ed., pp. 388-407). St. Louis, MO: Mosby.

Campinha-Bacote, J. (2013). People of African American heritage. In L.D. Purnell (Ed.), *Transcultural health care* (4th ed., pp. 91-114). Philadelphia: F.A. Davis.

Catalano, J.T., & Catalano, S. (2015). Bioethical issues. In J. T. Catalano, *Nursing now! Today's issues, tomorrow's trends.* Philadelphia: F.A. Davis.

Chang, K. (2017). Chinese Americans. In J.N. Giger (Ed.), *Transcultural nursing: Assessment and intervention* (7th ed., pp. 388-407). St. Louis, MO: Mosby.

Corr, C.A., & Corr, D.M. (2013). *Death and dying: Life & living* (7th ed.). Belmont, CA: Wadsworth.

Hazell, L. (2016). Cross-cultural funeral service rituals. Retrieved from https://www.funeralwise.com/customs/cross-cultural-funerals/

Hensley, P.L., & Clayton, P.J. (2013). Why the bereavement exclusion was introduced in DSM-III. *Psychiatric Annals, 43*(6), 256-260.

Ito, M., & Hattori, K. (2013). People of Japanese heritage. In L. D. Purnell (Ed.), *Transcultural health care: A culturally competent approach* (4th ed., pp. 319-338). Philadelphia: F.A. Davis.

Kearns, C. (2014). PTSD and the bereaved parent. Retrieved from http://carolkearns.com/columns/col_ptsd-bereaved.html

King, M., Vasanthan, M., Petersen, I., Jones, L., Marston, L., & Nazareth, I. (2013). Mortality and medical care after bereavement: A practical cohort study. *PloS ONE, 8*(1), 1-7. doi:10.1371/journal.pone.0052561

Mattson, S. (2013). People of Vietnamese heritage. In L.D. Purnell (Ed.), *Transcultural health care: A culturally competent approach* (4th ed., pp. 479-480). Philadelphia: F.A. Davis.

McMurry, L., Song, H., Owen, D.C., Gonzalez, E.W., & Esperat, C.R. (2017). Mexican Americans. In J.N. Giger (Ed.), *Transcultural nursing: Assessment and intervention* (7th ed., pp. 208-241). St. Louis, MO: Mosby.

MedlinePlus. (2015). Bereavement. Retrieved from https://www.nlm.nih.gov/medlineplus/bereavement.html

Moriarty, J., Maguire, A., O'Reilly, D., & McCann, M. (2015). Bereavement after informal caregiving: Assessing mental health burden using linked population data. *American Journal of Public Health, 105*(8), 1630-1637. doi:10.2105/AJPH.2015.302597

Morrow, A. (2016). Grief and mourning: What's normal and what's not? Retrieved from https://www.verywell.com/grief-and-mourning-process-1132545

Munoz, C.C. (2013). People of Filipino Heritage. In L. D. Purnell (Ed.), *Transcultural health care: A culturally competent approach* (4th ed., pp. 228-249) Philadelphia: F.A. Davis.

Parris, R.J. (2011). Initial management of bereaved relatives following trauma. *Trauma, 14*(2), 139-155. doi:10.1177/1460408611420352

Peacock, S.C., Hammond-Collins, K., & Ford, D.A. (2014). The journey with dementia from the perspective of bereaved caregivers: A qualitative descriptive study. *BioMed Central Nursing, 13*(42), 1-10. doi:10.1186/s12912-014-0042-x

Pies, R.W. (2013). Grief and depression: The sages knew the difference. *Psychiatric Times,* April 29, 2013. Retrieved from www.psychiatrictimes.com/display/article/10168/2140230

Purnell, L.D. (2013). The Purnell model for cultural competence. In L.D. Purnell (Ed.), *Transcultural health care: A culturally competent approach* (4th ed.). Philadelphia: F.A. Davis

Purnell, L.D. (2014). People of Navajo Indian heritage. *Guide to culturally competent health care* (3nd ed.). Philadelphia: F.A. Davis.

Sadock, B.J., Sadock, V.A., & Ruiz, P. (2015). *Synopsis of psychiatry: Behavioral sciences/clinical psychiatry* (11th ed.). Philadelphia: Lippincott Williams & Wilkins

Sealey, M., Breen, L.J., O'Connor, M., & Aoun, J.M. (2015). A scoping review of bereavement risk assessment measures: Implications for palliative care. *Palliative Medicine, 29*(7), 577-589. doi:10.1177/0269216315576262

Selekman, J. (2013). People of Jewish heritage. In L.D. Purnell (Ed.), *Transcultural health care: A culturally competent approach* (4th ed., pp. 339-356). Philadelphia: F.A. Davis.

Shah, S.M., Carey, I.M., Harris, T., DeWilde, S., Victor, C.R., & Cook, D.G. (2013). The effect of unexpected bereavement on mortality in older couples. *American Journal of Public Health, 103*(6), 1140-1145. doi:10.2105/AJPH.2012.301050

Tousley, M. (2013). Coping with cumulative losses. *Grief Healing.* Retrieved from www.griefhealingblog.com/2013/02/coping-with-cumulative-losses.html

Tsai, Hsiu-Min. (2013). People of Chinese heritage. In L.D. Purnell (Ed.), *Transcultural health care: A culturally competent approach* (4th ed., pp. 178-196). Philadelphia: F.A. Davis.

Worden, J. W. (2009). *Grief counseling and grief therapy: A handbook for the mental health practitioner* (4th ed.). New York: Springer.

Zoucha, R., & Zamarripa, C.A. (2013). People of Mexican heritage. In L.D. Purnell (Ed.), *Transcultural health care: A culturally competent approach* (4th ed., pp. 374-390). Philadelphia: F.A. Davis.

Classical References

Bowlby, J. (1961). Processes of mourning. *International Journal of Psychoanalysis, 42,* 22.

Engel, G. (1964). Grief and grieving. *American Journal of Nursing, 64*(9), 93.

Kübler-Ross, E. (1969). *On death and dying.* New York: Macmillan.

Military Families

38

KEY TERMS

deployment

posttraumatic stress disorder (PTSD)

traumatic brain injury

veterans

OBJECTIVES

After reading this chapter, the student will be able to:

1. Discuss historical aspects and epidemiological statistics related to members and veterans of the U.S. military.
2. Describe the lifestyle of career military families.
3. Discuss the impact of deployment on families of service members.
4. Discuss concerns of women in the military.
5. Describe combat-related illnesses common in members and veterans of the U.S. military.
6. Apply steps of the nursing process in care of veterans with traumatic brain injury and posttraumatic stress disorder.
7. Discuss various modalities relevant to treatment of traumatic brain injury and posttraumatic stress disorder.

HOMEWORK ASSIGNMENT

Please read the chapter and answer the following questions:

1. Name some positives and negatives associated with the military lifestyle.
2. Describe behaviors that may be exhibited by school-aged children in response to deployment of a parent.
3. How do feelings about leaving their children during a deployment differ between male and female service members?
4. Name some symptoms of posttraumatic stress disorder.

Because of U.S. involvement in Iraq and Afghanistan, perhaps at no time in modern history has so much attention been given to what individuals and families experience as a result of their lives in the military. There is an ongoing effort by organizations that provide services for active-duty military personnel and **veterans** of military combat to keep up with the growing demand, and resources for these services will be required for many years to come. The need for mental health care practitioners will rise as the increasing number of veterans and their family members struggle to cope with the effects of military deployment.

This chapter addresses issues associated with the lives of military families and veterans of military combat. A discussion of nursing care for these individuals is presented, and selected medical treatment modalities are described.

Historical Aspects

"To care for him who shall have borne the battle and for his widow and his orphan."
—Abraham Lincoln, 1865

There is little doubt that individuals who survive military combat return from battle with scars—physical, psychological, or both. Reports of war-related psychological symptoms have existed in writing throughout the centuries, identified by terms such as "shell shock" and "battle fatigue." Many veterans of World War I and World War II were expected to be stoic, to lock up their feelings, and to never speak of the scenes of carnage and combat that they witnessed. The abuse of alcohol became a common way to deal with the emotions that they did not feel comfortable discussing. **Posttraumatic stress disorder (PTSD)** has been related to the high rates of alcoholism among veterans, particularly those who have experienced active-duty combat. Only in recent history have the invisible wounds of combat veterans received the treatment they desperately require.

Very little was written about PTSD during the years between 1950 and 1970. This absence was followed in the 1970s and 1980s by an explosion in the amount of research and writing on the subject. Many of the papers written during this time were about Vietnam veterans. Clearly, the renewed interest in PTSD was linked to the psychological casualties of the Vietnam War. The diagnostic category of PTSD did not appear until the third edition of the *Diagnostic and Statistical Manual of Mental Disorders (DSM-III)* in 1980, after a need was indicated by increasing numbers of problems with Vietnam veterans and victims of multiple disasters.

Epidemiological Statistics

Currently, more than 1.3 million individuals serve on active duty in the U.S. armed forces in more than 150 countries around the world, along with 736,964 civilian personnel and another 777,114 serving in the National Guard and Reserve forces (Department of Defense [DoD], 2015a). Approximately 16.1 percent of those in active duty are women. Veterans currently number more than 20 million, about 9 percent of whom are women (U.S. Census Bureau, 2016).

Since the beginning of the wars in Afghanistan and Iraq in 2001, more than 2.2 million U.S. military personnel have been deployed in 3 million tours of duty lasting more than 30 days as part of Operation Enduring Freedom (OEF) and Operation Iraqi Freedom (OIF) (Institute of Medicine [IOM], 2013). According to the IOM report (2013) *Returning Home from Iraq and Afghanistan: Readjustment Needs of Veterans, Service Members, and Their Families*, 44 percent of these military personnel identify difficulty readjusting to daily living upon return from deployment, and 30 percent report unemployment after returning—twice the percentage of their nonveteran counterparts. The cost in deaths and physical and psychological injuries cannot be measured.

Application of the Nursing Process

Assessment

The Military Family

The military lifestyle offers both positive and negative aspects for those who choose this way of life. Hall (2011) summarizes a number of pros and cons about what is sometimes called the Warrior Society. Some advantages include:

- Early retirement compared to civilian counterparts
- A vast resource system to meet family needs
- Job security with a guaranteed paycheck
- Health-care benefits
- Opportunities to see the world
- Educational opportunities

Some disadvantages include:

- Frequent familial separations and reunions
- Regular household relocations
- Living life under the maxim of "the mission must always come first"
- A pattern of rigidity, regimentation, and conformity in family life
- Feelings of detachment from nonmilitary community
- The social effects of "rank"
- The lack of control over pay, promotion, and other benefits

Mary Wertsch (1996), who conducted a vast amount of research on the culture of the military family, stated, "The great paradox of the military is that its members, the self-appointed frontline guardians of our cherished American democratic values, do not live in democracy themselves" (p. 15). The military is maintained by a rigid authoritarian structure, and these characteristics often extend into the structure of the home.

A class system is strikingly evident in the military, with two distinct subcultures: that of the officer and that of the enlisted ranks. Hall (2011) states:

> The United States has made great strides in the past five decades to affirm and equalize the differences in society, but the assumption of all military systems in the world is that it is essential for the functioning of the organization to maintain a rigid hierarchical system based on dominance and subordination. (p. 38)

Isolation and alienation are common facets of military life. To compensate for the extreme mobility, the focus of this lifestyle turns inward to the military world rather than outward to the local community. Children of military families almost always report that no matter what school they attend, they feel "different" from the other students (Wertsch, 1996).

These descriptions apply principally to "career" military families. Another type of military family, those in the all-volunteer military, have become a familiar part of the American culture in recent years. The OEF and OIF military campaigns together make up the longest sustained U.S. military operation since the Vietnam War, and they are the first extended conflicts to depend on an all-volunteer military (IOM, 2013). There has been heavy dependence on the National Guard and Reserves and an escalation in the pace, duration, and number of deployments and redeployments experienced by these individuals. Many joined the National Guard or Reserves as a second job for financial reasons or for the educational opportunities available to them. Little thought had been given to the possibility of actually fighting in a war. As one anonymous reservist posted on his blog:

> The active forces have the harder role. They're required to be fully ready 24/7/365, and to deploy and fight on much shorter notice than the Reserve [forces]. It's their livelihood and (for many) their career. They're serving full-time; reservists aren't. That was once clearly true. But not really quite true anymore. Many reservists in critically needed specialties have already served multiple years on active duty since 9/11, and this situation doesn't look to change anytime soon. (Kelly Temps in Uniform, 2012)

In recent years, enlistees in the National Guard and Reserves are told that they should expect to serve an interval of active duty. The Iraq and Afghanistan conflicts have engaged more National Guard and Reserve forces members than previous conflicts, and more women and parents of young children are being deployed as well (IOM, 2013). Most individuals in the National Guard and Reserves are willing to serve when and where they are needed but consider themselves "part-timers." The extended OEF and OIF campaigns have changed this part-time concept for many who have served multiple tours of duty, creating a hardship on their families and their civilian careers. The IOM reports that, in general, recent military tours of duty are marked by longer deployments and shorter intervals at home. Many of these "temporary citizen soldiers," as well as their full-time military counterparts, now carry the physical and psychological scars of battle.

Military Spouses and Children

A military spouse inherently knows and lives with the concept of "mission first." Devries and colleagues (2012) state, "While the military works hard to value the family lives of service members and their welfare, the nature of the job is that the mission trumps all other concerns" (p. 11). However, times have changed from the days when life in the military was viewed as a two-person career, in which a woman was expected to "create the right family setting so that her husband's work reflected his life at home, by staying positive, being interested in his duty, and being flexible and adaptable" (Hall, 2012, p. 148). Many of today's military spouses have their own careers or are pursuing higher levels of education. They do not view the military as a joint career with their service member spouse.

The lives of military spouses and children are clearly affected when the service member's active-duty assignments require frequent family moves. Wakefield (2007) has stated, "The many short-term relationships, complications of spousal employment, university transfer issues, escalated misbehavior of the children, day care arrangements, spousal loneliness, and increased financial obligations are just some of the issues military personnel face that can lead to frustration." In most instances, when the service member receives orders for a new geographical assignment, the spouse's education, career, or both are put on hold, and the entire family is relocated. Other occasions may arise when the family is unable to immediately follow the service member to the new location. In certain instances, such as when a student may be about to complete a semester or is about to graduate, the service member may proceed to the new assignment without the family. This is difficult for the military spouse who is left alone to care for the children, as well as to deal with all aspects of the move.

Military children face unique challenges. There are almost 1.9 million children in military families, and the largest percentage (37.4%) are ages 5 and younger (DoD, 2013). Clever and Segal (2013) note that while the Department of Defense (DoD) collects substantial demographic research, more is needed on the effects of military family life on infants and toddlers. School-aged children primarily attend civilian public schools where they form a unique subculture among staff and peers who often do not understand their life experiences. Children who grow up in a career military family learn to adapt to changing situations very quickly and to hide a certain level of fear associated with the nomadic lifestyle. Hall (2008) states:

> It is not just a fear of what might happen to their family or their military parents but a fear of the unknown, of not being accepted, of being behind, of not finding friends, or of not being cool. One of the most common concerns expressed by students when they arrive in a new school is who they will eat lunch with. Another reality for student athletes is that a student could be the star of the basketball team in one school and be sitting on the bench at the next. (p. 103)

The Impact of Deployment

Not since the Vietnam War have so many U.S. military families been affected by deployment-related family separation, combat injury, and death. Many service members have been deployed multiple times. Those who are deployed most frequently describe their greatest fear as having to leave their spouse and children. Lengthy separations pose many challenges to all members of the family. Spouses undertake all the challenges of managing the household in addition to assuming the role of the single parent. The pressure and stress are intense as the spouse attempts to maintain an atmosphere of strength for the children, while experiencing the fears and anxiety associated with the life-threatening conditions facing his or her service member partner.

Approximately 2 million American children have experienced the **deployment** of a parent to Iraq or Afghanistan. More than 48,000 children either have lost a parent or have a parent who was wounded in these conflicts. Smith (2012) states:

> The stress that comes when a family member is deployed is significant, and that stress is multiplied when a loved one is wounded or killed. When parents return from deployment, they are not always the same as they were before. Major injuries, such as loss of a limb, traumatic brain injury, or posttraumatic stress disorder are life-altering, and children often have a hard time understanding the reason for a significant change in the appearance, personality, or behavior of a parent.

The following behaviors have been reported in children in response to the deployment of a parent (American Academy of Child & Adolescent Psychiatry, no date):

■ Infants (birth to 12 months): May respond to disruptions in their schedule with decreased appetite, weight loss, irritability, and/or apathy.

■ Toddlers (1 to 3 years): May become sullen, tearful, throw temper tantrums, or develop sleep problems.

■ Preschoolers (3 to 6 years): May regress in areas such as toilet training, sleep, separation fears, physical complaints, or thumb sucking. May assume blame for parent's departure.

■ School-age children (6 to 12 years): Are more aware of potential dangers to parent. May exhibit irritable behavior, aggression, or whininess. May become more regressed and fearful about parent's safety.

■ Adolescents (13 to 18 years): May be rebellious, irritable, or more challenging of authority. Parents need to be alert to high-risk behaviors, such as problems with the law, sexual acting out, and drug or alcohol abuse.

Pincus and associates (2013) describe the cycle of deployment in five distinct stages: predeployment, deployment, sustainment, redeployment, and postdeployment.

Predeployment The time frame for this stage is variable, beginning with the receipt of the orders and ending when the service member departs. Family members alternate between feelings of denial and anticipation of loss. The soldier and family get their affairs in order, extended training periods result in long hours apart, and the anxiety of the anticipated departure promotes stress and irritability among family members.

Deployment This stage includes the time from actual deployment through the first month of separation. Military spouses report feeling disoriented and overwhelmed, and experience a range of emotions including numbness, sadness, loneliness, and abandonment. It is a time of disorganization as the spouse struggles to take charge of the details of living without his or her partner.

Sustainment Sustainment begins about 1 month into the deployment until about a month before the service member's expected return. During this stage, the spouse and children establish new support systems and institute new family routines. Technology makes it possible for the family and service member to keep in touch with each other by phone, video, and e-mail. Despite the difficulties and obstacles encountered, most military families successfully negotiate this stage and anxiously anticipate their loved one's return.

Redeployment This stage is defined as the month before the service member is scheduled to return home. There is excitement and apprehension associated with the homecoming. Pincus and associates (2013) identify concerns such as, "Will he (she) agree with the changes I have made?" "Will I have to give up my independence?" "Will we get along?"

Postdeployment This stage typically lasts 3 to 6 months and begins with the return of the service member to the home station. There is a period of adjustment beginning with the "honeymoon" period, when the spouses reconnect physically, but not necessarily emotionally. The returning service member may desire to "pick up where he or she left off," only to encounter resistance from the spouse who expresses a reluctance to relinquish the degree of independence and autonomy to which he or she has become accustomed during the separation. Pincus and associates (2013) state:

> Postdeployment is probably the most important stage for both soldier and spouse. Patient communication, going slow, lowering expectations, and taking time to get to know each other again is critical to the task of successful reintegration of the soldier back into the family.

Counseling may be required in the event that the service member has been injured or experiences a traumatic stress reaction.

Women in the Military

Women make up approximately 15 percent of the U.S. military and 18 percent of National Guard and Reserve members (CNN, 2013). Women have been serving in the military since the time of the Civil War, mostly as nurses, spies, and support persons. In recent years, the Pentagon has relaxed its ban on women serving in combat roles, and "women began to fly combat aircraft, staff missile placements, drive convoys in the desert, and participate in other roles that involved potential combat exposure" (Mathewson, 2011, p. 217). Early in 2013, the Secretary of Defense lifted the ban on combat jobs to women, gradually opening direct combat units to female troops. At the present time, certain specialty positions continue to remain off limits, although the plan is to eventually integrate women into these positions. Flexibility in the new law exists for exemptions to occur if further assessment reveals that some jobs are inappropriate for women.

Special Concerns of Women in the Military

A number of issues are of special concern to women in the military, including sexual harassment, sexual assault, differential treatment and conditions, and being a parent.

Sexual Harassment Sexual harassment is defined as "unwanted, unwelcome comments or physical contact of a sexual nature occurring in the workplace" (Mathewson, 2011, p. 221). From statements such as "you look nice this morning" or "hey, you smell good" to blatant suggestions or requests for sexual interactions, Wolfe and associates (1998), in a study of women on active duty during the Persian Gulf War, found that both physical and sexual harassment were higher than typically found in peacetime military samples. Reports by military therapists conveyed that women who were sexually harassed while in the military suffer higher than average rates of a range of problems following discharge, including poor self-image, relationship issues, drug use, depression, and PTSD.

Sexual Assault The DoD (2015b) reported 6,131 cases of active service member sexual assaults in 2014. They define this as "unwanted sexual contact" and now track reports annually. From 2012 to 2013, a 53 percent increase in reporting incidents was identified, a trend that continued in 2014 with an 11 percent annual increase. Despite that more incidents are now being reported, 62 percent of those who reported an incident expected professional or social retaliation.

Only an estimated 25 percent of sexual assaults in the military are reported. Reasons for not reporting include fear of causing trouble in their units, that their commanders and fellow soldiers would turn against them, that they would be passed over for well-deserved promotions, or that they would be transferred and removed from duty altogether (Vlahos, 2012). Some women who have reported incidents to their commanding officers have been told to "forget about it," "buckle up," or "pretend it didn't happen," and are made to feel as though they are perpetrators instead of victims. Wolf (2012) describes the way the military deals with rape as "a culture of cover-up."

In 2000, following incidents of military sexual assaults that were made public, the Veteran's Health Administration mandated universal health screening for sexual trauma among military personnel. But despite the efforts within the DoD to identify and correct this problem, incidents continue, suggesting that sexual assault remains a part of military culture (Burgess, Slattery, & Herlihy, 2013).

Some women who report their sexual assaults are discharged from the service with psychiatric diagnoses of personality disorder or adjustment disorder. Vlahos (2012) reports:

> For the veteran, getting a personality disorder or adjustment disorder discharge can be catastrophic. Not only does it carry a stigma for future employers, it cuts the veteran off from a series of benefits, including health care and service-related disability compensation.

Although they compose only 15 percent of military personnel, women constitute almost one-fourth of all personality disorder discharges. Survivors of sexual assault in the military report long-lasting effects, including PTSD, depression, suicidal ideation and attempts, eating disorders, anxiety disorders, relationship difficulties, and substance abuse. Wolf (2012) notes that among military veterans, the leading cause of PTSD for men is combat trauma, whereas for women it is sexual trauma. She states, "Our women veterans are more likely to be traumatized by a sexual assault by a fellow soldier or a commander than by their own battlefield or war experiences."

Differential Treatment and Conditions Although their numbers have increased, women still constitute a minority in the military. One female officer accounted that because of the small number of women in any given unit, officers and enlisted personnel are often housed together. She indicated that she missed being with other officers to discuss work and spend time with her peers. She also reported that the enlisted women were uncomfortable with an officer in their presence. Burgess and associates (2013) add that when sexual trauma occurs among military personnel, it is occurring in the workplace, and as such, the victim often has ongoing contact with the perpetrator and may also be in a dependent position if the perpetrator was in a supervisory role.

Women's military careers are often limited by their exclusions from occupational specialties. These sanctions often preclude female officers and enlisted personnel from the most prestigious units and occupations in the military, their participation in which is essential to ascending in the ranks should they choose to make the military a career. Fear of additional occupational discrimination may prevent women from reporting sexual harassment and assault. Many bans have been lifted, and occupations that historically have been off limits are now open to women. However, the manner in which the culture within the military will respond to those changes remains to be seen.

Parenting Issues Women's feelings associated with leaving their children often differ from those of men. Women seem to struggle more with guilt feelings for "abandoning" their children, whereas men have stronger emotions tied to a sense of doing their duty. Although men also experience regret at leaving their children, they often rely on the assurance that the children have their mothers to care for them.

Veterans

Most veterans returning from a combat zone undergo a period of adjustment. A recent study of young veterans (Pedersen, Marshall, & Kurz, 2016) identified that 70 percent screened as positive for behavioral health problems, less than a third of whom received adequate psychotherapy or psychotropic treatment. Many veterans suffer from migraine headaches and experience cognitive difficulties such as memory loss. Hypervigilance, insomnia, and jitteriness are common. The Substance Abuse and Mental Health Services Administration (Substance Abuse and Mental Health Services Administration [SAMHSA], 2012) states, "Veterans may struggle to concentrate; engage in aggressive behavior, such as aggressive driving; and use alcohol, tobacco, and drugs excessively. However, the intensity and duration of these and other worrisome behaviors can indicate a more serious problem and the need for professional treatment" (p. 1). Plach and Sells (2013) identified in a study of veterans that over 50 percent screened positive for problem drinking and over 90 percent had engaged in hazardous drinking (Cogan, 2014).

Traumatic Brain Injury

The incidence of **traumatic brain injury (TBI)** is a significant consequence of the Iraq and Afghanistan conflicts. Mild TBI is so frequent that it has been referred to as the "signature injury" of the wars in these countries (Cogan, 2014). The Defense and Veterans Brain Injury Center (DVBIC) report a total of 339,462 TBIs since 2000 and over 18,000 cases in 2015 alone (2016).

The Department of Veterans Affairs (VA) and the DoD offer the following definition of TBI:

> A traumatically induced structural injury and/or physiological disruption of brain function as a result of an external force that is indicated by new onset or worsening of at least one of the following clinical signs, immediately following the event:

■ Any period of loss of or a decreased level of consciousness

■ Any loss of memory for events immediately before or after the injury (posttraumatic amnesia)

■ Any alteration in mental state at the time of the injury (confusion, disorientation, slowed thinking, etc.) (Alteration of consciousness/mental state)

■ Neurological deficits (weakness, loss of balance, change in vision, praxis, paresis/plegia, sensory loss, aphasia, etc.) that may or may not be transient

■ Intracranial lesion (VA/DoD, 2016, pp. 4–5)

Symptoms may be classified as mild, moderate, or severe. In the civilian population, the most common causes of TBI include child abuse in infants and toddlers, motor vehicle accidents in adolescents and young adults, and falls and associated subdural hematomas in older adults (Strong & Donders, 2012). Blasts from explosive devices are the leading cause of TBI for active-duty military personnel in combat (Birk, 2010; Cogan, 2014). While the mechanism of damage from explosive blasts is not completely understood, researchers believe that it is "the pressure wave passing through the brain that significantly disrupts brain function" (Mayo Clinic, 2014). TBI also results from penetrating wounds, severe blows to the head with shrapnel or debris, and falls or bodily collisions with objects following a blast. Symptoms of TBI according to level of severity are presented in Table 38–1.

Most soldiers who have sustained a mild TBI improve with no lasting clinical complications (VA/DoD, 2016). Many recover within hours, days, or at most, weeks. In a small minority, symptoms persist from 6 months to a year. The location and severity of the injury are factors that determine the long-term outcome for individuals with TBI. Severity is determined by the nature, speed, and location of the impact and the presence of complications such as hypoxemia, hypotension, intracranial hemorrhage, or increased intracranial pressure (Ribbers, 2013).

The most common long-term consequences of TBI include problems with cognition (e.g., thinking, memory, and reasoning) and behavior or mental

TABLE 38–1 Criteria and Symptomatology of Traumatic Brain Injury According to Level of Severity

MILD	MODERATE	SEVERE
CRITERIA	**CRITERIA**	**CRITERIA**
Structural imaging = normal	Structural imaging = normal or	Structural imaging = normal or abnormal
Loss of consciousness 0–30 min	abnormal	Loss of consciousness >24 hrs
Alteration of consciousness/mental	Loss of consciousness >30 min	Alteration of consciousness/mental
state = a moment up to 24 hrs	and <24 hrs	state = >24 hours. Severity based
Posttraumatic amnesia = 0–1 day	Alteration of consciousness/mental	on other criteria.
Glasgow Coma Scale = 13–15	state = >24 hours. Severity based	Posttraumatic amnesia = >7 days
	on other criteria.	Glasgow Coma Scale = <9
	Posttraumatic amnesia = >1 and	
	<7 Days	
	Glasgow Coma Scale = 9–12	
SYMPTOMS	**SYMPTOMS**	**SYMPTOMS**
Headache	Any of the symptoms of mild TBI	Any of the symptoms of mild TBI
Dizziness, ringing in the ears	Headache that gets worse or does	Headache that gets worse or does
Nausea	not go away	not go away
Trouble concentrating, confusion	Repeated nausea and vomiting	Repeated nausea and vomiting
Blurred vision	Seizures	Seizures
Changes in sleep patterns	Difficulty awakening from sleep	Inability to awaken from sleep
Mood changes	Dilation of one or both pupils of	Dilation of one or both pupils of
Sensitivity to light or sound	the eyes	the eyes
	Slurred speech	Slurred speech
	Weakness or numbness in the	Weakness or numbness in the
	extremities	extremities
	Loss of coordination	Loss of coordination
	Increased confusion	Profound confusion
	Restlessness	Restlessness
	Agitation	Agitation

SOURCE: Department of Veterans Affairs & Department of Defense. (2016). Clinical practice guideline for management of concussion/mild traumatic brain injury. Retrieved from www.healthquality.va.gov/guidelines/Rehab/mtbi/mTBICPGClinicianSummary50821816.pdf; Mayo Clinic. (2014). Traumatic brain injury. Retrieved from www.mayoclinic.com/health/traumatic-brain-injury/DS00552; and National Institute of Neurological Disorders and Stroke. (2016). Traumatic brain injury: Hope through research. Retrieved from www.ninds.nih.gov/disorders/tbi/tbi.htm.

health (e.g., depression, anxiety, personality changes, aggression, acting out, and social inappropriateness) (Ribbers, 2013). Seizures occur in about 15 to 20 percent of individuals with TBI and commonly develop within the first 24 hours following the injury. With mild TBI, seizures usually subside within a week after the initial trauma. The potential for chronic epilepsy increases with severity of the injury.

Language and communication problems, such as aphasia, dysarthria, and dysphasia, can result from TBI (Safaz et al., 2008). Difficulties may also exist in the subtle aspects of communication, such as body language and nonverbal expression.

Studies show that TBI has long-term adverse effects on social functioning and productivity. Temkin and associates (2009) stated:

Penetrating head injury sustained in wartime is clearly associated with increased unemployment. TBI also adversely affects leisure and recreation, social relationships, functional status, quality of life, and independent living. Although there is a dose-response relationship between severity of injury and social

outcomes, there is insufficient evidence to determine at what level of severity the adverse effects are demonstrated. (p. 460)

Neurocognitive disorders, such as Alzheimer's disease (AD) and Parkinson's disease, are related to TBI (Ribbers, 2013). The risk for AD in individuals with moderate TBI is 2.3 times greater than that of the general population. An association between Parkinson's disease and TBI has also been established. The disorder may develop years after TBI as a result of damage to the basal ganglia (Ribbers, 2013).

Several factors have been identified that may worsen the condition of military personnel sustaining a TBI. Being in a high-stress environment, extreme temperatures such as the 120-degree heat common in Iraq, and delay of TBI recognition until the postdeployment period may all interfere with healing (Cogan, 2014). The prevalence as well as potential short- and long-term consequences suggest that screening for TBI should be conducted for any military personnel returning from active duty who presents with physical, cognitive, or emotional symptoms.

Posttraumatic Stress Disorder

PTSD is the most common mental disorder among veterans returning from military combat. The VA cites statistics that identify the lifetime prevalence for PTSD in the general population at 6.8 percent (Gradus, 2017). In comparison, they identify the following prevalence estimates for military veterans:

■ Veterans of OEF and OIF, 13.8 to 18.5 percent
■ Gulf War veterans, 10 percent
■ Vietnam veterans, 30 percent

The diagnostic criteria for PTSD from the *Diagnostic and Statistical Manual of Mental Disorders, Fifth Edition* (*DSM-5,* 2013) are presented in Chapter 28, Trauma- and Stressor-Related Disorders, of this text. The disorder can occur when an individual is exposed to an accident or violence in which death or serious injury to others or oneself occurs or is threatened. Symptoms of PTSD include:

■ Reliving the trauma through flashbacks, nightmares, and intrusive thoughts
■ Intensive efforts to avoid activities, people, places, situations, or objects that arouse recollections of the trauma
■ Chronic negative emotional state and diminished interest or participation in significant activities
■ Aggressive, reckless, or self-destructive behavior
■ Hypervigilance and exaggerated startle response
■ Angry outbursts, problems with concentration, and sleep disturbances

Symptoms of PTSD may be delayed, in some instances for years. When emotions regarding the trauma are constricted, they may suddenly appear in the future following a major life event, stressor, or an accumulation of stressors over time that challenge the person's defenses. Symptoms also may be masked by other physical or mental health problems. In some instances, the symptoms do not appear to be problematic until the individual begins a readjustment to routine occupational or social functioning.

Reports indicate that some World War II veterans are only now, decades after returning from combat, being diagnosed with PTSD. At the time of their return, these veterans rarely spoke of their war experiences. But for many, the visions of horror have seeped to the surface in nightmares, flashbacks, anxiety, and emotional numbness. In a study at the University of Michigan, Dr. Helen Kales found that in a group of World War II veterans being treated for depression, 38 percent met the criteria for PTSD (Albrecht, 2009). Langer (2011) reported that the PTSD symptoms for these veterans seemed to become more prominent in midlife and that the most significant precipitant was retirement. For many, their work gave meaning to their lives, and without it the symptoms of depression, anxiety, substance abuse, and PTSD began to emerge. Langer (2011) stated:

> Besides retirement, other precipitants [to PTSD in midlife] include the deaths of friends, one's own deteriorating health, children becoming autonomous, divorce, and other losses associated with aging. Other precipitants include current events that trigger memories of one's own combat experience, e.g., 9/11, and other wars.

Veterans with PTSD experience marital and relationship difficulties, including higher rates of physical and verbal aggression against their partners and children and higher rates of divorce (Monson, Fredman, & Adair, 2008). In its report on the readjustment needs of veterans, the IOM (2013) identified a significant rise in domestic violence among veterans of the Iraq and Afghanistan wars and recommended this as a high priority for assessment and intervention. The burden of caregiving to a partner with PTSD has been noted as an etiological factor in relationship difficulties. The caregiver's perception of how caring for the impaired partner affects their social life, health, or financial status is directly associated with the degree of difficulty experienced in the relationship (Lavender & Lyons, 2012). Some caregivers may experience what has been termed *secondary trauma* or *vicarious traumatization,* a condition in which somatic symptoms and emotional distress occur as a response to caring for an individual who exhibits the symptoms of PTSD. Secondary symptoms are also common in children with a parent suffering from PTSD. Family members sometimes report having nightmares that mimic feelings and experiences of the veteran, difficulty sleeping, depression, and even visual hallucinations that are similar to the veteran's flashbacks.

Co-occurring disorders are common in individuals with PTSD, including major depressive disorder, substance use disorders, and anxiety disorders. Individuals with TBI also may develop PTSD, depending on the degree of amnesia experienced immediately following the cerebral trauma.

Depression and Suicide

Depressive disorders have been identified as a growing problem among Americans in general, with an estimated 16 million adults reporting at least one depressive episode each year (National Alliance on Mental Illness [NAMI], 2016). Depression has been identified as a significant problem among veterans as well. SAMHSA (2014) reports that 18.5 percent of veterans returning from Iraq or Afghanistan are diagnosed with depression or PTSD; the two are often comorbidities. Impairments are observed in the domains of home management, interpersonal relationships, and occupational and social functioning. The

Veteran's Health Administration (2015) reports that older adult veterans are a high-risk group for depression as well; 11 percent (twice that in the general population) have major depressive disorder, and 40 percent of veterans older than age 60 with depression also have PTSD. This finding highlights the importance of asking older veterans about past trauma.

Reports by the DoD and VA indicate that the number of suicides among veterans and active-duty military has risen dramatically since 2001, the year that detailed record-keeping began. This number reached an all-time high in 2012 with a rate of 22.7 suicides per 100,000 (319) active-duty military personnel. While that number declined somewhat in 2013 to 18.7 per 100,000 (259), the number of suicides among reservists and National Guard personnel remained alarmingly high at 23.4 to 28.9 per 100,000 respectively (Kime, 2015). When suicides among veterans are added to the numbers, the incidence is even higher. The IOM report (2013) identified that the VA policy against restricting access to privately owned weapons compounds suicide risk. In 2014, VA policies were expanded to allow commanders to discuss access to firearms with at-risk populations and provide for voluntary surrender of their firearms if they request it (Kime, 2015).

Suicide among military personnel is closely associated with the diagnoses of substance use disorder, major depressive disorder, PTSD, and TBI. A common theme among investigations of suicide attempts and completed suicides by military service members is marital/relationship distress. Devries and associates (2012) stated:

> From 2005 to 2009, relationship problems were a factor in over 50 percent of the suicides in the Army. The health of our military fighting force is directly related to the health of our military marriages. What we see in the military is a common drama of relationship problems played out in an environment of uncommon stressors. (p. 7)

A study by Jakupcak and associates (2010) concluded that veterans who are unmarried or report lower satisfaction with their social support networks are at increased risk for suicide.

The multiplicity of factors influencing these dramatic suicide rates makes it hard to pinpoint a specific cause, but it has captured the attention of the government and the general public. In 2015, President Obama signed into law the Clayton Hunt SAV (suicide prevention for American veterans) Act, which intends to expand peer support for troubled veterans, streamline transitions for exiting servicemen, and mandate annual surveying of VA mental health and suicide prevention programs, among other initiatives (NAMI, 2015). Clayton Hunt was a decorated Marine who struggled with PTSD and depression after returning home from active duty and took his own life in 2011.

Substance Use Disorder

In addition to rising suicide rates, substance use disorder has also been on the rise in the military. The Army Suicide Prevention Task Force reported that 29 percent of active-duty military suicides between 2005 and 2009 involved alcohol or drugs, and in 2009 about one-third involved prescription drugs (National Institute on Drug Abuse [NIDA], 2013). Substance use disorder is a common co-occurring condition with PTSD. One study reports that almost 22 percent of veterans with PTSD also receive a diagnosis of substance use disorder (Brancu, Straits-Troster, & Kudler, 2011). The combination of substance use, PTSD, depression, and TBI all contribute to a significant risk for mental health, relationship problems, difficult readjustment to home life, and in many cases risk for suicide.

Among veterans who sought treatment for substance use disorder, 65 percent (almost double that of the nonveteran population) identified alcohol as their primary substance of abuse, 10 percent identified heroin as their primary drug, and 6.2 percent primarily used cocaine (SAMHSA, 2015). As with U.S. civilians, opioid pain medication use and abuse among military personnel has been on the rise. NIDA (2013) reported that from 2005 to 2009, prescriptions for pain medications by military physicians quadrupled. Crosby (2015) reports that smoking tobacco among military personnel is also higher (24 percent) than in the general population. The IOM report (2013) on readjustment needs of veterans identified that as many as 39 percent of veterans are struggling with substance use issues. Their recommendations include supporting research to identify evidence-based treatments for substance use disorders as well as reevaluating policies about access to abused substances within the military. A firsthand account of what it was like for Sean, a soldier who served in Iraq, and his experiences afterward is presented in "Real People, Real Stories: The Military Experience."

Diagnosis and Outcome Identification

Nursing diagnoses are formulated from the data gathered during the assessment phase and with background knowledge regarding predisposing factors to the disorder. Table 38–2 presents a list of selected client behaviors and the NANDA nursing diagnoses that correspond to those behaviors, which may be used in planning assistance for families as they confront the unique challenges associated with military life. Outcome criteria are presented for each.

Real People, Real Stories: The Military Experience

(The individual requested that his real name not be used.)

Karyn: What was it like for you when you returned from your tour of duty?

Sean: I was in Iraq for 360 days, and when we landed in the U.S., there was a little welcome home ceremony, and then we went to hang out at the NCO club. The next day, there was a lot of paper to process for benefits and release forms. There was an assessment by a doctor that was about 5 minutes. Basically, they ask if you're okay and they take your word for it. If you say you're not okay, then you can't leave with everyone else. The third day, they encouraged us to join the American Legion and VFW clubs and then bussed us home.

Karyn: You've mentioned before that you had postconcussion headaches and some nightmares. Were you still having these symptoms when you got home?

Sean: Yeah, I had been in an area, during my tour of duty, where a roadside bomb detonated. At the time, I was having extreme headaches, and I got pain medications, but no one talked about what had happened or how I was handling that. The role of the military was to make the soldier mission-capable, so that meant just treating the symptoms. When I got home, I was still having some nightmares and headaches, but I couldn't talk about it. My wife was in the military too, so we had both learned not to talk about emotions. Within a year, I was drinking heavily and separated from my wife. I sought out treatment at the VA, but I only went three times. I felt like they were primarily trying to validate my story as if they wanted to defend themselves against a potential claim. They never asked about alcohol use. I felt angry, and I had some aggression. I felt abandoned. Then I found out my mom had stolen my military checks and had spent them. At that point, I lost faith in everything. All of my core beliefs were gone. The only thing I had faith in was my fellow soldiers, and now that we were back home, they weren't there.

Karyn: Do you get together with any fellow vets?

Sean: Mostly people connect over Facebook, so they don't really get together. The military clubs are all about drinking, so there aren't any healthy options. I do know, though, that sometimes when vets have gotten wind through Facebook that one of us is suicidal, they've traveled across the country to track them down and try to get them help.

Karyn: The suicide rates have been tragically high among vets. Have you ever had thoughts yourself about suicide?

Sean: I have. I was in a very dark place. I thought I was such an awful person that the best option was to kill myself. I was drinking, I was making bad moral decisions, and I was nasty to friends. I didn't care about anything or any consequences. I just wanted momentary relief, so I drank more, but, of course, that increased the depression. And it seems like every time we go to military exercises, we hear of another loss of someone to suicide. Last week, it was a fellow soldier who was a decorated hero for saving the lives of many of our guys. [Tearful.] So how do you rectify that someone saved all those lives and then comes home and takes their own life?

Karyn: It does seem like senseless, tragic loss. What has helped you get out of that dark place?

Sean: I have a brother who, even though he couldn't understand what I was going through, he kept checking in on me and repeatedly told me he was praying for me. He just kept showing up and telling me I had to get God back in my life. I knew he cared. I had a DUI and an accident, but I kept thinking, "I just have to suck it up and be stronger than this." Instead, the drinking just increases exponentially faster than you can respond or try to control it. One night, I went home and trashed my house. I was ripping sinks out of walls. I remember a neighbor came over and told me I just needed to sober up, but I called the police and told them to take me in. I knew I was out of control. When I got to the psych unit, I knew I wanted "fixed," but that mainly meant I wanted to be under control. I don't remember being asked if I wanted pills, but they gave me pills, and I didn't want to take them because it just made me feel less in control. There was an LPN there who told me that her husband was a vet and that she knew he was a good person. She said she never let his behavior define who he was. That gave me a lot of hope, like maybe I wasn't such an awful person. I reached out to God, and things started to change. I acknowledged that drinking was a primary issue, I cut ties with several unhealthy relationships, and there were supportive friends who came to visit me in the hospital, so I started to see that there were people who genuinely cared about me.

Karyn: What do you want health-care providers and fellow soldiers to learn from your experience?

Sean: First, a soldier is not who you are; it's a job you do. I wish I had spent more time before my deployment literally writing down all those things that define who I am, like, I'm a loving father and a good friend and what is most important to me; what am I willing to die for. I think it would have helped me, when I came back home, to concretely remind myself of who I am. It's easy to lose all sense of that in the military. Second, no mood-altering chemicals. There are a lot of things within the military that promote the use of chemicals such as alcohol and pain medication, and while it may keep people mission-ready or temporarily numb you, it becomes disastrous. Third, reach out for support or, if you are a health-care provider, help someone identify those people who will provide ongoing support. Supportive people and reaching out to God have been my lifelines.

Table 38–2 | NURSING DIAGNOSES: PLANNING CARE FOR MILITARY FAMILIES

RISK FACTORS/DEFINING CHARACTERISTICS	NURSING DIAGNOSES	OUTCOME CRITERIA
PTSD		
Rage reactions, aggression, irritability, substance use, flashbacks, startle reaction	Risk for other-directed violence	Client will demonstrate appropriate coping behaviors. Client will not harm others.
Depression, perception of lack of social support, physical disabilities from combat injuries, feelings of hopelessness	Risk for suicide	Client will not harm self.
Anger, aggression, depression, difficulty concentrating, flashbacks, guilt, headaches, hypervigilance, intrusive thoughts and dreams, nightmares, emotional numbness, panic attacks, substance abuse	Posttrauma syndrome related to having experienced the trauma of military combat	Client will begin a healthy grief resolution, initiating the process of psychological healing. Client will demonstrate ability to deal with emotional reactions in an individually appropriate manner.
Substance abuse	Ineffective coping; ineffective denial	Client will verbalize understanding of the destructiveness of substance abuse and demonstrate a more adaptive method of coping.
Confusion, fear, and anxiety among family members and their inability to deal with the affected member's unpredictable behavior; ineffective family decision-making process	Interrupted family processes related to crisis associated with veteran member's illness	Family will verbalize understanding of trauma-related illness, demonstrate ability to maintain anxiety at manageable level, and make appropriate decisions to stabilize family functioning.
TRAUMATIC BRAIN INJURY		
Impaired physical mobility, limited range of motion, decreased muscle strength and control, perceptual or cognitive impairment, seizures	Risk for injury	Client will remain free of physical injury.
Memory deficits; distractibility; altered attention span or concentration; impaired ability to make decisions, problem-solve, reason or conceptualize; personality changes	Disturbed thought processes*	Client will regain cognitive ability to execute mental functions realistic with the extent of the injury.
Inability to perform desired or appropriate activities of daily living	Self-care deficit (specify)	Client performs self-care activities within level of own ability.
Confusion, fear, and anxiety among family members and the inability to adapt to changes associated with veteran member's injury; difficulty accepting/receiving help; inability to express or to accept each other's feelings	Interrupted family processes related to situational transition and crisis; uncertainty about expectations and ultimate outcome	Family will verbalize understanding of trauma-related illness, demonstrate ability to maintain anxiety at manageable level, and make appropriate decisions to stabilize family functioning.
FAMILY MEMBERS' ISSUES		
Regressive behaviors, loss of appetite, temper tantrums, clinging behaviors, guilt and self-blame, sleep problems, irritability, aggression (children)	Risk for delayed development related to feelings of abandonment associated with parent's deployment	Parent/caregiver will identify behaviors at risk and initiate interventions to promote appropriate development.

Continued

Table 38–2 | NURSING DIAGNOSES: PLANNING CARE FOR MILITARY FAMILIES—cont'd

RISK FACTORS/DEFINING CHARACTERISTICS	NURSING DIAGNOSES	OUTCOME CRITERIA
		Child will develop healthy coping strategies and resume normal developmental progression.
Rebelliousness, irritability, acting out behaviors, promiscuity, substance use (adolescents)	Ineffective coping related to feelings of abandonment associated with parent's deployment	Client will work through stages of grief associated with the perceived loss and demonstrate healthy, age-appropriate coping strategies.
Depression, anxiety, loneliness, fear, feeling overwhelmed and powerless, anger (spouse/partner)	Risk for complicated grieving related to military deployment of spouse/partner	Client will work through stages of grief, achieve a healthy acceptance, and express a sense of control over the present situation and future outcome.
Anger, anxiety, frustration, ineffective coping, sleep deprivation, somatic symptoms, fatigue (spouse/partner/caregiver)	Caregiver role strain related to complexity of care-giving responsibilities; lack of respite	Caregiver will demonstrate effective problem-solving skills and develop adaptive coping mechanisms to regain equilibrium.

*This diagnosis has been resigned from the NANDA-I list of approved diagnoses. It is used in this instance because it is most compatible with the identified behaviors.

Planning, Implementation, and Evaluation

Nurses provide care for service members, veterans, and their families in a variety of settings, including general hospitals, VA hospitals, community health centers, doctors' offices, long-term care centers, and community-based clinics. The care required by veterans returning from combat in the war on terrorism is complex and multifaceted. War-related physical injuries are often striking and conspicuous in their visibility. However, it is the veterans' *invisible* injuries that psychiatric-mental health nurses are most often called upon to treat. The need for nurses to provide care for the increasing number of veterans with these invisible injuries is intensifying, and the VA continues to search for more effective ways to ensure that military veterans and families receive the care that they desperately need and deserve. Clever and Segal (2013) caution that even though military families have some unique challenges, including compounding issues when both spouses are in the military, they are a diverse group and their needs are dynamic as they move through transitions in their military career and family life.

Interventions for a selected number of nursing diagnoses relevant to veterans and military families are presented in Table 38–3. Evaluation is conducted by reassessing to determine if the nursing actions have been successful in meeting the outcome criteria.

Treatment Modalities

Posttraumatic Stress Disorder

Psychosocial Therapies

Cognitive therapy, prolonged exposure therapy, group and family therapy, and eye movement desensitization and reprocessing have all been used successfully in the treatment of PTSD.

Psychopharmacology

Selective serotonin reuptake inhibitors (SSRIs) are now considered the first-line treatment of choice for PTSD because of their efficacy, tolerability, and safety ratings. Other antidepressants that have been effective include trazadone, the tricyclics amitriptyline and imipramine, and the monoamine oxidase inhibitor phenelzine. Benzodiazepines are sometimes prescribed for their antipanic effects, although their addictive properties make them less desirable. Antihypertensives, such as propranolol and clonidine, have been successful in alleviating symptoms such as nightmares, intrusive recollections, hypervigilance, insomnia, startle responses, and angry outbursts. More recently, intravenous ketamine infusions (in combination with psychotherapy) have demonstrated efficacy in treating PTSD (Chaverneff, 2016). While these findings are still under further investigation, the researcher identifies that ketamine binds at N-methyl-D-aspartate receptors, which impacts fear learning and extinction.

TABLE 38-3 Nursing Interventions for Veteran Clients and Military Families

Posttrauma syndrome (PTSD)	Stay with the client during periods of flashbacks and nightmares and offer reassurance of personal safety.
	Encourage the client to talk about the traumatic experience at his or her own pace.
	Discuss maladaptive coping mechanisms being employed. Assist the client in his or her effort to use more adaptive strategies.
	Include available support systems, and make referrals for additional assistance where required.
	Help client understand that use of substances merely numbs feelings and delays healing. Refer for treatment of substance use disorder.
	Discuss use of stress-management techniques, such as deep breathing, meditation, relaxation, and exercise.
	Administer medications as prescribed, and provide medication education.
Risk for suicide (PTSD, TBI)	Assess degree of risk according to seriousness of threat, existence of a plan, and availability and lethality of the means.
	Ask directly if person is thinking of acting on thoughts or feelings.
	Ascertain presence of significant others for support.
	Determine whether substance use is a factor.
	Encourage expression of feelings, including appropriate expression of anger.
	Ensure that environment is safe.
	Help client identify more appropriate solutions and offer hope for the future.
	Collaborate with the client to develop a plan for ongoing safety.
	Involve family/significant others in the planning.
Disturbed thought processes (TBI)	Evaluate mental status, including extent of impairment in thinking ability; remote and recent memory; orientation to person, place, and time; insight and judgment; changes in personality; attention span, distractibility, and ability to make decisions or problem-solve; ability to communicate appropriately; anxiety level; evidence of psychotic behavior.
	Report to physician any cognitive changes that become obvious.
	Note behavior indicative of potential for violence and take appropriate action to prevent harm to client and others.
	Provide safety measures as required. Institute seizure precautions if indicated. Assist with limited mobility issues.
	Monitor medication regimen.
	Refer to appropriate rehabilitation providers.
Interrupted family processes (PTSD; TBI)	Encourage the importance of continuous, open communication between family members to facilitate ongoing problem-solving.
	Assist the family to identify and use previously successful coping strategies.
	Encourage family participation in multidisciplinary team conference or group therapy.
	Involve family in social support and community activities of their interest and choice.
	Encourage use of stress-management techniques.
	Make necessary referrals (e.g., parent effectiveness training, specific disease or disability support groups, self-help groups, clergy, psychological counseling, or family therapy).
	Assist family to identify situations that may lead to fear or anxiety.
	Involve family in mutual goal-setting to plan for the future.
	Identify community agencies from which family may seek assistance (e.g., Meals on Wheels, visiting nurse, trauma support group, American Cancer Society, Veterans Administration).
Risk for complicated grieving (family of deployed service member)	Help family members to realize that all of the feelings they are having are a normal part of the grieving process.
	Validate their feelings of anger, loneliness, fear, powerlessness, dysphoria, and distress at separation from their loved one.

Continued

TABLE 38-3 **Nursing Interventions for Veteran Clients and Military Families—cont'd**	
	Help parent to understand that children's and adolescents' problematic behaviors are symptoms of grieving, and that they should not be deemed unacceptable and result in punishment, but rather be recognized as having their basis in grief.
	Children should be allowed an appropriate amount of time to grieve. Some experts believe children need at least 4 weeks to adjust to a parent's deployment (Gabany & Shellenbarger, 2010). Refer for professional help if improvement is not observed in a reasonable period of time.
	Assess if maladaptive coping strategies, such as substance abuse, are being used.
	Identify and encourage clients to employ previously used successful coping strategies.
	Encourage resuming involvement in usual activities.
	Caution against spending too much time alone.
	Suggest keeping a journal of experiences and feelings.
	Refer to other resources, as needed, such as psychotherapy, family counseling, religious references or pastor, or grief support group.
Caregiver role strain (spouse/caregiver of injured service member)	Assess the spouse/caregiver's ability to anticipate and fulfill the injured service member's unmet needs. Provide information to assist the caregiver with this responsibility.
	Ensure that the caregiver encourages the injured service member to be as independent as possible.
	Encourage the caregiver to express feelings and to participate in a support group.
	Provide information or demonstrate techniques for dealing with acting out, violent, or disoriented behavior by the injured service member.
	Identify additional needs and ensure that resources are provided (e.g., physical therapy, occupational therapy, nutritionist, financial and legal help, and respite care).
	Assess for abuse of substances as a coping strategy.
	Refer to counseling or psychotherapy as needed.

Keizer (2016; the researcher cited by Chaverneff) indicates that these treatments allow veterans to remember what happened to them but with less fear. He further notes that 50 percent of military veterans with PTSD also have chronic pain. The use of ketamine demonstrated efficacy in treating both issues.

Complementary Therapies

Acupuncture and pet therapy have been successful adjuncts to treatment for individuals with PTSD. Relaxation techniques have been shown to alleviate symptoms associated with physiological hyperreactivity, and hypnosis may be helpful for symptoms such as pain, anxiety, dissociation, and nightmares (Brancu et al., 2011).

Traumatic Brain Injury

The type of care for the client with TBI depends on severity of the injury and area of the brain involved. Brancu and associates (2011) state, "Since 90 percent of patients have mild cases and experience full recovery, early intervention involving education and a focus on recovery is strongly recommended" (p. 59).

Psychosocial Therapies

Cognitive-behavioral therapy (CBT) has been shown to be helpful to individuals with TBI. Scorer (2013) states,

"An advantage of [CBT] interventions is that, given their highly structured content, they are amenable to specialized adaptation for memory, attention, and problem-solving impairments, reflecting the difficulties people with TBI often experience." Chard and associates (2011), as cited by Cogan (2014), found that cognitive processing therapy, a modification of CBT, was effective in reducing psychological symptoms for individuals with comorbid PTSD and mild traumatic brain injury. Other therapies, such as prolonged exposure therapy, may also work well for veterans with mild TBI and emotional trauma (Brancu et al., 2011).

Rehabilitation Therapies

Rehabilitation therapy is multifaceted and determined by severity and location of the brain damage. Specialists in the care of the individual with TBI may include any or all of the following (Mayo Clinic, 2014):

- **Physiatrist:** A physician trained in the medical specialty of physical medicine and rehabilitation. This physician oversees other professionals involved in the rehabilitation process.
- **Occupational therapist:** Helps the individual learn, relearn, or improve skills for everyday living.
- **Physical therapist:** Assists the veteran with mobility and relearning movement patterns, balance, and walking.

- **Recreational therapist:** Assists with leisure activities.
- **Speech and language pathologist:** Helps the person improve communication skills and use assistive communication devices, if necessary.
- **Neuropsychologist or psychiatrist:** Helps the veteran manage behaviors or learn coping strategies, provides talk therapy as needed for emotional and psychological well-being, and prescribes medication as needed.
- **Social worker or case manager:** Coordinates access to services, assists with care decisions and planning, and facilitates communication among various professionals, care providers, and family members.

Psychopharmacology

Medications for the individual with TBI are given to ameliorate specific symptoms. Antidepressants are prescribed for depression, which is very prevalent in individuals with TBI. SSRIs are commonly the antidepressants of choice, although tricyclics and others, such as venlafaxine, trazodone, bupropion, and duloxetine, are also used. Benzodiazepines or SSRIs may be administered for treatment of anxiety symptoms, and antipsychotics are prescribed if aggression, agitation, or psychotic behaviors occur. Anticonvulsants are given if seizures are a problem, and the physician may prescribe skeletal muscle relaxants for muscle spasms or spasticity. Methylphenidate or modafinil has been used to treat attention deficits and hyperactivity, and donepezil has been shown to be effective in enhancing cognitive performance of individuals with TBI (Foster & Spiegel, 2008).

Summary and Key Points

- More than 3 million individuals are serving in the U.S. armed forces in more than 150 countries around the world.
- Veterans currently number 20.6 million.
- Since the beginning of the wars in Afghanistan and Iraq in 2001, more than 2.2 million U.S. military personnel have been deployed in 3 million tours of duty.
- The military lifestyle offers both positive and negative aspects for those who choose this way of life.
- To compensate for the extreme mobility, the focus of the military lifestyle turns inward to the military world rather than outward to the local community.
- In the OEF and OIF campaigns, there has been heavy dependence on the National Guard and Reserves and an escalation in the pace, duration,

and number of deployments and redeployments experienced by these individuals.

- Military families face unique challenges, including frequent moves and many separations.
- Children and adolescents exhibit a number of problematic behaviors in response to the separation from a deployed parent.
- The cycle of deployment is described in five distinct stages: predeployment, deployment, sustainment, redeployment, and postdeployment.
- Special concerns of women in the military include sexual harassment, sexual assault, differential treatment and conditions, and issues related to being a parent.
- Evidence supports that a majority of young veterans screen positive for behavioral health problems and a third or less of those have had adequate health care treatment. Returning from a combat zone causes feelings and reactions that may contribute to difficulties with reintegration into civilian life.
- Traumatic brain injury (TBI) is a trauma-induced structural injury and/or physiological disruption of brain function as a result of an external force to the head.
- Symptoms of TBI are related to the severity of the injury and the area of the brain that has been injured.
- The most common long-term consequences of TBI include problems with cognition and behavior or mental health.
- PTSD is the most common mental disorder among veterans returning from military combat.
- Symptoms of PTSD may occur shortly after the trauma or may be delayed, in some instances for years.
- Depression among military veterans is quite common, and suicide rates among veterans and service members have continued to rise.
- Substance use disorder is a common co-occurring condition with PTSD.
- Nursing care of military families and veterans is multifaceted and requires reassessment over time using the six steps of the nursing process. Treatment modalities for PTSD and TBI include psychosocial therapies, psychopharmacology, complementary therapies, and rehabilitation therapies.

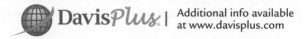

DavisPlus | Additional info available at www.davisplus.com

Review Questions
Self-Examination/Learning Exercise

Select the answer that is most appropriate for each of the following questions.

1. Dana's husband, who was deployed to Afghanistan a year ago, is returning home this week. Which of the following postdeployment situations may be likely to occur during the first few months of his return? (Select all that apply.)
   a. A honeymoon period of physical reconnection
   b. Resistance from the spouse regarding possible loss of autonomy
   c. Rejection by the children for perceived abandonment
   d. A period of adjustment to reconnect emotionally

2. Which of the following is the leading cause of TBI in active-duty military personnel in combat?
   a. Military vehicle accidents
   b. Blasts from explosive devices
   c. Falls
   d. Blows to the head from falling debris

3. Shane, a veteran of the war in Iraq, has been diagnosed with PTSD. He is a client of the VA outpatient clinic. He tells the nurse that he experiences panic attacks. Which of the following medications may be prescribed for Shane to treat his panic attacks?
   a. Alprazolam
   b. Lithium
   c. Carbamazepine
   d. Haldol

4. Shane, a veteran of the war in Iraq, has been diagnosed with PTSD. He has been hospitalized after swallowing a handful of his antipanic medication. His physical condition was stabilized in the emergency department, and he has been admitted to the psychiatric unit. In developing his initial plan of care, which is the priority nursing diagnosis that the nurse selects for Shane?
   a. Posttrauma syndrome
   b. Risk for suicide
   c. Complicated grieving
   d. Disturbed thought processes

5. Mike was injured during combat in Afghanistan. He has a diagnosis of TBI. Which of the following medications might the physician prescribe to improve Mike's memory and thinking capability?
   a. Carbamazepine
   b. Duloxetine
   c. Donepezil
   d. Bupropion

6. Juan, a veteran of the war in Iraq, has been diagnosed with PTSD. He has been hospitalized on the psychiatric unit following an attempted suicide. In the middle of the night, he wakes up yelling and tells the nurse he was having a flashback to when his unit transport drove over an improvised explosive device (IED) and most of his fellow soldiers were killed. He is breathing heavily, perspiring, and his heart is pounding. The nurse's most appropriate *initial* intervention is which of the following?
   a. Contact the doctor on call to report the incident.
   b. Administer the prn order for chlorpromazine.
   c. Stay with Juan and reassure him of his safety.
   d. Have Juan sit outside the nurses' station until he is calm.

Review Questions—cont'd
Self-Examination/Learning Exercise

7. Mike, a veteran of combat in Afghanistan, has a diagnosis of mild TBI. The psychiatric home health nurse from the VA medical center is assigned to make home visits to Mike and his wife, Marissa, who is his caregiver. Which of the following would be an appropriate nursing intervention by the home health nurse? (Select all that apply.)
   a. Assess for use of substances by Mike or Marissa.
   b. Encourage Marissa to do everything for Mike to prevent further deterioration in his condition.
   c. Assess Marissa's level of stress and potential for burnout.
   d. Encourage Marissa to allow Mike to be as independent as possible.
   e. Suggest that Marissa ask the physician for a nursing home placement for Mike.

8. Which of the following psychosocial therapies has been shown to be helpful for clients with TBI?
   a. Eye movement desensitization
   b. Psychoanalysis
   c. Reality therapy
   d. Cognitive-behavioral therapy

9. Amy's husband of 1 year left 2 weeks ago for a year-long deployment in Afghanistan. Amy makes an appointment with the psychiatric nurse practitioner at the community mental health clinic. She tells the nurse that she can't sleep, has no appetite, is chronically fatigued, and thinks about her husband constantly and fears for his life. Which of the following might the nurse suggest/prescribe for Amy? (Select all that apply.)
   a. A prescription for sertraline, 50 mg/day
   b. Participation in a support group
   c. Resuming involvement in usual activities
   d. Regular relaxation exercises

 MOVIE CONNECTIONS

The Best Years of Our Lives (1946) • *The Deer Hunter* (1978) • *Jarhead* (2005) • *In the Valley of Elah* (2007) • *The Lucky Ones* (2008) • *A Walk in My Shoes* (2010)

References

Albrecht, B. (2009, July 16). Post-traumatic stress disorder hitting World War II veterans. *Cleveland Plain Dealer*, p. A1. Retrieved from www.cleveland.com/news/plaindealer/index.ssf?/base/cuyahoga/1247733140222090.xml&coll=2

American Academy of Child & Adolescent Psychiatry. (no date). Military families resource center. Retrieved from www.aacap.org/aacap/families_and_youth/resource_centers/Military_Families_Resource_Center/FAQ.aspx#question4

Birk, M. (2010). Traumatic brain injury. *Army Medicine*. Retrieved from www.armymedicine.army.mil/hc/healthtips/08/201003mtbi.cfm

Brancu, M., Straits-Troster, K., & Kudler, H. (2011). Behavioral health conditions among military personnel and veterans: Prevalence and best practices for treatment. *North Carolina Medical Journal, 72*(1), 54-60.

Burgess, A.W., Slattery, D.M., & Herlihy, P.A. (2013). Military sexual trauma: A silent syndrome. *Journal of Psychosocial Nursing, 51*(2), 20-26. doi:10.3928/02793695-20130109-03

Chard, K.M., Schumm, J.A., McIlvain, S.M., Bailey, G.W., & Parkinson, R.B. (2011). Exploring the efficacy of a residential treatment program incorporating cognitive processing therapy-cognitive for veterans with PTSD and traumatic brain injury. *Journal of Traumatic Stress, 24*, 347-351. doi:10.1002/jts.20644

Chaverneff, F. (2016). Ketamine shows signs of efficacy in treating PTSD. Retrieved from www.clinicalpainadvisor.com/aapmanagement-2016/ketamine-to-treat-both-complex-regional-pain-syndrome-and-post-traumatic-stress-disorder/article/524792

Clever, M., & Segal, D.R. (2013). The demographics of military children and families. *The Future of Children, 23*(2), 13-39. doi:10.1353/foc.2013.0018

CNN. (2013). By the numbers: Women in the U.S. military. Retrieved from www.cnn.com/2013/01/24/us/military-women-glance

Cogan, A.M. (2014). Occupational needs and intervention strategies for military personnel with mild traumatic brain injury and persistent post-concussion symptoms: A review. *OTJR: Occupation, Participation, and Health, 34*(3), 150-159. doi:10.3928/15394492-20140617-01

Crosby, K. (2015). FDA and the Department of Defense: A joint force to reduce tobacco use in the military (FDA blog,

September 2015). Retrieved from http://blogs.fda.gov/fdavoice/index.php/2015/09/fda-and-the-department-of-defense-a-joint-force-to-reduce-tobacco-use-in-the-military-2/?utm_source=CTPtwitter&utm_medium=social-media&utm_campaign=HealthyBase

Defense and Veterans Brain Injury Center. (2016). DoD worldwide numbers for TBI. Retrieved from http://dvbic.dcoe.mil/dod-worldwide-numbers-tbi

Department of Defense. (2017). *DoD personnel, workforce reports & publications.* Retrieved from https://www.dmdc.osd.mil/appj/dwp/dwp_reports.jsp

Department of Defense. (2015). *Department of Defense annual report on sexual assault in the military, fiscal year 2014.* Washington, DC: Department of Defense.

Department of Defense. (2013). 2013 demographics: Profile of the military community. Retrieved from http://download.militaryonesource.mil/12038/MOS/Reports/2013-Demographics-Report.pdf

Department of Veterans Affairs & Department of Defense (VA/DoD). (2016). Clinical practice guideline for management of concussion/mild traumatic brain injury. Retrieved from www.healthquality.va.gov/guidelines/Rehab/mtbi/mTBICPGClinicianSummary50821816.pdf

Devries, M.R., Hughes, H.K., Watson, H., & Moore, B.A. (2012). Understanding the military culture. In B.A. Moore (Ed.), *Handbook of counseling military couples* (pp. 7-18). New York: Routledge.

Foster, M., & Spiegel, D.R. (2008). Use of donepezil in the treatment of cognitive impairments of moderate traumatic brain injury. *Journal of Neuropsychiatry and Clinical Neurosciences, 20*(1), 106. doi:10.1176/appi.neuropsych.20.1.106

Gabany, E., & Shellenbarger, T. (2010). Caring for families with deployment stress: How nurses can make a difference in the lives of military families. *American Journal of Nursing, 110*(11), 36-41. doi:10.1097/01

Gradus, J.L. (2017). Epidemiology of PTSD. Retrieved from www.ptsd.va.gov/professional/PTSD-overview/epidemiological-facts-ptsd.asp

Hall, L.K. (2008). *Counseling military families.* New York: Taylor & Francis.

Hall, L.K. (2011). The military culture, language, and lifestyle. In R.B. Everson & C.R. Figley (Eds.), *Families under fire* (pp. 31-52). New York: Routledge.

Hall, L.K. (2012). The military lifestyle and the relationship. In B.A. Moore (Ed.), *Handbook of counseling military couples* (pp. 137-156). New York: Routledge.

Institute of Medicine. (2013). Returning home from Iraq and Afghanistan: Readjustment needs of veterans, service members, and their families. Retrieved from http://iom.nationalacademies.org/~/media/Files/Report%20Files/2013/Returning-Home-Iraq-Afghanistan/Returning-Home-Iraq-Afghanistan-RB.pdf

Jakupcak, M., Vannoy, S., Imel, Z., Cook, J.W., Fontana, A., Rosenheck, R., & McFall, M. (2010). Does PTSD moderate the relationship between social support and suicide risk in Iraq and Afghanistan war veterans seeking mental health treatment? *Depression and Anxiety, 27*(11), 1001-1005. doi:10.1002/da.20722

Keizer, B. (2016). Interdisciplinary treatment for the war on comorbid CRPS and PTSD. Presented at AAPM 2016, September 21-25, San Antonio, TX.

Kelly Temps in Uniform. (2012). This ain't Hell, but you can see it from here. Retrieved from http://thisainthell.us/blog/?p=30410

Kime, P. (2015). DoD military suicide rate declining. *Military Times.* Retrieved from www.militarytimes.com/story/military/pentagon/2015/01/16/defense-department-suicides-2013-report/21865977/

Langer, R. (2011). Combat trauma, memory, and the World War II veteran. *War, Literature & the Arts, 23*(1). Retrieved from http://wlajournal.com/23_1/images/langer.pdf

Lavender, J.M., & Lyons, J.A. (2012). Posttraumatic stress disorder. In B.A. Moore (Ed.), *Handbook of counseling military couples* (pp. 183-200). New York: Routledge.

Mathewson, J. (2011). In support of military women and families. In R.B. Everson & C.R. Figley (Eds.), *Families under fire* (pp. 215-235). New York: Routledge.

Mayo Clinic. (2014). Traumatic brain injury. Retrieved from www.mayoclinic.com/health/traumatic-brain-injury/DS00552

Monson, C.M., Fredman, S.J., & Adair, K.C. (2008). Cognitive-behavioral conjoint therapy for posttraumatic stress disorder: Application to Operation Enduring and Iraqi Freedom veterans. *Journal of Clinical Psychology, 64*(8), 958-971. doi:10.1002/jclp.20511

National Alliance on Mental Illness. (2015). President Obama signs Veterans Suicide Prevention Act [blog]. Retrieved from https://www.nami.org/Search?searchtext=Clayton+Hunt+Act&searchmode=anyword

National Alliance on Mental Illness. (2016). Tell me about depression. Retrieved from www.nami.org/Videos/Tell-Me-About-Depression

National Institute of Neurological Disorders and Stroke (NINDS). (2016). Traumatic brain injury: Hope through research. Retrieved from www.ninds.nih.gov/disorders/tbi/tbi.htm

National Institute on Drug Abuse. (2013). Drug facts: Substance abuse among the military. Retrieved from https://www.drugabuse.gov/publications/drugfacts/substance-abuse-in-military.

Pedersen, E.R., Marshall, G.N., & Kurz, J. (2016). Behavioral health treatment receipt among a community sample of young adult veterans. *Journal of Behavioral Health Services & Research.* doi:10.1007/s11414-016-9534-7

Pincus, S.H., House, R., Christenson, J., & Alder, L.E. (2013). The emotional cycle of deployment: A military family perspective. Retrieved from https://msrc.fsu.edu/system/files/The%20Emotional%20Cycle%20of%20Deployment%20-%20A%20Military%20Family%20Perspective.pdf

Plach, H.L., & Sells, C.H. (2013). Occupational performance needs of young veterans. *American Journal of Occupational Therapy, 67,* 73-81. doi:10.5014/ajot.2013.003871

Ribbers, G.M. (2013). Brain injury: Long-term outcome after traumatic brain injury. In J.H. Stone & M. Blouin (Eds.), *International Encyclopedia of Rehabilitation.* Retrieved from http://cirrie.buffalo.edu/encyclopedia/en/article/338

Safaz, I., Yasar, A.R., Tok, F., & Yilmaz, B. (2008). Medical complications, physical function, and communication skills in patients with traumatic brain injury. *Brain Injury, 22:* 733-739. doi:10.1080/02699050802304714

Scorer, R. (2013). Psychological therapies for victims of traumatic brain injury. Retrieved from www.pannone.com/media/articles/clinical-negligence/medical-negligence/psychological-therapies-for-victims-of-traumatic-brain-injury-and-how-medical-evidence-plays-a-crucial-role

Smith, R. (2012). Military children and families. *Helping Hands for Freedom.* Retrieved from http://helpinghandsforfreedom.org/remaining-programs-2012-arizona-military-children-families/#more-567

Strong, C.H., & Donders, J. (2012). Traumatic brain injury. In B.A. Moore (Ed.), *Handbook of counseling military couples* (p. 279-294). New York: Routledge.

Substance Abuse and Mental Health Services Administration. (2012). Behavioral health issues among Afghanistan and Iraq U.S. war veterans. *SAMHSA In Brief, 7*(1).

Substance Abuse and Mental Health Services Administration. (2014). Veterans and military families. Retrieved from www.samhsa.gov/veterans-military-families

Substance Abuse and Mental Health Services Administration. (2015). Veterans' primary substance of abuse is alcohol in treatment admissions. *The CBHSQ Report.* Retrieved from www.samhsa.gov/data/sites/default/files/report_2111/Spotlight-2111.pdf

Temkin, N.R., Corrigan, J.D., Dikmen, S.S., & Machamer, J. (2009). Social functioning after traumatic brain injury. *Journal of Head Trauma Rehabilitation, 24*(6), 460-467. doi:10.1097/HTR.0b013e3181c13413

U.S. Census Bureau. (2016). Quick Facts United States. Retrieved from www.census.gov/quickfacts/table/PST045215/00

Veteran's Health Administration. (2015). One in ten older vets is depressed. Retrieved from www.va.gov/health/NewsFeatures/20110624a.asp

Vlahos, K.B. (2012). The rape of our military women. *Anti-War.Com.* Retrieved from http://original.antiwar.com/vlahos/2012/05/14/the-rape-of-our-military-women

Wakefield, M. (2007). Guarding the military home front. *Counseling Today.* Retrieved from http://ct.counseling.org/2007/01/from-the-president-guarding-the-military-home-front

Wolf, N. (2012). A culture of cover-up: Rape in the ranks of the U.S. military. *The Guardian.* Retrieved from www.guardian.co.uk/commentisfree/2012/jun/14/culture-coverup-rape-ranks-us-military

Wolfe, J., Sharkansky, E.J., Read, J.P., Dawson, R., Martin, J.A., & Oimette, P.C. (1998). Sexual harassment and assault as predictors of PTSD symptomatology among U.S. female Persian Gulf military personnel. *Journal of Interpersonal Violence, 13*(1), 40-57. doi:10.1177/088626098013001003

Classical References

Wertsch, M.E. (1996). *Military brats: Legacies of childhood inside the fortress.* St. Louis, MO: Brightwell.

Appendix A

Answers to Chapter Review Questions

CHAPTER 1. The Concept of Stress Adaptation
1. b **2.** d **3.** a **4.** b **5.** c **6.** a, b, c

CHAPTER 2. Mental Health and Mental Illness: Historical and Theoretical Concepts
1. c **2.** d **3.** b **4.** a **5.** b **6.** d **7.** c
8. a, b, c, d **9.** c **10.** b

CHAPTER 3. Concepts of Psychobiology
1. d **2.** d **3.** a **4.** b **5.** c **6.** a **7.** d **8.** c
9. b **10.** a **11.** a, b, c **12.** b, c, d

CHAPTER 4. Psychopharmacology
1. a **2.** c **3.** d **4.** b **5.** c **6.** b **7.** a **8.** b
9. a **10.** b

CHAPTER 5. Ethical and Legal Issues in Psychiatric-Mental Health Nursing
1. b **2.** a **3.** c **4.** b **5.** c **6.** d **7.** a, b, d
8. b, d **9.** a, b **10.** c **11.** a

CHAPTER 6. Cultural and Spiritual Concepts Relevant to Psychiatric-Mental Health Nursing
1. c **2.** d **3.** a **4.** d **5.** b **6.** c **7.** b **8.** b
9. a **10.** d

CHAPTER 7. Relationship Development
1. c **2.** a **3.** a, b, c **4.** b, e **5.** b **6.** d **7.** c
8. b **9.** d **10.** a, c, d

CHAPTER 8. Therapeutic Communication
1. b **2.** a **3.** d **4.** c **5.** a **6.** b **7.** d **8.** a
9. a, b, d **10.** b

CHAPTER 9. The Nursing Process in Psychiatric-Mental Health Nursing
1. b **2.** a **3.** d **4.** a **5.** c **6.** b **7.** a, b, c, d
8. d **9.** c **10.** a, c, d

CHAPTER 10. Therapeutic Groups
1. b **2.** d **3.** a **4.** c **5.** c **6.** d **7.** c **8.** b
9. d **10.** a **11.** b, c, e

CHAPTER 11. Intervention With Families
1. b **2.** c **3.** a **4.** b **5.** d **6.** c **7.** b **8.** c
9. d **10.** a

CHAPTER 12. Milieu Therapy—The Therapeutic Community
1. a, b, c **2.** b **3.** c **4.** b **5.** a **6.** d **7.** c
8. b **9.** a, b, d, e **10.** a, b, c

CHAPTER 13. Crisis Intervention
1. c **2.** d **3.** a **4.** b **5.** c **6.** a **7.** d **8.** b
9. b **10.** d **11.** c **12.** c **13.** e

CHAPTER 14. Assertiveness Training
1. c **2.** a **3.** b **4.** a **5.** a **6.** c **7.** d **8.** a
9. c **10.** b

CHAPTER 15. Promoting Self-Esteem
1. b **2.** a **3.** d **4.** c **5.** a **6.** c **7.** b **8.** d
9. b **10.** a **11.** a, b, d, e

CHAPTER 16. Anger and Aggression Management
1. b, c **2.** c **3.** a **4.** a, b, d **5.** c **6.** a, b, c
7. c **8.** b **9.** b, c, d, e **10.** a, b, c

CHAPTER 17. Suicide Prevention
1. a **2.** a, c, d, e **3.** c **4.** a **5.** d **6.** c **7.** b
8. b, e **9.** a, b, c **10.** b

CHAPTER 18. Behavior Therapy
1. a **2.** a **3.** b **4.** c **5.** a **6.** b **7.** d
8. f, b, d, a, e, c

CHAPTER 19. Cognitive Therapy
1. c **2.** a **3.** d **4.** b **5.** c **6.** a **7.** d **8.** a
9. b **10.** c

CHAPTER 20. Electroconvulsive Therapy
1. c **2.** b **3.** a, b, c, d **4.** b **5.** d **6.** a **7.** c
8. d **9.** b **10.** c

CHAPTER 21. The Recovery Model
1. b, d **2.** c **3.** d **4.** a **5.** c

CHAPTER 22. Neurocognitive Disorders
1. c, e **2.** d **3.** b **4.** a, b, e **5.** b **6.** a, c, e
7. d **8.** c **9.** a **10.** b **11.** c, e

CHAPTER 23. Substance-Related and Addictive Disorders
1. a **2.** c **3.** b **4.** b **5.** a **6.** c **7.** a **8.** b
9. d **10.** a **11.** a, b, c, d, e

CHAPTER 24. **Schizophrenia Spectrum and Other Psychotic Disorders**
1. b **2.** b **3.** c **4.** d **5.** d **6.** a **7.** c **8.** b
9. c **10.** d **11.** c **12.** a, b, e

CHAPTER 25. **Depressive Disorders**
1. c **2.** b **3.** a **4.** d **5.** a, b, d **6.** a, b, c, e
7. a **8.** c **9.** b **10.** a, b, d

CHAPTER 26. **Bipolar and Related Disorders**
1. b **2.** c **3.** a **4.** a, c, d **5.** b **6.** d **7.** b
8. c **9.** a = 3, b = 1, c = 4, d = 2 **10.** c

CHAPTER 27. **Anxiety, Obsessive-Compulsive, and Related Disorders**
1. d **2.** c **3.** d **4.** a **5.** b **6.** c **7.** a, b, c
8. c **9.** a **10.** b

CHAPTER 28. **Trauma- and Stressor-Related Disorders**
1. b **2.** c **3.** a **4.** d **5.** b **6.** b **7.** c **8.** a
9. a **10.** d **11.** a, c

CHAPTER 29. **Somatic Symptom and Dissociative Disorders**
1. a **2.** b **3.** d **4.** b **5.** c **6.** d **7.** b **8.** a
9. b **10.** d

CHAPTER 30. **Issues Related to Human Sexuality and Gender Dysphoria**
1. b **2.** c **3.** a, b, c, d **4.** a **5.** b **6.** d **7.** b
8. c **9.** a, b, d, e

CHAPTER 31. **Eating Disorders**
1. c **2.** a **3.** b **4.** b **5.** c **6.** b **7.** c **8.** b
9. c **10.** a, b, c, d

CHAPTER 32. **Personality Disorders**
1. d **2.** a **3.** b **4.** d **5.** a **6.** b **7.** c **8.** a
9. d **10.** b

CHAPTER 33. **Children and Adolescents**
1. b **2.** c **3.** a **4.** b **5.** b **6.** b, c, d **7.** c
8. d **9.** a **10.** b

CHAPTER 34. **The Aging Individual**
1. c **2.** d **3.** b **4.** a **5.** c **6.** d **7.** a **8.** a
9. c **10.** a

CHAPTER 35. **Survivors of Abuse or Neglect**
1. b **2.** c **3.** a **4.** d **5.** b **6.** d **7.** a **8.** b
9. b **10.** d

CHAPTER 36. **Community Mental Health Nursing**
1. a **2.** b **3.** a **4.** c **5.** d **6.** b **7.** c **8.** d
9. a **10.** a, b, c, d

CHAPTER 37. **The Bereaved Individual**
1. a, b, c, d **2.** c **3.** c **4.** d **5.** a **6.** a **7.** b
8. c **9.** a **10.** c

CHAPTER 38. **Military Families**
1. a, b, d **2.** b **3.** a **4.** b **5.** c **6.** c **7.** a, c, d
8. d **9.** a, b, c, d

Bonus Chapters on DavisPlus

Complementary and Psychosocial Therapies
1. a, c, e, f **2.** a, b, d **3.** c, d **4.** a, d, e **5.** c
6. d **7.** a **8.** b **9.** a, b, c **10.** c

Relaxation Therapy
1. a, b, e **2.** a, b, d **3.** a **4.** c **5.** d

Theoretical Models of Personality Development
1. b **2.** c **3.** d **4.** b **5.** b **6.** b **7.** a **8.** c
9. a **10.** b

Forensic Nursing
1. c **2.** b **3.** a, b, e **4.** a, d, e **5.** c **6.** d
7. d **8.** b **9.** a, c, d, e **10.** c

Appendix B

Examples of Answers to Communication Exercises

Chapter 13. Crisis Intervention

1. "I'll try to help you to the best of my ability. Please tell me what is upsetting you." Establish rapport, convey respect, and assess precipitating events.

2. "Hi Shelley, my name is Mrs. Smith, and I am a registered nurse here to help you. I'm so glad you came in to seek help. I'd like to ask you some questions about the events you've experienced. All right?" (Convey respect, provide reassurance of help, and empower the client to be involved in decision-making.)

3. "Thomas, last evening you became very upset, stating you thought the FBI was trying to kill you, and you struck another patient." (Giving information.) "Do you remember any of those events?" (Assessing the patient's perception and memory.) "Restraint is an intervention that we only use when other efforts have failed to protect your safety and the safety of others." (Giving information.) "Let's talk about what you think would be helpful in preventing that from happening again." (Formulating a plan, empowering the client to be involved in problem-solving.)

Chapter 17. Suicide Prevention

1. "Mr. J., it sounds like you have been feeling hopeless; this is a common symptom of depression." (Giving information.) "Have you been having any thoughts of taking your own life?" (Closed-ended, directive questioning to assess for the presence of suicide ideation.)

2. Communication at this point should be focused on thorough assessment of Mr. J.'s expressed suicide ideas. Assessment questions include (but are not comprehensive): "When you have these ideas, do you have a plan in mind?" "How strong is your intention to die?" "Do you have access to the means for implementing this plan?"

3. "It sounds like you are grieving. That must be very painful. Tell me more about your experience and feelings related to losing your wife." (Empathy, exploring and encouraging description.)

Chapter 21. The Recovery Model

1. Because inability to sit still may be a side effect of many antipsychotic medications, one response is to assess the client's medications, assess the client's symptoms, and educate him about akathisia as appropriate. This response supports the principle that recovery should empower the client to make informed decisions through providing information and resources. Asking the client how he wishes to proceed supports the principle that recovery is person-driven.

   For example:

   "Joshua, I see that you are taking Thorazine, and the inability to sit still may be a side effect of this medication. There are other medications that will treat your symptoms and that don't have the same risk for this side effect. Would you like to explore these options further?"

2. Using the recovery model principles of respect and the importance of support through peers and allies, one possible response may be, "Kelly, I haven't been in an active combat situation, but I hope to earn your trust as a mental health professional and try to understand, to the best of my ability, the issues you've been struggling with. Many veterans identify, as you have, that fellow veterans are better able to provide ongoing support with an appreciation for the shared experiences you've endured. Are you interested in exploring some of those options, too?"

Chapter 22. Neurocognitive Disorders

1. "Mrs. B., you are not in a restaurant. This is the General Hospital. I am your nurse, Mary. How may I help you?" (Reality orientation.)

2. "Mrs. B., you have already eaten your breakfast. Would you like a snack?"

   "Please tell me what it was like when you lived on the farm." (Reminiscing.)

Chapter 23. Substance-Related and Addictive Disorders

1. "Tom, you are here because it has been determined that drinking alcohol is causing problems for you at home and at your work." (Confronting reality.)

2. "Tom, you are experiencing symptoms related to your body's withdrawal from alcohol. When did you have your last drink?" (Confrontation with caring.)

3. "You are feeling angry toward your boss and your wife, but your drinking is apparently interfering with your job and your marriage. Unless you abstain from alcohol, you are at risk of losing both." (Confronting reality.)

Chapter 24. Schizophrenia Spectrum and Other Psychotic Disorders

1. "I know that you believe what you are saying is true, but I find it very hard to accept." (Voicing doubt.)
"Please understand that you are safe here." (Reassurance of safety.)

2. The nurse should slowly and carefully approach Hal so that he is not startled by his or her presence. "Hal, are you hearing the voices again? What do you hear the voices saying to you?" (Encouraging description of perceptions. This type of information may help to protect the client and others from potential violence associated with command hallucinations.)
"I know the voices seem real to you, but I do not hear any voices speaking." (Presenting reality.)

3. "I don't understand what you are saying, Hal. What message do you want to give me? Might you be telling me that you are lonely?" (Seeking clarification; attempting to translate words into feelings.)

Chapter 25. Depressive Disorders

1. "You have had a lot of losses. You are feeling very much alone right now." (Verbalizing the implied.)

2. "You feel sad because you can no longer do the things that you used to do . . . the things that made you feel good about yourself." (Statement that focuses on feelings.)

3. Direct questions assessing suicide potential: "Are you or have you been thinking about harming yourself? Do you have a plan for doing so? Have you ever acted on that plan?"
Demonstrations of genuine concern and caring: "I care about you, Carrie. I will stay here with you." Expressions of empathy: "It must be frightening to feel so all alone. But you are not alone. There are many people who care about you, and I am one of those people."

Chapter 26. Bipolar and Related Disorders

1. "Bob, I'm not sure I understand what you are saying. Are your thoughts racing?" (Clarifying, assessing.)

2. "John, I have an activity in the next room that I could use your help with. Would you please come with me?" (Offering an alternative activity, redirecting, reducing stimulation.)

Chapter 27. Anxiety, Obsessive-Compulsive, and Related Disorders

1. "John, I'd like to check your vital signs and then discuss how I can best help you feel more comfortable." (Giving information, physical assessment is a priority. Informing the client about nursing intervention with a matter-of-fact approach may facilitate anxiety reduction; offering self.)

2. "Often, when people become very anxious, they develop irrational thinking patterns that contribute to worsening their mood and impacting their behavior in negative ways. By becoming aware of thought patterns that increase your anxiety you can learn how to replace those automatic thoughts with more rational patterns in a way that improves your mood symptoms and behavior." (Giving information. The nurse in this example provides information and identifies how that is relevant to the client's recovery.)

Chapter 30. Issues Related to Human Sexuality and Gender Dysphoria

1. "Are you having thoughts of taking your own life?" (Assessment for suicide ideation and intentions are the priority because Jamie has expressed feeling that he wants to die.)

2. "I'd be glad to discuss with you the benefits and disadvantages of this option. What do you already know about hormone treatments?" (Conveys respect, collaboration, assessment.)

Chapter 31. Eating Disorders

1. "Helena, we've established a treatment plan that limits going to the restroom immediately after a meal because we are trying to help you avoid the urge to purge the food you just ate. Let's talk about how you are feeling right now and see if we can identify some other options for your behaviors before and after meals." (Setting limits, formulating a plan.)

2. "John, many people with this kind of eating disorder report feeling a loss of control, and I understand how that can alter your self-esteem. These are symptoms of an illness with many contributing factors. I want to support you in your efforts to manage this illness, and there is good evidence that recovery is achievable." (Validation of client's feelings, empathy, giving information, offering self.)

Chapter 32. Personality Disorders

1. "My name is Nancy. I am your nurse on this shift, and you will be in my care until 11 p.m. You may ask for me by my name if you have any requests." (Giving information.)
2. "You were arrested because you broke the law." (Confronting reality.)
3. "I do not give out personal information to patients, and I do not go out with patients. I hope that you will be able to get your life straightened out in a positive way." (Confrontation with caring.)

Chapter 35. Survivors of Abuse or Neglect

1. "You are not to blame, Sarah. You do not deserve to be abused in this way. He is responsible for his behavior." (Presenting reality, empathy.)
2. "There are places you can go where you and your children will be safe. I will give you that information." (Giving information.)
"You will need to consider whether you want to press charges against him." (Encouraging formulation of a plan.)

3. "You must consider the safety of yourself and your children. You have the phone number of the Safe House. It is your decision what to do now." (Patient-centered care involves communicating important information and empowering the client to make their own decisions.)

Chapter 37. The Bereaved Individual

1. "I believe we did everything we could to provide care for your husband, and it's so hard to lose someone you love to a terminal illness. I'll stay with you and try to answer any questions you have." (The nurse uses "I" communication to respond assertively with empathy; offering self.)
2. "Yes, John, it's probable that you are in the end stage of life. Let's talk about how to prepare for this." (Giving information; offering self; encouraging formulation of a plan.)
3. "Nancy, those are difficult spiritual questions. Would you like to talk more with the chaplain?" (Verbalizing the implied; formulating a plan.)

Appendix C

Mental Status Assessment

Gathering the correct information about the client's mental status is essential to the development of an appropriate plan of care. The mental status examination is a description of all the areas of the client's mental functioning. The following are the components that are considered critical in the assessment of a client's mental status. Examples of interview questions and criteria for assessment are included.

Identifying Data

1. Name
2. Gender
3. Age
   a. How old are you?
   b. When were you born?
4. Race/culture
   a. What country did you (your ancestors) come from?
5. Occupational/financial status
   a. How do you make your living?
   b. How do you obtain money for your needs?
6. Educational level
   a. What was the highest grade level you completed in school?
7. Significant other
   a. Are you married?
   b. Do you have a significant relationship with another person?
8. Living arrangements
   a. Do you live alone?
   b. With whom do you share your home?
9. Religious preference
   a. Do you have a religious preference?
10. Allergies
    a. Are you allergic to anything?
    b. Foods? Medications?
11. Special diet considerations
    a. Do you have any special diet requirements?
    b. Diabetic? Low sodium?
12. Chief complaint
    a. For what reason did you come for help today?
    b. What seems to be the problem?
13. Medical diagnosis

General Description

Appearance

1. Grooming and dress
   a. Note unusual modes of dress.
   b. Evidence of soiled clothing?
   c. Use of makeup?
   d. Neat; unkempt?
2. Hygiene
   a. Note evidence of body or breath odor.
   b. Note condition of skin, fingernails.
3. Posture
   a. Note if standing upright, rigid, slumped over.
4. Height and weight
   a. Perform accurate measurements.
5. Level of eye contact
   a. Intermittent?
   b. Occasional and fleeting?
   c. Sustained and intense?
   d. No eye contact?
6. Hair color and texture
   a. Is hair clean and healthy-looking?
   b. Greasy, matted, tangled?
7. Evidence of scars, tattoos, or other distinguishing skin marks
   a. Note any evidence of swelling or bruises.
   b. Birth marks?
   c. Rashes?
8. Evaluation of client's appearance compared with chronological age

Motor Activity

1. Tremors
   a. Do hands or legs tremble?
      • Continuously?
      • At specific times?
2. Tics or other stereotypical movements
   a. Any evidence of facial tics?
   b. Jerking or spastic movements?
3. Mannerisms and gestures
   a. Specific facial or body movements during conversation?
   b. Nail biting?
   c. Covering face with hands?
   d. Grimacing?

4. Hyperactivity
   a. Gets up and down out of chair.
   b. Paces.
   c. Unable to sit still.
5. Restlessness or agitation
   a. Lots of fidgeting.
   b. Clenching hands.
6. Aggressiveness
   a. Overtly angry and hostile.
   b. Threatening.
   c. Uses sarcasm.
7. Rigidity
   a. Sits or stands in a rigid position.
   b. Arms and legs appear stiff and unyielding.
8. Gait patterns
   a. Any evidence of limping?
   b. Limitation of range of motion?
   c. Ataxia?
   d. Shuffling?
9. Echopraxia
   a. Evidence of mimicking the actions of others?
10. Psychomotor retardation
   a. Movements are very slow.
   b. Thinking and speech are very slow.
   c. Posture is slumped.
11. Freedom of movement (range of motion)
   a. Note any limitation in ability to move.

Speech Patterns

1. Slowness or rapidity of speech
   a. Note whether speech seems very rapid or slower than normal.
2. Pressure of speech
   a. Note whether speech seems frenzied.
   b. Unable to be interrupted?
3. Intonation
   a. Are words spoken with appropriate emphasis?
   b. Are words spoken in monotone, without emphasis?
4. Volume
   a. Is speech very loud? Soft?
   b. Is speech low-pitched? High-pitched?
5. Stuttering or other speech impairments
   a. Hoarseness?
   b. Slurred speech?
6. Aphasia
   a. Difficulty forming words.
   b. Use of incorrect words.
   c. Difficulty thinking of specific words.
   d. Making up words (neologisms).

General Attitude

1. Cooperative/uncooperative
   a. Answers questions willingly.
   b. Refuses to answer questions.

2. Friendly/hostile/defensive
   a. Is sociable and responsive.
   b. Is sarcastic and irritable.
3. Uninterested/apathetic
   a. Refuses to participate in interview process.
4. Attentive/interested
   a. Actively participates in interview process.
5. Guarded/suspicious
   a. Continuously scans the environment.
   b. Questions motives of interviewer.
   c. Refuses to answer questions.

Emotions

Mood

1. Depressed; despairing
   a. An overwhelming feeling of sadness.
   b. Loss of interest in regular activities.
2. Irritable
   a. Easily annoyed and provoked to anger.
3. Anxious
   a. Demonstrates or verbalizes feeling of apprehension.
4. Elated
   a. Expresses feelings of joy and intense pleasure.
   b. Is intensely optimistic.
5. Euphoric
   a. Demonstrates a heightened sense of elation.
   b. Expresses feelings of grandeur ("Everything is wonderful!").
6. Fearful
   a. Demonstrates or verbalizes feeling of apprehension associated with real or perceived danger.
7. Guilty
   a. Expresses a feeling of discomfort associated with real or perceived wrongdoing.
   b. May be associated with feelings of sadness and despair.
8. Labile
   a. Exhibits mood swings that range from euphoria to depression or anxiety.

Affect

1. Congruence with mood
   a. Outward emotional expression is consistent with mood (e.g., if depressed, emotional expression is sadness, eyes downcast, may be crying).
2. Constricted or blunted
   a. Minimal outward emotional expression is observed.
3. Flat
   a. There is an absence of outward emotional expression.

4. Appropriate
   a. The outward emotional expression is what would be expected in a certain situation (e.g., crying upon hearing of a death).
5. Inappropriate
   a. The outward emotional expression is incompatible with the situation (e.g., laughing upon hearing of a death).

Thought Processes
Form of Thought

1. Flight of ideas
   a. Verbalizations are continuous and rapid, and flow from one to another.
2. Associative looseness
   a. Verbalizations shift from one unrelated topic to another.
3. Circumstantiality
   a. Verbalizations are lengthy and tedious, and because of numerous details, are delayed reaching the intended point.
4. Tangentiality
   a. Verbalizations that are lengthy and tedious, and never reach an intended point.
5. Neologisms
   a. The individual is making up nonsensical-sounding words, which only have meaning to him or her.
6. Concrete thinking
   a. Thinking is literal; elemental.
   b. Absence of ability to think abstractly.
   c. Unable to translate simple proverbs.
7. Clang associations
   a. Speaking in puns or rhymes; using words that sound alike but have different meanings.
8. Word salad
   a. Using a mixture of words that have no meaning together; sounding incoherent.
9. Perseveration
   a. Persistently repeating the last word of a sentence spoken to the client (e.g., Nurse: "George, it's time to go to lunch." George: "lunch, lunch, lunch, lunch").
10. Echolalia
    a. Persistently repeating what another person says.
11. Mutism
    a. Does not speak (either cannot or will not).
12. Poverty of speech
    a. Speaks very little; may respond in monosyllables.
13. Ability to concentrate and disturbance of attention
    a. Does the person hold attention to the topic at hand?
    b. Is the person easily distractible?
    c. Is there selective attention (e.g., blocks out topics that create anxiety)?

Content of Thought

1. Delusions (Does the person have unrealistic ideas or beliefs?)
   a. Persecutory: A belief that someone is out to get him or her in some way (e.g., "The FBI will be here at any time to take me away").
   b. Grandiose: An idea that he or she is all-powerful or of great importance (e.g., "I am the king—and this is my kingdom! I can do anything!").
   c. Reference: An idea that whatever is happening in the environment is about him or her (e.g., "Just watch the movie on TV tonight. It is about my life").
   d. Control or influence: A belief that his or her behavior and thoughts are being controlled by external forces (e.g., "I get my orders from Channel 27. I do only what the forces dictate").
   e. Somatic: A belief that he or she has a dysfunctional body part (e.g., "My heart is at a standstill. It is no longer beating").
   f. Nihilistic: A belief that he or she, or a part of the body, or even the world does not exist or has been destroyed (e.g., "I am no longer alive").
2. Suicidal or homicidal ideas
   a. Is the individual expressing ideas of harming self or others?
   b. Does the individual express plans and intentions to die? Or plans and intentions to harm another?
3. Obsessions
   a. Is the person verbalizing about a persistent thought or feeling that he or she is unable to eliminate from their consciousness?
4. Paranoia/suspiciousness
   a. Continuously scans the environment.
   b. Questions motives of interviewer.
   c. Refuses to answer questions.
5. Magical thinking
   a. Is the person speaking in a way that indicates his or her words or actions have power? (e.g., "If you step on a crack, you break your mother's back!")
6. Religiosity
   a. Is the individual demonstrating obsession with religious ideas and behavior?
7. Phobias
   a. Is there evidence of irrational fears (of a specific object, or a social situation)?
8. Poverty of content
   a. Is little information conveyed by the client because of vagueness or stereotypical statements or clichés?

Perceptual Disturbances

1. Hallucinations (Is the person experiencing unrealistic sensory perceptions?)
   a. Auditory (Is the individual hearing voices or other sounds that do not exist?)
   b. Visual (Is the individual seeing images that do not exist?)
   c. Tactile (Does the individual feel unrealistic sensations on the skin?)
   d. Olfactory (Does the individual smell odors that do not exist?)
   e. Gustatory (Does the individual have a false perception of an unpleasant taste?)
2. Illusions
   a. Does the individual misperceive or misinterpret real stimuli within the environment? (Sees something and thinks it is something else?)
3. Depersonalization (altered perception of the self)
   a. The individual verbalizes feeling "outside the body;" visualizing him- or herself from afar.
4. Derealization (altered perception of the environment)
   a. The individual verbalizes that the environment feels "strange or unreal." A feeling that the surroundings have changed.

Sensorium and Cognitive Ability

1. Level of alertness/consciousness
   a. Is the individual clear-minded and attentive to the environment?
   b. Or is there disturbance in perception and awareness of the surroundings?
2. Orientation. Is the person oriented to the following?
   a. Time.
   b. Place.
   c. Person.
   d. Circumstances.

3. Memory
   a. Recent (Is the individual able to remember occurrences of the past few days?)
   b. Remote (Is the individual able to remember occurrences of the distant past?)
   c. Confabulation (Does the individual fill in memory gaps with experiences that have no basis in fact?)
4. Capacity for abstract thought
   a. Can the individual interpret proverbs correctly?
      • "What does 'no use crying over spilled milk' mean?"

Impulse Control

1. Ability to control impulses. (Does psychosocial history reveal problems with any of the following?)
   a. Aggression.
   b. Hostility.
   c. Fear.
   d. Guilt.
   e. Affection.
   f. Sexual feelings.

Judgment and Insight

1. Ability to solve problems and make decisions
   a. What are your plans for the future?
   b. What do you plan to do to reach your goals?
2. Knowledge about self
   a. Awareness of limitations.
   b. Awareness of consequences of actions.
   c. Awareness of illness.
      • "Do you think you have a problem?"
      • "Do you think you need treatment?"
3. Adaptive/maladaptive use of coping strategies and ego defense mechanisms (e.g., rationalizing maladaptive behaviors, projection of blame, displacement of anger)

Appendix D

DSM-5 Classification: Categories and Codes*

International Classification of Diseases, 10th revision, Clinical Modification (ICD-10-CM) codes are provided.

Neurodevelopmental Disorders

Intellectual Disabilities

	Intellectual Disability (Intellectual Developmental Disorder)
	Specify current severity:
70	Mild
71	Moderate
72	Severe
73	Profound
F88	Global Developmental Delay
F79	Unspecified Intellectual Disability (Intellectual Developmental Disorder)

Communication Disorders

F80.9	Language Disorder
F80.0	Speech Sound Disorder
F80.81	Childhood-Onset Fluency Disorder (Stuttering) Note: Later-onset cases are diagnosed as F98.5 adult-onset fluency disorder.
F80.89	Social (Pragmatic) Communication Disorder
F80.9	Unspecified Communication Disorder

Autism Spectrum Disorder

F84.0	Autism Spectrum Disorder *Specify* if: Associated with a known medical or genetic condition or environmental factor; Associated with another neurodevelopmental, mental, or behavioral disorder *Specify* current severity for Criterion A and Criterion B: Requiring very substantial support, Requiring substantial support, Requiring support *Specify* if: With or without accompanying intellectual impairment, With or without accompanying language impairment, With catatonia (use additional code F06.1)

Attention-Deficit/Hyperactivity Disorder

	Attention-Deficit/Hyperactivity Disorder *Specify* whether:
F90.2	Combined presentation
F90.0	Predominantly inattentive presentation
F90.1	Predominantly hyperactive/impulsive presentation *Specify* if: In partial remission *Specify* current severity: Mild, Moderate, Severe
F90.8	Other Specified Attention-Deficit/Hyperactivity Disorder
F90.9	Unspecified Attention-Deficit/Hyperactivity Disorder

Specific Learning Disorder

	Specific Learning Disorder *Specify* if:
F81.0	With impairment in reading (*specify* if with word reading accuracy, reading rate or fluency, reading comprehension)
F81.81	With impairment in written expression (*specify* if with spelling accuracy, grammar and punctuation accuracy, clarity or organization of written expression)
F81.2	With impairment in mathematics (*specify* if with number sense, memorization of arithmetic facts, accurate or fluent calculation, accurate math reasoning) *Specify* current severity: Mild, Moderate, Severe

---

*Reprinted with permission from the *Diagnostic and Statistical Manual of Mental Disorders, Fifth Edition.* (Copyright 2013). American Psychiatric Association.

Motor Disorders

F82	Developmental Coordination Disorder
F98.4	Stereotypic Movement Disorder

Specify if: With self-injurious behavior, Without self-injurious behavior
Specify if: Associated with a known medical or genetic condition, neurodevelopmental disorder, or environmental factor
Specify current severity: Mild, Moderate, Severe

Tic Disorders

F95.2	Tourette's Disorder
F95.1	Persistent (Chronic) Motor or Vocal Tic Disorder

Specify if: With motor tics only, With vocal tics only

F95.0	Provisional Tic Disorder
F95.8	Other Specified Tic Disorder
F95.9	Unspecified Tic Disorder

Other Neurodevelopmental Disorders

F88	Other Specified Neurodevelopmental Disorder
F89	Unspecified Neurodevelopmental Disorder

Schizophrenia Spectrum and Other Psychotic Disorders

The following specifiers apply to Schizophrenia Spectrum and Other Psychotic Disorders where indicated:

[a]*Specify* if: The following course specifiers are only to be used after a 1-year duration of the disorder: First episode, currently in acute episode; First episode, currently in partial remission; First episode, currently in full remission; Multiple episodes, currently in acute episode; Multiple episodes, currently in partial remission; Multiple episodes, currently in full remission; Continuous; Unspecified

[b]*Specify* if: With catatonia (use additional code F06.1)

[c]*Specify* current severity of delusions, hallucinations, disorganized speech, abnormal psychomotor behavior, negative symptoms, impaired cognition, depression, and mania symptoms

F21	Schizotypal (Personality) Disorder
F22	Delusional Disorder[a, c]

Specify whether: Erotomanic type, Grandiose type, Jealous type, Persecutory type, Somatic type, Mixed type, Unspecified type
Specify if: With bizarre content

F23	Brief Psychotic Disorder[b, c]

Specify if: With marked stressor(s), Without marked stressor(s), With postpartum onset

F20.81	Schizophreniform Disorder[b, c]

Specify if: With good prognostic features, Without good prognostic features

F20.9	Schizophrenia[a, b, c]
	Schizoaffective Disorder[a, b, c]

Specify whether:

F25.0	Bipolar type
F25.1	Depressive type
	Substance/Medication-Induced Psychotic Disorder[c]

Note: See the criteria set and corresponding recording procedures for substance-specific codes and ICD-10-CM coding.
Specify if: With onset during intoxication, With onset during withdrawal

Psychotic Disorder Due to Another Medical Condition[c]
Specify whether:

F06.2	With delusions
F06.0	With hallucinations
F06.1	Catatonia Associated With Another Mental Disorder (Catatonia Specifier)
F06.1	Catatonic Disorder Due to Another Medical Condition
F06.1	Unspecified Catatonia

Note: Code first 781.99 (R29.818) other symptoms involving nervous and musculoskeletal systems.

F28	Other Specified Schizophrenia Spectrum and Other Psychotic Disorder
F29	Unspecified Schizophrenia Spectrum and Other Psychotic Disorder

Bipolar and Related Disorders

The following specifiers apply to Bipolar and Related Disorders where indicated:

[a]*Specify*: With anxious distress (*specify* current severity: mild, moderate, moderate-severe, severe); With mixed

features; With rapid cycling; With melancholic features; With atypical features; With mood-congruent psychotic features; With mood incongruent psychotic features; With catatonia (use additional code F06.1); With peripartum onset; With seasonal pattern

	Bipolar I Disorder[a]
	Current or most recent episode manic
F31.11	Mild
F31.12	Moderate
F31.13	Severe
F31.2	With psychotic features
F31.73	In partial remission
F31.74	In full remission
F31.9	Unspecified
F31.0	Current or most recent episode hypomanic
F31.73	In partial remission
F31.74	In full remission
F31.9	Unspecified
	Current or most recent episode depressed
F31.31	Mild
F31.32	Moderate
F31.4	Severe
F31.5	With psychotic features
F31.75	In partial remission
F31.76	In full remission
F31.9	Unspecified
F31.9	Current or most recent episode unspecified
F31.81	Bipolar II Disorder[a]

Specify current or most recent episode: Hypomanic, Depressed

Specify course if full criteria for a mood episode are not currently met: In partial remission, In full remission

Specify severity if full criteria for a mood episode are not currently met: Mild, Moderate, Severe

F34.0	Cyclothymic Disorder

Specify if: With anxious distress

Substance/Medication-Induced Bipolar and Related Disorder

Note: See the criteria set and corresponding recording procedures for substance-specific codes and ICD-10-CM coding.

Specify if: With onset during intoxication, With onset during withdrawal

	Bipolar and Related Disorder Due to Another Medical Condition

Specify if:

F06.33	With manic features
F06.33	With manic- or hypomanic-like episode
F06.34	With mixed features
F31.89	Other Specified Bipolar and Related Disorder
F31.9	Unspecified Bipolar and Related Disorder

Depressive Disorders

The following specifiers apply to Depressive Disorders where indicated:

[a]*Specify*: With anxious distress (*specify* current severity: mild, moderate, moderate-severe, severe); With mixed features; With melancholic features; With atypical features; With mood-congruent psychotic features; With mood-incongruent psychotic features; With catatonia (use additional code F06.1); With peripartum onset; With seasonal pattern

F34.8	Disruptive Mood Dysregulation Disorder
	Major Depressive Disorder[a]
	Single episode
F32.0	Mild
F32.1	Moderate
F32.2	Severe
F32.3	With psychotic features
F32.4	In partial remission
F32.5	In full remission
F32.9	Unspecified
	Recurrent episode
F33.0	Mild
F33.1	Moderate
F33.2	Severe
F33.3	With psychotic features
F33.41	In partial remission
F33.42	In full remission
F33.9	Unspecified
F34.1	Persistent Depressive Disorder (Dysthymia)[a]

Specify if: In partial remission, In full remission

Specify if: Early onset, Late onset

Specify if: With pure dysthymic syndrome; With persistent major depressive episode; With intermittent major depressive episodes, with current episode; With intermittent major

depressive episodes, Without current episode
Specify current severity: Mild, Moderate, Severe

N94.3	Premenstrual Dysphoric Disorder

Substance/Medication-Induced Depressive Disorder
Note: See the criteria set and corresponding recording procedures for substance-specific codes and ICD-10-CM coding.
Specify if: With onset during intoxication, With onset during withdrawal
Depressive Disorder Due to Another Medical Condition
Specify if:

F06.31	With depressive features
F06.32	With major depressive-like episode
F06.34	With mixed features
F32.8	Other Specified Depressive Disorder
F32.9	Unspecified Depressive Disorder

Anxiety Disorders

F93.0	Separation Anxiety Disorder
F94.0	Selective Mutism
	Specific Phobia

Specify if:

F40.218	Animal
F40.228	Natural environment
	Blood-injection-injury
F40.230	Fear of blood
F40.231	Fear of injections and transfusions
F40.232	Fear of other medical care
F40.233	Fear of injury
F40.248	Situational
F40.298	Other
F40.10	Social Anxiety Disorder (Social Phobia)

Specify if: Performance only

F41.0	Panic Disorder
	Panic Attack Specifier
F40.00	Agoraphobia
F41.1	Generalized Anxiety Disorder

Substance/Medication-Induced Anxiety Disorder
Note: See the criteria set and corresponding recording procedures for substance-specific codes and ICD-10-CM coding.

Specify if: With onset during intoxication, With onset during withdrawal, With onset after medication use

F06.4	Anxiety Disorder Due to Another Medical Condition
F41.9	Unspecified Anxiety Disorder

Obsessive-Compulsive and Related Disorders

The following specifier applies to Obsessive-Compulsive and Related Disorders where indicated:
aSpecify if: With good or fair insight, With poor insight, With absent insight/delusional beliefs

F42	Obsessive-Compulsive Disordera
	Specify if: Tic-related
F45.22	Body Dysmorphic Disordera
	Specify if: With muscle dysmorphia
F42	Hoarding Disordera
	Specify if: With excessive acquisition
F63.3	Trichotillomania (Hair-Pulling Disorder)
L98.1	Excoriation (Skin-Picking) Disorder

Substance/Medication-Induced Obsessive-Compulsive and Related Disorder
Note: See the criteria set and corresponding recording procedures for substance-specific codes and ICD-9-CM and ICD-10-CM coding.
Specify if: With onset during intoxication, With onset during withdrawal, With onset after medication use

F06.8	Obsessive-Compulsive and Related Disorder Due to Another Medical Condition

Specify if: With obsessive-compulsive disorder-like symptoms, With appearance preoccupations, With hoarding symptoms, With hair-pulling symptoms, With skin-picking symptoms

F42	Other Specified Obsessive-Compulsive and Related Disorder
F42	Unspecified Obsessive-Compulsive and Related Disorder

Trauma- and Stressor-Related Disorders

F94.1	Reactive Attachment Disorder *Specify* if: Persistent *Specify* current severity: Severe
F94.2	Disinhibited Social Engagement Disorder *Specify* if: Persistent *Specify* current severity: Severe
F43.10	Posttraumatic Stress Disorder (includes Posttraumatic Stress Disorder for Children 6 Years and Younger) *Specify* whether: With dissociative symptoms *Specify* if: With delayed expression
F43.0	Acute Stress Disorder
	Adjustment Disorders *Specify* whether:
F43.21	With depressed mood
F43.22	With anxiety
F43.23	With mixed anxiety and depressed mood
F43.24	With disturbance of conduct
F43.25	With mixed disturbance of emotions and conduct
F43.20	Unspecified
F43.8	Other Specified Trauma- and Stressor-Related Disorder
F43.9	Unspecified Trauma- and Stressor-Related Disorder

Dissociative Disorders

F44.81	Dissociative Identity Disorder
F44.0	Dissociative Amnesia *Specify* if:
F44.1	With dissociative fugue
F48.1	Depersonalization/Derealization Disorder
F44.89	Other Specified Dissociative Disorder
F44.9	Unspecified Dissociative Disorder

Somatic Symptom and Related Disorders

F45.1	Somatic Symptom Disorder *Specify* if: With predominant pain *Specify* if: Persistent *Specify* current severity: Mild, Moderate, Severe
F45.21	Illness Anxiety Disorder *Specify* whether: Care seeking type, Care avoidant type
	Conversion Disorder (Functional Neurological Symptom Disorder)

	Specify symptom type:
F44.4	With weakness or paralysis
F44.4	With abnormal movement
F44.4	With swallowing symptoms
F44.4	With speech symptom
F44.5	With attacks or seizures
F44.6	With anesthesia or sensory loss
F44.6	With special sensory symptom
F44.7	With mixed symptoms
	Specify if: Acute episode, Persistent *Specify* if: With psychological stressor (*specify* stressor), Without psychological stressor
F54	Psychological Factors Affecting Other Medical Conditions *Specify* current severity: Mild, Moderate, Severe, Extreme
F68.10	Factitious Disorder (includes Factitious Disorder Imposed on Self, Factitious Disorder Imposed on Another) *Specify* Single episode, Recurrent episodes
F45.8	Other Specified Somatic Symptom and Related Disorder
F45.9	Unspecified Somatic Symptom and Related Disorder

Feeding and Eating Disorders

The following specifiers apply to Feeding and Eating Disorders where indicated:

[a]*Specify* if: In remission
[b]*Specify* if: In partial remission, In full remission
[c]*Specify* current severity: Mild, Moderate, Severe, Extreme

	Pica[a]
F98.3	In children
F50.8	In adults
F98.21	Rumination Disorder[a]
F50.8	Avoidant/Restrictive Food Intake Disorder[a]
	Anorexia Nervosa[b, c] *Specify* whether:
F50.01	Restricting type
F50.02	Binge-eating/purging type
F50.2	Bulimia Nervosa[b, c]
F50.8	Binge-Eating Disorder[b, c]
F50.8	Other Specified Feeding or Eating Disorder
F50.9	Unspecified Feeding or Eating Disorder

Elimination Disorders

F98.0	Enuresis *Specify* whether: Nocturnal only, Diurnal only, Nocturnal and diurnal
F98.1	Encopresis *Specify* whether: With constipation and overflow incontinence, Without constipation and overflow incontinence
	Other Specified Elimination Disorder
N39.498	With urinary symptoms
R15.9	With fecal symptoms
	Unspecified Elimination Disorder
R32	With urinary symptoms
R15.9	With fecal symptoms

Sleep-Wake Disorders

The following specifiers apply to Sleep-Wake Disorders where indicated:

[a]*Specify* if: Episodic, Persistent, Recurrent
[b]*Specify* if: Acute, Subacute, Persistent
[c]*Specify* current severity: Mild, Moderate, Severe

G47.00	Insomnia Disorder[a] *Specify* if: With non-sleep disorder mental comorbidity, With other medical comorbidity, With other sleep disorder
G47.10	Hypersomnolence Disorder[b, c] *Specify* if: With mental disorder, With medical condition, With another sleep disorder
	Narcolepsy[c] *Specify* whether:
G47.419	Narcolepsy without cataplexy but with hypocretin deficiency
G47.411	Narcolepsy with cataplexy but without hypocretin deficiency
G47.419	Autosomal dominant cerebellar ataxia, deafness, and narcolepsy
G47.419	Autosomal dominant narcolepsy, obesity, and type 2 diabetes
G47.429	Narcolepsy secondary to another medical condition

Breathing-Related Sleep Disorders

G47.33	Obstructive Sleep Apnea Hypopnea[c]
	Central Sleep Apnea *Specify* whether:
G47.31	Idiopathic central sleep apnea
R06.3	Cheyne-Stokes breathing
G47.37	Central sleep apnea comorbid with opioid use Note: First code opioid use disorder, if present. *Specify* current severity
	Sleep-Related Hypoventilation *Specify* whether
G47.34	Idiopathic hypoventilation
G47.35	Congenital central alveolar hypoventilation
G47.36	Comorbid sleep-related hypoventilation *Specify* current severity
	Circadian Rhythm Sleep-Wake Disorders[a] *Specify* whether:
G47.21	Delayed sleep phase type *Specify* if: Familial, Overlapping with non-24-hour sleep-wake type
G47.22	Advanced sleep phase type *Specify* if: Familial
G47.23	Irregular sleep-wake type
G47.24	Non-24-hour sleep-wake type
G47.26	Shift work type
G47.20	Unspecified type

Parasomnias

	Non-Rapid Eye Movement Sleep Arousal Disorders *Specify* whether:
F51.3	Sleepwalking type *Specify* if: With sleep-related eating, With sleep-related sexual behavior (sexsomnia)
F51.4	Sleep terror type
F51.5	Nightmare Disorder[b, c] *Specify* if: During sleep onset *Specify* if: With associated non-sleep disorder, With associated other medical condition, With associated other sleep disorder
G47.52	Rapid Eye Movement Sleep Behavior Disorder
G25.81	Restless Legs Syndrome
	Substance/Medication-Induced Sleep Disorder Note: See the criteria set and corresponding recording procedures for substance-specific codes and ICD-10-CM coding.

Specify whether: Insomnia type, Daytime sleepiness type, Parasomnia type, Mixed type
Specify if: With onset during intoxication, With onset during discontinuation/withdrawal

G47.09	Other Specified Insomnia Disorder
G47.00	Unspecified Insomnia Disorder
G47.19	Other Specified Hypersomno-lence Disorder
G47.10	Unspecified Hypersomnolence Disorder
G47.8	Other Specified Sleep-Wake Disorder
G47.9	Unspecified Sleep-Wake Disorder

Sexual Dysfunctions

The following specifiers apply to Sexual Dysfunctions where indicated:

ª*Specify* whether: Lifelong, Acquired
ᵇ*Specify* whether: Generalized, Situational
ᶜ*Specify* current severity: Mild, Moderate, Severe

F52.32	Delayed Ejaculationª, ᵇ, ᶜ
F52.21	Erectile Disorderª, ᵇ, ᶜ
F52.31	Female Orgasmic Disorderª, ᵇ, ᶜ
	Specify if: Never experienced an orgasm under any situation
F52.22	Female Sexual Interest/Arousal Disorderª, ᵇ, ᶜ
F52.6	Genito-Pelvic Pain/Penetration Disorderª, ᶜ
F52.0	Male Hypoactive Sexual Desire Disorderª, ᵇ, ᶜ
F52.4	Premature (Early) Ejaculationª, ᵇ, ᶜ
	Substance/Medication-Induced Sexual Dysfunctionᶜ
	Note: See the criteria set and corresponding recording procedures for substance-specific codes and ICD-10-CM coding.
	Specify if: With onset during intoxication, With onset during withdrawal, With onset after medication use
F52.8	Other Specified Sexual Dysfunction
F52.9	Unspecified Sexual Dysfunction

Gender Dysphoria

	Gender Dysphoria
F64.2	Gender Dysphoria in Children

Specify if: With a disorder of sex development

F64.1	Gender Dysphoria in Adolescents and Adults

Specify if: With a disorder of sex development
Specify if: Posttransition
Note: Code the disorder of sex development if present, in addition to gender dysphoria.

F64.8	Other Specified Gender Dysphoria
64.9	Unspecified Gender Dysphoria

Disruptive, Impulse-Control, and Conduct Disorders

F91.3	Oppositional Defiant Disorder
	Specify current severity: Mild, Moderate, Severe
F63.81	Intermittent Explosive Disorder Conduct Disorder
	Specify whether:
F91.1	Childhood-onset type
F91.2	Adolescent-onset type
F91.9	Unspecified onset
	Specify if: With limited prosocial emotions
	Specify current severity: Mild, Moderate, Severe
F60.2	Antisocial Personality Disorder
F63.1	Pyromania
F63.2	Kleptomania
F91.8	Other Specified Disruptive, Impulse-Control, and Conduct Disorder
F91.9	Unspecified Disruptive, Impulse-Control, and Conduct Disorder

Substance-Related and Addictive Disorders

The following specifiers and note apply to Substance-Related and Addictive Disorders where indicated:

ª*Specify* if: In early remission, In sustained remission
ᵇ*Specify* if: In a controlled environment
ᶜ*Specify* if: With perceptual disturbances
ᵈThe ICD-10-CM code indicates the comorbid presence of a moderate or severe substance use disorder, which must be present in order to apply the code for substance withdrawal.

Substance-Related Disorders

Alcohol-Related Disorders

	Alcohol Use Disorderª, ᵇ
	Specify current severity:
F10.10	Mild
F10.20	Moderate
F10.20	Severe

	Alcohol Intoxication
F10.129	With use disorder, mild
F10.229	With use disorder, moderate or severe
F10.929	Without use disorder
	Alcohol Withdrawal[c, d]
F10.239	Without perceptual disturbances
F10.232	With perceptual disturbances
	Other Alcohol-Induced Disorders
F10.99	Unspecified Alcohol-Related Disorder

Caffeine-Related Disorders

F15.929	Caffeine Intoxication
F15.93	Caffeine Withdrawal
	Other Caffeine-Induced Disorders
F15.99	Unspecified Caffeine-Related Disorder

Cannabis-Related Disorders

		Cannabis Use Disorder[a, b]
		Specify current severity
	F12.10	Mild
	F12.20	Moderate
	F12.20	Severe
		Cannabis Intoxication[c]
		Without perceptual disturbances
F12.129		With use disorder, mild
F12.229		With use disorder, moderate or severe
F12.929		Without use disorder
		With perceptual disturbances
F12.122		With use disorder, mild
F12.222		With use disorder, moderate or severe
F12.922		Without use disorder
	F12.288	Cannabis Withdrawal[d]
		Other Cannabis-Induced Disorders
	F12.99	Unspecified Cannabis-Related Disorder

Hallucinogen-Related Disorders

	Phencyclidine Use Disorder[a, b]
	Specify current severity:
F16.10	Mild
F16.20	Moderate
F16.20	Severe
	Other Hallucinogen Use Disorder[a, b]
	Specify the particular hallucinogen

	Specify current severity:
F16.10	Mild
F16.20	Moderate
F16.20	Severe
	Phencyclidine Intoxication
F16.129	With use disorder, mild
F16.229	With use disorder, moderate or severe
F16.929	Without use disorder
	Other Hallucinogen Intoxication
F16.129	With use disorder, mild
F16.229	With use disorder, moderate or severe
F16.929	Without use disorder
F16.983	Hallucinogen Persisting Perception Disorder
	Other Phencyclidine-Induced Disorders
	Other Hallucinogen-Induced Disorders
F16.99	Unspecified Phencyclidine-Related Disorder
F16.99	Unspecified Hallucinogen-Related Disorder

Inhalant-Related Disorders

	Inhalant Use Disorder[a, b]
	Specify the particular inhalant
	Specify current severity:
F18.10	Mild
F18.20	Moderate
F18.20	Severe
	Inhalant Intoxication
F18.129	With use disorder, mild
F18.229	With use disorder, moderate or severe
F18.929	Without use disorder
	Other Inhalant-Induced Disorders
F18.99	Unspecified Inhalant-Related Disorder

Opioid-Related Disorders

		Opioid Use Disorder[a]
		Specify if: On maintenance therapy, In a controlled environment
		Specify current severity:
	F11.10	Mild
	F11.20	Moderate
	F11.20	Severe
		Opioid Intoxication[c]
		Without perceptual disturbances
F11.129		With use disorder, mild

F11.229	With use disorder, moderate or severe	
F11.922	Without use disorder	
F11.23	Opioid Withdrawal[d]	
	Other Opioid-Induced Disorders	
F11.99	Unspecified Opioid-Related Disorder	

Sedative-, Hypnotic-, or Anxiolytic-Related Disorders

	Sedative, Hypnotic, or Anxiolytic Use Disorder[a, b]
	Specify current severity:
F13.10	Mild
F13.20	Moderate
F13.20	Severe
	Sedative, Hypnotic, or Anxiolytic Intoxication
F13.129	With use disorder, mild
F13.229	With use disorder, moderate or severe
F13.929	Without use disorder
	Sedative, Hypnotic, or Anxiolytic Withdrawal[c, d]
F13.239	Without perceptual disturbances
F13.232	With perceptual disturbances
	Other Sedative-, Hypnotic-, or Anxiolytic-Induced Disorders
F13.99	Unspecified Sedative-, Hypnotic-, or Anxiolytic-Related Disorder

Stimulant-Related Disorders

	Stimulant Use Disorder[a, b]	
	Specify current severity:	
	Mild	
F15.10		Amphetamine-type substance
F14.10		Cocaine
F15.10		Other or unspecified stimulant
	Moderate	
F15.20		Amphetamine-type substance
F14.20		Cocaine
F15.20		Other or unspecified stimulant
	Severe	
F15.20		Amphetamine-type substance
F14.20		Cocaine
F15.20		Other or unspecified stimulant
	Stimulant Intoxication[c]	

	Specify the specific intoxicant
	Amphetamine or other stimulant, Without perceptual disturbances
F15.129	With use disorder, mild
F15.229	With use disorder, moderate or severe
F15.929	Without use disorder
	Cocaine, Without perceptual disturbances
F14.129	With use disorder, mild
F14.229	With use disorder, moderate or severe
F14.929	Without use disorder
	Amphetamine or other stimulant, With perceptual disturbances
F15.122	With use disorder, mild
F15.222	With use disorder, moderate or severe
F15.922	Without use disorder
	Cocaine, With perceptual disturbances
F14.122	With use disorder, mild
F14.222	With use disorder, moderate or severe
F14.922	Without use disorder
	Stimulant Withdrawal[d]
	Specify the specific substance causing the withdrawal syndrome
F15.23	Amphetamine or other stimulant
F14.23	Cocaine
	Other Stimulant-Induced Disorders
	Unspecified Stimulant-Related Disorder
F15.99	Amphetamine or other stimulant
F14.99	Cocaine

Tobacco-Related Disorders

	Tobacco Use Disorder[a]
	Specify if: On maintenance therapy, In a controlled environment
	Specify current severity:
Z72.0	Mild
F17.200	Moderate
F17.200	Severe
F17.203	Tobacco Withdrawal[d]
	Other Tobacco-Induced Disorders
F17.209	Unspecified Tobacco-Related Disorder

Other (or Unknown) Substance-Related Disorders

	Other (or Unknown) Substance Use Disorder[a, b]
	Specify current severity:
F19.10	Mild
F19.20	Moderate
F19.20	Severe
	Other (or Unknown) Substance Intoxication
F19.129	With use disorder, mild
F19.229	With use disorder, moderate or severe
F19.929	Without use disorder
F19.239	Other (or Unknown) Substance Withdrawal[d]
	Other (or Unknown) Substance-Induced Disorders
F19.99	Unspecified Other (or Unknown) Substance-Related Disorder

Non-Substance-Related Disorders

F63.0	Gambling Disorder[a]
	Specify if: Episodic, Persistent
	Specify current severity: Mild, Moderate, Severe

Neurocognitive Disorders

	Delirium[a]
	Note: See the criteria set and corresponding recording procedures for substance-specific codes and ICD-10-CM coding.
	Specify whether:
	Substance intoxication delirium[a]
	Substance withdrawal delirium[a]
	Medication-induced delirium[a]
F05	Delirium due to another medical condition
F05	Delirium due to multiple etiologies
	Specify if: Acute, Persistent
	Specify if: Hyperactive, Hypoactive, Mixed level of activity
R41.0	Other Specified Delirium
R41.0	Unspecified Delirium

Major and Mild Neurocognitive Disorders

Specify whether due to: Alzheimer's disease, Frontotemporal lobar degeneration, Lewy body disease, Vascular disease, Traumatic brain injury, Substance/medication use, HIV infection, Prion disease, Parkinson's disease, Huntington's disease, Another medical condition, Multiple etiologies, Unspecified

[a]*Specify* Without behavioral disturbance, With behavioral disturbance. For possible major neurocognitive disorder and for mild neurocognitive disorder, behavioral disturbance cannot be coded but should still be indicated in writing.

[b]*Specify* current severity: Mild, Moderate, Severe. This specifier applies only to major neurocognitive disorders (including probable and possible).

Note: As indicated for each subtype, an additional medical code is needed for probable major neurocognitive disorder or major neurocognitive disorder. An additional medical code should *not* be used for possible major neurocognitive disorder or mild neurocognitive disorder.

Major or Mild Neurocognitive Disorder Due to Alzheimer's Disease

	Probable Major Neurocognitive Disorder Due to Alzheimer's Disease[b]
	Note: Code first G30.9 Alzheimer's disease.
F02.81	With behavioral disturbance
F02.80	Without behavioral disturbance
G31.9	Possible Major Neurocognitive Disorder Due to Alzheimer's Disease[a, b]
G31.84	Mild Neurocognitive Disorder Due to Alzheimer's Disease[a]

Major or Mild Frontotemporal Neurocognitive Disorder

	Probable Major Neurocognitive Disorder Due to Frontotemporal Lobar Degeneration[b]
	Note: Code first G31.09 frontotemporal disease.
F02.81	With behavioral disturbance
F02.80	Without behavioral disturbance
G31.9	Possible Major Neurocognitive Disorder Due to Frontotemporal Lobar Degeneration[a, b]
G31.84	Mild Neurocognitive Disorder Due to Frontotemporal Lobar Degeneration[a]

Major or Mild Neurocognitive Disorder With Lewy Bodies

	Probable Major Neurocognitive Disorder With Lewy Bodies[b]
	Note: Code first G31.83 Lewy body disease.
F02.81	With behavioral disturbance
F02.80	Without behavioral disturbance

G31.9   Possible Major Neurocognitive Disorder With Lewy Bodies[a, b]

G31.84   Mild Neurocognitive Disorder With Lewy Bodies[a]

Major or Mild Vascular Neurocognitive Disorder

Probable Major Vascular Neurocognitive Disorder[b]
Note: No additional medical code for vascular disease.

F01.51   With behavioral disturbance

F01.50   Without behavioral disturbance

G31.9   Possible Major Vascular Neurocognitive Disorder[a, b]

G31.84   Mild Vascular Neurocognitive Disorder[a]

Major or Mild Neurocognitive Disorder Due to Traumatic Brain Injury

Major Neurocognitive Disorder Due to Traumatic Brain Injury[b]
Note: For ICD-9-CM, code first 907.0 late effect of intracranial injury without skull fracture. For ICD-10-CM, code first S06.2X9S diffuse traumatic brain injury with loss of consciousness of unspecified duration, sequela.

F02.81   With behavioral disturbance

F02.80   Without behavioral disturbance

G31.84   Mild Neurocognitive Disorder Due to Traumatic Brain Injury[a]

Substance/Medication-Induced Major or Mild Neurocognitive Disorder[a]

Note: No additional medical code. See the criteria set and corresponding recording procedures for substance-specific codes and ICD-10-CM coding.
    Specify if: Persistent

Major or Mild Neurocognitive Disorder Due to HIV Infection

Major Neurocognitive Disorder Due to HIV Infection[b]
Note: Code first B20 HIV infection.

F02.81   With behavioral disturbance

F02.80   Without behavioral disturbance

G31.84   Mild Neurocognitive Disorder Due to HIV Infection[a]

Major or Mild Neurocognitive Disorder Due to Prion Disease

Major Neurocognitive Disorder Due to Prion Disease[b]
Note: Code first A81.9 prion disease.

F02.81   With behavioral disturbance

F02.80   Without behavioral disturbance

G31.84   Mild Neurocognitive Disorder Due to Prion Disease[a]

Major or Mild Neurocognitive Disorder Due to Parkinson's Disease

Major Neurocognitive Disorder Probably Due to Parkinson's Disease[b]
Note: Code first 332.0 (G20) Parkinson's disease.

F02.81   With behavioral disturbance

F02.80   Without behavioral disturbance

G31.9   Major Neurocognitive Disorder Possibly Due to Parkinson's Disease[a, b]

G31.84   Mild Neurocognitive Disorder Due to Parkinson's Disease[a]

Major or Mild Neurocognitive Disorder Due to Huntington's Disease

Major Neurocognitive Disorder Due to Huntington's Disease[b]
Note: Code first G10 Huntington's disease.

F02.81   With behavioral disturbance

F02.80   Without behavioral disturbance

G31.84   Mild Neurocognitive Disorder Due to Huntington's Disease[a]

Major or Mild Neurocognitive Disorder Due to Another Medical Condition

Major Neurocognitive Disorder Due to Another Medical Condition[b]
Note: Code first the other medical condition.

F02.81   With behavioral disturbance

F02.80   Without behavioral disturbance

G31.84   Mild Neurocognitive Disorder Due to Another Medical Condition[a]

Major or Mild Neurocognitive Disorder Due to Multiple Etiologies

	Major Neurocognitive Disorder Due to Multiple Etiologies[b] Note: Code first all the etiological medical conditions (with the exception of vascular disease).
F02.81	With behavioral disturbance
F02.80	Without behavioral disturbance
G31.84	Mild Neurocognitive Disorder Due to Multiple Etiologies[a]

Unspecified Neurocognitive Disorder

R41.9	Unspecified Neurocognitive Disorder[a]

Personality Disorders

Cluster A Personality Disorders

F60.0	Paranoid Personality Disorder
F60.1	Schizoid Personality Disorder
F21	Schizotypal Personality Disorder

Cluster B Personality Disorders

F60.2	Antisocial Personality Disorder
F60.3	Borderline Personality Disorder
F60.4	Histrionic Personality Disorder
F60.81	Narcissistic Personality Disorder

Cluster C Personality Disorders

F60.6	Avoidant Personality Disorder
F60.7	Dependent Personality Disorder
F60.5	Obsessive-Compulsive Personality Disorder

Other Personality Disorders

F07.0	Personality Change Due to Another Medical Condition *Specify* whether: Labile type, Disinhibited type, Aggressive type, Apathetic type, Paranoid type, Other type, Combined type, Unspecified type
F60.89	Other Specified Personality Disorder
F60.9	Unspecified Personality Disorder

Paraphilic Disorders

The following specifier applies to Paraphilic Disorders where indicated:

   [a]*Specify* if: In a controlled environment, In full remission

F65.3	Voyeuristic Disorder[a]
F65.2	Exhibitionistic Disorder[a]

	Specify whether: Sexually aroused by exposing genitals to prepubertal children, Sexually aroused by exposing genitals to physically mature individuals, Sexually aroused by exposing genitals to prepubertal children and to physically mature individuals.
F65.81	Frotteuristic Disorder[a]
F65.51	Sexual Masochism Disorder[a] *Specify* if: With asphyxiophilia
F65.52	Sexual Sadism Disorder[a]
F65.4	Pedophilic Disorder *Specify* whether: Exclusive type, Nonexclusive type *Specify* if: Sexually attracted to males, Sexually attracted to females, Sexually attracted to both *Specify* if: Limited to incest
F65.0	Fetishistic Disorder[a] *Specify*: Body part(s), Nonliving object(s), Other

Other Mental Disorders

F06.8	Other Specified Mental Disorder Due to Another Medical Condition
F09	Unspecified Mental Disorder Due to Another Medical Condition
F99	Other Specified Mental Disorder
F99	Unspecified Mental Disorder

Medication-Induced Movement Disorders and Other Adverse Effects of Medication

G21.11	Neuroleptic-Induced Parkinsonism
G21.19	Other Medication-Induced Parkinsonism
G21.0	Neuroleptic Malignant Syndrome
G24.02	Medication-Induced Acute Dystonia
G25.71	Medication-Induced Acute Akathisia
G24.01	Tardive Dyskinesia
G24.09	Tardive Dystonia
G25.71	Tardive Akathisia
G25.1	Medication-Induced Postural Tremor

G25.79	Other Medication-Induced Movement Disorder Antidepressant Discontinuation Syndrome
T43.205A	Initial encounter
T43.205D	Subsequent encounter
T43.205S	Sequelae
	Other Adverse Effect of Medication
T50.905A	Initial encounter
T50.905D	Subsequent encounter
T50.905S	Sequelae

Other Conditions That May Be a Focus of Clinical Attention

Relational Problems

Problems Related to Family Upbringing

Z62.820	Parent-Child Relational Problem
Z62.891	Sibling Relational Problem
Z62.29	Upbringing Away From Parents
Z62.898	Child Affected by Parental Relationship Distress

Other Problems Related to Primary Support Group

Z63.0	Relationship Distress With Spouse or Intimate Partner
Z63.5	Disruption of Family by Separation or Divorce
Z63.8	High Expressed Emotion Level Within Family
Z63.4	Uncomplicated Bereavement

Abuse and Neglect

Child Maltreatment and Neglect Problems

Child Physical Abuse, Confirmed

T74.12XA	Initial encounter
T74.12XD	Subsequent encounter

Child Physical Abuse, Suspected

T76.12XA	Initial encounter
T76.12XD	Subsequent encounter

Other Circumstances Related to Child Physical Abuse

Z69.010	Encounter for mental health services for victim of child abuse by parent
Z69.020	Encounter for mental health services for victim of non-parental child abuse
Z62.810	Personal history (past history) of physical abuse in childhood
Z69.011	Encounter for mental health services for perpetrator of parental child abuse

Z69.021	Encounter for mental health services for perpetrator of nonparental child abuse
F65.1	Transvestic Disorder[a] *Specify* if: With fetishism, With autogynephilia
F65.89	Other Specified Paraphilic Disorder
F65.9	Unspecified Paraphilic Disorder

Child Sexual Abuse, Confirmed

T74.22XA	Initial encounter
T74.22XD	Subsequent encounter

Child Sexual Abuse, Suspected

T76.22XA	Initial encounter
T76.22XD	Subsequent encounter

Other Circumstances Related to Child Sexual Abuse

Z69.010	Encounter for mental health services for victim of child sexual abuse by parent
Z69.020	Encounter for mental health services for victim of non-parental child sexual abuse
Z62.810	Personal history (past history) of sexual abuse in childhood
Z69.011	Encounter for mental health services for perpetrator of parental child sexual abuse
Z69.021	Encounter for mental health services for perpetrator of non-parental child sexual abuse

Child Neglect, Confirmed

T74.02XA	Initial encounter
T74.02XD	Subsequent encounter

Child Neglect, Suspected

T76.02XA	Initial encounter
T76.02XD	Subsequent encounter

Other Circumstances Related to Child Neglect

Z69.010	Encounter for mental health services for victim of child neglect by parent
Z69.020	Encounter for mental health services for victim of non-parental child neglect
Z62.812	Personal history (past history) of neglect in childhood
Z69.011	Encounter for mental health services for perpetrator of parental child neglect

Z69.021	Encounter for mental health services for perpetrator of non-parental child neglect

Child Psychological Abuse, Confirmed

T74.32XA	Initial encounter
T74.32XD	Subsequent encounter

Child Psychological Abuse, Suspected

T76.32XA	Initial encounter
T76.32XD	Subsequent encounter

Other Circumstances Related to Child Psychological Abuse

Z69.010	Encounter for mental health services for victim of child psychological abuse by parent
Z69.020	Encounter for mental health services for victim of non-parental child psychological abuse
Z62.811	Personal history (past history) of psychological abuse in childhood
Z69.011	Encounter for mental health services for perpetrator of parental child psychological abuse
Z69.021	Encounter for mental health services for perpetrator of nonparental child psychological abuse

Adult Maltreatment and Neglect Problems

Spouse or Partner Violence, Physical, Confirmed

T74.11XA	Initial encounter
T74.11XD	Subsequent encounter

Spouse or Partner Violence, Physical, Suspected

T76.11XA	Initial encounter
T76.11XD	Subsequent encounter

Other Circumstances Related to Spouse or Partner Violence, Physical

Z69.11	Encounter for mental health services for victim of spouse or partner violence, physical
Z91.410	Personal history (past history) of spouse or partner violence, physical
Z69.12	Encounter for mental health services for perpetrator of spouse or partner violence, physical

Spouse or Partner Violence, Sexual, Confirmed

T74.21XA	Initial encounter
T74.21XD	Subsequent encounter

Spouse or Partner Violence, Sexual, Suspected

T76.21XA	Initial encounter
T76.21XD	Subsequent encounter

Other Circumstances Related to Spouse or Partner Violence, Sexual

Z69.81	Encounter for mental health services for victim of spouse or partner violence, sexual
Z91.410	Personal history (past history) of spouse or partner violence, sexual
Z69.12	Encounter for mental health services for perpetrator of spouse or partner violence, sexual

Spouse or Partner Neglect, Confirmed

T74.01XA	Initial encounter
T74.01XD	Subsequent encounter

Spouse or Partner Neglect, Suspected

T76.01XA	Initial encounter
T76.01XD	Subsequent encounter

Other Circumstances Related to Spouse or Partner Neglect

Z69.11	Encounter for mental health services for victim of spouse or partner neglect
Z91.412	Personal history (past history) of spouse or partner neglect
Z69.12	Encounter for mental health services for perpetrator of spouse or partner neglect

Spouse or Partner Abuse, Psychological, Confirmed

T74.31XA	Initial encounter
T74.31XD	Subsequent encounter

Spouse or Partner Abuse, Psychological, Suspected

T76.31XA	Initial encounter
T76.31XD	Subsequent encounter

Other Circumstances Related to Spouse or Partner Abuse, Psychological

Z69.11	Encounter for mental health services for victim of spouse or partner psychological abuse
Z91.411	Personal history (past history) of spouse or partner psychological abuse

Z69.12	Encounter for mental health services for perpetrator of spouse or partner psychological abuse

Adult Physical Abuse by Nonspouse or Nonpartner, Confirmed

T74.11XA	Initial encounter
T74.11XD	Subsequent encounter

Adult Physical Abuse by Nonspouse or Nonpartner, Suspected

T76.11XA	Initial encounter
T76.11XD	Subsequent encounter

Adult Sexual Abuse by Nonspouse or Nonpartner, Confirmed

T74.21XA	Initial encounter
T74.21XD	Subsequent encounter

Adult Sexual Abuse by Nonspouse or Nonpartner, Suspected

T76.21XA	Initial encounter
T76.21XD	Subsequent encounter

Adult Psychological Abuse by Nonspouse or Nonpartner, Confirmed

T74.31XA	Initial encounter
T74.31XD	Subsequent encounter

Adult Psychological Abuse by Nonspouse or Nonpartner, Suspected

T76.31XA	Initial encounter
T76.31XD	Subsequent encounter

Other Circumstances Related to Adult Abuse by Nonspouse or Nonpartner

Z69.81	Encounter for mental health services for victim of nonspousal adult abuse
Z69.82	Encounter for mental health services for perpetrator of nonspousal adult abuse

Educational and Occupational Problems

Educational Problems

Z55.9	Academic or Educational Problem

Occupational Problems

Z56.82	Problem Related to Current Military Deployment Status
Z56.9	Other Problem Related to Employment

Housing and Economic Problems

Housing Problems

Z59.0	Homelessness
Z59.1	Inadequate Housing
Z59.2	Discord With Neighbor, Lodger, or Landlord
Z59.3	Problem Related to Living in a Residential Institution

Economic Problems

Z59.4	Lack of Adequate Food or Safe Drinking Water
Z59.5	Extreme Poverty
Z59.6	Low Income
Z59.7	Insufficient Social Insurance or Welfare Support
Z59.9	Unspecified Housing or Economic Problem

Other Problems Related to the Social Environment

Z60.0	Phase of Life Problem
Z60.2	Problem Related to Living Alone
Z60.3	Acculturation Difficulty
Z60.4	Social Exclusion or Rejection
Z60.5	Target of (Perceived) Adverse Discrimination or Persecution
Z60.9	Unspecified Problem Related to Social Environment

Problems Related to Crime or Interaction With the Legal System

Z65.4	Victim of Crime
Z65.0	Conviction in Civil or Criminal Proceedings Without Imprisonment
Z65.1	Imprisonment or Other Incarceration
Z65.2	Problems Related to Release From Prison
Z65.3	Problems Related to Other Legal Circumstances

Other Health Service Encounters for Counseling and Medical Advice

Z70.9	Sex Counseling
Z71.9	Other Counseling or Consultation

Problems Related to Other Psychosocial, Personal, and Environmental Circumstances

Z65.8	Religious or Spiritual Problem
Z64.0	Problems Related to Unwanted Pregnancy

Z64.1	Problems Related to Multiparity
Z64.4	Discord With Social Service Provider, Including Probation Officer, Case Manager, or Social Services Worker
Z65.4	Victim of Terrorism or Torture
Z65.5	Exposure to Disaster, War, or Other Hostilities
Z65.8	Other Problem Related to Psychosocial Circumstances
Z65.9	Unspecified Problem Related to Unspecified Psychosocial Circumstances

Other Circumstances of Personal History

Z91.49	Other Personal History of Psychological Trauma
Z91.5	Personal History of Self-Harm
Z91.82	Personal History of Military Deployment
Z91.89	Other Personal Risk Factors

Z72.9	Problem Related to Lifestyle
Z72.811	Adult Antisocial Behavior
Z72.810	Child or Adolescent Antisocial Behavior

Problems Related to Access to Medical and Other Health Care

| Z75.3 | Unavailability or Inaccessibility of Health Care Facilities |
| Z75.4 | Unavailability or Inaccessibility of Other Helping Agencies |

Nonadherence to Medical Treatment

Z91.19	Nonadherence to Medical Treatment
E66.9	Overweight or Obesity
Z76.5	Malingering
Z91.83	Wandering Associated With a Mental Disorder
R41.83	Borderline Intellectual Functioning

Appendix E

Assigning NANDA International Nursing Diagnoses to Client Behaviors

Following is a list of client behaviors and the NANDA-I nursing diagnoses that correspond to the behaviors and that may be used in planning care for the client exhibiting the specific behavioral symptoms.

BEHAVIORS	NANDA-I NURSING DIAGNOSES
Aggression; hostility	Risk for injury; Risk for other-directed violence
Anorexia or refusal to eat	Imbalanced nutrition: Less than body requirements
Anxious behavior	Anxiety (Specify level)
Confusion; memory loss	Confusion (acute/chronic); Impaired memory; Disturbed thought processes*
Delusions	Disturbed thought processes*
Denial of problems	Ineffective denial
Depressed mood or anger turned inward	Complicated grieving; Risk for self-directed violence
Detoxification; withdrawal from substances	Risk for injury
Difficulty accepting new diagnosis or recent change in health status	Risk-prone health behavior
Difficulty making important life decision	Decisional conflict
Difficulty sleeping	Insomnia; Disturbed sleep pattern
Difficulty with interpersonal relationships	Impaired social interaction; Ineffective relationship
Disruption in capability to perform usual responsibilities	Ineffective role performance
Dissociative behaviors (depersonalization; derealization)	Disturbed sensory perception (kinesthetic)*
Expresses feelings of disgust about body or body part	Disturbed body image
Expresses anger at God	Spiritual distress
Expresses lack of control over personal situation	Powerlessness
Fails to follow prescribed therapy	Ineffective health management; Noncompliance
Flashbacks, nightmares, obsession with traumatic experience	Post-trauma syndrome
Hallucinations	Disturbed sensory perception (auditory; visual)*
Highly critical of self or others	Low self-esteem (chronic; situational)
HIV positive; altered immunity	Ineffective protection; Risk for infection
Inability to meet basic needs	Self-care deficit (feeding; bathing; dressing; toileting); Impaired home maintenance; Self-neglect
Loose associations or flight of ideas	Impaired verbal communication

BEHAVIORS	NANDA-I NURSING DIAGNOSES
Loss of a valued entity, recently experienced	Risk for complicated grieving
Manic hyperactivity	Risk for injury; Insomnia; Sleep deprivation
Manipulative behavior	Ineffective coping
Multiple personalities	Disturbed personal identity
Orgasm, problems with; lack of sexual desire; erectile dysfunction	Sexual dysfunction
Overeating, compulsive	Risk for overweight; Overweight; or Obesity
Phobias	Fear; Ineffective coping
Physical symptoms as coping behavior	Ineffective coping
Potential or anticipated loss of significant entity	Risk for complicated grieving
Projection of blame; rationalization of failures; denial of personal responsibility	Defensive coping
Ritualistic behaviors	Anxiety (severe); Ineffective coping
Seductive remarks; inappropriate sexual behaviors	Impaired social interaction
Self-inflicted injuries (non-life-threatening)	Self-mutilation; Risk for self-mutilation
Sexual behaviors (difficulty, limitations, or changes in; reported dissatisfaction)	Ineffective sexuality pattern
Stress from caring for chronically ill person	Caregiver role strain
Stress from locating to new environment	Relocation stress syndrome
Substance use as a coping behavior	Ineffective coping
Substance use (denies use is a problem)	Ineffective denial
Suicidal gestures/threats; suicidal ideation	Risk for suicide; Risk for self-directed violence
Suspiciousness	Ineffective coping; Disturbed thought processes*
Vomiting, excessive, self-induced	Risk for deficient fluid volume; Risk for electrolyte imbalance
Withdrawn behavior	Social isolation

*These diagnoses have been resigned from the NANDA-I list of approved nursing diagnoses.

Glossary

A

abandonment. A unilateral severance of the professional relationship between a health-care provider and a client without reasonable notice at a time when there is still a need for continuing health care.

abreaction. "Remembering with feeling"; bringing into conscious awareness painful events that have been repressed, and reexperiencing the emotions that were associated with the events.

abuse. To use wrongfully or in a harmful way. Improper treatment or conduct that may result in injury.

acculturation. The cultural modification of a group or individual through borrowing traits of another culture, often through prolonged contact.

acupoints. In Chinese medicine, acupoints represent areas along the body that link pathways of healing energy.

acupressure. A technique in which the fingers, thumbs, palms, or elbows are used to apply pressure to certain points along the body. This pressure is thought to dissolve any obstructions in the flow of healing energy and to restore the body to a healthier functioning.

acupuncture. A technique in which hair-thin, sterile, disposable, stainless-steel needles are inserted into points along the body to dissolve obstructions in the flow of healing energy and restore the body to a healthier functioning.

adaptation. Restoration of the body to homeostasis following a physiological and/or psychological response to stress.

adaptive responses. Behaviors that contribute to maintaining an individual's health and integrity.

addiction. A compulsive or chronic requirement. The need is so strong as to generate distress (either physical or psychological) if left unfulfilled.

adjustment. The process of modifying one's behavior in changed circumstances or an altered environment in order to fulfill psychological, physiological, and social needs.

adjustment disorder. A maladaptive reaction to an identifiable psychosocial stressor that occurs within 3 months after onset of the stressor. The individual shows impairment in social and occupational functioning or exhibits symptoms that are in excess of a normal and expectable reaction to the stressor.

advance directive. A legal document that a competent individual may sign to convey wishes regarding future health-care decisions intended for a time when the individual is no longer capable of informed consent. It may include one or both of the following: (1) a living will, in which the individual identifies the type of care that he or she does or does not wish to have performed, and (2) a durable power of attorney for health care, in which the individual names another person who is given the right to make health-care decisions for the individual who is incapable of doing so.

advocacy. The act of pleading for, supporting, or representing a cause or individual. Advocacy in nursing applies to any act in which the nurse is serving in the best interests of the patient, from simple procedures such as hand washing to protect the patient from infection to complex ethically and morally charged issues in which certain clients are unable to advocate for themselves. Nurses also advocate for their patients indirectly by serving in organizations that support and serve to improve health care for all individuals, and by participating in policy-making legislation that affects health care of the public.

affect. The behavioral expression of emotion; may be appropriate (congruent with the situation); inappropriate (incongruent with the situation); constricted or blunted (diminished range and intensity); or flat (absence of emotional expression).

affective domain. A category of learning that includes attitudes, feelings, and values.

aggression. Harsh physical or verbal actions intended (either consciously or unconsciously) to harm or injure another.

aggressiveness. Behavior that defends an individual's own basic rights by violating the basic rights of others (as contrasted with **assertiveness**).

agoraphobia. The fear of being in places or situations from which escape might be difficult (or embarrassing) or in which help might not be available in the event of a panic attack.

agranulocytosis. Extremely low levels of white blood cells. Symptoms include sore throat, fever, and malaise. This may be a side effect of long-term therapy with some antipsychotic medications.

akathisia. Restlessness; an urgent need for movement. A type of extrapyramidal side effect associated with some antipsychotic medications.

akinesia. Muscular weakness; or a loss or partial loss of muscle movement; a type of extrapyramidal side effect associated with some antipsychotic medications.

Alcoholics Anonymous (AA). A major self-help organization for the treatment of alcoholism. It is based on a 12-step program to help members attain and maintain sobriety. Once individuals have achieved sobriety, they in turn are expected to help other alcoholic persons.

allopathic medicine. Traditional medicine. The type traditionally, and currently, practiced in the United States and taught in U.S. medical schools.

alternative medicine. Practices that differ from usual traditional (allopathic) medicine.

altruism. One therapeutic factor of group therapy (identified by Yalom) in which individuals gain self-esteem through mutual sharing and concern. Providing assistance and support to others creates a positive self-image and promotes self-growth.

altruistic suicide. Suicide that occurs in response to the expectations of a group to which an individual is excessively integrated.

amenorrhea. Cessation of the menses; may be a side effect of some antipsychotic medications.

amnesia. An inability to recall important personal information that is too extensive to be explained by ordinary forgetfulness.

amnesia, generalized. The inability to recall anything that has happened during the individual's entire lifetime.

amnesia, localized. The inability to recall all incidents associated with a traumatic event for a specific time period following the event.

amnesia, selective. The inability to recall only certain incidents associated with a traumatic event for a specific time period following the event.

amphetamine. A racemic sympathomimetic amine that acts as a central nervous system stimulant. It (and its derivatives, such as methamphetamine and dextroamphetamine) is a commonly abused substance, but has therapeutic use in the treatment of narcolepsy and attention-deficit/hyperactivity disorder.

andropause. A term used to identify the male climacteric. Also called *male menopause.* A syndrome of symptoms related to the decline of testosterone levels in men. Some symptoms include depression, weight gain, insomnia, hot flashes, decreased libido, mood swings, decreased strength, and erectile dysfunction.

anger. An emotional response to one's perception of a situation. Anger has both positive and negative functions.

anger management. The use of various techniques and strategies to control responses to anger-provoking situations. The goal of anger management is to reduce both the emotional feelings and the physiological arousal that anger engenders.

anhedonia. The inability to experience or even imagine any pleasant emotion.

anomic suicide. Suicide that occurs in response to changes that occur in an individual's life that disrupt cohesiveness from a group and cause that person to feel without support from the formerly cohesive group.

anorexia. Loss of appetite.

anorexiants. Drugs that suppress appetite.

anorgasmia. Inability to achieve orgasm.

anosmia. Inability to smell.

anosognosia. An individual's lack of awareness of having any illness or disorder even when symptoms appear obvious to others.

anticipatory grief. A subjective state of emotional, physical, and social responses to an anticipated loss of a valued entity. The grief response is repeated once the loss actually occurs, but it may not be as intense as it might have been if anticipatory grieving has not occurred.

antisocial personality disorder. A pattern of socially irresponsible, exploitative, and guiltless behavior, evident in the tendency to fail to conform to the law, develop stable relationships, or sustain consistent employment; exploitation and manipulation of others for personal gain is common.

anxiety. Vague diffuse apprehension that is associated with feelings of uncertainty and helplessness.

aphasia. Inability to communicate through speech, writing, or signs, caused by dysfunction of brain centers.

aphonia. Inability to speak.

apraxia. Inability to carry out motor activities despite intact motor function.

arbitrary inference. A type of thinking error in which the individual automatically comes to a conclusion about an incident without the facts to support it, or even sometimes despite contradictory evidence to support it.

ascites. Excessive accumulation of serous fluid in the abdominal cavity, occurring in response to portal hypertension caused by cirrhosis of the liver.

assault. An act that results in a person's genuine fear and apprehension that he or she will be touched without consent. Nurses may be guilty of assault for threatening to place an individual in restraints against his or her will.

assertive behavior. Behavior that enables individuals to act in their own best interests, to stand up for themselves without undue anxiety, to express their honest feelings comfortably, or to exercise their own rights without denying those of others.

assessment. A systematic process of collecting and analyzing data relevant to planning, providing, and evaluating patient care. Assessment may include several dimensions of the client's history and present functioning including physical, emotional, cognitive, social, sexual, cultural, environmental, occupational, and spiritual.

assimilation. The process by which a minority individual or group adapts to the cultural norms of the majority culture.

ataxia. Muscular incoordination.

attachment theory. The hypothesis that individuals who maintain close relationships with others into old age are more likely to remain independent and less likely to be institutionalized than those who do not.

attention-deficit/hyperactivity disorder. A disorder that is characterized by a persistent pattern of inattention and/or hyperactivity and impulsivity, or both. Motor activity is excessive, and the ability to concentrate is impaired.

attitude. A frame of reference around which an individual organizes knowledge about his or her world. It includes an emotional element and can have a positive or negative connotation.

autism. A focus inward on a fantasy world, while distorting or excluding the external environment; common in schizophrenia.

autism spectrum disorder. A disorder that is characterized by impairment in social interaction skills and interpersonal communication, and a restricted repertoire of activities and interests.

autocratic. A leadership style in which the leader makes all decisions for the group. Productivity is very high with this type of leadership, but morale is often low because of the lack of member input and creativity.

autoimmunity. A condition in which the body produces a disordered immunological response against itself. In this situation, the body fails to differentiate between what is normal and what is a foreign substance. When this occurs, the body produces antibodies against normal parts of the body to such an extent as to cause tissue injury.

automatic thoughts. Thoughts that occur rapidly in response to a situation, and without rational analysis. They are often negative and based on erroneous logic.

autonomy. Independence; self-governance. An ethical principle that emphasizes the status of persons as autonomous moral agents whose right to determine their destinies should always be respected.

aversive stimulus. A stimulus that follows a behavioral response and decreases the probability that the behavior will recur; also called punishment.

axon. The cellular process of a neuron that carries impulses away from the cell body.

B

battering. A pattern of repeated physical assault, usually of a woman by her spouse or intimate partner. Men are also battered, although this occurs much less frequently.

battery. The unconsented touching of another person. Nurses may be charged with battery should they participate in the treatment of a client without his or her consent and outside of an emergency situation.

behavior modification. A treatment modality aimed at changing undesirable behaviors, using a system of reinforcement to bring about the modifications desired.

behavior therapy. A form of psychotherapy, the goal of which is to modify maladaptive behavior patterns by reinforcing more adaptive behaviors.

behavioral objectives. Statements that indicate to an individual what is expected of him or her. Behavioral objectives are a way of measuring learning outcomes, and are based on the affective, cognitive, and psychomotor domains of learning.

belief. A belief is an idea that one holds to be true. It can be rational, irrational, taken on faith, or a stereotypical idea.

beneficence. An ethical principle that refers to one's duty to benefit or promote the good of others.

bereavement overload. An accumulation of grief that occurs when an individual experiences many losses over a short period of time and is unable to resolve one before another is experienced. This phenomenon is common among the elderly.

binge and purge. A syndrome associated with eating disorders, especially bulimia nervosa, in which an individual consumes thousands of calories of food at one sitting, and then purges through the use of laxatives or self-induced vomiting.

bioethics. The term used with ethical principles that refer to concepts within the scope of medicine, nursing, and allied health.

biofeedback. The use of instrumentation to become aware of processes in the body that usually go unnoticed and to bring them under voluntary control (e.g., the blood pressure or pulse); used as a method of stress reduction.

bipolar disorder. Characterized by mood swings from profound depression to extreme euphoria (mania), with intervening periods of normalcy. Psychotic symptoms may or may not be present.

body image. One's perception of his or her own body. It may also be how one believes others perceive his or her body. (See also **physical self.**)

borderline personality disorder. A disorder characterized by a pattern of intense and chaotic relationships, with affective instability, fluctuating and extreme attitudes regarding other people, impulsivity, direct and indirect self-destructive behavior, and lack of a clear or certain sense of identity, life plan, or values.

boundaries. The level of participation and interaction between individuals and between subsystems. Boundaries denote physical and psychological space individuals identify as their own. They are sometimes referred to as limits. Boundaries are appropriate when they permit appropriate contact with others while preventing excessive interference. Boundaries may be clearly defined (healthy) or rigid or diffuse (unhealthy).

bulimia. Excessive, insatiable appetite.

C

cachexia. A state of ill health, malnutrition, and wasting; extreme emaciation.

cannabis. The dried flowering tops of the hemp plant. It produces euphoric effects when ingested or smoked and is commonly used in the form of marijuana or hashish.

carcinogen. Any substance or agent that produces or increases the risk of developing cancer in humans or lower animals.

case management. A health-care delivery process, the goals of which are to provide quality health care, decrease fragmentation, enhance the client's quality of life, and contain costs. A case manager coordinates the client's care from admission to discharge and sometimes following discharge. Critical pathways of care are the tools used for the provision of care in a case management system.

case manager. The individual responsible for negotiating with multiple health-care providers to obtain a variety of services for a client.

catastrophic thinking. Always thinking that the worst will occur without considering the possibility of more likely, positive outcomes.

catatonia. A type of psychological disturbance that is typified by stupor or excitement. Stupor is characterized by extreme psychomotor retardation, mutism, negativism, and posturing; excitement by psychomotor agitation, in which the movements are frenzied and purposeless. Catatonic symptoms may be associated with other mental or physical disorders.

catharsis. One therapeutic factor of group therapy (identified by Yalom), in which members in a group can express both positive and negative feelings in a nonthreatening atmosphere.

cell body. The part of the neuron that contains the nucleus and is essential for the continued life of the neuron.

Centers for Medicare and Medicaid Services (CMS). The division of the U.S. Department of Health and Human Services responsible for Medicare funding.

child sexual abuse. Any sexual act, such as indecent exposure or improper touching to penetration (sexual intercourse), that is carried out with a child.

chiropractic medicine. A system of alternative medicine based on the premise that the relationship between structure and function in the human body is a significant health factor and that such relationships between the spinal column and the nervous system are important because the normal transmission and expression of nerve energy are essential to the restoration and maintenance of health.

Christian ethics. The ethical philosophy that states one should treat others as moral equals, and recognize the equality of other persons by permitting them to act as we do when they occupy a position similar to ours; sometimes referred to as "the ethic of the golden rule."

circadian rhythm. A 24-hour biological rhythm controlled by a "pacemaker" in the brain that sends messages to other systems in the body. Circadian rhythm influences various regulatory functions, including the sleep-wake cycle, body temperature regulation, patterns of activity such as eating and drinking, and hormonal and neurotransmitter secretion.

circumstantiality. In speaking, the delay of an individual to reach the point of a communication, owing to unnecessary and tedious details.

civil law. Law that protects the private and property rights of individuals and businesses.

clang association. A pattern of speech in which the choice of words is governed by sounds. Clang associations often take the form of rhyming.

classical conditioning. A type of learning that occurs when an unconditioned stimulus (UCS) that produces an unconditioned response (UCR) is paired with a conditioned stimulus (CS), until the CS alone produces the same response, which is then called a conditioned response (CR). Pavlov's example: food (i.e., UCS) causes salivation (i.e., UCR); ringing bell (i.e., CS) with food (i.e., UCS) causes salivation (i.e., UCR), ringing bell alone (i.e., CS) causes salivation (i.e., CR).

codependency. An exaggerated dependent pattern of learned behaviors, beliefs, and feelings that make life painful. It is a dependence on people and things outside the self, along with neglect of the self to the point of having little self-identity.

cognition. Mental operations that relate to logic, awareness, intellect, memory, language, and reasoning powers.

cognitive. Relating to the mental processes of thinking and reasoning.

cognitive development. A series of stages described by Piaget through which individuals progress, demonstrating at each successive stage a higher level of logical organization than at each previous stage.

cognitive domain. A category of learning that involves knowledge and thought processes within the individual's intellectual ability. The individual must be able to synthesize information at an intellectual level before the actual behaviors are performed.

cognitive maturity. The capability to perform all mental operations needed for adulthood.

cognitive therapy. A type of therapy in which the individual is taught to control thought distortions that are considered to be a factor in the development and maintenance of emotional disorders.

collectivist culture. A culture that values close dependence on and interconnectedness with family and tribe. AI/AN groups are collectivist cultures.

colposcope. An instrument that contains a magnifying lens and to which a 35-mm camera can be attached. A colposcope is used to examine for tears and abrasions inside the vaginal area of a sexual assault victim.

common law. Laws that are derived from decisions made in previous cases.

communication. An interactive process of transmitting information between two or more entities.

community. A group of people living close to and depending to some extent on each other.

compensation. An ego defense mechanism in which an individual covers up a real or perceived weakness by emphasizing a trait one considers more desirable.

complementary medicine. Practices that differ from usual traditional (allopathic) medicine, but may in fact supplement it in a positive way.

compounded rape reaction. Symptoms that are in addition to the typical rape response of physical complaints, rage, humiliation, fear, and sleep disturbances. They include depression and suicide, substance abuse, and even psychotic behaviors.

compulsions. Unwanted repetitive behavior patterns or mental acts (e.g., praying, counting, repeating words silently) that are intended to reduce anxiety, not to provide pleasure or gratification (APA, 2013). They may be performed in response to an obsession or in a stereotyped fashion.

concept mapping. A diagrammatic teaching and learning strategy that allows students and faculty to visualize interrelationships between medical diagnoses, nursing diagnoses, assessment data, and treatments. A diagram of client problems and interventions.

concrete thinking. Thought processes that are focused on specifics rather than on generalities and immediate issues rather than eventual outcomes. Individuals who are experiencing concrete thinking are unable to comprehend abstract terminology.

conditioned response. In classical conditioning, a response that is a *learned* response (not reflexive) following repeated exposure to a target stimulus.

conditioned stimulus. In classical conditioning, an unrelated stimulus that is presented to a subject with a target stimulus, and that, with repeated exposure, comes to elicit the same response as the original target stimulus.

confabulation. Creating imaginary events to fill in memory gaps.

confidentiality. The right of an individual to the assurance that his or her case will not be discussed outside the boundaries of the health-care team.

contextual stimuli. Conditions present in the environment that support a focal stimulus and influence a threat to self-esteem.

contingency contracting. A written contract between individuals used to modify behavior. Benefits and consequences for fulfilling the terms of the contract are delineated.

controlled response pattern. The response to rape in which feelings are masked or hidden, and a calm, composed, or subdued affect is seen.

counselor. One who listens as the client reviews feelings related to difficulties he or she is experiencing in any aspect of life; one of the nursing roles identified by H. Peplau.

countertransference. In psychoanalytic theory, countertransference refers to the counselor's behavioral and emotional response to the client. These responses may be related to unresolved feelings toward significant others from the counselor's past, or they may be generated in response to the client's behavior toward the counselor.

covert sensitization. An aversion technique used to modify behavior that relies on the individual's imagination to produce unpleasant symptoms. When the individual is about to succumb to undesirable behavior, he or she visualizes something that is offensive or even nauseating in an effort to block the behavior.

criminal law. Law that provides protection from conduct deemed injurious to the public welfare. It provides for punishment of those found to have engaged in such conduct.

crisis. Psychological disequilibrium in a person who confronts a hazardous circumstance that constitutes an important problem which for the time he or she can neither escape nor solve with usual problem-solving resources.

crisis intervention. An emergency type of assistance in which the intervener becomes a part of the individual's life situation. The focus is to provide guidance and support to help mobilize the resources needed to resolve the crisis and restore or generate an improvement in previous level of functioning. Usually lasts no longer than 6 to 8 weeks.

critical pathways of care. An abbreviated plan of care that provides outcome-based guidelines for goal achievement within a designated length of time.

cultural syndromes. Medical and psychiatric symptoms that are specific to a cultural group and do not share an exact correlation to any *DSM-5* diagnostic category.

culture. A particular society's entire way of living, encompassing shared patterns of belief, feeling, and knowledge that guide people's conduct and are passed down from generation to generation.

curandera. A female folk healer in Latino culture.

curandero. A male folk healer in Latino culture.

cycle of battering. Three phases of predictable behaviors that are repeated over time in a relationship between a batterer and a victim: tension-building phase; the acute battering incident; and the calm, loving, respite (honeymoon) phase.

cyclothymic disorder. A chronic mood disturbance involving numerous episodes of hypomania and depressed mood, of insufficient severity or duration to meet the criteria for bipolar disorder.

D

date rape. A type of acquaintance rape in which the rapist is known to the victim through dating.

decatastrophizing. In cognitive therapy, with this technique the therapist assists the client to examine the validity of a negative automatic thought. Even if some validity exists, the client is then encouraged to review ways to cope adaptively, moving beyond the current crisis situation.

defamation of character. An individual may be liable for defamation of character by sharing with others information about a person that is detrimental to that person's reputation.

defense mechanisms. Mechanisms used by the ego in efforts to relieve anxiety posed by threats to biological or psychological integrity.

deinstitutionalization. The removal of mentally ill individuals from institutions and the subsequent plan to provide care for these individuals in the community setting.

delayed grief. The absence of evidence of grief when it ordinarily would be expected.

delayed ejaculation. Delayed or absent ejaculation, even though the man has a firm erection and has had more than adequate stimulation.

delirious mania. A grave form of mania characterized by severe clouding of consciousness and representing an intensification of the symptoms associated with mania. The symptoms of delirious mania have become relatively rare since the availability of antipsychotic medications.

delirium. A state of mental confusion and excitement characterized by disorientation for time and place, often with hallucinations, incoherent speech, and a continual state of aimless physical activity.

delusions. False personal beliefs, not consistent with a person's intelligence or cultural background. The individual continues to have the belief in spite of obvious proof that it is false and/or irrational.

dementia. See **neurocognitive disorder.**

democratic. A leadership style in which the leader promotes shared decision making. The leader provides guidance and expertise as needed.

dendrites. The cellular processes of a neuron that carry impulses toward the cell body.

denial. Refusal to acknowledge the existence of a real situation and/or the feelings associated with it.

density. The number of people in a given environmental space, influencing interpersonal interaction.

depersonalization. An alteration in the perception or experience of the self so that the feeling of one's own reality is temporarily lost.

depression. An alteration in mood that is expressed by feelings of sadness, despair, and pessimism. There is a loss of interest in usual activities, and somatic symptoms may be evident. Changes in appetite and sleep patterns are common.

derealization. An alteration in the perception or experience of the external world so that it seems strange or unreal.

detoxification. The process of withdrawal from a substance to which one has become addicted.

diagnosis related groups (DRGs). A system used to determine prospective payment rates for reimbursement of hospital care based on the client's diagnosis.

Diagnostic and Statistical Manual of Mental Disorders, Fifth Edition (DSM-5). Standard nomenclature of emotional illness published by the American Psychiatric Association (APA) and used by all healthcare practitioners. It classifies mental illness and presents guidelines and diagnostic criteria for various mental disorders.

dichotomous thinking. In this type of thinking, situations are viewed in all-or-nothing, black-or-white, good-or-bad terms.

directed association. A technique used to help clients bring into consciousness events that have been repressed. Specific thoughts are guided and directed by the psychoanalyst.

disaster. A natural or man-made occurrence that overwhelms the resources of an individual or community, and increases the need for emergency evacuation and medical services.

discriminative stimulus. A stimulus that precedes a behavioral response and predicts that a particular reinforcement will occur. Individuals learn to discriminate between various stimuli that will produce the responses they desire.

disengagement. In family theory, disengagement refers to extreme separateness among family members. It is promoted by rigid boundaries or lack of communication among family members.

disengagement theory. The hypothesis that there is a process of mutual withdrawal of aging persons and society from each other that is correlated with successful aging. This theory has been challenged by many investigators.

displacement. Feelings are transferred from one target to another that is considered less threatening or neutral.

dissociation. The splitting off of clusters of mental contents from conscious awareness, a mechanism central to hysterical conversion and dissociative disorder.

distance. The means by which various cultures use space to communicate.

distraction. In cognitive therapy, when dysfunctional cognitions have been recognized, activities are identified that can be used to distract the client and divert him or her from the intrusive thoughts or depressive ruminations that are contributing to the client's maladaptive responses.

disulfiram. A drug that is administered to individuals who abuse alcohol as a deterrent to drinking. Ingestion of alcohol while disulfiram is in the body results in a syndrome of symptoms that can produce a great deal of discomfort, and can even result in death if the blood alcohol level is high.

domains of learning. Categories in which individuals learn or gain knowledge and demonstrate behavior. There are three domains of learning: affective, cognitive, and psychomotor.

double-bind communication. An emotionally distressing situation in which an individual receives conflicting messages in the communication process, whereby one message is negated by another. This creates a condition in which a successful response to one message results in a failed response to the other.

dual diagnosis. A client has a dual diagnosis when it is determined that he or she has a coexisting substance disorder and mental illness. Treatment is designed to target both problems.

dysthymia. A depressive neurosis. The symptoms are similar to, if somewhat milder than, those ascribed to major depression. There is no loss of contact with reality.

dystonia. Involuntary muscular movements (spasms) of the face, arms, legs, and neck; may occur as an extrapyramidal side effect of some antipsychotic medications.

E

echolalia. The parrot-like repetition, by an individual with loose ego boundaries, of the words spoken by another.

echopraxia. An individual with loose ego boundaries attempting to identify with another person by imitating movements that the other person makes.

ego. One of the three elements of the personality identified by Freud as the rational self or "reality principle." The ego seeks to maintain harmony between the external world, the id, and the superego.

ego defense mechanisms. Strategies employed by the ego for protection in the face of threat to biological or psychological integrity. (See individual defense mechanisms.)

egoistic suicide. The response of an individual who feels separate and apart from the mainstream of society.

electroconvulsive therapy (ECT). A type of somatic treatment in which electric current is applied to the brain through electrodes placed on the temples. A grand mal seizure produces the desired effect. This is used with severely depressed patients refractory to antidepressant medications.

emaciated. The state of being excessively thin or physically wasted.

emotional abuse. A pattern of behavior on the part of the parent or caretaker that results in serious impairment of the child's social, emotional, or intellectual functioning.

emotional intelligence (EI). A set of competencies related to one's emotional health that includes self-awareness, empathy, emotional self-control, and effective relationship management.

emotional neglect. A chronic failure by the parent or caretaker to provide the child with the hope, love, and support necessary for the development of a sound, healthy personality.

empathy. The ability to see beyond outward behavior, and sense accurately another's inner experiencing. With empathy, one can accurately perceive and understand the meaning and relevance in the thoughts and feelings of another.

enculturation. The process of acquiring cultural behavior through socialization.

enmeshment. Exaggerated connectedness among family members. It occurs in response to diffuse boundaries in which there is overinvestment, overinvolvement, and lack of differentiation between individuals or subsystems.

esophageal varices. Veins in the esophagus become distended because of excessive pressure from defective blood flow through a cirrhotic liver.

essential hypertension. Persistent elevation of blood pressure for which there is no apparent cause or associated underlying disease.

ethical dilemma. A situation that arises when on the basis of moral considerations an appeal can be made for taking each of two opposing courses of action.

ethical egoism. An ethical theory espousing that what is "right" and "good" is what is best for the individual making the decision.

ethics. A branch of philosophy dealing with values related to human conduct, to the rightness and wrongness of certain actions, and to the goodness and badness of the motives and ends of such actions.

ethnicity. The concept of people identifying with each other because of a shared heritage.

evaluation. The process of determining the progress toward attainment of expected outcomes, including the effectiveness of care (ANA, 2010).

exhibitionistic disorder. A paraphilic disorder characterized by a recurrent urge to expose one's genitals to a stranger.

expressed response pattern. Pattern of behavior in which the victim of rape expresses feelings of fear, anger, and anxiety through such behavior as crying, sobbing, restlessness, and tenseness; in contrast to the rape victim who withholds feelings in the **controlled response pattern.**

extinction. In behavior therapy, the gradual decrease in frequency or disappearance of a response when the positive reinforcement is withheld.

extrapyramidal symptoms (EPS). A variety of symptoms that originate outside the pyramidal tracts and in the basal ganglion of the brain. Symptoms may include tremors, chorea, dystonia, akinesia, akathisia, and others. May occur as a side effect of some antipsychotic medications.

F

factitious disorder. Factitious disorders involve conscious, intentional feigning of physical or psychological symptoms. Individuals with factitious disorder pretend to be ill in order to receive emotional care and support commonly associated with the role of "patient."

false imprisonment. The deliberate and unauthorized confinement of a person within fixed limits by the use of threat or force. A nurse may be charged with false imprisonment by placing a patient in restraints against his or her will in a non-emergency situation.

family. Two or more individuals who depend on one another for emotional, physical, and economical support. The members of the family are self-defined (Kaakinen, Hanson, & Denham, 2010).

family structure. Family structure is founded on a set of invisible principles that influence the interaction among family members. These principles are established over time and become the "laws" that govern the conduct of various family members.

family system. The entirety of the family as a unit that includes patterns for social and emotional interaction, interdependence, and the subsystems within the family. These subsystems may include a marital dyad, parent-child dyad, and sibling groups.

family therapy. A type of therapy in which the focus is on relationships within the family. The family is viewed as a system in which the members are interdependent, and a change in one creates change in all.

fetishistic disorder. A paraphilic disorder characterized by recurrent sexual urges and sexually arousing fantasies involving the use of nonliving objects.

fight-or-flight syndrome. A syndrome of physical symptoms that results from an individual's real or perceived notion that harm or danger is imminent.

flexible boundary. A personal boundary is flexible when, because of unusual circumstances, individuals can alter limits that they have set for themselves. Flexible boundaries are healthy boundaries.

flooding. Sometimes called *implosion therapy*, this technique is used to desensitize individuals to phobic stimuli. The individual is "flooded" with a continuous presentation (usually through mental imagery) of the phobic stimulus until it no longer elicits anxiety.

focal stimulus. A situation of immediate concern that results in a threat to self-esteem.

Focus Charting®. A type of documentation that follows a data, action, and response (DAR) format. The main perspective is a client "focus," which can be a nursing diagnosis, a client's concern, a change in status, or a significant event in the client's therapy. The focus cannot be a medical diagnosis.

folk medicine. A system of health care within various cultures that is provided by a local practitioner, not professionally trained, but who uses techniques specific to that culture in the art of healing.

forensic. Pertaining to the law; legal.

forensic nursing. The application of forensic science combined with the bio-psychological education of the registered nurse, in the scientific investigation, evidence collection and preservation, analysis, prevention and treatment of trauma and/or death related medical-legal issues.

free association. A technique in psychoanalytic therapy used to help individuals bring to consciousness material that has been repressed. The individual is encouraged to verbalize whatever comes into his or her mind, drifting naturally from one thought to another.

frotteuristic disorder. A paraphilic disorder characterized by the recurrent preoccupation with intense sexual urges or fantasies involving touching or rubbing against a nonconsenting person.

fugue. A sudden unexpected travel away from home or customary work locale with the assumption of a new identity and an inability to recall one's previous identity; usually occurring in response to severe psychosocial stress.

G

Gamblers Anonymous (GA). An organization of inspirational group therapy, modeled after Alcoholics Anonymous (AA), for individuals who desire to, but cannot, stop gambling.

gay. The term used to describe males in same-sex relationships.

gender. The condition of being either male or female.

gender dysphoria. A sense of discomfort associated with an incongruence between biologically assigned gender and subjectively experienced gender.

general adaptation syndrome. The general biological reaction of the body to a stressful situation, as described by Hans Selye. It occurs in three stages: the alarm reaction stage, the stage of resistance, and the stage of exhaustion.

generalized anxiety disorder. A disorder characterized by chronic (at least 6 months), unrealistic, and excessive anxiety and worry.

genetics. Study of the biological transmission of certain characteristics (physical and/or behavioral) from parent to offspring.

genogram. A graphic representation of a family system. It may cover several generations. Emphasis is on family roles and emotional relatedness among members. Genograms facilitate recognition of areas requiring change.

genotype. The total set of genes present in an individual at the time of conception, and coded in the DNA.

genuineness. The ability to be open, honest, and "real" in interactions with others; the awareness of what one is experiencing internally and the ability to project the quality of this inner experiencing in a relationship.

geriatrics. The branch of clinical medicine specializing in the care of the elderly and concerned with the problems of aging.

gerontology. The study of normal aging.

geropsychiatry. The branch of clinical medicine specializing in psychopathology of the elderly.

granny-dumping. Media-generated term for abandoning elderly individuals at emergency departments, nursing homes, or other facilities—literally leaving them in the hands of others when the strain of caregiving becomes intolerable.

grief. A subjective state of emotional, physical, and social responses to the real or perceived loss of a valued entity. Change and failure can also be perceived as losses. The grief response consists of a set of relatively predictable behaviors that describe the subjective state that accompanies mourning.

grief, exaggerated. A reaction in which all of the symptoms associated with normal grieving are exaggerated out of proportion. Pathological depression is a type of exaggerated grief.

grief, inhibited. The absence of evidence of grief when it ordinarily would be expected.

group. A collection of individuals whose association is founded on shared commonalities of interest, values, norms, or purpose. Membership in a group is generally by chance (born into the group), by choice (voluntary affiliation), or by circumstance (the result of life-cycle events over which an individual may or may not have control).

group therapy. A therapy group, founded in a specific theoretical framework, led by a person with an advanced degree in psychology, social work, nursing, or medicine. The goal is to encourage improvement in interpersonal functioning.

gynecomastia. Enlargement of the breasts in men; may be a side effect of some antipsychotic medications.

H

hallucinations. False sensory perceptions not associated with real external stimuli. Hallucinations may involve any of the five senses.

hepatic encephalopathy. A brain disorder resulting from the inability of the cirrhotic liver to convert ammonia to urea for excretion. The continued rise in serum ammonia results in progressively impaired mental functioning, apathy, euphoria or depression, sleep disturbances, increasing confusion, and progression to coma and eventual death.

HIV-associated neurocognitive disorder. A neuropathological syndrome, possibly caused by chronic HIV encephalitis and myelitis and manifested by cognitive, behavioral, and motor symptoms that become more severe with progression of the disease.

home care. A wide range of health and social services that are delivered at home to recovering, disabled, chronically or terminally ill persons in need of medical, nursing, social, or therapeutic treatment and/or assistance with essential activities of daily living.

homocysteine. An amino acid produced by the catabolism of methionine. Elevated levels may be linked to increased risk of cardiovascular disease.

homosexuality. A sexual preference for persons of the same gender.

hope. A foundational principle in the recovery model stressing that recovery emerges from the client's sense that recovery is attainable.

hospice. A program that provides palliative and supportive care to meet the special needs arising out of the physical, psychosocial, spiritual, social, and economic stresses that are experienced during the final stages of illness and during bereavement.

humors. The four body fluids described by Hippocrates: blood, black bile, yellow bile, and phlegm. Hippocrates associated insanity and mental illness with dysequilibrium among these four fluids.

hypersomnia. Excessive sleepiness or seeking excessive amounts of sleep.

hyperactivity. Excessive psychomotor activity that may be purposeful or aimless, accompanied by physical movements and verbal utterances that are usually more rapid than normal. Inattention and distractibility are common with hyperactive behavior.

hypertensive crisis. A potentially life-threatening syndrome that results when an individual taking monoamine oxidase (MAO) inhibitors eats a product high in tyramine. Symptoms include severe occipital headache, palpitations, nausea and vomiting, nuchal rigidity, fever, sweating, marked increase in blood pressure, chest pain, and coma. Foods with tyramine include aged cheeses or other aged, overripe, and fermented foods; broad beans; pickled herring; beef or chicken liver; preserved meats; beer and wine; yeast products; chocolate; caffeinated drinks; canned figs; sour cream; yogurt; soy sauce; and some over-the-counter cold medications and diet pills.

hypnosis. A treatment for disorders brought on by repressed anxiety. The individual is directed into a state of subconsciousness and assisted, through suggestions, to recall certain events that he or she cannot recall while conscious.

hypomania. A mild form of mania. Symptoms are excessive hyperactivity, but not severe enough to cause marked impairment in social or occupational functioning or to require hospitalization.

hysteria. A polysymptomatic disorder characterized by recurrent, multiple somatic complaints often described dramatically.

I

id. One of the three components of the personality identified by Freud as the "pleasure principle." The id is the locus of instinctual drives; is present at birth; and compels the infant to satisfy needs and seek immediate gratification.

identification. An attempt to increase self-worth by acquiring certain attributes and characteristics of an individual one admires.

illusion. A misperception of a real external stimulus.

implosion therapy. See **flooding**.

impulsive. The urge or inclination to act without consideration to the possible consequences of one's behavior.

incest. Sexual exploitation of a child under 18 years of age by a relative or non-relative who holds a position of trust in the family.

individualist culture. A culture that values independence, self reliance, and freedom.

informed consent. Permission granted to a physician by a client to perform a therapeutic procedure, prior to which information about the procedure has been presented to the client with adequate time given for consideration about the pros and cons.

insomnia. Difficulty initiating or maintaining sleep.

insulin coma therapy. The induction of a hypoglycemic coma aimed at alleviating psychotic symptoms; a dangerous procedure, questionably effective, no longer used in psychiatry.

integration. The process used with individuals with dissociative identity disorder in an effort to bring all the personalities together into one; usually achieved through hypnosis.

intellectualization. An attempt to avoid expressing actual emotions associated with a stressful situation by using the intellectual processes of logic, reasoning, and analysis.

interdisciplinary care. A concept of providing care for a client in which members of various disciplines work together with common goals and shared responsibilities for meeting those goals.

intimate distance. The closest distance that individuals will allow between themselves and others. In the United States, this distance is 0 to 18 inches.

intoxication. A physical and mental state of exhilaration and emotional frenzy or lethargy and stupor.

introjection. The beliefs and values of another individual are internalized and symbolically become a part of the self, to the extent that the feeling of separateness or distinctness is lost.

isolation. The separation of a thought or a memory from the feeling, tone, or emotions associated with it (sometimes called *emotional isolation*).

J

justice. An ethical principle reflecting that all individuals should be treated equally and fairly.

K

Kantianism. The ethical principle espousing that decisions should be made and actions taken out of a sense of duty.

kleptomania. A recurrent failure to resist impulses to steal objects not needed for personal use or monetary value.

Korsakoff's psychosis. A syndrome of confusion, loss of recent memory, and confabulation in alcoholics, caused by a deficiency of thiamine. It often occurs together with Wernicke's encephalopathy and may be termed *Wernicke-Korsakoff syndrome*.

L

laissez-faire. A leadership style in which the leader lets group members do as they please. There is no direction from the leader. Member productivity and morale may be low, owing to frustration from lack of direction.

lesbian. The term used to describe females in same-sex relationships.

libel. An action with which an individual may be charged for sharing with another individual, in writing, information that is detrimental to someone's reputation.

libido. Freud's term for the psychic energy used to fulfill basic physiological needs or instinctual drives such as hunger, thirst, and sexuality.

limbic system. A system of brain structures under the cortex sometimes called the "emotional brain." It is associated with feelings of fear and anxiety; anger and aggression; love, joy, and hope; and with sexuality and social behavior.

long-term memory. Memory for remote events, or those that occurred many years ago. The type of memory that is preserved in the elderly individual.

loose association. A thinking process characterized by speech in which ideas shift from one unrelated subject to another. The individual is unaware that the topics are unconnected.

loss. The experience of separation from something of personal importance.

luto. In Mexican culture, the period of mourning following the death of a loved one which is symbolized by wearing black, black and white, or dark clothing and by subdued behavior.

M

magical thinking. A primitive form of thinking in which an individual believes that thinking about a possible occurrence can make it happen.

magnification. A type of thinking in which the negative significance of an event is exaggerated.

maladaptation. A failure of the body to return to homeostasis following a physiological and/or psychological response to stress, disrupting the individual's integrity.

maladaptive responses. Behaviors that are considered unhealthy and destructive to one's integrity.

malpractice. The failure of one rendering professional services to exercise that degree of skill and learning commonly applied under all the circumstances in the community by the average prudent reputable member of the profession with the result of injury, loss, or damage to the recipient of those services or to those entitled to rely upon them.

managed care. A concept purposefully designed to control the balance between cost and quality of care. Examples of managed care are health maintenance organizations (HMOs) and preferred provider organizations (PPOs). The amount and type of health care that the individual receives is determined by the organization providing the managed care.

mania. A manifestation of bipolar disorder in which the predominant mood is elevated, expansive, or irritable. Motor activity is frenzied and excessive. Psychotic features may or may not be present.

marital rape. Sexual violence directed at a marital partner against that person's will.

marital schism. A state of severe chronic disequilibrium and discord within the marital dyad, with recurrent threats of separation.

marital skew. A marital relationship in which there is lack of equal partnership. One partner dominates the relationship and the other partner.

Medicaid. A system established by the federal government to provide medical care benefits for indigent Americans. The Medicaid program is jointly funded by state and federal governments, and coverage varies significantly from state to state.

Medicare. A system established by the federal government to provide medical care benefits for elderly Americans.

meditation. A method of relaxation in which an individual sits in a quiet place and focuses total concentration on an object, word, or thought.

melancholia. A severe form of major depressive episode. Symptoms are exaggerated, and interest or pleasure in virtually all activities is lost.

menopause. The period marking the permanent cessation of menstrual activity; usually occurs at approximately 48 to 51 years of age.

mental health. The successful adaptation to stressors from the internal or external environment, evidenced by thoughts, feelings, and behaviors that are age-appropriate and congruent with local and cultural norms.

mental illness. Maladaptive responses to stressors from the internal or external environment, evidenced by thoughts, feelings, and behaviors that are incongruent with the local and cultural norms, and interfere with the individual's social, occupational, and/or physical functioning.

mental imagery. A method of stress reduction that employs the imagination. The individual focuses imagination on a scenario that is particularly relaxing to him or her (e.g., a scene on a quiet seashore, a mountain atmosphere, or floating through the air on a fluffy white cloud).

meridians. In Chinese medicine, pathways along the body in which the healing energy (qi) flows, and which are links between acupoints.

migraine personality. Personality characteristics that have been attributed to the migraine-prone person. The characteristics include perfectionistic, overly conscientious, somewhat inflexible, neat and tidy, compulsive, hard worker, intelligent, exacting, and places a very high premium on success, setting high (sometimes unrealistic) expectations on self and others.

milieu. French for "middle"; the English translation connotes "surroundings, or environment."

milieu therapy. Also called therapeutic community, or therapeutic environment, this type of therapy consists of a scientific structuring of the environment in order to effect behavioral changes and to improve the individual's psychological health and functioning.

minimization. A type of thinking in which the positive significance of an event is minimized or undervalued.

mobile outreach units. Programs in which volunteers and paid professionals drive or walk around and seek out homeless individuals who need assistance with physical or psychological care.

modeling. Learning new behaviors by imitating the behaviors of others.

mood. An individual's sustained emotional tone, which significantly influences behavior, personality, and perception.

moral behavior. Conduct that results from serious critical thinking about how individuals ought to treat others; reflects respect for human life, freedom, justice, or confidentiality.

moral-ethical self. That aspect of the personal identity that functions as observer, standard setter, dreamer, comparer, and most of all evaluator of who the individual says he or she is. This component of the personal identity makes judgments that influence an individual's self-evaluation.

motivational interviewing. An evidence-based, patient-centered style of communicating that promotes behavior change by guiding clients to explore their own motivation for change and the advantages and disadvantages of their decisions.

mourning. The psychological process (or stages) through which the individual passes on the way to successful adaptation to the loss of a valued entity.

multidisciplinary care. A concept of providing care for a client in which individual disciplines provide specific services for the client without formal arrangement for interaction between the disciplines.

Munchausen syndrome. See **factitious disorder.**

N

narcissism. Self-love or self-admiration.

narcissistic personality disorder. A disorder characterized by an exaggerated sense of self-worth. These individuals lack empathy and are hypersensitive to the evaluation of others.

narcolepsy. A disorder in which the characteristic manifestation is sleep attacks. The individual cannot prevent falling asleep, even in the middle of a sentence or performing a task.

natural law theory. The ethical theory that has as its moral precept to "do good and avoid evil" at all costs. Natural law ethics are grounded in a concern for the human good that is based on people's ability to live according to the dictates of reason.

negative reinforcement. Increasing the probability that a behavior will recur by removal of an undesirable reinforcing stimulus.

negativism. Strong resistance to suggestions or directions; exhibiting behaviors contrary to what is expected.

neglect of a child. *Physical neglect* of a child includes refusal of or delay in seeking health care, abandonment, expulsion from the home or refusal to allow a runaway to return home, and inadequate supervision. *Emotional neglect* refers to a chronic failure by the parent or caretaker to provide the child with the hope, love, and support necessary for the development of a sound, healthy personality.

negligence. The failure to do something that a reasonable person, guided by those considerations that ordinarily regulate human affairs, would do, or doing something that a prudent and reasonable person would not do.

neologism. New words that an individual invents that are meaningless to others, but have symbolic meaning to the psychotic person.

neurocognitive disorder. Global impairment of cognitive functioning that is progressive and interferes with social and occupational abilities.

neuroendocrinology. The study of hormones functioning within the neurological system.

neuroleptic. Antipsychotic medication used to prevent or control psychotic symptoms.

neuroleptic malignant syndrome (NMS). A rare but potentially fatal complication of treatment with neuroleptic drugs. Symptoms include severe muscle rigidity, high fever, tachycardia, fluctuations in blood pressure, diaphoresis, and rapid deterioration of mental status to stupor and coma.

neuron. A nerve cell; consists of a cell body, an axon, and dendrites.

neurosis. An unconscious conflict that produces anxiety and other symptoms and leads to maladaptive use of defense mechanisms.

neurotic disorder. A psychiatric disturbance, characterized by excessive anxiety and/or depression, disrupted bodily functions, unsatisfying interpersonal relationships, and behaviors that interfere with routine functioning. There is no loss of contact with reality.

neurotransmitter. A chemical that is stored in the axon terminals of the presynaptic neuron. An electrical impulse through the neuron stimulates the release of the neurotransmitter into the synaptic cleft, which in turn determines whether or not another electrical impulse is generated.

nonassertive. A communication and behavioral approach (sometimes called passive) in which the individual seeks to please others at the expense of denying their own basic human rights.

nonmaleficence. The ethical principle that espouses abstaining from negative acts toward another, including acting carefully to avoid harm.

nursing diagnosis. A clinical judgment about individual, family, or community responses to actual and potential health problems/life processes. Nursing diagnoses provide the basis for selection of nursing interventions to achieve outcomes for which the nurse is accountable.

Nursing Interventions Classification (NIC). A comprehensive, research-based, standardized classification of interventions that nurses perform.

Nursing Outcomes Classification (NOC). A comprehensive, standardized classification of patient/client outcomes developed to evaluate the effects of nursing interventions.

nursing process. A dynamic, systematic process by which nurses assess, diagnose, identify outcomes, plan, implement, and evaluate nursing care. It has been called "nursing's scientific methodology." Nursing process gives order and consistency to nursing intervention.

O

obesity. The state of having a body mass index of 30 or above.

object constancy. The phase in the separation/ individuation process when the child learns to relate to objects in an effective, constant manner. A sense of separateness is established, and the child is able to internalize a sustained image of the loved object or person when out of sight.

obsessions. Unwanted, intrusive, persistent ideas, thoughts, impulses, or images that cause marked anxiety or distress. Common ones include repeated thoughts about contamination, doubts, a need to have things in a particular order, aggressive or sexual impulses, and fears of harm to oneself or others (APA, 2013).

obsessive-compulsive disorder. Recurrent thoughts or ideas (obsessions) that an individual is unable to put out of his or her mind, and actions that an individual is unable to refrain from performing (compulsions). The obsessions and compulsions are severe enough to interfere with social and occupational functioning.

oculogyric crisis. An attack of involuntary deviation and fixation of the eyeballs, usually in the upward position. It may last for several minutes or hours and may occur as an extrapyramidal side effect of some antipsychotic medications.

operant conditioning. The learning of a particular action or type of behavior that is followed by a reinforcement.

opioids. A group of compounds that includes opium, opium derivatives, and synthetic substitutes.

orgasm. A peaking of sexual pleasure, with release of sexual tension and rhythmic contraction of the perineal muscles and pelvic reproductive organs.

osteoporosis. A reduction in the mass of bone per unit of volume that interferes with the mechanical support function of bone. This process occurs because of demineralization of the bones, and is escalated in women about the time of menopause.

outcomes. End results that are measurable, desirable, and observable, and translate into observable behaviors.

overgeneralization. Also called "absolutistic thinking." With overgeneralization, sweeping conclusions are made based on one incident—an "all or nothing" type of thinking.

overt sensitization. A type of aversion therapy that produces unpleasant consequences for undesirable behavior. An example is the use of disulfiram therapy with alcoholics, which induces an undesirable physical response if the individual has consumed any alcohol.

P

palilalia. Repeating one's own sounds or words (a type of vocal tic associated with Tourette's disorder).

panic. A sudden overwhelming feeling of terror or impending doom. This most severe form of emotional anxiety is usually accompanied by behavioral, cognitive, and physiological signs and symptoms considered to be outside the expected range of normalcy.

panic disorder. A disorder characterized by recurrent panic attacks, the onset of which are unpredictable, and manifested by intense apprehension, fear, or terror, often associated with feelings of impending doom, and accompanied by intense physical discomfort.

paradoxical intervention. In family therapy, "prescribing the symptom." The therapist requests that the family continue to engage in the behavior that they are trying to change. Tension is relieved, and the family is able to view more clearly the possible solutions to their problem.

paralanguage. The gestural component of the spoken word. It consists of pitch, tone, and loudness of spoken messages, the rate of speaking, expressively placed pauses, and emphasis assigned to certain words.

paranoia. A term that implies extreme suspiciousness. In schizophrenia, paranoia is characterized by persecutory delusions and hallucinations of a threatening nature.

paraphilic disorder. Repetitive behaviors or fantasies that involve nonhuman objects, real or simulated suffering or humiliation, or nonconsenting partners.

parasomnia. Unusual or undesirable behaviors that occur during sleep (e.g., nightmares, sleep terrors, and sleepwalking).

passive-aggressive behavior. Behavior that defends an individual's own basic rights by expressing resistance to social and occupational demands. Sometimes called *indirect aggression*, this behavior takes the form of sly, devious, and undermining actions that express the opposite of what the person is really feeling.

pathological gambling. A failure to resist impulses to gamble, and gambling behavior that compromises, disrupts, or damages personal, family, or vocational pursuits.

pedophilic disorder. Recurrent urges and sexually arousing fantasies involving sexual activity with a prepubescent child.

peer assistance programs. A program established by the American Nurses Association to assist impaired nurses. The individuals who administer these efforts are nurse members of the state associations, as well as nurses who are in recovery themselves.

perseveration. Persistent repetition of the same word or idea in response to different questions.

personal distance. The distance between individuals who are having interactions of a personal nature, such as a close conversation. In the U.S. culture, personal distance is approximately 18 to 40 inches.

personal identity. An individual's self-perception that defines his or her functions as observer, standard setter, and self-evaluator. It strives to maintain a stable self-image and relates to what the individual strives to become.

personal self. See **personal identity.**

personality. Deeply ingrained patterns of behavior, which include the way one relates to, perceives, and thinks about the environment and oneself.

personalization. Taking complete responsibility for situations without considering that other circumstances may have contributed to the outcome.

pharmacoconvulsive therapy. The chemical induction of a convulsion, used in the past for the reduction of psychotic symptoms; a type of therapy no longer used in psychiatry.

phencyclidine. An anesthetic used in veterinary medicine; used illegally as a hallucinogen, referred to as PCP or angel dust.

phenotype. Characteristics of physical manifestations that identify a particular genotype. Examples of phenotypes include eye color, height, blood type, language, and hairstyle. Phenotypes may be genetic or acquired.

phobia. An irrational fear.

physical neglect of a child. The failure on the part of the parent or caregiver to provide for a child's basic needs, such as food, clothing, shelter, medical-dental care, and supervision.

PIE charting. More specifically called "APIE," this method of documentation has an assessment, problem, intervention, and evaluation (APIE) format and is a problem-oriented system used to document the nursing process.

positive reinforcement. A reinforcement stimulus that increases the probability that the behavior will recur.

postpartum depression. Depression that occurs during the postpartum period. It may be related to hormonal changes, tryptophan metabolism, or alterations in membrane transport during the early postpartum period. Other predisposing factors may also be influential.

posttraumatic stress disorder (PTSD). A syndrome of symptoms that develop following a psychologically distressing event that is outside the range of usual human experience (e.g., rape, war). The individual is unable to put the experience out of his or her mind, and has nightmares, flashbacks, and panic attacks.

posturing. The voluntary assumption of inappropriate or bizarre postures.

preassaultive tension state. Behaviors predictive of potential violence. They include excessive motor activity, tense posture, defiant affect, clenched teeth and fists, and other arguing, demanding, and threatening behaviors.

precipitating event. A stimulus arising from the internal or external environment that is perceived by an individual as taxing or exceeding his or her resources and endangering his or her well-being.

predisposing factors. A variety of elements that influence how an individual perceives and responds to a stressful event. Types of predisposing factors include genetic influences, past experiences, and existing conditions.

Premack principle. This principle states that a frequently occurring response (R1) can serve as a positive reinforcement for a response (R2) that occurs less frequently. For example, a girl may talk to friends on the phone (R2) only if she does her homework (R1).

premature ejaculation. Ejaculation that occurs with minimal sexual stimulation or before, upon, or shortly after penetration and before the person wishes it.

premenstrual dysphoric disorder. A disorder that is characterized by depressed mood, anxiety, mood swings, and decreased interest in activities during the week prior to menses and subsiding shortly after the onset of menstruation.

priapism. Prolonged painful penile erection; may occur as an adverse effect of some antidepressant medications, particularly trazodone.

primary neurocognitive disorder (NCD). NCD, such as Alzheimer's disease, in which the NCD itself is the major sign of some organic brain disease not directly related to any other organic illness.

primary gain. The receipt of positive reinforcement for somaticizing by being able to avoid difficult situations because of physical complaint.

primary prevention. Reduction of the incidence of mental disorders within the population by helping individuals to cope more effectively with stress and by trying to diminish stressors within the environment.

privileged communication. A doctrine common to most states that grants certain privileges under which health-care professionals may refuse to reveal information about and communications with clients.

problem-oriented recording (POR). A system of documentation that follows a subjective data, objective data, assessment, plan, implementation, and evaluation (SOAPIE) format. It is based on a list of identified patient problems to which each entry is directed.

prodromal syndrome. A syndrome of symptoms that often precede the onset of aggressive or violent behavior. These symptoms include anxiety and tension, verbal abuse and profanity, and increasing hyperactivity.

progressive relaxation. A method of deep muscle relaxation in which each muscle group is alternately tensed and relaxed in a systematic order with the person concentrating on the contrast of sensations experienced from tensing and relaxing.

projection. Attributing to another person feelings or impulses unacceptable to oneself.

prospective payment. The program of cost containment within the health-care profession directed at setting forth preestablished amounts that would be reimbursed for specific diagnoses.

pseudocyesis. A condition in which an individual has nearly all the signs and symptoms of pregnancy but is not pregnant; a conversion reaction.

pseudodementia. Symptoms of depression that mimic those of neurocognitive disorder (NCD).

pseudohostility. A family interaction pattern characterized by a state of chronic conflict and alienation among family members. This relationship pattern allows family members to deny underlying fears of tenderness and intimacy.

pseudomutuality. A family interaction pattern characterized by a facade of mutual regard with the purpose of denying underlying fears of separation and hostility.

pseudoparkinsonism. A side effect of some antipsychotic medications. Symptoms mimic those of Parkinson's disease, such as tremor, shuffling gait, drooling, and rigidity.

psychiatric home care. Care provided by psychiatric nurses in the client's home. Psychiatric home care nurses must have physical and psychosocial nursing skills to meet the demands of the client population they serve.

psychobiology. The study of the biological foundations of cognitive, emotional, and behavioral processes.

psychodrama. A specialized type of group therapy that employs a dramatic approach in which patients become "actors" in life situation scenarios. The goal is to resolve interpersonal conflicts in a less-threatening atmosphere than the real-life situation would present.

psychodynamic nursing. Being able to understand one's own behavior, to help others identify felt difficulties, and to apply principles of human relations to the problems that arise at all levels of experience.

psychoimmunology. The study of the implications of the immune system in psychiatry.

Psychological Recovery model. A recovery model which identifies five stages of recovery: moratorium (despair and confusion), awareness (that recovery is possible), preparation (begins the work of recovery), rebuilding (taking steps toward one's goals for recovery), and growth (some outcomes have been met and there is recognition that growth is a dynamic, lifelong process).

psychomotor domain. A category of learning in which the behaviors are processed and demonstrated. The information has been intellectually processed, and the individual is displaying motor behaviors.

psychomotor retardation. Extreme slowdown of physical movements. Posture slumps; speech is slowed; digestion becomes sluggish. Common in severe depression.

psychophysiological. Referring to psychological factors contributing to the initiation or exacerbation of a physical condition. Either a demonstrable organic pathology or a known pathophysiological process is involved.

psychosis. A mental state in which there is a severe loss of contact with reality. Symptoms may include delusions, hallucinations, disorganized speech patterns, and bizarre or catatonic behaviors.

psychosomatic. See **psychophysiological.**

psychotic disorder. A serious psychiatric disorder in which there is a gross disorganization of the personality, a marked disturbance in reality testing, and the impairment of interpersonal functioning and relationship to the external world.

psychotropic medication. Medication that affects psychic function, behavior, or experience.

public distance. Appropriate interactional distance for speaking in public or yelling to someone some distance away. U.S. culture defines this distance as 12 feet or more.

purging. The act of attempting to rid the body of calories by self-induced vomiting or excessive use of laxatives or diuretics.

purpose. A foundational principle in the recovery model which stresses that recovery is facilitated when an individual is able to find purpose and meaning in life.

pyromania. An inability to resist the impulse to set fires.

Q

qi. In Chinese medicine, the healing energy that flows through pathways in the body called *meridians.* (Also called "chi.")

R

rape. The expression of power and dominance by means of sexual violence, most commonly by men over women, although men may also be rape victims. Rape is considered an act of aggression, not of passion.

rapport. The development between two people in a relationship of special feelings based on mutual acceptance, warmth, friendliness, common interest, a sense of trust, and a nonjudgmental attitude.

rationalization. Attempting to make excuses or formulate logical reasons to justify unacceptable feelings or behaviors.

reaction formation. Preventing unacceptable or undesirable thoughts or behaviors from being expressed by exaggerating opposite thoughts or types of behaviors.

receptor sites. Molecules that are situated on the cell membrane of the postsynaptic neuron that will accept only molecules with a complementary shape. These complementary molecules are specific to certain neurotransmitters that determine whether an electrical impulse will be excited or inhibited.

reciprocal inhibition. Also called counterconditioning, this technique serves to decrease or eliminate a behavior by introducing a more adaptive behavior, but one that is incompatible with the unacceptable behavior (e.g., introducing relaxation techniques to an anxious person; relaxation and anxiety are incompatible behaviors).

reframing. Changing the conceptual or emotional setting or viewpoint in relation to which a situation is experienced and placing it in another frame that fits the "facts" of the same concrete situation equally well or even better, and thereby changing its entire meaning. The behavior may not actually change, but the consequences of the behavior may change because of a change in the meaning attached to the behavior.

regression. A retreat to an earlier level of development and the comfort measures associated with that level of functioning.

relaxation. A decrease in tension or intensity, resulting in refreshment of body and mind. A state of refreshing tranquility.

religion. A set of beliefs, values, rites, and rituals adopted by a group of people. The practices are usually grounded in the teachings of a spiritual leader.

religiosity. Excessive demonstration of or obsession with religious ideas and behavior; common in schizophrenia.

reminiscence therapy. A process of life review by elderly individuals that promotes self-esteem and provides assistance in working through unresolved conflicts from the past.

repression. The involuntary blocking of unpleasant feelings and experiences from one's awareness.

residual stimuli. Certain beliefs, attitudes, experiences, or traits that may contribute to an individual's low self-esteem.

retrograde ejaculation. Ejaculation of the seminal fluid backwards into the bladder; may occur as a side effect of antipsychotic medications.

right. That which an individual is entitled (by ethical, legal, or moral standards) to have, or to do, or to receive from others within the limits of the law.

rigid boundaries. A person with rigid boundaries is "closed" and difficult to bond with. Such a person has a narrow perspective on life, sees things one way, and cannot discuss matters that lie outside his or her perspective.

ritualistic behavior. Purposeless activities that an individual performs repeatedly in an effort to decrease anxiety (e.g., hand washing); common in obsessive-compulsive disorder.

S

safe house or shelter. An establishment set up by many cities to provide protection for battered women and their children.

scapegoating. Occurs when hostility exists in a marriage dyad and an innocent third person (usually a child) becomes the target of blame for the problem.

schemas (also called *core beliefs*). Cognitive structures that consist of the individual's fundamental beliefs and assumptions, which develop early in life from personal experiences and identification with significant others. These concepts are reinforced by further learning experiences and in turn, influence the formation of other beliefs, values, and attitudes.

schizotypal personality disorder. A disorder characterized by odd and eccentric behavior, not decompensating to the level of schizophrenia.

secondary gain. The receipt of positive reinforcement for somaticizing through added attention, sympathy, and nurturing.

secondary NCD. Neurocognitive disorder (NCD) that is caused by or related to another disease or condition, such as HIV disease or a cerebral trauma.

secondary prevention. Health care that is directed at reduction of the prevalence of psychiatric illness by shortening the course (duration) of the illness. This is accomplished through early identification of problems and prompt initiation of treatment.

selective abstraction (sometimes referred to as "mental filter"). A type of thinking in which a conclusion is drawn based on only a selected portion of the evidence.

self-concept. The composite of beliefs and feelings that one holds about oneself at a given time, formed from perceptions of others' reactions. The self-concept consists of the physical self, or body image; the personal self or identity; and the self-esteem.

self-consistency. The component of the personal identity that strives to maintain a stable self-image.

self-esteem. The degree of regard or respect that individuals have for themselves. It is a measure of worth that they place on their abilities and judgments.

self-ideal. The component of the personal identity that is the individual's perception of what he or she wants to be, to do, or to become.

sensate focus. A therapeutic technique used to treat individuals and couples with sexual dysfunction. The technique involves touching and being touched by another and focusing attention on the physical sensations encountered thereby. Clients gradually move through various levels of sensate focus that progress from nongenital touching to touching that includes the breasts and genitals; touching done in a simultaneous, mutual format rather than by one person at a time; and touching that extends to and allows eventually for the possibility of intercourse.

serotonin syndrome. A syndrome of symptoms related to excessive levels of serotonin in the body as a result of certain drugs or drug interactions. Symptoms may include diarrhea, nausea, vomiting, tremors, headache, agitation, restlessness, diaphoresis, and in severe cases, muscle rigidity, high fever, irregular heartbeat, seizures, unconsciousness and death, if left untreated.

sexual assault nurse examiner (SANE). A clinical forensic registered nurse who has received specialized training to provide care to the sexual assault victim.

sexual exploitation of a child. The inducement or coercion of a child into engaging in sexually explicit conduct for the purpose of promoting any performance (e.g., child pornography).

sexual masochism disorder. Sexual stimulation derived from being humiliated, beaten, bound, or otherwise made to suffer.

sexual sadism disorder. Recurrent urges and sexually arousing fantasies involving acts (real, not simulated) in which the psychological or physical suffering (including humiliation) of the victim is sexually exciting.

sexuality. Sexuality is the constitution and life of an individual relative to characteristics regarding intimacy. It reflects the totality of the person and does not relate exclusively to the sex organs or sexual behavior.

shaman. A medicine man (or woman) who uses a variety of practices which may include healing ceremonies, herbs, crystals, and other remedies with healing properties.

shaping. In learning, one shapes the behavior of another by giving reinforcements for increasingly closer approximations to the desired behavior.

shelters. A variety of places designed to help the homeless, ranging from converted warehouses that provide cots or floor space on which to sleep overnight to significant operations that provide a multitude of social and health-care services.

shiva. In the Jewish-American culture, following the death of a loved one, *shiva* is the 7-day period following the burial. During this time, mourners do not work, and no activity is permitted that diverts attention from thinking about the deceased.

short-term memory. The ability to remember events that occurred very recently. This ability deteriorates with age.

silent rape reaction. The response of a rape victim in which he or she tells no one about the assault.

slander. An action with which an individual may be charged for orally sharing information that is detrimental to a person's reputation.

social distance. The distance considered acceptable in interactions with strangers or acquaintances, such as at a cocktail party or in a public building. U.S. culture defines this distance as 4 to 12 feet.

social phobia. The fear of being humiliated in social situations.

social skills training. Educational opportunities through role play for the person with schizophrenia to learn appropriate social interaction skills and functional skills that are relevant to daily living.

Socratic questioning (also called *guided discovery*). When the therapist questions the client with Socratic questioning, the client is asked to describe feelings associated with specific situations. Questions are stated in a way that may stimulate in the client a recognition of possible dysfunctional thinking and produce a dissonance about the validity of the thoughts.

somatization. A method of coping with psychosocial stress by developing physical symptoms.

specific phobia. A persistent fear of a specific object or situation, other than the fear of being unable to escape from a situation (agoraphobia) or the fear of being humiliated in social situations (social phobia).

spirituality. The human quality that gives meaning and sense of purpose to an individual's existence. Spirituality exists within each individual regardless of belief system and serves as a force for interconnectedness between the self and others, the environment, and a higher power.

splitting. A primitive ego defense mechanism in which the person is unable to integrate and accept both positive and negative feelings. In the view of these individuals, people—including themselves—and life situations are either all good or all bad. This trait is common in borderline personality disorder.

statutory law. A law that has been enacted by legislative bodies, such as a county or city council, state legislature, or the U.S. Congress.

statutory rape. Unlawful intercourse between a person who is over the age of consent and a person who is under the age of consent. Legal age of consent varies from state to state. An individual can be arrested for statutory rape even when the interaction has occurred between consenting individuals.

stereotyping. The process of classifying all individuals from the same culture or ethnic group as identical.

stimulus. In classical conditioning, that which elicits a response.

stimulus generalization. The process by which a conditioned response is elicited from all stimuli *similar* to the one from which the response was learned.

store-front clinics. Establishments that have been converted into clinics that serve the homeless population.

stress. A state of disequilibrium that occurs when there is a disharmony between demands occurring within an individual's internal or external environment and his or her ability to cope with those demands.

stress management. Various methods used by individuals to reduce tension and other maladaptive responses to stress in their lives; includes relaxation exercises, physical exercise, music, mental imagery, or any other technique that is successful for a person.

stressor. A demand from within an individual's internal or external environment that elicits a physiological and/or psychological response.

sublimation. The rechanneling of personally and/or socially unacceptable drives or impulses into activities that are more tolerable and constructive.

subluxation. The term used in chiropractic medicine to describe vertebrae in the spinal column that have become displaced, possibly pressing on nerves and interfering with normal nerve transmission.

substance abuse. Use of psychoactive drugs that poses significant hazards to health and interferes with social, occupational, psychological, or physical functioning.

substance addiction. Physical addiction is identified by the inability to stop using a substance despite attempts to do so; a continual use of the substance despite adverse consequences; a developing tolerance; and the development of withdrawal symptoms upon cessation or decreased intake. Psychological addiction is said to exist when a substance is perceived by the user to be necessary to maintain an optimal state of personal well-being, interpersonal relations, or skill performance.

substitution therapy. The use of various medications to decrease the intensity of symptoms in an individual who is withdrawing from, or experiencing the effects of excessive use of, substances.

subsystems. The smaller units of which a system is composed. In family systems theory, the subsystems are composed of husband-wife, parent-child(ren), or sibling-sibling.

sundowning. A phenomenon in neurocognitive disorder (NCD) in which the symptoms seem to worsen in the late afternoon and evening.

superego. One of the three elements of the personality identified by Freud that represents the conscience and the culturally determined restrictions that are placed on an individual.

suppression. The voluntary blocking from one's awareness of unpleasant feelings and experiences.

surrogate. One who serves as a substitute figure for another.

symbiotic relationship. A type of "psychic fusion" that occurs between two people; it is unhealthy in that severe anxiety is generated in either or both if separation is indicated. A symbiotic relationship is normal between infant and mother.

sympathy. The actual sharing of another's thoughts and behaviors. Differs from **empathy** in that with empathy one experiences an objective understanding of what another is feeling, rather than actually sharing those feelings.

synapse. The junction between two neurons. The small space between the axon terminals of one neuron and the cell body or dendrites of another is called the synaptic cleft.

systematic desensitization. A treatment for phobias in which the individual is taught to relax and then asked to imagine various components of the phobic stimulus on a graded hierarchy, moving from that which produces the least fear to that which produces the most.

T

tangentiality. The inability to get to the point of a story. The speaker introduces many unrelated topics, until the original topic of discussion is lost.

tardive dyskinesia. Syndrome of symptoms characterized by bizarre facial and tongue movements, a stiff neck, and difficulty swallowing. It may occur as an adverse effect of long-term therapy with some antipsychotic medications.

technical expert. Peplau's term for one who understands various professional devices and possesses the clinical skills necessary to perform the interventions that are in the best interest of the client.

temperament. A set of inborn personality characteristics that influence an individual's manner of reacting to the environment, and ultimately influences his or her developmental progression.

territoriality. The innate tendency of individuals to own space. Individuals lay claim to areas around them as their own. This phenomenon can have an influence on interpersonal communication.

tertiary gain. The receipt of positive reinforcement for somaticizing by causing the focus of the family to switch to the individual and away from conflict that may be occurring within the family.

tertiary prevention. Health care that is directed toward reduction of the residual effects associated with severe or chronic physical or mental illness.

therapeutic communication. Caregiver verbal and nonverbal techniques that focus on the care receiver's needs and advance the promotion of healing and change. Therapeutic communication encourages exploration of feelings and fosters understanding of behavioral motivation. It is nonjudgmental, discourages defensiveness, and promotes trust.

therapeutic community. Also called *milieu therapy*, this approach strives to manipulate the environment so that all aspects of the client's hospital experience are considered therapeutic.

therapeutic group. Differs from group therapy in that there is a lesser degree of theoretical foundation. Focus is on group relations, interactions between group members, and the consideration of a selected issue. Leaders of therapeutic groups do not require the degree of educational preparation required of group therapy leaders.

therapeutic relationship. An interaction between two people (usually a caregiver and a care receiver) in which input from both participants contributes to a climate of healing, growth promotion, and/or illness prevention.

thought-stopping. A self-taught technique that an individual uses each time he or she wishes to eliminate intrusive or negative, unwanted thoughts from awareness.

Tidal model. A recovery focused treatment approach in which the individual is encouraged to tell their story and take an active role in deciding what changes need to occur to promote recovery.

time out. An aversive stimulus or punishment during which the individual is removed from the environment where the unacceptable behavior is being exhibited.

token economy. In behavior modification, a type of contracting in which the reinforcers for desired behaviors are presented in the form of tokens, which may then be exchanged for designated privileges.

tolerance. The need for increasingly larger or more frequent doses of a substance in order to obtain the desired effects originally produced by a lower dose.

tort. The violation of a civil law in which an individual has been wronged. In a tort action, one party asserts that wrongful conduct on the part of the other has caused harm, and compensation for harm suffered is sought.

transcendence. Erikson's last developmental stage (added in the 1990's), following the stage of integrity versus despair, in which the individual develops a broader world view that transcends oneself and enhances one's sense of meaning and purpose in life.

transference. Transference occurs when a client unconsciously displaces (or "transfers") to the nurse or therapist feelings formed toward a person from his or her past.

transgender. The individual, despite having the anatomical characteristics of a given gender, has the self-perception of being of the opposite gender, and may seek to have gender changed through surgical intervention.

transvestic disorder. Recurrent urges and sexually arousing fantasies involving dressing in the clothes of the opposite gender.

triangles. A three-person emotional configuration that is considered the basic building block of the family system. When anxiety becomes too great between two family members, a third person is brought in to form a triangle. Triangles are dysfunctional in that they offer relief from anxiety through diversion rather than through resolution of the issue.

trichotillomania (hair-pulling disorder). The recurrent failure to resist impulses to pull out one's own hair.

type A personality. The personality characteristics attributed to individuals prone to coronary heart disease, including excessive competitive drive, chronic sense of time urgency, easy anger, aggressiveness, excessive ambition, and inability to enjoy leisure time.

type B personality. The personality characteristics attributed to individuals who are not prone to coronary heart disease; includes characteristics such as ability to perform even under pressure but without the competitive drive and constant sense of time urgency experienced by the type A personality. Type Bs can enjoy their leisure time without feeling guilty, and they are much less impulsive than type A individuals; that is, they think things through before making decisions.

type C personality. The personality characteristics attributed to the cancer-prone individual. Includes characteristics such as suppression of anger, calm, passive, puts the needs of others before his or her own, but holds resentment toward others for perceived "wrongs."

type D personality. Personality characteristics attributed to individuals who are at increased risk of cardiovascular morbidity and mortality. The characteristics include a combination of negative emotions and social inhibition.

tyramine. An amino acid found in aged cheeses or other aged, overripe, and fermented foods; broad beans; pickled herring; beef or chicken liver; preserved meats; beer and wine; yeast products; chocolate; caffeinated drinks; canned figs; sour cream; yogurt; soy sauce; and some over-the-counter cold medications and diet pills. If foods high in tyramine content are consumed while an individual is taking MAO inhibitors, a potentially life-threatening syndrome called hypertensive crisis can result.

U

unconditional positive regard. Carl Rogers's term for the respect and dignity of an individual regardless of his or her unacceptable behavior.

unconditioned response. In classical conditioning, an unconditioned response refers to a reflexive response to a specific target stimulus.

unconditioned stimulus. In classical conditioning, a specific stimulus that elicits an unconditioned, reflexive response.

undoing. A mechanism used to symbolically negate or cancel out a previous action or experience that one finds intolerable.

universality. One therapeutic factor of groups (identified by Yalom) in which individuals realize that they are not alone in a problem and in the thoughts and feelings they are experiencing. Anxiety is relieved by the support and understanding of others in the group who share similar experiences.

utilitarianism. The ethical theory that espouses "the greatest happiness for the greatest number." Under this theory, action would be taken based on the end results that will produce the most good (happiness) for the most people.

V

values. Personal beliefs about the truth, beauty, or worth of a thought, object, or behavior, that influence an individual's actions.

values clarification. A process of self-discovery by which people identify their personal values and their value rankings. This process increases awareness about why individuals behave in certain ways.

velorio. In Mexican culture, following the death of a loved one, the *velorio* is a festive watch by family and friends over the body of the deceased person before burial.

veracity. An ethical principle that refers to one's duty to always be truthful.

voyeuristic disorder. Recurrent urges and sexually arousing fantasies involving the act of observing unsuspecting people, usually strangers, who are either naked, in the process of disrobing, or engaging in sexual activity.

W

waxy flexibility. A condition by which the individual with schizophrenia passively yields all movable parts of the body to any efforts made at placing them in certain positions.

Wernicke's encephalopathy. A brain disorder caused by thiamine deficiency and characterized by visual disturbances, ataxia, somnolence, stupor, and, without thiamine replacement, death.

withdrawal. The physiological and mental readjustment that accompanies the discontinuation of an addictive substance.

word salad. A group of words that are put together in a random fashion without any logical connection.

WRAP model (Wellness Recovery Action Plan). A recovery model that focuses on developing a system for monitoring distressing symptoms and planned responses to minimize or eliminate distress.

Y

yin and yang. The fundamental concept of Asian health practices. Yin and yang are opposite forces of energy such as negative/positive, dark/light, cold/hot, hard/soft, and feminine/masculine. Food, medicines, and herbs are classified according to their yin and yang properties and are used to restore a balance, thereby restoring health.

yoga. A system of beliefs and practices, the ultimate goal of which is to unite the human soul with the universal spirit. In Western countries, yoga uses body postures, along with meditation and breathing exercises, to achieve a balanced, disciplined workout that releases muscle tension, tones the internal organs, and energizes the mind, body, and spirit, so that natural healing can occur.

Page numbers followed by f denote figures; those followed by t denote tables; those followed by b denote boxes; those followed by *e* denote online chapters.

Hypothalamic-pituitary-adrenocortical axis, in depression, 501
Hypothalamic-pituitary-thyroid axis, in depression, 501, 503
Hypothalamus, 30t, 31–32
in appetite regulation, 673
pituitary gland and, 42f
Hysterical neuroses, 615. *See also* Somatic symptom disorders

I

Id, 941*e*
Identification, 19t
Identifying oneself in personality development, 953t*e*, 954–955*e*
Identity disorder, dissociative
prevalence of, 616
treatment modalities for, 635
Identity vs. role confusion, in development of self-esteem, 269
Identity vs. role confusion, in psychosocial theory of development, 946t*e*, 947*e*
Illness anxiety disorder
background assessment data, 617–618
case study and sample care plan on, 636–637
diagnostic criteria for, 618b
learning theory and, 621
prevalence of, 616
Illusions, in schizophrenia, 470
Iloperidone, 485t
psychotropic medication effects on, 58t
Imagery, mental, 923*e*
to achieve relaxation, 935*e*
Imaginative activity, impaired, in autism spectrum disorder, 738
Imitative behavior, in therapeutic groups, 191
Immune system
age-related changes in, 780
in psychiatric illness, 48–49
response of, normal, 48–49
Implementation (nursing process), 174–175
anger/aggression, 285
in antisocial personality disorder, 719–720
of assertiveness training, 261
attention-deficit/hyperactivity disorder, 746–748t
autism spectrum disorder, 740–741t
behavior therapy, 323–324
for bereaved individuals, 873–875t
borderline personality disorder, 710–714
in conduct disorder, 760, 761–762t
cultural implications for, 116, 120
depression, 513–517, 514–515t
in disaster nursing, 242, 243–249t
dissociative disorders, 625–632
in eating disorders, 680, 682–683t, 684–686
elderly clients, 792, 793–797t
electroconvulsive therapy, 344–346
in family therapy case study, 218–219
gender dysphoria in children, 647, 648–649t
intellectual disability, 734
neurocognitive disorders, 392–393

oppositional defiant disorder, 755, 756–757t
schizophrenia, 472–479
for self-esteem issues, 274
in separation anxiety disorder, 765, 765t
substance-related and addictive disorders, 435–436t, 437–438
Tourette's disorder, 752–753t
Implementation (nursing process), relaxation therapy, 937*e*
Implosion therapy, 581–582. *See also* Flooding
Implosive therapy, in behavior modification, 322
Imprisonment, false, 98
Impulse control, ineffective, planning and implementation for client with, 578
Impulsiveness, definition of, 742
Impulsivity
in attention deficit/hyperactivity disorder, 742, 745b
in borderline personality disorder, 709
Inattention, in attention-deficit/hyperactivity disorder, 745b
Incest, 814–815
definition of, 814
Incomprehensibility, mental illness and, 16
Indian Americans, cultural phenomena related to, 111–112, 117t
Indigenous systems (of medicine), traditional, 905t*e*
Individuality
in American culture, 110b
of family members, ignoring, 206
Industry vs. inferiority, in development of self-esteem, 269
Industry vs. inferiority, in psychosocial theory of development, 946t*e*, 947*e*
Infants, reaction of, to death in family, 869
Infection, viral, schizophrenia and, 461–462
Inference, arbitrary, 330
Informality, in American culture, 110b
Information, imparting of, in therapeutic groups, 191
Information sharing, as group function, 189
Informed consent, as legal issue, 96–97
Inhalants, symptoms associated with intoxication and withdrawal, 428t
Inhalant use disorder, 416–417
central nervous system effects, 417
effects on body, 417
gastrointestinal effects, 417
historical aspects, 416
intoxication, 417
patterns of use, 416–417
profile of substance, 416
renal system effects, 417
respiratory effects, 417
Inhibition, reciprocal, in behavior modification, 322
Inhibitory amino acids, 38
Inhibitory response, 33
Initiative vs. guilt, in development of self-esteem, 269
Initiative vs. guilt, in psychosocial theory of development, 946–947*e*, 946t*e*

Injury, risk of, in attention-deficit/hyperactivity disorder, care plan for, 746t
Insight, lack of, in schizophrenia, 470
Institutionalization, risk factors for, 787–788
Instrumental relativist orientation stage of moral development, 951*e*, 951t*e*
Insulin coma therapy, 341
Integration, in dissociative identity disorder, 635
Intellectual disability, 733–737, 733b, 735–736t
care plans for, 735–736t
developmental characteristics in, by degree of severity, 735t
diagnostic criteria, 733b
DSM-5 classification of, 753
nursing process applied to, 734, 735–737t
predisposing factors, 733–734
Intellectual functioning, age-related changes in, 781
Intellectualization, 19t
Interdisciplinary treatment team, in milieu therapy, 226, 227–229t
Interests, restricted, in autism spectrum disorder, 738–739
International Society of Psychiatric-Mental Health Nurses and American Nurses Association: Scope and Standards of Practice, 87
Interneurons, 33
Interpersonal communication, as adaptive coping strategy, 8–9
Interpersonal concordance orientation stage of moral development, 951–952*e*, 951t*e*
Interpersonal learning, in therapeutic groups, 191
Interpersonal psychotherapy, 921–922*e*
Interpersonal security, in interpersonal theory of personality development, 944*e*
Interpersonal theory of suicide, 299
Interpreter, using, 107b
Interpreting, in nontherapeutic communication, 156t
Intersexual, definition of, 645
Intervention(s) (nursing process)
crisis, 241
with families, 199–222
recovery model of, in standards of practice, 165
for veteran clients and military families, 895–896t
Interviewing, motivational, 156–157, 157–158b
Intimacy vs. isolation, in development of self-esteem, 269
Intimacy vs. isolation, in psychosocial theory of development, 946t*e*, 947*e*
Intimate distance, 107
Intimate partner violence, 809–812
Intoxication
alcohol, 407
cannabis, 424
CNS stimulants, substitution therapy for, 447
hallucinogen, 422
inhalant, 417
opioid, 420
PCP, 422